FOURTH EDITION

ROGERS' HANDBOOK OF PEDIATRIC INTENSIVE CARE

FOURTH EDITION

ROGERS' HANDBOOK OF PEDIATRIC INTENSIVE CARE

Editors

Mark A. Helfaer, MD, FCCM
Professor of Anesthesiology, Critical Care,
 Pediatrics and Nursing
University of Pennsylvania Schools of
 Medicine and Nursing
Chief, Critical Care Medicine
Endowed Chair Critical Care
 Medicine
Children's Hospital of Philadelphia
Philadelphia, Pennsylvania

**David G. Nichols, MD, MBA,
FAAP, FCCM**
Professor
Department of Anesthesiology and
Department of Critical Care Medicine
 and Pediatrics
Vice Dean for Education
The Johns Hopkins University School
 of Medicine
Baltimore, Maryland

Wolters Kluwer | Lippincott Williams & Wilkins
Health
Philadelphia · Baltimore · New York · London
Buenos Aires · Hong Kong · Sydney · Tokyo

Acquisitions Editor: Brian Brown
Managing Editor: Nicole Dernoski
Project Manager: Jennifer Harper
Manufacturing Coordinator: Kathleen Brown
Marketing Manager: Angela Panetta/Jennifer Kuklinski
Design Coordinator: Terry Mallon
Production Services: Aptara, Inc.

Library of Congress Cataloging-in-Publication Data

Rogers' handbook of pediatric intensive care / editors, Mark A. Helfaer, David G. Nichols.—4th ed.
   p. ; cm.
  Companion to: Rogers' textbook of pediatric intensive care / editor, David G. Nichols. 4th ed. c2008.
  Rev. ed. of: Handbook of pediatric intensive care / edited by Mark C. Rogers, Mark A. Helfaer. 3rd ed. c1999.
  Includes index.
  ISBN-13: 978-0-7817-8705-5
  ISBN-10: 0-7817-8705-X
  1. Pediatric intensive care—Handbooks, manuals, etc. 2. Pediatric emergencies—Handbooks, manuals, etc.
I. Helfaer, Mark A. II. Nichols, David G. (David Gregory), 1951– III. Rogers, Mark C. IV. Rogers' textbook of pediatric intensive care. V. Handbook of pediatric intensive care. VI. Title: Handbook of pediatric intensive care.
  [DNLM: 1. Critical Care—Handbooks. 2. Child. 3. Emergencies—Handbooks. 4. Infant. WS 39 R726 2009]
  RJ370.H36 2009
  618.92′0028—dc22

2008027535

■ PREFACE

The purpose of the *Rogers' Handbook of Pediatric Critical Care* is to be a companion to, not a replacement for, the *Rogers' Textbook of Pediatric Critical Care*. It is designed to be smaller and more economical than the *Textbook*, and in making it so, only essential information for the treatment of patients has been included in the *Handbook*. In addition to the references, we have omitted the first section of the *Textbook*, which contained chapters on the larger context of critical care medicine. The remaining chapters have been distilled to include the vital information needed for bedside care. It is the sound *practice of pediatric critical care* that is captured in the *Handbook*. Readers are encouraged to refer to the *Textbook* for a more comprehensive review of the material, as well as the references.

We thank the authors and section editors who submitted the full chapters for the *Textbook*. A special thanks also goes to Ms. Tzipora Sofare for her invaluable editorial assistance. As always, we are also indebted to the international patients, families, doctors, nurses, respiratory therapists, social workers, pharmacists, case managers, child-life specialists, nutritionists, and other members of the team who ensure the highest level of care for critically ill children. In addition, we thank our wives and children, who are always near and dear to our hearts.

M. A. Helfaer
D. G. Nichols

■ CONTRIBUTORS

Nicholas S. Abend, MD
Department of Neurology
University of Pennsylvania School of Medicine
Philadelphia, Pennsylvania

Mateo Aboy, PhD
Department of Electronics Engineering
    & Technology
Oregon Institute of Technology
Portland, Oregon

Kareem Abu-Elmagd, MD
Thomas E. Starzl Transplantation Institute
University of Pittsburgh
Pittsburgh, Pennsylvania

Meredith L. Allen, MB, BS, FRACP, PhD
Portex Department of Anaesthesia, Intensive
    Therapy, and Respiratory Medicine
Institute of Child Health, University College
London, United Kingdom

John H. Arnold, MD
Department of Anaesthesia (Pediatrics)
Harvard Medical School
Boston, Massachusetts

Stephen Ashwall, MD
Department of Pediatrics
Loma Linda University School of Medicine
Loma Linda, California

John Scott Baird, MD
Department of Pediatrics
Columbia University, College of Physicians
    and Surgeons
New York, New York

Aristides Baltodano, MD
Departamento de Pediatriay Cuidados Criticos
Universidad de Costa Rica, Escuela de Medicina
San José, Costa Rica

Kenneth J. Banasiak, MD
Department of Pediatrics
Yale University School of Medicine
New Haven, Connecticut

Arun Bansal, MD
Department of Pediatrics
Postgraduate Institute of Medical Education
    and Research
Chandigarh, India

Hülya Bayir, MD
Departments of Critical Care Medicine and
    Environmental and Occupational Health
University of Pittsburgh School of Medicine
Pittsburgh, Pennsylvania

Robert A. Berg, MD, FAAP, FCCM
Departments of Anesthesiology & Critical Care
University of Pennsylvania School of Medicine
Philadelphia, Pennsylvania

Katherine Biagas, MD
Department of Pediatrics
Columbia University, College of Physicians
    and Surgeons
New York, New York

Michael T. Bigham, MD
Pediatric Critical Care Medicine
Cincinnati Children's Hospital Medical Center
Cincinnati, Ohio

Mark S. Bleiweis, MD
Departments of Surgery and Pediatrics
University of Florida College of Medicine
Gainesville, Florida

Jeffrey L. Blumer, PhD, MD
Department of Pediatrics
Case Western Reserve University
Cleveland, Ohio

Clifford W. Bogue, MD
Department of Pediatrics
Yale University School of Medicine
New Haven, Connecticut

Geoffrey J. Bond, MD, FRACS
Department of Pediatrics
University of Pittsburgh School of Medicine
Pittsburgh, Pennsylvania

Brigid M. Bradley, MD
Department of Pediatrics
Columbia University, College of Physicians
   and Surgeons
New York, New York

Kenneth M. Brady, MD
Department of Anesthesiology & Critical
   Care Medicine
The Johns Hopkins University School of Medicine
Baltimore, Maryland

John Philip Breinholt, III, MD
Department of Pediatrics
Baylor College of Medicine
Houston, Texas

Richard J. Brilli, MD
Department of Pediatrics
University of Cincinnati College of Medicine
Cincinnati, Ohio

Deborah L. Brown, MD
Department of Pediatrics
The University of Texas School of Medicine
Houston, Texas

Werther Brunow de Carvalho, MD
Departamento de Pediatria
Universidade Federal de São Paulo
Escola Paulista de Medicina
São Paulo, Brasil

Timothy E. Bunchman, MD
Department of Pediatric Nephrology
Michigan State University, College of Human
   Medicine
East Lansing, Michigan

**Warwick W. Butt, MB, BS, FRACP,
   FJFICM**
Department of Pediatrics
Melbourne University, Faculty of Medicine,
   Dentistry, and Health Sciences
Melbourne, Victoria, Australia

Mitchell S. Cairo, MD
Department of Pediatrics
Columbia University, College of Physicians
   and Surgeons
New York, New York

James D. Campbell, MD, MS
Department of Pediatrics
Center for Vaccine Development
University of Maryland School of Medicine
Baltimore, Maryland

Michael F. Canarie, MD
Department of Pediatrics
Yale University School of Medicine
New Haven, Connecticut

G. Patricia Cantwell, MD
Department of Critical Care Medicine
University of Miami, Miller School of Medicine
Miami, Florida

Joseph A. Carcillo, MD
Departments of Critical Care Medicine
   and Pediatrics
University of Pittsburgh School of Medicine
Pittsburgh, Pennsylvania

Todd Carpenter, MD
Department of Pediatrics
University of Colorado at Denver and Health
   Sciences Center
Denver, Colorado

Thomas O. Carpenter, MD
Department of Pediatrics
Yale University School of Medicine
New Haven, Connecticut

Ira M. Cheifetz, MD, FCCM, FAARC
Department of Pediatrics
Duke University School of Medicine
Durham, North Carolina

Wendy K. Chung, MD, PhD
Departments of Pediatrics and Medicine
Columbia University, College of Physicians
   and Surgeons
New York, New York

Robert S.B. Clark, MD
Departments of Pediatrics and Critical
   Care Medicine
University of Pittsburgh School of Medicine
Pittsburgh, Pennsylvania

Steven A. Conrad, MD, PhD, FCCM
Departments of Pediatrics, Medicine, Emergency
    Medicine, and Anesthesiology
Louisiana State University Health Sciences Center
Shreveport, Louisiana

Arthur Cooper, MD, MS
Department of Surgery
Columbia University, College of Physicians
    and Surgeons
New York, New York

Mehrengise K. Cooper, MD, FRCPCH
Department of Paediatrics
Imperial College School of Medicine
London, United Kingdom

Ashraf H. Coovadia, MD
Department of Paediatrics and Child Health
University of The Witwatersrand
Johannesburg, Gauteng, South Africa

Jose A. Cortes, MD
Departments of Pediatrics and Anesthesiology
    & Critical Care Medicine
The University of Texas School of Medicine
Houston, Texas

Heidi J. Dalton, MD
Department of Pediatrics
George Washington University School of Medicine
    and Health Sciences
Washington, DC

Sally L. Davidson Ward, MD
Department of Pediatrics
University of Southern California, Keck School
    of Medicine
Los Angeles, California

Allan de Caen, MD, FRCPC
Department of Pediatrics
University of Alberta, Faculty of Medicine
    & Dentistry
Edmonton, Alberta, Canada

Susan W. Denfield, MD
Department of Pediatrics
Baylor College of Medicine
Houston, Texas

Denis J. Devictor, MD, PhD
Département de Pédiatrie
Université Paris-Sud 11
Le Kremlin-Bicêtre, France

Troy E. Dominguez, MD
Department of Anesthesiology and Critical Care
University of Pennsylvania School of Medicine
Philadelphia, Pennsylvania

Aaron J. Donoghue, MD, MSCE
Departments of Anesthesiology and Critical Care
    and Pediatrics
University of Pennsylvania School of Medicine
Philadelphia, Pennsylvania

Lesley Doughty, MD
Department of Pediatrics
University of Cincinnati School of Medicine
Cincinnati, Ohio

William J. Dreyer, MD
Department of Pediatrics
Baylor College of Medicine
Houston, Texas

Jonathan Duff, MD, FRCPC
Pediatric Intensive Care Unit
Stollery Children's Hospital
Edmonton, Alberta, Canada

R. Blaine Easley, MD
Department of Anesthesiology and Critical
    Care Medicine
The Johns Hopkins University School of Medicine
Baltimore, Maryland

Ori Eyal, MD
Pediatric Endocrinology and Diabetes Unit
The Chaim Sheba Medical Center
Tel Aviv University Sackler School of Medicine
Tel Hashomer, Israel

Edward Vincent S. Faustino, MD
Department of Pediatrics
Yale University School of Medicine
New Haven, Connecticut

Kathryn A. Felmet, MD
Department of Critical Care Medicine
University of Pittsburgh School of Medicine
Pittsburgh, Pennsylvania

Pamela Feuer, MD
Department of Pediatrics
Columbia University, College of Physicians
    and Surgeons
New York, New York

Alan I. Fields, MD, FCCM
Departments of Pediatrics and Anesthesiology
    & Critical Care Medicine
The University of Texas School of Medicine
Houston, Texas

Jeffrey R. Fineman, MD
Department of Pediatrics
Cardiovascular Research Institute
University of California, San Francisco
San Francisco, California

Ericka L. Fink, MD
Department of Critical Care Medicine
Children's Hospital of Pittsburgh
Pittsburgh, Pennsylvania

George L. Foltin, MD
Departments of Pediatrics and Emergency
    Medicine
New York University School of Medicine
New York, New York

Marcelo Cunio Machado Fonseca, MD
Departamento de Pediatria
Universidade Federal de São Paulo
Escola Paulista de Medicina
São Paulo, Brasil

Alain Fraisse, MD, PhD
Départment de Cardiologie
Université de la Méditerranée
Marseille, France

Philippe S. Friedlich, MD, Ms, Epi, MBA
Department of Pediatrics
University of Southern California, Keck School
    of Medicine
Los Angeles, California

Muraya Gathinji, MS
The Johns Hopkins University School of Medicine
Baltimore, Maryland

**Jonathan Gillis, MB, BS, PhD, FRACP,
    FJFICM**
Department of Paediatric Intensive Care
Children's Hospital at Westmead
Sydney, New South Wales, Australia

Brahm Goldstein, MD, FCCM
Novo Nordisk, Inc.
Princeton, New Jersey

Salvatore R. Goodwin, MD
Department of Anesthesiology & Critical Care
Mayo Clinic, College of Medicine
Rochester, Minnesota

Ana Lia Graciano, MD, FAAP
Department of Pediatrics
University of California at San Francisco
Fresno, California

Alan Graham, MD
Department of Pediatrics
Oregon Health & Science University
Portland, Oregon

Philip L. Graham III, MD, MSc
Department of Pediatrics
Columbia University College of Physicians
    and Surgeons
New York, New York

Bruce M. Greenwald, MD
Department of Pediatrics
Weill Medical College of Cornell University
New York, New York

Brandt P. Groh, MD
Department of Pediatrics
Penn State College of Medicine
Hershey, Pennsylvania

Richard Hackbarth, MD
Department of Pediatrics and Human Development
Michigan State University, College of Human
    Medicine
East Lansing, Michigan

Gabriel G. Haddad, MD
Departments of Pediatrics and Neurosciences
University of California, San Diego, School
    of Medicine
San Diego, California

Mark W. Hall, MD
Department of Pediatrics
The Ohio State University College of Medicine
Columbus, Ohio

Gillian C. Halley, MBChB
Paediatric Intensive Care Unit
Royal Brompton Hospital
London, United Kingdom

Donna S. Hamel, RRT, RCP, FAARC
Department of Pediatric Critical Care Medicine
Duke University Medical Center
Durham, North Carolina

Z. Leah Harris, MD
Department of Anesthesiology & Critical
    Care Medicine
The Johns Hopkins University School of Medicine
Baltimore, Maryland

Abeer Hassoun, MD
Department of Pediatrics
Columbia University, College of Physicians
    and Surgeons
New York, New York

Jan A. Hazelzet, MD, PhD, FCCM
Pediatric Intensive Care Unit
Sophia Childrens Hospital, Erasmus Medical
    Center
Rotterdam, The Netherlands

Mary Fran Hazinski, RN, MSN, FAAN
Departments of Surgery and Pediatrics
Vanderbilt University School of Medicine
Nashville, Tennessee

Gregory P. Heldt, MD
Department of Pediatrics
University of California, San Diego, School
of Medicine
San Diego, California

Mark A. Helfaer, MD
Departments of Anesthesiology and Critical Care
University of Pennsylvania School of Medicine
Philadelphia, Pennsylvania

Mark J. Heulitt, MD
Departments of Pediatrics, Physiology
and Biophysics
University of Arkansas for Medical Sciences,
College of Medicine
Little Rock, Arkansas

Siew Yen Ho, MD
Imperial College, National Heart & Lung Institute
London, United Kingdom

Julien I. Hoffman, MD
Department of Pediatrics
University of California, San Francisco
San Francisco, California

Joy D. Howell, MD
Department of Pediatrics
Weill Medical College of Cornell University
New York, New York

S. Adil Husain, MD
Department of Surgery
University of Indiana
Indianapolis, Indiana

Tomas Iölster, MD
Departamento de Pediatria
Universidad Austral School of Medicine
Pilar, Buenos Aires, Argentina

Ronald Jaffe, MD
Department of Pathology
University of Pittsburgh School of Medicine
Pittsburgh, Pennsylvania

M. Jayashree, MB, BS, MD
Department of Pediatrics
Advanced Pediatric Centre
Post Graduate Institute of Medical Education
and Research
Chandigarh, India

John Lynn Jefferies, MD, MPH
Department of Pediatrics
Baylor College of Medicine
Houston, Texas

Larry W. Jenkins, PhD
Departments of Neurological Surgery
and Neurobiology
Safar Center for Resuscitation Research
University of Pittsburgh School of Medicine
Pittsburgh, Pennsylvania

Sachin S. Jogal, MD
Department of Pediatric Hematology/Oncology/
Bone Marrow Transplantation
Medical College of Wisconsin
Milwaukee, Wisconsin

Cíntia Johnston, RRT
Departamentos da Medicina e Pediatria
Universidade Federal de São Paulo
Escola Paulista de Medicina
São Paulo, Brasil

Phillippe Jouvet, MD, PhD
Department of Pediatrics
University of Montreal, Faculty of Medicine
Montreal, Quebec, Canada

Sushil K. Kabra, MD, DNB
Department of Pediatrics
All India Institute of Medical Sciences
New Delhi, India

Jonathan R. Kaltman, MD
Department of Cardiology
University of Pennsylvania School of Medicine
Philadelphia, Pennsylvania

Thomas G. Keens, MD
Departments of Pediatrics, Physiology
and Biophysics
University of Southern California, Keck School
of Medicine
Los Angeles, California

Lisa K. Kelly, MD
Department of Pediatrics
University of Southern California, Keck School
of Medicine
Los Angeles, California

Andrea Kelly, MD
Department of Pediatrics
University of Pennsylvania School of Medicine
Philadelphia, Pennsylvania

Sudha Kilaru V. Kessler, MD
Department of Neurology
University of Pennsylvania School of Medicine
Philadelphia, Pennsylvania

Alka Khadwal, MD
Department of Pediatrics
Postgraduate Institute of Medical Education
& Research
Chandigarh, India

Praveen Khilnani, MD, FCCM
Department of Pediatrics
Ipapollo Hospital
New Delhi, India

Jeffrey J. Kim, MD
Department of Pediatrics
Baylor College of Medicine
Houston, Texas

Carroll J. King, MD
Departments of Pediatrics and Anesthesiology
& Critical Care Medicine
The University of Texas School of Medicine
Houston, Texas

Fenella Kirkham, MBBChir
Neurosciences Unit
Institute of Child Health, University College
London
London, United Kingdom

**Niranjan "Tex" Kissoon, MD, FAAP,
FRCP(C), FCCM, FACPE, CPE**
Department of Pediatrics
University of British Columbia, Faculty of Medicine
Vancouver, British Columbia, Canada

Nigel J. Klein, MB, BS, MD
Infectious Diseases and Microbiology Unit
Institute of Child Health
London, United Kingdom

Monica E. Kleinman, MD
Department of Anaesthesia
Harvard Medical School
Boston, Massachusetts

Patrick M. Kochanek, MD
Safar Center for Resuscitation Research
Departments of Critical Care Medicine,
Anesthesiology, and Pediatrics
University of Pittsburgh School of Medicine
Pittsburgh, Pennsylvania

Keith C. Kocis, MD, MS
Department of Pediatric Critical Care Medicine
The University of North Carolina
Chapel Hill, North Carolina

Karen L. Kotloff, MD
Department of Pediatrics
University of Maryland School of Medicine
Baltimore, Maryland

Sheila S. Kun, RN, BSN, MS
Division of Pediatric Pulmonology
Childrens Hospital Los Angeles
Los Angeles, California

Jacques Lacroix, MD, FRCPC
Département de pédiatrie
Université de Montréal, Faculté de Médicine
Montréal, Quebec, Canada

Miriam K. Laufer, MD
Department of Pediatrics
Center for Vaccine Development
University of Maryland School of Medicine
Baltimore, Maryland

Matthew B. Laurens, MD, MPH
Department of Pediatrics
University of Maryland School of Medicine
Baltimore, Maryland

Heitor Pons Leite, MD, PhD
Departamento de Pediatria
Universidade Federal de São Paulo
Escola Paulista de Medicina
São Paulo, Brasil

Daniel L. Levin, MD
Departments of Pediatrics and Anesthesia
Dartmouth Medical School
Hanover, New Hampshire

Daniel J. Licht, MD
Department of Neurology
University of Pennsylvania School of Medicine
Philadelphia, Pennsylvania

Rakesh Lodha, MD
Department of Pediatrics
All India Institute of Medical Sciences
Ansari Nagar, New Delhi, India

David M. Loeb, MD, PhD
Departments of Pediatrics and Oncology
The Johns Hopkins University School of Medicine
Baltimore, Maryland

Anne Lortie, MD
Department of Pediatrics
University of Montreal, Faculty of Medicine
Montreal, Quebec, Canada

Naomi L.C. Luban, MD
Departments of Pediatrics and Pathology
George Washington University School of Medicine
and Health Sciences
Washington, DC

Robert Luten, MD
Department of Emergency Medicine
University of Florida College of Medicine
Jacksonville, Florida

Duncan J. Macrae, BMSc, MBChB, FRCA, FRCPCH
Department of Pediatrics
University of London, Imperial College
London, United Kingdom

Mioara D. Manole, MD
Department of Pediatrics
University of Pittsburgh School of Medicine
Pittsburgh, Pennsylvania

Bruno Maranda, MD, MSc
Service of Medical Genetics
Ste. Justine Hospital
Montreal, Quebec, Canada

Bradley S. Marino, MD, MPP, MSCE
Department of Pediatrics
University of Cincinnati College of Medicine
Cincinnati, Ohio

Michele M. Mariscalco, MD
Department of Pediatrics
Baylor College of Medicine
Houston, Texas

Dolly Martin, RN
Intestinal Rehabilitation and Transplant Center
Thomas E. Starzl Transplantation Institute
Pittsburgh, Pennsylvania

Norma Maxvold, MD
Department of Pediatric Critical Care
DeVos Children's Hospital
Grand Rapids, Michigan

George V. Mazariegos, MD, FACS
Department of Pediatrics
University of Pittsburgh School of Medicine
Pittsburgh, Pennsylvania

Jennifer A. McArthur, DO
Department of Pediatrics
Medical College of Wisconsin
Milwaukee, Wisconsin

Rodrigo Mejia, MD, FAAP
Departments of Pediatrics and Anesthesiology
& Critical Care Medicine
The University of Texas School of Medicine
Houston, Texas

Jon N. Meliones, MD
Department of Pediatric Critical Care
Duke University School of Medicine
Durham, North Carolina

David Joshua Michelson, MD
Department of Pediatrics, Division of
Child Neurology
Loma Linda University School of Medicine
Loma Linda, California

Johnny Millar, MBChB, PhD
Pediatric Intensive Care Unit
Royal Children's Hospital
Melbourne, Australia

Katsuyuki Miyasaka, MD, PhD, FAAP, FCCP
Nagano Children's Hospital
Toyoshina, Nagano, Japan

Thomas Moshang, Jr., MD
Department of Pediatrics
University of Pennsylvania School of Medicine
Philadelphia, Pennsylvania

Simon Nadel, FRCP
Paediatric Intensive Care Unit
Department of Paediatrics
St. Mary's Hospital
London, United Kingdom

Vinay M. Nadkarni, MD
Departments of Anesthesiology & Critical
Care and Pediatrics
University of Pennsylvania School of Medicine
Philadelphia, Pennsylvania

David P. Nelson, MD
Department of Pediatrics
Baylor College of Medicine
Houston, Texas

Charle RJC Newton, MBChB, MD, MRCP, FRCPCH
Department of Neurosciences
University College of London
London, United Kingdom

David G. Nichols, MD
Departments of Anesthesiology & Critical Care
Medicine and Pediatrics
The Johns Hopkins University School of Medicine
Baltimore, Maryland

Sharon E. Oberfield, MD
Department of Pediatrics
Columbia University, College of Physicians
   and Surgeons
New York, New York

George Ofori-Amanfo, MD
Department of Pediatrics
University of Pennsylvania School of Medicine
Philadelphia, Pennsylvania

Peter E. Oishi, MD
Department of Pediatrics
University of California, San Francisco
San Francisco, California

Richard A. Orr, MD
Departments of Critical Care Medicine
   and Pediatrics
University of Pittsburgh School of Medicine
Pittsburgh, Pennsylvania

John Pappachan, MA, MBBChir, FRCA
Paediatric Intensive Care Unit
Southampton University Hospitals Trust
Southampton, England

Robert I. Parker, MD
Department of Pediatrics
SUNY at Stony Brook School of Medicine
Stony Brook, New York

Mark J. Peters, MD, PhD
Portex Unit
Institute of Child Health
London, United Kingdom

Frank L. Powell, PhD
Department of Medicine
University of California, San Diego, School
   of Medicine
San Diego, California

Jack F. Price, MD
Department of Pediatrics
Baylor College of Medicine
Houston, Texas

Gerardo Quezada, MD, FAAP
Department of Pediatrics
The University of Texas School of Medicine
Houston, Texas

Elisabeth L. Raab, MD
Department of Pediatrics
University of Southern California, Keck School
   of Medicine
Los Angeles, California

Surender Rajasekaran, MD, MPH
Department of Pediatrics
University of Tennessee Health Science Center
Memphis, Tennessee

Rangasamy Ramanathan, MD, FAAP
Department of Pediatrics
University of Southern California, Keck School
   of Medicine
Los Angeles, California

Suchitra Ranjit, MD, DCH
Pediatric Intensive Care Unit
Apollo Hospitals
Chennai, India

Thyyar M. Ravindranath, MD
Department of Pediatrics
Columbia University, College of Physicians
   and Surgeons
New York, New York

Chitra Ravishankar, MD
Department of Pediatrics
University of Pennsylvania
Philadelphia, Pennsylvania

Antonio Rodriguez-Nuñez, MD, PhD
Department of Pediatrics
University of Santiago de Compostela
Santiago de Compostela, Spain

Susan R. Rose, MD
Division of Pediatric Endocrinology
University of Cincinnati College of Medicine
Cincinnati, Ohio

Joseph W. Rossano, MD
Department of Pediatrics
Baylor College of Medicine
Houston, Texas

Daniel Russo, MD
Departamento de Pediatria
Universidad Austral School of Medicine
Pilar, Buenos Aires, Argentina

**Monique M. Ryan, MB, BS, MMed,
   FRACP**
Department of Paediatrics
Royal Children's Hospital
Parkville, Victoria, Australia

Michael E. Rytting, MD, FAAP
Department of Pediatrics
The University of Texas School of Medicine
Houston, Texas

Stephen M. Schexnayder, MD
Department of Pediatrics
University of Arkansas College of Medicine
Little Rock, Arkansas

Charles L. Schleien, MD
Departments of Pediatrics and Anesthesiology
Columbia University, College of Physicians
    and Surgeons
New York, New York

Eduardo Schnitzler, MD
Departamento de Pediatria
Universidad Austral School of Medicine
Pilar, Buenos Aires, Argentina

Steven M. Schwartz, MD
Department of Pediatrics
University of Toronto
Toronto, Ontario, Canada

Istvan Seri, MD
Professor of Pediatrics
University of Southern California, Keck School
    of Medicine
Los Angeles, California

Donald H. Shaffner, MD
Department of Anesthesiology & Critical
    Care Medicine
The Johns Hopkins University School of Medicine
Baltimore, Maryland

**R. Lara Shekerdemian, MBChB, MD,
MRCP (UK), FRACP, FRCPCH**
Paediatric Intensive Care Unit
The Royal Children's Hospital
Melbourne, Victoria, Australia

Naoki Shimizu, MD, PhD
Department of Anaesthesia and Intensive Care
National Centre for Child Health and Development
Tokyo, Japan

Jakub Simon, MD
Department of Pediatrics
University of Maryland School of Medicine
Baltimore, Maryland

Rakesh Sindhi, MD, FACS
Department of Pediatrics
University of Pittsburgh School of Medicine
Pittsburgh, Pennsylvania

Sunit C. Singhi, MB, BS, MD
Department of Pediatrics
Postgraduate Institute of Medical Education
    and Research
Chandigarh, India

Pratibha D. Singhi, MB, BS, MD
Department of Pediatrics
Postgraduate Institute of Medical Education
    and Research
Chandigarh, India

**Peter W. Skippen, MD, FANZCA,
FJFICM, FRCPC**
Department of Pediatrics
University of British Columbia
Vancouver, British Columbia, Canada

Zdenek Slavik, MD, DM, FRCPCH
Department of Pediatrics
Charles University
Pilsen, Czech Republic

Arthur Smerling, MD
Departments of Pediatrics and Anesthesiology
Columbia University, College of Physicians
    and Surgeons
New York, New York

Kyle A. Soltys, MD
Department of Pediatrics
University of Pittsburgh School of Medicine
Pittsburgh, Pennsylvania

Meridith F. Sonnett, MD
Department of Pediatrics
Columbia University, College of Physicians
    and Surgeons
New York, New York

Robert H. Squires, Jr., MD
Department of Pediatrics
University of Pittsburgh School of Medicine
Pittsburgh, Pennsylvania

Kimberly D. Statler, MD, MPH
Departments of Pediatrics and Neurology
University of Utah School of Medicine
Salt Lake City, Utah

Kurt R. Stenmark, MD
Department of Pediatric Critical Care
Developmental Lung Biology Laboratory
University of Colorado at Denver and Health
    Sciences Center
Denver, Colorado

Caron Strahlendorf, MD
Divisions of Hematology, Oncology,
    & Bone Marrow Transplantation
University of British Columbia
Vancouver, British Columbia, Canada

John P. Straumanis, MD
Department of Pediatrics
University of Maryland School of Medicine
Baltimore, Maryland

Kevin J. Sullivan, MD
Department of Anesthesiology & Critical Care
Mayo Clinic, College of Medicine
Rochester, Minnesota

William V. Tamborlane, MD
Department of Pediatrics
Yale University School of Medicine
New Haven, Connecticut

Robert F. Tamburro, MD, MSc
Department of Pediatrics
Pennsylvania State University College of Medicine
Hershey, Pennsylvania

Ronn E. Tanel, MD
Department of Pediatrics
University of Pennsylvania School of Medicine
Philadelphia, Pennsylvania

Robert C. Tasker, MB, BS, MD, FRCP
Department of Paediatrics
Cambridge University, School of Clinical Medicine
Cambridge, United Kingdom

David F. Teitel, MD
Department of Pediatrics
Cardiovascular Research Institute
University of California, San Francisco
San Francisco, California

Neal J. Thomas, MD, MSc
Pediatrics and Health Evaluation Sciences
Pennsylvania State University College of Medicine
Hershey, Pennsylvania

Ann E. Thompson, MD
Department of Critical Care Medicine
University of Pittsburgh School of Medicine
Pittsburgh, Pennsylvania

James Tibballs, BMedSc, MB, BS, MEd, MBA, MD, FANZCA, FJFICM, FACTM
Australian Venom Research Unit
University of Melbourne
Melbourne, Victoria, Australia

Shane M. Tibby, MBChB, MRCP, MSc
Department of Paediatric Intensive Care
Evelina Children's Hospital
Guy's and St. Thomas' NHS Foundation Trust
London, United Kingdom

Pierre Tissières, MD, MSc
Départment de Pédiatrie
Hôpital de Bicêtre
Le Kremlin-Bicêtre, France

Joseph D. Tobias, MD
Department of Anesthesiology
University of Missouri School of Medicine
Columbia, Missouri

Philip Toltzis, MD
Department of Pediatrics
Case Western Reserve University
Cleveland, Ohio

Jeffrey A. Towbin, MD
Department of Pediatrics
Baylor College of Medicine
Houston, Texas

Colin B. Van Orman, MD
Department of Pediatrics
University of Utah School of Medicine
Salt Lake City, Utah

John S. Venglarcik, III, MD
Department of Pediatrics
Northeastern Ohio Universities, College of Medicine
Rootstown, Ohio

Shekhar T. Venkataraman, MD
Departments of Critical Care Medicine and Pediatrics
University of Pittsburgh School of Medicine
Pittsburgh, Pennsylvania

Kathleen M. Ventre, MD
Department of Pediatrics
University of Utah School of Medicine
Salt Lake City, Utah

Prof.-Dr. med. Hans-Dieter Volk
Charité Institut für Medizinische Immunologie
Berlin, Germany

Steven A. Webber, MBChB, MRCP
Department of Pediatrics
University of Pittsburgh School of Medicine
Pittsburgh, Pennsylvania

Stuart A. Weinzimer, MD
Department of Pediatrics
Yale University School of Medicine
New Haven, Connecticut

Richard S. Weisman, PharmD, ABAT
Department of Pediatrics
University of Miami, Miller School of Medicine
Miami, Florida

David L. Wessel, MD
Division of Critical Care Medicine
Children's National Medical Center
Washington, DC

Randall C. Wetzel, MB, BS, MS Bus., FAAP, FCCM
Departments of Pediatrics and Anesthesiology
University of Southern California, Keck School of Medicine
Los Angeles, California

Michael Wilhelm, MD
Department of Pediatrics
Columbia University, College of Physicians and Surgeons
New York, New York

Kenneth D. Winkel, MB, BS, PhD
Australian Venom Research Unit
Department of Pharmacology
University of Melbourne
Melbourne, Australia

Gerhard K. Wolf, MD
Department of Anaesthesia
Harvard Medical School
Boston, Massachusetts

Edward C.C. Wong, MD
Departments of Pediatrics and Pathology
George Washington University School of Medicine and Health Sciences
Washington, DC

Angela T. Wratney, MD, MHSc
Department of Pediatrics
George Washington University School of Medicine
Washington, DC

Roger W. Yurt, MD
Department of Surgery
Weill Medical College of Cornell University
New York, New York

Arno L. Zaritsky, MD
Department of Pediatrics
University of Florida College of Medicine
Gainesville, Florida

David Zideman, QHP(C), BSc, MB, BS, FRCA, FIMC
Department of Anaesthetics
Hammersmith Hospital
London, United Kingdom

■CONTENTS

CHAPTER 1 ■ AIRWAY MANAGEMENT

ALLAN DE CAEN, JONATHAN DUFF, ASHRAF COOVADIA,
ROBERT LUTEN, ANN THOMPSON, MARY FRAN HAZINSKI

The major differences between the pediatric and the adult airway are size, shape, and position in the neck (**Table 1.1**). Because the diameter of the pediatric trachea is small, relatively small compromise in airway radius can significantly increase resistance to airflow and work of breathing. When respiratory distress is present, providers should attempt to keep the child as quiet as possible, minimizing agitation to reduce turbulent flow, airway resistance, and work of breathing. The infant's tongue is large in proportion to the rest of the oral cavity and is closer to the palate; therefore, it can easily obstruct the airway. Upper airway obstruction (e.g., caused by croup, epiglottitis, or extrathoracic foreign body) can produce tracheal collapse and stridor. The epiglottis is proportionally larger in the child than in the adult, and the ligamentous connection between the base of the tongue and the epiglottis is not as strong in the young child as in the adult. These differences can influence the selection of laryngoscope blade (straight versus curved) for intubation of young children. Although most of the child's laryngeal mucosa is loosely connected to the underlying tissues, it is tightly connected in the area of the vocal cords and at the laryngeal surface of the epiglottis. Subglottic inflammation is typically contained below this level; however, with little room to accommodate even modest inflammation at the level of the vocal cords or epiglottis, such inflammation can lead to a gross distortion of tissue planes and anatomic positions.

The glottic opening lies at approximately the level of C-2 or C-3 in the infant or child and at the level of C-3 or C-4 in the adolescent or adult (**Fig. 1.1**). The position of the pediatric airway has been described as "*anterior*" when compared to the mature airway, because the airway may become "hidden" behind the tongue on laryngoscopy.

The pediatric airway is actually more *superior* (i.e., higher or more cephalad) *and* more *anterior* than the adult airway. Airway webcam videos are available at http://www.airwaycam.com/vol2.html. The characteristics of the child's larynx are summarized in **Fig. 1.1** and **Table 1.2**.

Oral intubation with direct laryngoscopy requires alignment of 3 axes: the oral, pharyngeal, and laryngeal axes. The rescuer aligns the 3 axes in an older child or adult by placing a towel or other support beneath the occiput to tilt the neck forward (from the shoulders) and by lifting the chin to extend the neck. A technique to align the axes in younger children is placing them in the *sniffing position* (**Fig. 1.2**).

The basic components of the oropharyngeal examination include evaluation of atlanto-occipital joint extension and measurement of the potential mandibular displacement area. The degree of mouth opening is assessed by asking the cooperative patient to open the mouth to the widest extent possible and to protrude the tongue as far as possible, enabling assessment of the palate, the range of motion of the temporomandibular joint, and the size of the tongue relative to the oral cavity. The *Mallampati assessment* (**Fig. 1.3**) classifies the degree of airway difficulty based on the ability to visualize the faucial pillars, soft palate, and uvula with exposure of the glottis. With a Class 1 airway (i.e., all 3 pharyngeal structures can be visualized), laryngoscopy yields adequate "laryngeal exposure" in >99% of adult patients, while with a Class 3 airway (i.e., glottis cannot be exposed), laryngoscopy yields "adequate exposure" in only 7% of adult patients.

The size of the potential space (defined by the lateral and anterior aspects of the mandible to the hyoid bone) can be estimated with the neck extended by evaluating the *thyromental distance*, the distance

TABLE 1.1

TRACHEAL DIMENSIONS

Age (yrs)	Tracheal diameter (mm)	Superior tracheal limb length (mm)	Inferior tracheal limb length (mm)	Combined tracheal length (mm)
0–1	4.91 ± 0.88	27.94 ± 5.75	16.74 ± 7.78	44.68
1–2	6.68 ± 3.37	30.54 ± 5.74	20.11 ± 10.01	50.65
2–4	6.38 ± 1.86	31.87 ± 5.92	26.36 ± 5.91	58.23
4–6	8.4 ± 0.98	35.88 ± 14.03	27.84 ± 11.98	63.72
6–8	8.88 ± 1.51	35.45 ± 11.34	29.43 ± 10.80	64.88
8–10	9.35 ± 1.70	39.53 ± 6.95	35.48 ± 9.19	75.00
10–12	9.55 ± 1.14	38.53 ± 6.97	34.03 ± 7.31	72.56
12–14	10.46 ± 2.32	41.81 ± 9.28	40.19 ± 12.99	82.00
≥ 14	12.99 ± 1.35	47.21 ± 13.56	44.30 ± 17.14	91.51

Measurements are listed ± sample standard deviation.
From Reed JM, O'Conner DM, Myer CM 3rd. Magnetic resonance imaging determination of tracheal orientation in normal children. Practical implications. *Arch Otolaryngol Head Neck Surg* 1996; 122(6):605–8, with permission.

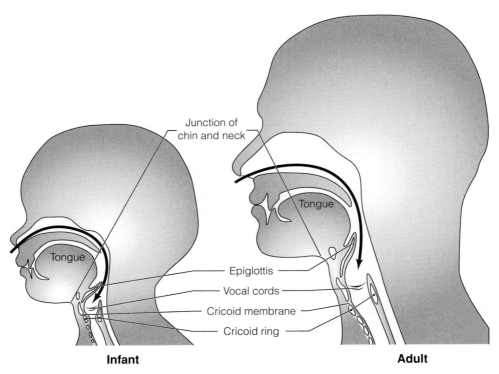

Infant   **Adult**

FIGURE 1.1. The anatomic differences particular to children are these: **1.** Higher, more anterior position of the glottic opening. (Note the relationship of the vocal cords to the chin/neck junction.) **2.** Relatively larger tongue in the infant, which lies between the mouth and glottic opening. **3.** Relatively larger and more floppy epiglottis in the child. **4.** The cricoid ring is the narrowest portion of the pediatric airway versus the vocal cords in the adult. **5.** Position and size of the cricothyroid membrane in the infant. **6.** Sharper, more difficult angle for blind nasotracheal intubation. **7.** Larger relative size of the occiput in the infant. Adapted from Luten RC, Kissoon NJ. In: Wallis R, Luten LC, Murphy MF et al., eds. *Manual of Emergency Airway Management*, 2nd ed., Philadelphia: Lippincott Williams & Wilkins, 2004: 217.

TABLE 1.2

ANATOMIC DIFFERENCES BETWEEN ADULT AND PEDIATRIC AIRWAYS

Anatomy	Clinical significance
Tongue occupies relatively large portion of the oral cavity.	High anterior airway position of the glottic opening compared with that in adults.
High tracheal opening (relative to cervical vertebrae): C-1 in infancy C-3 to C-4 at 7 years of age C-4 to C-5 in the adult	Straight blade preferred over curved blade to push distensible anatomy out of the way to visualize the larynx.
Large occiput may cause flexion of the airway, and large tongue can fall against the posterior pharynx when child is supine.	Sniffing position opens the airway. The larger occiput actually elevates the head toward the sniffing position in most infants and children (neck must be extended). A towel may be required under shoulders to elevate torso relative to head in small infants.
Cricoid ring is the narrowest portion of the child's trachea (vocal cords are the narrowest portion in the adult).	Uncuffed tubes may provide adequate seal, as they can fit snugly at the level of the cricoid ring. Selection of correct tube size is essential because use of excessively large tube may cause mucosal injury.
Consistent anatomic variations with age, with fewer anatomic abnormal variations related to body habitus, arthritis, and chronic disease.	Age-related variations: <2 years: high anterior airway 2–8 years: transition >8 years: small adult
Large tonsils and adenoids may bleed. More acute angle between epiglottis and laryngeal opening makes endotracheal intubation difficult.	Blind nasotracheal intubation not indicated in children. May cause failure of attempted nasotracheal intubation.
Small cricothyroid membrane.	Needle cricothyrotomy difficult; surgical cricothyrotomy impossible in infants and small children.

Adapted from Luten RC, Kissoon NJ. Approach to the pediatric airway. In: Walls R, ed. *Manual of Emergency Airway Management*, 2nd ed. Philadelphia: Lippincott Williams & Wilkins, 2004.

between the upper aspect of the thyroid cartilage/hyoid bone and the lower aspect of the mandible. When this distance is small, the angle between the pharyngeal and laryngeal axes will be more acute, making it difficult to align these axes to visualize the larynx. The potential mandibular displacement area is considered adequate for the adult and child if, with the head in neutral position, 2 fingers (3 cm) can be placed between the hyoid bone and the anterior ramus of the mandible. The minimum hyoid-to-mandible distance for an infant is 1.5 cm.

INITIAL MANEUVERS TO CLEAR AIRWAY

If the child is awake, with mild-to-moderate airway obstruction and no suspected cervical spine injury, he/she should be allowed to assume a position of comfort. The airway is suctioned as needed, and oxygen is administered. If the child is obtunded, the airway can become obstructed by a combination of neck flexion, jaw relaxation, displacement of the tongue against the posterior pharyngeal wall, and collapse of the hypopharynx. A simple jaw-thrust maneuver is the most effective method of opening the airway, although a head tilt-chin lift may also be successful. Providers should use the jaw thrust to open the airway if cervical spine injury is suspected, and they must perform the jaw thrust to provide effective bag-mask ventilation. If no cervical spine injury is suspected or if the airway cannot be opened using the jaw thrust, the provider should open the airway using a head tilt-chin lift maneuver.

Oropharyngeal Airway

The *oropharyngeal airway* (OPA) consists of a flange, a short bite-block segment, and a curved plastic body that provides an airway and suction channel through the mouth to the pharynx. It is designed to relieve

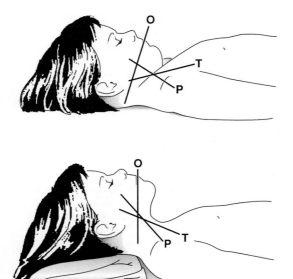

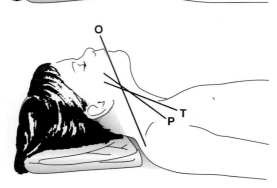

FIGURE 1.2. The 3 airway axes. The oral, pharyngeal, and laryngeal axes are optimally aligned for intubation when the child is placed in the "sniffing" position. For children <2 years of age, this requires slight extension of the neck. The prominent occiput of the infant or young child often provides the needed movement of the head forward of the shoulders. In the child over 2 years of age, a small towel is placed under the head (to lift the head forward) and the neck is slightly extended. The opening of the ear canal should be above or just anterior to the front of the child's shoulder. **A.** Resting position; **B.** Proper forward movement of head relative to shoulders; **C.** Proper positioning with both head position and neck extension for intubation: the oral, pharyngeal, and laryngeal axes are aligned. Adapted from Pediatric Advanced Life Support. American Heart Association, Inc., 2002.

airway obstruction by fitting over the tongue to hold it and the soft hypopharyngeal structures away from the posterior wall of the pharynx. An OPA may be used in the *unconscious* child if manual attempts to open the airway (e.g., head tilt-chin lift or jaw thrust) fail to provide and maintain a clear, unobstructed

airway. Use of an OPA in patients with intact cough or gag reflexes may stimulate gagging and vomiting; therefore, it is not recommended. A correctly sized OPA will extend from the corner of the mouth to the angle of the jaw. If the OPA is too large, it may obstruct the pharynx; if it is too small, it may push the base of the tongue back against the posterior pharynx. A tongue depressor may be used to insert the OPA directly into place. The OPA may also be inserted sideways and then rotated (90 degrees) into position. Upside-down insertion with 180-degree rotation is not routinely recommended because it may injure tissues or push the tongue posteriorly.

Nasopharyngeal Airway

A *nasopharyngeal airway* (NPA) is a soft rubber or plastic tube (a shortened ETT can be used) that provides an airway and channel for suctioning between the nares and the pharynx. NPAs may be used in patients with or without an intact cough and gag reflex. NPAs are available in sizes 12–36 French. A 12-French NPA (approximately the size of a 3-mm ETT) will generally fit the nasopharynx of a full-term infant. The NPA should be smaller than the inner aperture of the nares, and its proper length is approximately equal to the distance from the tip of the nose to the tragus of the ear. If the NPA is too long, it may cause vagal stimulation and bradycardia, or it may injure the epiglottis or vocal cords.

BAG-MASK VENTILATION

The most common technique for single-rescuer bag-mask ventilation involves the "E-C clamp" technique. The rescuer tilts the child's head and uses the last 3 fingers of one hand (forming a capital letter "E") to lift the jaw while pressing the mask against the face with the thumb and forefinger of the same hand (creating a "C"). The second hand squeezes the bag to deliver each breath over 1 sec to produce visible chest rise. It is important that the jaw is lifted to open the airway and the mask is simultaneously held tightly against the face.

General Indications for an Advanced Airway

The indications for advanced airway placement include loss of airway protection from impaired central nervous system function; need for hyperventilation to treat increased intracranial pressure (ICP); and

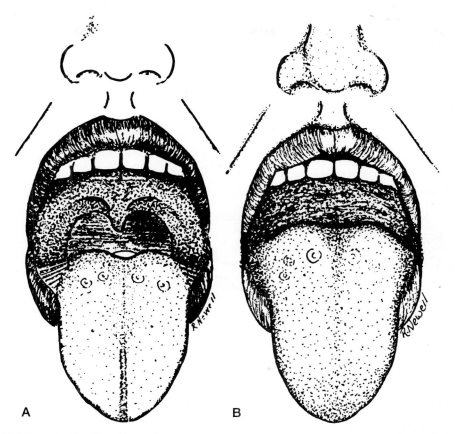

FIGURE 1.3. A. Tonsillar pillars, soft palate, and uvula are clearly visualized—a Class 1 airway. **B.** None of the pharyngeal structures are visualized—a Class IV airway. From Mallampati SR, Gatt SP, Gugino LD, et al. A clinical sign to predict difficult tracheal intubation: A prospective study. *Can Anaesth Soc J* 1985;32:429–34, with permission.

inadequate ventilation or ventilatory drive despite oxygen administration. Advanced airway placement may be appropriate if deterioration of the patient's respiratory status is anticipated or if a "borderline" patient must be moved into a poorly monitored or poorly controlled environment (e.g., sedation of a patient in the CT scanner or the interhospital transport of a child).

Choice of Advanced Airway

Placement of an advanced airway during attempted cardiopulmonary resuscitation (CPR) requires interruption of life-saving interventions such as cardiac compressions, and it may cause hypoxemia, reflux, and aspiration. Unrecognized tube misplacement is likely to be fatal. The intubator should always have a second strategy to provide oxygenation and ventilation if the initial airway approach fails. Bag-mask ventilation may provide this second strategy.

Endotracheal Intubation

After establishing that the airway can be intubated, the provider should assemble the necessary equipment and personnel and establish monitoring (**Table 1.3**). Although the use of age-based formulas (**Table 1.4**) to estimate the initial choice of cuffed and uncuffed tracheal tubes is more reliable than estimates based on the size of the fifth finger, these formulas are not as accurate as length-based tapes in predicting appropriate ETT size. The intubator should avoid manipulation of the neck if a risk exists of cervical spinal instability. Proceduralmonitoring is essential during ETI, including the monitoring of heart rate, blood pressure, oxygen saturation, and end-tidal capnometry/capnography prior to and immediately following ETI. Children may rapidly become hypoxemic during the procedure, so the intubator must provide adequate oxygenation before attempting the intubation. The intubator should

---

TABLE 1.3

EQUIPMENT FOR ENDOTRACHEAL INTUBATION

Monitoring Equipment (apply before intubation if at all possible)
Cardiorespiratory monitor (including monitoring of blood pressure, if possible)
Pulse oximeter

Length-based Tape to Estimate Tube and Equipment Sizes
Suction Equipment
Tonsil-tipped suction device or large-bore suction to suction pharynx
Suction catheter of appropriate size to suction endotracheal tube
Suction canister and device capable of generating –80 to –120 mm Hg
(a wall-suction device capable of generating –300 mm Hg is preferred)

Bag and Mask
Check size and oxygen connections
Connected to high-flow oxygen source with reservoir (capable of providing ~100% oxygen)

Medications
Anticholinergics (atropine)
Sedatives
Paralytics
Appropriate IV equipment and syringes for administration of medications

Intubation Equipment
Stylet
Cuffed and uncuffed tubes of estimated size and cuffed and uncuffed tubes that are 0.5 mm larger and smaller than
    estimated sizes
Laryngoscope blades (curved and straight) and handle with working light (with extra batteries and bulb ready)
Water-soluble lubricant
Syringe to inflate tube cuff (if appropriate)
Towel or pad to place under patient (if appropriate)

Confirmation Device(s)
Exhaled CO_2 detector (pediatric size for patients <15 kg and adult size for patients >15 kg)
Esophageal detector device may be used for children who are >20 kg with a perfusing rhythm

Tape/device to Secure Tube
Tape and tincture of benzoin or
Commercial device

TABLE 1.4

**FORMULAS FOR ESTIMATION OF
ENDOTRACHEAL TUBE SIZE AND DEPTH
OF INSERTION**

Size
Uncuffed tubes for children >2 years: Endotracheal Tube (internal diameter in mm) $= \dfrac{\text{Age (yrs)}}{4} + 4$
Cuffed tubes for children >2 years Endotracheal Tube (internal diameter in mm) $= \dfrac{\text{Age (yrs)}}{4} + 3$
Depth of insertion Depth of insertion (cm) = (age in years/2) + 12 Depth of insertion = (ETT internal diameter) × 3

terminate ETI efforts and initiate bag-mask ventilation if the patient's heart rate, oxygenation, or clinical appearance deteriorate. The laryngoscope blade is used to deflect the tongue and lift the supraglottic structures (or tent the epiglottis) to visualize the glottis. The ETT is inserted through the vocal cords. Both curved and straight laryngoscope blades should be available.

If, despite appropriate head positioning, the intubator cannot see the glottis during the attempt, an assistant should perform external laryngeal manipulation (backward, upward, and rightward push—BURP) to attempt to bring the glottis into view. If the provider can only visualize the posterior aspects of the glottis, successful intubation may be possible by using a stylet to create a bend (a "hockey stick") in the end of the tracheal tube. Intubators must ensure that the tip of the stylet does not protrude beyond the end of the tracheal tube. The tracheal tube should be positioned with the tube's marker line placed at or distal to the vocal cords. Cuffed tubes should be placed so that the cuff is positioned immediately below the level of the cords. Correct depth of insertion can be estimated from formulas using the child's age or the ETT size (**Table 1.4**). To perform clinical confirmation of tube position, bag-tube ventilation is provided while the intubator observes for chest rise, auscultating bilaterally over the anterior chest, both axillae, and the stomach and observing for water vapor in the tracheal tube on exhalation. Either exhaled CO_2 detectors or an esophageal detector device is used for device confirmation. In a child with a perfusing rhythm, the detection of exhaled CO_2 using a colorimetric detector or capnometer is both sensitive and specific for ETT placement. In cardiac arrest, or with a large pulmonary embolus, pulmonary blood flow may be extremely low; therefore, inadequate CO_2 may be detected despite correct tracheal tube placement. When time permits, a chest x-ray should be obtained to confirm proper depth of tube insertion.

After confirmation of correct tube position, it should be taped in place and the depth of insertion should be recorded (in cm) at the lip or gum. Hand ventilation is provided using a bag with attached manometer to assess for the presence of leak around the tracheal tube. Absence of a leak with pressures of 15–25 cm H_2O suggests that the tube is too large or that the cuff inflation pressure is too high; either condition can cause tracheal mucosal injury.

Nasotracheal Intubation

To perform nasotracheal intubation, the lubricated tube is passed through one of the nares and guided through the larynx with McGill forceps. Care is taken to avoid lacerating or rupturing the laryngeal tube balloon during manipulation of the tube with the forceps. Blind nasotracheal intubation as taught for awake intubation of adults is generally difficult to perform in children. Relative contraindications to nasotracheal intubation include coagulopathy, maxillofacial injury, or basilar skull fracture. Complications of nasotracheal intubation include nose bleed (especially problematic if no other airway is in place), pressure-induced ischemic injury to the rim of the nares, and nasal deformity due to nasal septal pressure necrosis (more likely when a tube is in place for long periods of time in premature infants). In older children, nasal intubation may be associated with a greater risk of sinusitis or otitis media than is oral intubation.

Rapid-sequence Intubation

Rapid-sequence intubation (RSI) is a technique used to secure the airway in the patient who presents with full (or presumed full) stomach, where even moderate preintubation gastric insufflation by bag-mask ventilation may cause gastric regurgitation and pulmonary aspiration. The steps of the classic RSI include (18):

- A basic airway assessment, including relevant patient history using the *SAMPLE* mnemonic (*s*igns and *s*ymptoms, *a*llergies, *m*edications, *p*ast history, *l*ast meal, *e*vents leading to intubation) to assess risk/suitability for the use of anesthetics or paralytics.
- Preparation of personnel and equipment and establishment of monitoring.
- Preoxygenation for 2–3 mins with 100% O_2, delivered via a tight-fitting mask.
- Administration of an IV anesthetic/sedative/analgesic and almost simultaneous delivery muscle relaxant.
- Application of cricoid pressure (once patient is deeply sedated).
- A period of apnea until the patient has full muscle relaxation.
- Tracheal intubation.
- Removal of cricoid pressure only after tube position is confirmed and the tube cuff (if present) is inflated.

Some patients who require emergent intubation (e.g., those with intracranial or pulmonary hypertension) will be intolerant of even brief periods of hypercapnia associated with apnea. For these reasons, a "modified RSI technique" is often used in the intubation of critically ill children. After establishment of monitoring, some degree of bag-mask ventilation is provided while cricoid pressure is applied to minimize gastric distention. This technique should prevent or delay the onset of hypoxia and hypercarbia and their sequelae. Some patients have tenuous airways that allow for some oxygenation during spontaneous ventilation. Administration of sedatives and paralytics will remove spontaneous respiratory effort.

Several types of medications are used during RSI (**Table 1.5**). No perfect combination of drugs exists for all patients; providers should select drugs based on the patient's condition and the provider's expertise. Bradycardia can develop during RSI as the result of airway manipulation and as a side effect of some RSI drugs. Atropine should be administered to children who undergoing RSI are <1 year of age, for children 1–5 years of age who are receiving succinylcholine,

TABLE 1.5

RAPID-SEQUENCE INTUBATION DRUGS AND DOSES

Drug	Dose/Route	Duration	Comments
Cardiovascular adjuncts			
Atropine	IV: 0.01–0.02 mg/kg (min: 0.1 mg max: 1 mg)	>30 min	■ Inhibits bradycardic response to hypoxia; may cause tachycardia ■ May cause pupil dilation
Glycopyrrolate	IV: 0.005–0.01 mg/kg (max: 0.2 mg)	>30 min	■ Inhibits bradycardic response to hypoxia; may cause tachycardia
Sedative hypnotic agents/analgesics			
Diazepam	IV: 0.1–0.2 mg/kg (max: 4 mg)	30–90 min	■ May cause respiratory depression or potentiate depressant effects of narcotics and barbiturates
Lorazepam	IV: 0.05–0.1 mg/kg (max: 4 mg)	4–6 hr	■ May cause hypotension Minimal cardiac depression
Midazolam	IV: 0.1–0.3 mg/kg (max: 4 mg)	1–2 hr	■ Occasional respiratory depression ■ No analgesic properties
Fentanyl citrate	IV, IM: 2–4 mcg/kg	IV: 30–60 min IM: 1–2 hrs	■ May cause respiratory depression, hypotension, chest wall rigidity with high-dose (>5 mg/kg) infusions. ■ May elevate ICP
Anesthetic agents (in doses indicated)			
Thiopental	IV: 2–5 mg/kg	5–10 min	■ Negative inotropic effects and often causes hypotension ■ Decreases cerebral metabolic rate and ICP ■ Potentiates respiratory depressive effects of narcotics and benzodiazepines ■ No analgesic properties
Etomidate	IV: 0.2–0.4 mg/kg	5–15 min	■ Decreases cerebral metabolic rate and ICP ■ May cause respiratory depression ■ Minimal cardiovascular effects ■ Causes myoclonic activity; may lower seizure threshold ■ Causes cortisol suppression; contraindicated in patients dependent on endogenous cortisol response ■ No analgesic properties
Lidocaine	IV: 1–2 mg/kg	~30min	■ Causes myocardial and CNS depression with high doses ■ May decrease ICP during RSI ■ Hypotension occurs infrequently
Ketamine	IV: 1–2 mg/kg IM: 3–5 mg/kg	30–60 min	■ May increase blood pressure, heart rate, cardiac output ■ May cause increased secretions, laryngospasm ■ Causes limited respiratory depression ■ Bronchodilator ■ May cause hallucinations, emergence reactions

(Continued)

TABLE 1.5

CONTINUED

Propofol	IV: 2 mg/kg (up to 3 mg/kg in young children)	3–5 min	■ May cause hypotension, especially in hypovolemic patients ■ May cause pain on injection ■ Highly lipid soluble ■ Causes less airway reactivity than barbiturates
Neuromuscular blocking agents			
Succinylcholine	Infant IV: 2 mg/kg Child IV: 1–1.5 mg/kg IM: Double the IV dose	3–5 min	■ Depolarizing muscle relaxant; causes muscle fasciculation ■ May cause rise in ICP and intraocular and intragastric pressures ■ May cause rise in serum potassium ■ May cause hypertension ■ Avoid in renal failure, burns, crush injuries, or hyperkalemia
Atracurium	IV: 0.5 mg/kg	30–40 min	■ Metabolized by plasma hydrolysis ■ May cause mild histamine release
Cis-Atracurium	IV: 0.1 mg/kg, then 1–5 mg/kg/min	20–35 min	■ Metabolized by plasma hydrolysis ■ May cause mild histamine release
Rocuronium	IV: 0.6–1.2 mg/kg	30–60 min	Few cardiovascular effects
Vecuronium	IV: 0.1–0.2 mg/kg	30–60 min	Few cardiovascular effects

ICP, intracranial pressure; RSI, rapid-sequence intubation.
Adapted from Hazinski M, Zaritsky A, Nadkarni V, et al. Rapid sequence intubation. In: *PALS Provider Manual*. Dallas: American Heart Association, 2002, and Venkataraman ST, Khan N, Brown A. Validation of predictors of extubation success and failure in mechanically ventilated infants and children. *Crit Care Med* 2000; 28:2991–6.

and for adolescents who are receiving a second dose of succinylcholine.

Anesthesia can be achieved in high doses with *benzodiazepines* (midazolam, lorazepam, and diazepam). Any of the *opioids* can provide anesthesia at high doses but usually at a hemodynamic (i.e., hypotensive) cost. Fentanyl (a synthetic opioid) is commonly used during RSI. High bolus doses of fentanyl (≥ 5 mcg/kg) can cause acute onset of chest wall rigidity, which can be prevented by coadministration of a paralytic agent. *Anesthetic agents* used during RSI include ketamine, propofol, thiopental, and etomidate. IV or endotracheal lidocaine may be given to suppress reflex autonomic and airway responses to laryngoscopy. Clinical indications of adequate paralysis after administration *neuromuscular blocking* include lack of spontaneous movements, respiratory effort, and blink reflex, as well as jaw relaxation, manifested by the ability to fully open the patient's mouth without resistance.

Complications associated with succinylcholine include a modest rise in serum potassium (typically 0.5–1 mEq/L); malignant hyperthermia; masseter spasm with subsequent airway obstruction and significant hyperkalemia in specific at-risk patients, who include patients with burns; peripheral nerve injury; renal failure; neuromuscular disease; or major trauma with rhabdomyolysis. The risk of acute hyperkalemia in the child with previously undiagnosed neuromuscular disease triggered a US Food and Drug Administration warning that succinylcholine is contraindicated in pediatric intubation "except when used for emergency tracheal intubation or in instances where immediate securing of the airway is necessary." High-dose nondepolarizing neuromuscular blockers (e.g., rocuronium and atracurium) can create adequate conditions for intubation in times to onset similar to those of succinylcholine. The provider must be ready to assume control of the airway and ventilation when a priming dose is used in children.

Cricoid Pressure

The "Sellick Maneuver" puts direct pressure on the cricoid cartilage, compressing the upper esophageal sphincter, preventing reflux of gastric contents from the esophagus into the airway and preventing the insufflation of air into the stomach during positive-pressure ventilation (PPV). Cricoid pressure can distort the upper airway, preventing effective visualization of the airway and effective bag-mask ventilation. The use of cricoid pressure in patients with laryngeal or cervical spine pathology is controversial because it may cause cervical spine movement. It is contraindicated in patients with a cough or gag reflex.

Laryngeal Mask Airway

The laryngeal mask airway (LMA) consists of a small mask with an inflatable cuff that is connected to a plastic tube with a universal adaptor. It is designed to be placed in the oropharynx with its tip in the hypopharynx and the base of the mask at the epiglottis. When the cuff of the mask is inflated, it creates a seal with the supraglottic area, allowing air flow between the tube and the trachea. The LMA can be used with spontaneously breathing patients to deliver PPV or as a guide for insertion of another airway device, such as an ETT, airway-exchange catheter, lighted stylet, or flexible fiberoptic bronchoscope. The original LMA (the LMA Classic) is a multiuse device with sizes for neonates through adults (**Table 1.6**). The combined widths of the patient's index, middle, and ring fingers can be used to estimate the size of the LMA. The LMA can be inserted with the cuff fully deflated and lubricated; it is advanced with the aperture of the mask facing toward the tongue until the rescuer feels resistance, and the cuff then is inflated. Cuff inflation

may push the LMA slightly out of the mouth. The LMA may also be inserted with the cuff partially inflated (i.e., with half of the recommended volume) and the LMA mask inverted or turned to the side. Once the LMA is fully inserted, it is rotated to normal position, and the cuff is fully inflated. LMAs will not prevent aspiration of refluxed gastric contents.

The Esophagotracheal Combitube

The *Combitube* is a dual-lumen, dual-cuff airway device that is blindly placed. When the 2 cuffs are inflated (one distal in the esophagus and the second in the oropharynx), the larynx is trapped between them, and ventilation can be provided through the first (pharyngeal) lumen. If the tip of the tube is placed in the trachea (<5% of insertions), the second lumen must be used for ventilation. The provider must accurately determine the location of the distal tip to ensure ventilation through the correct lumen. In that the smallest size is designed for patients taller than 4 feet, its use in children is limited.

Gum Elastic Bougie and Airway-exchange Catheter

The *gum elastic bougie* can be inserted blindly into the airway and used as a guide for insertion of an ETT. The *airway-exchange catheter* was designed to be placed through an existing ETT and used as a guide for exchanging that ETT for a new one. It can also be used to intubate the larynx directly if an ETT will not pass through the larynx; the ETT is then threaded over the airway-exchange catheter into the airway. Some airway-exchange catheters have

---

TABLE 1.6

LMA AIRWAY SELECTION AND CUFF INFLATION VOLUMES

LMA airway size	Patient size	Maximum cuff inflation volumes (mL)
1	Neonates/infants up to 5 kg	4
1½	Infants 5–10 kg	7
2	Infants/children 10–20 kg	10
2½	Children 20–30 kg	14
3	Children 30–50 kg	20
4	Adults 50–70 kg	30
5	Adults 70–100 kg	40
6	Adults >100 kg	50

Note: These are maximum clinical volumes that should never be exceeded. It is recommended that the cuff be inflated to 60 cm H_2O intracuff pressures.
From LMA. Available at: http://www.lmana.com/faqs.php#faq03. Accessed March 26, 2007.

a central lumen, allowing oxygenation or insertion over a guidewire.

Fiberoptic Intubation

Endotracheal intubation over a flexible fiberoptic bronchoscope has become an important method by which to secure the airway in patients when direct ETI is impossible. Very small, ultra-thin broncho-scopes are available for tube sizes as small as 3.0 mm, although most of these scopes do not have a suction port, are very delicate, and are difficult to control. Cooperative older children may tolerate flexible laryngoscopy awake, but most patients will require sedation to minimize gagging and laryngospasm. Topical anesthesia can be given through the scope to attenuate airway protective reflexes. Ideally, the child will be breathing spontaneously, which allows dynamic visualization of the glottic structures to identify malacia or vocal cord paralysis and provides a margin of safety if ETI is unsuccessful. Other inexpensive and easy-to-use fiberoptic devices, such as the *optical stylet* and the GlideScope, have been used in neonates and children.

The tip of the tube should be in mid-trachea, at approximately the level of the third or fourth thoracic vertebra. Most commercially available ETTs have marks that indicate depth of insertion; the depth marker at the child's teeth or lips should be noted before the tube is secured and throughout intubation. Position of the tip of the tube will move with changes in head position; the tube will move further into the trachea when the neck is flexed.

Lighted Intubation Stylet

The lighted intubation stylet, also known as the *light wand*, is essentially a rigid stylet with a fiberoptic light at the tip. Blind placement of an ETT over the stylet can be very useful in cases of limited neck and/or jaw mobility because it does not require full mouth opening or neck extension. The lighted stylet can be used when large amounts of blood and secretions are present, unless they are sufficiently thick to disrupt transillumination. It is relatively contraindicated in the "impossible-to-intubate, impossible-to-oxygenate" scenario. As the procedure requires that the airway be midline, it is contraindicated in conditions where the glottis is deviated laterally or when laryngeal pathology is present. Any condition that limits transmission of light through the anterior neck (e.g., mass lesions, scarring, or massive edema or obesity) will also interfere with use of the stylet.

Percutaneous Needle Cricothyrotomy/Tracheostomy

Needle cricothyrotomy/tracheostomy is indicated as a life-saving procedure in patients who present or progress to the "cannot intubate, cannot ventilate" scenario, with obstruction proximal to the glottic opening, or in patients with abnormal anatomy that precludes laryngoscopic visualization of the glottic opening. Bag-catheter ventilation can provide effective oxygenation but not ventilation. The use of potentially harmful and rarely employed procedures, such as jet ventilation through a catheter, has high potential for complications. The simplest equipment, appropriate for use in infants, consists of a 14-gauge over-the-needle catheter, a 3.0-mm ETT adapter, and a 5-mL syringe. Although it is ideal to puncture the cricothyroid membrane, this membrane may be difficult to palpate in infants, and insertion of the catheter through adjacent structures is unlikely to cause life-threatening complications. The upper trachea should be considered functionally as a large palpable vein, which should be isolated and cannulated, with the catheter directed at the shallowest angle practical. For this reason, the procedure is probably better called *percutaneous needle tracheostomy*; the priority is to quickly establish adequate airway and oxygenation through a needle placed in the trachea. Once the catheter is in place, the 3.0-mm ETT adapter and a ventilation bag with oxygen are attached, and bag-catheter ventilation is begun. Placement is confirmed by clinical examination (chest rise and breath sounds may be difficult to appreciate) and detection of exhaled CO_2.

Complications of Endotracheal Intubation

Immediate complications of intubation can result from the medications required for intubation, from trauma to (e.g., laceration of) airway structures or injury to the cervical spine, and from the physiologic effects of laryngoscopy and PPV. Laryngoscopy can cause increased intracranial and intraocular pressures, coughing, regurgitation, aspiration, and laryngospasm, especially in the patient with inadequate sedation. The potential for airway and dental injury increases with a difficult airway and with multiple intubation attempts. Mainstem bronchus intubation (more commonly right sided) can result in atelectasis, hypoxia, and pneumothorax.

While the tube is in place, providers should assess the nares, lip, and tongue for signs of pressure injury.

Ulcers may develop on the arytenoids, posterior vocal cords, subglottic area, anterior tracheal wall, and epiglottis. Unplanned extubation, oropharyngeal aspiration, ventilator-associated pneumonia and sinusitis can be sources of morbidity in intubated patients. ETI results in hyperemia, edema, and mucosal hemorrhage, which can progress to ulceration, erosion, and eventual chronic fibrosis. Fibrosis typically develops in the subglottic region and is circumferential but may be asymmetric and result in granuloma formation, especially posteriorly.

Weaning from the ventilator and extubation may be attempted after the patient has adequate airway protective reflexes, oral and gastric feeding is suspended for 4–6 hrs prior to extubation, the cuff is deflated, and oxygen (100%) is provided.

THE DIFFICULT AIRWAY: ASSESSMENT AND MANAGEMENT

Caregivers should be questioned and old records obtained to determine whether previous intubations have been difficult. The American Society of Anesthesiologists has developed an algorithm for approach and management of the difficult airway. Often, the most difficult decision is whether to attempt conventional intubation or to proceed directly to more advanced techniques. A kit with the equipment necessary to deal with the difficult airway should be readily available and should include different types and sizes of laryngoscope blades, ET tubes and LMAs, forceps, stylets, a needle cricothyrotomy/tracheostomy kit, and an intubating bronchoscope. If a surgical airway is anticipated, notify personnel skilled at emergent cricothyrotomy and tracheostomy. If sedation is necessary for airway management, use of short-acting and/or reversible agents is preferred, but the safety of the airway is the priority.

Management of Specific Problems

Cervical spine abnormalities may be associated with conditions such as Goldenhar, Down, and Klippel-Feil syndromes, juvenile idiopathic arthritis, spondyloarthropathies, and neuromuscular scoliosis. Airway management in these patients is further complicated if the disease process affects the temporomandibular joint, limiting mouth opening. A history of neurologic symptoms and flexion/extension cervical spine x-rays can help to screen for these patients. In cases of uncertainty, it is prudent to treat all children with Trisomy 21 as if they have unstable cervical spines. In trauma patients, cervical spine instability is assumed to be present in all patients with a head or neck injury or a consistent mechanism of injury.

The provider should assume that the child in shock has a full stomach and should use an RSI technique for placement of an advanced airway. Potential bradycardia (as a result of vagal or drug-related effects) should be anticipated, and prophylactic use of atropine should be considered.

Inhalation injury should be anticipated in any burn patient with facial burns, singed nasal hairs, carbonaceous debris in the airway, or a history of closed-space exposure. Caustic ingestion can have a similar effect on airway structures. Anaphylaxis and hereditary angioedema are abrupt reactions that can result in severe airway edema, obstruction, and cardiovascular collapse.

When a child has a penetrating eye injury, extrusion of vitreous contents can occur during intubation. Rises in ocular pressure, produced by any Valsalva maneuver (such as crying, coughing, gagging, or straining), will exacerbate this risk. The best combination of drugs to facilitate the intubation of such a patient is RSI with adequate amounts of analgesia and sedation. IV lidocaine may be helpful in preventing the rise in intraocular pressure. Succinylcholine and ketamine have historically been associated with vitreous extrusion in this setting.

The anterior mediastinal space can occasionally be occupied malignant lesions such as lymphoma (Hodgkins or non-Hodgkins), but nonmalignant lesions can occur as well. The diagnosis may be made during preanesthesia respiratory function testing, with a finding of partial intrathoracic airway obstruction. The diagnosis may also be made through the use of chest x-rays, CT scans, echocardiography, or MRI. Although the airway may be intubatable, the mass may compress the trachea distal to the end of the tracheal tube, precluding effective oxygenation and ventilation even after intubation. The basic principle of management of the patient with a mediastinal mass is to keep the patient breathing spontaneously. The lateral or even prone position may minimize airway compression. Anesthetic agents with minimal hemodynamic effects (e.g., ketamine) should be used. Preload should be optimized with IV fluids to counteract the mass compression of vascular structures. Acute airway obstruction may be successfully managed with the use of rigid bronchoscopy or median sternotomy and extracorporeal life support. These solutions will only be possible if this complication is anticipated and equipment and personnel are prepared in advance.

Craniofacial anomalies, such as gross macrocephaly, midface hypoplasia, maxillary protrusion, facial asymmetry, high arched palate, a small mouth, a short muscular/immobile neck, facial clefts, Pierre Robin, Treacher-Collins, and Goldenhar, are associated with challenges of visualization of the glottis by direct laryngoscopy. The LMA can provide an effective airway for children with craniofacial anomalies.

Macroglossia is an enlargement of the tongue, present in patients with Beckwith-Wiedemann syndrome and Trisomy 21. These syndromes are also characterized by hypotonia, and the combination can make bag-mask ventilation difficult. Infiltration of the soft tissues from hemangiomas and cystic hygromas require early detection and possible insertion of an advanced airway.

The obese child can present challenges during basic (noninvasive) and advanced airway and ventilation support. Fatty infiltration may distort the airway. Superimposed infection, even from "benign" upper respiratory viral illnesses, or altered airway tone with sleep, anesthesia, or muscle relaxation can further compromise the airway. Two rescuers or insertion of a nasal/oral airway may be required. Positioning of the obese child's airway may be complicated by the presence of fatty infiltration of the posterior thorax.

The deposition of mucopolysaccharides in the airway leads to macroglossia, tonsillar hypertrophy, thickening of the oral mucosa, and obstruction of nasal passages. A short neck is common. The temporal-mandibular joints and cervical spine may be involved, limiting jaw and neck mobility. Patients with Morquio syndrome are at risk for atlantoaxial subluxation. The airway infiltration worsens with age; therefore, intubation becomes more difficult (and sometimes impossible) as the child ages. This situation can occur with Hurler syndrome at as early as 2 years of age. The use of an LMA to aid fiberoptic intubation has been described in this population though it is not always successful.

Foreign-body aspiration is a common cause of airway obstruction in children <2 years of age. Food, especially nuts and seeds, are the most commonly aspirated foreign objects. They can lodge in any part of the airway from the nasal passage to the lung parenchyma. The trachea and the main-stem bronchi are common sites of foreign body deposition. A high index of suspicion is necessary to diagnose foreign-body aspiration because many choking episodes are not witnessed and findings in physical and radiographic exams are nonspecific. Cervical and chest x-rays should be obtained, especially in the case of a radio-opaque foreign body. If the inspiratory chest x-ray is normal, an expiratory chest x-ray can demonstrate air trapping due to endobronchial foreign bodies causing partial bronchial obstruction. If foreign-body aspiration is at all suspected, endoscopy is indicated. Back slaps/chest thrusts in responsive infants and abdominal thrusts in responsive older children can be attempted if endoscopy is not immediately available. Flexible bronchoscopy can be used for diagnosis, but a rigid scope is almost always required for removal.

Symptoms of infections of the deep neck space (parapharyngeal, retropharyngeal, and peritonsillar) include fever, neck swelling, pain, torticollis, limited neck movement, drooling, and trismus. A protruding tongue can suggest infection in the submandibular or sublingual space (Ludwig angina). Therapy includes early antibiotics and surgical evaluation.

Laryngotracheobronchitis (croup) presents with hoarseness, barky cough, and stridor and is almost always viral in origin. Only the most severe cases that are not responsive to steroids and nebulized racemic epinephrine require intubation. Subglottic narrowing may necessitate use of a much smaller ETT than predicted. Bacterial laryngotracheobronchitis (bacterial tracheitis) is most commonly caused by *Staphylococcus aureus*. It often begins with a viral prodrome similar to croup but progresses rapidly with high fever, severe stridor, and respiratory distress.

Acute epiglottis is marked by sudden onset of fever, dysphagia, drooling, a "hot-potato voice," and toxemia. Unlike croup and bacterial tracheitis, cough is rarely present. Older patients often present in the "tripod" position to maximize air entry. Antibiotic therapy should be instituted as soon as possible. Patients with impending airway obstruction from upper airway infection or any other rapidly progressive process have an urgent consultation with pediatric anesthesia and otolaryngology specialists. It is imperative to keep the child calm and allow the child to remain in the position of comfort; placing the child supine or performing unnecessary procedures, such as blood sampling, can trigger laryngospasm and irreversible airway obstruction. Examinations should be limited until all necessary equipment and personnel are available to treat airway collapse. Patients should always be accompanied by a physician skilled in airway procedures. The utility of a lateral neck x-ray in these patients is controversial and can agitate them, resulting in further airway compromise. Intubation in the operating room using an inhalational anesthetic is preferred.

Resolution of acute airway obstruction can result in postobstructive pulmonary edema. It usually develops within a few minutes to a few hours following the onset of obstruction and usually resolves in ≤72 hrs.

CHAPTER 2 ■ PEDIATRIC CARDIOPULMONARY RESUSCITATION

ROBERT A. BERG • KATSUYUKI MIYASAKA • ANTONIO RODRIGUEZ-NUÑEZ
• MARY FRAN HAZINSKI • DAVID ZIDEMAN • VINAY M. NADKARNI

The strongest accessible central arterial pulse to palpate in an adult is the carotid pulse; however, the short, fleshy neck of a baby with potential to compress the airway and impede respiration limits the appropriateness of using the carotid location to assess central pulse presence in infants. Early detection of impending cardiac arrest is essential because lack of prompt recognition and effective intervention results in death or profound neurologic devastation. Cardiac arrest is the end result of diverse etiologies and pathophysiologic mechanisms, ultimately leading to an electrical or mechanical cardiac arrest due to progressive hypoxic-ischemic events or metabolic disturbances. Arrhythmogenic ("electrical") cardiac arrests are typically due to ventricular fibrillation (VF) or rapid ventricular tachycardia (VT). These arrhythmias can result from (a) *congenital cardiac abnormalities* associated with myocardial ischemia (e.g., coronary artery anomalies), genetic channelopathies associated with prolonged QT syndrome, familial cardiomyopathies (e.g., hypertrophic, dilated, arrhythmogenic right ventricular dysplasia), or mitochondrial diseases or from (b) *acquired cardiomyopathies* from drugs and toxins (e.g., doxorubicin cardiomyopathy, drug-induced prolonged QT syndrome), an hypoxic-ischemic event with inadequate myocardial oxygen delivery, cardiac surgical injury, commotio cordis, mechanically induced VF, ischemia during cardiopulmonary resuscitation (CPR), and inappropriate unsynchronized cardioversion shock. Mechanical ("pump") cardiomyopathic arrests are due to inadequate myocardial oxygen delivery from asphyxial, ischemic, metabolic (e.g., hypoglycemia, hypocalcemia, severe acidosis), or pharmacologic (e.g., β blocker, calcium channel blocker, or barbiturate toxicity) problems.

PHASES OF CARDIAC ARREST AND CARDIOPULMONARY RESUSCITATION

Cardiac arrest has at least four "phases": prearrest, no flow (untreated cardiac arrest), low flow (CPR), and postresuscitation. Interventions during the no-flow phase of untreated, pulseless cardiac arrest focus on early recognition of cardiac arrest and initia-tion of basic and advanced life support (**Table 2.1**). The goal of effective CPR is to optimize coronary perfusion pressure and blood flow to critical organs during the low-flow phase. Basic life support with continuous, effective chest compressions (i.e., push hard, push fast, allow full chest recoil, minimize interruptions, and do not overventilate) is the emphasis in this phase. When cardiac arrest is witnessed and of short duration, excellent outcomes *can* occur after various types of bystander CPR, including mouth-to-mouth rescue breathing alone, chest compressions alone, or standard chest compressions and mouth-to-mouth rescue breathing.

Recently published Utstein style reports of in-hospital pediatric cardiac arrests are derived from the multicentered National Registry of Cardiopulmonary Resuscitation (NRCPR) of the American Heart Association. The NRCPR is a prospective, multicentered observational registry of in-hospital cardiac arrests and resuscitations. The large size, scope, and quality of the NRCPR distinguish these North American data, which characterize the process and outcome of pediatric in-hospital CPR events. Summaries of these important characteristics are presented in **Table 2.2**. In these NRCPR reports, a cardiac arrest was explicitly defined as cessation of cardiac mechanical activity, determined by the absence of a reported palpable central pulse, unresponsiveness, and apnea.

Despite the diverse and complex clinical circumstances that led to their arrests, 52% attained sustained restoration of spontaneous circulation (ROSC), 36% survived for 24 hours, and 27% survived to hospital discharge. Outcomes for these children were substantially better than reported outcomes for adults in this registry (adjusted odds ratio [OR], 2.3; 95% confidence interval [CI], 2.0 to 2.7). Importantly, 65% of these children had good neurologic outcome.

Outcomes following pediatric out-of-hospital arrests appear to be worse than those following in-hospital arrests. These poor outcomes are in part due to prolonged periods of "no flow" and in part due to specific diseases with especially poor outcomes. Two common types of out-of-hospital cardiac arrests have especially poor outcomes: traumatic arrests and those associated with sudden infant death syndrome (SIDS).

TABLE 2.1

PHASES OF CARDIAC ARREST AND RESUSCITATION

Phase	Intervention
Prearrest phase (protect)	Optimize community education regarding child safety.
	Optimize patient monitoring and rapid emergency response.
	Recognize and treat respiratory failure and/or shock to prevent cardiac arrest.
Arrest (no-flow) phase (preserve)	Minimize interval to BLS and ALS (organized response).
	Minimize interval to defibrillation, when indicated.
Low-flow (CPR) phase (resuscitate)	"Push hard, push fast."
	Allow full-chest recoil.
	Minimize interruptions in compressions.
	Avoid overventilation.
	Titrate CPR to optimize myocardial blood flow (coronary perfusion pressures and exhaled CO_2).
	Consider adjuncts to improve vital organ perfusion during CPR.
	Consider ECMO if standard CPR/ALS are not promptly successful.
Postresuscitation phase: short-term rehabilitation	Optimize cardiac output and cerebral perfusion.
	Treat arrhythmias, if indicated.
	Avoid hyperglycemia, hyperthermia, hyperventilation.
	Consider mild postresuscitation systemic hypothermia.
	Debrief to improve future responses to emergencies.
Postresuscitation phase: longer-term rehabilitation (regenerate)	Early intervention with occupational and physical therapy
	Bioengineering and technology interface
	Possible future role for stem cell transplantation

BLS, basic life support; ALS, advanced life support; ECMO, extracorporeal membrane oxygenation; CPR, cardiopulmonary resuscitation

PEDIATRIC VENTRICULAR FIBRILLATION

VF is an uncommon but not rare electrocardiographic rhythm during out-of-hospital pediatric cardiac arrests. In special circumstances, such as tricyclic antidepressant overdose, cardiomyopathy, post–cardiac surgery, and prolonged QT syndromes, VF is a more likely rhythm during cardiac arrest. Commotio cordis, or mechanically initiated VF due to relatively low-energy chest-wall impact during a narrow window of repolarization, is reported predominantly in children 4–16 years old. Out-of-hospital VF cardiac arrest, uncommon in infants, occurs more frequently in children and adolescents.

Recent studies indicate that VF and VT (shockable rhythms) occur in 27% of in-hospital cardiac arrests at some time during the arrest and resuscitation. Although the rhythms during most in-hospital cardiac arrests (both in children and adults) are asystole and pulseless electrical activity (PEA), in many arrests, the rhythms are VF or pulseless VT. Traditionally, VF and VT have been considered "good" cardiac arrest rhythms, resulting in better outcomes than asystole and PEA. Of note, survival to discharge was much more common among children with an initial shockable rhythm than among children with shockable rhythms that occurred later during the resuscitation.

Termination of Ventricular Fibrillation: Defibrillation

Defibrillation (defined as termination of VF) is necessary for successful resuscitation from VF cardiac arrest. Note that termination of fibrillation can result in asystole, PEA, or a perfusing rhythm. The goal of defibrillation is return of an organized electrical rhythm with pulse. When prompt defibrillation is provided soon after the induction of VF in a cardiac catheterization laboratory, the rates of successful defibrillation and survival approach 100%. When automated external defibrillators are used within 3 mins of adult-witnessed VF, long-term survival can occur in >70%. In general, the mortality increases by 7%–10% per minute of delay to defibrillation. Early and effective, near-continuous chest compressions can attenuate the incremental increase in mortality with delayed defibrillation.

Successful termination of VF (defibrillation) is achieved by attaining current flow adequate to

TABLE 2.2

CHARACTERISTICS OF PEDIATRIC IN-HOSPITAL CARDIAC ARRESTS FROM THE NATIONAL REGISTRY OF CARDIOPULMONARY RESUSCITATION OF THE AMERICAN HEART ASSOCIATION

Characteristic	Pediatric cardiac arrest ($n = 880$) (100%)
Age, years	
Mean (SD)	5.6 (6.4)
Median (range)	1.8 (0–17.0)
Sex	
Male	473 (54)
Female	407 (46)
Race/ethnicity	
White	447 (51)
Black	226 (26)
Hispanic	105 (12)
Other/unknown	102 (12)
Patient type	
Inpatient	750 (85)
Emergency department	121 (14)
Other (outpatient, visitor, or employee)	9 (1)
Illness category	
Medical, cardiac	158 (18)
Medical, noncardiac	402 (46)
Surgical, cardiac	150 (17)
Surgical, noncardiac	62 (7)
Trauma	91 (10)
Other[a]	17 (2)
Preexisting Conditions	
Respiratory insufficiency	511 (58)
Hypotension/hypoperfusion	319 (36)
Congestive heart failure	273 (31)
Pneumonia/septicemia/other infection	259 (29)
Arrhythmia	182 (21)
Renal insufficiency	104 (12)
Diabetes mellitus	11 (1)
Metabolic/electrolyte abnormality	178 (20)
Baseline depression in CNS function	151 (17)
Metastatic or hematologic malignancy	43 (5)
Myocardial infarction	21 (2)
None[b]	69 (8)
Hepatic insufficiency	55 (6)
Acute CNS nonstroke event	94 (11)
Acute stroke	5 (1)
Major trauma	97 (11)
Toxicologic problem	12 (1)

Data are expressed as number (%) unless otherwise specified. Because of rounding, percentages may not all total 100. Preexisting conditions total more than the total number of patients due to patients having more than one preexisting condition present at the time of admission to hospital.
[a]All 17 were obstetrics.
[b]No documented preexisting conditions.
SD, standard deviation; CNS, central nervous system
Data from Nadkarni VM, Larkin GL, Peberdy MA, et al. First documented rhythm and clinical outcome from in-hospital cardiac arrest among children and adults. *JAMA* 2006;295:50–7.

depolarize a critical mass of myocardium. Current flow (amperes) is primarily determined by the shock energy (joules), which is selected by the operator, and the patient's transthoracic impedance (ohms). The AHA recommends that "pediatric" or "small" paddles only be used in infants.

Defibrillation is typically achieved with biphasic defibrillators, and the 150-J or 200-J biphasic adult automated external defibrillator (AED) dosage is nearly 90% successful at terminating prolonged VF (much better than the ~60% effectiveness with 200-J monophasic defibrillation). The presently recommended pediatric VF dose of 2 J/kg by monophasic waveform is safe.

Interventions During the Cardiac Arrest (No-Flow) Phase and Cardiopulmonary (Low-Flow) Phase: Cardiopulmonary Resuscitation

Airway and Breathing

One of the most common precipitating events for cardiac arrest in children is respiratory insufficiency. Adequate oxygen delivery to meet metabolic demands and removal of carbon dioxide are the goals of initial assisted ventilation. Effective bag-mask ventilation skills remain the cornerstone of providing effective emergency ventilation. Effective ventilation does not necessarily require a tracheal tube. Overventilation during CPR is common and can substantially compromise venous return and cardiac output. Most concerning, these adverse hemodynamic effects during CPR combined with the interruptions in chest compressions that are typically necessary to provide airway management and rescue breathing can contribute to worse survival outcomes. Although airway and breathing are prioritized in the ABC assessment approach, special circumstances may impact that priority order. Asphyxia results in significant arterial hypoxemia and acidemia prior to resuscitation in contrast to VF. In this circumstance, rescue breathing can be life saving.

Circulation

The most critical element to providing basic life support with continuous effective chest compressions is to *push hard* and *push fast*. Because no flow occurs without chest compressions, it is important to minimize interruptions in chest compressions. To allow good venous return in the decompression phase of external cardiac massage, it is important to allow full-chest recoil and to avoid overventilation. In smaller infants, it is often possible to encircle the

chest with both hands and depress the sternum with the thumbs, while compressing the thorax circumferentially. Duty cycle is the ratio of time of compression phase to the entire compression-relaxation cycle (a duty cycle of 40%–50% if 120 compressions are delivered per min) correlated with improved cerebral perfusion pressure when compared to shorter duty cycles of 30%.

Excellent standard closed-chest CPR generates ~10%–25% of baseline myocardial blood flow and a cerebral blood flow that is ~50% of normal. By contrast, open-chest CPR can generate a cerebral blood flow that approaches normal.

Ratio of Compressions to Ventilation

Mathematical models of compression-ventilation ratios suggest that matching the amount of ventilation to the amount of reduced pulmonary blood flow during closed-chest cardiac compressions should favor very high compression-to-ventilation ratios: of 15 chest compressions to 2 ventilations in children.

Intraosseous Vascular Access

The intraosseous (IO) needle is typically inserted into the anterior tibial bone marrow; alternative sites include the distal femur, medial malleolus or the anterior superior iliac spine, and the distal tibia. In adults and older children, the medial malleolus, distal radius, and distal ulna are optional locations. Resuscitation drugs, fluids, continuous catecholamine infusions, and blood products can be safely administered by the IO route. Complications have been reported in <1% of patients following IO infusion and include tibial fracture, lower-extremity compartment syndrome, severe extravasation of drugs, and osteomyelitis. Most of these complications may be avoided by careful technique.

Endotracheal Drug Administration

Epinephrine, atropine, naloxone, and lidocaine are commonly administered via the endotracheal route. Sodium bicarbonate and calcium may be very irritating to the airways and lung parenchyma and are not recommended for endotracheal administration.

Absorption of drugs into the circulation after endotracheal administration depends on dispersion over the respiratory mucosa, pulmonary blood flow, and the matching of the ventilation (drug dispersal) to perfusion. The small volumes of drug that remain as droplets in the tracheal tube are obviously not effective. Inadequate chest compressions that result in poor pulmonary blood flow will also limit absorption of the drug and prevent its delivery to the heart and systemic circulation. Preexisting patho-physiologic conditions such as pulmonary edema, pneumonitis, and airway disease also affect the pharmacokinetics of endotracheally administered drugs. Another confounding factor is that the vasoconstrictive effects of epinephrine may limit local pulmonary blood flow, thereby diminishing drug uptake and delivery. It is therefore not surprising that drug absorption varies greatly and that optimal drug doses have not been determined. Animal studies reveal a wide variability in plasma epinephrine levels and physiologic effects after endotracheal administration. On average, 10 times as much endotracheal epinephrine is required to attain peak plasma levels comparable to IV administration. Moreover, a prolonged depot effect typically occurs after endotracheal epinephrine administration, which can lead to postresuscitation hypertension, tachycardia, and ventricular arrhythmias.

Medication Use During Cardiac Arrest

Although animal studies indicate that epinephrine can improve initial resuscitation success after both asphyxial and VF cardiac arrests, no single medication has been shown to improve survival outcome from pediatric cardiac arrest.

Vasopressors

During CPR, epinephrine's α-adrenergic effect on vascular tone is most important. The α-adrenergic action increases systemic vascular resistance, increasing diastolic blood pressure, which in turn increases coronary perfusion pressure and blood flow and increases the likelihood of ROSC. Epinephrine also increases cerebral blood flow during CPR because peripheral vasoconstriction directs a greater proportion of flow to the cerebral circulation. The β-adrenergic effect increases myocardial contractility and heart rate and relaxes smooth muscle in the skeletal muscle vascular bed and bronchi, although this effect is of less importance. Epinephrine also increases the vigor and intensity of ventricular fibrillation, increasing the likelihood of successful defibrillation.

High-dose epinephrine (0.05–0.2 mg/kg) improves myocardial and cerebral blood flow during CPR more than standard-dose epinephrine (0.01–0.02 mg/kg) and may increase the incidence of initial ROSC. Administration of high-dose epinephrine, however, can worsen a patient's postresuscitation hemodynamic condition with increased myocardial oxygen demand, ventricular ectopy, hypertension, and myocardial necrosis. Prospective and retrospec-

tive studies indicate that use of high-dose epinephrine in adults or children does not improve survival and may be associated with a worse neurologic outcome.

A randomized, controlled trial of rescue high-dose epinephrine versus standard-dose epinephrine following failed initial standard-dose epinephrine for pediatric in-hospital cardiac arrest demonstrated a worse 24-hr survival in the high-dose epinephrine group (1/27 vs. 6/23; $p < 0.05$). In particular, high-dose epinephrine seemed to worsen the outcome of patients with asphyxia-precipitated cardiac arrest. High-dose epinephrine cannot be recommended routinely for initial therapy or rescue therapy.

Wide variability in catecholamine pharmacokinetics and pharmacodynamics dictates individual titration. A life-saving dose during CPR for one patient may be life-threatening to another. High-dose epinephrine should be considered as an alternative to standard-dose epinephrine in special circumstances of refractory pediatric cardiac arrest (e.g., patient on high-dose epinephrine infusion prior to cardiac arrest) and/or when continuous direct arterial blood pressure monitoring allows titration of the epinephrine dosage to diastolic (decompression phase) arterial pressure during CPR. Nevertheless, high-dose epinephrine has not been demonstrated to improve outcome and should only be used with caution.

Vasopressin is a long-acting endogenous hormone that acts at specific receptors to mediate systemic vasoconstriction (V_1 receptor) and reabsorption of water in the renal tubule (V_2 receptor). In experimental models of cardiac arrest, vasopressin increases blood flow to the heart and brain and improves long-term survival compared to epinephrine. Vasopressin may decrease splanchnic blood flow during and following CPR. In randomized, controlled trials of in-hospital and out-of-hospital arrests in adults, vasopressin had comparable efficacy to epinephrine. Vasopressin did not improve outcome compared with epinephrine.

In a piglet model of prolonged VF, the use of vasopressin and epinephrine in combination resulted in higher left ventricular blood flow than either pressor alone, and both vasopressin alone and vasopressin plus epinephrine resulted in superior cerebral blood flow than epinephrine alone. By contrast, in a piglet model of *asphyxial* cardiac arrest, return of spontaneous circulation was more likely in piglets treated with epinephrine than in those treated with vasopressin. A case series of 4 children who received vasopressin during 6 prolonged cardiac arrest events suggests that the use of bolus vasopressin may result in return of spontaneous circulation when standard medications have failed. Vasopressin has also been reported to be useful in low-cardiac-output states associated with sepsis syndrome and organ recovery in children. While vasopressin will not likely replace epinephrine as a first-line agent in pediatric cardiac arrest, preliminary data suggest that its use in conjunction with epinephrine in pediatric cardiac arrest deserves further investigation.

Calcium

For in-hospital pediatric cardiac arrests, hypocalcemia is not uncommon. Although calcium administration is only recommended during cardiac arrest for hypocalcemia, hyperkalemia, hypermagnesemia, and calcium-channel-blocker overdose, it is commonly used for in-hospital pediatric cardiac arrests, especially those that occur post–cardiac surgery. The administration of calcium has not been demonstrated to improve outcome in cardiac arrest. Animal studies suggest that calcium administration may worsen reperfusion injury.

Buffer Solutions

Cardiac arrest results in lactic acidosis from inadequate organ blood flow and poor oxygenation. Acidosis depresses myocardial function, reduces systemic vascular resistance, and inhibits defibrillation. Nevertheless, the routine use of sodium bicarbonate for a child in cardiac arrest is not recommended. Clinical trials that involved critically ill adults with severe metabolic acidosis did not demonstrate a beneficial effect of sodium bicarbonate. However, as the presence of acidosis may depress the action of catecholamines, the use of sodium bicarbonate seems rational in an acidemic child who is refractory to catecholamine administration. The administration of sodium bicarbonate is more clearly indicated in the patient with a tricyclic antidepressant overdose, hyperkalemia, hypermagnesemia, or sodium-channel-blocker poisoning.

The buffering action of bicarbonate occurs when a hydrogen cation and a bicarbonate anion combine to form carbon dioxide and water. If carbon dioxide is not effectively cleared through ventilation, its build-up will counterbalance the buffering effect of bicarbonate. Other side effects with sodium bicarbonate include hypernatremia, hyperosmolarity, and metabolic alkalosis. THAM is a non–carbon-dioxide-generating buffer that can be used during cardiac arrest. Note that excessive alkalosis decreases calcium and potassium concentration and shifts the oxyhemoglobin dissociation curve to the left.

Antiarrhythmic Medications: Lidocaine and Amiodarone

Administration of antiarrhythmic medications should not delay administration of a shock for a patient with VF. However, after unsuccessful attempts at electrical defibrillation, medications to increase the effectiveness of defibrillation should be considered. In both pediatric and adult patients, the medication first administered for ventricular fibrillation is epinephrine. If epinephrine with or without vasopressin and a subsequent repeat attempt to defibrillate are unsuccessful, the antiarrhythmic agents amiodarone or lidocaine should be considered.

Lidocaine has been recommended traditionally for shock-resistant VF in adults and children. However, the only antiarrhythmic agent that has been prospectively determined to improve survival to hospital admission in the setting of shock-resistant VF when compared to placebo is amiodarone. Furthermore, patients who received amiodarone for shock-resistant out-of-hospital ventricular fibrillation had a higher rate of survival to hospital admission than did patients who received lidocaine alone. Neither of these randomized, controlled trials included children. Although no comparisons of antiarrhythmic medications for pediatric refractory VF have been published, extrapolation of the adult studies has led to the recommendation of amiodarone as the preferred antiarrhythmic agent for children.

POSTRESUSCITATION INTERVENTIONS

Temperature Management

Mild induced hypothermia is a promising goal-directed, postresuscitation therapy for adults. Two seminal articles established that induced hypothermia (32°C–34°C) could improve outcome for comatose adults after resuscitation from VF cardiac arrest. In both of these randomized, controlled trials, the inclusion criteria were patients older than 18 years who were persistently comatose after successful resuscitation from nontraumatic VF. The multicentered European study had a goal of 32°C–34°C for the first 24 hrs postarrest. The mean time until attainment of this temperature goal was 8 hrs. Six-month survival with good neurologic outcome was superior in the hypothermic group (75/136 vs. 54/137; RR, 1.40; CI, 1.08–1.81). Similarly, death at 6 months postevent occurred less often in the hypothermic group (56/137 vs. 76/138; RR, 0.74; CI, 0.58–0.95). The second study reported good outcomes in 21/43 (49%) of the hypothermic group versus 9/34 (26%) of the control group; $p = 0.046$; OR, 5.25; CI, 1.47–18.76). Importantly, hypotension occurred among over half of the patients in both groups and was aggressively treated with vasoactive infusion in the European study. Similarly, more than half of Bernard's patients received epinephrine infusions during the first 24 hrs postresuscitation.

Interpretation and extrapolation of these studies to children is difficult. Fever following cardiac arrest, brain trauma, stroke, and other ischemic conditions are associated with poor neurologic outcome. Hyperthermia following cardiac arrest is common in children. It is reasonable to believe that mild, induced, systemic hypothermia may benefit children who are resuscitated from cardiac arrest. However, benefit from this treatment deserves to be rigorously studied in children and in adult patients with non-VF arrests. At a minimum, it is advisable to avoid even mild hyperthermia in children following CPR. Scheduled administration of antipyretic medications *and* use of external cooling devices are often necessary to avoid hyperthermia in this population. Emerging neonatal trials of selective brain cooling and systemic cooling may show promise in neonatal hypoxic-ischemic encephalopathy, suggesting that induced hypothermia may improve outcomes.

Postresuscitation Myocardial Support

Postarrest myocardial stunning occurs commonly after successful resuscitation in animals, adults, and children. In addition, most adults who survive to hospital admission after an out-of-hospital cardiac arrest die in the postresuscitation phase, many due to progressive myocardial dysfunction. Animal studies demonstrate that postarrest myocardial stunning is characterized by a global biventricular systolic and diastolic dysfunction and typically resolves after 1 or 2 days. Postarrest myocardial stunning is pathophysiologically similar to sepsis-related myocardial dysfunction and postcardiopulmonary bypass myocardial dysfunction, including increases in inflammatory mediator and nitric oxide production. Postarrest myocardial stunning is worse after a more prolonged untreated cardiac arrest, after more prolonged CPR, after defibrillation with higher-energy shocks, and after a greater number of shocks.

Optimal treatment of postarrest myocardial dysfunction has not been rigorously established. As noted above, this myocardial dysfunction has been treated with various continuous inotropic/vasoactive agents, including dopamine, dobutamine, and epinephrine, in both children and adults. In addition, milrinone improves the hemodynamic status of children with postcardiopulmonary bypass myocardial dysfunction and septic shock. Finally, the new inotropic agent levosimendan has also been effective in treatment of animal models of postresuscitation myocardial dysfunction, treatment of myocardial stunning in adults, and pediatric low-cardiac output.

Although prospective, controlled trials in animals have demonstrated that the myocardial dysfunction can be effectively treated with vasoactive agents, no data demonstrate improvements in outcome. Nevertheless, because myocardial dysfunction is common and can lead to secondary ischemic injuries to other organ systems or even cardiovascular collapse, treatment with vasoactive medications is a rational therapeutic choice that may improve outcome. The hemodynamic benefits in animal studies of postarrest myocardial dysfunction, pediatric studies of postcardiopulmonary bypass myocardial dysfunction, and pediatric sepsis-related myocardial dysfunction support the use of inotropic/vasoactive agents in this setting. In addition, adult studies document the common occurrence of postarrest hypotension and/or poor myocardial function "requiring" inotropic/vasoactive agents.

In summary, because treatment of postarrest myocardial dysfunction with inotropic/vasoactive infusions can improve the patient's hemodynamic status, such treatment should be routinely considered and titrated to effect. Unfortunately, evidence-based therapeutic targets for goal-directed therapy are ill defined.

Blood Pressure Management

It has been demonstrated that 55% of adults who survived out-of-hospital cardiac arrests required in-hospital vasoactive infusions for hypotension unresponsive to volume boluses. Compared to healthy volunteers, adults resuscitated from cardiac arrest have impaired autoregulation of cerebral blood flow. Hence, they may not maintain cerebral perfusion pressure in the face of systemic hypotension and, likewise, may not be able to protect the brain from acutely increased blood flow in the face of systemic hypertension. It is rational to presume that blood pressure variability should be minimized as much as possible following resuscitation from cardiac arrest.

A brief period of hypertension following resuscitation from cardiac arrest may diminish the no-reflow phenomenon. In animal models, brief, induced hypertension following resuscitation results in improved neurologic outcome compared to normotension. In a retrospective human study, postresuscitative hypertension was associated with a better neurologic outcome after controlling for age, gender, duration of cardiac arrest, duration of CPR, and preexisting diseases. It seems reasonable to aggressively treat and prevent hypotension. Moreover, severe sustained hypertension is not desirable.

Glucose Control

Hyperglycemia following adult cardiac arrest is associated with worse neurologic outcome after controlling for duration of arrest and presence of cardiogenic shock. In animal models of asphyxial and ischemic cardiac arrest, administration of insulin and glucose, but not administration of glucose alone, improved neurologic outcome compared to administration of normal saline. Data for evidence-based titration of specific end points are not available.

Extracorporeal Membrane Oxygenation: Cardiopulmonary Resuscitation

Perhaps the ultimate technology to control postresuscitation temperature and hemodynamic parameters is extracorporeal membrane oxygenation (ECMO). The concomitant administration of heparin may optimize microcirculatory flow. The use of veno-arterial ECMO to reestablish circulation and provide controlled reperfusion following cardiac arrest has been published, but prospective, controlled studies are lacking. Nevertheless, these series have reported extraordinary results with the use of ECMO as a rescue therapy for pediatric cardiac arrests, especially from potentially reversible acute postoperative myocardial dysfunction or arrhythmias. In one study, 11 children who suffered cardiac arrest in the PICU after cardiac surgery were placed on ECMO during CPR after 20–110 mins of CPR. Prolonged CPR was continued until ECMO cannulae, circuits, and personnel were available. Six of these 11 children were long-term survivors without apparent neurologic sequelae. More recently, 2 centers have reported an additional remarkable 8 pediatric cardiac patients who were provided with mechanical cardiopulmonary support during CPR within 20 mins of the initiation of CPR. All 8 survived to hospital discharge. CPR and ECMO are not curative treatments. They are simply cardiopulmonary supportive measures that may allow tissue perfusion and viability until recovery from the precipitating disease process. As such, they can be powerful tools. Most remarkably, in a report of 66 children who were placed on ECMO during CPR over 7 yrs, the median duration of CPR prior to establishment of ECMO was 50 mins, and 35% (23/66) of these children survived to hospital discharge. Additional centers corroborate this find-ing. It is important to emphasize that these children had brief periods of "no flow," excellent CPR during the "low-flow" period, and a well-controlled postresuscitation phase.

Potential advantages of ECMO come from its ability to maintain tight control of physiologic parameters after resuscitation: blood flow rates, oxygenation, ventilation, anticoagulation, and body temperature can be manipulated precisely through the ECMO circuit. As we learn more about the processes of secondary injury following cardiac arrest, ECMO might enable controlled perfusion and temperature management to minimize reperfusion injury and maximize cell recovery.

POSTRESUSCITATION OUTCOMES

The most important postresuscitation outcomes are survival with favorable neurologic outcome and acceptable quality of life. Many studies report end points of return of sustained circulation or survival to hospital discharge. Information about neurologic outcomes and predictors of neurologic outcome after both adult and pediatric cardiac arrests is limited. Barriers to assessment of neurologic outcomes of children after cardiac arrests include the constantly changing developmental context that occurs with brain maturation. Prediction or prognosis for future neuropsychologic status is a complex task, particularly after an acute neurologic insult. Little information is available regarding the predictive value of clinical neurologic examinations, neurophysiologic diagnostic studies (e.g., electroencephalogram or somatosensory-evoked potentials), biomarkers, or imaging (CT, MRI, or positron-emission tomography) on eventual outcomes following cardiac arrest or other global hypoxic-ischemic insults in children. CT scans are not sensitive in detecting early neurologic injury. The value of MRI studies following pediatric cardiac arrest is not yet clear. However, MRI with diffusion weighting should provide valuable information about hypoxic/ischemic injury in the subacute and recovery phases. Emerging data suggest that burst-suppression pattern on postarrest electroencephalogram is sensitive and specific for poor neurologic outcome. One study showed somatosensory-evoked potential was highly sensitive and specific in pediatric patients after cardiac arrest. However, somatosensory-evoked potentials are not standardized in the pediatric population and are difficult to interpret. Many children who suffer a cardiac arrest have substantial preexisting neurologic problems. For example, 17% of the children with in-hospital cardiac arrests from the NRCPR were neurologically abnormal before the arrest. Thus, comparison to pre-arrest neurologic function of a child is difficult and adds another dimension/barrier to the assessment and prediction of postarrest neurologic status.

Biomarkers are emerging tools with which to predict neurologic outcome. In an adult study, serum level of neuron-specific enolase and S100b protein showed prognostic value. Neuron-specific enolase >33 mcg/L and S100b >0.7 mcg/L were highly sensitive and specific for poor neurologic outcome (death or persisting unconsciousness). The validation of those biomarkers in pediatric postarrest patients requires further study.

Most pediatric cardiac arrest outcome studies have not included neurologic outcomes. Investigations that include neurologic outcomes have generally used the Pediatric Cerebral Performance Category, a gross outcome scale. Many neuropsychologic tests can detect more subtle, clinically important neuropsychologic sequelae from neurologic insults. Neuropsychologic outcomes are important issues for future pediatric cardiac arrest outcome studies.

QUALITY OF CARDIOPULMONARY RESUSCITATION AND RESUSCITATION INTERVENTIONS

Despite evidence-based guidelines, extensive provider training, and provider credentialing in resuscitation medicine, the quality of CPR is typically poor. Slow compression rates, inadequate depth of compression, and substantial pauses are the norm. A mantra must be "push hard, push fast, minimize interruptions, allow full-chest recoil, and don't overventilate"; it can markedly improve myocardial, cerebral, and systemic perfusion and improve outcomes. Quality of postresuscitative management has also been demonstrated to be critically important to improve resuscitation survival outcomes.

CONCLUSIONS AND FUTURE DIRECTIONS

Outcomes from pediatric cardiac arrest and CPR appear to be improving. Evolving understanding of the pathophysiology of events and titration of the interventions to the timing, etiology, duration, and intensity of the cardiac arrest event can improve resuscitation outcomes. Exciting discoveries in basic and applied science are on the immediate horizon for study in specific populations of cardiac arrest victims. By strategically focusing therapies to specific phases of cardiac arrest and resuscitation and to evolving pathophysiology, critical care interventions hold great promise to lead the way to more successful cardiopulmonary and cerebral resuscitation in children. Treatment of sudden death in children in the future requires more evidence-based and less anecdotal interventions. Timing of therapeutic interventions to prevent arrest and to protect, preserve, and promote restoration of intact neurologic survival is of the highest priority. Emerging technology interfaced with evolving teams and systems of postresuscitative care will likely facilitate high-quality interventions and ensure optimal odds for survival.

Exciting new epidemiologic studies, such as the NRCPR for in-hospital cardiac arrests and the large-scale, multicentered Resuscitation Outcome Consortium funded by the National Heart, Lung, and Blood Institute, are providing new data to guide our resuscitation practices and generate hypotheses for new approaches to improve outcomes. It is increasingly clear that excellent basic life support is often not provided. Innovative technical advances, such as directive and corrective real-time feedback, can increase the likelihood of effective basic life support. In addition, team dynamic training and debriefing can substantially improve self-efficacy and operational performance.

Induced hypothermia is a promising neuroprotective and cardioprotective postarrest intervention. Experimental data suggest that it can and should be considered as an intra-arrest intervention, especially during prolonged CPR efforts. Even chemical hibernation, controlled reanimation, and emergency preservation and resuscitation techniques are being considered.

Mechanical interventions, such as ECMO or other cardiopulmonary bypass systems, are already commonplace interventions during prolonged in-hospital cardiac arrests. Technical advances are likely to further improve our ability to provide such mechanical support.

In the past, the concept of evidence-based pediatric cardiac arrest recommendations seemed fanciful. Recommendations were based on extrapolated animal and adult data. These suboptimal approaches are no longer acceptable. Pediatric cardiac arrest clinical trials have started with the randomized controlled trial of high-dose epinephrine versus standard-dose epinephrine as rescue therapy for in-hospital pediatric cardiac arrests. Clinical trials are necessary for appropriate evidence-based recommendations for treatment of pediatric cardiac arrests. It is likely that the evolution of systems, such as "cardiac arrest centers," similar to trauma, stroke and myocardial infarction centers, is likely to facilitate the appropriate intensive care to patients who require specialized postresuscitation care.

CHAPTER 3 ■ TRANSPORT

MONICA E. KLEINMAN • AARON J. DONOGHUE • RICHARD A. ORR
• NIRANJAN "TEX" KISSOON

Transport is a neglected aspect of care in many areas of the world owing to lack of resources (trained personnel, vehicles, resources to pay personnel, lack of roads, and attacks on transport vehicles during conflicts). Under these circumstances, adverse events are high and improvement in outcomes is not demonstrated. Deciding whether developing and transitional countries should have PICU transport involves a balance of the overall health priorities of that community, and decisions can only be made locally with full knowledge of continuous quality improvement data.

Pediatric critical care transport programs are part of the continuum of care of emergency medical services (EMS) for children and are intended to provide a safe environment during transport between healthcare institutions. EMS includes all aspects of basic life support, advanced life support, and critical care transport in which emergency care is provided at a scene and/or in a vehicle. EMS encompasses the prehospital and interfacility components of transport and includes hospital-based specialty teams. Prehospital care providers have variable educational backgrounds and experience in the care of critically ill or injured children. Limited provider exposure to critically ill children leads to a problem in maintaining pediatric assessment and treatment skills. The federally funded EMS for Children (EMS-C, www.ems-c.org) program, founded in 1984, has as its mission to ensure that all children and adolescents receive state-of-the-art emergency care throughout the EMS system, from prevention through rehabilitation.

THE TRANSPORT ENVIRONMENT

Both ground and air transport result in noise levels that can prohibit auscultation of lung and heart sounds. Vehicular motion and vibration can result in artifacts in pulse oximetry, electrocardiography, and oscillometric blood pressure monitoring. It is possible to perform advanced procedures in a mobile environment. The threshold for establishing a secure airway is lower when interfacility transport is required. Handheld devices enable point-of-care testing through the use of rapid assays, permitting analysis of whole-blood chemistries and blood gases. Most therapies that are available in the ICU can be employed during critical care transport, includ-

ing mechanical ventilation (invasive and noninvasive), continuous infusions, administration of inhaled nitric oxide, and cardiac pacing.

Advantages of ground transport include virtually ubiquitous access, low cost, and ability to respond in most weather conditions. Ambulances are more spacious than most aeromedical transport vehicles and provide the option to perform procedures or clinical interventions in a stationary setting when necessary. Disadvantages of ground transport include severe winter weather, traffic congestion, and road and highway conditions. The use of sirens to facilitate the navigation of traffic, while helpful in expediting transports in urban areas, can impair the ability of the team to perform any clinical tasks dependent on auscultation.

Aeromedical transport is widely available in the US and other developed countries. Both rotor-wing (helicopter) and fixed-wing (airplane) aircraft can be adapted for use as critical care transport vehicles. Use of aeromedical services requires an understanding of the unique physiologic stresses and logistic issues associated with rotor- and fixed-wing transport.

Barometric pressure is defined as the sum of the partial pressures of each of the component gases in the atmosphere and represents the force or weight exerted by the atmosphere at any given altitude. Barometric pressure at sea level is 760 mm Hg and decreases as altitude increases. At altitudes that are within the physiologic range, the component gases exist in constant proportions: nitrogen (78%), oxygen (21%).

Dalton's Law states that the total pressure of a gas represents the sum of the partial pressures of the different gas components:

$$P_T = P_1 + P_2 + P_3 \cdots \qquad [3.1]$$

As total barometric pressure decreases with increasing altitude, the partial pressure of each gas is reduced. Likewise, the addition of another gas to the mixture decreases the partial pressure of all other gases.

The partial pressure of any inspired gas is determined by the barometric pressure (P_B) and the fraction of the atmospheric gas it represents. In the case of oxygen, for example, P_{IO_2} at sea level can be calculated as follows:

$$\begin{aligned} P_{IO_2} &= P_B \times F_{IO_2} \\ &= 760\,\text{mm Hg} \times 0.21 \\ &= 159\,\text{mm Hg} \qquad [3.2] \end{aligned}$$

At an altitude of 8000 feet, the partial pressure of inspired oxygen is reduced as follows:

$$P_{IO_2} = P_B \times F_{IO_2}$$
$$= 565 \, mm\,Hg \times 0.21$$
$$= 118 \, mm\,Hg \qquad [3.3]$$

While P_{IO_2} represents the partial pressure of inspired oxygen, the actual partial pressure of oxygen at the alveolar level is affected by the presence of water vapor and carbon dioxide, both of which reduce the partial pressure of oxygen in accordance with Dalton's Law. The amount of carbon dioxide in the alveolar space is, in part, determined by, *the respiratory quotient*.

The *alveolar gas equation* defines the relationship between the alveolar partial pressure of oxygen (P_{AO_2}), P_B, fraction of oxygen in inspired gas (F_{IO_2}), alveolar partial pressure of carbon dioxide (P_{aCO_2}), and the respiratory quotient (R), as follows:

$$P_{AO_2} = (P_B - P_{H_2O}) \times F_{IO_2} - (P_{aCO_2}/R) \qquad [3.4]$$

Assuming that R is 0.8, P_{aCO_2} is normal (i.e., ~40 mm Hg), and the partial pressure of water vapor at body temperature (37°C) is 47 mm Hg, the P_{AO_2} while breathing room air at sea level is calculated as follows:

$$P_{AO_2} = (760 \, mm\,Hg - 47 \, mm\,Hg) \times 0.21 - (40/0.8)$$
$$= 99 \, mm\,Hg \qquad [3.5]$$

Thus, with increasing altitude and decreasing P_B, the resultant P_{AO_2} will decrease. P_{AO_2} can be restored to baseline values by increasing the F_{IO_2}. If other factors remain constant, the F_{IO_2} required to maintain the same P_{AO_2} at a lower barometric pressure can be calculated as follows:

$$F_{IO_2(1)} \times P_{B(1)} = F_{IO_2(2)} \times P_{B(2)} \qquad [3.6]$$

The maintenance of a specific barometric pressure in the cabin of an aircraft (i.e., cabin pressurization) ameliorates this effect to some extent, but this is possible only in fixed-wing aircraft and not in helicopters.

A decrease in the ambient barometric pressure has the potential to affect any gas-filled compartment in the body. *Boyle's Law* states that an inverse relationship exists between volume and pressure of a gas; therefore, a decrease in pressure results in an increase in volume. The formula for Boyle's law is:

$$P_1 V_1 = P_2 V_2 \qquad [3.7]$$

where: P_1 = pressure at altitude 1
        V_1 = volume at altitude 1
        P_2 = pressure at altitude 2
        V_2 = volume at altitude 2

The significance of decreased barometric pressure is dependent on the altitude at which an unpressurized aircraft operates. Most medical helicopters travel at between 1500 and 5000 feet above ground level. If ground level represents sea level, then barometric pressure will decrease by 20% at 5000 feet, with a consequent 20% increase in gas volume. Most commercial aircraft will maintain a cabin pressure that is equivalent to ~8000 feet above sea level, corresponding to a 30% decrease in barometric pressure and a 30% increase in the volume of air-filled spaces. It is essential to anticipate and address the potential for gas expansion by such interventions as gastric drainage, pleural decompression, and replacement of air in an endotracheal tube cuff (using saline) prior to transport.

Rotor-wing transport can be deployed and complete a trip quickly—an important advantage in densely populated urban areas, where traffic can impede expeditious ground-based transport. Disadvantages of helicopter transport include a high level of noise, which impairs or sometimes totally eliminates the ability to use a stethoscope, and vibration, which can interfere with evaluation of the patient.

Fixed-wing transport is typically reserved for travel over long distances. It has the advantage of the fastest speed of the three commonly used transport modalities. Additional advantages include cabin pressurization, minimizing the adverse physiologic effects of altitude, and the ability to fly in weather conditions that may not be favorable for helicopter transport. Disadvantages of fixed-wing transport include the same considerations with regard to noise and movement as encountered in a helicopter.

INTRAHOSPITAL TRANSPORT

For any given procedure or test that requires travel outside of the ICU, the clinician must weigh the risks and benefits to the patient. Monitoring, at a minimum, must include electrocardiography, pulse oximetry, and noninvasive blood pressure. Most portable monitors are also equipped with the capability to measure arterial blood pressure, intracardiac or pulmonary artery pressure, central venous pressure, and intracranial pressure. Capnography during transport is essential for the intubated patient, both to provide a noninvasive measure of ventilation and to ensure early recognition of a displaced or obstructed endotracheal tube. Equipment and medications for emergent airway management should be available for all patients who have an artificial airway or who may require assisted ventilation.

By its nature, interfacility transport carries additional potential risks for healthcare providers and other individuals (i.e., parents). Collisions during air and ground interfacility transport are uncommon but can result in injury to, and death of, patients, clinicians, and vehicle operators, as well as disruption of care delivery systems due to loss of work days and damage to vehicles and equipment.

PRINCIPLES OF TRANSPORT MEDICINE

It is the responsibility of the referring hospital to use its best available resources to stabilize a child prior to transport. In the interest of time, the referring physician may initiate the transport process during ongoing efforts at patient stabilization. It must be determined by the referring physician that the benefit of transferring a child to another center for further management outweighs the risk of the transport itself. It may be helpful for the referring physician to consult with the medical control physician at the receiving hospital regarding the advantages of transfer for a particular patient.

Initial communication should include a direct conversation between the referring physician and the receiving physician. Information provided by the referring facility should include the patient's history, the clinical status, including a complete set of vital signs, and an assessment of respiratory, cardiovascular, and neurologic function. The patient's management through the time of the call should be described completely.

The receiving physician may be asked for medical advice pertaining to the ongoing treatment of the patient. Such advice should be clearly documented. Giving medical advice to a referring facility, depending on the level of comfort and capability of the referring facility with respect to critically ill or injured children, can be fraught with potential difficulty. The risks and benefits of interfacility transfer must be explained and consent obtained, either in person or by phone.

Family and Ethical Considerations

The existence of a do-not-attempt-resuscitation (DNAR) order or advance directive does not imply that the child should not receive any treatment. Children for whom a DNAR order has been written may still present for emergency care due to issues with pain management, fear or uncertainty about the trajectory of deterioration, or unanticipated changes in condition. Many factors may lead to a request for transfer: desire for end-of-life care by familiar caretakers, uncertainty as to whether the patient is actually at end of life, or inability to control symptoms such as pain or anxiety.

Death on Transport

By policy, most critical care transport programs will not depart from the referring facility with active cardiopulmonary resuscitation in progress. In most states in the US, it is illegal for anyone other than authorized funeral homes and the medical examiner's office staff to transport a patient who has been pronounced dead. Transporting a child's body to the referring facility for autopsy, for instance, requires that the child be sent to the referring hospital's morgue and then transported by an authorized party. In general, if cardiac arrest occurs after the team departs from the referring facility, the team should continue resuscitative efforts until arrival at the receiving facility.

Special considerations related to the presence of a family member or caretaker during interfacility transport include the effect on care delivery, safety, and the emotional milieu for patients, parents, and staff. Additional seats for passengers are present in most ambulances and ~one-half of helicopters used for transport in the US, but opinions and policies regarding the presence of parents during critical care transport vary greatly. Possible advantages associated with parental presence include emotional benefit to the patient, decreased parental anxiety, caretaker availability for procedural consent when necessary, and improved public relations. Disadvantages include limitations of space, distraction or increased anxiety for the crew, and increased parental or patient anxiety.

TRANSPORT CONSIDERATIONS FOR SPECIFIC POPULATIONS

The American Academy of Pediatrics and American College of Emergency Physicians have jointly published guidelines for the care of children in the emergency department, addressing leadership, personnel, equipment, and policies and procedures.

Trauma is the leading cause of death for children between the ages of 6 months and 14 years; consequently, the interfacility transport of critically injured children is a frequent occurrence. The American College of Surgeons Committee on Trauma has developed a classification system for trauma center levels based on predefined criteria for staffing, facilities, and other resources; it designates an individual institution through a process called *verification* (http://www.amtrauma.org/tiep/reports/ACSClassification.html). Level 1 trauma centers may be classified as Level 1 pediatric and/or adult trauma centers. As expected, to be so designated, these facilities must meet additional requirements for specially trained pediatric medical and surgical specialists. Most pediatric trauma patients suffer blunt injuries that are typically managed nonoperatively. Pediatric trauma resuscitation focuses on airway management, ventilatory support, and restoration of intravascular volume. A small percentage of injured children (e.g., patients with expanding epidural hematomas) will require immediate surgery on arrival at the trauma center. Components of a "direct-to-the-OR" protocol include a communication system to notify the appropriate surgical service(s) and other essential personnel (e.g., anesthesia, operating room nursing, blood bank, radiology). In most cases, eligible patients should already have a secure airway and any imaging that would be considered essential (e.g., CT scan) prior to surgery. Given the nonoperative nature of most pediatric trauma cases, trauma specialists and transport providers debate regarding whether direct transfer from the scene of the injury to a trauma center is preferable to secondary transfer after stabilization at a nontertiary hospital. Proponents of the former method cite rapid access to diagnostic and surgical services, while proponents of the latter emphasize the importance of early airway and shock management. Stabilization at a community hospital prior to transfer to a trauma center may improve survival for injured children.

Guidelines for PICUs have been updated by the AAP and the Society of Critical Care Medicine. Level I facilities are those that provide a full range of pediatric subspecialty services and meet specific requirements for availability of personnel, equipment, and support services on a 24-hr basis. For Level II facilities, some of these resources are considered optional, with continued minimum requirements for staffing and other services.

While adult burn units are commonly found at major medical centers, specialized care for pediatric burn patients is concentrated among a small number of facilities, such as the nationwide Shriner's Hospital system. The American Burn Association (www.ameriburn.org) has developed guidelines for the transfer of pediatric patients to a pediatric burn center.

Unlike trauma centers or PICUs, NICUs are typically licensed by the individual state to provide a specific level of services for neonatal patients. The level of NICU care is usually designated by the state's hospital regulatory agency, such as the Department of Public Health, whose definitions may vary from state to state. The AAP recommends a uniform classification and subclassification of NICUs based on their capabilities.

Extracorporeal membrane oxygenation (ECMO), a form of extracorporeal life support, is provided at ~115 centers in the US, a number that has decreased over the past 10 years, reflecting the decreased demand for ECMO due to the use of therapies such as HFOV, inhaled nitric oxide (iNO), and surfactant replacement. The initiation of iNO therapy in a non-ECMO center is controversial, as it may delay transfer to a facility with ECMO capability. A few select programs have the capability to respond to requests for transport by mobilizing an ECMO team that is capable of cannulating the patient at the referring facility, then transporting while on ECMO to the base institution. While it is labor intensive, expensive, and associated with high risk, this practice has been carried out safely and successfully in both civilian and military programs. The Extracorporeal Life Support Organization recommends that a neonate whose condition is deteriorating be transferred at a time when the conversion to conventional ventilation can still be tolerated and suggests that an infant who has not improved after 6 hrs of HFOV be considered a candidate for expedient transfer. Individual institutions may use the alveolar-arterial oxygen difference, the oxygenation index, or the persistence of a PaO_2 of <50 torr as predictors of the need for ECMO.

ADMINISTRATIVE AND TRAINING ISSUES

Emergency medical care for critically ill or injured children should be provided regardless of the patient's insurance status or ability to pay. Most costs (e.g., equipment and personnel costs) associated with operating a transport service are fixed. Significant expenses include vehicle maintenance, insurance, and repairs; durable equipment; and disposable supplies. As in other areas of healthcare, personnel salaries and benefits compose most of a transport team's budget. In the current financial climate, many smaller hospitals are reducing pediatric subspecialty services and referring sicker children to tertiary facilities. The EMS-C program has published sample pediatric transfer guidelines for adoption by different states or programs (www.ems-c.org).

The practice of interfacility patient transfer is regulated by federal laws that serve to protect patients who present to a hospital facility with an emergency condition. The Consolidated Omnibus Budget Reconciliation Act was first passed in 1986; one component of this legislation was the Emergency Medical Transportation and Labor Act (EMTALA). EMTALA was created to prevent "patient dumping" (i.e., transfer of an individual who does not have the ability to pay for services to another facility without assessment or stabilizing treatment). (www.cms.hhs.gov/EMTALA).

Unlike personnel who function solely within a hospital environment, transport team members are exposed to a higher risk of accidents and injuries during ground and air transports. Because transport team members tend to be young with many productive years ahead of them, disability coverage is important to provide financial security following an accident or work-related injury.

A quality improvement (QI) program should establish criteria to ensure that the standards of care are practiced by individuals and groups, linking the transport team with the medical director, administrative team, risk management, and other pertinent disciplines to identify opportunities to improve care. The medical director serves in various capacities as a resource, supervisor, moderator, evaluator, and educator. Activities for the medical director related to QI include interviewing, hiring, educating personnel, developing treatment protocols, and directing the overall transport system. Supervision of patient care during transport (i.e., on-line medical control) via direct communication is another important component of ensuring quality of care. The medical director should oversee the post-transport case-review process, including audits of charts, recorded audiotapes, and morbidity and mortality conferences.

Within the transport arena, the Commission on Accreditation of Medical Transport Systems (www.camts.org) is an organization that aims to improve the quality of patient care and safety of the transport environment through its voluntary accreditation process. Multiple standardized life-support courses provide certification in specialty areas such as neonatal resuscitation, pediatric resuscitation, advanced trauma care, and disaster management. Regarding procedural skills, skill acquisition is accomplished through initial training, and performance evaluation occurs in a precepted setting. The term "scope of practice" describes the clinical abilities and skill set for each team member, and may vary depending on an individual's educational background or experience, even among staff with the same professional degree. Healthcare providers are licensed by the state in which they practice, usually through the Department of Health or related state agency. Transport team members must be licensed for their professional practice according to the regulations of the state in which their service is based. Paramedics also have the option of national certification but still require state

licensure. Many transport teams provide services in multiple states or even in multiple countries. It is not necessary for each transport team professional to be licensed in every jurisdiction in which they provide patient care; instead, they are considered to be practicing within their home state for purposes of licensure, regardless of the patient's location. Transport team members are typically credentialed by the institution where they are based or with which they are primarily affiliated.

Transport represents an excellent educational opportunity for residents in training but may conflict with the efficiency and effectiveness of a dedicated transport team. The Residency Review Committee of the Accreditation Council for Graduate Medical Education refers to pediatric resident involvement in critical care transport in its program requirements for residency education in pediatrics as follows: (a) participation in decision making in the admitting, discharging, and transferring of patients to the ICU and (b) resuscitation, stabilization, and transportation of patients to the ICU and within the hospital (www.acgme.org).

Several scoring systems have been developed based on pretransport data, but their utility is limited by the subjective nature and variable accuracy of referring physicians' assessments. The risk of mortality correlated with the likelihood of deterioration and the need for major interventions or procedures during transport.

Pediatric critical care transport teams may be staffed with a variety of personnel combinations including registered nurses or nurse practitioners, physicians, respiratory therapists, and paramedics. In many European countries and Australia, it is commonplace for physicians to serve as team members for both prehospital and interhospital transports. With adequate pretransport stabilization, most pediatric transports occur without the need for advanced procedures. Inadequate stabilization and adverse events are reduced when transport team members receive specialized pediatric training.

One obvious justification for the use of critical care transport services is the need for evaluation by experts who are located in another facility. New technology makes it possible for patient assessment or test interpretation to be performed remotely, potentially improving pretransport care or, at the other extreme, obviating the need for patient transfer. A specific area in which the benefits of telemedicine have been demonstrated is the use of remote echocardiography interpretation.

CHAPTER 4 ■ INVASIVE PROCEDURES

STEPHEN M. SCHEXNAYDER • PRAVEEN KHILNANI • NAOKI SHIMIZU • ARNO L. ZARITSKY

CENTRAL VENOUS CATHETERIZATION

Indications for placement of central venous catheters (CVC) include reliable venous access for medication administration, monitoring of central venous pressure, hemodialysis, hemofiltration, apheresis, central venous oxygen saturation, parenteral nutrition, and frequent blood sampling. Increased use of CVCs and decreased use of pulmonary artery catheters are used for goal-directed therapies in the ICU.

Contraindications for the procedure are based on balancing the benefits and risks: bleeding, infection, thrombosis, air or clot embolus, vessel puncture or injury, nerve or lymphatic injury, catheter malfunction, wire-induced arrhythmia, or catheter displacement. Bleeding complications may be the most common adverse associated events, and subclavian catheters are frequently avoided in very young and coagulopathic patients due to inability to effectively compress the subclavian vessels. Vessel cannulation complications can be reduced using visualization techniques, such as bedside ultrasound. Recent advances demonstrate that catheter-related bloodstream infection, the most common complication of CVC, can be substantially reduced by a "bundle" of practices advocated as part of the "Saving 100,000 Lives" campaign of the Institute of Health Care Improvement.

Three sites are commonly used for pediatric CVC placement: femoral, internal jugular, and subclavian. Increasingly, peripherally inserted central catheters are used from both upper- and lower extremity sites, often by interventional radiologists in infants and children. Adults have a lower risk of infection from subclavian sites. Recommended insertion techniques for all sites include strict hand scrubbing prior to placement, skin antisepsis with chlorhexidine, and full barrier precautions (operator wearing hair covering, mask, sterile gown, and gloves, and use of a large sterile-field drape). Sedation and analgesia plus local anesthesia should be routinely used for pediatric CVC placement, both for patient comfort and to facilitate placement and reduce complications related to patient movement.

Most CVCs are placed using the wire-guided (Seldinger) technique, in which a needle or catheter-over-needle unit is introduced into the desired vein, blood is aspirated, and a guidewire is placed through the needle or catheter. Advancing the guidewire through the veins into the chambers of the heart, particularly into the ventricle, may cause cardiac arrhythmias. With multi-lumen catheters and soft single-lumen catheters, a dilation step is frequently required next and is performed by passing the dilator over the guidewire after the needle has been removed. Care must be taken to insert the dilator only to the estimated depth of the vessel, as the stiffness of the dilator may penetrate the posterior wall of the vessel. Catheters should be flushed with saline or diluted heparin flush solution prior to insertion, and their lumens should be occluded to reduce the chance of air embolism. In hypovolemic patients, volume resuscitation through a peripheral or intraosseous site prior to attempted CVC placement will facilitate successful cannulation for all central veins. In patients with low venous pressures, a fluid and air column from unoccluded tubing at 10 cm above the body surface will frequently flow into the patient, and extreme care should be taken to avoid air embolism. A sterile pressure transducer set can be attached to the tubing to verify pressures and differentiate arterial and venous waveforms. Suggested placement of the catheter tip is at or above the junction of the superior vena cava and right atrium for upper body catheters.

Femoral Venous Catheterization

For femoral venous cannulation, the lower extremity should be positioned with slight external rotation at the hip and flexion at the knee (frog-leg appearance). A rolled towel under the buttock may facilitate successful venous access, particularly in smaller children. Restraining the leg in the desired position will help to maintain optimal conditions. The femoral artery should be located by palpation or ultrasound or, in the pulseless patient, assumed to be at the midpoint between the pubic symphysis and anterior superior iliac spine. The area over the intended puncture site should be infiltrated with local anesthetic. During cardiopulmonary resuscitation, pulsations may be felt in the femoral vein or artery; therefore if cannulation is not successful medial to the pulsations, one should aim for the pulsation during cardiopulmonary resuscitation. The needle should be inserted 1–2 cm below the inguinal ligament just medial to the femoral artery and slowly advanced while negative pressure is applied to a syringe attached to the introducer needle. The needle should be directed at a 15–45-degree angle toward the umbilicus, depending on the size of the child, with a flatter approach used in infants than in older children. Once free flow of venous blood is observed, the syringe should be removed while the needle is carefully stabilized and the guidewire is introduced gently. Some manufacturers (e.g., Raulerson) include a specially designed syringe that allows the guidewire to pass through the syringe without removing the needle when placing larger catheters. The guidewire should pass easily with minimal resistance; *force should not be applied* to overcome a great deal of resistance. Once the guidewire is in place, the Seldinger technique as described above should be employed. Some experts recommend a lateral abdominal x-ray when femoral venous catheters are placed to document that the catheter has not been placed in the lumbar venous placement. Lumbar venous placement is more common from the left versus the right femoral vein. The catheter should be secured with suture or a special sutureless catheter securement device (Stat-lock, Venetec International, San Diego, CA).

Subclavian Venous Catheterization

For cannulation of the subclavian vein, positioning of the patient in a head-down position (Trendelenburg) of ~30 degrees increases upper body venous pressures, which causes distention of the central veins. This positioning also minimizes risk for introduced air embolism to travel to the brain. The patient's neck should be extended, and a rolled towel should be placed beneath the patient along the axis of the thoracic spine. However, some authorities recommend keeping the head in a neutral (midline) position in children to optimize the diameter of the vein or slightly flexing the neck and turning the head toward the puncture site when using the right side approach in infants. The shoulders should be maintained in neutral position with the arms at the patient's side.

In the smaller intubated patient, sedation, analgesia, and temporary neuromuscular blockade will facilitate proper patient positioning and reduce complications related to patient movement. In intubated patients, care should be taken to avoid kinking, disconnection, or dislodgement of the endotracheal tube. Bilateral breath sounds should be verified after proper patient positioning. Both the left and right sides have been advocated as preferable, although no clear-cut evidence exists for one side versus the other. The junction of the middle and proximal thirds of the clavicle should be located, and a small (25-gauge) needle should be used to infiltrate local anesthesia. The needle should be introduced just under the clavicle at the junction of the middle and medial thirds and slowly advanced while negative pressure is applied with an attached syringe. The needle should be

inserted parallel with the frontal plane and directed medially and slightly cephalad, under the clavicle toward the lower end of the fingertip in the sternal notch. When patients are mechanically ventilated, the needle is advanced while someone holds the ventilator in an expiratory hold position to minimize the risk of pneumothorax. When free flow of venous blood is obtained, the needle should be stabilized and the syringe removed while a fingertip is placed over the needle hub to prevent air entrainment. The guidewire should be introduced during inspiration in a patient on positive-pressure ventilation or during exhalation in a spontaneously breathing patient (to avoid air embolus). The Seldinger technique as described above should then be followed. Once the CVC is placed, the catheter should be secured with sutures and a chest x-ray should be obtained to verify catheter location prior to using the catheter and to rule out complications, such as pneumothorax or hemothorax.

Internal Jugular Catheterization

Internal jugular catheterization can be achieved via multiple approaches. Right-sided approaches are preferred due to potential injury to the thoracic duct on the left side. The carotid artery should be palpated, as it lies medial to the internal jugular vein within the carotid sheath. For all approaches, the patient should be positioned supine and in a slight (15–30 degree) Trendelenburg position, with a roll under the shoulders and with the head turned away from puncture site.

In the anterior approach, the needle is introduced along the anterior margin of the sternocleidomastoid halfway between the mastoid process and sternum and directed toward the ipsilateral nipple. In all approaches, the needle should be advanced during exhalation to minimize the chance of pneumothorax, and the syringe should be aspirated as the needle is advanced. When the vein is entered and free flow of venous blood is established, the needle should be stabilized and the syringe removed while the hub of the needle is covered to prevent air entrainment. The guidewire should then be introduced and advanced a distance that approximates the distance to the junction of the superior vena cava and right atrium.

Complications

Early complications include early perforations (vessels and other structures) that may be related to the needle, guidewire, dilator, or catheter or later perforations related to catheter erosion. Hemothorax, hydrothorax, and pericardial tamponade may occur with upper body CVCs or long femoral CVCs.

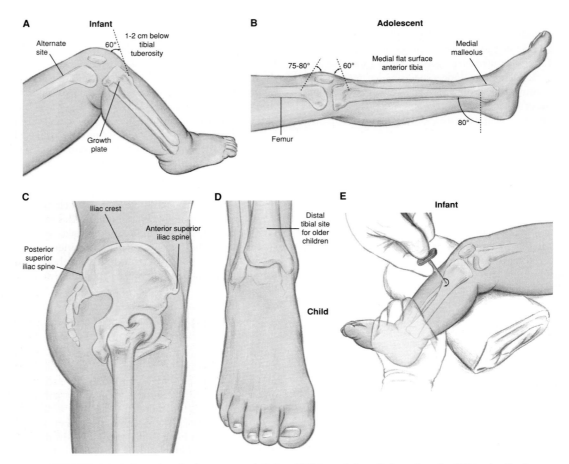

FIGURE 4.1. A: Locations for intraosseous infusion (IOI) in an infant. **B:** Locations for IOI in the distal tibia and the femur in older children. **C:** Location for IOI in the iliac crest. **D:** Location for IOI in the distal tibia. **E:** Technique for IOI infusion needle.

Pneumothoraces may occur with the subclavian and internal jugular approaches. Hemorrhagic complications may be reduced through the correction of coagulopathies prior to CVC attempts. Catheter-related bloodstream infection (CRBSI) is the most common complication of CVC and can be reduced by employing strict attention to the insertion technique.

Ultrasound guidance reduces complications in infants and children while vessels are being cannulated. Higher success rates are generally found when real-time images are obtained and used to guide needle and catheter insertion during the procedure. To train providers on CVC placement, anatomic models are available (Blue Phantom, Kirkland, WA).

INTRAOSSEOUS INFUSION

Recent guidelines recommend intraosseous infusion (IO) access for all ages and during cardiopulmonary

arrest when no vascular access is present. IO infusions have drug delivery times equivalent to peripheral and central IVs and can be used to administer all medications that can be given IV. Blood can be drawn for laboratory analyses and culture, and this route can deliver continuous medication infusions. The IO route is preferred for drug delivery during cardiopulmonary resuscitation compared with endotracheal drug delivery. IO placement options are summarized in **Figure 4.1** and **Figure 4.2**.

ARTERIAL CATHETERIZATION

Arterial access is frequently used in the care of critically ill infants and children for arterial blood gas and other blood sampling, as well as continuous blood pressure monitoring. Like central venous catheterization, sedation and analgesia plus local anesthesia facilitate the successful placement of arterial lines. To

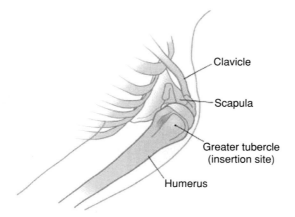

FIGURE 4.2. Placement of intraosseous needle in the humerus.

minimize infection risks, sterile technique should be employed in the placement of arterial catheters. The femoral artery is occasionally used in hemodynamically unstable patients when other access sites are difficult. Both the dorsalis pedis and posterior tibial arteries can be cannulated in the foot. The posterior tibial artery is best approached with the foot dorsiflexed, while the dorsalis pedis artery is cannulated with the foot in mid-plantar flexion.

THORACENTESIS/TUBE THORACOSTOMY

Tube thoracostomy or thoracentesis may be rapidly required for patients in extremis or may be performed in a purely elective manner. Both procedures may be required to drain abnormal accumulations of matter within the chest, which may include air (pneumothorax), blood (hemothorax), fluids (hydrothorax), or pus (empyema). Any abnormal collection in the pleural space may interfere with respiratory function and, in severe cases, will impair cardiovascular function. The usual site for a thoracentesis to obtain fluid is the posterior axillary line near the tip of the scapula, which represents the seventh intercostal space during full inspiration. For classic chest tube placement, a skin incision in an axis parallel to the rib is made through the area and blunt dissection is performed using a curved hemostat or Kelly clamp through the incision site and directed up to the superior intercostal space that has been chosen for chest wall entry. A number of percutaneous chest drainage systems are available, including pigtail catheters and tube-over-obturator systems (ThalQuik, Cook Critical Care, Bloomington, IN). In general, when tube drainage has fallen to less than 2–3 mL/kg over 24 hrs, the tube may

be considered for removal. If the tube was placed for a pneumothorax and no active air leak is present, a several-hour trial of observation without suction (water seal) is recommended, obtaining another x-ray to assess reaccumulation of the pneumothorax prior to removing the tube. Not all pneumothoraces require drainage. In small pneumothoraces in spontaneously breathing patients, observation alone may be sufficient. Breathing 100% oxygen may be helpful in facilitating reabsorption of the pneumothorax.

NEEDLE THORACOSTOMY

Emergent decompression is indicated when a tension pneumothorax is suspected in a deteriorating patient. In these circumstances, awaiting a confirmatory chest x-ray is unnecessary. A needle or catheter-over-needle unit (IV catheter) is inserted perpendicular to the chest wall and advanced along the superior border of the third rib (second intercostal space) in the midclavicular line until a rush of air is heard. A syringe may also be attached to the end of the needle-catheter unit and air may be aspirated as the procedure is completed. When a catheter over the needle unit is used, the needle is removed, and the catheter is left in place. When spontaneous respirations are present, a stopcock should be attached to prevent air entry into the chest. Repeated aspiration of air through a syringe attached to the stopcock may be required until a tube thoracostomy can be performed.

PERICARDIOCENTESIS

The classic clinical presentation of "paradoxical pulse" and severe hypotension with distended neck veins is seen in adults and children. The pathophysiology of cardiac tamponade results from reduced filling of the right heart during diastole because of the pressure of blood within the contained pericardium exceeds venous return pressures, causing a decrease in cardiac output and, ultimately, hypotension. Any sick children with signs of elevated venous pressures (jugular venous distension, hepatomegaly, pulmonary edema), tachycardia, hypotension, and a prominent "paradoxical pulse" must be suspected of having pericardial tamponade. If the physical findings and signs suggest tamponade, confirmation of the diagnosis is ideally obtained by echocardiography, although in some cases immediate intervention without delay may be required. Immediate complications associated with pericardiocentesis include puncture and laceration of the ventricular epicardium or myocardium, laceration of a coronary artery or vein, and hemopericardium secondary to laceration of the ventricle, coronary vessels, or great vessels. Lethal arrhythmias, pneumothorax pneumopericardium, diaphragm perforation, peritoneal puncture with subsequent peritonitis or false-positive aspirate, esophageal puncture with subsequent mediastinitis, pericardial leakage and development of a cutaneous fistula, and local infection may occur. Recommended needle sizes are a 20-gauge needle (1 inch, or 2.5 cm) for infants, a 20-gauge needle (1.5–2 inches, or 3–5 cm) for children, and an 18- or 20-gauge needle (3 inches, or 7.5 cm) for adolescents. Some operators prefer an electrocardiogram (ECG) lead attached to the needle to detect epicardial contact of the needle. Over-the-needle IV catheters may also be used in smaller children, but most do not allow attachment of an ECG lead. If time allows, the xiphoid and subxiphoid areas and thorax should be disinfected. The child should be placed in a head-up position, if possible, to promote anterior pooling of the effusion. The overlying skin should be infiltrated with lidocaine, and a small stab incision should be made with a blade just below and to the left of tip of the xiphoid process to facilitate easier passage of the needle. Some experts prefer to enter the chest just to the right of the xiphoid tip. An 18- or 20-gauge pericardiocentesis needle is ideal for percutaneous drainage. A small syringe containing 1% lidocaine without epinephrine is attached to the needle via a 3-way stopcock so that local anesthetics may be administered as the needle is advanced. The 3-way stopcock is also attached to tubing, which may be used to monitor intrapericardial pressure. Although many sources advocate the use of an ECG lead clipped to the pericardiocentesis needle with an alligator clamp, this feature may not be essential. The needle should be inserted into the skin incision site at a 45-degree angle to the skin and directed toward the left nipple or the tip of the left scapula. The needle is advanced slowly, aspirating and injecting lidocaine until pericardial fluid is aspirated. Once pericardial fluid is obtained, the intrapericardial pressure is recorded if the system is being transduced. In the setting of pericardial tamponade, the intrapericardial pressure should be equal to the central venous pressure. If an ECG lead is attached to the needle, contact with the ventricular wall is indicated by ECG changes. If ECG changes are seen, the needle should be withdrawn slightly until the ECG change disappears. If the ECG tracing does not normalize, the needle should be removed completely. In addition, a recording of the intrapericardial pressure could identify intraventricular placement if a ventricular waveform is documented. Once the needle tip is in the correct position, the stopcock is disconnected and a J-tipped guidewire is introduced into the pericardial space. Often, a dilator is then inserted over the wire, a pigtail pericardial catheter is advanced over the guidewire, and then the guidewire is removed before evacuation of the pericardial fluid.

Blood aspirated from the pericardial sac will not clot; blood aspirated from the heart chambers will clot within 4–6 mins, although this is not universally accepted. If the cause of the pericardial tamponade is catheter perforation of a heart chamber, the pericardial blood will often clot even though it is not drawn directly from the heart chamber. As much fluid as possible should be aspirated, and the intrapericardial pressure following the procedure should be less than 3 mm Hg, with negative deflections during spontaneous inspiration. Echocardiography should be performed following the procedure to document evacuation of the fluid and to determine catheter position.

TRANSPYLORIC FEEDING TUBE PLACEMENT

Whenever possible, enteral nutrition is the method of choice, as it reduces complication rates and maintains gut integrity. Nasogastric tube feeding is the first choice of enteral nutrition, but it may be poorly tolerated in critically ill children as a result of gastroparesis. In this setting, transpyloric placement of a feeding tube into the duodenum or jejunum is often recommended to support early feeding, improve tolerance of enteral nutrition, and decrease the risk of aspiration pneumonia. Blind insertion of a transpyloric tube is usually performed at bedside with a weighted or unweighted tube. Prokinetic agents, such as metoclopramide or erythromycin, are occasionally used. Ultrasonography can also be used for placement confirmation. If a child is stable and requires early establishment of feeding, fluoroscopic-guided insertion may be considered, although if bedside fluoroscopy is not available, the risks of moving critically ill children to the radiology suite should be considered. Various alternative bedside techniques, including pH-assisted, endoscopic, magnet/endoscope guided, and spontaneous passage with or without motility (prokinetic) agents have been suggested as alternative techniques to facilitate tube passage through the pylorus. Malplacement of a nasogastric tube, such as tracheal intubation, may occur during feeding tube placement. Gastric feeding with erythromycin as a prokinetic may be equivalent to transpyloric feeding in meeting the nutritional goals of the critically ill.

ABDOMINAL PARACENTESIS

Therapeutic indications for abdominal paracentesis include an increase in intra-abdominal pressure (IAP) that causes some combination of significant respiratory distress, cardiovascular compromise, oliguria, acidosis, or raised intracranial pressure. In the PICU, common etiologies of massive ascites include fluid resuscitation for treatment of shock (e.g., in meningococcemia), viral hemorrhagic shock (e.g., Dengue shock syndrome), trauma, severe burns, and multiple-organ dysfunction with fluid overload from capillary leak syndromes. Diagnostic indications include new onset ascites, chronic ascites with clinical deterioration and suspected peritonitis, pancreatitis, and intraperitoneal bleeding. Various causes of ascites include portal hypertension, inferior vena cava obstruction, heart failure, nephrotic syndrome, lymphomas, leukemias or neoplasms that involve liver or mediastinum, chronic pancreatitis, or cirrhosis of the liver. Special caution is necessary in patients with severe bowel distension, history of previous abdominal or pelvic surgery, coagulopathy, or distended bladder not adequately drained by a Foley catheter. In ascites, the bowel tends to float in the nondependent midline area. Therefore, the area of needle insertion should be dependent and lateral in children. The patient should be placed in a supine position, with head elevated and the bladder empty. Lateral insertion can be accomplished preferably in the left lower quadrant a few centimeters above the inguinal ligament, lateral to the rectus abdominis muscle. A Z-track method minimizes the risk of fluid leak, compared with a direct linear-track insertion. The Z-track can be applied by placing caudal traction on skin after the needle has been inserted perpendicular to the abdominal wall. Once the initial needle insertion is made through the skin and subcutaneous tissues, negative pressure is maintained with the syringe, while the needle is advanced further until a "pop" is felt as the needle enters the peritoneal cavity and free fluid is aspirated. If a catheter-over-needle system is used, the catheter is advanced over the needle into the peritoneal cavity and the needle is Ascitic fluid may be sent for cell count with differential count, specific gravity, glucose, total protein, alkaline phosphatase, albumin, amylase, LDH, ammonia, creatinine, potassium, bilirubin, triglycerides, cellular morphology, aerobic and anaerobic cultures, viral, fungal cultures, acid fast bacilli stain and culture, and gram stain, as clinically indicated. Corresponding serum chemistries should also be sent. A large volume drained quickly can result in shock and hypotension; therefore, no more than 15–20 mL/kg should be drained at one time. Positional change may be necessary to facilitate drainage of the ascitic fluid. A pigtail catheter may be used if drainage is required over the following 24–48 hrs, leaving the catheter in place. After the removal of the needle or the catheter, a sterile pressure dressing should be applied.

Complications include bowel or bladder perforation, bleeding, subcutaneous hematoma, infection, persistent leak, scrotal edema, and hypotension. Perforation of the bladder can be prevented if care is taken to empty the bladder prior to the procedure. As the risk of bowel perforation is high in patients with a history of previous surgery and adhesions, it can be prevented by avoiding old scars at the insertion site to prevent injury to an adherent bowel loop. Ultrasound-guided paracentesis will also reduce risk in this setting. A comparison of ascitic fluid composition in different types of ascites is shown in **Table 4.1**.

TRANSURETHRAL BLADDER CATHETER PLACEMENT AND BLADDER PRESSURE MONITORING

The measurement of bladder pressure as a surrogate for IAP is used to detect intra-abdominal hypertension (IAH), leading to abdominal compartment syndrome (ACS). Among the common clinical situations in which IAP can increase is trauma that leads to accumulation of blood, fluid, or edema; nontraumatic bowel ischemia, infarction, and gastrointestinal hemorrhage can also lead to increased IAP due to edema or fluid collection. IAP increases in the PICU are commonly seen in (a) children with septic shock with capillary leak, (b) children with multiple organ dysfunction syndrome, (c) severely burned or trauma patients with ischemia/reperfusion injury following fluid resuscitation, and (d) those who are post-liver transplantation or post-surgical closure of an abdominal wall defect. Patients at risk for significant increases in IAP include (a) those with blunt abdominal injury, (b) those with multiple organ dysfunction syndrome, meningococcemia, dengue shock syndrome, severe burns, or high cumulative fluid balance who are mechanically ventilated, and (c) those who are postoperative with abdominal packing. Signs of ACS include abdominal distension, oliguria, hypoxia, hypotension, and acidosis. Early monitoring of IAP should be considered in situations in which the patient is already exhibiting signs of ACS or is at high risk of developing it.

To monitor intravesical pressure, the urinary catheter must have a closed drainage system, and the patient must be in the supine position. The transducer system should be connected to the monitor, with connection to a bag of saline. A 30-mm or 60-mm pressure scale on the monitor is selected, a 60-mL syringe is attached to the distal stopcock, and the symphysis pubis is taken as the zero

TABLE 4.1

COMPARISON OF ASCITIC FLUID OF DIFFERENT ETIOLOGIES

Spontaneous bacterial peritonitis	>250 cells/mL Total protein is >1 g/dL LDH and glucose may be normal pH may be low or normal Culture and Gram stain may be negative Serum-ascitic albumin gradient is usually >1.1 g
Secondary bacterial peritonitis	Total protein is >3 g/dL LDH is >serum LDH Glucose is <50 mg/dL >500 cells/mL with polymorphonuclear predominance Gram stain is positive Serum-ascitic albumen gradient is <1.1 g/dL pH is not a reliable correlate of bacterial peritonitis
Chylous ascites	Milky or yellow fluid, but may be clear WBC = 1000–5000, with lymphocytic predominance (usually >90%) Triglyceride level >> serum triglycerides (>1500 g/dL) Total protein is <3 g/dL
Pancreatic ascites	Turbid, tea-colored, or bloody fluid Elevated total WBC count and protein Amylase and lipase are > serum levels; in patients <4–6 months of age, amylase may be low, but lipase is always higher
Tuberculous ascites	Bloody or yellow fluid, firm clots Total protein is >2.5 g/dL WBC >1000 with predominant lymphocytes Glucose is <30 mg/dL
Urine ascites	Protein is <1 g/dL Potassium and creatinine are >serum
Malignant ascites	Bloody fluid ⇑ Protein and LDH ⇓ Glucose Serum-ascitic albumen gradient is <1.1 g/dL
Nephrotic syndrome	Total protein is <2.5 g/dL
Biliary ascites	Bile-stained fluid Bilirubin >> serum bilirubin (100–400 mg/dL)

LDH, lactate dehydrogenase; WBC, white blood count

reference point. The bladder drainage system is clamped distal to the catheter and drainage bag connection. The sampling port of the catheter is cleaned with an antiseptic swab, and a large (18-gauge) needle is inserted into sampling port. The stopcock attached to the syringe is turned off to the patient. The saline bag is then opened toward the syringe, and the syringe is filled with saline flush. The stopcock is turned off to the pressure bag, and 1 mL/kg of saline from the syringe is injected into the bladder. Any air seen between the clamp and the urinary catheter should be expelled by opening the clamp and allowing the saline to flow back past the clamp before reapplying the clamp. The pressure waveform typically shows a small variation between inspiration and expiration, with the end-expiratory pressure taken as the IAP. A printed strip facilitates measurement of the IAP. Once the pressure measurement is made, the needle is removed from the sampling port, and the catheter drainage tubing is unclamped. When a transducer is not available, the catheter tubing is simply raised vertically above the symphysis pubis at a 90-degree angle to the patient's pelvis, and tubing is unclamped. The distance in centimeters between the symphysis pubis zero point and the maximal height of the fluid column is recorded. This minimally invasive technique is popular in some institutions because it is quick and can be easily performed by the staff without the need for a transducer set-up. A closed commercial monitoring and drainage system that utilizes an inline valve allows monitoring without the need to use a needle to connect to the sampling port of the catheter (AbViser, Wolfe Tory Medical Inc., Salt Cake City, UT). Based on adult data, normal range of IAP is

considered to be 0–12 mm Hg. IAH is defined as an IAP of >12 mm Hg. ACS may occur with an IAP of >20 mm Hg. Various interventions to reduce IAP include gastric suction, enemas, diuretics, muscle relaxants, paracentesis, and surgical decompression, as clinically indicated.

CHAPTER 5 ■ RECOGNITION AND INITIAL MANAGEMENT OF SHOCK

SIMON NADEL • NIRANJAN "TEX" KISSOON • SUCHITRA RANJIT

Shock is divided into three major categories: hypovolemic, cardiogenic, and distributive, with a degree of overlap. Hypovolemic shock is a result of inadequate circulating blood volume owing to blood or fluid loss or of insufficient fluid intake. Cardiogenic shock occurs when cardiac compensatory mechanisms fail and may occur in infants and young children and in patients with preexisting myocardial disease or injury. Distributive shock, such as septic and anaphylactic shock, is associated with peripheral vasodilatation, arterial and capillary shunting past tissue beds with pooling of venous blood, and decreased venous return to the heart. Shock is a clinical diagnosis, but its recognition remains problematic in children. Shock may be present long before hypotension occurs. Children will often maintain their blood pressure until late stages of shock; therefore, the presence of systemic hypotension is not required to make the diagnosis of shock in children, as it is in adults. For example, septic shock in pediatric patients has been defined as tachycardia (which may be absent in the hypothermic patient) with signs of decreased perfusion, including decreased peripheral pulses compared with central pulses, altered alertness, flash capillary refill or capillary refill >2 secs, mottled or cool extremities, and decreased urine output. Hypotension is a sign of late and decompensated shock in children if present in a child with these other features.

CLASSIFICATION OF SHOCK

Decreased Flow (Hypovolemic, Cardiogenic Shock)

Decreased flow may be the consequence of either decreased circulating volume (absolute or relative hypovolemia) or failure of the cardiac pump. Cardiac

failure resulting in shock can be due to myocardial injury (infectious or ischemic) or obstructive lesions (increased right ventricular afterload, increased pulmonary vascular resistance, increased left ventricular afterload, increased systemic vascular resistance), and/or from lack of ventricular filling (decreased right ventricular or left ventricular preload, valvular lesions, decrease in filling time due to tachycardia).

Decreased Oxygen Content (Hemorrhagic Shock, Acute Hypoxemic Respiratory Failure, Poisoning)

Decreased oxygen-carrying capacity (CaO_2), of hemoglobin (Hb), and therefore inadequate DO_2, may also result in shock. For instance, with carbon monoxide poisoning, a decrease in DO_2 results from competitive binding of carbon monoxide in preference to O_2 and is exacerbated by abnormal O_2 utilization, as carbon monoxide interferes with oxidative phosphorylation, resulting in a decreased oxygen extraction ratio (O_2ER). In any respiratory cause of acute hypoxia, decreased arterial oxygen saturation (SaO_2) leads to a decrease in DO_2 as soon as cardiac output is unable to compensate for metabolic needs.

Distributive Shock (Decreased Oxygen Extraction)

Distributive shock occurs when blood is redistributed among organs such as secondary to sepsis, anaphylaxis, or vasodilating agents. In addition, especially in sepsis, a decrease in capillary recruitment secondary to altered vascular reactivity, disseminated intravascular coagulation, endothelial cell dysfunction, or

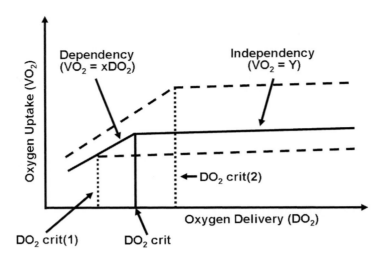

FIGURE 5.1. Relationship of oxygen uptake (VO_2) to oxygen delivery (DO_2): When VO_2 is supply independent (Independency), whole-body O_2 needs are met. When VO_2 becomes dependent on DO_2 (Dependency), VO_2 becomes linearly dependent on DO_2 at the critical DO_2 (DO_2crit), which corresponds to the definition of "dysoxia." DO_2crit is influenced by global oxygen requirements: When VO_2 is decreased (i.e., during sedation and hypothermia), the DO_2crit is also decreased [DO_2crit(1)]. When VO_2 is increased (i.e., agitation, hyperthermia, sepsis), DO_2crit is increased [DO_2crit(2)].

increased blood cell adhesiveness and abnormal mitochondrial function (mitochondrial injury or dysfunction) may be present. These changes contribute to the inability to fully utilize oxygen that is delivered. Spinal cord injury is a specific form of distributive shock that leads to profound hemodynamic changes. Sudden loss of sympathetic outflow from the spinal cord leads to a sudden decrease in total peripheral resistance and cardiac output, while central venous pressure (CVP) remains unchanged.

During circulatory shock or hypoxemia, as DO_2 declines, VO_2 is maintained by a compensatory increase in O_2ER; VO_2 and DO_2, therefore, remain independent. However, if DO_2 falls further, a critical point is reached (DO_2crit). O_2ER can no longer increase to compensate for the fall in DO_2, and at this point, VO_2 becomes dependent on DO_2. If VO_2 is higher, this DO_2crit is also higher (**Fig. 5.1**).

MIXED VENOUS OXYGEN SATURATION

In the clinical setting, mixed venous O_2 saturation (SvO_2) can be useful in assessing whole-body VO_2-DO_2 relationships.

SvO_2 is proportional to $SaO_2 - VO_2/(CO \times Hb \times 1.39)$.

Four conditions may cause SvO_2 to decrease: hypoxemia (decrease in SaO_2), increase in VO_2 (oxygen consumption), reduction in CO, and decrease in Hb concentration. At DO_2crit, SvO_2 is ~40% (SvO_2crit), with an O_2ER of 60% and SaO_2 of 100%. A 40% SvO_2 can be taken as an imbalance between arterial blood O_2 supply and tissue O_2 demand, with evident risk of dysoxia. In the clinical setting, a decrease in

SvO_2 of 5% from its normal value (65%–77%) represents a significant fall in DO_2 and/or an increase in O_2 demand. If treatment is instituted to restore SvO_2 to the normal range (such as fluid resuscitation, inotropic therapy, or red cell transfusion), measurement of CO, as well as SaO_2 and Hb, should be instituted to choose and monitor response to therapy.

ASSESSMENT

Good data are not available for selection of threshold blood pressures that should be maintained in these situations, particularly in children. Arbitrary values of a systolic of 90 mm Hg or a mean arterial pressure (MAP) of 60 mm Hg in adults have been chosen, with population standards for age in children. The hemodynamic variables important in shock also relate to flow to vital organs. Flow (Q) varies directly with perfusion pressure (dP) and inversely with resistance (R):

$$CO = MAP - CVP/\text{systemic vascular resistance}$$

This relationship also holds for organ perfusion. Some organs, including the kidney and brain, have vasomotor autoregulation that maintains flow in low-pressure states. However, even in organs with autoregulation capabilities, at some critical point, perfusion pressure is reduced below the ability to maintain blood flow.

Because the kidney receives the second highest blood flow of any organ in the body, measurement of urine output can be used as an indicator of adequate perfusion pressure (with the exception of patients with hyperosmolar states leading to osmotic diuresis). In this regard, maintenance of MAP with norepinephrine has been shown to improve urine output and creatinine clearance in hyperdynamic sepsis. However, maintenance of supranormal MAP above this point is likely of no benefit.

Measurement of cardiac output and oxygen consumption, Cardiac Index (CI) × (arterial oxygen content – mixed venous oxygen), has been proposed as being of benefit in patients with persistent shock, because a CI between 3.3 and 6.0 $L/min/m^2$ and oxygen consumption >200 $mL/min/m^2$ are associated with improved survival. Assuming a hemoglobin concentration of 10 g/dL and 100% arterial oxygen saturation, a CI of >3.3 $L/min/m^2$ would correlate to a mixed venous oxygen saturation of 70% in a patient with a normal oxygen consumption of 150 $mL/min/m^2$. Oxygen consumption is the product of CI, arterial oxygen content, and oxygen extraction. Therefore, an oxygen consumption of 150 $mL/min/m^2 = 3.3 \ L/min/m^2 \times [1.36 \times 10 \ g/dL \times 100 + PaO_2 \times 0.003] \times [100\%–70\%]$.

Body temperature gradients have long been used as a parameter of peripheral perfusion. At physiologic concentrations, the molecules that absorb most light are hemoglobin, myoglobin, cytochrome, melanins, carotenes, and bilirubin. The assessment of tissue oxygenation is based on the specific absorption spectrum of oxygenated Hb (HbO_2), deoxygenated Hb, and cytochrome aa3 ($Cytaa3$). Commonly used optical methods for peripheral monitoring are perfusion index, near-infrared spectroscopy, laser-Doppler flowmetry, and orthogonal polarization spectral. The peripheral perfusion (flow) index (PFI) is derived from the photoelectric plethysmographic signal of pulse oximetry and has been used as a noninvasive measure of peripheral perfusion in critically ill patients. Deoxygenated Hb absorbs more light at 660 nm, and HbO_2 absorbs more light at 940 nm. The PFI is calculated as the ratio of the light that reaches the detector of the oximeter between the pulsatile component (arterial compartment) and the nonpulsatile component (other tissues) and is calculated independently of the patient's oxygen saturation.

Near-infrared spectroscopy (NIRS) uses the principles of light transmission and absorption to measure the concentrations of hemoglobin, oxygen saturation (StO_2), and Cytaa3 in tissues. Cytaa3 is the end receptor in the oxygen transport chain that reacts with oxygen to form water, and most cellular energy is derived from this reaction. Monitoring changes in the Cytaa3 redox state can provide a measure of the adequacy of oxidative metabolism.

Orthogonal polarization spectral (OPS) is a noninvasive technique that uses reflected light. As the light reaches the tissue, the depolarized light is reflected back through the lenses to a second polarizer or analyzer and forms an image of the microcircula-

tion, which can be recorded. OPS produces images of the sublingual microcirculation by placement of the probe under the tongue. The use of OPS to assess the sublingual tissues provides information about the dynamics of microcirculatory blood flow and, therefore, has been used to monitor the perfusion during clinical treatment of circulatory shock.

Continuous noninvasive measurement of oxygen and carbon dioxide tension is possible because the sensor heats the skin to 43°–45°C, which causes dermal capillary hyperemia and enable the estimation of arterial oxygen pressure (PaO_2) and arterial carbon dioxide pressure ($PaCO_2$) in both neonates and in adults. When blood flow is adequate, $PtcO_2$ and PaO_2 values are almost equal, and the tc-index is close to 1. During low flow states, such as shock, the $PtcO_2$ drops and becomes dependent on the PaO_2 value, and tc-index decreases. $PtcO_2$ and $PtcCO_2$ have also been used as early indicators of tissue hypoxia and subclinical hypovolemia. The sensor position must be changed every 1–2 hrs to avoid burns.

Measurement of the tissue-arterial CO_2 tension gradient has been used to reflect the adequacy of tissue perfusion. Gastric and ileal mucosal CO_2 clearance has been the primary reference for measurements of regional PCO_2 gradient during circulatory shock. The regional PCO_2 gradient represents the balance between regional CO_2 production and clearance. In low flow states, tissue CO_2 increases as a result of a stagnation phenomenon. Comparable decreases in tissue blood flow during circulatory shock have also been demonstrated by measuring the sublingual tissue PCO_2 ($PslCO_2$).

CLINICAL ASSESSMENT

Children who are febrile, who have an identifiable source of infection, or who are hypovolemic are at increased risk of developing shock. In neonates, the maternal and birth histories are required, especially with regard to timing and duration of rupture of membranes, maternal fever, blood loss, fetal distress, and other obstetric information. In the case of trauma, history regarding the mechanism and timing of injury, whether excessive blood loss has occurred, and the level of consciousness before hospital arrival is vital. A history of immunodeficiency, use of immunosuppressive agents, duration and height of fever, and associated features, such as lethargy, vomiting, diarrhea, decreased oral intake, and decreased level of consciousness or awareness, may suggest infection and the possibility of septic shock or dehydration. Other details, such as environmental exposure, drug ingestion, previous medical history, and allergies, are also important.

As children often will maintain their blood pressure until they are severely ill, the presence of systemic hypotension is not required to make the diagnosis of shock, as in adults. In guidelines published by the American College of Critical Care Medicine, shock in pediatric patients is defined as tachycardia (which may be absent in the hypothermic patient) with signs of decreased organ or peripheral perfusion, including decreased peripheral pulses compared with central pulses, altered alertness, flash capillary refill or capillary refill >2 secs, mottled or cool extremities, or decreased urine output. Hypotension is a sign of late shock and should not be relied on to make the diagnosis. Moreover, the classifications of shock in children (e.g., warm and cold shock, fluid-refractory shock, or catecholamine-resistant shock) are not helpful for diagnosis but may dictate therapy. Shock in children can be recognized before hypotension occurs by clinical and laboratory signs that include altered mental status, tachypnea and tachycardia, hypothermia or hyperthermia, and changes in peripheral perfusion [vasodilation (warm shock) or cool extremities (cold shock)], together with reduction of urine output, metabolic acidosis, or increased blood lactate. The physical examination may reveal a decrease in tissue perfusion, which is identified by changes in body surface temperature, prolonged capillary refill time, and impaired organ function.

Serial blood gas and arterial lactate evaluation are widely used to complement the clinical assessment of systemic perfusion by quantifying the extent of tissue hypoperfusion and providing useful trends with which to titrate therapy. Mixed venous O_2 saturation (SvO_2) can be useful in assessing whole-body VO_2-DO_2 relationships. While lactate and base deficit estimations together with $ScvO_2$ measurement are invaluable for detection and monitoring of global O_2 deficiency, regional and tissue perfusion may not be accurately assessed using these indices.

Apart from repeated clinical examinations, the minimal monitoring appropriate for patients who are either in incipient or actual shock includes continuous electrocardiography, pulse oximetry, continuous invasive or rapid and regular noninvasive blood pressure, and urine catheter for continuous measurement of urine output. A central venous catheter allows CVP monitoring, which may indicate the need for fluid if the CVP is <8 mm Hg. In addition, the catheter allows rapid infusion of drugs and fluids and monitoring of $ScvO_2$ (a surrogate for mixed SvO_2). However, a central venous catheter insertion for CVP monitoring is not essential in the early stages of management of a child in shock.

Supplemental O_2 and respiratory support should be titrated in response to acute respiratory failure (whether primary respiratory failure, as in acute lung injury, or secondary, as a result of shock). Acute circulatory failure should be initially treated by fluid challenge. If intravascular volume is optimized and myocardial contractility remains reduced, support with vasoactive agents will be necessary. In the case of distributive shock (e.g., anaphylaxis or acute vasodilation), adrenaline or vasoconstrictors should be considered. Suggested protocols for management in the emergency department and shortly after transition to the ICU are outlined in **Figure 5.2** and **Figure 5.3**.

Fluid challenge is the first step in therapy. 60 mL/kg of fluid may be given in the first hour of therapy to children with septic shock, without increasing the risk of pulmonary edema. In septic shock, it is widely accepted that maximal preload and, thus, cardiac output are obtained at a pulmonary artery occlusion pressure of 12–15 mm Hg. Clinical fluid requirement is usually determined in the emergency situation by clinical parameters, such as a combination of heart rate, blood pressure, peripheral perfusion, and urine output, and these are supplemented by invasive monitoring of CVP and arterial pressure, as well as biochemical parameters of global perfusion, such as venous oxygen saturation, serum lactate, strong ion gap, and base deficit. The choice of fluid for resuscitation is also a subject of intense debate. The use of normal saline as the initial fluid for shock resuscitation is reasonable.

Ample evidence suggests that early administration of appropriate antibiotics reduces mortality in critically ill patients with bloodstream infections. The choice of antibiotics is vital and should be guided by the susceptibility of likely pathogens in the community and the hospital, as well as any specific knowledge about the patient, including underlying disease and the clinical syndrome. The regimen should cover all likely pathogens. A guide to aid in the selection of the most appropriate early antibiotic based on the suspected source can be found in **Table 5.1**.

Although restricting the use of antibiotics is important for decreasing the development of antibiotic-resistant pathogens, critically ill children with severe sepsis or septic shock warrant broad-spectrum therapy until the causative organism and its antibiotic susceptibilities are available. The antimicrobial regimen should always be reassessed after 48–72 hrs on the basis of microbiologic and clinical data, with the aim of narrowing the antibiotic spectrum to reduce (a) the risk of development of antimicrobial resistance, (b) toxicity, and (c) costs.

Usually, blood replacement is not required unless shock is due to acute hemorrhage or anemia. However, an Hb of >8–10 g/dL is thought to be useful in patients with severe sepsis and/or decreased cardiac contractility. In these patients, the decreased

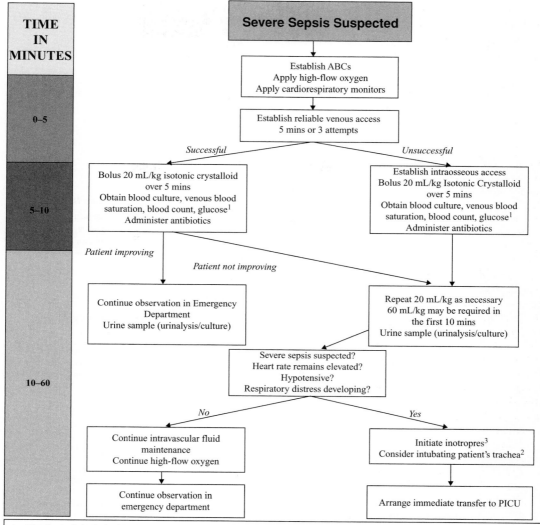

FIGURE 5.2. Suggested emergency department sepsis protocol.

1. Blood sample includes blood culture, complete blood count with differential, electrolytes, BUN, creatinine, venous blood saturation, lactate, ionized calcium, glucose.

2. Consider: Vagolytic (atropine 20 mcg/kg); Induction agent with minimal hypotensive effect (ketamine 1 mg/kg); Paralytic (rocuronium 1 mg/kg or succinylcholine 2 mg/kg).

3. Recommended inotropes if peripheral access only: dopamine 10 mcg/kg/min, epinephrine 0.1–0.2 mcg/kg/min.
   Recommended inotropes if central access: dopamine 10 mcg/kg/min, epinephrine 0.05–2 mcg/kg/min, norepinephrine (0.05–2 mcg/kg/min).

Hb concentration is not compensated by an increase in cardiac output, and DO_2crit is reached more rapidly.

Catecholamines help in restoration of perfusion pressure and augmentation of cardiac output to ensure sufficient DO_2, which should allow regional flow distribution and improved O_2ER. All catecholamines are inotropic agents and can be classified as (a) *inodilators* when they combine inotropic properties with vasodilation (e.g., dobutamine and milrinone, which agents increase flow) and (b) *inoconstictors* when they combine inotropic properties with vasoconstricting effects (e.g., dopamine, adrenaline, noradrenaline, which agents increase perfusion pressure).

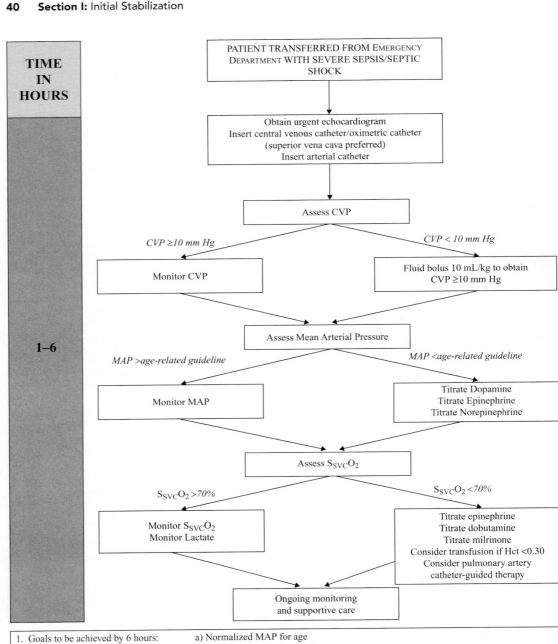

TIME IN HOURS	
1–6	

PATIENT TRANSFERRED FROM EMERGENCY DEPARTMENT WITH SEVERE SEPSIS/SEPTIC SHOCK

Obtain urgent echocardiogram
Insert central venous catheter/oximetric catheter
(superior vena cava preferred)
Insert arterial catheter

Assess CVP

CVP ≥10 mm Hg   *CVP < 10 mm Hg*

Monitor CVP   Fluid bolus 10 mL/kg to obtain CVP ≥10 mm Hg

Assess Mean Arterial Pressure

MAP >age-related guideline   *MAP <age-related guideline*

Monitor MAP   Titrate Dopamine
                           Titrate Epinephrine
                           Titrate Norepinephrine

Assess $S_{SVC}O_2$

$S_{SVC}O_2 >70\%$ $S_{SVC}O_2 <70\%$

Monitor $S_{SVC}O_2$ Titrate epinephrine
Monitor Lactate   Titrate dobutamine
                                   Titrate milrinone
                                   Consider transfusion if Hct <0.30
                                   Consider pulmonary artery
                                   catheter-guided therapy

Ongoing monitoring
and supportive care

1. Goals to be achieved by 6 hours:
   a) Normalized MAP for age
   b) Normalized CVP for age
   c) $S_{SVC}O_2 >70\%$
   d) Resolving lactic acidemia

FIGURE 5.3. Suggested PICU sepsis protocol. CVP, central venous pressure; MAP, mean arterial pressure.

Due to variations in individual sensitivities, dose titration of inotropes is mandatory.

More potent vasoactive agents, such as vasopressin and its derivatives, and inhibitors of nitric oxide synthase are now being used in children with shock. These agents cause a rise in blood pressure. However, just as a low blood pressure is not nec-

essary to diagnose shock in children, restoration of blood pressure may not necessarily be a surrogate for clinical benefit in any patient.

Infectious source control and its eradication are vital. In addition, treatment of hypoxia and identification and treatment of ongoing fluid losses or occult hemorrhage are mandatory. The importance

TABLE 5.1

A GUIDE FOR SELECTION OF EARLY ANTIBIOTICS BASED ON SUSPECTED SOURCE OF INFECTION

	NEONATE (<1 mo)	INFANT (1–3 mos)	PEDIATRIC (>3 mos)
Sepsis Unknown Source	Ampicillin + [gentamicin or cefotaxime] Ampicillin 50 mg/kg/dose IV and q6h (q8h if <1 week old) **plus** Gentamicin 2.5 mg/kg/dose IV q8 hrs (q12 hrs if <1 week old) and Acyclovir 20 mg/kg/dose IV q8 hrs **OR** Ampicillin 50 mg/kg/dose IV and q6h (q8 hrs if <1 wk old) **plus** Cefotaxime 50 mg/kg/dose IV and q8 hrs (q12 hrs if <1 wk old)	Ampicillin + cefotaxime Ampicillin 50 mg/kg/dose IV & q6 hrs **plus** Cefotaxime 50 mg/kg/dose & IV q6 hrs	Cloxacillin + Cefotaxime Cloxacillin 50 mg/kg/dose IV and q6 hrs (Max 2 g/dose) **plus** Cefotaxime 50 mg/kg/dose IV and q6 hrs (Max 2 g/dose)
CNS Suspected Source			Cefotaxime ± Vancomycin Cefotaxime 75 mg/kg/dose IV and q6 hrs (Max 2 g/dose) **plus** Vancomycin 20 mg/kg IV × 1 dose, then 15 mg/kg/dose IV q6 hrs
		Shunt/EVD Meropenem 40 mg/kg dose IV and q8 hrs (Max 2g/dose) plus Vancomycin 20 mg/kg IV × 1 dose, then 15 mg/kg/dose IV q6 hrs	
Pneumonia Suspected Source		Cloxacillin + Cefotaxime Cloxacillin 50 mg/kg/dose IV and q6 hrs (Max 2 g/dose) **plus** Cefotaxime 50 mg/kg/dose IV and q6 hrs (Max 2 g/dose)	Cloxacillin + Cefotaxime +/- azithromycin Cloxacillin 50 mg/kg/dose IV and q6 hrs (Max 2 g/dose) **plus** Cefotaxime 50 mg/kg/dose IV and q6 hrs (Max 2 g/dose) **plus** Azithromycin 10 mg/kg/dose PO/IV × 1 dose (Max 500 mg), then 5 mg/kg/dose PO/IV q24 hrs (max 250 mg/dose) × 5 days
GU Suspected Source	**No known anatomic abnormalities or first presentation:** Ampicillin + gentamicin Ampicillin 50 mg/kg/dose IV and q6 hrs (q8 hrs if <1 wk old) **plus** Gentamicin 2.5 mg/kg/dose IV NOW and q8 hrs (q12 hrs if <1 wk old) **Known abnormality of GU tract:** Piperacillin + gentamicin Piperacillin 75 mg/kg/dose IV q6 hrs (q8 hrs if <1 wk old) **plus** Gentamicin 2.5 mg/kg/dose IV q8 hrs (q12 hrs if <1 wk old)	**> 1 mo old:** **No known anatomic abnormalities or first presentation:** Ampicillin + gentamicin Ampicillin 50 mg/kg/dose IV and q6 hrs (Max 3g/dose) **plus** Gentamicin 7 mg/kg/dose IV and every q24 hrs **Known abnormality of GU tract:** Piperacillin/ tazobactam + gentamicin Piperacillin/tazobactam 75 mg/kg/dose piperacillin component IV q6 hrs (Max 4 g/dose) plus Gentamicin 7 mg/kg/dose IV **NOW** and every q24 hrs	
Skin/ Soft Tissue Suspected Source	Clindamycin + Penicillin + Gentamicin **OR** Clindamycin + Cefotaxime Clindamycin 5 mg/kg/dose IV and q6 hrs (q8 hrs if <1 wk old) **plus** Penicillin 50,000 units/kg/dose IV and q6 hrs (q8 hrs if <1wk old) **plus** Gentamicin 2.5 mg/kg/dose IV and q8 hrs (q12 hrs if <1wk old) **OR** Clindamycin 5 mg/kg/dose IV **NOW** and q6 hrs (q8 hrs if <1wk old) **plus** Cefotaxime 50 mg/kg/dose IV **NOW** and q8 hrs (q12 hrs if <1 wk old)	**> 1 mo old:** Clindamycin + Penicillin + Gentamicin **OR** Clindamycin + Cefotaxime Clindamycin 13 mg/kg/dose IV and q8 hrs (Max 900 mg/dose) **plus** Penicillin 65,000 units/kg/dose IV and q4 hrs (Max 4 million units/dose) **plus** Gentamicin 7 mg/kg/dose IV and q24 hrs **OR** Clindamycin 13 mg/kg/dose IV and q8 hrs (Max 900 mg/dose) **plus** Cefotaxime 50 mg/kg/dose IV and q6 hrs (Max 2 g/dose) **if Group A Strep suspected** **Add IV immunoglobulin (IVIG) 1 g/kg/dose IV q24 hrs × 2 doses** ****ordered from blood bank**	
Immunocompromised/Febrile Neutropenic Patient		> 1 mo old: Piperacillin/tazobactam + gentamicin Piperacillin/tazobactam 75 mg/kg/dose piperacillin component IV NOW and q6 hrs (Max 4 g/dose) **plus** Gentamicin 7 mg/kg/dose IV and q24 hrs	

of correction of metabolic abnormalities has been emphasized in anecdotal guidelines in children with meningococcal shock. However, clinical studies of the use of bicarbonate therapy to correct shock-induced metabolic acidosis failed to show any improvement in cardiac output or reduction in inotrope requirement, regardless of the degree of acidemia. Treatment for adults has moved toward goal-directed therapies. Replacement low-dose steroid therapy has been shown to be beneficial in patients with septic shock and evidence of adrenal hyporesponsiveness, especially in those with high or increasing requirements for inotropes. This benefit has not yet been demonstrated in pediatric patients. However, similar adrenal hyporesponsiveness has been shown in children, and stress doses of steroids are now commonly used in children who require high-dose inotropes.

SECTION II ■ ENVIRONMENTAL CRISES

CHAPTER 6 ■ MULTIPLE TRAUMA

JOHN SCOTT BAIRD • ARTHUR COOPER

Most pediatric deaths from trauma are associated with motor vehicles. The National Safe Kids Campaign (www.safekids.org) and the Injury Free Coalition for Kids (www.injuryfree.org) have both proven effective in reducing the burden of childhood injury. Intracranial injuries are the cause of most pediatric trauma deaths. Blunt injuries outnumber penetrating injuries in children by a ratio of 12:1, a ratio that has decreased in recent years. While blunt injuries are more common, penetrating injuries are more lethal. The automobile is responsible for ~75% of all childhood deaths, which are split between those resulting from pedestrian trauma and those resulting from occupant injuries. Injury mechanism is the main predictor of injury pattern (**Table 6.1**). Pedestrian motor vehicle trauma may result in the Waddell triad of injuries to the head, torso, and lower extremities, while occupant injuries include head, face, and neck trauma in unrestrained passengers and cervical spine injuries, bowel disruption or hematoma, and Chance fractures of the spine in restrained passengers. Bicycle trauma results in head injury in unhelmeted riders, as well as upper extremity and upper abdominal injuries, the latter the result of contact with the handlebar. Low falls, the most common cause of childhood injury, rarely produce significant trauma, but high falls (from the second story or higher) are associated with serious head injuries, with the addition of long-bone fractures (at the third story), and intrathoracic and intra-abdominal injuries (at the fifth-story, the height from which 50% of children can be expected to die following a high fall).

Persistent unopposed hypermetabolic state may occur in severely injured children and is characterized by prolonged catabolism with resultant impaired healing and immunodeficiency. A shift in protein production to acute-phase proteins, including α1-antitrypsin, C-reactive protein, complement components, fibrinogen, and haptoglobin, among others, is common and appears to be mediated by cytokines. Inflammation remote to the site of injury may occur and manifest as systemic inflammatory response syndrome and/or multiple organ dysfunction syndrome. The different functions of acute-phase proteins include bacterial killing and phagocytosis, thrombosis and fibrinolysis, control of proteolysis, and various repair processes; these proteins thus work to restore homeostasis following inflammation or injury and are part of a carefully orchestrated response The trauma-associated hypermetabolic state in children also involves a shift in the hormonal milieu from anabolic to catabolic mediators, including an increase in cortisol, epinephrine, and glucagon concentrations, concurrently with a decrease in activity of insulin and the somatotropic axis hormones. Both insulin and growth hormone resistance occur in critically ill children, including those with major trauma, and contribute to the trauma-associated hypermetabolic state. Stress hyperglycemia (serum glucose >200 mg/dL) is common following pediatric trauma and is related to insulin and growth

TABLE 6.1

COMMON INJURY MECHANISMS AND CORRESPONDING INJURY PATTERNS IN CHILDHOOD TRAUMA

Injury mechanism	Details	Injury pattern
Motor vehicle injury—occupant	Unrestrained	Head/neck injuries Scalp/facial lacerations
	Restrained	Abdomen injuries Lower spine fractures
Motor vehicle injury—pedestrian	Single injury	Lower extremity fractures
	Multiple injuries	Head/neck injuries Chest/abdomen injuries Lower extremity fractures
Fall from height	Low	Upper extremity fractures
	Medium	Head/neck injuries Scalp/facial lacerations Upper extremity fractures
	High	Head/neck injuries Scalp/facial lacerations Chest/abdomen injuries Extremity fractures
Fall from bicycle	Unhelmeted	Head/neck injuries Scalp/facial lacerations Upper extremity fractures
	Helmeted	Upper extremity fractures
	Handlebar impact	Abdomen injuries

Adapted from Cooper A. Early assessment and management of trauma. In: Ashcroft KW, Holcomb GW, Murphy JP, eds. *Pediatric Surgery*. Philadelphia: Elsevier, 2005:168–84.

hormone resistance in the presence of enhanced gluconeogenesis.

PRINCIPLES OF MANAGEMENT

The emphasis in pediatric prehospital trauma care is on aggressive support of vital functions during what has been called the "platinum half-hour" of early pediatric trauma care. Prehospital transport of critically injured children frequently presents a critical choice to emergency medical personnel—"scoop and run or stay and play." Trauma centers are hospitals with special expertise in trauma care, and centers verified by the American College of Surgeons are classified as Level One (with the most comprehensive array of specialists and services, Level Two (with most but not all of the specialists and services available in Level One), and Level Three (only core specialists and services are available). In addition, hospitals and clinics without trauma center designation (nontrauma centers) are still part of the regional trauma system and should be capable of routine resuscitation and

stabilization of injured patients. The Injury Severity Score and the Revised Trauma Score (**Table 6.2**) do not specifically address the pediatric population. The Glasgow Coma Scale (GCS) is used to assess gross neurologic status following injury (and requires modification for infants and small children), while the Pediatric Risk of Mortality III and Pediatric Index of Mortality II are focused on the outcome of all patients admitted to a PICU. Among the scores utilized to assess and predict outcome in critically injured children, the Pediatric Trauma Score (PTS; **Table 6.2**) is acceptable for outcome assessment as well as field use and carries the endorsement of the American College of Surgeons Committee on Trauma and the American Pediatric Surgical Association Trauma Committee. A PTS score <9 is consistent with significant risk of mortality.

Because most pediatric trauma is blunt trauma involving the head, it is primarily a disease of airway and breathing, rather than circulation, bleeding, and shock. The primary survey—the ABCs: Airway, Breathing, and Circulation (D may be added for disability or gross neurologic impairment)—is

TABLE 6.2

TRAUMA SCORES COMMONLY USED IN CHILDREN

PEDIATRIC TRAUMA SCORE

Points	+2	+1	−1
Size (kg)	>20	10–20	<10
Airway	Normal	Maintained	Unmaintained
Systolic blood pressure (mm Hg)	>90	50–90	<50
Central nervous system	Awake	Obtunded	Coma
Open wound	None	Minor	Major
Skeletal trauma	None	Closed	Open-Multiple

REVISED TRAUMA SCORE

Glasgow coma scale	Systolic blood pressure (mm Hg)	Respiratory rate (breaths/min)	Points
13–15	>89	10–29	4
9–12	76–89	>29	3
6–8	50–75	6–9	2
4–5	1–49	1–5	1
3	0	0	0

addressed concurrently with the primary survey in a continuous cycle of assessment, intervention, and re-assessment. The primary survey is generally accompanied by undressing the injured child to more fully assess injury: in an environment at room temperature, avoiding hypothermia.

Airway control and cervical spine stabilization are of prime concern. When endotracheal intubation is required for respiratory failure, rapid sequence (oral) intubation is reasonable following appropriate cervical spine protection, working under the assumption that each patient has a full stomach. Intubation will be additionally necessary for the child in decompensated shock. All patients undergoing a primary survey should receive supplemental oxygen with a FiO$_2$ of 1. An airway obstructed by soft tissues and secretions is opened (utilizing the modified jaw thrust maneuver with or without an oropharyngeal airway to displace the mandible) while taking proper cervical spine precautions (maintaining the cervical spine in a neutral position with bimanual cervical spine stabilization followed by application of an semirigid cervical extrication collar and long backboard), then cleared (utilizing a large-bore Yankauer-type suction device) before its patency can be confirmed and assessment can proceed to the next step. A head tilt is avoided in patients with possible cervical spine injury.

Important considerations regarding pediatric endotracheal intubation include: (a) nasal intubation is contraindicated in patients with severe facial or head trauma, including in particular those with cerebrospinal fluid leak, and blind intubation is discouraged; (b) trauma patients should be considered to have a full stomach, independent of their last documented meal, as gastric emptying time may be delayed in this setting; (c) children are more likely to develop respiratory failure than are adults with equivalent injury; (d) the patient's hemodynamic status will help determine the most appropriate therapeutic approach; and (e) a cuffed endotracheal tube may be indicated, particularly if respiratory compliance appears to be diminished during bag valve mask ventilation. The routine use of noninvasive ventilation in injured children, particularly those with head, face, or neck injury, is contraindicated. Infants may tolerate only 30 secs of apnea, even if fully denitrogenated. Denitrogenation is thus essential in children and is accomplished by 3–5 mins of tidal breathing at an FiO$_2$ of 1. When endotracheal intubation is unsuccessful, or in patients with significant facial, head, neck and/or airway injury, the laryngeal mask airway is of limited use in this setting, as it is inserted blindly; in addition, it may not completely seal the airway, so that aspiration remains a possibility. Fiberoptic-assisted intubation may be helpful in patients with injury to the upper airway; indeed, endoscopy is mandatory for suspected injury to the larynx, trachea, or bronchi. A needle cricothyrotomy is appropriate for trauma patients with upper airway obstruction (above the larynx) after failed orotracheal intubation or because significant upper airway injury renders an attempt at intubation futile, but it is contraindicated in the presence of laryngotracheal injury, as it may exacerbate the injury. A needle cricothyrotomy is merely a temporary expedient, and plans for the next step should be made concurrently. An emergent tracheostomy is indicated for trauma patients with significant laryngeal injury or following failed procedures to secure an airway; some practitioners also perform a tracheostomy emergently for acute, posttraumatic asphyxia.

As soon as a patent airway is assured, an FiO_2 of 1 should continue to be made available to the patient. If ventilation is inadequate, positive pressure ventilatory assistance should be offered. Inadequate ventilation is characterized by decreased breath sounds, an abnormal respiratory pattern, and clinical evidence of hypercarbia; hypoxia occurs late in the course. Hypercarbia may rise rapidly without obvious signs, though decreased responsiveness is the rule.

Laboratory examinations, often helpful in this setting, should not be relied upon to determine therapy: Waiting for the chest radiograph to drain a tension pneumothorax (indicated by decreased breath sounds, deviated trachea, progressive respiratory distress, and hemodynamic compromise) in a patient with multiple trauma is not helpful, nor is it helpful to rely on the arterial blood gas to decide whether or not to intubate a patient: that decision is a clinical one, dependent not just on the patient's ability to adequately exchange gas but equally to maintain and protect the airway.

Attention devoted to the maintenance of adequate circulation will help attenuate the stress response and thus may prevent delayed inflammatory complications of major trauma. The basic steps in the management of hemorrhagic shock are control of active hemorrhage, placement of IV lines, and volume replacement.

Control of active hemorrhage involves the principles of hemostasis. The first and most important step is to apply direct pressure over all actively bleeding wounds. Tourniquet techniques are rarely advocated or used, though the MAST suit may be helpful in selected patients. Most children in hypotensive shock following traumatic injury are victims of unrecognized hemorrhage, which can be reversed only if promptly recognized and appropriately treated by means of rapid blood transfusion and immediate surgical intervention. The MAST suit may be a valuable tool in the prehospital stabilization of patients. When confronted with a MAST-suited patient, careful attention is mandatory; deflation should not be attempted until the primary survey is complete and a plan for possible surgical intervention is formulated. In addition, deflation should be carried out sequentially: The abdominal portion is deflated first, followed by each of the lower extremity compartments, and blood pressure and perfusion must be stabilized following each deflation.

Coagulopathies in injured children typically are related to dilution of platelet and plasma coagulation factors during extensive resuscitation and transfusion, though hypothermia may also contribute. When platelets fall below $50,000/mm^3$ and clinical evidence of bleeding is observed, it is appropriate to begin a platelet transfusion. A general rule of thumb is to administer 6 units to an adult or 0.1–0.2 units/kg to a child. Consideration of empiric platelet and fresh frozen plasma transfusions is reasonable when more than two blood volumes (or 15 units of stored blood in an adult) have been replaced during resuscitation. Laboratory tests of the coagulation system are used to guide specific replacement: The prothrombin time, partial thromboplastin time, and platelet count are routinely monitored. If fibrinolysis is suspected, an appropriate laboratory assessment is also indicated (d-dimer, fibrinogen). Efficacious therapies for hemorrhage with coagulopathy include the replacement of specific coagulation components, avoiding inhibition of coagulation factors, and consideration of aprotinin and aminocaproic acid if excessive fibrinolysis is contributing to hemorrhage. In addition, as activated factor VII is sufficient to initiate the activation of thrombin from prothrombin and thus initiate coagulation, therapy with recombinant activated factor VII offers another potential treatment for severe, unresponsive hemorrhage.

The child who presents with major trauma will require volume resuscitation if signs of hypovolemic shock are present (rapid thready pulse, cool mottled skin, prolonged capillary refill, decreased pulse pressure, and altered sensorium). Shock is less obvious in children. Frank hypotension is a late sign of pediatric shock and may not develop until 30%–35% of circulating blood volume is lost, leading to a "deceptive" presentation of shock in children. Even in the absence of signs of (hypovolemic) shock, vascular access should be immediately available. Resuscitation is best achieved by means of large bore peripheral catheters placed percutaneously. In the event that access cannot be established rapidly in younger children, intraosseous access may be utilized. Access by central venous catheter or by cut down is helpful during resuscitation if experienced operators are immediately available and other means of vascular access are inadequate. Following acute resuscitation, arterial and central venous catheterization are indicated for children with ongoing cardiorespiratory compromise. Simple hypovolemia usually responds to 20–40 mL/kg of warmed isotonic solution, but frank hypotension (clinically defined by a systolic blood pressure <70 mm Hg plus twice the age in years) typically requires in addition 10–20 mL/kg warmed packed red blood cells. Any injured child who cannot be stabilized using this regimen likely has internal bleeding and needs emergency surgery.

If a child presents in shock, has no signs of intrathoracic, intra-abdominal or intrapelvic bleeding, but fails to improve despite seemingly adequate

TABLE 6.3

CLASSIFICATION OF ESTIMATED BLOOD VOLUME LOSS BY CLINICAL SIGNS

System	Mild[a] 15%–30% total blood volume loss	Moderate[b] 30%–45% total blood volume loss	Severe[c] >45% total blood volume loss
Cardiovascular	Tachycardia with weak, thready pulses	Tachycardia with absent peripheral pulses and weak, thready central pulses; mild hypotension with narrow pulse pressure	Tachycardia followed by bradycardia; hypotension
Central nervous system	Anxious, irritable, confused	Lethargic, dulled response to pain	Comatose
Skin	Cool, mottled; prolonged capillary refill	Cyanotic unless anemic; markedly prolonged capillary refill	Pale, cold
Urine output	Minimally decreased	Minimal	None

[a]Corresponds to Class I/II blood loss in adults.
[b]Corresponds approximately to Class III blood loss in adults.
[c]Corresponds approximately to Class IV blood loss in adults.
Adapted from *Advanced Trauma Life Support*, 7th ed. Chicago: American College of Surgeons, 2004.

volume resuscitation, other forms of shock (obstructive, cardiogenic, neurogenic) should be considered. Causes include tension pneumothorax, cardiac tamponade, unrecognized myocardial contusion, or a spinal cord injury. Over-resuscitation contributing to hemorrhage or edema in injured children is not as much of a problem as insufficient or delayed resuscitation. Close attention to the estimated blood volume as a function of size is essential and may help to provide valuable estimates of the severity of hemorrhage (**Table 6.3**). Most injured children will not become hypotensive until nearly one-third of their estimated blood volume is lost. Outcome following resuscitation with albumin or other colloid solutions is no different when compared to crystalloid solutions. Crystalloid solutions are cheaper than colloids and are immediately available. Colloid solutions in this setting may have theoretical advantages. Resuscitation with hypotonic solution is contraindicated. Isotonic crystalloid solutions commonly utilized for resuscitations (often while blood products are being prepared) include normal saline and Ringer's lactate. The excessive use of normal saline may lead to a hyperchloremic metabolic acidosis that can obscure underlying metabolic acidosis secondary to hypoperfusion. The lactate in Ringer lactate provides a buffer so long as hepatic function remains intact. In patients with severe hepatic injury, it may be reasonable to limit lactate intake. Plasmalyte is another isotonic solution that provides buffer as acetate and gluconate. Hypertonic saline may offer some benefits in hemorrhagic shock, including a redistribution of extracellular water due to tonicity changes: As hypertonic saline increases extracellular fluid osmolality, a tonicity

gradient helps pull water from the intracellular compartment. In some patients with multiple trauma, including neurologic injury, the judicious use of hypertonic (3%) saline may be appropriate.

Albumin is a human blood product that is heat-treated to remove infectious disease risks. Both 5% and 25% (or "salt poor") albumin have been used in resuscitation of pediatric trauma patients; other colloid solutions include 6% hydroxyethyl starch and low-molecular-weight dextran; the latter agent is seldom used in the trauma setting, as it induces platelet dysfunction, interferes with cross-matching of blood, and may be filtered by the renal tubules leading to renal failure. Hydroxyethyl starch expands the plasma volume for only 24–36 hrs. Adverse effects include inhibition of platelet aggregation following the administration of more than 15–20 mL/kg.

The treatment of hemorrhagic shock must include transfusion of blood products, particularly in patients with moderate to severe blood volume loss. The hematocrit of a unit of packed red blood cells will depend on the anticoagulant used. With citrate phosphate dextrose, the average hematocrit is 65%–75%, while the more commonly used adenine anticoagulants are associated with hematocrits of 50%–60%. In the emergent resuscitative phase, time may not allow a full type and cross-match to be accomplished before transfusion. When using uncross-matched blood, it is best to obtain at least an ABO and Rh type and partial cross-match. If time does not permit even a preliminary screen, ABO and Rh type-specific, uncross-matched blood is still preferable (and more abundant) than type O negative, Rh negative uncross-matched blood. In the absence of type specific blood, the latter can be used, though cross-matching may still be helpful to ensure the absence of A and/or B antibodies. Blood warmers should be used whenever possible, especially if the volumes delivered are great or if the patient is small. Although the majority of patients will respond to timely intravascular repletion of volume and hemoglobin, some severely injured patients have persistent perfusion defects that will not correct without immediate surgical intervention. Rarely infusion of vasoactive medications like epinephrine or the use of a MAST suit may help bridge the time from primary resuscitation to operating room.

Assessment of disability and the neurologic status completes the primary survey ("ABCD") and relies on the use of the GCS, evaluation of pupillary responses (to exclude mass lesions), and evidence of an altered mental status. Traumatic coma (GCS ≤8) and pupillary asymmetry mandate immediate involvement of neurosurgical consultants. It is important to make at least a preliminary assessment of the neurologic status while the severely injured patient is being prepared for endotracheal intubation.

The most sensitive monitor of cardiac output and volume status in a child is the heart rate. The adequacy of circulation is assessed by noting the quality, rate, and regularity of the pulse and secondarily by obtaining the blood pressure. Progressively weakening pulses, particularly with other signs of poor perfusion, suggest an impending cardiac arrest. On the other hand, bounding pulses with an active precordium do not guarantee that all will be well in patients with a stress response following severe trauma. Respiratory rates in children generally require careful assessment, as a cursory examination over a few seconds is likely to miss periods of apnea, intermittent distress, or progressive deterioration. Perfusion of distal extremities is monitored by assessing capillary refill, skin turgor, as well as looking for cyanosis or other signs of circulatory embarrassment. A capillary refill of more than 2 secs suggests poor distal perfusion. The central venous pressure may be a helpful marker of intravascular volume, particularly in patients with extensive fluid resuscitation. It is measured from a catheter within the vena cava, as near to the right atrium as possible, and when measured at end-expiration/end-diastole offers a good estimate of right atrial and right ventricular pressure (in the absence of pericardial or other cardiovascular disease). The Weil criteria for central venous pressure change with hypovolemia following intravascular fluid bolus therapy is also known as the "2-5° rule." If the response to a fluid bolus within 10 minutes of starting the bolus is an increase in central venous pressure <2 mm Hg or >5 mm Hg, it is continued or discontinued, respectively. Urinary output should be measured in all seriously injured children as an indicator of renal perfusion, as this may be a surrogate for perfusion of other vital organs and should be at least 0.5–1 mL/kg/hr. Additional helpful markers of adequate resuscitation include mixed venous oxygen saturation, arterial lactic acid concentration, and the base deficit. Lack of improvement in arterial lactic acid concentration and/or base deficit in spite of appropriate volume resuscitation may indicate ongoing hemorrhage.

Once the primary survey is complete, resuscitation is ongoing, and shock is being effectively treated, a secondary survey is undertaken for definitive evaluation of the injured child. The primary survey and associated resuscitation efforts should be well advanced within 15 mins. The secondary survey consists of a "SAMPLE" history (*s*ymptoms, *a*llergies, *m*edications, *p*ast illnesses, *l*ast meal, *e*vents and environment) and a complete head-to-toe examination addressing all body regions and organ systems, along with a complete history of the injury. Continued reassessment and resuscitation must proceed with the secondary survey. In examining the child, the first responsibility is to identify life-threatening injuries that may have been overlooked during the primary survey, such as tension pneumothorax, massive hemothorax, and gastric dilatation. If the head demonstrates any sign of drainage from the nose or ears or any evidence of mid-face instability, it suggests the presence of a basilar skull fracture (which precludes the passage of a nasogastric tube) or an oromaxillofacial fracture (which may threaten the airway). Hemotympanum and Battle sign point toward a basilar skull fracture. Following the lateral cervical spine radiograph, the neck is examined for tenderness, swelling, torticollis, or spasm suggesting the presence of a cervical spine fracture (which may not be detected on lateral cervical spine films; that is, spinal cord injury without radiologic abnormality, or SCIWORA). The trachea should be midline, and the large vessels of the neck should be examined. A chest that discloses point tenderness; palpable bony deformity; crepitus; subcutaneous emphysema on inspection or palpation; inadequate chest rise or air entry on auscultation or percussion; or asymmetry in excursion suggests the presence of a rib fracture or air or blood in the thorax (mandating a search for a pneumothorax or hemothorax). Muffled or distant heart sounds with jugular venous distention may suggest cardiac tamponade. An abdomen that remains distended following gastric decompression suggests the presence of intra-abdominal bleeding (most often from the spleen or liver) or a disrupted hollow viscus (especially if fever, tenderness, or guarding is found together with abdominal distention or nasogastric aspirate stained with blood or bile).

All skeletal components should be palpated for evidence of instability or discontinuity, especially bony prominences such as the anterior superior iliac spines, which commonly are injured in major blunt trauma. In the absence of obvious deformities, fractures should be suspected in the presence of bony point tenderness (or hematoma or spasm of overlying muscles), an unstable pelvic girdle, or perineal swelling or discoloration. The integrity of the pelvic ring may be tested by pressing simultaneously on the anterior superior iliac spines to see whether the pelvic wings "spring" apart due to separation of the public symphysis. Most long-bone fractures will be selfevident, but such injuries are occasionally missed during the secondary survey, emphasizing the need to assume a fracture is present on the basis of history alone (even if no deformity is obvious) until proven otherwise; in addition, frequent reexamination of all injured extremities is necessary for evidence of pain, pallor, pulselessness, paresthesias, and paralysis (the classic signs of associated neurovascular trauma). The back should be completely examined.

Arterial blood gases are of paramount importance in determining the adequacy of ventilation ($PaCO_2$), oxygenation (PaO_2), and perfusion (base deficit), although the critically important determinant of blood oxygen content, hence tissue oxygen delivery (assuming the PaO_2 exceeds 60 mm Hg), is the blood hemoglobin concentration. Serial hematocrits are essential to the management of severely injured children. In the presence of abdominal injury or occult hemorrhage, elevations in serum transaminases or amylase and lipase suggest injury to the liver or pancreas. Coagulopathy is more common in children with extensive resuscitation or traumatic brain injury, and a screen that includes the prothrombin time and partial thromboplastin time should be performed in these patients. Urinalysis should be performed on children with suspected abdominal injury: Urine that is grossly bloody or is positive for blood by dipstick (of note, myoglobin may yield false positive results) or microscopy (which shows 20 or more red blood cells per high power field) suggests renal trauma, hence damage to adjacent organs (owing to the high incidence of associated injuries). A pregnancy test is advisable for injured adolescent females.

Radiologic examinations are an integral part of the secondary survey. At no time should imaging studies take precedence over resuscitation from life-threatening injuries, nor should an unstable patient be taken to the radiology department, nor should the physician and nurse fail to accompany and continuously monitor a critically injured child. CTs of the head should be obtained whenever the patient has had loss of consciousness or suspected neurologic injury. CTs of the abdomen should be obtained whenever signs are present of internal bleeding (abdominal tenderness, distention, bruising, or gross hematuria), a history of hypotensive shock (which has responded to volume resuscitation), penetrating injury, or major trauma, to the extent that hemodynamic stability permits. Generally, patients with severe, multiple trauma preventing a complete examination benefit from routine CT of the head, thorax, abdomen, and pelvis, though normal results do not rule out injury; spiral or helical scanners in this setting may allow for optimal use of IV contrast, given the increased rapidity and resolution of such scans. Angiography is reasonable for further study of injuries to large vessels in some patients, often following preliminary identification of such injury by CT. Interventional radiologists may then be able to offer an alternative to surgical intervention, including embolization and stenting.

Though the incidence of SCIWORA is low, it is a frequent cause of spinal cord injury in children. SCIWORA is a result of high-energy injuries, usually associated with automobile accidents, and is characterized by normal radiographic studies (either plain films or CTs) with demonstrable defects on MRI. Focused assessment by sonography in trauma (FAST) may be useful in detecting intra-abdominal blood, but it is not sufficiently reliable to exclude blunt abdominal injury in hemodynamically stable children, and like diagnostic peritoneal lavage (which it has largely supplanted), it adds little to the management of pediatric abdominal trauma (as unstable patients with suspected intra-abdominal injuries are candidates for immediate operation, while stable patients are managed nonoperatively without regard to the presence of intra-abdominal blood). However, a detailed sonographic examination may be useful for those cases in which intra-abdominal injury is suspected and CT cannot be obtained. Echocardiography is helpful in the evaluation of thoracic injury, as it may reveal anatomic or functional cardiovascular injury or injury adjacent to cardiovascular structures.

Any child who requires resuscitation should initially receive no oral intake (because of the temporary paralytic ileus that often accompanies major blunt abdominal trauma and because general anesthesia may later be required), but should receive isotonic IV fluid at a maintenance rate (assuming both normal hydration at the time of the injury and normalization of both vital signs and perfusion status following resuscitation). Gastric tube decompression and a urinary catheter should be placed unless proscribed by signs of a craniofacial or pelvic fracture, respectively. With few exceptions, hypotensive pediatric trauma patients require immediate operation, while nonoperative management of blunt visceral trauma is often successful. Penetrating injuries of the head, neck, and abdomen also require surgical intervention, but most intrathoracic injuries, whether blunt or penetrating, require only tube thoracostomy. Resuscitative emergency department thoracotomy has a dismal outcome in children. It is thus not required, except in cases of massive hemothorax (20 mL/kg), ongoing (2–4 mL/kg/hr) hemorrhage from the chest tube, persistent massive air leak, or food or salivary drainage from the chest tube. Laparotomy is always required for gunshot wounds to the abdomen and for penetrating abdominal injury associated with hemorrhagic shock, peritonitis, or evisceration. Thoracoabdominal injury should be suspected whenever the torso is penetrated between the nipple line and the costal margin, if peritoneal irritation develops following thoracic penetration, if food or chyme is recovered from the chest tube, or if injury-trajectory imaging studies suggest the possibility of diaphragmatic penetration and mandate tube thoracostomy, followed by laparotomy or laparoscopy for repair of the diaphragm and damaged organs. Skeletal injuries constitute the majority of cases in which surgical intervention is necessary. All penetrating wounds are contaminated and must be treated as infected, while accessible missile fragments should be removed (once swelling has subsided) to prevent the development of lead poisoning.

Analgesia appropriate for the injury is essential and may require frequent titration. Most children with multiple trauma benefit from parenteral opiate therapy. Age-appropriate rating devices to assess for pain are available and should be monitored frequently during the first few days following injury. Physician staff should be notified when increasing needs for analgesia are noted. Patient-controlled analgesia (also with parenteral opiate) is indicated for capable older children and adolescents with significant injury-associated pain. Alternative methods of analgesia that may be valuable for some patients include local anesthesia, epidural analgesia, and nonopioid analgesia; adjunctive use of sedative-hypnotic agents may also be helpful in some injured children.

It appears reasonable to avoid glucose supplementation in non-infant trauma victims, at least during the first day of therapy following major trauma, unless hypoglycemia or underlying disease is noted, and close monitoring of patients who are receiving supplemental glucose as well as those with an increased risk for hyperglycemia (i.e., a history of diabetes) is also a reasonable goal.

Early involvement of social services, psychiatric support, pastoral care, and responsible law enforcement and child-protective agencies is mandatory, especially in cases of nonaccidental injury. The care of children with major traumatic injury also involves nutritional support, of nitrogen even more than energy and, in patients who are not eating, antacid ther-

apy to avoid gastric stress ulcer bleeding. Tetanus-prone wounds require tetanus toxoid, with or without tetanus immune globulin, depending upon immunization status and degree of contamination.

Critical care of the respiratory insufficiency that accompanies severe thoracic injury emphasizes avoidance of further injury related to atelectrauma, barotrauma, biotrauma, and volutrauma, using the least amount of oxygen and respiratory support necessary to maintain the PaO_2 at 70–80 mm Hg (hence a S_pO_2 of 90%–100%). Normocarbia is a reasonable goal unless the patient has evidence of acute lung injury (PaO_2/FiO_2, 200–300). Avoiding volutrauma by using tidal volumes of 6–8 mL/kg and permissive hypercapnia are also reasonable for most patients, as long as head injury is not present, to attenuate further lung injury and lessen progression to acute respiratory distress syndrome (ARDS). Positive end-expiratory pressure sufficient to prevent end-expiratory collapse of small airways should be used, in order to minimize atelectrauma. If peak inspiratory pressure cannot be maintained below 30 cm H_2O with minimal attendant barotraumas (less in the presence of air leak syndromes or fresh bronchial or pulmonary suture lines), alternative strategies should be considered such as high frequency oscillatory ventilation, pronation, and lung surfactant. Pulmonary parenchymal injury due to blunt trauma is characterized by alveolar hemorrhage, consolidation, and edema, leading to decreased gas exchange and pulmonary compliance. It may manifest as hemoptysis, subcutaneous emphysema, and respiratory distress and occurs commonly in children with thoracic injury. Persistent hemorrhage from a laceration or contusion may result in a pulmonary hematoma; distinction of this entity from a simple contusion is not clearly defined.

Secondary complications of pulmonary contusion include aspiration, infection, and ARDS. Careful attention to fluid intake is essential in patients with pulmonary contusion. Pulmonary contusions uncomplicated by aspiration, overhydration, or infection can be expected to resolve in 7–10 days, mandating the judicious use of pulmonary toilet, crystalloid fluid (i.e., avoiding overhydration), loop diuretics, and antibiotic therapy to preclude development of ARDS. Fluid and blood in lung parenchyma provide an excellent "culture medium" for bacterial infection, and care must be taken to recognize early signs of superinfection of a pulmonary contusion.

Blunt or penetrating trauma leading to a communication between the pleural space and the atmosphere results in an immediate accumulation of air (and possibly blood) into the pleural space, with contralateral mediastinal shift. Often these injuries are associated with rib fractures. Initial therapy of hemo-pneumothorax in this setting includes a sterile, occlusive dressing to convert the open injury to a closed injury. A tube thoracostomy inserted via the fifth intercostal space in the mid-axillary line via open or Seldinger technique is then connected to a collection chamber with an applied pressure of negative 20 cm H_2O; a water-seal chamber connected in series will facilitate the identification of air leaks in the system. CPR is rarely associated with anterior rib fractures. When present, fracture of a first rib may be a marker of major vascular injury in children. Treatment of isolated rib fractures includes adequate analgesia and chest physiotherapy to prevent atelectasis and pneumonia. Older children may be able to use incentive spirometry and deep breathing exercises. A flail chest is rare in children and is characterized by a chest wall segment that has lost continuity with the thorax and moves paradoxically with changes in intrathoracic pressure: in with inspiration and out with expiration. This injury is the result of major thoracic blunt trauma and is usually associated with multiple rib fractures, such that contiguous ribs have two or more fractures and a pulmonary contusion. Definitive management includes controlled mechanical ventilation: The inflated lung acts as a splint, stabilizes the rib fractures, and decreases pain associated with the chest wall injury. Epidural analgesia may be helpful.

Symptoms of myocardial contusion include chest pain, dysrhythmias, and myocardial dysfunction. Signs on physical examination include tachycardia or dysrhythmia, a gallop rhythm, and findings consistent with cardiogenic pulmonary edema. Laboratory examinations may reveal the presence of cardiomegaly, myocardial dysfunction on electrocardiography and/or echocardiography, and elevated myocardial enzymes. Treatment is primarily supportive. Because children with myocardial contusion are at risk for sudden and lethal dysrhythmias, even if the initial electrocardiogram is unremarkable, they require admission to a PICU and continuous cardiac monitoring. Sudden death that occurs with a relatively minor blunt injury to the chest is known as *commotio cordis* and occurs principally in male adolescents in association with athletic events.

Pericardial contusions and lacerations may lead to hemopericardium and subsequent cardiac tamponade. Rising pericardial pressure obstructs both venous return and cardiac output, leading to Beck's triad (pulsus paradoxus, a quiet precordium, and distended neck veins); shock is the result. Additional data from the physical examination that may be helpful include a jugular venous pressure tracing with absent y descent and, occasionally, the presence of pulsus alternans. Laboratory tests that are helpful include chest x-ray, electrocardiography, and echocardiography (in

particular, the presence of right atrial diastolic collapse in patients with a pericardial effusion). Expansion of intravascular volume is a helpful temporizing measure as the patient is prepared for a pericardiocentesis. As most anesthetic agents are associated with a decrease in systemic vascular resistance and a subsequent fall in preload, local anesthesia is often the best choice, particularly when hemodynamic effects of tamponade are severe. Positive-pressure ventilation with or without intubation is not well tolerated in these patients, either, until at least partial decompression has occurred. Sedation with agents that permit spontaneous ventilation without significant decreases in myocardial contractility and systemic vascular resistance are helpful in some patients unable to tolerate the procedure: Ketamine and etomidate are reasonable choices in this setting. Bedside pericardiocentesis with contemporaneous placement of a drainage catheter via Seldinger technique may help temporize until definitive repair in the operating room can be undertaken.

Traumatic rupture of the diaphragm results from severe compression forces over the lower chest and upper abdomen, and patients generally have severe associated injuries. It has been recognized with increased frequency in the pediatric trauma patient following blunt trauma or with lap-belt injuries. A small tear in the diaphragm may not cause immediate symptoms but eventually results in progressive herniation of abdominal contents through the diaphragmatic defect. The diagnosis should be suspected when the left diaphragm is not clearly visualized or is abnormally elevated or shaped, abdominal visceral shadows are abnormally located on the initial chest radiograph, or a nasogastric tube terminates in the hemithorax.

Although injury to the aorta is uncommon in children, it may occur following severe deceleration injuries and/or a fall from extreme heights. It is characterized by a heart murmur and back pain, as well as hemorrhagic shock; a widened mediastinum, loss of the aortic knob, deviation of the trachea to the right, fracture of the first or second ribs, and apical capping may suggest its presence in this setting. Arch aortography, as well as a chest CT or MRI scan and transesophageal echocardiography, are frequently needed to adequately delineate the injury. Preoperative β blockade may be reasonable in selected patients. Treatment is emergent thoracotomy and surgical repair.

Rupture of the tracheobronchial tree due to blunt or penetrating thoracic trauma is often difficult to diagnose: Most patients with major tracheobronchial tears die at the scene. Those who survive often have symptoms and signs of airway obstruction (dyspnea, bronchi, and stridor), sometimes with subcutaneous emphysema. Occasionally a persistent air leak following tube thoracostomy suggests the presence of a tracheobronchial tear. Bronchoscopy is usually needed to confirm the diagnosis. Fiberoptic intubation may be helpful when this injury is suspected, and blind airway suctioning is contraindicated. As positive-pressure ventilation may exacerbate the leak, careful management of airway pressures and fluid intake is essential. Conservative management is often successful in children with laryngotracheal injury, at least in the absence of a persistent air leak. High-frequency oscillatory ventilation may be helpful.

Physical signs of significant abdominal injury in children include diminished bowel sounds, tenderness to palpation, guarding, rebound tenderness, and other signs of peritoneal irritation; depending on the mechanism of injury, some children may develop an abdominal wall hematoma (i.e., the "seatbelt sign" due to a restraint). Though the physical examination usually is abnormal in children with significant intraabdominal injury, the findings may not be specific. Frequent reexamination is essential, as the possible need for intervention does not abate immediately following the injury. Laboratory examinations that should be reviewed in the child with abdominal injury include serial hematocrits, a type and crossmatch, a complete blood count, serum transaminases, a coagulation screen (prothrombin time and partial thromboplastin time), urinalysis, and amylase and lipase in patients at increased risk. Abdominal radiographs should be assessed for evidence of free air. Following plain abdominal radiographs in children with suspected abdominal injury, CT scanning is the imaging study of choice; it is readily available, noninvasive, and has helped reduce the need for acute surgical interventions. As the extent of abdominal injury may be more difficult to appreciate from the pediatric physical examination than is the extent of thoracic injury, imaging results often help guide resuscitation. Key findings on abdominal CT scans with IV contrast include vascular blush and other signs of contrast extravasation. Oral contrast may be helpful in selected cases but is not routinely indicated. A FAST examination may be useful to confirm abnormalities in children too unstable to undergo a CT scan but is less helpful when negative.

Most solid visceral injuries are successfully treated nonoperatively, Bleeding from renal, splenic, and hepatic injuries is mostly self limited and resolves spontaneously, unless the patient presents in hypotensive shock or the transfusion requirement exceeds 40 mL/kg of body weight (half the circulating blood volume) within 24 hrs of injury. Vascular injury in children is associated with a high mortality, whether in the thorax or abdomen. The role of peritoneal lavage to diagnose intra-abdominal hemorrhage in children has declined with an increased reliance on radiologic imaging and nonoperative management. The indications for immediate abdominal surgery in pediatric trauma patients include evidence of ongoing intra-abdominal hemorrhage, suspicion of hollow viscus perforation, and major pancreatic ductal disruption. When hemorrhage is ongoing, transfusion of blood products requires careful attention; rapid transfusions may be best accomplished with specific devices and catheters, warming of blood products is essential, and close monitoring of blood chemistry will help to prevent or treat resultant electrolyte problems and metabolic acidosis. Appreciation of the likelihood of multiple injuries in children mandates prioritization (e.g., "uncontrolled intraabdominal hemorrhage takes precedence over a stable thoracic aorta tear"). Angiographic interventional radiology may be useful in selected cases, particularly where bleeding is severe and easily accessible. Nevertheless, extravasation of IV contrast in the abdomen generally mandates a laparotomy. A grading system for anatomic findings in solid-organ injury has been developed by the American Association for the Surgery of Trauma (**Table 6.4**). Of particular importance in the evaluation of patients for potential surgical intervention is hemodynamic stability. If the hematocrit is stable, hemorrhage may have stopped.

Lacerations of the kidney are not uncommon and result mostly from crush injuries against the ribs or spine. Gross hematuria remains the most reliable indicator of serious urologic injury and mandates radiographic examination. As rhabdomyolysis following crush injury may present with pigmented urine and a urinalysis positive for heme, it is important to distinguish this entity: Red blood cells on microscopic analysis of urine suggest urologic hemorrhage instead of myoglobinuria. An abdominal CT scan with contrast is the most appropriate test for hemodynamically stable children with suspected renal trauma. Conservative management of renal injury in grades I to III is routine (**Table 6.5**). In children with grades IV and V renal injury, indications for surgical exploration include persistent hemorrhage, expanding or uncontained retroperitoneal hematoma, or suspected renal pedicle avulsion. The ureters are rarely injured, though ureteropelvic junction disruption may occur following severe abdominal trauma. Pelvic fractures are also associated with urethral injury, particularly in males, and blood is generally present at the urethral meatus of affected patients. Diagnosis mandates retrograde urethrography. Rhabdomyolysis secondary to crush injuries may be associated with renal dysfunction and failure; serum muscle enzymes are dramatically elevated, and early treatment with urinary alkalinization is helpful. Renal replacement therapy

TABLE 6.4

GRADING SYSTEM FOR HEPATIC AND SPLENIC INJURIES[a]

Injury	Grade I	Grade II	Grade III	Grade IV	Grade V	Grade VI
Hematoma: liver, spleen	Subcapsular, <10% surface area	Subcapsular, 10%–50% surface area; intraparenchymal diameter <10 cm (liver) vs. <5 cm (spleen)	Subcapsular, >50% surface area or expanding; ruptured subcapsular or parenchymal hematoma; intraparenchymal hematoma >10 cm (liver) vs.>5 cm (spleen) or expanding			
Laceration: liver	Capsular tear <1 cm parenchymal depth	1–3 cm parenchymal depth, <10 cm in length (liver) vs not involving a trabecular vessel (spleen)	>3 cm parenchymal depth or involving trabecular vessels (spleen)	Parenchymal disruption of 25%–75% of hepatic lobe, or 1–3 segments within a lobe	Parenchymal disruption >75% of hepatic lobe, or >3 segments within a lobe	
Laceration: spleen				Involvement of hilar vessels with >25% devascularization	Shattered spleen	
Vascular injury: liver					Juxtahepatic venous injuries	Hepatic avulsion
Vascular injury: spleen					Hilar injury with devascularization	

[a]Advance one grade for multiple injuries, up to grade III.
Adapted from Moore EE, Cogbill TH, Jurkovich GJ, et al. Organ injury scaling: spleen and liver (1994 revision). *J Trauma* 1995;38:323–4.

GRADING SYSTEM FOR RENAL INJURY[a]

Injury	Grade I	Grade II	Grade III	Grade IV	Grade V
Contusion	Microscopic or gross hematuria, normal urologic studies				
Hematoma	Subcapsular, nonexpanding	Nonexpanding perirenal hematoma confined to renal retroperitoneum			
Laceration		<1 cm parenchymal depth (renal cortex) without urinary extravasation	>1 cm parenchymal depth (renal cortex) without urinary extravasation	Extending through renal cortex, medulla and collecting system	Shattered kidney
Vascular injury				Main renal artery or vein injury with contained hemorrhage	Avulsion of renal hilum

[a]Advance one grade for multiple injuries to the same organ.
Adapted from Moore EE, Shackford SR, Pachter HL, et al. Organ injury scaling: Spleen, liver, and kidney. *J Trauma* 1989;29:1664–6.

is appropriate for patients with trauma-associated renal failure, regardless of whether rhabdomyolysis is present.

Blunt injuries to the gastrointestinal tract may follow several patterns, including crush injury, burst injury, and shear injury. Subsequent damage may include hematoma, laceration, perforation, or transection of the gastrointestinal tract, and symptomatology may change over hours or days. Blunt stomach injury results in a perforation or "blowout" injury along the greater curvature. Nasogastric drainage may be bloody, and radiographic studies are generally positive for free air. Duodenal injuries are not frequent. Hematomas and/or perforations involving the remainder of the small bowel may be difficult to diagnose early, as peritoneal signs may take several hours to develop. The pancreas may be injured with severe blunt abdominal trauma, and a delay in diagnosis may occur; affected children generally have multiple associated injuries. Diagnosis depends mainly on CT scan results, though clinical and laboratory data may also be useful

Trauma-associated abdominal compartment syndrome may occur following massive fluid resuscitation. The syndrome is recognized by increasing intraabdominal pressure, leading to hypoperfusion injury that leads to organ dysfunction. Oliguria and respiratory insufficiency are common clinical findings in children. Diagnosis involves instilling 1 mL/kg of sterile saline via the bladder catheter and measuring the pressure: pressure >25 mm Hg (or

~18 cm H_2O) is diagnostic (the reference point is the symphysis pubis).

As immature bone is also more elastic, fractures in children are often incomplete or nondisplaced. Fractures in childhood are also unique as a result of the presence of growth plates, the rapid rate of healing, a tendency to remodel in the plane of the fracture, and a high incidence of ischemic vascular injuries. Diaphyseal fractures of the long bones cause significant overgrowth, while physeal (growth plate) fractures, particularly if severe (SalterHarris types 3 and 4), cause significant undergrowth. Because isolated long-bone and pelvic fractures are rarely associated with significant hemorrhage, a diligent search must be made for another source of bleeding if signs of hypotensive shock are observed: This search frequently leads to the abdomen, though infants and children may also lose substantial amounts of blood in the thorax or head Closed treatment predominates for fractures of the clavicle, upper extremity, and tibia, while fractures of the femur increasingly involve use of fixation. Careful inspection of all wounds is necessary, as an open fracture may be associated with an innocuous-appearing puncture wound. Open fractures significantly increase the risk of developing a compartment syndrome. Operative treatment is required for open fractures, displaced supracondylar fractures, and major or displaced physeal fractures. Critical care of skeletal injuries consists of careful immobilization as appropriate, with emphasis on prevention of immobilization related complications (such as friction burns and decubitus ulcers) through use of supportive and assistive devices (such as egg crate or similar mattresses and a trapeze to permit limited freedom of movement). Prolonged skeletal traction in children with fractures may be associated with hypertension and hypercalcemia; both respond to mobilization. Frequent neurovascular checks are essential to assess for the development of arterial insufficiency, a hallmark of the compartment syndrome. Care of open fractures includes antibiotics, generally a first-generation cephalosporin unless significant comminuted bone from a high-energy injury is present. Complications, including traumatic fat embolism following long-bone fracture and rhabdomyolysis following severe crush injury, are rare but require aggressive care when present. The former may be associated with the acute respiratory distress syndrome and/or emboli to other organs, and early stabilization of long bone fractures is helpful.

Fracture-associated arterial insufficiency is recognized by the presence of a pulse deficit on serial examination, but detection of the compartment syndrome usually requires the measurement of compartment pressures. This syndrome can develop occasionally even in the absence of trauma with extravasation of IV fluid. Symptoms include the five Ps: pallor, pulselessness, paresthesia, paralysis, and pain. The last— pain—is the earliest sign of the syndrome, is often out of proportion to the injury, and may be difficult to treat, even with opiates. Frequent, repeated neurovascular checks of multiply traumatized children are essential to detect this devastating complication early. Fasciotomy is indicated when the compartment pressure is >40 cm water, though lower pressures may mandate treatment if the child is symptomatic or the capillary perfusion pressure reduced.

When the history of injury in a child is insufficient to account for the severity of injury, child abuse must be considered. Child abuse may be suspected whenever an unexplained delay in obtaining treatment has occurred, when the history is vague or otherwise incompatible with the observed physical findings, when the caretaker blames siblings or playmates or other third parties, or when the caretaker protects other adults rather than the child. While the recognition and sociomedicolegal management of suspected cases of child abuse require a team approach, assessment and medical treatment of physical injuries is no different than for any other mechanism of injury. Confrontation and accusation hinder treatment and rehabilitation and have no place in the management of any injured child, regardless of the nature of the injury (although reports of suspected child abuse must be filed with local child-protective services in every state and territory). The "shaken baby syndrome"

comprises a unique set of symptoms and signs peculiar to nonaccidental trauma; this entity is also known as the "whiplash shaken infant syndrome." These patients have intracranial and intraocular hemorrhages in the absence of external trauma to the head or fracture of the calvaria. Ophthalmologic examination often reveals retinal hemorrhages of varying severity, occasionally with retinal detachment. Additional patterns of injury secondary to physical abuse include burns and contusions, particularly in patterns suggesting a mechanism such as cigarette or hot iron burns or fingerprint contusions, as well as asphyxiation, blunt abdominal injury, multiple fractures of various ages, and sexual abuse. Findings on physical examination may include signs of general neglect such as poor skin hygiene, malnutrition, failure to thrive, hematomas and petechiae of various ages and distribution (though the color of cutaneous contusions is not generally a sensitive and specific indicator of contusion age), bite marks, burn injuries, abrasions, strap or belt injuries, and soft-tissue swelling. An ophthalmologic examination is mandatory in infants who are possible abuse victims. Particular attention should also be directed at evidence of sexual abuse such as condylomata, perianal and genital hematoma, other venereal disease (oral and genital), and pain in the anogenital area. In addition to requiring routine laboratory examinations for childhood trauma, infant victims of abuse also require an examination for skeletal injury: Either a skeletal survey with chest x-ray or a bone scan is commonly used. Radiographic manifestations of child abuse include new and old injuries, subperiosteal hemorrhages, epiphyseal separations, periosteal shearings, metaphyseal fragmentations, previously healed periosteal calcifications, and shearing of the metaphysis. The diagnosis of child abuse is rarely made with absolute certainty on the initial presentation, and the physician's role is to serve as an advocate for children: The possibility of abuse should therefore be investigated expeditiously, as it is equally important to protect siblings still in the home. Involvement of social services and the state child welfare departments allows the PICU staff to attend to the child's medical problems.

The anxiety and stress associated with pediatric traumatic injury impact the patient, the family, and often the community. Referral to behavioral health specialists with expertise treating families after traumatic events is reasonable for these families. When symptoms are present more than a month following a traumatic event, posttraumatic stress disorder may be diagnosed: This is suggested by avoidance of reminders of the event, persistent hyperarousal symptoms, and unwanted recollections of the event.

As fever, leukocytosis, and other signs of inflammation are commonly observed in injured children during the acute-phase response, they are neither sensitive nor specific to infection: Resorption of large hematomas, atelectasis, long-bone fractures, and retained necrotic tissue all may contribute to or suggest an inflammatory response. Trauma-related infections typically involve the wound, abdomen, or central nervous system. Broad-spectrum IV antibiotics are often prescribed following significant penetrating trauma and/or open fractures but not after blunt trauma. Routine antibiotic therapy following trauma, including burn injury, is not indicated, as it may lead to the selection of resistant organisms and does not seem to prevent infection.

Significant deep venous thromboses and/or pulmonary emboli are rare following pediatric traumatic injury. As a result, routine prophylaxis is not indicated for infants and children. Compression stockings and pneumatic devices are reasonable in older adolescents likely to require prolonged bed rest or in the presence of other risk factors in those able to tolerate these devices. Assuming that hemorrhage has been controlled, further therapy to prevent thrombotic complications may be considered for those adolescents with a history of venous stasis and/or injury, or prothrombotic conditions. Both therapeutic anticoagulation and vena cava filters have been used successfully in injured pediatric patients.

CHAPTER 7 ■ DROWNING AND NEAR DROWNING: SUBMERSION INJURIES

KATHERINE BIAGAS

Three groups of children are at particular risk for submersion injuries: the very young, adolescent males, and nonwhites. Submersion events that involve infants and toddlers commonly occur in sources of water in the home. Infants who are 6–11 months of age largely drown in bathtubs, and the use of infant bathtub seats does not prevent such events. Older infants and toddlers may drown as the result of a fall into a shallow body of water such as a wading pool, spa, or bathtub. Certain medical conditions may predispose children to submersion (**Table 7.1**). Screening of relatives is recommended for anyone suspected of having a swimming-related arrhythmia syndrome. Counseling regarding safe water-related activities and β-blockade therapy are recommended for affected individuals. Submersion injuries in older children and adolescents may be associated with cervical spine injury. Radiographs of the cervical spine may be normal despite debilitating cord injury, and MR imaging may be necessary to confirm the clinical suspicion.

The initial sequence of events in drowning consists of the following: initial struggle sometimes with a surprise inhalation, suspension of movement and exhalation of a little air frequently followed by swallowing, violent struggle, convulsions with spasmodic respiratory efforts through an open mouth, loss of reflexes, and death. During the initial seconds of submersion, small amounts of fluid are aspirated, often

causing laryngospasm. Victims who are resuscitated at this phase will have little water aspiration, but ventilation by rescue breathing may be difficult because of glottic closure. If the victim loses muscle tone, larger quantities of fluid may be aspirated. In addition, a victim may swallow a large amount of fluid and may vomit, aspirating gastric contents. The development of hypothermia is extremely common with submersion. Hypothermia is usually secondary to rapid radiant heat losses in tepid water. As core temperature drops below the mid-30°C, the victim may develop muscular weakness, and aspiration is facilitated. At lower core temperatures, unconsciousness ensues. Atrial fibrillation occurs with core temperatures in the low 30°C and ventricular fibrillation or asystole with severe hypothermia (core temperature lower than 28°C). Coagulopathy, platelet dysfunction, and immunologic dysfunction also may occur with severe hypothermia.

Postmortem examination has demonstrated mild-to-moderate hyponatremia of victims who drowned in fresh water and moderate hypernatremia and hyperchloremia in those who drowned in salt water. However, clinically important abnormalities in serum electrolyte concentrations usually are not found in patients who survive the event. Submersion victims experience some period of hypoxia. For those with brief episodes, hypoxemia is limited to the duration of hypopnea or apnea and may resolve with rescue or

TABLE 7.1

MEDICAL CONDITIONS THAT PREDISPOSE CHILDREN TO SUBMERSION EVENTS

Seizure disorder
Long QT syndrome or other "channelopathies"
Use of alcohol or other illicit substances
Other conditions that less frequently predispose to
  drowning:
  Depression
  Coronary artery disease
  Cardiomyopathy
  Hypoglycemia
  Hypothermia

initial resuscitation efforts. However, many patients, even those with hypoxia of relatively short duration, may develop increased permeability of pulmonary capillaries, with alveolar fluid leak and dysfunction of surfactant. In patients with longer hypoxic episodes or alveolar aspiration, these processes are more aggressive, with resultant lung collapse, alveolar derecruitment, intrapulmonary shunting, raised pulmonary vascular resistance, and ventilation-perfusion mismatching. Additional cardiac dysfunction may lead to left atrial hypertension and pulmonary-capillary engorgement, furthering pulmonary capillary leak. Large- and small-airway dysfunction may occur, exacerbating gas exchange problems by trapping gas. In combination, these processes create the clinical syndromes of acute lung injury and, later, acute respiratory distress syndrome. Aspiration of gastric contents may add caustic injury to airways and alveoli, worsening gas trapping and hypoxemia. Neurogenic pulmonary edema may contribute to deficits in gas exchange and lung function. The hallmark of cardiovascular dysfunction with submersion injury is shock. Systemic and pulmonary vascular resistances are raised with hypothermia and sympathetic activity associated with the "diving reflex." With these processes, ventricular end-diastolic pressures are raised, as are atrial pressures, with resultant congestion of central and pulmonary veins. Myocardial contractility is diminished with hypoxia. Poor myocardial contractility, in combination with raised systemic vascular resistance, results in lower cardiac output. The clinical examination is one of "cold" shock, with poor perfusion and end-organ dysfunction. The degree to which such derangements are reversible with resuscitation efforts is related to the duration of hypoxemia and low-flow states. Important end-organ (kidneys, liver, etc.) dysfunctions may be demonstrable during the patient's hospitalization but usually fully recover with supportive care.

In the brain, disruption of neuronal and glial functions and architecture occurs. The vascular end zones are particularly vulnerable, and "watershed" infarctions may be appreciated on CT scans. With a more extensive hypoxic-ischemic insult, CT scan of the brain may show a "reversal sign" or global "ground glass" appearance, with attenuation of signal in the supratentorial intracranial contents or entire brain, respectively. While the functional outcome after submersion injury is usually related to the duration and depth of the hypoxic-ischemic insult, brain function may be preserved in "cold water drowning," with good and even normal neurologic outcomes observed despite extensive submersions. The term *cold water drowning* is a misnomer in that the submersion must occur in ice-cold water and, with very rare exceptions, is a phenomenon restricted to northern climates. Patients who have drowned in more temperate water but who have become hypothermic should be considered to have hypothermia from prolonged submersion. Such secondary hypothermia is often a poor prognostic sign. Young children are particularly susceptible to rapid cooling of the brain in icy water because of little subcutaneous fat insulation and large head-to-body ratio. Moreover, activation of the "diving reflex" slows metabolism and preserves some perfusion to the heart and brain. Additionally, neurologic preservation can be seen when the lower body is submersed in ice water and the head remains above water, allowing the victim to continue to breathe. The result is rapid brain cooling in the face of residual perfusion and provision of brain substrates.

MANAGEMENT

Management at the scene should focus on rapid restoration of oxygenation and spontaneous circulation with basic cardiopulmonary resuscitation. Emergency medicine services should be summoned as quickly as possible. No attempts should be made to drain water from the lungs before initiation of rescue breathing. Bystanders should perform mouth-to-mouth breathing even before the victim is removed from the water. Trained rescuers, equipped with a buoyant rescue aid, should attempt in-water rescue breathing of the victim found in deep water. Once on solid ground, chest compressions should be performed unless the presence of a pulse is established. Cervical spine immobilization should be performed in cases with history of diving or when the cause of drowning is not known. Spinal immobilization is otherwise unnecessary and should not interfere with resuscitative efforts. Advanced life support should be initiated by paramedics for victims who do not regain spontaneous breathing and consciousness with rescue breaths. Bag-valve mask ventilation with supplemental oxygen is sufficient to restore circulation in some victims. Endotracheal intubation with manual ventilation, administration of fluid boluses, defibrillation, and administration of bolus vasoactive medications may be required in others; however, these efforts should not be pursued to the extent that transportation of the victim to a hospital is delayed.

Definitive management of submersion injuries begins in the emergency department. Advanced life support should focus on establishment of adequate oxygenation and ventilation, adequate circulation, and determination of neurologic functioning (**Table 7.2**). In the emergency department, definitive warming should be initiated for all but mild hypothermia (35°–36°C) and performed in concert with resuscitation efforts. The simplest warming techniques include the use of warmed IV fluids, external radiant heat, ventilation with heated gas, and immersion in a warm bath.

TABLE 7.2

IMPORTANT PRINCIPLES FOR THE MANAGEMENT OF CHILDREN WITH SUBMERSION INJURY

IN THE EMERGENCY DEPARTMENT

Establish adequate oxygenation and ventilation	Intubate airway of unconscious or hypoventilating children
	Provide supplemental oxygen
Establish normal circulation	Bolus IV fluids (NS) for hypotension
	Initiate use of vasopressor infusions (epinephrine, consider addition of vasopressin) for continued hypotension
Neurologic examination	Determine Glasgow Coma Scale score
	Control seizures with bolus administration of anticonvulsants (lorazepam, phenobarbital, or fosphenytoin)
Rewarming of hypothermia, unless mild (35°–36°C)	Use warmed fluids and ventilation with heated gas
	Consider bladder washes with warmed fluids
	Consider cardiopulmonary bypass
Transfer patient for definitive care	Transfer to inpatient unit for observation if full neurologic and cardiovascular function are rapidly restored
	Transfer to a PICU if full function not restored

IN THE PICU

Employ ventilator strategies for ALI/ARDS	Limit ventilator peak pressures to <25 torr
	Limit tidal volumes to 6–8 mL/kg
	Limit fraction of inspired oxygen to <0.60
	Liberal use of PEEP
	Consider the use of exogenous surfactant or ECMO for continued hypoxemia
Treat myocardial dysfunction	Titrate vasoactive infusions to normal cardiac output and adequate end-organ perfusion
Employ brain-protective strategies	Avoid hyperthermia
	Treat clinical and subclinical seizures
	Use mild systemic cooling (35°–36°C) for 24–48 hrs
	Frequent neurologic reassessments and adjunct studies of function as indicated
Refer to a rehabilitation facility for persistent neurologic injury upon recovery	

NS, normal saline; ALI, acute lung injury; ARDS, acute respiratory distress syndrome; PEEP, positive end-expiratory pressure; ECMO, extracorporeal membrane oxygenation

More aggressive efforts are necessary for moderate hypothermia: warmed peritoneal lavage or dialysis fluids and/or bladder washes with warm fluids. For severe hypothermia, passive rewarming can induce "rewarming shock," with peripheral vasodilatation and impaired cardiac output. The use of cardiopulmonary bypass has been advocated for core rewarming in severe hypothermia. Failure to restore circulation after 30 minutes of rewarming to at least 32°C suggests that further resuscitation efforts will not be successful. Consideration should be given to maintaining mild hypothermia (core temperature of 32°–35°C) in children who remain comatose after submersion for the possibility of neuroprotection.

Management in the PICU

Cardiorespiratory dysfunction should be aggressively treated. An "open lung" strategy should be employed for patients with acute lung injury or acute respiratory distress syndrome. Usual ventilator settings include limiting ventilator peak pressures to 25 torr, tidal volumes to 6–8 mL/kg, and fraction of inspired oxygen to <0.60. Liberal use of positive end-expiratory pressure may improve oxygenation dramatically. Administration of exogenous surfactant can be used successfully to treat severe acute respiratory distress syndrome following submersion injury when surfactant wash out/dysfunction is suspected. Extracorporeal membrane oxygenation can be considered. Continuous vasoactive infusions may be required to treat myocardial dysfunction and correct abnormal peripheral vascular resistance. Treatment should concentrate on normalizing blood pressure, organ perfusion, and gas exchange as quickly as possible.

The other focus of ICU care is restoration of cerebral function, though no definitive treatment exists to reverse the neuronal injury processes previously discussed. Instead, care of the brain is supportive. Normal cardiorespiratory function should be maintained. Hypermetabolic states such as seizures and fevers should be aggressively treated. Routine electroencephalography should be used to detect subclinical seizures and to titrate antiepileptic therapy. In cases of severe global brain injury, consideration should be given to maintaining mild hypothermia for 24 to 48 hours. To maintain a hypothermic state, patients may require the use of neuromuscular blocking agents, which will interfere with performance of the neurologic examination. In addition, intracranial hypertension may be found in cases of severe brain injury. Monitoring and treatment of intracranial pressure does not affect ultimate outcome. Raised intracranial pressure is a marker of poor neurologic prognosis.

A reasonable approach is to avoid determining which patients should receive initial treatment based on prognostic factors. Rather, the "treat-them-all approach" applies, with aggressive efforts despite initial lack of heartbeat. The adage "You're not dead until you're warm and dead" applies with vigorous resuscitative efforts, including rewarming, as needed. Prognosis is deferred until circulation is restored and perfusion optimized. At that time, the patient can be more completely examined. CT is used in the initial assessment of patients, especially in patients with a history of possible associated traumatic injury. Repeated brain CT scans often add little more information. MRI and MR spectroscopy can detect more subtle injury. Serial MR scans obtained 3–4 days after submersion can provide predictive outcome value. Electrophysiologic studies may provide additional information. The early use of electroencephalography may be limited by the need for sedatives in the initial recovery phase, but persistent low attenuation of the electroencephalogram is a poor prognostic sign. Brainstem auditory-evoked responses have been used to evaluate function in prolonged outcome with some success. Use of a series of electrophysiologic modalities, including sleep recordings, brainstem auditory-evoked responses, somatosensory-evoked potentials, and polysomnography to generate a more complete picture of functioning in 5 comatose children after near-drowning events suggested that better prediction could be attained using all of these modalities over the use of electroencephalography alone. No single prognostic test or assessment can reliably discriminate good from poor functional outcomes in all victims of submersion injury; moreover, no indicator is sufficiently reliable to be the sole determinant of whether to withdraw or withhold therapy in a victim of submersion injury.

PREVENTION

The outcome of a drowning event is determined in the first few minutes of submersion. Prevention strategies have focused on calling attention to the common causes of childhood drowning, specifically bathtub drowning and recreation-related incidents. Slogans such as "Don't Turn Your Back On Me" alert parents to the proper supervision of infants and toddlers. Other alerts focus on specific events (e.g., the installation of a home pool). Most pool-related submersions occur within the first 6 months of pool exposure. The absence of proper pool fencing may increase the odds of pool-related drowning by as much as three- to five-fold. Written alerts about drowning risks are generally distributed to customers upon purchase of a new pool. Additional prevention campaigns have focused on the family pediatrician. The American Academy of Pediatrics issued a policy statement in 2003 to guide pedi-

atricians in incorporating regular, age-appropriate teaching about water safety in their anticipatory guidance to families. Their recommendations can be found at The Injury Prevention Program Web site, www.aap.org/family/tippmain.htm. Additional prevention tips are available at the Consumer Product Safety Commission Web site, http://www.cpsc.gov/.

CHAPTER 8 ■ BURNS, ELECTRICAL INJURIES, AND SMOKE INHALATION

ROGER W. YURT • JOY D. HOWELL • BRUCE M. GREENWALD

The loss of integrity of the skin exposes the child to the exterior environment of bacterial, fungal, and viral pathogens. At the same time, the wounds provide a portal for loss of fluid and body heat. The extent of tissue injury caused by a burn is quantified by the surface area and the depth of injury. Determination of the extent of injury provides a basis for estimation of fluid requirements for resuscitation and for determining an overall care plan. For estimation of the extent of surface area involved, a Lund & Browder chart or Berkow's formula should be used. The "rule of nines" cannot be used in children younger than age 15. The distribution of surface area by age is shown in the chart that is in use at the William Randolph Hearst Burn Center (**Table 8.1**). A first-degree burn is characterized as erythematous, painful, and dry, while a third-degree burn, also known as a full-thickness burn, is leathery, dry, and insensate. Burn injuries at an intermediate depth of partial thickness are more difficult to assess. They are divided into superficial and deep partial-thickness wounds. Whether superficial or deep, these wounds appear very similar on physical examination. They are erythematous, moist, and sensate. Evaluation of these wounds is complicated by the fact that they evolve over time, are frequently not homogenous with regard to depth, and are dynamic over the first days after injury. The importance of differentiating these depths of injury relates to the fact that a superficial partial-thickness burn will re-epithealize in 2 weeks, whereas a deep partial-thickness wound heals by epithelialization and contraction. To avoid scarring, the deeper wound must be treated by skin grafting. Except for small surface area wounds, full-thickness wounds should be either excised and closed primarily or grafted with the patient's skin. A cross-

section of skin with indication of the various depths of injury is depicted in **Figure 8.1**.

Three zones of injury have been identified in burn-injured skin. The outer zone of coagulative necrosis includes necrotic tissue that is irreversibly damaged by heat or chemical. Below that is the zone of stasis in which some viable tissue remains. This dynamic region is subject to further necrosis if it is not protected from further physical damage The zone adjacent to the zone of stasis has been termed the zone of hyperemia, given the increased blood flow and local inflammatory response to the injury.

Chemical burns cause denaturation of protein and disruption of cellular integrity. The degree of injury is dependent on the time of exposure, the strength of the agent, and the solubility of the agent in tissue. Alkaline agents tend to penetrate deeper into tissues than do acids.

The major concern in evaluating patients who sustain electrical injuries is that the surface injury, which may appear similar to other burn injuries, is often not indicative of the extent of injury. Electrical current follows the path of least resistance and will pass through nerve and blood vessels preferentially and cause injury to these tissues. Injury of the heart is primarily associated with arrhythmia. Practice guidelines for the management of electrical injury suggest that patients who contact a low voltage (<1000 volts) source can be cared for as outpatients if they have no electrocardiographic abnormalities, no history of loss of consciousness, and no other reason for admission. Patients who contact high-voltage sources are usually admitted and placed on cardiac monitoring. Creatine kinase levels, including the MB subunit, do not reliably indicate extent of myocardial injury. Late sequelae of electrical injury, which may occur months

TABLE 8.1

DISTRIBUTION OF BODY SURFACE AREA BY AGE AS PERCENTAGE OF TOTAL BODY SURFACE AREA

Area	Age in years				
	0–1	1–4	5–9	10–14	15
Head	19	17	13	11	9
Neck	2	2	2	2	2
Anterior trunk	13	13	13	13	13
Posterior trunk	13	13	13	13	13
Each buttock	2.5	2.5	2.5	2.5	2.5
Genitalia	1	1	1	1	1
Each upper arm	4	4	4	4	4
Each lower arm	3	3	3	3	3
Each hand	2.5	2.5	2.5	2.5	2.5
Each thigh	5.5	6.5	8	8.5	9
Each leg	5	5	5.5	6	6.5
Each foot	3.5	3.5	3.5	3.5	3.5

or even years after injury, include the development of cataracts and transverse myelitis of the spinal cord.

Injury caused by exposure to ionizing radiation may be limited to the skin but is often deeper. Because these wounds do not heal well, care must be taken to avoid additional damage of the tissue. The vasculitis that is associated with these injuries is usually a life-long problem.

The index of suspicion should be high when a child is injured by burning. The determination of whether abuse or neglect has occurred is based on the characteristics of the wounds and the history provided. A history that is inconsistent with the findings on physical exam is sufficient reason to launch a deeper investigation into the injury. Conflicting histories should also lead to a search for additional information about the incident. Well-defined lines of demarcation between burned and unburned skin in a scald burn and the absence of splash burns are suggestive of intentional injury. However, splash burns can also be seen in intentional scald-burning cases. In addition, sparing of areas of skin may be suggestive of an intentional injury, particularly seen when the

extremity is held in flexion and the area around the joint is protected and spared.

Upper airway injury edema associated with aspiration of hot liquid at the time of a scald injury is an injury rarely seen in children. Signs of upper airway obstruction will often lead to intubation of the airway in this group of patients. In the management of burn and trauma patients, airway evaluation and management are of paramount importance and begin with an assessment of airway patency and quality of respirations. Chest radiography, arterial blood gas determination, and pulmonary function testing are usually normal during the first 3 days following injury. Patients who sustain injury in a closed space have burns above the clavicle, singeing of facial hair, hoarseness, or carbonaceous sputum should be assumed to have sustained an inhalation injury. Elevated carboxyhemoglobin levels will confirm exposure to carbon monoxide but are not diagnostic for injury to the lung. Because the primary concern early after inhalation injury is obstruction of the airway, the upper airway should be evaluated immediately, usually in the emergency department. Flexible

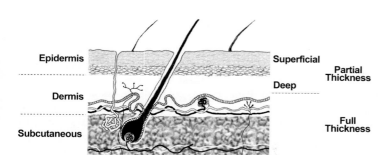

FIGURE 8.1. Schematic depiction of a cross-section through skin. The epidermis, dermis, and subcutaneous layers are shown. The levels of burn injury are divided into partial thickness, which may be superficial or deep, and full thickness.

CRITERIA FOR REFERRAL FOR CARE OF A PATIENT WITH A BURN INJURY TO A REGIONAL BURN CENTER

For adults and pediatric patients with second- and third-degree cutaneous burns, burn center candidates are identified according to the following:
1. Any burn >15% of the body surface area
2. Any burn in patients with significant preexisting disease that may complicate or retard recovery
3. Any burn >9% of the body surface area in patients ≤5 years of age or ≥60 years of age
4. Any burn that involves critical body parts, such as eyes, face, hands, feet, ears, or genital area
5. Any third-degree burn of >5% of the body surface area
6. Inhalation injuries, electrical burns, and burn injuries complicated by underlying fractures or other trauma

bronchoscopy provides the opportunity to confirm the diagnosis. Xenon ventilation/perfusion scans show air trapping when parenchymal injury is present; however, this test does not provide quantitative information on the extent of injury.

Although travel time and distance to a burn center are of concern, transfer of burn-injured patients after initial evaluation has been shown to be safe, especially if initiated early after injury. Patients with burns over more than 30% of their body surface area (BSA), those at the extremes of age, those with injury of critical body parts, such as genitalia, and those with significant preexisting disease should be cared for in a burn center. Specific guidelines have been published by the American Burn Association (**Table 8.2**).

PRINCIPLES OF CLINICAL MANAGEMENT

Peripheral venous cannulation is preferred over central venous access and may be performed through burn-injured tissue if access through uninjured sites is not available. Children with >15% total BSA injury require IV fluid resuscitation and should have a urinary catheter. In addition, patients who have sustained a major injury should have a nasogastric tube placed to decompress the stomach. During transport and resuscitation, every effort should be made to maintain body temperature. Patients should be wrapped in clean sheets or blankets, and in the initial phase in the emergency care area, the room should be warmed. Resuscitation fluids should be warmed. Burn injury leads to intravascular volume depletion

because fluid is lost into burn-injured tissue, through the wound, and into noninjured tissue. The major losses occur during the first 24 hrs following the injury, and it is generally agreed that during this period, crystalloid solutions should be used. As fluid shifts from the vascular space are massive in major injuries, formulae have been developed to provide an estimate of the fluid requirements.

The Parkland formula is the crystalloid-based formula and calls for the initiation of resuscitation with lactated Ringer solution at a rate based on the BSA of burn injury and the patient's body weight. The calculated resuscitation volume for the first 24 hrs is:

$$(4\,mL/kg \times \%\,BSA\,burn) + maintenance\,fluids \quad [8.1]$$

Maintenance fluids (5% dextrose in lactated Ringer solution) should be estimated (100 mL/kg for the first 10 kg, 50 mL/kg for the second 10 kg, and 20 mL/kg above 20 kg body weight) for children who weigh <40 kg. For adults and children who weigh >40 kg, maintenance fluids are not included in the estimate of fluid requirements. Half of this volume is given in the first 8 hrs after injury, and the other half is given in the following 16 hrs.

At the Shriners Burn Center in Galveston, Texas, an alternative formula used for calculating resuscitation fluid for the first 24 hrs after injury calls for lactated Ringer solution based upon surface area of injury in square meters (SA) with maintenance fluid (5% dextrose in lactated Ringer's) based on total BSA in square meters:

$$(5000\,mL \times SA\,burn) + (2000\,mL \times total\,BSA) \quad [8.2]$$

After the first 24 hrs, fluids are given to meet maintenance requirements and to replace ongoing losses. The hourly evaporative fluid loss from the patient's wounds can be estimated as:

$$(25 + \%\,BSA\,burn) \times total\,BSA \quad [8.3]$$

The evaporative losses are primarily free water. However, to avoid rapid changes in sodium concentration in children, this loss is replaced with a salt-containing solution, such as 5% dextrose in 0.2% normal saline. The loss of serum protein is clinically significant when the burn injury exceeds 40% BSA. When the injury is this size or larger, the loss is replaced in the second 24 hrs after injury with 5% albumin solution. The volume required can be estimated as:

$$0.3 - 0.4\,mL/kg \times \%\,BSA\,burn \quad [8.4]$$

The ultimate goal in the post-resuscitation period is to maintain normal blood pressure, heart rate, urine output, and serum sodium. In burn patients, hypoalbuminemia is a frequent finding. Mild-to-moderate hypoalbuminemia is well tolerated in previously healthy patients. Routine albumin repletion may not be warranted, but the present practice in the William Randolph Hearst Burn Center is to ensure appropriate caloric delivery, preferably by the enteral route, as quickly as possible and—in critically ill pediatric patients—replete with 25% albumin if the serum level is below 3 mg/dL.

The majority of injuries to the lung are caused by inhalation of toxic chemical products of combustion, in particular, aldehydes. Carbon monoxide and cyanide poisoning may occur as well. The local edema, infiltration of the tissue with polymorphonuclear leukocytes, and sloughing of bronchial mucosa can lead to the formation of an endobronchial cast and obstruction of terminal bronchioles. The obstruction of the small airways and the accumulation of carbonaceous material and necrotic debris provide a fertile ground for the development of infection. Therapy consists of aggressive pulmonary toilet, use of mucolytics, and early identification and treatment of infection and supportive care. The level of support that is required may range from supplemental oxygen to advanced modes of assisted ventilation and hyperbaric oxygen therapy. For patients with evidence of inhalation, injury supplemental oxygen should be provided via nasal cannula or simple facemask, both of which will add additional humidification. If stridor due to upper airway inflammation and edema is present, racemic epinephrine may be employed to transiently relieve the obstruction to airflow. Helium/oxygen admixtures reduce resistance to turbulent airflow and, in turn, improve work of breathing in situations of upper airway obstruction. Heliox is most frequently used to treat upper airway obstruction following extubation. When the airway is compromised, these patients should be intubated to permit definitive assessment and airway control.

The use of cuffed endotracheal tubes in the management of pediatric burns and smoke inhalation has increased. The size of the endotracheal tube when using a cuffed tube should be 0.5 cm smaller than an uncuffed tube. The current Pediatric Advanced Life Support guidelines recommend use of the formulas: $(Age/4) + 3$ for cuffed endotracheal tubes and $(Age/4) + 4$ for uncuffed tubes. Acute lung injury and acute respiratory distress syndrome (ARDS) represent significant clinical challenges, especially in very young patients. Pressure control ventilation and synchronized intermittent mandatory ventilation are the modes most frequently used, while more advanced modes are reserved for patients with severe restrictive lung disease. The use of lung-protective strategies, include low tidal volume/high positive end-expiratory pressure (PEEP), airway pressure release ventilation (APRV) and high frequency oscillatory ventilation (HFOV). Early excision and closure of the burn wound and lung-protective ventilation strategies are the 2 main priorities in the management of burn patients with ARDS. High-frequency percussive ventilation has been used in adult burn patients with ARDS. APRV has been used in the management of burn victims with inhalational injury and/or ARDS. APRV provides continuous positive airway pressure with time-cycled releases. Oxygenation is accomplished by maintenance of airway pressure, typically at 20–30 cm H_2O (P_{high}) for several seconds (T_{high}), thereby achieving a mean airway pressure equivalent to or higher than conventional mechanical ventilation but with lower peak pressures. Ventilation is achieved by pressure releases, spontaneous breathing, and maximizing time spent at T_{high}. APRV is associated with several physiologic benefits, including improved recruitment of diseased lung units with long time constants, maintenance of spontaneous ventilation, augmentation of the thoracic pump, and decreased risk of alveolar over distension. Cuffed endotracheal tubes and lung protective ventilator strategies should be employed in patients at risk for acute lung injury. Low tidal volume with high PEEP is used initially and progresses to HFOV or APRV in patients who require PEEP in excess of 10 cm of H_2O. Tracheostomy is classically utilized in patients following a prolonged course of endotracheal intubation. However, early tracheostomy has also been used safely in a cohort of pediatric burn patients. Currently, tracheostomy is generally reserved for patients who have failed extubation or for those projected to require chronic mechanical ventilation (i.e., neurologically devastated patients).

The objective of wound care is to avoid infection and protect the wound from further injury. Inpatient wound care is provided in a warm environment in an area reserved for wound care in a burn center. Systemic antimicrobial prophylaxis is not used in patients who are admitted to the hospital. The wounds are closely observed for infection, and treatment is initiated if infection occurs. The advent of effective topical antimicrobial agents has substantially reduced the mortality associated with burn wound infection. The commonly used agents and their advantages and disadvantages are listed in **Table 8.3**. Due to concern that kernicterus is associated with exposure to sulfonamides, silver sulfadiazine is not used in infants <2 months of age or in patients who are near-term pregnant.

Excision and closure of wounds has the advantage of reducing the extent of injury and eliminating the risk of wound infection. One of the major advances in burn care has been the recognition that patients

TABLE 8.3

TOPICAL ANTIMICROBIAL AGENTS FOR TREATMENT OF BURN INJURY BY TYPE

	Application	Advantages	Disadvantages
OINTMENT			
Bacitracin	2nd degree burns, small areas	Not water soluble, good on face	Not indicated for large surface area
CREAM			
Silver sulfadiazine	2nd and 3rd degree burns	Soothing, good for range of motion	Possible neutropenia; little penetration
Mafenide acetate	2nd and 3rd degree burns	Penetrates eschar	Painful, metabolic acidosis
SOLUTION			
Aqueous silver nitrate (0.5%)	2nd and 3rd degree burns	Good antimicrobial	Hyponatremia, stains wound; little penetration
Mafenide acetate (5%)	Graft dressing, open wound soak	Broad activity, moist dressing	Not used for unexcised wound
IMPREGNATED DRESSINGS			
Acticoat	2nd degree burns	Dressing change every 3 days	Only 2nd degree
Aquacel Ag	2nd degree burns	Leave on for 21 days	Less flexibility and ease of motion; only 2nd degree burns

in whom the wounds are excised early after injury have fewer complications. The usual approach is to begin excision within the first 3–4 days after injury. In the patient with wounds that will require grafting (i.e., deep partial- and full-thickness) over >40% of the BSA, a strategy for surgical intervention must be developed that accounts for available donor sites, with a goal of reducing the amount of open wound as quickly as possible. The closure of the excised wound requires the use of autograft. When donor sites are limited, autograft can be expanded by passing it through a mechanical meshing device. Closure of the excised wound may be staged by temporarily covering it with biologic or manufactured dressings. Allograft provides for closure of the wound and may also be used as a test graft in areas where infection is of concern or when the adequacy of the excised wound bed is suspect. Integra Life Sciences Corporation provides a temporary epidermis as an outer layer of silastic and an inner-layer matrix for the growth of a neodermis. *AlloDerm* is human dermis that has been processed to extract cells and their components. This nonantigenic matrix provides a scaffold for a new dermis upon which a thin epidermal graft may be placed. The advantage that these products offer for patients with large surface areas of injury is that donor sites are available in shorter time frames for recropping of epidermis for further grafting. Immediate application of other products, such as pigskin or *Biobrane* (a synthetic membrane composed of silastic and a chondroitin sulfate–coated surface), on partial-thickness

wounds moderates pain and eliminates the need to change dressings.

All extremities with circumferential full-thickness burns should be elevated to minimize edema formation and should be evaluated hourly for the classic signs of vascular compromise: pallor, pain, paresthesia, paralysis, and poikilothermia. Because these signs are often difficult to evaluate in a burn-injured extremity, additional assessment of Doppler-measured blood flow in the distal extremity should also be performed. Loss of Doppler signals may not be seen until after damage has occurred; therefore, the threshold for performing an escharotomy to release subeschar pressure should be low. Decompression of the hand should be performed when full-thickness burn injury leads to compromise of blood flow and function. Escharotomies are performed in fingers in the midaxial line on the ulnar side and on the radial side of the thumb, so as to preserve tactile sensation of the surfaces of opposition of the fingers and thumb. In a similar way, a "compartment syndrome" can occur in the chest or abdomen in patients with circumferential full-thickness burn injury in these areas. A decrease in pulmonary compliance in these patients may indicate that decompression is necessary. Escharotomy of the chest in the anterior axillary line will often decrease the inspiratory pressures required to maintain tidal volume.

The systemic inflammatory response that is associated with a major burn ignites a cascade of events that presents as a clinical syndrome that is difficult to distinguish from infection. Virtually all children who sustain burn injury have fever; severely burn-injured patients often have core body temperatures of 39°–39.5°C, and they frequently develop an intestinal ileus, become disoriented, develop hyperglycemia, and sustain changes in fluid balance. The burn wound has been described as a "black box" in which a local inflammatory process occurs that leads to introduction of mediators of inflammation into the systemic circulation.

Impetigo "involves the loss of epithelium from a previously reepithelialized surface such as a grafted burn, a partial-thickness burn allowed to heal by secondary intention, or a healed donor site." This infection, which has also been termed *melting graft syndrome*, is not necessarily associated with systemic signs of infection, fever, or an elevated white blood cell count. Though it is often caused by streptococcal or staphylococcal species, it may be caused by other organisms as well. Burn wound surface cultures, which give no insight into what is occurring within the wound, are helpful in determining the inciting organism in these infections. Treatment consists of local care of the wound and systemic antibiotics.

Open surgical wound infections are associated with a surgical intervention that has not healed. They may occur in an ungrafted, excised burn or at unhealed donor sites and are associated with culture-positive purulent exudates. In addition, at least one of the following conditions is present:

- Loss of synthetic or biologic covering of the wound
- Changes in wound appearance, such as hyperemia
- Erythema in the uninjured skin surrounding the wound
- Systemic signs, such as fever or leukocytosis

These infections require a change in local wound care, usually the addition of a topical antimicrobial, more frequent dressing changes, and the administration of systemic antibiotics. Burn-associated cellulitis must be differentiated from the normal local inflammatory response to a burn injury that is manifest as erythema at the margin of the wound. This finding differs from cellulitis by its localized nature (usually <1–2 cm from the margin of the wound) and by the lack of extension beyond that zone. The guidelines suggest that in addition to a requirement for antibiotic treatment the definition of cellulitis requires at least one of the following:

- Localized pain, tenderness, swelling, or heat at the affected site
- Systemic signs of infection, such as hyperemia, leukocytosis, or septicemia
- Progression of erythema and swelling
- Signs of lymphangitis, lymphadenitis, or both

The diagnosis of invasive burn wound infection rests on the recognition of changes in the wound, which include black, purple, or reddish discoloration, maceration, or early separation of eschar and systemic manifestations of infection. In addition to the clinical assessment of the wound, biopsy may be performed for quantitative culture or histologic evaluation. A tissue culture with >100,000 organisms is cultured from a gram of tissue. The topical antimicrobials, with the exception of mafenide acetate, which may be used in preparation for excision, are not used for therapy for invasive burn wound infection because they do not penetrate eschar. The criteria for diagnosis of invasive infection, as outlined in the American Burn Association guidelines, include the following:

- Inflammation of the surrounding uninjured skin
- Histologic examination that shows invasion by the infectious organism into adjacent viable tissue
- Isolation of an organism from the blood in the absence of other infection
- Signs of the systemic inflammatory response syndrome (such as hyperthermia, hypothermia, leukocytosis, tachypnea, hypotension, oliguria, or hyperglycemia at a previously tolerated level of carbohydrate intake) and mental status changes

The use of effective topical antimicrobials for prevention and therapy of wound infection, along with earlier surgical intervention in wound care, has led to a decrease in the incidence of wound infection, and respiratory failure is now the leading cause of death in the patient with thermal injury. Although inhalation injury is a prominent cause of respiratory complications in these patients, the incidence of pneumonia and acute respiratory distress syndrome is high, even when direct lung injury is not present

Bacterial colonization of venous catheters in patients in ICUs and, in particular, of central catheters in burn-injured patients is high. Some centers suggest peripheral, central venous and arterial catheters be changed over a guidewire on day 3 and that a new site be used on day 6. Others have suggested that once-a-week catheter replacement is sufficient to maintain an acceptable rate of catheter-related bloodstream infection in children. The reason for concern, especially in burn-injured individuals, is that suppurative thrombophlebitis can be an insidious and life-threatening infection. The only findings may be persistent fever and a bacteremia that continues despite appropriate antibiotic treatment. The classic findings (edema, erythema, pain, and a palpable cord at an IV site) that are associated with phlebitis may not be identifiable. Diagnosis is confirmed by aspiration of purulent material from the affected vein, and treatment consists of excision of the involved vein to the point at which bleeding is encountered and the vessel is normal.

The cartilage of the ear has minimal protection and blood supply and is highly susceptible to infection when the overlying tissue is damaged. Dressings should not be applied to the ear, and pillows should not be used. The topical agent of choice is mafenide acetate because it penetrates eschar and avascular cartilage. When suppurative chondritis occurs, systemic antibiotics are of little value due to the avascular nature of the tissue.

It appears that the incidence of bacteremia following wound manipulation is related to the extent of injury. Bacteremia related to burn care, especially in patients with a large burn injury, may seed distant sites, such as cardiac valves or the brain, and it is likely that in this population of patients, perioperative administration of antibiotics that are active against the flora of the wound is of benefit. Burn-injured patients have a high incidence of urinary tract infections and pneumonia. They may also develop other infections, such as appendicitis, but often do not present with classic features due to a suppressed inflammatory response. One source of sepsis that is frequently overlooked in the burn patient is nosocomial sinusitis. Factors that predispose to sinusitis are indwelling catheters for nasogastric or nasoduodenal feeding and nasotracheal intubation, especially in patients with inhalation injury. The diagnosis is made by culture of drainage fluid and by CT scan of the sinuses. Once the diagnosis is made, treatment consists of removal of all tubes and catheters, initiation of appropriate antibiotic therapy, and drainage. If a nasal endotracheal tube is present, it should be changed to orotracheal. In some cases, it may be necessary to perform a tracheostomy.

Immune compromise, recurrent bacteremia, and the frequent use of central venous catheters in the patient with burn injury are risk factors for the development of endocarditis. The association of central venous and pulmonary artery catheters with the development of bacterial endocarditis in burn-injured patients is well documented. Similar to suppurative thrombophlebitis, bacterial endocarditis is insidious and should be suspected when blood cultures are positive without an obvious source. The presence of a new cardiac murmur supports the diagnosis, which should be confirmed by echocardiography.

The classic description of the metabolic response to injury includes an early ebb phase that is characterized by low cardiac output and a decreased metabolic rate followed by a hypermetabolic phase that starts at 24–36 hrs after injury. An approximate 50% increase in protein metabolism and energy expenditure occurs due to hypermetabolism, fluid losses, sepsis, and inflammation in children following a large burn injury, and this catabolic state can persist for 9–12 months. The stress hormones (cortisol, epinephrine, and glucagon) all increase, mediating increased gluconeogenesis, glycogenolysis, muscle breakdown, and bone loss. Furthermore, the anabolic effects of insulin and growth hormone are antagonized in patients with burns. Early and aggressive nutritional support has been shown to reduce the elevated resting energy expenditure (REE) in burn victims. The use of the Harris benedict formula, the World Health Organization formula, or the Schofiel-HW equation showed poor correlation with REE in children after major burn injury. Nutritional support in the burn patient is usually guided by a formula, such as that used at the Shriners Burn Center, especially when indirect calorimetry is not available. The formula is:

- Infants (0–12 months): 2100 kcal/m^2 plus 1000 kcal/m^2 burn
- Children 1–11 years: 1800 kcal/m^2 plus 1300 kcal/m^2 burn
- Children 12 years and older: 1500 kcal/m^2 plus 1500 kcal/m^2 burn

The enteral route is the preferred route for administration of nutrition. A nasogastric or nasoduodenal tube should be placed as soon as the initial evaluation and burn resuscitation are complete and, in the absence of contraindications, enteral feeds should be initiated within 24 hrs of injury. However, feeding intolerance as evidenced by significant gastric residual volume and diarrhea may limit use of the gastrointestinal tract for caloric delivery. Diarrhea is a commonly encountered problem in the burn population. Factors associated with a decreased incidence of diarrhea in burn victims include fat intake <20% of overall caloric intake, vitamin A intake >10,000 IU/day in adults, and early implementation of enteral feeds (<48 hrs postburn). In addition to vitamin A, other vitamins, minerals, and trace elements may be required in excess of recommended daily allowances, including calcium, magnesium, vitamin D, zinc, copper, and other micronutrients. The hypermetabolism can be blunted to some extent by propranolol given via nasogastric tube in doses of 0.3–1.0 mg/kg body weight every 4–6 hrs. Muscle wasting, decreased bone mineralization, and retarded linear growth can be quite profound. A synthetic testosterone analog, oxandrolone, may contribute to an earlier normalization of serum albumin, prealbumin, and retinol-binding protein and to improve lean body mass and bone mineral content in pediatric patients with burns of ≥40% BSA.

Protein metabolism and energy expenditure increase by ~50% in children following a large burn injury. Hyperglycemia in burn patients is associated with increased morbidity and mortality. Administration of exogenous insulin can overcome insulin resistance, retard protein catabolism, and promote normoglycemia. The combined benefits of glycemic control and the favorable effects of insulin in promoting protein synthesis and preventing protein catabolism support the use of insulin administration to achieve glycemic control in the burn patient. Careful attention must be paid to avoiding hypoglycemia.

Advances in medical care leading to increased survival from thermal injury have led to a renewed emphasis on quality of life after these injuries. Rehabilitation of the patient with a burn injury begins from the time of initial medical care, requires intense care in the first year after injury and—often—continued lifelong care. Splinting of injured extremities begins as soon as the patient is stabilized, and range-of-motion exercises begin within the first 24 hrs. As soon as wounds have a stable epidermal closure, usually within 2 weeks after grafting or primary healing has occurred, attention is turned to wound and scar management. Garments that apply pressure to the wounds are tailor-made for the patient and worn 24 hr/day. The opportunity to modulate the development of cicatrix is restricted to the time when the wound is immature and actively remodeling.

CHAPTER 9 ■ TERRORISM AND MASS CASUALTY EVENTS

PHILIP L. GRAHAM III • GEORGE L. FOLTIN • F. MERIDITH SONNETT

PEDIATRIC-SPECIFIC DISASTER PREPAREDNESS

The vulnerabilities that are unique to pediatric disaster victims are highlighted in **Table 9.1**. Children are disproportionately affected by terrorism-related events and require prolonged and extensive medical care that substantially exceeds the needs of adult victims. The unique physiology of children dictates that they will be overly represented among the victims of a chemical or biological incident. Advance planning for a mass-casualty event must include comprehensive evaluation and preparation for implementation of systems to support communication, staffing, supplies, capacity, infection control, availability of durable equipment, assessment of current patient status, and clinical standards.

Specific clinicians who live close to the hospital and who have family situations that allow them to report to the hospital on short notice should be predesignated as "first responders." The healthcare workers who support the first responder pool are expected to perform their function when communication systems may be inoperable. It is critical to hold a second wave of responders "on reserve," with a plan to have them report later (e.g., 12 hrs) after the start of the incident. Periodic disaster drills must be conducted so that these systems can be tested and adjustments in the execution can be made, as necessary. Pre-event planning for increased supply needs is an important element of a comprehensive emergency preparedness plan. The Joint Commission of Accreditation of Health Care Organizations currently recommends 48–72 hrs of supplies, including ventilators, but this may be expanded in the future. Critical care bed capacity may be expanded by using stretchers, cots, or additional beds in existing PICU locations. Additionally, critical care may be provided in alternative locations, such as postoperative holding areas, catheterization laboratories, procedure rooms, the NICU, and the emergency department.

Infection control precautions can be divided into a 2-tiered approach, with *standard precautions* as the first tier, or foundation, for the prevention of transmission of infectious pathogens. Standard precautions include hand hygiene, which is the single most effective tool for minimizing disease transmission, and use of personal protective equipment for all contacts with blood, body fluids, nonintact skin, and mucous membranes. The second tier of precautions is termed *extended precautions*, the use of which is recommended when specific pathogens are known or suspected, and includes *contact precautions*, *droplet precautions*, and *airborne infection isolation precautions*. In a biological event, standard precautions will continue to be critically important, but expanded precautions may also be necessary. The provision of multiple *airborne infection isolation environments* (i.e., negative pressure rooms) is

---

TABLE 9.1

PEDIATRIC-SPECIFIC VULNERABILITIES FROM EXPOSURE TO TERRORISM-RELATED AGENTS

Increased respiratory exposure (higher minute ventilation, live "closer to the ground")
Increased dermal exposure (less fat, thinner, more permeable skin; larger body surface area/mass ratio)
Increased risk of dehydration due to toxin-induced vomiting and diarrhea (decreased intravascular volume, larger body surface area/mass ratio)
Increased risk of hypothermia during decontamination procedures (larger body surface area/mass ratio)
Immunologic immaturity, resulting in more virulent disease manifestations; greater permeability of blood-brain barrier
Developmentally less capable of escaping attack and taking appropriate protective actions (developmental immaturity, dependence on adult caregivers who may be severely injured or dead)
Increased incidence of multiple-organ injury (thoracic cage not as well developed, less protection of visceral organs)
Increased incidence of head injury (head is larger proportionally; calvarium is thinner and offers less protection of brain matter, more susceptible to penetrating and blunt trauma)

Adapted from Henretig FM, Ciesiak TJ, Eitzen EM Jr. Biologic and chemical terrorism. *J Pediatr* 2002; 141:311–26.

---

beyond the capability of most hospitals. Alternative processes, such as portable high-efficiency particulate air filtration and isolation tents, may mitigate risk.

In the event of increased demand for critical care, it will be possible to transfer some patients out of the PICU to general medical or surgical units; a few may be stable enough to be discharged home. Transferring patients to other facilities is also an option to help increase ICU capacity; however, in a mass-casualty event, most healthcare facilities will be equally overwhelmed. *Emergency mass critical care* is a term used to define the level of care that would be required in the event of a mass casualty that results in enormous numbers of people needing medical and surgical treatment. The vast number of victims who require critical care would overwhelm existing medical delivery systems that would not be able to maintain traditional standards of care. A plan for *emergency mass critical care* must be developed and should include the following strategies:

a. Provide only the most basic critical care interventions.
b. Expand the scope of noncritical care-trained providers.
c. Provide critical care in noncritical care settings.
d. Alter triage decision making, including withholding of care.

TERRORIST-RELATED EVENTS

Information compiled following the 1995 Oklahoma City bombing provided important data about the injuries that were sustained by the pediatric victims. Explosives can be categorized according to speed, size, weight, TNT equivalents, source, original purpose, and adulterant components ("dirty bomb," bolts, nails). Typically, explosives are categorized as high-order explosives (HE) and low-order explosives (LE). HE create supersonic overpressurization shock waves and require detonation. Examples of HE are all military bombs, TNT, ammonium nitrate fuel oil, and C-4 "plastic" explosives. HE explosions result in primary blast injury (PBI). LE produce subsonic explosions and do not create the shock wave characterized by HE. They are composed of propellants and undergo deflagration rather than the detonation caused by HE. In comparison to HE, the release of energy from LE is slower. Although LE explosions are associated with significant mortality and morbidity, they rarely result in the characteristic pulmonary and central nervous system injuries unique to PBI from HE. LE primarily result in penetrating injuries from shrapnel and flying debris, crush, blunt, and burn injuries, and they include pipe bombs, gunpowder, and pure petroleum-based bombs (Molotov cocktails).

The severity of injury from blast trauma is related almost exclusively to 3 main factors: the distance of the victim from the site of explosion, the environment in which the explosion occurs (open versus confined space), and the proximity to solid surfaces (blast waves are reflected off of solid surfaces and increase the victim's level of exposure). The mechanisms of injury from blast exposures are reviewed in CDC Mass Trauma Preparedness and Response website at http://www.bt.cdc.gov/masscasualties/explosions.asp#classification. Accessed September 2006.

The injuries of PBI are directly related to the effects on air-filled organs. The organ systems most commonly affected are pulmonary, GI, and auditory. Brain, cardiothoracic, and ocular structures are affected as well. Pulmonary barotrauma that results in pulmonary contusion and air embolism represents the most common cause of death from PBI. The

TABLE 9.2

OVERVIEW OF BLAST-RELATED INJURY

System	Injury or condition
Auditory	Traumatic tympanic membrane rupture, disruption of middle and inner ear structures (ossicles and cochlea)
Respiratory	Blast lung, pulmonary barotrauma, hemothorax, pneumothorax, pulmonary hemorrhage, arteriovenous fistula from air embolism, aspiration pneumonitis
Gastrointestinal	Bowel perforation, organ rupture, mesenteric ischemia from air embolism
Cardiovascular/circulatory	Cardiac contusion; air embolism, which causes myocardial infarction, cardiogenic shock, peripheral vascular injury
Ocular	Globe rupture, foreign bodies, orbital fractures, air embolism
Neurologic	Closed brain injury, concussion, cerebral and spinal cord infarcts from air embolism
Renal/genitalia	Renal contusion, laceration, fracture, testicular rupture
Musculoskeletal	Bony fractures, traumatic amputations, crush injuries, compartment syndrome, burns, lacerations

Adapted from: CDC Mass Trauma Preparedness and Response website at http://www.bt.cdc.gov/masscasualties/explosions.asp# classification. Accessed on September 2006.

clinical triad of apnea, bradycardia, and hypotension is usually evident immediately after explosion. Chest x-ray reveals a classic white butterfly pattern. The diagnosis of blast lung injury (BLI) should be considered in any victim with dyspnea, cough, chest pain, or hemoptysis following exposure to a blast. The signs and symptoms associated with BLI are listed in **Table 9.2**.

The development of air emboli, a specific and particularly ominous complication of BLI, is directly related to the degree of injury sustained. It may be difficult to diagnose because other serious clinical conditions have similar presenting signs and symptoms. Initial treatment consists of administration of 100% oxygen therapy and maintaining a patent airway. Most victims will require mechanical ventilation. Prophylactic chest tube placement is recommended prior to induction of anesthesia and/or inter-institutional transport. Massive hemoptysis is managed with endotracheal intubation and selective ventilation of the uninvolved lung. Diagnostic imaging or medical interventions may aid in confirming the diagnosis of air embolism. Echocardiography, CT scan, and bronchoscopy can provide direct visualization of air bubbles. Transesophageal echocardiography allows visualization of air particles as small as 2 mcm. Suspicion of coronary artery air emboli must be managed aggressively with oxygen and attempts to stop the further passage of air. A tight-fitting mask with 100% oxygen must be applied immediately. Rapid and aggressive treatment to stop air entry into the circulation system is indicated. Thoracotomy on the affected side is usually recommended;

however, blast injuries may be associated with multiple sites of injury, and selective thoracotomy may not be effective. The safest management strategy is to place the patient in either a modified left lateral decubitus/prone position or injured-lung side down position to increase venous pressure on that side and reduce/minimize embolization. An additional mode of therapy that has theoretic potential for treating air emboli is hyperbaric oxygen therapy. The use of positive pressure ventilation (PPV) has been recommended but is controversial and should be considered only in circumstances of severe respiratory failure or massive hemoptysis. Mechanical ventilation for patients with BLI who require intubation presents a similar challenge, as does the use of PPV.

Injury to the GI tract is the second most common lethal injury from exposure to a blast. As with other air-filled organs, the overpressurization wave from a blast attack causes extensive compression and distortion of the GI tract. The manifestations of "blast-abdomen" are generally delayed, presenting from 8–36 hrs after exposure. The terminal ileum and colon are especially vulnerable to blast effects. These areas are at significant risk for perforation. Fractures of the liver and spleen, ruptured testicle, and subcapsular and retroperitoneal hematomas represent high-morbidity injuries following blast trauma. The signs and symptoms associated with intra-abdominal injury are listed in **Table 9.3**. The initial management of these patients in the emergency department includes meticulous attention to the ABCs of Advanced Trauma Life Support protocols (airway with C-spine control, breathing, and circulation). CT scan,

TABLE 9.3

SIGNS AND SYMPTOMS ASSOCIATED WITH BLAST ABDOMINAL INJURY

Absence of bowel sounds
Abdominal pain
Abdominal distension
Hematochezia
Hypotension
Involuntary guarding
Rebound tenderness
Nausea and vomiting
Orthostasis/syncope
Testicular pain
Tenesmus

Adapted from: Foltin GL, Schoenfeld D, Shannon M. Pediatric terrorism and disaster preparedness a resource for pediatricians. AHRQ Publication Nos. 06(07)-0056 and 06(07)-0056-1, October 2006. Agency for Healthcare Research and Quality, Rockville, MD. http://www.ahrq.gov/research/pedprep/resource.htm. Accessed May 2007.

ultrasonography, and diagnostic peritoneal lavage are the most reliable methods used to detect intra-abdominal injury. CT scan provides excellent data on intra-abdominal hemorrhage, organ injury, free intraperitoneal air, and intramural hematomas, but CT is not reliable for detecting hollow viscus perforation in early stages. For patients who may be compromised from other significant injuries, it is reasonable to begin prophylactic antibiotics until such time that a definitive intervention/procedure can confirm an intact bowel and GI tract. Exploratory laparotomy may be required to identify a peritoneal source of bleeding in the hemodynamically unstable patient.

NONCONVENTIONAL WEAPONS

The acronym CBRN is commonly used for nonconventional terror weapons: chemical-biological-radiological-nuclear.

Chemical

Chemical agents include nerve, asphyxiant, choking/pulmonary, and blistering/vesicant. The single most important first step for treating all chemical exposures is the initial decontamination strategy. Immediate removal of patient clothing can eliminate ~90% of contaminants. After the clothing is removed, the patient's skin and eyes may require decontamination. In most cases, decontamination of skin can be accomplished by gentle and thorough washing with water and soap, if available. Thorough decon-tamination should occur before a patient enters the hospital (**Table 9.4**).

Nerve Agents

Nerve agents are similar to organophosphate insecticides and include cholinesterase inhibitors, such as Sarin, Soman, and VX. These agents are generally colorless, odorless, tasteless, and nonirritating to the skin. Nerve agent vapors are denser than air and tend to accumulate in low-lying areas, putting children at risk for higher exposure. The agents used in terrorist attacks are inhaled and absorbed through skin and mucous membranes. Symptoms are characteristic of muscarinic excess (rhinorrhea, bronchorrhea, bronchospasm, vomiting, diarrhea) as well as nicotinic excess (respiratory muscle paralysis and peripheral muscle fasciculation, followed by paralysis). Ocular symptoms include miosis, eye pain, vision changes, and tearing. Tachycardia or bradycardia may be present. CNS toxicity includes headache, agitation, and seizures. Emergent treatment of nerve agent toxicity is described in **Table 9.4**. Initial treatment includes administration of atropine followed by pralidoxime, with liberal use of benzodiazepines. Autoinjector kits ("Mark 1" kits contain a 2-mg dose of atropine and a 600-mg dose of pralidoxime) ("AtroPen" is produced in 3 sizes: 0.25 mg, 0.5 mg, and 1 mg of atropine), but corresponding pralidoxime autoinjectors are not available. If pediatric patients survive a nerve agent attack and arrive at a critical care environment, they will likely need atropine and benzodiazepines for several days. Adult survivors of nerve agent exposure have required up to 20 mg of atropine over the first 24 hrs and have received pralidoxime doses repeated hourly or by infusion (500 mg/hr). Topical cycloplegics may reduce nerve agent-induced ocular pain.

Asphyxiants

Asphyxiants are toxic compounds that inhibit cytochrome oxidase, causing cellular anoxia and lactic acidosis (high anion gap). Hydrogen cyanide, the most commonly known toxicant in this class, is a colorless liquid or gas that smells like bitter almonds Exposure to hydrogen cyanide produces rapid onset of tachypnea, tachycardia, and flushed skin, followed by nausea, vomiting, confusion, weakness, trembling, seizures, and death. Death may occur as quickly as 8 mins after exposure. "Classic" signs of cyanide poisoning include severe dyspnea without cyanosis. Cyanide exposure results in seizure activity that begins within seconds of inhalation, and death occurs within minutes, generally with little cyanosis or other findings. Initial management is reviewed in **Table 9.4**.

TABLE 9.4

CENTERS FOR DISEASE CONTROL CATEGORY A CHEMICAL AGENTS

Agent	Findings	Treatment
Nerve agents Sarin, Soman, VX	Rhinorrhea, bronchorrhea, bronchospasm, respiratory muscle paralysis, eye pain	Airway, breathing, circulation support, 100% oxygen Atropine: 0.05–0.1 mg/kg (0.1–5 mg) IM, IV, ETT, IO q2–5 mins for secretions and respiratory symptoms *THEN* Pralidoxime (2-PAM): 25–50 mg/kg IM or IV (max 1 g IV, 2 g IM) repeat in 30 mins, then every 60 mins for weakness and/or high atropine requirement Diazepam: 0.3 mg/kg (max 10 mg) IV OR equivalent benzodiazepine IM, IV, IO*ᵃ*
Asphyxiants Cyanide	"Cherry red skin," tachypnea, seizures	Airway, breathing, circulation support, 100% oxygen If conscious: No antidote If unconscious: Sodium nitrate 3%: 0.12–0.33 mL/kg (max 10 mL) slowly IV (minimum 5 mins). Often causes orthostatic hypotension. Sodium thiosulfate: 25%: 1.65 mL/kg over 10–20 mins (max 50 mL). Sodium bicarbonate for acidosis after above if unresponsive.
Choking agents Chlorine, phosgene	Eye, nose, throat irritation (especially chlorine); bronchospasm, pulmonary edema (especially phosgene)	Symptomatic care, possible bronchoscopy, aggressive management of pulmonary edema
Blistering/vesicant "Mustard" Lewisite	Skin erythema; vesicle and ocular inflammation; respiratory tract inflammation	Symptomatic care, "burn" care, possible use of hematopoietic growth factors British Anti-Lewisite (BAL) (if available) 3 mg/kg IM q4–6 hrs for systemic effects in severe cases.

IM, intramuscularly; ETT, endotracheal tube; IO, intraosseous
*ᵃ*Some authorities recommend seizure prophylaxis with benzodiazepines, others suggest use for treatment.

Choking/Pulmonary Agents

Choking agents include chlorine and phosgene, which are in the gaseous form at room temperature. Phosgene smells like "freshly mown hay." Chlorine has a strong, characteristic odor. When inhaled, these agents produce massive mucosal irritation and edema, as well as significant damage to lung parenchyma. Chlorine acts primarily on the tracheobronchial tree at the level of the respiratory epithelium of the bronchi and larger bronchioles. After initial decontamination, management follows the standard recommendations for acute lung injury, including administration of oxygen and bronchodilators. Corticosteroids are often added to the treatment regimen.

Blistering/Vesicant Agents

Blistering agents include sulfur mustard and Lewisite. Both were employed during World War I as maiming agents. Symptoms generally begin 12 hrs after exposure and include eye, skin, and pulmonary irritation, as well as blister formation and are summarized in **Table 9.4.**

Biological Agents

The Centers for Disease Control has categorized potential agents of bioterror into 3 groups based on their potential threat. Category A agents, which constitute the highest threat, include anthrax, plague, tularemia, smallpox, the viral hemorrhagic fevers, and botulism. Clusters of patients with acute respiratory distress with fever (signs and symptoms consistent with anthrax, plague, tularemia), similar characteristic rash with fever (signs and symptoms consistent with smallpox and viral hemorrhagic fevers), or neurologic syndromes (botulism) should

TABLE 9.5

CENTERS FOR DISEASE CONTROL CATEGORY A BIOLOGICAL AGENTS

Agent	Findings	Treatment
Inhalational: Anthrax	Febrile, widened mediastinum, effusions, sepsis	Ciprofloxacin: (10 mg/kg/dose) IV (max 400 mg) q12 hrs *OR* doxycycline: 2.2 mg/kg/dose IV (max 100 mg) q12 hrs *AND* 1–2 other drugs[a]
Plague	Pneumonia, sepsis	Gentamicin: 2.5 mg/kg/dose IV q8 hrs *OR* doxycycline: 2.2 mg/kg/dose IV (max 100 mg) q12 hrs *OR* ciprofloxacin: (10 mg/kg/dose) IV (max 400 mg) q12 hrs *OR* chloramphenicol 25 mg/kg q6 hrs IV (max 4 g/ day)[b]
Tularemia	Pneumonia, hilar adenopathy	Gentamicin: 2.5 mg/kg/dose IV q8 hrs *OR* doxycycline: 2.2 mg/kg/dose IV (max 100 mg) q12 hrs *OR* ciprofloxacin: (10 mg/kg/dose) IV (max 400 mg) q12 hrs
Smallpox	Multiple firm pustules all in the same stage of evolution, fever	Vaccination for exposure within 96 hrs. Potential use of cidofovir or analogs.
Viral hemorrhagic fevers	Fever, bleeding, shock	Supportive, ribavirin for some etiologies (Lassa)
Botulism	Flaccid afebrile descending paralysis	Anti-toxin, supportive care

[a]Penicillin, amoxicillin, clindamycin. Most authorities would treat with 3–4 drugs for 2 weeks, then switch to monotherapy or dual therapy to complete 60 days when sensitivities are known. Anthrax may have either natural or engineered resistance elements.
[b]Recommended for plague meningitis. Serum levels and hematologic adverse events must be monitored.

prompt immediate notification of hospital infection control teams and public heath authorities (**Table 9.5**).

Anthrax

Three types of anthrax affect humans: cutaneous anthrax, which is acquired when a spore enters the skin through a cut or an abrasion; GI tract anthrax, contracted from eating contaminated food, primarily meat from an animal that died of the disease; and pulmonary, or inhalation anthrax, which results from breathing in airborne anthrax spores. Cutaneous lesions in the form of papules appear 1–7 days after exposure. Papules progress to form vesicles and then ulcerate, resulting in a black eschar that covers the lesion. The incubation time of inhalational anthrax is most commonly thought to be 1–7 days, but periods of up to 2 months have been described. Inhalational illness is biphasic; 1–6 days after exposure, victims develop nonspecific upper respiratory infection–type symptoms; they then appear to recover. Later-appearing symptoms include high fever, respiratory distress, shock, and death (75% fatality rate if untreated). The chest x-ray may be notable for

mediastinal widening and may lack infiltrates. Specific multiagent antimicrobial therapy is required, as well as aggressive ventilatory and intravascular support for the multiorgan system failure that occurs in severely affected patients. Antimicrobial treatment is detailed in **Table 9.5**. Person-to-person transmission of anthrax is not possible; therefore, standard precautions are the only required infection control measures.

Yersinia Pestis

Yersinia pestis causes plague, which can naturally occur in septicemic, bubonic, or pneumonic forms. Like anthrax, a bioterrorist incident that involves plague would likely occur through aerosolization and result in pneumonic involvement. Direct inhalation of the bacillus results in pneumonic plague and subsequent bacteremia and septicemia. The bacillus causes a multilobar hemorrhagic and necrotizing bronchopneumonia. After an incubation period of 2–8 days (less for aerosolized exposure), rapidly progressive pulmonary disease with hemoptysis and cyanosis develops. Cough with purulent sputum (Gram-negative rods may be seen) may be present. Pneumonia is evident on chest x-ray. Immediate early treatment (**Table 9.5**) with an aminoglycoside or doxycycline is critical. Chloramphenicol is the recommended treatment regimen when plague-induced meningitis occurs. Patients with pneumonic plague should be cared for using droplet precautions until they have received 72 hrs of antibiotic therapy (21).

Francisella Tularensis

Francisella tularensis is a highly virulent, small, non-motile, aerobic, Gram-negative coccobacillus that causes tularemia after host contact with infected animal carcasses or fluids, in glandular, oculoglandular, oropharyngeal, septicemic, typhoidal, and pneumonic forms. A bioterror aerosol release of *F. tularensis* primarily causes pulmonary disease, though other forms are possible. After 1–14 days after exposure, victims develop an influenza-like illness and atypical pneumonia; chest x-ray may show hilar adenopathy. After inhalational exposure, hemorrhagic inflammation of the airways develops and progresses to necrotizing pneumonia. Pleural disease is common. Treatment (**Table 9.5**) with gentamicin or doxycycline reduces mortality from 30% to 10% (31). Person-to-person spread of tularemia is not possible; therefore, standard precautions are the only infection control measure required.

Variola Virus—Smallpox

Since naturally occurring smallpox disease no longer exists, a single case of smallpox (Variola virus) anywhere in the world would be considered evidence that a bioterror attack has occurred.

Individuals infected with smallpox present clinically with a general viral prodrome that is characterized by high fever and constitutional symptoms. The characteristic rash of smallpox begins on the face and rapidly spreads centrifugally. The patient's fever decreases with the onset of rash, and infectivity begins. Lesions progress as a group through stages of being macular, papular, vesicular, and finally as deep, hard, large pustules that crust after 8–10 days. Treatment is primarily supportive. Appropriate antibiotic coverage for bacterial superinfections will likely be required. Cidofovir has been shown to have a beneficial effect in animal models, but its efficacy in humans is unknown. If smallpox occurs, mass vaccination campaigns must take place; vaccination within 72–96 hrs after exposure provides good protection against disease and excellent protection against fatal disease. Vaccinia immune globulin has no clinical benefit for patients who are infected with smallpox. Persons hospitalized with smallpox should be cared for in a negative-pressure environment, with staff using both airborne and contact precautions. Ideally, only staff previously vaccinated for smallpox should care for victims.

Viral Hemorrhagic Fevers

The viral hemorrhagic fevers are a group of infections caused by a variety of agents (e.g., Ebola and Lassa). The clinical manifestations are similar and include rash and fever. Bleeding diathesis that can progress into severe hemorrhagic disease can occur, manifested as bleeding from internal organs and mucous membranes. After an incubation period ranging from 2 to 28 days, victims of the viral hemorrhagic fevers develop rash and fever, variable bleeding diatheses, petechiae, mucosal hemorrhages, hematuria, and GI bleeding. Diagnosis of the specific agents is made epidemiologically or by acute and convalescent titers. Treatment advice must be obtained from public health authorities; ribavirin might be effective for several of the viruses. Florid cases will require extensive amounts of blood products to support victims. Empiric isolation should include airborne and contact precautions, unless the exact nature of the virus is known.

Clostridium botulinum is a spore-forming anaerobe that produces the most lethal toxin that exists, with an LD50 in humans estimated at 0.000001 mg/kg. Botulism occurs naturally in 3 main forms: food-borne botulism, wound botulism, and infant botulism. An intentional release of botulism toxin would result in cases of inhalational disease. The seven known serotypes of botulism toxin act by inhibiting acetylcholine release, thereby decoupling the nervous system from skeletal muscle, causing death from aspiration and respiratory arrest. Close monitoring of the respiratory effort of botulism victims is critical; bedside pulmonary function testing allows for the decision of ventilatory support to be made efficiently. There are equine antisera that can considerably reduce the amount of time that victims require ICU care. Human-to-human spread of botulism does not occur; therefore, standard precautions are the only infection control measures required.

Radiological/Nuclear

Radiological and nuclear terrorism have a wide spectrum of possible effects. Regardless of the magnitude of the damage or contamination, widespread panic will occur within the affected geographic area. Radiological terror involves exposing portions of the population to radioactive materials, most likely with a radiological dispersal device (or "dirty bomb"). Such devices use conventional explosives to disperse radioactive materials that have potential to contaminate limited geographic areas. Acute radiation syndrome (or "radiation sickness") can occur in the survivors of a nuclear attack. Despite widespread concerns over potential attacks on nuclear power plants, such an attack would likely cause radiological exposure, as opposed to a full blown nuclear event. Unlike some of the biological and chemical scenarios above, decontamination of radiological victims is less time sensitive. Critical and life-threatening conditions should be treated before decontamination occurs. As with chemical exposures, removal of clothing will eliminate 90% of contamination. If a patient is exposed to radioactive material and is alive upon arrival at a hospital, he is very unlikely to be sufficiently contaminated to cause harm to healthcare workers. After stabilization of conventional injuries, the patient can be disrobed and washed with soap and water (run-off should be contained). The eyes may then be flushed. Standard precautions are the only measures required for healthcare workers who do not come into direct contact with radioactive dust or debris.

Victims of radiation exposure are likely to initially have a nonspecific prodrome (hours to days of nausea, vomiting, and fatigue) followed by a latent period and culminating in illness that can occur from days to weeks after exposure. All cell lines of the hematopoietic system are the first to be affected. Severely affected patients have total loss of their hematopoietic system, much like a bone marrow transplant patient who has had a fully ablative preparative regimen. Hemorrhage and sepsis are common. The GI system is affected, causing mucosal sloughing, hemorrhage, obstruction, and sepsis. Radiation pneumonitis can occur and requires aggressive ventilatory support. Treatment is supportive (fluids, nutrition, antimicrobials, skin care, hematopoietic growth factors).

While all PICUs will be able to treat one or more victims of severe radiation exposure, these patients will require tremendous resource utilization, and surge capacity may be quickly overwhelmed. Expert nuclear medicine and health physicist advice and guidance will be critical in determining which victims are most likely to benefit from critical care interventions. This expertise will help to determine if exposure-specific treatments are available.

CHAPTER 10 ■ POISONING

G. PATRICIA CANTWELL • RICHARD S. WEISMAN

Management of childhood poisoning is challenging due to the existence of hundreds of prescription medications, household chemicals, stings and envenomations, illicit and designer drugs, and increased use of nonprescription and herbal medications. Pediatric fatalities are most often associated with the following agents: analgesics, hydrocarbons, antidepressants, gases and fumes, stimulants and street drugs, cardiovascular drugs, anticonvulsants, sedatives/hypnotics/antipsychotics, and chemicals.

CLINICAL APPROACH TO THE POISONED CHILD

Urgent priorities include the focus on a primary survey that involves attention to the patient's airway, breathing, and circulation (ABCs). Following the establishment of life-saving supportive care, a detailed evaluation can be meticulously performed. Toxins may cause respiratory failure by depression of the respiratory drive, hypoperfusion of the central nervous system (CNS), coma with impaired/absent protective airway reflexes, or direct toxic effects on the pulmonary system. Airway management mandates a low threshold for rapid-sequence intubation due to the potential for loss of protective airway reflexes and expectation of a full stomach, with risk for aspiration. Many toxins may cause extreme hemodynamic instability due to dysrhythmias and/or hypotension. Comprehensive stabilization involves attention to respiratory, cardiovascular, neurologic, and metabolic aberrancies.

A comprehensive history for the potential of toxic exposure may be obtained from witnesses, family members, friends, and emergency medical services personnel. It is helpful to estimate the quantity of liquid toxins by quantifying a swallow: 5–10 mL in a young child and 10–15 mL in an adolescent. Extremely dangerous single medications are summarized in **Table 10.1**. After obtaining the history, early contact with the regional poison control center (1-800-222-1222) provides rapid access to a toxicology consult.

TOXICITY LEVELS OF SELECTED MEDICATIONS AND MEDICATION CLASSES

Agents	Minimum potential lethal dose	Maximum dose available	Potentially fatal units in a 10-kg child
Antimalarials			
Chloroquine	20 mg/kg	500 mg	1
Hydroxychloroquine	20 mg/kg	200 mg	1
Camphor	100 mg/kg	200 mg/mL	5 mL
Imidazolines			
Clonidine	0.01 mg/kg	0.3 mg; 7.5 mg/patch	1
Tetrahydrozoline	2.5–5 mL	0.1%	2.5–5 mL
Methyl Salicylates	150–200 mg/kg	1400 mg/mL	1.1–1.4 mL
Sulfonylureas			
Glipizide	0.1 mg/kg	5 mg	1
Glyburide	0.1 mg/kg	10 mg	1

From Matteucci MJ. One pill can kill: Assessing the potential for fatal poisonings in children. *Pediatr Ann* 2005;34:964–8, with permission.

A comprehensive physical examination can be crucial in determining which agents are involved in causing toxic symptoms. The signs and symptoms that suggest specific classes of poisoning are generally grouped into syndromes and referred to as toxidromes. The classic toxidromes may be grouped into 4 categories: sympathomimetic, cholinergic, anticholinergic, and opiate-sedative-ethanol syndromes. Herbal poisoning and dietary supplements have also been implicated with a host of typical symptomatology (**Table 10.2, Table 10.3**). The specific physical findings are summarized in **Table 10.4**.

EXAMPLES OF KNOWN HERBAL PRODUCTS AND THEIR ASSOCIATED TOXIC EFFECTS

Herbal product	Toxic chemicals	Effect or target organ
Monkshood (*Aconitum* sp.)	Aconite	Cardiac arrhythmias, shock, weakness, seizures, coma, paresthesias, nausea, emesis
Wormwood (*Artemisia absinthium*)	Thujone	Seizures, dementia, tremors, headache, ataxia
Chaparral (*Larrea divaricata*)	Nordihydro-guaiaretic acid	Nausea, emesis, hepatitis
Cinnamon oil (*Cinnamomum* sp.)	Cinnamaldehyde	Dermatitis, abuse syndrome
Comfrey (*Symphytum officinale*)	Pyrrolizidines	Hepatic veno-occlusive disease
Crotalalaria sp.	Pyrrolizidines	Hepatic veno-occlusive disease
Eucalyptus (*Eucalyptus globules*)	1,8 cineol	Drowsiness, ataxia, seizures, nausea, vomiting, coma
Garlic (*Allium sativum*)	Allicin	Nausea, emesis, anorexia, weight loss, bleeding, platelet dysfunction
Heliotropium sp.	Pyrrolizidines	Hepatic veno-occlusive disease
Jin bu huan	Tetrahydropalmatine	Hepatitis
Kava (*Piper methysticum*)	Kavapyrones	Hepatitis, cirrhosis
Laetrile	Cyanide	Coma, seizures, death, respiratory failure
Licorice (*Glycyrrhiza glabra*)	Glycyrrhetic acid	Hypertension, hypokalemia, dysrhythmias
Ma Huang (*Ephedra sinica*)	Ephedrine	Hypertension, dysrhythmias, stroke, seizures
Nutmeg (*Myristica fragrans*)	Myristacin, eugenol	Hallucinations, emesis, headache
Strychnos nux-vomica	Strychnine	Seizures, abdominal pain, respiratory failure
Pennyroyal (*Mentha pulegium*; *Hedeoma* sp.)	Pulegone	Centrilobular liver necrosis, fetotoxicity, abortion
Senecio sp.	Pyrrolizidines	Hepatic veno-occlusive disease

From Woolf AD. Herbal remedies and children: Do they work? Are they harmful? *Pediatrics* 2003;112:240–6, with permission.

TABLE 10.3

TWELVE MOST DANGEROUS DIETARY SUPPLEMENTS

Name (also known as)	Dangers
DEFINITELY HAZARDOUS *Documented organ failure and known carcinogenic properties*	
ARISTOLOCHIC ACID *Aristolochia* sp. (birthwort, snakeroot, snakeweed, sangree root, sangrel, serpentary, serpentaria); *Asarun canadense* (wild ginger)	Potent human carcinogen; can cause kidney failure and death
VERY LIKELY HAZARDOUS *Banned in some countries, FDA warning, or adverse effects in studies*	
COMFREY *Symphytun officinale* (ass ear, black root, blackwort, bruisewort, consolidate radix, consound, gum plant, healing herb, knitback, knitbone, salsify, slippery root, symphytum radix, wallwort)	Abnormal liver function or irreversible damage; deaths reported
ANDROSTENEDIONE *4-androstene-3* (17-dione, andro, androstene)	Increased cancer risk; decrease in HDL cholesterol
CHAPARRAL *Larrea divaricate* (creosote bush, greasewood, hediondilla, jarilla, larreastat)	Abnormal liver function or irreversible damage; deaths reported
GERMANDER *Teucrium chamaedrys* (wall germander, wild germander)	Abnormal liver function or irreversible damage; deaths reported
KAVA *Piper methysticum* (ava, awa, gea, gi, intoxicating pepper, kao, kavain, kawa-pfeffer, kew, long pepper, malohu, maluk, meruk, milik, rauschpfeffer, sakau, tonga, wurzelstock, yagona, yangona)	Abnormal liver function or irreversible damage; deaths reported
LIKELY HAZARDOUS *Adverse events reported, theoretical risks*	
BITTER ORANGE *Citrus aurantium* (green orange, kijitsu, neroli oil, Seville orange, and shangzhou zhiqiao, sour orange, zhi oiao, zhi xhi)	High blood pressure; risk of arrhythmias, heart attack, and stroke
LOBELIA *Lobelia inflata* (asthma weed, bladderpod, emetic herb, gagroot, lobelie, indian tobacco, pukeweed, vomit wort, wild tobacco)	Breathing difficulty, rapid heartbeat, low blood pressure, diarrhea, dizziness; possible related deaths reported
ORGAN/GLANDULAR EXTRACTS Brain, adrenal, pituitary, placenta, other gland "substance," or "concentrate"	Theoretical risk of mad cow disease, especially from brain extracts
PENNYROYAL OIL *Hedeoma pulegioides* (lurk-in-the-ditch, mosquito plant, piliolerial, pudding grass, pulegium, run-by-the-ground, squaw balm, squawmint, stinking balm, tickweed)	Liver and kidney failure, nerve damage, convulsions, abdominal tenderness, burning of the throat; deaths reported
SCULLCAP *Scutellaria lateriflora* (blue pimpernel, helmet flower, hoodwort, mad weed, mad-dog herb, mad-dog weed, quaker bonnet, scutelluria, skullcap)	Abnormal liver function or damage
YOHIMBE *Pausinystalia yobimbe* (johimbi, yohimbehe, yohimbine)	Changes in blood pressure, arrhythmias, respiratory depression, myocardial infarction; deaths reported

From Natural Medicines Comprehensive Database 2004 and Consumers Union's medical and research consultants. Data extracted from *Consumer Reports*, May 2004.

TABLE 10.4

CLINICAL MANIFESTATIONS OF POISONING

SKIN

Cyanosis (unresponsive to oxygen-methemoglobinemia)	Nitrates, nitrites, phenacetin, benzocaine
Red flush	Carbon monoxide, cyanide, boric acid, anticholinergics
Sweating	Amphetamines, LSD, organophosphates, cocaine, barbiturates
Dry	Anticholinergics
Bullae	Barbiturates, carbon monoxide
Jaundice	Acetaminophen, mushrooms, carbon tetrachloride, iron, phosphorus
Purpura	Aspirin, warfarin, snakebite

TEMPERATURE

Hypothermia	Sedative hypnotics, ethanol, carbon monoxide, phenothiazines, TCAs, clonidine
Hyperthermia	Anticholinergics, salicylates, phenothiazines, TCAs, cocaine, amphetamines, theophylline

BLOOD PRESSURE

Hypertension	Sympathomimetics (especially phenylpropanolamine in over-the-counter cold remedies) organophosphates, amphetamines, PCP
Hypotension	Narcotics, sedative hypnotics, TCAs, phenothiazines, clonidine, β-blockers, calcium channel blockers

PULSE RATE

Bradycardia	Digitalis, sedative hypnotics, β-blockers, ethchlorvynol, calcium channel blockers
Tachycardia	Anticholinergics, sympathomimetics, amphetamines, alcohol, aspirin, theophylline, cocaine, TCAs
Arrhythmias	Anticholinergics, TCAs, organophosphates, phenothiazines, digoxin, β-blockers, carbon monoxide, cyanide, theophylline

MUCOUS MEMBRANES

Dry	Anticholinergics
Salivation	Organophosphates, carbamates
Oral lesions	Corrosives, paraquat
Lacrimation	Caustics, organophosphates, irritant gases

RESPIRATION

Depressed	Alcohol, narcotics, barbiturates, sedative/hypnotics
Tachypnea	Salicylates, amphetamines, carbon monoxide
Kussmaul	Methanol, ethylene glycol, salicylates
Wheezing	Organophosphates
Pneumonia	Hydrocarbons
Pulmonary edema	Aspiration, salicylates, narcotics, sympathomimetics

CENTRAL NERVOUS SYSTEM

Seizures	TCAs, cocaine, phenothiazines, amphetamines, camphor, lead, salicylates, isoniazid, organophosphates, antihistamines, propoxyphene, strychnine
Pupils, miosis	Narcotics (except Demerol and Lomotil), phenothiazines, organophosphates, diazepam, barbiturates, mushrooms (muscarine types)
Mydriasis	Anticholinergics, sympathomimetics, cocaine, TCAs, methanol, glutethimide, LSD
Blindness, optic atrophy	Methanol
Fasciculation	Organophosphates
Nystagmus	Diphenylhydantoin, barbiturates, carbamazepine, PCP, carbon monoxide, glutethimide, ethanol
Hypertonus	Anticholinergics, strychnine, phenothiazines
Myoclonus, rigidity	Anticholinergics, phenothiazines, haloperidol
Delirium, psychosis	Anticholinergics, sympathomimetics, alcohol, phenothiazines, PCP, LSD, marijuana, cocaine, heroin, methaqualone, heavy metals
Coma	Alcohols, anticholinergics, sedative hypnotics, narcotics, carbon monoxide, tricyclic antidepressants, salicylates, organophosphates, barbiturates
Weakness, paralysis	Organophosphates, carbamates, heavy metals

GASTROINTESTINAL SYSTEM

Vomiting, diarrhea, abdominal pain	Iron, phosphorus, heavy metals, lithium, mushrooms, fluoride, organophosphates, arsenic

Adapted from Guzzardi L, Bayer MJ. Emergency management of the poisoned patient. In: Bayer M, Rumack BH, Wanke LA, eds. *Toxicologic Emergencies.* Bowie, MD: Robert J. Brady, 1984.

TABLE 10.5

TOXINS ASSOCIATED WITH CHARACTERISTIC BREATH ODORS

Toxin	Characteristic odor
Acetone	Acetone
Arsenic	Garlic
Camphor	Mothballs
Chloroform	Sweet
Cyanide	Bitter almond
Ethanol	Ethanol
Hydrogen sulfide	Rotten eggs
Isopropanol	Acetone
Methyl salicylate	Wintergreen
Nicotine	Stale tobacco
Organophosphates	Garlic
N-Pyridylmethylnitrophenylurea (Vacor rat poison)	Peanuts
Paraldehyde, chloral hydrate	Pears (urine)
Phenol, cresol	Phenolic
Phosphorus	Garlic
Salicylates	Acetone
Thallium	Garlic
Turpentine	Violets

From Woolf AD. Principles of toxin assessment and screening. In: Fuhrman BP, Zimmerman J, eds. *Pediatric Critical Care*, 3rd ed. Philadelphia: Mosby, Elsevier, 2006:1511–31, with permission.

Symmetrical pupillary changes are typical of toxic exposures, with asymmetry most commonly evidencing a structural or focal neurologic abnormality. Management based on the isolated evaluation of pupil size may lead to misdiagnosis. Drug withdrawal may be heralded by agitation, abnormal vital signs, irritability, and an altered sensorium. Nystagmus, tinnitus, and visual disturbances are commonly observed neurologic findings in selected intoxications.

Dermatologic examination may yield the identification of varied toxins. Inhalant abuse may lead to skin rashes around the nose and mouth. Needle tracks or characteristic tattooing are suggestive of IV drug use. Telltale odors are another means of compartmentalizing a variety of toxins (**Table 10.5**).

LABORATORY EVALUATION

In some circumstances, important decisions about therapy will be made based upon quantitative drug/toxin levels in blood specimens. These include acetaminophen, ethanol, methanol, ethylene glycol, lithium, salicylates, iron, lead, mercury, arsenic, phenobarbital, carbon monoxide, methemoglobin, and theophylline. Most laboratories routinely screen for

acetaminophen, ethanol, barbiturates, opiates, anticonvulsants, benzodiazepines, phenothiazines, and salicylates. A "negative" toxicology screen by no means excludes the possibility of a toxic exposure. Opioids, such as hydrocodone, oxycodone, methadone, fentanyl, meperidine, and propoxyphene, may not be detected by some opiate screening methodology, such as the immunoassay. In certain instances, toxins may be better detected in urine than in blood. Analysis of gastric contents may be helpful in elucidating a particular toxin if they are collected before absorption is likely. Consultation with a toxicologist at the regional poison control center (800-222-1222) is helpful in selecting and interpreting test results. The National Institute for Drug Abuse has established the commonly employed "drug of abuse screen" (NIDA-5), which utilizes immunoassay for amphetamines, marijuana, cocaine, opiates, and phencyclidine.

Electrolytes and blood urea nitrogen (BUN)/creatinine ratio allow for the determination of an anion gap acidosis, basic electrolytes, and the assessment of renal function. The anion gap calculation is:

$$Na(mEq/L) - [Cl(mEq/L) + HCO_3(mEq/L)]$$

The normal anion gap is generally 3–16 mEq/L. Agents that cause an elevated anion gap metabolic acidosis are listed in **Table 10.6**.

The 12-lead electrocardiogram is an invaluable tool in the evaluation of potential intoxication, particularly in detecting dysrhythmias and conduction abnormalities, such as widening of the QRS complex or prolongation of the QT interval. Cardiovascular toxicity is a common cause of death that results from antidepressant overdose and can manifest as myocardial depression, ventricular fibrillation, and ventricular tachycardia. The electrocardiogram is useful both in diagnosis and in management.

Urine color may be helpful in the identification of a number of toxins (**Table 10.7**). It is important to obtain urine pregnancy tests on any patient of

TABLE 10.6

METABOLIC ACIDOSIS [Na − (Cl + HCO₃)]: MUDPILES

*M*ethanol
*U*remia
*D*iabetic ketoacidosis
*P*araldehyde and phenformin
*I*soniazid and iron
*L*actic acidosis
*E*thanol and ethylene glycol
*S*alicylates

TABLE 10.7

CHARACTERISTIC URINE COLOR CHANGES

Orange to red-orange
Rifampin, deferoxamine, mercury, phenazopyridine, chronic lead poisoning
Pink
Cephalosporins or ampicillin
Brown
Chloroquine or carbon tetrachloride
Green to blue
Amitriptyline

child-bearing age. Urinalysis may reveal specific crystals (calcium oxalate crystals in ethylene glycol poisoning) or myoglobinuria. The presence of myoglobinuria is suggestive of rhabdomyolysis, which is followed by determination of serum creatinine phosphokinase. A positive urine ferric chloride test (phenylpyruvic acid) is indicative of a phenothiazine or salicylate overdose.

Intoxication with methanol, ethanol, ethylene glycol, acetone, and isopropanol can be recognized due to their propensity to increase serum osmolality. Calculated serum osmolality is determined by the following:

$$2 \times Na\,(mEq/L) + blood\ urea\ nitrogen\,(g/L)/2.8 + glucose\,(mg/dL)/18$$

The osmolar gap is evaluated by subtracting the calculated osmolality from the measured osmolality. Normal osmolar gap is 3–10 mOsm/kg H_2O. Calculation of the osmolar gap may be confounded by the presence of lipemia or other osmotically active agents often used in the ICU, such as mannitol or contrast for diagnostic imaging procedures.

Radiographic evaluation is particularly useful in detecting ingestion of certain foreign bodies, as well as in the instance of a number of radiopaque drugs, metals, and chemicals. In the event of the ingestion of disc batteries, it is warranted to obtain serial chest/abdominal x-rays to document the movement of the foreign body through the GI tract. Radiographic evaluation has identified efforts at drug smuggling via body packing with cocaine-filled containers. Chest and abdominal x-rays are extremely helpful in locating a number of radiopaque pills or tablets and in elucidating aspiration or pulmonary edema. Pill bezoars may be identified when contrast is utilized for the study. Radiopaque compounds may be grouped by the mnemonic "COINS": chloral hydrate and cocaine packets, opiate packets, iron and heavy metals (lead, arsenic, mercury), neuroleptics, and sustained–release or enteric coated tablets.

MANAGEMENT

Toxicokinetics focuses on the dynamics of the processes of absorption, distribution, metabolism, and elimination of drugs or toxins. Prevention of absorption is a mainstay of toxicology. Washing a toxin from the skin or removing a victim from an environment with a toxic gas may dramatically reduce toxicity. Preventing absorption from the GI tract is more complex, as the drug or toxin must dissolve in aqueous gastric fluids and transverse several lipophilic membranes prior to reaching the vascular compartment. Consequently, factors such as pH and pKa of the toxin and lipid solubility of the drug may alter absorption. Timely administration of activated charcoal may allow the drug or toxin an opportunity to be adsorbed to activated charcoal within the GI lumen. Enteric-coated tablets and sustained-release formulations have been designed to delay and sustain the absorption process. Kinetically, this delayed absorption results in a lengthier time to achieve peak serum concentrations, which prolongs the duration of action of the drug. Whole-bowel irrigation may allow enteric-coated tablets or sustained-release formulations to transit the GI tract before absorption begins. Drugs with complex or slow dissolution or absorption are most amenable to activated charcoal. Many enzymes involved in metabolism have specific isoenzymes that can be induced (cigarette smoke, omeprazole, rifampin) or inhibited (amiodarone, cimetidine, erythromycin, grapefruit juice, ketoconazole), resulting in toxicity or subtherapeutic levels. Renal elimination is the most common route of elimination. Many drugs are metabolized in the liver to water-soluble metabolites so that they may be renally cleared.

Syrup of ipecac leads to vomiting by means of central chemotactic stimulation and local effects on the gastric mucosa. The American Academy of Clinical Toxicology and the European Association of Poisons Centres and Clinical Toxicologists issue recommendations that are incorporated below for syrup of ipecac as well as other interventions: "Syrup of ipecac should not be administered routinely in the management of poisoned patients...its routine administration in the emergency department should be abandoned."

A mainstay of gastric decontamination has been the utilization of gastric lavage. The proper technique of gastric lavage involves the insertion of a large-bore orogastric tube into the stomach, followed by administration and aspiration of fluid, with the intent of recovering newly ingested toxins. This technique can be particularly traumatizing to a young child and is truly associated with risk in a patient with any degree of impaired airway protection. Contraindications

TABLE 10.8

AGENTS NOT ADSORBED BY CHARCOAL

Common electrolytes
Iron
Mineral acids or bases
Alcohols
Cyanide
Most solvents
Most water insoluble compounds (hydrocarbons)
Pesticides
Lithium

to gastric lavage include compromised upper airway protection, ingestion of corrosive substances or hydrocarbons, and patients at risk for GI perforation or hemorrhage. Gastric lavage should not be employed routinely in the management of poisoned patients. Gastric lavage should not be considered unless a patient has ingested a potentially life-threatening amount of a poison and the procedure can be undertaken within 60 mins of ingestion.

Activated charcoal is a particularly efficacious therapy in the management of most poisonings, as it can potentially decrease the absorption of a broad array of toxins and is only ineffective in a small number of cases (**Table 10.8**). "Activated charcoal should not be routinely administered in the management of poisoned patients . . . the greatest benefit is within one hour of ingestion . . . " The usual dosage for unquantified ingestions is 1 g/kg. Activated charcoal is contraindicated in the event of an inadequately protected airway, heralded by absent gag reflex or extreme somnolence. If the administration of activated charcoal is deemed to be ideal, the patient may undergo rapid-sequence intubation to attain a protected airway. Extreme caution must be utilized when the toxic agent is known to slow GI motility (e.g., tricyclic antidepressants, calcium channel blockers, and opiates). Activated charcoal may be found in preparation with sorbitol, a common cathartic. The consensus is that the isolated use of cathartics has no role in the management of the poisoned patient, and a sound recommendation is lacking regarding the routine use of a cathartic in combination with activated charcoal.

The technique of whole-bowel irrigation utilizing osmotically balanced polyethylene glycol electrolyte solutions (PEG-ES) appears attractive in that it can enhance the elimination of toxins prior to their absorption. A definite theoretical benefit can be gained in aiding elimination following ingestions of heavy metals, iron, sustained-release or enteric-coated tablets, and illegal drug packets. Recommendations regarding dosing of PEG-ES have proposed target goals of 1500–2000 mL/hr in adults, 1000

mL/hr in children ages 6–12 years, and 500 mL/hr in children 9 months to 6 years of age. Utilization of this technique has absolutely no role in the management of patients with an unprotected airway, hemodynamic compromise, intractable vomiting, and GI hemorrhage, ileus, perforation, or obstruction. Emergent surgical GI decontamination may prove useful in rare cases.

Antidotal therapy is a vital component of management, as it may prove useful in initiating therapy and in definitively identifying a particular toxin (**Table 10.9, Table 10.10**). The major adverse reactions reported with flumazenil use are seizures and dysrhythmias. Naloxone, an opiate-receptor antagonist, proves particularly useful in effecting rapid reversal of narcotic toxicity.

Aggressive supportive therapies to enhance toxin elimination have included hemoperfusion and hemodialysis. Hemodialysis is indicated for the management of severe salicylate and lithium exposures, following toxic exposures to methanol and ethylene glycol. Consultation with the Poison Control Center and a nephrologist is often helpful in determining whether hemodialysis is indicated. Hemoperfusion involves the passage of blood through an extracorporeal circuit and cartridge, which contains an adsorbent, and return of the detoxified blood to the patient. Using hemoperfusion is advantageous over using hemodialysis for a few drugs (e.g., theophylline). One must weigh the risk-benefit ratio of these therapies when considering their use.

Drug elimination may be facilitated by ensuring adequate renal flow: 2–5 mL/kg/hr. Drugs and toxins with which alkalinization of the urine has shown to be effective in enhancing elimination include salicylate, phenobarbital, chlorpropamide, and the chlorophenoxy herbicides. Alkalinization of the urine may be achieved by adding sodium bicarbonate (50–75 mEq/L) to the IV fluids. It is imperative to ensure vigilance in following serum potassium and sodium levels as alkalinization is accomplished.

Several agents are particularly useful to employ as diagnostic trials in elucidating the presence of a particular toxin (**Table 10.10**).

TOXIDROMES

Sympathomimetic/Adrenergic Agents

Common sympathomimetic adrenergic agents are listed in **Table 10.11**. Signs and symptoms of sympathomimetic toxicity (**Table 10.12**) are dependent upon the target receptor sites. Benzodiazepines are useful in reducing CNS catecholamine release and

SELECTED ANTIDOTES AND METHODS OF ENHANCING TOXIN ELIMINATION

Antidote	Toxin
Antivenoms	
Crotalidae	North American Pit Viper envenomation
Polyvalent (ACP)	
Polyvalent immune Fab	
Micruris sp.	Eastern or Texas coral snake envenomations
Latrodectus mactans	Black widow spider envenomation
Atropine	Organophosphate (OP), carbamate poisoning, bradydysrhythmias, Centruroides envenomation
Calcium (chloride or gluconate)	Calcium-channel blocker overdose, hydrofluoric acid ingestion/exposure
Cyanide antidote package	Cyanide, acetonitrile (artificial nail remover), amygdalin (peach, apricot pits), nitroprusside (thiosulfate only)
Amyl nitrite	
Sodium nitrite	
Sodium thiosulfate	
Deferoxamine	Iron
Digoxin-specific antibody fragments	Digoxin, digitoxin, natural cardiac glycosides (e.g., oleander, red squill, Bufo toad venom)
Flumazenil	Benzodiazepines
Fomepizole	Toxic alcohols (ethylene glycol, methanol)
Glucagon	Calcium-channel blocker, β-blocker toxicity
Glucose (dextrose)	Sulfonylureas, insulin, hypoglycemia (multiple toxins)
Hydroxocobalamin (vitamin B_{12})[a]	Cyanide, acetonitrile, amygdalin, nitroprusside
Insulin (high dose)/euglycemia[b]	Calcium-channel blocker, β-blocker toxicity
Methylene blue	Methemoglobinemia
N-acetylcysteine	Acetaminophen, pennyroyal oil, carbon tetrachloride
Naloxone	Opioid toxicity
Octreotide	Sulfonylurea toxicity
Physostigmine	Antimuscarinic delirium (as a diagnostic tool only)
Pralidoxime	OP poisoning (insecticides, nerve agents)
Protamine sulfate	Heparins
Pyridoxine	Isoniazid, monomethylhydrazine (rocket fuel), gyromitra mushrooms
Thiamine	Deficiency states (e.g., alcoholism, anorexia nervosa)
Sodium bicarbonate	Sodium channel blocking cardiotoxins, salicylates

Method of removal	Indication
Dialysis	Toxic alcohols, salicylates, lithium, theophylline, valproic acid, atenolol, sotalol, others
Urinary alkalinization with sodium bicarbonate	Salicylates, phenobarbital, chlorpropamide, chlorophenoxy herbicides, methotrexate

[a]Not FDA approved for this use.
[b]Anecdotal experience.
From Barry JD. Diagnosis and management of the poisoned child. *Pediatr Ann* 2005;34:937–46, with permission.

thereby are effective in controlling severe hypertension, tachycardia, agitation, and extreme muscle activity. It is essential to recognize that use of a β-blocking agent to control tachycardia and hypertension may result in unopposed α-receptor stimulation. For this reason, β-blockers are best avoided, and a benzodiazepine alone or with nitroprusside or phentolamine should be used when control of hypertension and tachycardia becomes necessary. Cocaine toxicity can result in depletion of catecholamines, which may cause late cardiovascular collapse. It follows that short-acting antihypertensive agents are preferred for treating these overdoses. The sympathomimetic toxidrome is not seen with toxicity due to such centrally acting α agonists as clonidine. These agents result in decreased sympathetic outflow and cause reflex bradycardia, hypotension, and CNS and respiratory depression.

TABLE 10.10

USEFUL DIAGNOSTIC TRIALS

Agent suspected	Agent administered	Dose	Positive results
Benzodiazepines	Flumazenil	0.2–0.3 mg/kg IV (maximum 3 mg)	Improved consciousness
Iron	Deferoxamine	40 mg/kg IM (maximum 2 g)	"Vin rosé" urine color
Opiates	Naloxone hydrochloride	0.03 mg/kg (up to 4 mg)	Improved consciousness
Organophosphate	Atropine	0.1 mg/kg	Mydriasis, less secretions
Phenothiazine (dystonia)	Diphenhydramine	1–2 mg/kg IV (maximum 25 mg)	Resolution
Phenothiazine (neuroleptic malignant syndrome)	Dantrolene	1–3 mg/kg IV	Resolution
Insulin reaction	Dextrose	1 g/kg IV	Improved consciousness
Isoniazid	Pyridoxine	5 g IV	Seizures abate; improved consciousness

From Woolf AD. Principles of toxin assessment and screening. In: Fuhrman BP, Zimmerman J, eds. *Pediatric Critical Care*. 3rd ed. Philadelphia, PA: Mosby Elsevier, 2006:1511–31, with permission.

Cholinergic Agents

Muscarinic agents act at postganglionic, parasympathetic nerve endings and in sweat glands. The direct acting muscarinic agonists result in excessive parasympathetic activity. Nicotinic agents act at sympathetic and parasympathetic autonomic ganglia. Cholinesterase inhibitors result in an accumulation of acetylcholine at the cholinergic synapse (**Table 10.13**).

This toxidrome is effectively managed with atropine. Organophosphate pesticides and nerve agents are examples of cholinesterase inhibitors. It is possible to have a mixed toxicity, but parasympa-

thetic toxicity is most commonly seen. Carbamates, which are also used as pesticides, reversibly bind to acetylcholinesterase and ultimately undergo spontaneous hydrolysis, which results in a restoration of cholinesterase activity within hours. Topical decontamination with utilization of personal protective equipment is essential. Inhalational exposure is marked by upper airway involvement and subsequent respiratory distress. Vomiting and drooling are most commonly seen following ingestion. Seizures and severe CNS toxicity occur following large exposures to household products or small exposures to industrial pesticides and "nerve agents."

Management of organophosphate toxicity involves expeditious administration of atropine to reverse the muscarinic effects, an oxime (Pralidoxime) to facilitate reactivation of acetylcholinesterase, which reverses the neuromuscular blockade, and benzodiazepines to control seizures.

TABLE 10.11

SYMPATHOMIMETIC AGENTS

Albuterol
Amphetamines
Caffeine
Catecholamines
Cocaine
Ephedrine
Ketamine
Lysergic acid diethylamide (LSD)
Methamphetamine
Phencyclidine (PCP)
Phenylephrine
Phenylpropanolamine
Pseudoephedrine
Terbutaline
Theophylline

TABLE 10.12

SYMPATHOMIMETIC TOXIDROME

Agitation
Seizures
Mydriasis
Tachycardia
Hypertension
Diaphoresis
Pallor
Cool Skin
Fever

TABLE 10.13

CHOLINERGIC TOXIDROME FEATURES

Muscarinic effects (DUMBBELS)
  Diarrhea
  Urinary incontinence
  Miosis
  Bradycardia
  Bronchorrhea
  Emesis
  Lacrimation
  Salivation
Nicotinic effects
  Fasciculations
  Weakness
  Paralysis
  Tachycardia
  Hypertension
  Agitation
Central effects
  Lethargy
  Coma
  Agitation
  Seizures

Anticholinergic Agents

Agents that produce antimuscarinic properties result in a constellation of symptoms and signs referred to as the anticholinergic toxidrome (**Table 10.14, Table 10.15**). Sympathomimetic toxicity results in diaphoresis and cool skin, while anticholinergic toxicity is notoriously marked by impaired sweating and warm, dry skin. Sympathomimetics result in hyperactive bowel sounds, while anticholinergics cause diminished bowel sounds and even ileus. Tachycardia, mydriasis, urinary retention, flushing, and hyperthermia are found with both sympathomimetic and anticholinergic toxicity. Benzodiazepines may be

TABLE 10.14

ANTICHOLINERGIC AGENTS

Antihistamines—diphenhydramine, hydroxyzine
Atropine
Benztropine mesylate
Carbamazepine
Cyclic antidepressants
Cyclobenzaprine
Hyoscyamine
Jimsonweed
Oxybutynin
Phenothiazines
Scopolamine
Trihexyphenidyl

TABLE 10.15

ANTICHOLINERGIC TOXIDROME

Agitation
Delirium
Coma
Mydriasis
Dry mouth
Warm, dry, flushed skin
Tachycardia
Hypertension
Fever
Urinary retention
Decreased bowel sounds
Associated expressions
"Mad as a Hatter"
"Blind as a Bat"
"Red as a Beet"
"Hot as a Hare"
"Dry as a Bone"

extremely helpful in managing symptoms. Physostigmine, a cholinesterase inhibitor, may be employed with the intent of reversing central and peripheral manifestations of the anticholinergic toxidrome; however, it is not recommended for management of tricyclic antidepressant toxicity because of reported convulsions and asystole.

Opioid Agents

Most opioids and opiates cause a triad of respiratory depression, coma, and miosis. An exception is meperidine, with which toxicity is manifested by respiratory depression, coma, and mydriasis; additionally, seizures are reported to occur with meperidine toxicity. Physical findings often include bradycardia, hypotension, and decreased GI motility. Diphenoxylate and methadone present a particular hazard to toddlers due to low-dose ingestions. Management involves administration of naloxone, an opiate-receptor antagonist that results in rapid reversal of toxicity. Naloxone is generally initiated at 0.1 mg/kg/dose IV in children and 1–2 mg/dose in adolescents and adults to achieve reversal of respiratory depression. If a partial response is observed, up to 10 mg may be necessary. Alternate administration can be accomplished by a variety of routes: subcutaneous, intramuscular, and endotracheal. It is critical to note that administration of naloxone may precipitate an acute withdrawal syndrome in opiate-dependent patients. If opiate dependency is suspected, it is prudent to initiate therapy with lower doses. Naloxone has been associated with the development of pulmonary edema, though this condition may occur as a result of opiate toxicity. Nalmefene is a longer-acting opiate-receptor antagonist. Clonidine is a centrally acting α-agonist that is often included in the opiate toxidrome due to the diminished sympathetic tone, its ability to cause miosis and CNS and respiratory depression in overdose, and its occasional reversal with naloxone. Many opiates (e.g., codeine, hydrocodone, oxycodone, and propoxyphene) are formulated in combination with acetaminophen or aspirin. Therefore, it is extremely important to maintain a high index of suspicion for toxicity from such compounds. Fentanyl patches contain a high concentration of drug per patch; significant toxicity can result from ingestion as well as inhalation.

Acetaminophen

Acetaminophen presents a significant concern due to its toxicity, which can result in fulminant hepatic failure. The clinical manifestations of acetaminophen intoxication are commonly described in 4 stages.

The initial presentation of an acetaminophen overdose is usually heralded by nausea and vomiting within 12–24 hrs, although some patients may be completely asymptomatic (Stage I). This is clearly a reason to screen for acetaminophen levels in all ingestions. Acidosis may be present in extreme overdoses. The liver transaminases usually are noted to be elevated by 24 hrs following ingestion (Stage II), at which time clinical symptoms often abate. Liver function abnormalities peak at 48–72 hrs following ingestion, and symptomatology returns with nausea, vomiting, and anorexia (Stage III). The clinical course may result in complete recovery or fulminant hepatic failure. The recovery phase (Stage IV) generally lasts ~7–8 days. It is important to know that cases of fulminant hepatic failure with jaundice, encephalopathy, and bleeding occur infrequently. The most efficacious therapy involves the administration of N-acetylcysteine (NAC), which serves as a precursor to facilitate the synthesis of glutathione. Initiation of NAC is usually recommended within 10 hrs following ingestion; however, it has been beneficial when administered up to 24 hrs following ingestion. A decision to employ this therapy is based upon application of the Rumack-Matthew nomogram (**Fig. 10.1**) in plotting a serum level of acetaminophen drawn at least 4 hrs following ingestion. In the event that blood levels are not immediately available, treatment decisions should be based upon a suggestive history. The therapy can be stopped if a nontoxic level is eventually obtained. Oral dosing of NAC begins with a loading dose of 140 mg/kg, followed by maintenance therapy of 70 mg/kg every 4 hrs for 17 doses. Therapy should continue until all doses are administered,

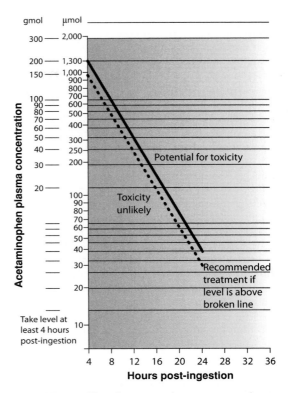

FIGURE 10.1. Use of nomogram in management of acute acetaminophen overdose. From Joshi P, Toxidromes and their treatment. Acetaminophen level is obtained at ≥4 hrs after ingestion. Level is then plotted on nomogram. Above the broken line = administer full course of acetylcysteine. Below the broken line = acetylcysteine not necessary. Adapted from Fuhrman BP, Zimmerman JJ, eds. *Pediatric Critical Care*, 3rd ed. Philadelphia: Mosby, Elsevier, 2006:1521–31.

even though the acetaminophen plasma level drops below the toxic range. NAC can also be administered IV in a 20-hr protocol. Initially, the patient receives a 150-mg/kg loading dose over 15 mins, followed by 50 mg/kg over 4 hrs, and then 100 mg/kg over the final 16 hrs. Care must be taken to ensure that the NAC is appropriately diluted and that the patient will not become fluid overloaded.

Salicylates

Acetylsalicylic acid, or aspirin, bismuth subsalicylate, sodium salicylate, and magnesium salicylate are often encountered in various drugs. Aspirin is contained in a wide variety of medications, including antihistamines, sympathomimetics, anticholinergics, opiates, and acetaminophen. Oil of wintergreen, comprised of 98% methylsalicylate, is a particularly dangerous compound. Another less commonly considered mode of intoxication occurs via exposure to topical aspirin-containing compounds that are ingested or absorbed cutaneously. In general, doses of <100 mg/kg produce minimal toxicity; however, doses that exceed 300 mg/kg can yield catastrophic clinical symptoms and often prove deadly. Respiratory alkalosis is often the first feature of salicylate intoxication. Nausea, vomiting, dehydration, and tinnitus are commonly seen. CNS manifestations include lethargy, coma, and seizures. Salicylate intoxication is quickly diagnosed by assessing the plasma salicylate concentration. Preliminary diagnosis may be rapidly made by utilizing the ferric chloride or Phenistix test. Ferric chloride added to a urine sample that contains salicylate will turn the specimen purple. Blood or urine that contains salicylate will turn the Phenistix brown. Determination of serum salicylate levels should be made 2 and 6 hrs following ingestion of immediate-release preparations. Targeted therapy in salicylate ingestion is directed at prevention of absorption early on with activated charcoal and alkalinization of the urine to enhance the elimination. Meticulous monitoring of urine pH is necessary to avoid significant alkalemia. Acetazolamide is not utilized to achieve an alkaline diuresis, as it results in a systemic metabolic acidosis. Hemodialysis is quite efficacious and is recommended for extremely elevated serum salicylate levels (>4100 mg/dL), presence of renal insufficiency, significant volume overload, and pulmonary edema or severe electrolyte aberrations.

Ethanol

Ethanol poses a hazard not only in beverage form but is contained in a variety of other products, such as mouthwash, perfume and cologne, and topical antiseptics. Children may present with nausea, vomiting, stupor, and ataxia. Infants and toddlers may dramatically develop coma, hypothermia, and hypoglycemia when ethanol levels exceed 50–100 mg/dL. Metabolic acidosis is typically found. Adolescents tend to have more typical signs of intoxication with levels of 100–150 mg/dL. Deaths directly attributed to alcohol ingestion are usually associated with alcohol concentrations >500 mg/dL. An ingestion of ~1 g/kg of ethanol will raise the blood alcohol level to 100 mg/dL. The following estimates of toxicity may be extrapolated: beer (5% alcohol), 10–15 mL/kg; wine (14% alcohol), 4–6 mL/kg; and 80-proof liquor (40% alcohol), 1–2 mL/kg. Binge drinking has been a catastrophic activity of adolescents and college students. Hemodialysis may increase the rate of elimination significantly, but it is rarely necessary.

Isopropyl Alcohol

Isopropyl alcohol is a component of many home products, including rubbing alcohol, aftershave lotions, perfumes, skin lotions, and antifreeze compounds. Ingestion is typically the most common route, but infants may be poisoned via inhalation of isopropyl vapors during sponging for a fever. The toxic dose is reported to be 1 mL/kg of 70% isopropyl alcohol; ingestion of more than a swallow is potentially toxic in children. Toxicity is manifested by vomiting, abdominal pain and, often, hematemesis due to gastritis. Neurologic manifestations include lethargy, dizziness, ataxia, and possible coma. In patients who have ingested isopropyl alcohol, the unusual finding of ketosis and ketonemia without an acidemia may be seen. Isopropyl alcohol is metabolized to acetone. Children are at extreme risk for hypoglycemia. Ethanol, fomepizole, and hemodialysis are usually not indicated in the management of isopropyl alcohol intoxication.

Methanol and Ethylene Glycol

Methanol and ethylene glycol are toxic alcohols most commonly found in antifreeze compounds, and both are known to cause CNS depression. Ingestions that exceed 0.5 mL/kg may result in significant toxicity, and ingestions >1 mL/kg may prove to be fatal. Determination of an elevated osmolal gap is helpful, as these compounds are osmotically active and may raise the measured serum osmolality. It must be recognized that the presence of a normal osmolal gap (−8 to +12) does not exclude significant levels of toxic alcohols. Toxicity may be documented with serum levels of the parent compounds; however, in the event of a late presentation, levels may be undetectable following complete metabolism. The laboratory hallmarks of ethylene glycol and methanol poisoning are a high anion gap metabolic acidosis and an elevated osmolal gap. The cornerstone of management has been aimed at blocking alcohol dehydrogenase to negate the formation of the toxic metabolites. Although ethanol has been utilized, it is fraught with difficulties in titration, as well as side effects of inebriation, CNS depression, hypoglycemia, and hypotension. Fomepizole has become the accepted drug of choice in blocking alcohol dehydrogenase. Thiamine and pyridoxine should be administered IV every 6 hrs to patients who have ingested ethylene glycol. Folic acid should be given to patients who have ingested methanol. Hemodialysis is recommended in the instance of high levels of methanol or ethylene glycol, especially with concomitant metabolic acidosis, electrolyte abnormalities, and renal impairment of visual disturbance.

CAUSTICS

Alkaline injury results from a liquefaction necrosis caused by saponification of cellular fats and protein degradation. Acid ingestion results in a superficial coagulation necrosis, with marked heat production and eschar formation. The clinical presentation may involve generalized systemic signs, including hyperpyrexia, respiratory distress, hemodynamic instability, hypocalcemia (with hydrofluoric acid ingestion), and metabolic acidosis (with acidic ingestion). Perforation may be marked by abdominal pain, subcutaneous emphysema, pneumothorax, pneumomediastinum, or peritonitis. Management of the caustic toxin involves aggressive decontamination, with washing and diluting of dermal or ocular exposures, fresh air and oxygen for inhalational injury, and removal of as much substance from the mouth as possible in the ingestion of a caustic solid. The pH of the ocular fluids should be determined following irrigation to ensure neutralization of caustics; normal pH of tears is 7. Alkali eye exposures mandate an urgent ophthalmologic consult. Serial radiographs are utilized to track swallowed button batteries. Button batteries lodged in the esophagus must be expeditiously removed; those in the stomach or intestines generally pass intact. If the patient can immediately drink a small amount of water or milk, it may help to reduce esophageal injury by washing the caustic into the stomach. Neutralization of a caustic substance is contraindicated, as the resultant exothermic reaction can yield more extensive tissue destruction. Ipecac, gastric lavage, and activated charcoal are not indicated. Endoscopy is recommended within the first 24 hrs following ingestion to quantify actual tissue damage. Risk for perforation if significant if endoscopy is delayed over 48 hrs due to loss of tissue integrity.

Carbon Monoxide

Carbon monoxide exposure results in significant tissue hypoxia due to the extremely high binding affinity with hemoglobin (200–300 times that of oxygen) and a leftward shift and change in shape (hyperbolic configuration) of the oxyhemoglobin dissociation curve. Definitive diagnosis is made by co-oximetry and determination of the carboxyhemoglobin level. Frequently reported signs and symptoms are associated with a specific level of carboxyhemoglobin (**Table 10.16**). Transcutaneous measurement of oxygen saturation by pulse oximetry will be falsely normal, as pulse oximetry cannot differentiate oxyhemoglobin from carboxyhemoglobin. The mainstay of therapy is directed at removing the patient from the source of contamination and expeditious delivery of 100% oxygen. The half-life of carboxyhemoglobin is dependent upon the mode of delivery of varying oxygen concentrations (**Table 10.17**). Strong consideration should be given to early consultation with a

TABLE 10.16

CARBON MONOXIDE INHALATION

Carboxyhemoglobin level	Intoxication classification	Symptoms
5%		Impaired judgment Altered fine motor skills
20%	Mild	Headache Dyspnea Visual changes Confusion
30%	Moderate	Drowsiness, dulled sensorium Faintness Nausea/vomiting Tachycardia
40%–60%	Moderate – severe	Weakness Poor coordination Loss of recent memory Impending cardiovascular and neurologic collapse
>60%	Severe	Coma Convulsion Death

TABLE 10.17

HALF-LIFE OF CARBOXYHEMOGLOBIN

Oxygen concentration	t 1/2
21%	5 hrs
100% (mask, ET)	90 min
Hyperbaric oxygen, 2–3 atmospheres	30 min

ET, endotracheal

hyperbaric oxygen therapy facility for patients who have experienced loss of consciousness or syncope or who continue to exhibit neurologic symptoms while receiving oxygen therapy. Complications associated with hyperbaric therapy include barotraumas (pneumomediastinum, pneumothorax, tympanic membrane rupture), oxygen toxicity (seizures), and claustrophobic reactions in a small chamber. It is disheartening that carbon monoxide poisoning that presents with loss of consciousness or syncope, even with initially low carboxyhemoglobin levels, may ultimately result in delayed or persistent neurologic sequelae.

Cyanide

Management is especially challenging, as the signs and symptoms are nonspecific but reflect profound hypoxia. Death often occurs within minutes of exposure. Patients do not present with cyanosis; venous oxygen saturation is elevated, which reflects the inability of the cells to utilize oxygen. Successful treatment requires rapid diagnosis and administration of the antidote. The antidote kit contains amyl nitrite ampules and IV sodium nitrite to produce methemoglobinemia. The amyl nitrite is administered by inhalation while IV access is obtained. Once an IV site is available, the sodium nitrite is given to produce an approximate 20% methemoglobinemia. Although cyanide toxicity may be present in fire victims, nitrite administration is particularly risky because the resultant methemoglobin formation would exacerbate the already diminished oxygen-carrying capacity due to carbon monoxide exposure.

Iron

Systemic toxicity usually does not occur unless the elemental iron dose exceeds 60 mg/kg. The first phase of iron intoxication usually occurs within 30 mins of ingestion and is marked by vomiting, diarrhea, and possible hematemesis or hematochezia.

This stage may require aggressive fluid resuscitation due to profound fluid and electrolyte losses. The latent period, or second phase, is heralded by a resolution of the GI manifestations, but the patient continues to have a nonspecific malaise. Tachycardia may be present following the previous fluid derangements, and metabolic acidosis may be developing. The third phase occurs 12 hrs following ingestion and is manifested by profound hemodynamic instability and shock. The fourth phase is depicted by liver failure. Scarring or strictures of the GI tract may occur due to the corrosive effect of the iron. Iron toxicity warrants serious consideration of GI lavage or whole-bowel irrigation because it is not effectively adsorbed by charcoal. Serum iron levels should be determined within 6 hrs of ingestion. If patients remain asymptomatic by 6 hrs following ingestion, it is highly unlikely that systemic illness will develop. Metabolic acidosis or acidemia correlates with toxicity. Deferoxamine chelation (gradually increasing to 15 mg/kg/hr IV) is indicated for serum iron levels >500 mcg/dL or in the event of hemodynamic collapse. Deferoxamine must be administered with caution for multiple reasons. Chelation therapy is continued until the serum iron level returns to normal, the metabolic acidosis resolves, the patient clinically improves, and the urine color returns to normal. Critical care management must focus upon the potential for cardiopulmonary failure with profound hypotension, extreme metabolic acidosis, hypo- or hyperglycemia, anemia and colloid losses due to GI hemorrhage, renal failure secondary to shock, and hepatic failure, which exacerbates the bleeding diathesis. Brisk urine output is essential for the excretion of the iron-deferoxamine complex.

CALCIUM CHANNEL BLOCKERS

The blockade of cardiac calcium channels causes negative inotropic, chronotropic, and dromotropic effects. Vasodilation results from the blockade of calcium channels in arteriolar smooth muscle. The dihydropyridine calcium channel antagonists (nifedipine, amlodipine, felodipine, nicardipine) may result in hypotension and reflex tachycardia. The life-threatening consequences of blocked calcium channels include bradydysrhythmias (pacemaker cell inhibition and AV block) and profound hypotension (vasodilatation and impaired contractility). Electrocardiographic changes include prolonged PR interval, inverted P waves, AV dissociation, AV block, ST-segment changes, sinus arrest, and asystole. Management considerations include reports of noncardiogenic pulmonary edema, which necessitates judicious fluid resuscitation and ventilatory support. GI hypomotility, ileus, and constipation may occur due to inhibition of GI motility hormone release. Fluid resuscitation is generally successful in symptomatic management. IV calcium and vasopressors may be employed in the instance of refractory hypotension. Activated charcoal should be administered and repeated if the calcium channel blocker is in a sustained-release formulation. Whole-bowel irrigation should also be considered for patients with ingestions of sustained-release calcium channel blockers.

Overdosage of verapamil and diltiazem is complicated by their propensity to cause cardiogenic shock/pump failure. Management in this case may be enhanced by the utilization of dobutamine or phosphodiesterase inhibitors (milrinone, amrinone). Glucagon has been considered a specific therapy for refractory hypotension: IV bolus 0.15 mg/kg, followed by an infusion of 0.05–0.1 mg/kg/hr. The utilization of high dose insulin has been proposed to offset the hyperglycemia. Hyperinsulinemia/euglycemia therapy has been reported to reverse cardiogenic shock in the instance of calcium channel blocker toxicity.

β-BLOCKERS

β–blocker toxicity results in bradycardia, hypotension, and conduction delay. Severe toxicity may result in arrhythmias, including torsades de pointes, ventricular fibrillation, and asystole. Patients may occasionally present with bronchospasm. Hypoglycemia is frequently seen in β-blocker toxicity. Propranolol not only causes hemodynamic compromise but, due to its lipid solubility, it has the potential to cross the blood–brain barrier and result in coma and seizures. Labetalol can have conflicting actions and may cause vasodilation and β-receptor blockade. Sotalol may cause dose-dependent prolongation of the QT interval and subsequent torsades de pointes. Acebutolol toxicity is one of the most severe, in that it predisposes to ventricular repolarization abnormalities, resulting in ventricular arrhythmias. Management may merely require hemodynamic monitoring if the patient presents with asymptomatic bradycardia. Atropine is often helpful to reverse bradycardia and hypotension. Contractility may also be enhanced by the action of glucagon.

Digoxin

Clinical manifestations of digoxin overdose include nausea, vomiting, altered sensorium, and cardiac dysrhythmias. Heart block or sinus bradycardia may be managed with atropine. It is absolutely essential to avoid any drugs whose action is to depress activity of the sinoatrial or atrioventricular nodes. Although calcium is employed in treating significant hyperkalemia, it should be avoided due to the action of digoxin, which causes an increase in intracellular calcium. Indications for utilization of Fab therapy (Digibind, DigiFab) in children include (a) a known ingestion of at least 0.1 mg/kg, (b) a digoxin level of >5 ng/mL and signs and symptoms of digoxin toxicity, (c) the occurrence of life-threatening arrhythmias, or (d) a serum potassium level of >6 mEq/L.

TRICYCLIC ANTIDEPRESSANTS

The tricyclic compounds have anticholinergic properties that result in the anticholinergic toxidrome. Their inhibition of α-adrenergic receptors can result in sedation and hypotension. Clinical symptoms have been related to the degree of QRS widening: seizures (QRS >100 ms) and arrhythmias (QRS >160 ms). Tricyclic toxicity often presents with the anticholinergic syndrome, hypotension, widening of the QRS complex, and seizures. Seizure management is generally accomplished with benzodiazepines. It is extremely important to avoid the use of flumazenil as reversal if a possibility of co-ingestion of benzodiazepines exists, as this may precipitate tricyclic-induced seizure activity. Sodium bicarbonate is utilized to achieve serum alkalinization (pH >7.4 and <7.55) when the QRS is widened or in the face of ventricular arrhythmias. Vasopressors (e.g., norepinephrine and epinephrine) may be needed to maintain adequate vascular tone and blood pressure. Carbamazepine toxicity may mirror the above constellation of symptoms and signs, as it is a benzodiazepine derivative structurally related to the tricyclic antidepressants. Toxicity has manifested following drug interactions with erythromycin, isoniazid, cimetidine, and propoxyphene.

HERBAL TOXICITY/NUTRITIONAL SUPPLEMENT TOXICITY

The 12 most dangerous supplements with alternate names and associated clinical manifestations are listed in **Table 10.3**. This information can be reviewed on the Consumer Reports website (www.consumerreports.org). A number of herbal remedies have been reported to carry significant toxicity and are listed in **Table 10.2**. Management of these poisonings can be summarized by aggressive supportive care and therapies directed at control of specific symptoms.

TABLE 10.18

COMMONLY ABUSED DRUGS AND THEIR STREET NAMES

Category substance name	Street names
Marijuana	Dope, ganja, joint, Mary Jane, pot, weed
Tobacco	Smoke, chew, beedi, snuff, cigar
Alcohol	Booze
Cocaine	Crack, candy, rock, Charlie, toot, snow
Methamphetamine	Crystal, meth, ice, speed, fire
Ritalin (methylphenidate)	MPH, Vitamin R, skippy
MDMA (methylenedioxy-methamphetamine)	Adam, clarity, ecstasy, XTC
GHB (gamma-hydroxybutyrate)	Georgia home boy, G, liquid ecstasy
Ketamine	Special K, K, Vitamin K
PCP (phencyclidine)	Angel dust
SD (lysergic acid diethylamide)	Acid, Big D, Blotters, cube
Heroin (diacetylmorphine)	Brown sugar, H, horse
OxyContin (oxycodone HCL)	Oxy, OC, killer
Vicodin (hydrocodone bitartrate with acetaminophen)	Vike, Watson-387
Benzodiazepines	Downers, sleeping pills
Rohypnol (flunitrazepam)	Roofies, roofinol, rope, R2
Anabolic steroids	Roids, juice
Inhalants	Poppers, snappers, whippets

From Nanda S, Konur N. Adolescent drug and alcohol use in the 21st Century. *Pediatr Ann* 2006; 35:193–9, with permission.

CLUB DRUGS

Common drugs of abuse, along with their respective street names are summarized in **Table 10.18**. A number of substances are abused via inhalation (**Table 10.19**). Clinical effects usually occur within seconds to minutes (**Table 10.20**). Inhalation of volatile compounds may result in chemical pneumonitis. CNS depression may result in depression of airway reflexes, which may lead to catastrophic aspiration and respiratory arrest.

Ecstasy (X, E, XTC, Adam) with or without commonly found contaminants include methylenedioxyamphetamine (MDA), paramethoxyamphetamine, phencyclidine (PCP), and heroin, can cause serious toxicity. Dehydration is a frequent manifestation of ecstasy toxicity. Mild cases may present with anxiety attacks, muscle cramping, severe trismus, or urinary retention due to spasm of the urethral sphincter. Acute intoxication with MDMA is heralded by hyperthermia, malignant hyperthermia, rhabdomyolysis, disseminated intravascular coagulation, acute renal failure, seizures, cardiac arrhythmias, intracranial hemorrhage, brain infarction, or death.

Gamma Hydroxy Butyrate (G, Liquid Ecstasy, Liquid E) is a CNS depressant that results in a state of euphoria, disinhibition, and heightened sexuality, making it a "date-rape drug." Dose-dependent side effects include drowsiness, dizziness, nausea, vomiting, amnesia, hallucinations, convulsions, respiratory

TABLE 10.19

COMMONLY ABUSED INHALANTS

Solvents	Commercial products	Medical gases	Aliphatic nitrites
Paint thinners	Butane lighters	Chloroform	Cyclohexyl nitrite
Gasoline	Whipping cream aerosols	Ether	Amyl nitrite
Glue	Spray paint	Halothane	Butyl nitrite
Felt-tip marker fluid	Hair and deodorant sprays	Nitrous oxide	
	Shoe polish		

Data from *Monitoring the Future National Results on Adolescent Drug Use: Overview of Key Findings.* Bethesda, MD: National Institute on Drug Abuse. 2004 NIH Publication No. 05-5726.

TABLE 10.20

EFFECTS OF INHALANTS

Effect	Inhalant
Hearing loss	Trichloroethylene, toluene
Peripheral neuropathies or limb spasms	Hexane, nitrous oxide
CNS or brain damage	Toluene
Bone marrow damage	Benzene
Liver and kidney damage	Toluene, chlorinated hydrocarbons
Blood oxygen depletion	Organic nitrates, methylene chloride

Data from *Monitoring the Future National Results on Adolescent Drug Use: Overview of Key Findings*. Bethesda, MD: National Institute on Drug Abuse. 2004 NIH Publication No. 05-5726.

failure, coma, and death. Aggressive supportive care is the mainstay of management.

Methamphetamines (Tina, Ice, Crystal Meth, Tweak, Crank, Glass) may be taken orally, rectally, or intravenously or may be smoked; it is most commonly snorted intranasally. This agent is extremely physically addictive. Symptomatology follows the pattern of the sympathomimetic toxidrome. Most patients do well with aggressive supportive care.

Cocaine toxicity is incorporated within the sympathomimetic toxidrome but deserves mention with the specific club drugs. It may be used by inhalation (cocaine alkaloid, or "crack"), nasal insufflation, or the IV or GI route. Cocaine results in an adrenergic storm by blocking reuptake of catecholamines at adrenergic nerve endings. Clinical manifestations include extreme CNS stimulation along with cardiovascular and respiratory effects. Seizures, hypertension, and hyperthermia may lead to cardiac ischemia, CNS bleeding and infarction; end-organ failure may progress to hemodynamic collapse, coma, and death. An acute coronary syndrome results from the combined effects of cocaine. Cocaine results in a variety of dysrhythmias (wide complex tachycardia and ventricular fibrillation). It is difficult to accurately identify a cocaine-related myocardial infarction, because the electrocardiogram may by abnormal even in the absence of myocardial infarction. Furthermore, serum creatine kinase concentrations are typically elevated without an accompanying myocardial infarction. This elevation is attributed to rhabdomyolysis, which mandates a need for aggressive diuresis. Serum troponin levels are helpful in the evaluation for cocaine related myocardial infarction. Management commonly includes the liberal use of benzodiazepines, which control seizure activity and have also been reported to be efficacious in reducing heart rate and systemic arterial pressure. Hypertensive crisis must be controlled to minimize cerebrovascular or myocardial injury. Management of pediatric acute coronary syndrome may be represented by the mnemonic MONA (morphine, oxygen, nitroglycerin, aspirin). Recommended dosing of nitroglycerine in children is by IV infusion: initial dose of 0.25–0.5 mcg/kg/min, titrated by 0.5–1 mcg/kg/min every 3–5 mins as needed; in general, the dose range is 1–3 mcg/kg/min. β-adrenergic blockers are contraindicated in the management of cocaine-induced acute coronary syndrome.

CHAPTER 11 ■ THERMOREGULATION

PAMELA FEUER • THYYAR M. RAVINDRANATH • DAVID G. NICHOLS

Body temperature consists of core and shell temperatures. Rectal, esophageal, and oral temperatures represent core temperature, while axillary and skin temperatures are examples of shell temperature. Core temperature determines the risk of injury to various organs in the body. Thermoreceptors for the shell reside in the skin. Core thermoreceptors exist in the cortex, hypothalamus, midbrain, medulla, spinal cord, and deep abdominal structures in addition to the skin. Upon sensing temperature change, these receptors transmit afferent impulses via the lateral spinothalamic tract to the central thermostat located in the preoptic/anterior hypothalamus, which maintains the temperature set point.

HYPERTHERMIA

Hyperthermia refers to body temperature elevation beyond the hypothalamic set point because of inadequate heat loss and/or excessive heat gain. *Fever* is a regulated temperature elevation (>38.5°C) to a new higher set point in the hypothalamus. Hyperthermia syndromes maybe be classified as environmental (or exertional), drug (or toxin) induced, or of genetic/unknown origin. In humans, hyperthermia may induce euphoria instead of discomfort, resulting in failure to seek prompt medical attention.

Heat Stroke (Environmental/Exertional Heat-related Illness)

Heat-related illnesses constitute a spectrum of diseases that range from heat stress—a benign condition—to heat stroke—a potentially fatal condition. The milder conditions (variously termed heat rash, heat cramps, heat edema, and heat exhaustion) generally do not require PICU management. Heat stroke is characterized by an elevation of core temperature >40°C. It is subdivided into classic or environmental and exertional heat stroke. Exertional heat stroke may be linked to a genetic predisposition. Children tend to become hyperthermic during physical activity in hot environments. Dehydration is a risk factor for heat-related illness. Hence, children should be encouraged to drink adequate quantities of fluids before and during physical activity. The risk factors are listed in **Table 11.1**.

A major portion of heat is lost from the body via the skin, and perspiration-induced evaporation is responsible for most heat loss. The skin's blood flow enhances heat loss through conduction and convection. The sympathetic nervous system controls blood flow through the skin by modulating adrenergic vasoconstrictor and vasodilator fibers. Acclimatization is an adaptation response that can take up to several weeks following exposure to a hot environment.

Serum levels of TNF-α, IL-1, IL-6 and endotoxin levels are increased following elevation in body temperature. Heat stress induces heat shock elements, which leads to an accelerated transcription of heat shock proteins. These proteins bestow cells with the ability to survive injury. The balance between proinflammatory mediators, such as TNF-α, IL-1β, interferon-γ, and anti-inflammatory mediators, such as sTNF-α and IL-10, determine the extent of tissue injury. Vasodilatation-induced shift of blood flow from the core to the peripheral circulation results in reduced blood flow to the gastrointestinal tract, with subsequent gut ischemia. The activation of coagulation cascade as a result of heat injury is supported by the presence of the thrombin-antithrombin complex and decreased levels of naturally synthesized anticoagulation proteins such as protein C, protein S, and antithrombin III.

TABLE 11.1	

RISK FACTORS FOR HEAT-RELATED ILLNESS

Factors	Description
Age	Elderly, children
Sex	Male due to increase in muscle mass and strenuous activity
Socioeconomic factors	Lack of access to air conditioners; individuals living in upper floors of apartment buildings especially with flat roof tops; social isolation; closed doors and windows during hot weather conditions
Weather conditions	Factors that prevent heat loss from the body: reduced wind, elevated barometric pressure, high humidity, high environmental temperature at or above body temperature for prolonged periods of time
Drugs	Alcohol, anticholinergics, amphetamines, anti-Parkinson medications, β-blockers, cocaine, diuretics, ecstasy, ephedra-containing diet supplements, neuroleptics, phenothiazines, tricyclic antidepressants
Body habitus	Obesity
Clothing	Thick, nonabsorbable clothing
Illnesses	Mental handicap; febrile illnesses; dehydrating illnesses such as diabetes insipidus, diabetes mellitus, diarrhea and vomiting; skin diseases such as anhidrosis; heat-producing illnesses such as thyrotoxicosis; lack of sleep, food, or water; diminished sweating as in cystic fibrosis; lack of acclimatization; previous heat stroke
Exertional heat illness	Athletes, military personnel, manual laborers

CLINICAL FEATURES

Individuals who suffer from heat exposure can present with delirium, seizures, lethargy, and coma due to metabolic disturbances, cerebral edema, or ischemia. The cerebellum is particularly sensitive to high temperatures. Neurologic complications include intracranial bleed, cerebral infarct, cerebral edema, central pontine myelinolysis, and Guillain-Barré syndrome.

Heat elimination by evaporation involves translocation of blood from central circulation to the periphery, which can lead to hypotension, especially in the presence of hypovolemia. Victims of heat stroke show electrocardiographic changes that include rhythm disturbances, conduction defects, and changes in the QT interval and the ST segment. Rhythm disturbances such as sinus tachycardia, supraventricular tachycardia, and atrial fibrillation are observed. Prolonged QT may be due to hypomagnesemia, hypocalcemia, or hypokalemia. The presence of ST segment changes indicates myocardial ischemia, which can lead to myocardial infarction.

Acute renal failure is attributed to hypovolemia, rhabdomyolysis, disseminated intravascular coagulation (DIC), and direct effects of thermal injury. *Lactic acidosis* with compensatory respiratory alkalosis occurs in exertional heat stroke. *Hyponatremia* is seen following sweat losses of >5 L/day and upon rehydration. *Hypokalemia* is seen initially as a consequence of respiratory alkalosis that is induced by hyperventilation secondary to hyperthermia, catecholamine secretion, sweat losses, and renal losses from hyperaldosteronism due to physical activity in a hot environment. Although hyperkalemia and hypokalemia occur in heat-related injury, hypokalemia is the predominant effect observed. Perturbations in phosphate levels, *hypocalcemia, hyperuricemia,* and *hypoglycemia* also occur.

Elevated serum creatine phosphokinase (CPK) indicates rhabdomyolysis. It occurs in most cases of heat stroke. The consequences of rhabdomyolysis include hyperkalemia leading to cardiotoxicity, myoglobinuria resulting in renal failure, shock from sequestration of fluid into injured muscle, and muscle necrosis of the diaphragm leading to respiratory failure.

DIFFERENTIAL DIAGNOSIS

Diagnosis of heat stroke should be suspected in anyone who presents with a core temperature of >40.6°C, hot, dry skin, and changes in mental status that include delirium, convulsions, and seizures. The differential diagnoses are listed in **Table 11.2**.

LABORATORY EVALUATION

Urine analysis may show elevated specific gravity with low urine output from dehydration and hypovolemia. Protein in the urine indicates muscle breakdown. The presence of red blood cells, myoglobin, and tubular casts denotes acute tubular necrosis as a consequence of hypovolemia and rhabdomyolysis. The finding of myoglobinuria is diagnostic of rhabdomyolysis. Urine drug screen is performed when drug ingestion is suspected. Serum chemistry typically reveals hyponatremia, hypokalemia followed by hyperkalemia, hyperphosphatemia, and hypocalcemia. Hypoglycemia is also noted in victims of heat stroke. Elevated blood urea nitrogen and creatinine levels can be observed as a consequence of dehydration and ensuing prerenal azotemia or renal failure. Increase in CPK follows rhabdomyolysis. Evaluation of arterial blood gases reveals respiratory alkalosis in cases of classic heat stroke and metabolic acidosis in cases of exertional heat strokes. A chest x-ray is useful in confirming the presence of acute respiratory distress syndrome (ARDS) and in detecting the presence of infective or aspiration pneumonia. CT imaging of the brain is performed to diagnose

TABLE 11.2

DIFFERENTIAL DIAGNOSES OF HEAT STROKE

Entities	Etiologies
Central nervous system	Meningitis, encephalitis, and hypothalamic infarction
Thyroid	Graves disease, thyroid storm
Infection	Sepsis
Drugs	Toxicity from anticholinergic, antidepressants, amphetamines, hallucinogens, cocaine, PCP, monoamine oxidase inhibitors, neuroleptics, and salicylates
Drug withdrawal	Narcotics, benzodiazepines
Metabolic	Diabetic ketoacidosis
Miscellaneous	Malignant hyperthermia

central nervous system complications of heat stroke victims such as cerebral infarction or edema. Patients with heat-related illnesses suffer from cardiac arrhythmias, which can be confirmed with a 12-lead electrocardiogram. An echocardiogram is indicated in patients who present with clinical suspicion of myocardial dysfunction. A spinal tap is useful in suspected cases of meningitis or encephalitis.

TREATMENT

Prompt attention to the ABCs of resuscitation is required. Various methods of cooling and their advantages and disadvantages are listed in **Table 11.3**. Those victims who had their airway controlled are placed on positive-pressure ventilation with supplemental oxygen to correct hypoxemia. Positive end-expiratory pressure should be titrated to treat hypoxemia and to keep FiO_2 below the toxic level of 0.5. Body cooling should be continued until core temperature is <39°C. Overhydration must be avoided. Hypocalcemia is corrected cautiously due to the risk of deposition of calcium carbonate and calcium phosphate in injured skeletal muscles. Rhabdomyolysis, identified by elevated creatine kinase and myoglobinuria, requires aggressive hydration to increase urine output to >3 mL/kg/hr. The addition of sodium bicarbonate to the IV fluids prevents tubular precipitation of myoglobin if the urine pH is raised to >6.5. In addition to volume expansion, mannitol 0.25 g/kg IV may be used as an osmotic diuretic to increase urine flow once adequate hydration has been assured. If meticulous monitoring of the electrocardiographic pattern shows signs of hyperkalemia (tall T waves, prolonged P-R interval, widened QRS, any dysrhythmia), the risk-benefit ratio argues for calcium administration. Aggressive lowering of the serum potassium level is paramount with (a) glucose 1 g/kg and insulin 0.1 unit/kg IV; (b) sodium polystyrene sulfonate (Kayexalate) 1 g/kg via nasogastric tube every 2–6 hrs; and/or (c) dialysis. Hyperphosphatemia is managed with phosphate binders (sevelamer) and dialysis. Hyperuricemia is managed with hydration, alkalinization, and drug therapy, including allopurinol and recombinant uricase (rasburicase). The most important aspect in the prevention of renal failure is to adequately hydrate patients.

TABLE 11.3

METHODS OF COOLING

Cooling method	Description	Advantages	Disadvantages
EXTERNAL COOLING			
Immersion	Immersion of body in ice water	Faster cooling, greater temperature gradient between core and periphery	Vasoconstriction; interferes with heat loss; shivering; interferes with resuscitative measures
Body-cooling unit	Spraying finely atomized water mixed with warm air to keep body temperature above 32°–33°C	Faster cooling (mean cooling rate of 0.31°C/min or 32.6°F/min); comfortable to the patient; heat is lost by evaporation and convection	Sophisticated unit that requires maintenance and storage
Wet sheet and fan	Patients are covered with a sheet, water is sprayed over the sheet, and fans are used to blow over the wet sheet	Heat lost by evaporation; heat loss is comparable to body-cooling unit; easy maintenance	
Ice packs	Ice packs are placed over the groin, axillae, and neck	Simple and readily available; inexpensive; shorter cooling time when combined with evaporative technique	Longer cooling time compared to evaporative technique
CORE COOLING			
Cold-water irrigation	Gastric, bladder, peritoneal lavage, extracorporeal technique	Not well studied	Invasive, especially peritoneal and extracorporeal techniques
IV fluids	Cold IV fluid administration	Not studied	Noninvasive

Shock can follow rhabdomyolysis from sequestration of large quantities of fluid into the injured muscles in the first 24 hrs following heat injury. The administered fluid may contribute to edema in injured muscles, which can lead to compartment syndrome in the extremities. Compartment syndrome generally occurs on the third or fourth day following injury and results in a secondary elevation of creatine kinase due to muscle necrosis from compression by trapped fluid. Fasciotomy is recommended if an increase in compartment pressures is documented or if clinical signs such as pulselessness, paresthesias, pain, or paralysis of the extremity, are present.

HYPERTHERMIA SYNDROMES

Malignant Hyperthermia

Malignant hyperthermia (MH) is a genetic syndrome that requires exposure to certain potent inhaled general anesthetics (halothane, isoflurane, sevoflurane) and/or the depolarizing muscle relaxant succinylcholine. Patients who are suspected to have MH should undergo testing at an MH testing center, wear a "medic alert" bracelet, and obtain up-to-date information from the Malignant Hyperthermia Association of the United States at www. mhaus.org. Patients with muscular dystrophy, myotonia, and central core disease are at increased risk. The cardinal features of MH include muscle rigidity. The sustained muscle contracture generates heat and greatly increased muscle metabolism, which in turn, lead to increased CO_2 production (increased end-tidal CO_2 concentration), acidosis, tachypnea, and tachycardia (including ventricular tachycardia). The body temperature often exceeds $41°C$. In the absence of prompt medical intervention, rhabdomyolysis supervenes, with the risk of hyperkalemia, ventricular tachycardia, myoglobinuric renal failure, and cardiac arrest. All patients who develop intraoperative MH must be admitted to an ICU because recrudescence of MH occurs in 20% of patients, especially in those with a muscular body type. The time between the initial onset of MH and recrudescence averages 13 hrs. Therapy for MH consists of immediate discontinuation of inhaled anesthesia and/or succinylcholine. The inspired gas is converted to 100% O_2 at high flow rates to wash out residual anesthetic as rapidly as possible. The muscle relaxant dantrolene, 2.5 mg/kg IV, is given as rapidly as possible. The dose may be repeated to control signs of hypermetabolism. Cold normal saline, 15 mL/kg, is administered rapidly if temperature is $>39°C$. Emergency laboratory testing involves serum potassium, creatine kinase, arterial blood gas, and coagulation tests to evaluate hyperkalemia, rhabdomyolysis, metabolic acidosis, and DIC, respectively.

In contrast to classic MH, patients with malignant hyperthermia-like syndrome (MHLS) are not exposed to anesthetics or succinylcholine; rather they present with type II diabetic coma and a hyperglycemic, hyperosmolar nonketotic state. Hyperthermia occurs typically after administration of insulin. The patients were usually obese African American males with acanthosis nigrans. Rhabdomyolysis, hemodynamic instability, and organ failure punctuate the course of this condition. Therapy for MHLS should include the immediate administration of dantrolene. Because dantrolene must be diluted in sterile water, a calculated dose of hypertonic saline can be administered concurrently to prevent a rapid decline in serum osmolality, which may precipitate cerebral edema. Cooling methods outlined in **Table 11.3** are indicated until temperature is $<39°C$.

Neurolept Malignant Syndrome

Neurolept malignant syndrome (NMS) is a rare clinical syndrome associated with the use of andipsychotic drugs and characterized classically by four cardinal signs: muscle rigidity, mental status changes (confusion, agitation, catatonia, encephalopathy, coma), hyperthermia, and autonomic instability (tachycardia, labile hypertension, diaphoresis). Risk factors for NMS appear to correlate with potent antipsychotics (e.g., haloperidol), rapid dose escalation, concomitant use of lithium, and comorbid diseases such as acute infection. Dantrolene, bromocriptine, and amantadine have been used to treat NMS.

Serotonin Syndrome

Serotonin syndrome (SS) is a clinical syndrome that exhibits signs of excess postsynaptic serotonergic neurotransmission, which may include hyperthermia. The classic triad of SS signs includes abnormalities of mental status (agitation, delirium), neuromuscular function, (hyperreflexia, clonus, hypertonicity, tremor), and autonomic function (hyperthermia, tachycardia, hypertension, diaphoresis, vomiting, diarrhea). Clonus may be spontaneous, inducible, or ocular. SS is often confused with NMS, but clonus is not a prominent finding in NMS. Furthermore, NMS develops over days and weeks, whereas SS usually develops within 24 hrs (**Table 11.4**). The Hunter Serotonin Toxicity Criteria incorporate the most important findings (clonus, agitation, diaphoresis, tremor, hyperreflexia, hypertonicity, hyperthermia) into a decision-making rule set. The

TABLE 11.4

DRUGS THAT INCREASE SEROTONIN LEVELS AND MAY PRECIPITATE SEROTONIN SYNDROME

Class	Mechanism	Examples
Dietary supplement	Increases serotonin formation	L-tryptophan
Illicit drug	Increases release of serotonin	Amphetamines, ecstasy, cocaine
Weight loss drug (amphetamine derivatives)	Increases release of serotonin	Phentermine, fenfluramine, dexfenfluramine
Herbal medication	Prevents reuptake of serotonin into the presynaptic neuron	St. John's Wort
Antidepressant: Selective serotonin re-uptake inhibitor	Prevents reuptake of serotonin into the presynaptic neuron	Citalopram, escitalopram, fluoxetine, paroxetine, sertraline
Antidepressant: Tricyclic antidepressant	Prevents reuptake of serotonin into the presynaptic neuron	Amitriptyline, amoxapine, desipramine, doxepin, imipramine, maprotiline, nortriptyline, protriptyline, trimipramine
Antidepressant: Selective serotonin/norepinephrine re-uptake inhibitor	Prevents reuptake of serotonin and norepinephrine into the presynaptic neuron	Bupropion, trazodone, nefazodone, venlafaxine
Antidepressant: Monoamine oxidase inhibitor	Inhibits metabolism of serotonin	Phenelzine, tranylcypromine, isocarboxazid
Antibiotic: Monoamine oxidase inhibitor (MAOI)	Inhibits metabolism of serotonin	Linezolid
Migraine drug	Activates serotonin 5-HT1 receptors	Almotriptan (Axert), naratriptan (Amerge), sumatriptan (Imitrex), zolmitriptan (Zomig)
Antiemetics	Prevents reuptake of serotonin into the presynaptic neuron	Ondansetron, granisetron
Antitussive	Prevents reuptake of serotonin into the presynaptic neuron	Dextromethorphan
Analgesic	Activates serotonin 5-HT1 receptors	Fentanyl

management of SS relies upon supportive care, as outlined for other hyperthermia syndromes. The serotonergic drug is discontinued immediately. Agitated patients should receive benzodiazepine sedation. If the triggering agent is a monoamine oxidase inhibitor (MAOI), which has caused hypotension, then it is prudent to avoid inotropes (e.g., dopamine) that are metabolized by monoamine oxidase inhibitors. After fluid volume resuscitation, a direct-acting vasoconstrictor such as phenylephrine is preferred to treat hypotension. The antidote for SS is cyproheptadine. Because cyproheptadine is only available as an oral formulation (tablet or syrup), it should be given via nasogastric tube at a total daily dose of 0.25 mg/kg divided every 6 hrs. The maximum daily dose is 12 mg for children 2–6 years and 16 mg for children 7–14 years old.

HYPOTHERMIA

Frostnip is a mild form of cold injury. It is a nonfreezing injury of skin tissues, usually of the face, fingertips, or toes of patients who are exposed to cold temperatures of ~15°C (59°F). A more significant nonfreezing injury is termed *chilblains*, which can occur as tissue temperature drops below 15°C (59°F). Treatment of frostnip and chilblains usually involves simple rewarming. *Frostbite* is the destruction of skin or other tissues caused by freezing between 6.1°C and –15°C. *Hypothermia* is defined as a core body temperature of <35°C (95°F). The degree of hypothermia has implications regarding expected pathophysiologic changes and appropriate therapeutic modalities. Thermogenesis, or heat production,

TABLE 11.5

ORGAN SYSTEM RESPONSES TO HYPOTHERMIA

Severity of hypothermia	Central nervous system	Cardiovascular	Respiratory	Metabolic, renal, endocrine	Neuromuscular
Mild (35°–32°C)	Depressed cerebral metabolism; confusion; amnesia; ataxia	Vasoconstriction; tachycardia followed by bradycardia; increased cardiac output; hypertension	Tachypnea followed by progressive decrease in minute ventilation; bronchospasm; impaired mucosal function	Increased metabolism; increased oxygen consumption; cold diuresis; impairment of renal-concentrating ability; hypovolemia	Increased tone with shivering, followed by muscle fatigue
Moderate (<32°–28°C)	Unconsciousness; papillary dilation; diminished gag reflex	Bradycardia; decreased contractility; slowed cardiac conduction; J waves on ECG; arrhythmias	Hypoventilation with acidosis despite decrease in CO_2 production; V/Q mismatch; decreased oxygen consumption	Decreased renal blood flow; no insulin activity	Extinction of shivering; hyporeflexia; muscle rigidity
Severe (<28°C)	Decreased or no EEG activity; nonreactive pupils; loss of ocular reflexes	Progressive decrease in BP, cardiac output, and heart rate; ventricular arrhythmias (fibrillation); asystole	Lung capillary damage; pulmonary edema; further decreased oxygen consumption; apnea	Decrease in basal metabolism; acidosis; renal failure	Areflexia; rhabdomyolysis

ECG, electrocardiogram; EEG, electroencephalogram; BP, blood pressure

TABLE 11.6

ETIOLOGIES OF HYPOTHERMIA

Increased heat loss	Decreased heat production	Impaired thermoregulation	Other clinical states
Environmental	**Neuromuscular insufficiency**	**Central nervous system failure or abnormalities**	Multisystem trauma
Immersion	Age extremes	Hemorrhage/infarction	Sepsis
Nonimmersion	Impaired shivering	Trauma	Shock
Iatrogenic	Lack of adaptation	Birth asphyxia	Systemic Acidoses
Exposure	**Insufficient fuel**	Tumors	Pancreatitis
Cold IV infusions	Hypoglycemia	Malformations	Uremia
Emergency deliveries	Malnutrition	Metabolic causes	Familial
Heat stroke treatment	Extreme physical exertion	Ethanol	dysautonomia
Dermatologic	Impaired mobility	Pharmacologic:	Water intoxication
Burns	**Endocrinologic failure**	barbiturates, narcotics,	Episodic
Exfoliative dermatitis	Hypothyroidism	phenothiazines, lithium	spontaneous
Induced vasodilation or	Hypopituitarism	**Peripheral nervous system**	hypothermia with
impaired peripheral	Hypoadrenalism	**failure**	hyperhidrosis
vasoconstriction		Neuropathies	
Ethanol		Diabetes	
Pharmacologic:		Acute spinal cord	
phenothiazines,		transection	
α-blockers			

normally occurs in obligatory ways, such as that due to basal metabolism and exercise. The conservation of heat occurs in response to cold stress. The response by the cutaneous circulation is a locally initiated and mediated vasoconstrictor response. The responses at different degrees of hypothermia are summarized in **Table 11.5**.

The organ system response to immersion in cold water versus exposure to cold air can be dramatically different at the onset of the insult. An initial "cold shock" results in uncontrolled respiratory gasping and hyperventilation, tachycardia, and hypertension. Respiratory alkalosis and cerebral vasoconstriction occur. Conditions that involve total immersion, including the head, initiate a "diving reflex" that consists of apnea, marked bradycardia, increased peripheral vascular resistance, and increased blood supply to the brain and heart.

Hypothermia may occur due to a variety of causes and can be accidental or nonaccidental and environmental or nonenvironmental (**Table 11.6**). The clinical features noted in mild, moderate, and severe hypothermia are listed in **Table 11.7**. Hypothermia leads to acidosis, altered blood clotting, and decreased kidney and renal function. Hypokalemia and hyperkalemia occur, and hyperkalemia becomes prominent with increased severity of hypothermia. Liver function tests are abnormal secondary to reduced cardiac output. Hyperglycemia occurs in acute hypothermia, but hy-

poglycemia may be seen in subacute or chronic hypothermic conditions. Hypothermia results in prolongation of prothrombin and partial thromboplastin times.

Clinical Management

Passive rewarming—the use of blankets to cover the head, neck, and body—reduces evaporative heat loss and can rewarm at a rate of 0.5°–4°C/hr. This method will be unsuccessful if shivering or other thermoregulatory mechanisms are absent. Passive external rewarming is usually an adequate treatment modality for patients with mild hypothermia.

Active external warming—the application of heat directly to the skin—is effective only if the patient has an intact circulation that can return peripherally rewarmed blood to the core. Warm blankets and heating blankets rewarm at variable rates and may also produce burns to the skin. Radiant warmers can also produce skin burns if patients are not covered with blankets. Forced-heated-air devices such as the Bair Hugger device can rewarm at a rate of 1°–2.5°C/hr by heat transfer via convection. Warm water immersion is not recommended because the patient cannot be monitored. External methods of rewarming are usually effective for mild-to-moderate hypothermia. Complications of active external warming are core temperature "after-drop."

TABLE 11.7

CLINICAL FEATURES OF HYPOTHERMIA

	Mild hypothermia (35°–32°C)	Moderate hypothermia (<32°–28°C)	Severe hypothermia (<28°C)
Thermoregulatory	Shivering	Extinction of shivering	No shivering
Respiratory	Tachypnea	Hypoventilation, respiratory acidosis, hypoxemia, aspiration pneumonia, atelectasis	Apnea, pulmonary edema, acute respiratory distress syndrome
Cardiovascular	Tachycardia, hypertension	Bradycardia, hypotension, prolonged QT interval, J wave, atrial arrhythmias	Pulseless electrical activity, atrial and ventricular fibrillation, asystole
Gastrointestinal	Ileus, nausea, vomiting	Pancreatitis, gastric erosions	Pancreatitis, gastric erosions
Renal/fluid/electrolyte	Cold diuresis, hypokalemia, alkalosis	Hyperkalemia, hyperglycemia, lactic acidosis	Hyperkalemia, hyperglycemia, lactic acidosis
Muscular	Hypertonia	Rigidity	Rhabdomyolysis
Hematologic		Hemoconcentration, hypercoagulability	Thrombocytopenia, disseminated intravascular coagulation, bleeding
Neurologic	Disorientation, impaired judgment, dysarthria, ataxia, hyperreflexia	Agitation, hallucination, unconsciousness, dilated pupils, diminished gag reflex, hyporeflexia	Coma, nonreactive pupils, areflexia, brain-dead-like state

Active internal warming methods include heated (42°C), humidified air via an endotracheal tube and heated (42°C) IV fluids via rapid infusion. Together, these methods can warm at a rate of 1°–2°C/hr. More invasive techniques include body cavity lavage (gastric, bladder, colon, pleural, peritoneal) with warmed saline, which can warm at a rate of 1°–4°C/hr. The most invasive methods of active internal rewarming are extracorporeal and include continuous arteriovenous or venovenous warming, hemodialysis and cardiopulmonary bypass. The first three require the presence of a pulse and adequate blood pressure. Cardiopulmonary bypass is highly effective and can increase core temperature by 1°–2°C every 3–5 mins. In addition, it provides the benefit of full circulatory support. Cardiopulmonary bypass is the method indicated for severe hypothermia associated with either the failure of less-invasive, active rewarming techniques, or severe hypothermia accompanied by cardiac arrest, or a nonperfusing cardiac rhythm. An algorithm for the rewarming approach to the hypothermic patient is shown in **Figure 11.1**.

Most dysrhythmias correct with rewarming alone. Hypothermic patients with cardiac arrest or nonperfusing rhythms require modification of conventional advanced life support protocols, as their hearts may be unresponsive to cardiovascular drugs, defibrillation, and pacemaker stimulation. For those with moderate hypothermia, cardiopulmonary resuscitation should be initiated and, if indicated, defibrillation should be attempted. However, IV resuscitative medications should be spaced at longer intervals. In the patient with severe hypothermia and cardiac arrest, cardiopulmonary resuscitation should be initiated, but attempts at ventricular fibrillation and administration of resuscitative medications should be withheld until the patient is rewarmed above 30°C with active internal rewarming methods. Resuscitative efforts in the severely hypothermic patient may be very prolonged, especially if extracorporeal warming is unavailable. Although a patient may appear clinically dead, resuscitative efforts should continue at least until the patient has been rewarmed to nearly normal core temperature.

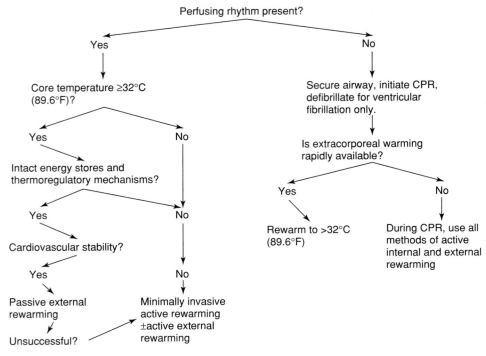

FIGURE 11.1. Rewarming approach for hypothermia.

Laboratory evaluation of the hypothermic patient may demonstrate numerous abnormalities to consider in the context of current acute and chronic conditions. Evaluation should include serum electrolytes, blood glucose, renal function tests, arterial blood gases and pH, complete blood cell count, and coagulation studies. Drug toxicology screens and blood alcohol level should be obtained when appropriate. The patient's hematocrit may be elevated. Aggressive volume resuscitation is warranted in hypothermic patients secondary to the dehydration caused by cold diuresis and the vascular expansion with vasodilatation upon rewarming.

CHAPTER 12 ◼ ENVENOMATION SYNDROMES

JAMES TIBBALLS • KENNETH D. WINKEL

SNAKEBITE

Venomous snakes can be classified into 2 major families: the *Elapidae* and the *Viperidae*. The elapids are front-fanged, terrestrial snakes (the taipan, brown, death adder, tiger, and black snakes); the cobras, mambas and kraits; and the coral snakes. The venoms of elapid species are highly neurotoxic, with an additional effect of cytotoxicity in some species (e.g., spitting cobras). Vipers have characteristically large front, foldable fangs and venom that is less toxic but notable for inducing bite-site swelling and tissue destruction. These snakes include the rattlesnakes and the old- and new-world vipers. A small number of venomous colubrids, a family of back-fanged snakes, such as the African Boomslang, are also medically important. A fourth family is the *Hydrophiidae*, or sea snakes, which are found along much of the IndoPacific coastline, predominantly in the tropics. Snake venom displays neurotoxic, myotoxic, procoagulant

TABLE 12.1

THE CLINICAL FEATURES OF VARIOUS MEDICALLY SIGNIFICANT VENOMOUS SNAKES OF THE WORLD

Region and species	Clinical features				
	Neurotoxic	Coagulopathic	Local cytotoxic	Myotoxic	Other
South America					
Bothrops spp (lance-headed vipers)	−	++	++	+	Shock, renal failure
Crotalus durrissus terrificus (pit vipers)	++	++	−	+++	Renal failure
North America					
Crotalus spp. (pit vipers)	+	++	++	+	Shock, renal failure
Micrurus spp. (coral snakes)	++			++	
Australia-Papua New Guinea					
Oxyuranus spp. (taipan)	+++	+++		+	Renal failure
Acanthophis spp. (death adder)	+++				
Notechis spp. (tiger)	+++	+++		++	Renal failure
Pseudechis spp. (black)	+	++	−	+++	Renal failure
Pseudonaja spp. (brown)	++	+++			Renal failure
Asia					
Daboia russelii (Russell's viper)	−/+	+++	++	+++	Shock, renal failure
Naja spp (cobras)	+++		+++		Shock
Naja philippinensis (Philippines cobra)	+++	−	+	−	Shock
Ophiophagus hannah (King cobra)	+++				
Echis carinatus (saw-scaled viper)	−	++	+++	−	Shock, renal failure
Bungaris spp. (kraits)	++		−	−	
Calloselasma rhodostoma (Malayan pit viper)		+++	+++		Shock, renal failure
Europe					
Vipera spp. (European adders)	+/−	++			Shock, renal failure
Africa					
Cerastes cerastes (Saharan horned viper)		+++	++		Shock
Echis ocellatus (carpet viper)		+++	++		Shock, renal failure
Naja spp (African spitting cobras)			+++		
Bitis gabonica (gaboon viper)	+	+++	+++		Cardiotoxic
Bitis arietans (puff adder)		++	+++		Cardiotoxic
Dendroaspis spp. (mambas)	+++		+/++		
Indopacific					
Hydrophids (sea snakes)	+++		+	++/+++	Renal failure

The symbols represent subjective degrees of severity: −, little clinical effect; +, mild effect of envenomation; ++, moderate effect; +++, severe effect. This is only an approximate guide as the extent of the envenomation syndrome varies with the species or subspecies. Adapted from Cheng AC, Currie BJ. *J Intensive Care Med* 2004;19:259–69, and Meier J, White J. *Clinical Toxicity of Animal Venoms and Poisons*. Florida: CRC Press, 1995.

and anticoagulant, and cytotoxic and hemolytic properties. The composition of venoms influences the clinical presentation of snakebites (**Table 12.1**).

A high index of suspicion should be maintained in children who suddenly become ill while unsupervised outside, particularly in rural areas and in the summer months. Signs of snakebite, but not necessarily envenomation, may include puncture marks and/or bleeding or oozing. Another sign of snakebite is regional tender lymphadenopathy, which may also be present after bites from nonvenomous snakes and is thus not by itself an indication for antivenom. The symptoms and signs of envenomation and the time course follow a predictable sequence (**Table 12.2**).

Laboratory investigations should include the following:

- Snake venom detection kit (SVDK) (preferably bite site, but secondarily urine or blood—only in Australia and Papua New Guinea)

TABLE 12.2

EXPECTED SEQUENCE OF MAJOR SYSTEMIC SYMPTOMS AND SIGNS AFTER
ENVENOMATION BY ELAPID SNAKE SPECIES

<1 hr after bite
Headache
Nausea, vomiting, abdominal pain
Transient hypotension associated with confusion or loss of consciousness
Coagulopathy (laboratory testing or whole-blood clotting time)
Regional lymphadenitis

1–3 hr after bite
Paresis/paralysis of cranial nerves, e.g., ptosis, double vision, external ophthalmoplegia, dysphonia,
  dysphagia, myopathic facies
Hemorrhage from mucosal surfaces and needle punctures secondary to DIC
Tachycardia, hypotension
Tachypnea, shallow tidal volume

>3 hr after bite
Paresis/paralysis of truncal and limb muscles
Paresis/paralysis of respiratory muscles (respiratory failure)
Peripheral circulatory failure (shock), hypoxemia, cyanosis
Rhabdomyolysis
Dark urine (due to myoglobinuria or hemoglobin)
Renal failure secondary to combinations of shock, hypoxemia, DIC, rhabdomyolysis and hemolysis
Coma secondary to cerebral hypoxemia or ischemia, occasionally due to hemorrhage

A more rapid illness may develop after multiple bites or in small child.
DIC, disseminated intravascular coagulation.

- Coagulation studies INR/PT, APTT, ACT, D-dimer, X-FDP, and fibrinogen. In remote areas where sophisticated clotting tests are unavailable, a simple test of coagulation may be performed by placing a sample of the patient's blood in a plain glass tube. It should clot within 10 mins in the absence of coagulopathy. If it remains unclotted at 20 mins (the "20-min whole-blood clotting test"), it is a highly sensitive and specific test of coagulopathy.
- Creatine kinase for myolysis
- Urinalysis for hemoglobin, myoglobin
- Renal function may be impaired secondary to myoglobinuria or other mechanisms
- Electrolytes—particularly K+, which may be elevated with rhabdomyolysis
- Full blood count—The white cell count is usually only mildly elevated; significant leukocytosis may indicate other pathology. Thrombocytopenia may occur with some snakebites both in isolation and as part of disseminated intravascular coagulation (DIC) or microangiopathic hemolytic anemia.

Venom may be injected quite deeply; consequently, little venom is removed by incision or excision (cutting or sucking). These practices are not recommended and may be dangerous, particularly in the coagulopathic patient. The use of arterial tourniquets, especially for prolonged periods, may also be dangerous and is no longer recommended for any type of venomous bite or sting. Suction devices are ineffective and may even worsen local tissue damage. Pressure-immobilization first aid for venomous bites and stings uses a continuous bandage applied, as tightly as binding a sprained ankle, to the whole limb; then a splint is applied to prevent movement. For example, for a bite on the ankle, the bandage is applied continuously from the toes upward to include the bite site and is extended above the knee, and a splint is applied to prevent use and movement of the limb. The rationale is compression of lymphatic channels and inactivation of the "muscle pump" by which lymph flows and by which venom reaches the circulation. Retarding the movement of venom from the bite site into the circulation "buys time" for the patient to reach medical care. Once an asymptomatic patient has reached a hospital that has appropriate antivenom, first aid measures may be removed. If, on removal of first aid measures, the patient's condition deteriorates, the bandages can be reapplied while antivenom is administered. If the patient has not developed any symptoms or signs of envenomation or any indication of coagulopathy or myolysis on blood taken 4–6 hrs after the removal of first aid (or after the bite if no first aid was used), then the patient has probably not sustained a significant envenomation, though delayed onset of symptoms up to 24 hrs after bites has been described. Particular care is required if a neurotoxic elapid bite is suspected, as few signs may be present apart from late-onset neurotoxicity. Overnight observation is desirable, especially if the patient is a young child or comes from a remote area. Ongoing evaluations of local tissue damage, coagulopathy, neurotoxicity, rhabdomyolysis, renal failure, shock, and cardiotoxicity will dictate ongoing therapies. All patients should receive appropriate tetanus and antibiotic prophylaxis if the bite wound is contaminated (but not otherwise).

Antivenom is the only specific treatment for bites by venomous snakes. Anticholinesterase inhibitors such as neostigmine may assist in the emergency management of predominantly post-junctional neurotoxic envenomations, due to the curare-like actions of neurotoxins. Antivenom is indicated if evidence is observed of systemic envenomation or progressive limb swelling or necrosis. If pressure-immobilization first aid is in place, symptoms or signs of envenomation, including laboratory signs, may only become apparent when first aid measures are removed. Antivenoms only neutralize the venoms used in their production. Australia and Papua New Guinea are the only countries that have a commercially available SVDK. This test is a rapid, two-step, enzyme immunoassay in which reactions occur with antibodies to the venoms of major Australian snake genera. If a reliable identification of the snake cannot be made, polyvalent antivenom or a selection of monovalent that covers likely species should be used. Skin testing for allergy to antivenom is not recommended. Antivenoms should be diluted in at least 100 mL of normal saline, 5% dextrose, or Hartmann solution immediately prior to administration. Initial administration should be slow, while the patient is observed for signs of allergic reaction. If no reaction is observed, the infusion may be run over 15–30 mins. If the patient reacts to the antivenom, the rate may be slowed or the infusion ceased temporarily. If reaction is severe, treatment with adrenaline, antihistamines, corticosteroids, or plasma volume expanders should be undertaken as required. For premedications, adults should receive 0.25 mg of epinephrine by the subcutaneous route (0.005 mg/kg for children). Serum sickness due to the deposition of immune complexes is a recognized complication of the administration of foreign protein solutions such as antivenoms. Symptoms include fever, rash, arthralgia, lymphadenopathy, and a flu-like illness. It usually occurs 7–10 days after antivenom administration. Both the incidence and severity of delayed serum sickness may be reduced by the administration of prednisolone, 1–2 mg/kg daily for 5 days after the administration of antivenoms.

SPIDER BITE

Funnel-web spiders are the most dangerous spiders in the world, as they have caused death within 2 hrs. Any dark-colored or brown spider that is 2–3 cm in body size on the eastern seaboard of Australia should be regarded, from a medical perspective, as if it were a funnel-web. Capture and formal identification of the spider is helpful. The characterization of Phases 1 and 2 of envenomation by the funnel-web spider, as well as its treatment, are listed in **Table 12.3**. If no symptoms or signs of envenomation have begun 4 hrs after the removal of first aid measures or after the bite, the patient may be discharged. Tetanus status should be assessed and prophylaxis provided if indicated.

The widow, button, koppie, or redback spiders are the most medically significant. Bites by widow spiders produce a recognizable syndrome, "latrodectism," that may necessitate antivenom administration. Usually the bite is painful, but it may be relatively painless and, unless the spider is seen, may initially go unnoticed. Puncture marks and swelling are uncommon. Effects may persist for weeks after an untreated bite and have been successfully treated with black widow or redback spider antivenom weeks or even months after the bite. Signs and symptoms include (a) local pain that radiates from the bite site and involves the entire limb, which increases over the first hour and typically persists for >24 hrs; (b) localized redness, piloerection, painful regional lymphadenopathy, and sweating (sometimes affecting only the bitten limb but sometimes occurring in a distribution unrelated to the bite site); (c) systemic features, including fever, hypertension, tachycardia, nausea and vomiting, abdominal pain, headache, lethargy, and insomnia; and (d) migratory arthralgia and paraesthesias. Children generally present with irritability and local pain, erythema, and nonspecific maculopapular rashes. Myalgia/neck spasms in children >4 years of age seem to be a prominent feature. Antivenom should be administered for pain that is unrelieved by simple analgesia (e.g., local application of ice or oral analgesics) and/or with systemic symptoms or signs of envenomation such as vomiting, severe headache, abdominal pain and collapse, hypertension, arthralgia, or myalgia. Typically, antivenom is effective within the first 2 hrs after injection, but occasionally symptoms can reappear, necessitating a further dose. The reaction rate to redback antivenom (manufactured by CSL, Ltd.) is low; therefore, premedication is usually not recommended, but patients with a history of horse allergy or prior exposure to equine immunoglobulin may be at higher risk for acute or delayed allergic reactions. The incidence of serum sickness is low; therefore, corticosteroids are not recommended routinely.

TABLE 12.3

EFFECTS AND TREATMENT OF ENVENOMATION BY FUNNEL-WEB SPIDERS

Phase I

Local Effects
- Bite site may be painful for days to weeks because of direct trauma and acidity of venom, but no local necrosis has been recorded.
- Local swelling and erythema

General Effects
- Numbness around the mouth, and spasms or fasciculation of the tongue
- Nausea and vomiting, abdominal pain, and acute gastric dilatation
- Profuse sweating, salivation, lacrimation, piloerection, and severe dyspnea
- Confusion progressing to coma
- Hypertension, tachycardia, and vasoconstriction (hypotension may occur later)
- Local and generalized muscle fasciculation and spasm, which may be prolonged and violent (facial, tongue, or intercostal muscles and including trismus)

Phase 2
- Hypotension
- Hypoventilation and apnea
- Acute noncardiogenic pulmonary edema
- Coma and, finally, irreversible cardiac arrest

Treatment
- Maintenance of airway, breathing, and circulation
- Prompt application of a PIB to affected limb, as for neurotoxic elapid snake bite. The PIB should be removed only after the patient has reached a location where appropriate resuscitation can be given and antivenom is available.
- If the PIB is removed and the patient deteriorates, it should be reapplied.
- If antivenom is not available, the PIB should be kept in place, because evidence from animal experiments suggests that venom may be inactivated at the bite site.
- Administration of IV antivenom
- Intubation and ventilation for respiratory failure and to reduce intracranial pressure (note: endotracheal intubation may be hindered by excessive salivary secretions and violent fasciculations)
- Supportive care (additional) may include:
  —Atropine in doses sufficient (20 mcg/kg initial dose) to reduce salivation and bronchorrhea
  —Nasogastric aspiration to relieve gastric dilatation
  —Muscle relaxants and sedatives to facilitate mechanical ventilation
  —Sympathetic blockade for hypertension and severe tachycardia
  —Fluid resuscitation in the event of hypotension, but with caution because of risk of noncardiogenic pulmonary edema

PIB, pressure-immobilization bandage.

Unlike most other antivenoms, administration of widow or redback spider antivenom may be effective even several weeks after a bite. Unlike snake antivenoms, redback and widow antivenom may be administered by the intramuscular route. However, if envenomation is severe or if response to intramuscular injection is poor, the IV route can be used. If given IV, the antivenom should be diluted in 100–500 mL of crystalloid solution (normal saline, Hartmann solution, or dextrose) and run over 15–30 mins. The redback antivenom is also effective against other widow spiders that cause latrodectism-like symptoms.

Loxosceles spiders cause "loxoscelism." Envenomation causes two syndromes: cutaneous loxoscelism and viscerocutaneous loxoscelism. Cutaneous loxoscelism is characterized by a dermonecrotic lesion at the bite site that can take weeks to heal. By day 3 or 4, the initial hemorrhagic areas degrade into a central area of blue necrosis, which eventually forms an eschar that sinks below the surface of the skin. This common pattern is referred to as the "red, white, and blue sign." This appearance of the wound differentiates this bite from non-necrotic ulcers, which tend to maintain a red lesion that remains raised above the surrounding skin. Viscerocutaneous loxoscelism is a severe systemic illness that sometimes occurs after *Loxosceles* envenomation in addition to the local damage. It consists of a low grade fever, arthralgia, diarrhea, vomiting, coagulopathy, disseminated intravascular coagulation, hemolysis, petechia, thrombocytopenia, urticaria, and sometimes rhabdomyolysis.

Despite the fact that loxoscelism is a leading cause of spider-bite morbidity in some regions, a definitive therapy is not established. Sulfones (i.e., dapsone) inhibit polymorphonuclear lymphocyte degranulation, reducing local tissue inflammation and subsequent destruction caused by these cells. Because of its side effects (including cholestatic jaundice, hepatitis, leukopenia, methemoglobinemia, hemolytic anemia, and rarely, peripheral neuropathy) and limited supporting data, the benefit-to-risk ratio of dapsone has been questioned. Nonetheless, its use is advocated in the US and Brazil. Early surgical management in general has been found to be ineffective and sometimes harmful as an initial management technique. Surgical excision only after a delay of 2–8 weeks allows dissipation of venom and the subsequent acute-phase reactants. The most important intervention might be wound irrigation. Various reviews indicate that, while systemic corticosteroids are not recommended for the cutaneous form of loxoscelism, they might have a role for viscerocutaneous loxoscelism. Necrotic lesions of any cause are usually treated with oral antibiotics to prevent infection, although this may be unnecessary if necrotic ulceration is highly likely to be due to envenomation. In a classic envenomation lesion, antibiotics are not indicated in the absence of evidence of infection. *Loxosceles* antivenoms are available through 4 sources (Institute Butantan in São Paulo and Centro de Produção e Pesquisa em Imunobiológicos in Paraná, both in Brazil; The Institutos Nacionales de Salud in Lima, Peru; and Instituto Bioclon in Mexico), but none are available in the US. The Brazilian Ministry of Health has the most extensive use of antibody treatment and has developed guidelines for its use in large cutaneous lesions and extensive necrosis or systemic illness. In most clinical investigations, a significant delay usually occurs between the actual bite and presentation for treatment. This delay does not negate the potential value of delayed use of antivenom to decrease lesion size and/or limit systemic illness.

The viscerocutaneous form of loxoscelismac causes renal failure resulting from hemolysis and from direct nephrotoxic effect, which may be more pronounced in children. Corticosteroids for viscerocutaneous loxoscelism are universally accepted as a means to help protect reticulocytes from the venom effect.

SCORPION STINGS

These nocturnally active creatures inhabit areas with warm or hot dry climates within a 45° latitude of either side of the Equator. Scorpion venom causes release of transmitters at sympathetic, parasympathetic,

and neuromuscular receptors. Life-threatening cardiovascular and neurotoxic effects are caused by most species. A systemic inflammatory response with cytokine release, kinin release, and complement activation may lead to multiorgan failure Although pain is the universal feature of envenomation by scorpions, bites may cause the following: coma, convulsions, cerebral edema, external ophthalmoplegia, mydriasis, meiosis, agitation, rigidity, tremor, twitching, tongue and muscle fasciculation, respiratory failure, gastric and pancreatic hypersecretion, bradycardia, tachycardia, salivation, sweating, abdominal pain, vomiting, and priapism. Myocardial ischemia or myocarditis with raised CPK-MB isoenzymes and cardiac troponin I levels may occur in children. Physicians experienced in treating scorpion envenomation suggest reserving antivenom therapy for patients with significant systemic toxicity, which includes arrhythmia, hypertension, hypotension, seizures, coma, or pulmonary edema. Intensive monitoring and titration of vasodilator and inotropic agents is required, along with judicious mechanical ventilation. In early envenomation, catecholamine release causes hypertension, but this may later culminate in cardiac failure and hypotension. Hydralazine, nifedipine, and oral prazosin have been used successfully clinically.

WASP STINGS

While reactions to most stings by Hymenoptera are mild and self-limiting, a life-threatening, immediate, hypersensitivity reaction (anaphylaxis) may occur for which the same treatment protocol should be adopted regardless of the responsible creature. Like bees, wasps are colony insects that construct large nests, often among the lower tree branches, where they can be accidentally disturbed, provoking an aggressive swarm attack. A wasp nest near a home or school should be destroyed, preferably at night when the wasps are less likely to attack, by experienced personnel wearing protective clothing. Despite some common components, wasp venom components vary greatly among species, with variable lethal doses. Hornets (*Vespa*) have potent venom (LD_{50} ranging from 1.6 to 4.1 mg/kg in four *Vespa* spp.) that can deliver lethal doses in as few as 50–200 stings. Social wasps (*Vespula* and *Dolichovespula*) have less potent venom.

ANT STINGS

The red imported fire ant, *Solenopsis invicta*, is of particular clinical significance. It forms super colonies and is an aggressive, territorial species that swarms onto an intruder before stinging. Stings are multiple, usually in the tens or hundreds.

ENVENOMATION BY BEE, WASP, AND ANT STINGS

Bee, wasp, and ant stings in nonallergic individuals produce immediate burning pain, redness, and swelling at the sting site. Pain usually subsides over some hours, while redness and swelling resolve more slowly. The effects of multiple stings cause systemic effects including headache, vomiting, thirst, pain, edema, discolored urine (hematuria and/or myoglobinuria), jaundice, and confusion. Rhabdomyolysis with resultant acute renal failure may occur. Intravascular hemolysis, coagulopathy, thrombocytopenia, metabolic disturbances, encephalopathy, liver dysfunction, and myocardial damage have also been reported. Hypersensitive patients may develop rapid catastrophic anaphylaxis that causes death in minutes.

The stinger should be removed as soon as possible (the method is unimportant) to limit the amount of venom injected. The majority of single bee stings do not require treatment, though cold packs and oral analgesia are valuable. Wasps and ants do not leave their sting behind; therefore, each individual may sting multiple times. Large, local reactions usually respond well to symptomatic treatment with nonsteroidal anti-inflammatory agents and topical steroid creams. Oral steroids and antihistamines are often used.

Treatment for anaphylaxis is based on administration of epinephrine as definitive therapy, supported by oxygen, β agonists for bronchoconstriction, steroids, and IV fluid (for hypotension). Individuals at risk for anaphylaxis from insect stings must carry, and be taught to use, injectable adrenaline (such as "EpiPen," an automated device for prehospital intramuscular injection of epinephrine) immediately after a sting. Two dosages are available (child, 150 mcg; adult, 300 mcg). Patients with serious systemic effects due to envenomation may require resuscitation. Renal function should be closely monitored. Prolonged hemofiltration or dialysis may be required. Permanent renal damage may necessitate long-term dialysis. Tetanus status should be addressed.

TICK BITE

A complex mixture of chemicals is secreted to enable long-term attachment to, and maintain blood flow from, the host. Such substances inhibit hemostasis, augment local blood flow, and suppress the inflammatory and immune responses of the host. Ticks cause a number of different problems, including allergy, transmission of infection (zoonoses), secondary infection, foreign-body granuloma if not removed in entirety, and paralysis. Ticks are vectors of rickettsial diseases, symptoms of which essentially consist of fever, rash, and myalgia. Lyme disease is a multisystem, infectious disease. The principle features of the syndrome are a rash, arthritis, various neurologic manifestations, and myocarditis.

In Europe, severe viral encephalitis and hemorrhagic fevers are caused by viruses of the genera *Flavivirus*, *Nairovirus*, and *Coltivirus*, which are transmitted by tick bite. Diseases such as tick-borne encephalitis, Omsk hemorrhagic fever, louping ill, and Crimean-Congo hemorrhagic fever have very low mortality.

Envenomation may cause progressive muscle weakness and ataxia. The tick may be above the hairline, in a skin fold, or in any body orifice. Local edema and inflammation may signal its presence, but it may also make it difficult to see and extract. Regional lymphadenopathy may be present. If a hypersensitivity to tick secretions has developed, local changes may be dramatic. Intoxication occurs after the tick has been feeding for 3 or more days. Usually, the child becomes subdued and sleepy and refuses food. The paralysis commences as ascending symmetrical weakness that progresses to involve the upper limbs and, terminally, the muscles involved with swallowing and breathing. Neurologic examination will reveal a paralysis of a lower motor neuron type. The deep tendon reflexes are diminished or absent, and the plantar response generally remains flexor in type. Early cranial nerve involvement, particularly both internal and external ophthalmoplegia, may occur. In older children and adults, the presenting complaint may be difficulty in reading. Double vision, photophobia, nystagmus, or pupillary dilation may be present. Once the possibility of tick paralysis is considered, a careful search for the culprit(s) may confirm the diagnosis. Other diagnoses to be considered are diphtheria, myasthenia, Guillain-Barré syndrome, botulism, myopathies, and a variety of inflammatory and toxic neuropathies. A facial nerve palsy may be mistaken for a viral infection. Hematologic investigations and lumbar puncture are not helpful. Eosinophilia does not occur. Plasma creatine kinase and troponin determinations should be made. Prompt and careful removal of the offending tick(s) is essential. The sprayed application of a personal insect repellent that contains pyrethrins or synthetic pyrethroid rapidly kills the tick and causes the hypostome and chelicerae (mouth parts) to lose turgidity and shrink away from the host tissue. Extrication is then easily effected by use of curved forceps, the points of which are pressed into position on either side of the tick's mouth parts, pressing well down into the skin, avoiding any pressure on the tick's body, and closing firmly on the hypostome before attempting to lift the tick out. The engorged body of the tick should not be grasped by the fingers or forceps, as this may result in incomplete removal and the expression of toxin. An alternative method of extraction is by gentle upward traction of a thread encircling the mouth parts. Surgical excision of the tick is not necessary, nor is application of a pressure-immobilization bandage after removal of the tick(s), as the onset of paralysis is slow. In Australia, an antitoxin prepared from the serum of infested dogs is available to treat both human and animal victims. However, it is used infrequently and only in significant paralysis, and it has a considerable incidence of adverse reaction.

Apart from neurotoxic effects, the likelihood of zoonosis and secondary infection must be considered, and tetanus prophylaxis should be brought up-to-date. The possibility of renal damage should be considered if rhabdomyolysis occurs.

JELLYFISH STINGS

Animals injected with a lethal venom dose die within 15 mins from cardiorespiratory arrest. *C. fleckeri* is rarely noticed by a victim until contact with tentacles occurs, usually while wading or swimming in shallow water. The tentacles are easily torn from the jellyfish by the encounter and, in adhering to the victim's skin, resemble earthworms of a pink, grey, or bluish hue. During the first 15 mins, pain increases in mounting waves despite removal of the tentacles. The victim may scream and become irrational. The lesions are distinctive and resemble marks made by a whip that is 8–10 mm wide with a "frosted ladder pattern" that matches the bands of nematocysts on the tentacles. Whealing is prompt and massive. Edema, erythema, and vesiculation soon follow, and when these subside (after some 10 days), patches of full-thickness necrosis leave permanent scars. Severity of injury is related to size of the jellyfish and the extent of tentacle contact. Most stings are quite minor.

C. fleckeri antivenom is the only jellyfish antivenom manufactured worldwide. It is concentrated immunoglobulin derived from the serum of sheep injected with *C. fleckeri* venom. Each vial contains sufficient activity to neutralize 20,000 IV LD$_{50}$ mouse doses. Antivenom is used in ~10% of envenomations. It is not effective against Australian *Chiropsalmus sp.* venom.

The severity and rapidity of envenomation necessitate decisive action, the mainstays of which include first aid, cardiopulmonary resuscitation, and antivenom administration. First aid measures include retrieval of the victim from the water to avoid further contact with the creature(s) and to prevent drowning; basic life support; inactivation of undischarged nematocysts by pouring vinegar (4%–6% acetic acid) over adhering tentacles for at least 30 secs to prevent further envenomation. (Alcohol in any form must not be used for this purpose). Vinegar-treated tentacles are harmless, but if vinegar is not available, tentacles may nonetheless be picked off safely by rescuers, as only a harmless prickling of the fingers may occur. Advanced cardiopulmonary resuscitation should be performed on the beach (if possible), during transportation and in the hospital. Three vials of antivenom should be administered. The use of verapamil is probably harmful due to its hypotensive effects. Magnesium may prove to be an important adjunctive therapy in envenomation. Mildly painful stings respond well to application of ice packs after they have been dowsed with vinegar.

Antivenom should be administered as soon as possible in the following circumstances: (a) unconsciousness, cardiorespiratory arrest, hypotension, dysrhythmia or hypoventilation; (b) difficulty with breathing, swallowing or speaking; (c) severe pain (parenteral analgesia is also usually required); and (d) possibility of significant skin scarring. The initial dose is 3 ampules infused IV, diluted 1 in 10 with a crystalloid solution.

Lesions produced by another highly dangerous Australian chirodropid jellyfish, *Chiropsalmus* sp. are narrower and milder, and the tentacular contact is far less than that of *Chironex fleckeri*. Chirodropids are found elsewhere in the world, including in the Gulf of Mexico and in Japanese waters.

C. rastoni is a 4-tentacled small jellyfish often found in swarms, with a very wide distribution in the Western Pacific Ocean and most Australian and Japanese waters. The bell is translucent and usually not much larger than 2 cm across. Its tentacles stretch ~5 cm to perhaps 30 cm.

Purified protein toxins cause vasoconstriction. Tentacles bear ovoid nematocysts. Stings are usually immediately painful, with linear lesions frequently 4 in number, ranging from 10 to 20 cm in length, and may blister. No specific management is recommended. Clumps of nematocysts (mammillations) appear as tiny red dots over the bell whereas on the tentacles, they are in tightly packed "collars" and in ring formations. The body and tentacles are almost completely transparent in water. The hyperadrenergic state may partially explain the clinical features of the "Irukandji syndrome." The victim rarely sees the offending jellyfish but is often aware of a sting, usually slight, to the upper body while swimming in deep water. Sometimes the sting is unnoticed, and it is the onset of symptoms that forces the victim to leave the water. The sting area contains no banding or puncture marks, just an oval area of barely perceptible erythema that measures ~5 cm by 7 cm. Irregularly spaced papules ("goose pimples") up to 2 mm in diameter develop within 20 mins of the sting and then fade, but erythema may last several days. From 5 mins to as late as 2 hrs after the sting, but usually after ~30 mins, a distinctive severe syndrome develops. Severe low back pain, cramping muscle pains, nausea, vomiting, profuse sweating, headache, restlessness, and agitation almost invariably occur, sometimes with hypertension. Abdominal pain is associated with spasm of the muscles of the abdominal wall, and cramps occur in the muscles of the limbs. Most stings are mild, but some cause "Irukandji syndrome." Pain relief is the most important feature of management in mild-to-moderate cases. Repeated doses of IV or intramuscular opiates may be required. IV magnesium salts provided pain relief and a reduction in blood pressure. Otherwise, treatment includes oxygen therapy, diuretics, vasodilators, inotropic support, and mechanical ventilation or application of continuous positive airway pressure. Antihypertensive therapy may be required in the initial phase of management. Infusions of phentolamine have been used successively for this purpose, although a "titratable" nitrate (nitroprusside) is preferred.

Portuguese Man-of-War "jellyfish" are the most frequent cause of significantly painful stings. The main lethal toxin causes cardiovascular toxicity. Upon contact, contracted tentacles produce a lesion, usually linear, like a row of beans or buttons, while uncontracted tentacles may give fine linear stings. Most stings are quite minor.

FISH STINGS

Stonefish are found throughout the entire IndoPacific region and, in Australia, stonefish are easily mistaken for a piece of rock or dead coral that has become encrusted with marine growth. When trodden on, venom is forced out of the tips of the spines into the victim's foot. Venom depresses the cardiovascular and neuromuscular systems and has a direct effect on muscle. Stings are extremely painful. The victim may become irrational. Stonefish antivenom, a pure equine $F(ab)_2$ preparation, is manufactured by Commonwealth Serum Laboratories (Pty) in Australia. The initial priority is pain relief. No attempt should be made to retard the movement of venom from the stung area, as this will only enhance local pain and tissue damage. Relief in minor cases may be achieved by bathing or immersing the sting with warm-to-hot water. Antivenom is recommended for all cases, except in those that involve only a single puncture wound with moderate discomfort. One vial (2000 units of antivenom in 2 mL) is sufficient for every 1–2 spine punctures. Antivenom is usually given intramuscularly. The injured limb should be comfortably immobilized. Administration of an antibiotic (e.g., trimethoprim-sulfamethoxazole, third-generation cephalosporins, or imipenem) active against pathogens found in salt or brackish water. Tetanus prophylaxis should be given according to the victim's immune status.

There are numerous other fish with stinging spines, such as Scorpion Fish Butterfly Cod, Waspfish, Scorpion Cods, South Australian Cobbler, Fortescue, Bullrout, Gurnard perch, Goblinfish, Ghoul, and numerous Catfish, Weeverfish, Rabbitfish, and Spinefeet. Many envenomations occur among amateur collectors. The mechanical penetration or laceration by spines is painful enough, but many also envenomate. There are no antivenoms. Otherwise, the management of a wound is as for Stonefish.

Stingrays have barbed tails that may inflict serious leg, abdominal, or chest wounds. Direct damage by penetration of the stinging barb is usually of greater importance than the introduction of the venom or a marine pathogen. A swimmer cruising the ocean floor is at risk of a serious chest wound when disturbing settled rays. Significant wounds require exploratory surgery because the wound track may contain a trail of glandular and integumentary sheath material as well as necrotic tissue. Penetrating wounds to the chest or abdomen must be explored because of likely internal damage. Tetanus and introduction of marine bacterial infection are possible.

Blue-ringed or Blue-lined octopuses are found around the coast of Australia. These small creatures, rarely larger than 20 cm from the tip of one arm to the tip of another, have characteristic dark brown or ochre bands over the body and arms with irregularly shaped blue circles, lines, and figures-of-8 superimposed. When the animal is disturbed, these markings become brilliant, iridescent, peacock blue. The saliva is highly venomous and is delivered when the octopus bites. The victim is generally unaware of any actual bite, but symptoms of envenomation occur within 5 or 10 mins and commence with weakness and numbness about the face and neck, combined with difficulty in breathing and nausea. No specific therapy is available. The pressure-immobilization method of first aid should be applied immediately to the bitten area, if accessible. Rescue breathing followed by mechanical ventilation must be instituted and continued until recovery, usually after several hours.

Cone snails fire a venom-laden miniature harpoon to rapidly paralyze prey such as fish. They inhabit the floor of tropical and subtropical seas. Venoms cause rapid disruption of neuronal transmission, neurotransmitter release (particularly acetylcholine), and neuroreceptor activation. A sharp, stinging pain is followed by local numbness or paresthesia. In serious envenomation, weakness and incoordination of voluntary muscles occurs rapidly and is accompanied by vision, swallowing, and speech disturbances. Respiratory failure due to paresis or paralysis may eventuate.

FISH THAT ARE POISONOUS TO EAT

Fish that are poisonous to eat contain a variety of toxins, including TTX, ciguatoxin (CTX), maitotoxin, and histamine, among others. Characteristic features of these fish are absence of scales, large eyes, and teeth arranged as 4 plates (tetraodontiformes). Examples include puffer fish, toad fish, globe fish, Toado, swell fish, and balloon fish. In Japan, the flesh of selected toad fish, "fugu," is a culinary delight, as traces of TTX produce a pleasant tingling gustatory sensation. TTX causes flaccid paralysis. The central effects are depression of spinal reflex pathways, induction of vomiting, and hypothermia. Hypoventilation is due to paralysis of peripheral nerves while hypotension is due to blockade of vasomotor nerves and direct suppression of vascular smooth muscle, causing vasodilation. The medullary vasomotor and respiratory centers are not affected. Myocardial cells are relatively insensitive to TTX. Signs and symptoms of poisoning develop within 10–45 mins of consumption. Most victims have some nausea, but vomiting is uncommon. Mildly poisoned victims usually experience only "tingling" sensations, but the severely poisoned rapidly develop serious illness. The diagnosis is usually straightforward, especially when a number of individuals have shared a meal. Although puffer fish are not ciguatoxic fish, the illness ciguatera may present in a similar fashion but later, usually 2–12 hrs after consumption of fish easily identified as not puffer fish. The ciguatera sufferer usually has reversed sensations; in particular, hot objects feel cold and vice versa, whereas this phenomenon is absent in tetrodotoxic poisoning. Apart from gastric lavage, TTX poisoning has no antidote or specific treatment; treatment is supportive. Vomiting should be induced, provided that the victim has no difficulty in swallowing or protection of the airway. Fluid administration should be regulated according to hemodynamic parameters. As TTX causes vasodilatation and cardiac depression in severe toxicity, plasma volume replace-

ment is necessary, along with an inotropic agent. Atropine may be ineffective in preventing bradycardia, which may respond to isoproterenol or epinephrine. Anticholinesterases are not recommended but, if administered, should be given in conjunction with an antimuscarinic agent to prevent bradycardia.

CTXs cause ciguatera characterized by diarrhea, increased peristalsis (treated with atropine), and increased mucus secretion. A typical case involves gastroenteritic symptoms for 1 or 2 days, weakness, myalgia and arthralgia for several days to a week, and paresthesias for several days to several weeks. Inability to discriminate temperatures and reversal of temperature perception (dysesthesia) are diagnostic. TTX poisoning is easily distinguished from ciguatera, and bacterial contamination of seafood will produce a very rapid onset of gastrointestinal symptoms without peripheral neurologic effects. This poison has no specific treatment or antidote. IV mannitol has been extolled as an effective treatment, but convincing clinical evidence of its efficacy has yet to be provided.

Maitotoxins are water-soluble polyether toxins that are distinct from CTXs in the gut of the "maito," the surgeonfish. Many of the in vitro effects of maitotoxin are prevented by calcium channel blockers such as verapamil.

Scombroid poisoning occurs when tuna or mackerel or other large oceanic fish become contaminated with enteric bacteria. Large amounts of histamine may develop in dead fish. Scombroid poisoning should be differentiated from "seafood allergy" and bacterial food poisoning by careful history elucidation. Typical symptoms in order of frequency are diarrhea, hot flushing or sweating, bright erythematous rash, nausea and vomiting, headache, abdominal pain, palpitations, burning in the mouth, fever, and dizziness. Facial edema is sometimes present. and respiratory distress may occur. Onset of illness is usually within 30 mins of fish ingestion and lasts only 8–12 hrs but is sometimes prolonged. Mild poisoning restricted to rash, flushing, sweating, tachycardia, palpitations, and headache may require a parenteral antihistamine (H1 and H2 antagonists).

Certain species of dinoflagellates (microalgae, plankton) produce toxins that are ingested by filter-feeding bivalve mollusks (e.g., mussels, clams, oysters, scallops, and cockles) that, in turn, may be ingested by crabs and lobsters. Life-threatening illnesses may result from ingesting the mollusks or other creatures that ingest them, with the most serious being paralytic shellfish poisoning and diarrhetic shellfish poisoning. Paralytic shellfish poisons affect neural and cardiac tissues, skeletal muscle, and vascular smooth muscle. Members of these genera bloom sporadically, creating "red tides" in sea or fresh waters. At such times, mollusks become heavily contaminated. Neurologic, respiratory, and cardiovascular symptoms usually develop within 30 mins.

Diarrhetic shellfish poisoning is characterized by gastroenteritis due to ingestion of shellfish, in particular mussels that have fed on marine dinoflagellates (plankton). Symptoms of nausea, vomiting, diarrhea, abdominal pain, and fever occur within 30 mins and last more than 8 hrs.

Amnestic shellfish poisoning is characterized by acute gastrointestinal symptoms and unusual neurologic abnormalities in people who have eaten mussels. Severely poisoned patients have experienced hemiparesis, seizures, hypotension, ophthalmoplegia, abnormalities of arousal ranging from agitation to coma, and residual severe anterograde memory deficits.

Brevetoxins are similar to CTXs and are associated with "red tide" algal blooms. They accumulate in filter-feeding shellfish such as oysters. Brevetoxins induce release of acetylcholine and catecholamines from central and peripheral neuronal sites and possible acetylcholine from neuromuscular junctions. No specific treatment is available.

SECTION III ■ LIFE-SUPPORT TECHNOLOGIES

CHAPTER 13 ■ MECHANICAL VENTILATION

MARK J. HEULITT • GERHARD K. WOLF • JOHN H. ARNOLD

Each ventilator is essentially a controller of pressure, volume, or flow. The manner in which each variable is controlled, described as the *mode of ventilation*, determines how the ventilator delivers the mechanical breath. Ventilators are classified as *pressure, volume, or flow* controllers (**Table 13.1**). It is important to recognize that any ventilator can directly control only one variable—pressure, volume, or flow—at a time. Thus, a ventilator is simply a technology that controls the airway pressure waveform, the inspired volume waveform, or the inspiratory flow waveform, and pressure, volume, and flow are referred to in this context as *control variables*.

Control variables relate to the elastic and resistive forces that must be overcome to allow gas delivery to the patient. If the clinician sets pressure as the control variable, volume varies directly with the compliance of the respiratory system. Thus, pressure is the independent variable set by the clinician, and volume is the dependent variable determined by the level of pressure. When the pressure pattern is preset by the clinician, the ventilator operates as a pressure controller. The volume becomes a function of compliance so that a decrease in compliance allows less volume to be delivered for the same pressure. During expiration, the elastic and resistive elements of the respiratory system are passive, and expiratory waveforms are not directly affected by the modes of ventilation or the controller. However, as the respiratory cycle is a set period of time, any change in the inspiratory time can influence expiratory time and, to a certain extent, the expiratory profile. When a ventilator operates as a constant pressure controller—for example, in pressure control (PC) mode, pressure-regulated volume control (PRVC) mode, and synchronized, intermittent mandatory ventilation-pressure control (SIMV-PC) mode—pressure is an independent, or controlled, variable (**Table 13.1**). The set pressure will be delivered and maintained constant throughout inspiration, independent of what resistive or elastic forces of the respiratory system might be. Even though pressure is constant, the delivered tidal volume (VT) will vary as a function of compliance and resistance, and the flow will also vary.

A waveform from a ventilator operating as a pressure controller is displayed in **Figure 13.1**. Under this condition, volume and flow become the dependent variables, and their patterns will depend upon compliance and resistance. When a pressure pattern is preset (constant in a PC mode), flow-time and volume-time waveforms vary exponentially with time and are a function of compliance and resistance. If the clinician sets flow as function of time, pressure then varies with resistance. Flow is the independent variable, and pressure is the dependent variable. When

TABLE 13.1

VENTILATOR CONTROLLERS

Flow controller (constant flow controller)	Pressure controller (constant pressure controller)	Volume controller (variable flow controller)
Modes	**Modes**	**Modes**
VC, SIMV-VC	PC, SIMV-PC, PRVC	VC
Equation	**Equation**	**Equation**
$Flow = \frac{Pressure}{Resistance}$	$Flow = \frac{Volume}{Compliance}$	$Flow = Pressure \times Compliance$
	$Pressure = Resistance \times Flow$	
Independent variables	***Independent variables***	***Independent variables***
Flow	Pressure	Volume
Dependent variables	***Dependent variables***	***Dependent variables***
Pressure	Volume Flow	Pressure
	Flow	
Limiting variables	***Limiting variables***	***Limiting variables***
Volume	Pressure	Volume
Trigger variables	***Trigger variables***	***Trigger variables***
Time	Time	Time
Pressure	Pressure	Pressure
Flow	Flow	Flow

VC, volume control; SIMV-VC, synchronized, intermittent mandatory ventilation-volume control; PC, pressure control; SIMV-PC, synchronized, intermittent mandatory ventilation-pressure control; PRVC, pressure-regulated volume control

a flow pattern is preset, the ventilator operates as a flow controller; pressure is a function of resistance. Volume increases linearly with time, although it does not have a direct relation to flow.

When a ventilator operates as a constant-flow controller (volume-controlled [VC] and SIMV-VC modes), flow is the independent variable. Regardless of the resistive or elastic forces of the respiratory system, the set flow will be delivered and maintained constant throughout inspiration. Pressure and VT will vary with time, depending on the compliance and resistance.

Waveforms from a ventilator operating as a flow controller are illustrated in **Figure 13.2**. Flow is the independent variable (controlled variable); pressure and volume are dependent variables. When a flow pattern is preset (constant in this case), pressure and volume are the dependent variables; they vary linearly with time and are functions of compliance and resistance. The modern ventilator can operate as a *flow controller* or as a *pressure controller*. As a flow controller, the most common pattern is *constant flow*, also referred to as a *square-wave flow* pattern. In this mode, the flow increases to a set level that is maintained for the duration of the inspiratory time. The pressure and volume that the patient receives are a function of compliance and resistance. The various ventilators are able to deliver various flow patterns. Flow

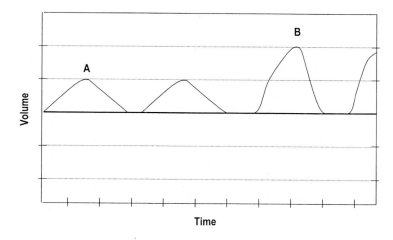

FIGURE 13.1. Volume-time wave form from a constant pressure mode of ventilation. **A:** Increased resistance. With inspiration, a decrease in inspired tidal volume occurs, as compared to tracing B (normal resistance). Expiration has an abnormal linear decay to baseline. **B:** Normal resistance. During inspiration, a normal exponential increase in tidal volume occurs. Expiration has a normal exponential decay to baseline.

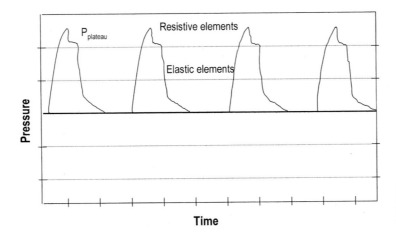

FIGURE 13.2. Pressure-time waveform from a constant flow mode illustrating resistive and elastic elements of the respiratory system.

patterns are most commonly constant and exponentially decelerating. In PC ventilation, the pressure pattern is "square," but flow increases rapidly at the beginning of the inspiratory phase to generate the set pressure limit and then decays exponentially over the inspiratory time. This flow pattern is described as *decelerating flow*. It is said that the major difference between volume and pressure ventilation is based on the "square wave" and the "decelerating" flow patterns observed. In PC mode, the initial "snap" of high flow to reach the set pressure limit has been thought to be potentially beneficial in opening stiff alveoli in conditions such as acute respiratory distress syndrome or surfactant deficiency. It has been proposed that a decelerating flow favors better gas exchange and improves distribution of ventilation among lung units with heterogeneous time constants. For this reason, clinicians often choose PC ventilation in patients with poor compliance, although the true benefit of PC versus other modes has not been well established in animal or clinical studies.

If the clinician sets volume as a function of time, pressure then varies with compliance. Volume is the independent variable, and pressure is the dependent variable.

VOLUME MEASUREMENT

Goals of modern mechanical ventilation in infants and children have focused on preventing overdistension of alveoli by limiting VT, thus reducing volutrauma. The inability to accurately measure VT in a conventional ventilator is caused by several factors, including (a) difficulty of compensating for volume loss in the ventilator circuit and (b) changes in temperature, humidification, and secretions. Air leaks around the ETT itself, especially in small patients with uncuffed tubes, are another source of volume measurement error. Given the importance of

knowing the true VT delivered to patients, it is essential to determine which is the most accurate, safe, and efficient site to monitor. Ventilator-displayed VT, without software compensation for circuit compliance, generally overestimates the true delivered VT. Conversely, when the circuit-compliance compensation feature is on, the ventilator-displayed VT generally underestimates the true delivered VT.

A patient on mechanical ventilation has the clinician-controlled mechanical pump of the ventilator and the patient's own respiratory muscle pump. Factors that affect patient-ventilator synchrony are listed in **Table 13.2** and can be subdivided into equipment factors, patient factors, and decision-making factors. Evaluation of patient-ventilator synchrony can also be subdivided into 4 phases that consist of issues of triggering, adequacy of flow delivery, adequate breath termination, and effects of positive end-expiratory pressure (PEEP) and/or PEEPi.

Mechanical ventilatory support can be subdivided into 3 phases: acute, maintenance, and weaning.

For patients with obstructive lung disease, such as asthma, lung protection strategy would include the prevention of high airway pressures and hyperinflation-associated complications. Initial settings would include a lower VT and prolonged exhalation times. Allowing such patients to breathe spontaneously in a support mode is ideal, as it allows the patient more control over the exhalation time. However, as some intubated asthmatics have elevated levels of $PaCO_2$, this strategy may result in agitation in the patient and, therefore, an increase in sedation. The level of PEEP in patients with obstructive disease has traditionally been set at minimal levels, secondary to the development of auto-PEEP, due to the patient's increased airway resistance with inadequate lung emptying during exhalation. However, some patients may require levels of PEEP to match the level of auto-PEEP to splint airways open, ensuring adequate oxygenation and improving

TABLE 13.2

VENTILATOR–PATIENT SYNCHRONY

Equipment factors
Trigger variables
Sensitivity settings
Response time of the ventilator
Inspiratory flow characteristics
Mode of ventilation
Expiratory valve design
Design of positive end-expiratory pressure valve and
    operation

Patient factors
Sedation and pain control
Patient's inspiratory effort and drive
Patient's disease process
Intrinsic positive end-expiratory pressure
Size of the airway
Presence of airway leak
Nutritional status
Patient homeostasis

Decision-making factors
Deleterious effects of patient-ventilator asynchrony
Patient fights the ventilator
Increased level of sedation
Higher work of breathing
Muscle damage
Ventilation-perfusion mismatch
Dynamic hyperinflation
Delayed or prolonged weaning
Prolonged intensive care or hospital stay
Higher costs

exhalation. Patients with decreased thoracic compliance must have ventilatory settings directed toward lung recruitment to reduce the severity of ventilator-induced lung injury. This lung protection strategy is primarily accomplished by limiting distending volume, the change in pressure to distend the alveoli, and the level of end-expiratory pressure. This strategy is directed toward reducing the cyclic collapse and reexpansion of the alveoli due to inadequate levels of PEEP and thus the inability to maintain the alveoli open throughout the respiratory cycle.

Lung recruitment is a strategy aimed at reexpanding collapsed lung tissue and maintaining high PEEP to prevent subsequent "derecruitment." The benefits of optimal lung recruitment and prevention of derecruitment involve (a) a reduction in the intrapulmonary shunt fraction with an improvement in arterial oxygenation, (b) an improvement in pulmonary compliance by shifting the compliance curve to the point where less pressure is required for the same change in volume, and (c) prevention of a cyclic opening, collapse, and reopening of alveolar units with each breath associated with ventilator-induced lung injury. To recruit collapsed lung tissue, sufficient pressure must be imposed to exceed the critical

opening pressure of the affected lung. Ideal patients for recruitment maneuvers are patients with putative acute respiratory distress syndrome in the early phase of the disease (before the onset of fibroproliferation). These patients will continue to be poorly oxygenated in spite of a high FiO_2. Preexisting focal lung disease that may predispose to barotrauma should be regarded as a relative contraindication to the maneuver (e.g., extensive apical bullous lung disease). Patients with "secondary" acute respiratory distress syndrome (e.g., following abdominal sepsis) are thought to be more likely to respond favorably to the maneuver than patients with "primary" lung disease and acute lung injury.

PEEP TITRATION

Cdyni may also be a useful parameter by which to find the appropriate level of PEEP that may prevent alveolar collapse during expiration, thereby helping to guide the titration of effective PEEP. This assessment may be performed by a stepwise decrease of the initial PEEP level and should be completed before the recruitment maneuver is performed. As PEEP is carefully decreased, the Cdyni will initially increase with each decrease of PEEP, indicating a relief of overdistended areas in the lung. Subsequently, the Cdyni will reach a plateau at which Cdyni no longer increases when the PEEP level is decreased. After further decrease in the PEEP level, the Cdyni will begin decreasing, indicating initial collapse of alveoli that can no longer be kept open at the current PEEP level. Effective PEEP should be set at 2–3 cm H_2O above the indicated collapse pressure as a safety margin after a preceding recruitment maneuver. Another method would be to identify the critical opening pressure of the airways by utilizing a static pressure-volume loop to generate the lower inflection point (**Fig. 13.3**). As the lung is inflated from zero end-expiratory pressure, the clinician attempts to identify the point at which the volume abruptly changes, termed the *lower inflection point*. As the lung is further inflated, the pressure-volume slope increases to the point at which the volume no longer changes with each change in pressure. This flattening of the pressure-volume loop is referred to as *beaking*, as in a bird's beak, and represents overdistension of the lung. The next phase of the pressure-volume loop is when expiration begins and the lung begins to deflate; the pressure point at which rapid loss of volume begins to occur has been termed the *deflection point*. Ideally, the clinician would utilize the identification of the inflection and defection points to select the PEEP level necessary to maintain the lung open throughout inspiration and expiration without allowing for overdistension.

Volume Pressure Loop

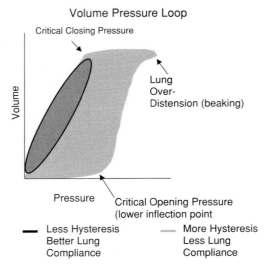

FIGURE 13.3. Two pressure volume loops superimposed on the same graph. The dark gray loop represents a lung with normal pulmonary compliance. The light gray loop demonstrates a lung with decreased pulmonary compliance. Illustrated on this loop is the critical opening pressure or point when volume increases once critical pressure is reached, point of lung over distention where there is pressure change without volume and the critical closing pressure.

Cdyni can be used as a measure of improvement in lung compliance during lung recruitment; however, other measures should be utilized to ensure recruitment without overdistension of the recruited alveoli. If the lung is recruited, oxygenation, pulmonary compliance, and ventilation should improve. It is important not to be misled by an improvement of oxygenation alone as a measure of lung recruitment. An increase in PEEP can reduce cardiac output and increase PaO_2 despite a decrease in oxygen delivery. The CO_2 concentration in expired air depends on alveolar ventilation, cardiac output, and the metabolic state. Alveoli already opened could be overdistended, thus decreasing the diffusion of the CO_2 into the alveoli. The effect of PEEP is as a distending pressure to increase the functional residual capacity (FRC) (volume of gas at the end of exhalation in the lung). By maintaining this pressure above the pressure in which the lungs collapse (closing pressure), atelectasis or alveolar collapse is minimized. The ultimate effect is decreased intrapulmonary shunting of blood and improved arterial oxygenation. PEEP increases intrathoracic pressure and causes potential hemodynamic consequences by transmission of the applied PEEP to transmural capillary pressure, which affects the right and left heart. The most dramatic effect of increased PEEP is decreased venous return to the right heart.

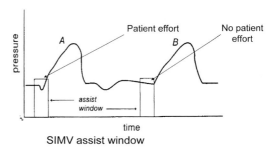

SIMV assist window

FIGURE 13.4. Two SIMV breaths. The first is patient triggered, and the second is machine triggered. If the patient does not trigger a breath in the assist window, the ventilator will deliver a machine breath at the start of the next window.

MODES OF VENTILATION

IMV is a mode of mechanical ventilation that allows the patient to breathe spontaneously between machine-cycled or clinician-controlled mandatory breaths. During intermittent mandatory ventilation (IMV), a preset number of positive-pressure (mandatory) breaths is delivered between which the patient can breathe spontaneously. The most common mode of IMV is SIMV, in which mandatory, or machine, breaths are synchronized via a timing window to the patient effort at the patient's intrinsic respiratory rate rather than the breaths being evenly spaced over each minute (**Fig. 13.4**). Commonly, this mode is combined with pressure support, which provides support to nonmandatory breaths. The main disadvantage of SIMV, as compared to assist control, is that the clinician may overestimate the amount of support, which leads to patient fatigue, as the WOB is increased.

Pressure-controlled Ventilation

During PC ventilation, a pressure-limited breath is delivered during a preset inspiratory time at the preset respiratory rate (**Fig. 13.5**). The VT is determined by the preset pressure limit and the compliance

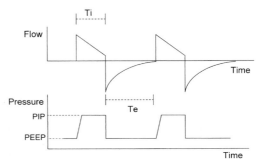

FIGURE 13.5. Pressure-controlled breath. Note the flow pattern is decelerating from high initial flow rapidly to baseline.

and resistance of the respiratory system. The flow waveform is always decelerating in PC. Gas flows into the chest along the pressure gradient. As the alveolar pressure rises with increasing alveolar volume, the rate of flow drops off (as the pressure gradient between the airway opening and the alveolar space narrows). The set pressure is maintained for the duration of inspiration. The higher initial flow associated with PC ventilation more easily meets the patient's flow demands, especially in patients with "stiff" lungs. The peak inspiratory pressure during PC ventilation is usually less compared to VC ventilation for the same obtained VT. During PC breaths, the distribution of ventilation may be more even in a lung with heterogeneous mechanical properties. That is, the initial high flow opens alveoli, and the constant pressure maintained during inspiration may allow gas to flow from more well-distended alveoli to more collapsed areas and thus distribute gas more efficiently throughout the lung. PC is also useful in the patient with an air leak. Although volume is lost through the leak, the ventilator will continue to attempt to compensate by maintaining the airway pressure for the duration of the inspiratory phase. PC ventilation also has several disadvantages. It does not guarantee minute ventilation.

Volume-controlled Ventilation

In the VC ventilation mode, the ventilator delivers a preset VT with a constant flow during a preset inspiratory time at the preset respiratory rate (**Fig. 13.6**). Airway and alveolar pressures are dependent variables and will rise or fall depending upon changes in lung mechanics or patient effort. By setting the volume to be delivered and the breath rate, the clinician has control over the patient's minute ventilation and CO_2 clearance, provided the presence of is only a small leak around the ETT. Ventilator-induced lung injury due to alveolar overdistension (volutrauma) can also be less in volume control. The constant-flow type

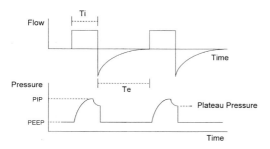

FIGURE 13.6. Volume-controlled breath. Note the flow pattern is square with an initial high flow that is maintained during inspiration and then quickly terminated at expiration.

of breath delivery in VC ventilation may not meet patient demands, especially if the patient has poorly compliant lungs that may benefit from the initial accelerated flow that occurs with PC ventilation, resulting in asynchrony between the patient's breathing efforts and the ventilator; this disadvantage leads to distress and often an increase in sedation requirement. The peak inspiratory pressure is higher in VC ventilation compared to PC ventilation for the same obtained VT.

Airway-pressure-release Ventilation

Airway-pressure-release ventilation (APRV) is essentially a high-level continuous positive-airway pressure (CPAP) mode that is terminated for a very brief period. The elevated baseline helps oxygenation, and the timed releases assist carbon dioxide removal. This mode allows the patient to spontaneously breathe during all phases of the cycle (**Fig. 13.7**). APRV is different from other modes of ventilation in that it is based on an intermittent decrease in airway pressure, rather than an increase. In addition to FiO_2, the operator-controlled parameters in APRV mode are: P_{high}, T_{high}, P_{low}, and T_{low}, where P and T equate to pressure and time. P_{high} should be set at a level equivalent to the plateau pressure being used in a conventional mode when transitioning to APRV. If APRV is the first mode to be used, P_{high} is set at ~20–30 cm H_2O, P_{low} at zero, T_{high} at ~4–6 sec, and T_{low} initially at ~0.2–0.6 sec. T_{low} should then be adjusted based on the expiratory gas flow waveform so that the expiratory flow falls to ~25%–75% of peak expiratory flow. Generally, T_{low} will be shortened in restrictive disease and lengthened in obstructive disease. To minimize derecruitment, the time (T_{low}) at P_{low} is brief. When the patient's underlying condition improves, APRV can gradually be weaned by lowering the P_{high} and extending the T_{high}. The goal is to arrive at straight CPAP. APRV may be less effective as a strategy to limit alveolar overdistension.

Pressure-regulated Volume Control

PRVC (or adaptive pressure ventilation, variable PC, Autoflow, or Volume Control Plus) is a dual-control, breath-to-breath mode. PRVC has a variable decelerating flow pattern, with breaths time cycled. During PRVC, the pressure and volume are regulated. Thus, all breaths are volume targeted, with pressure adjusted to reach that volume target. PRVC often incorporates a "compliance curve" that is developed within the ventilator computer, as it gives several initial breaths at varying VTs that increase incrementally up to the set value. From this

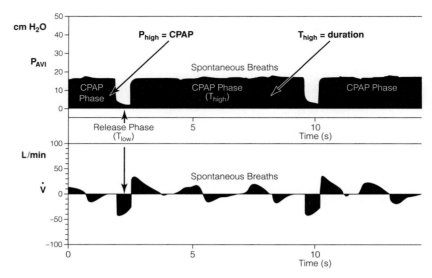

FIGURE 13.7. Patient breathing on airway-pressure-release ventilation. The CPAP phase (P_{high}) is intermittently released to a P_{low} for a brief duration (T_{low}) reestablishing the CPAP level on the subsequent breath. Spontaneous breathing may be superimposed at both pressure levels and is independent of time-cycling. (Adapted from Habashi, NM. Other approaches to open lung ventilation: airway pressure release ventilation. *Crit Care Med* 2005;33:S228–S240.

information, the ventilator computes the pressure target required to deliver the desired VT. Depending on the respiratory system compliance, the pressure associated with the tidal breath can vary over time. If the patient's compliance decreases, the pressure required to ensure the volume breath can be increased up to within 5 mm Hg of the set pressure alarm limit. If the patient's compliance improves, the pressure required to deliver the volume breath will be reduced. Thus, a specific VT and minute ventilation is assured, while pressure-induced lung damage is minimized. The proposed advantage of this mode is a constant V_E and VT with automatic weaning of the pressure limit as the patient's compliance improves.

Volume-assured Pressure Support

Volume-assured pressure support and pressure augmentation are described as a dual control within a breath mode, where the ventilator switches from PC to VC within the breath. In this mode, the clinician chooses a volume target and the breath begins as a pressure-limited, flow-cycled breath, either spontaneously (pressure support) or mechanically. When inspiratory flow has decelerated to the minimum set level, delivered volume is measured. If the target volume has been met or exceeded, the breath ends. If the delivered volume has not met the target, the breath is transitioned to a volume-targeted breath by prolonging inspiration at the minimum flow and increasing the inspiratory pressure until the delivered volume has been obtained.

Pressure-support Ventilation

PSV is a form of mechanical ventilatory support that delivers a clinician-selected amount of positive airway pressure to assist an intubated patient's spontaneous inspiratory effort. PSV is used either as low-level PSV to overcome the patient's work associated with the ETT or as high-level PSV as a stand-alone ventilatory support mode. If changes occur in the patient's resistance and/or compliance, the VT delivered may vary greatly and potentially underventilate or overventilate the patient.

Volume-support Ventilation

Volume-support ventilation is a volume-targeted mode of ventilation that is essentially pressure support with VT as a feedback. In this mode, the level of inspiratory pressure is adjusted with each breath to reach a targeted clinician-selected volume. All breaths are patient-triggered, pressure-limited, and flow-cycled.

Volume-assured Pressure Support/Pressure Augmentation

Volume-assured pressure support and pressure augmentation are described as dual-control-within-a-breath modes in which the ventilator switches from PC to VC within the breath. The theoretical advantage of these modes is their ability to maintain constant VT and minute volume with a resultant lower work of breathing (WOB). Little evidence is available on their use in infants and children, and no recent studies demonstrate its use.

High-frequency Ventilation

Tidal volumes of 1–3 mL/kg are delivered at rates from 3–20 Hz (180–1200 breaths/min). The limitation of delivered tidal volumes and optimization of alveolar recruitment, which minimizes atelectrauma and volutrauma, has become one of the main strategies of mechanical ventilation in patients with acute respiratory distress syndrome. A near-square waveform is generated either by a diaphragm or by a piston. Inspiration and expiration are active. Gas is forced into the lungs and actively withdrawn from the airways, as the diaphragm or piston travels forward and backward. Fresh gas flow pressurizes the system to the required mean airway pressure (MAP). The magnitude of the oscillations (often referred to as *delta P*) is controlled by the distance traveled by the piston or the diaphragm. The inspiratory time is set as a percentage of the respiratory cycle and determines the ratio of inspiratory-to-expiratory (I:E) time. An inspiratory time of 33% or 50%, resulting in an I:E ratio of 1:2 or 1:1, is frequently used in the clinical setting.

High-frequency Jet Ventilation

During high-frequency jet ventilation, a jet ventilator is combined with a conventional ventilator. The gas flows from two sources: The jet ventilator is the source of the small delivered tidal volumes, whereas the conventional ventilator is the source of the bias flow. Inspiration is active, whereas expiration is passive and driven by elastic recoil of the lungs and chest wall. Jet ventilation can be delivered during CPAP or conventional ventilation. The resulting tidal volume of the jet ventilator is a result of the driving pressure of the jet, resistance of the endotracheal tube (ETT), and the set inspiratory time. Inspiratory and expiratory times are variable in most devices. High-frequency jet ventilation has been evaluated in a number of neonatal trials.

High-frequency Flow Interrupters

With the use of high-frequency flow interrupters, a valve mechanism in the expiratory limb of the ventilator rapidly alters flow, causing a pulsating gas flow. Some conventional ventilators provide this mode as a back-up mode to transition to high-frequency flow interrupters without switching the ventilator. Due to their limited bias flow, high-frequency flow interruption devices are usually used in the neonatal setting.

The "Life Pulse High-Frequency Ventilator" (Bunnell, Salt Lake City, UT) is a jet-ventilator used in neonates. The ventilator is connected to a conventional ventilator at the patient's ETT with a special adapter. The jet ventilations are added to the conventional ventilation that the patient is receiving. The respiratory rate varies between 4 and 11 Hz (240–660 breaths/min), with airway pressure monitored at the ETT. The Babylog 8000 plus (Draeger Medical, Telford, PA) is a conventional ventilator with the option to ventilate in a high-frequency mode (high-frequency flow interruption). Small delivered tidal volumes are generated by rapidly switching the expiratory valve. The bias flow is up to 30 L/min. The ventilator can oscillate between 5 and 20 Hz (300–1200 breaths/min). High-frequency ventilation (HFV) can be applied during CPAP or SIMV.

The Sensormedics 3100 A/B (Viasys, Yorba Linda, CA) is a device used for high-frequency oscillation ventilation (HFOV). Oscillations are generated with a diaphragm. Fresh gas is provided by a bias flow system, with frequencies ranging from 3 to 15 Hz (180–900 breaths/min). The Sensormedics 3100 A is used for neonates and infants, with bias flow ranging from 0 to 40 L/min and MAPs ranging from 3 to 45 cm H_2O. The Sensormedics 3100 B is approved for adults and larger children who weigh >35 kg. In comparison to the 3100A, the 3100B has a more powerful diaphragm, can provide a larger bias flow (0–60 L/min), and can apply higher MAPs of up to 55 cm H_2O.

Optimal lung volume during HFV has been described as the lowest MAP that achieves oxygenating efficiency and maintains lung volume. Distal airway pressures vary in response to changes in the I:E ratio during HFV.

Tidal volume contributes more to CO_2 elimination than frequency does, as tidal volume is squared in the formula. In the clinical setting, it is appropriate to estimate alveolar ventilation as a product of the device frequency and the square of the delivered tidal volume. Any maneuver that alters tidal volume will alter CO_2 removal. Increasing the amplitude leads to increasing tidal volumes and improves CO_2 elimination. Conversely, decreasing the amplitude decreases CO_2 elimination by directly decreasing delivered tidal volume. With an increasing respiratory rate, the inspiratory time is decreased, and the oscillations of the diaphragm become less efficient, resulting in decreased delivered tidal volumes. As tidal volumes are more important than rate for CO_2 elimination, increasing the respiratory rate during HFV paradoxically diminishes CO_2 clearance. Conversely, decreasing the rate results in more efficient oscillations, larger tidal volumes, and improved CO_2 clearance. Creating an ETT cuff leak has been suggested as an alternative way to enhance CO_2 clearance in the setting of hypercarbia despite a maximized amplitude and a low rate. After the ETT cuff has been deflated to produce a cuff leak, the proximal MAP will decrease. The expiratory valve or bias flow should be adjusted to maintain the same MAP for this maneuver to be effective.

WEANING FROM MECHANICAL VENTILATORY SUPPORT

Extubation failure still occurs in up to 24% of cases. Standard indices for assessing patient weaning ability include (a) resolution of the etiology of respiratory failure and stable respiratory status; (b) decreased FiO_2 (usually to <50%) and decreased PEEP to 5 cm H_2O; (c) respiratory rate to <60 for infants <12 months of age, to <40 for preschool and school-aged children, and to <30 for adolescents; and (d) no acidosis (pH <7.35) or hypercapnia (PCO_2 >60 torr). Other parameters that indirectly assess oxygenation and compliance include a P:F ratio of >267 (PaO_2 >80 torr on FiO_2 of 0.3), SpO_2 >94% on FiO_2 ≤0.5, peak inspiratory pressure <20 cm H_2O, PEEP ≤5 cm H_2O, combined with adequate respiratory muscle function, and hemodynamic stability without evidence of shock. These criteria include good perfusion (e.g., capillary refill <3 secs), age-appropriate blood pressure (above −2 SD cut-off for age), and good cardiac function (e.g., no requirement of infusions of vasoactive and/or inotropic medications, with the exception of dopamine ≤5 mcg/kg^{-1}/min^{-1}). Patients must be easily arousable to verbal or physical stimulation (e.g., pediatric Glasgow Coma Scale score of ≥11) and must be capable of moving an uninjured upper and lower extremity against gravity. Patients must also have acceptable serum potassium, magnesium, and phosphorous concentrations.

Routine administration of corticosteroids is a frequent adjunct for extubation. Dexamethasone therapy may reduce stridor, but no definitive evidence suggests that it reduces reintubation.

After endotracheal extubation, upper and total airway reistances may frequently be increased, resulting in high inspiratory effort to breathe. A few patients, ranging from 5% to 16%, develop postextubation airway obstruction and frank respiratory distress. The use of HeO_2 mixture in adults and in children with upper airway obstruction has been reported in several anecdotal series and a few studies, and it has become one of the more accepted indications for HeO_2 use.

Noninvasive Mechanical Ventilatory Support

For noninvasive ventilatory support to function properly, the mask or nasal prongs must adequately seal to the patient. The varying physical sizes and the lack of tolerance of masks, or even prongs, can limit the utility of noninvasive ventilation in children. The variety of devices that is available for noninvasive support seems to be addressing some of these issues. Success with noninvasive techniques has been reported to avoid the need for tracheal intubation in some groups, such as immunosuppressed patients with asthma or respiratory insufficiency. One form of noninvasive ventilation that seems to be increasing in popularity is the use of high-flow, nasal cannula therapy.

Recognition of Weaning Failure

Failure of weaning can be categorized by increased respiratory load or decreased respiratory capacity. Increased respiratory load is represented by increased elastic load (unresolved lung disease, secondary pneumonia, abdominal distension, and hyperinflated lungs), increased resistive load (thickened airway secretions, partially occluded ETT, upper-airway obstruction), or increased minute ventilation (pain and irritability, sepsis/hyperthermia, metabolic acidosis). Decreased respiratory capacity is represented by decreased respiratory drive (sedation, central nervous system infection, traumatic brain injury, hypocapnia/alkalosis), muscular dysfunction (muscular catabolism and weakness [malnutrition], severe electrolyte disturbances), and neuromuscular disorder (diaphragmatic dysfunction, prolonged neuromuscular blockade, cervical spinal injury).

The rate of extrubation failure increases with the length of time patients received mechanical ventilation. Extubation failure increases significantly with decreasing VT indexed to body weight of a spontaneous breath, increasing FIO_2, increasing MAP, increasing oxygenation index, increasing fraction of total minute ventilation provided by the ventilator, increasing peak ventilatory inspiratory pressure, or decreasing mean inspiratory flow. Weaning from mechanical ventilation remains a complex and poorly standardized area of respiratory care. Technical advancements in integration of patient effort and mechanical response have great potential to revolutionize this field to the benefit of patients.

CHAPTER 14 ■ INHALED GASES

ANGELA T. WRATNEY • DONNA S. HAMEL • IRA M. CHEIFETZ

The nasal passages and upper airway warm, humidify, and filter air for the respiratory system. Thus, in the provision of inhaled gas therapies which bypass the upper airway or are administered with high pressure or flow, careful attention to temperature control, humidification, and infection control is warranted. Failure to do so may result in hypothermia, inspissated secretions, and airway injury and potentially contribute to the development of ventilator associated pneumonia.

OXYGEN

Oxygen is provided to patients with impaired respiratory function to improve arterial saturation, to vasodilate the pulmonary capillary bed, and to enhance systemic oxygen delivery. During the process of normal cellular metabolism, reactive oxygen species (ROS) such as the superoxide anion (O_2^-), oxygen radical (O_2^-), hydroxyl radical (OH^-), and hydrogen peroxide (H_2O_2) are produced. ROS cause oxidative injury to proteins, DNA, and lipids. Organs rich in lipids and proteins, such as the pulmonary and central nervous system, are especially at risk. Endogenous antioxidant enzyme systems such as superoxide dismutase (SOD), glutathione peroxidase, and catalase attempt to clear ROS to limit cellular injury **(Table 14.1)**.

Depending on the desired F_{IO_2}, a variety of devices exist for administering supplemental O_2 **(Table 14.2)**. High-flow delivery systems provide a more stable, measurable delivery of the F_{IO_2} independent of patient respiratory effort. High-flow delivery devices can be used with masks, tracheostomy collars, nebulizers, and oxygen tents or hoods. Low-flow systems include nasal cannula, simple face masks, or face masks with a reservoir (non-rebreather or partial rebreather). The nasal cannulae provides a comfortable, light-weight, and inexpensive method for low-flow oxygen delivery (0.1–6 L/min (LPM)). F_{IO_2} delivery ranges between 24% and 50%. Although variable in the actual F_{IO_2} delivered, a general "rule of thumb" states for each liter of supplemental oxygen provided, the inspired oxygen concentration increases by ~4%. Simple face masks fit over the patient's nose and mouth, providing an F_{IO_2} delivery between 35% and 55% oxygen. A non-rebreathing face mask consists of a simple face mask adapted with a reservoir bag and an inflow system for fresh gas

infusion to increase F_{IO_2} delivery close to 100% oxygen. Venturi masks are high-flow systems that provide fixed concentrations of 24%, 28%, 31%, 35%, 40%, or 50% oxygen. Oxygen hoods are transparent enclosures designed to surround the head of a neonate or small infant. Oxygen tents are available to allow the patient to move freely within a larger oxygen-rich environment.

Oxygen-mediated pulmonary toxicity is pathologically very similar to acute respiratory distress syndrome. Clinically, the patient may complain of chest pain, cough, and tracheal inflammation. Although an F_{IO_2} of 0.50 is commonly regarded as safe, a safe level or duration of F_{IO_2} exposure has not been established. When supplemental O_2 fails to improve the hypoxemia, other problems such as hypoventilation, airway obstruction, diffusion abnormalities, ventilation-perfusion mismatch (V/Q mismatch), or hemoglobinopathies may be present. Physiologic right-to-left shunts occur when pulmonary blood passes from systemic veins to systemic arteries without first exchanging gas with the alveoli. Patients with intrapulmonary shunts may benefit from invasive or noninvasive positive-pressure ventilation to improve lung volume and ventilation-perfusion (V/Q) matching. Patients with an anatomic right-to-left intracardiac shunt (i.e., cyanotic congenital heart disease) are hypoxemic and cannot increase their arterial oxygen content in response to supplemental O_2. Administering oxygen to patients with a chronically compensated respiratory acidosis will induce a mild increase in measured blood Pa_{CO_2}.

INHALED NITRIC OXIDE

Endogenous nitric oxide (NO) is an essential gaseous cell mediator in neurotransmission, inflammatory cell activation, and vascular smooth-muscle relaxation. Therapeutically, inhaled NO (iNO) is used as a selective pulmonary vasodilator to enhance V/Q matching, to treat pulmonary arteriolar hypertension, and to reduce pulmonary vascular resistance and right ventricular cardiac work. Endogenous NO is synthesized within most cells of the human body from arginine and oxygen by one of three isoforms of nitric oxide synthase (NOS). NO induces upregulation of cytosolic guanylyl cyclase triggering the activation of cGMP-dependent protein kinases . Ultimately, this cascade results in smooth muscle cell

TABLE 14.1

REACTIVE OXYGEN SPECIES AND THE ENDOGENOUS ANTIOXIDANT DEFENSE SYSTEMS

Reactive oxygen species	Chemical symbol	Antioxidant defense(s)
Superoxide anion	O_2^-	Superoxide dismutase
Hydrogen peroxide	H_2O_2	Glutathione peroxidase and catalase
Hydroxyl radical	OH•	Nonenzymatic mechanisms (e.g., vitamin C)

relaxation and pulmonary arteriolar vasodilation due to decreased intracellular calcium levels. iNO provides a therapeutic, selective pulmonary vasodilator. This selectivity results from NO reactions that limit movement and activity of iNO to the pulmonary vascular bed. Systemic uptake of NO is limited by scavenging mechanisms. NO can also react with free radicals when available to form nitrogen dioxide (NO_2) or peroxynitrite ($ONOO^-$). Protein nitration and oxidative lung injury can result from these toxic reactions and may underlie the pathologic mechanism for hyperoxic or ischemia-reperfusion injury. iNO is generally delivered during mechanical ventilation but can also be delivered to non-intubated patients via a tight-fitting face mask, transtracheal oxygen catheter, or nasal cannula. iNO should not be administered via an oxygen hood due to the potential for accumulation of toxic nitrogen dioxide byproducts within the hood. An integrated NO delivery unit and nitrogen dioxide monitoring system such as the Ohmeda IN-Ovent Nitric Oxide delivery system (Datex-Ohmeda, Madison, WI, USA) is generally used. iNO has an effective half-life of 15–30 secs. Therefore, to ensure that the iNO flow is not interrupted in the event the patient must be disconnected from the ventilator, a separate connector is used to facilitate iNO delivery via a manual bag system. During iNO administration, the appropriate monitoring and measurement of nitrogen dioxide and methemoglobin levels is necessary to prevent potential NO-induced toxicity. When administering iNO at doses <40 ppm,

toxic levels of NO_2 (>2 ppm) rarely occur. Methemoglobinemia may result in patients with inefficient methemoglobin reductase activity or in those who are exposed to high concentrations of iNO or oxygen. Blood methemoglobin levels should be monitored within 4 hrs of initiating iNO and after every 24 hrs of continued treatment. Abrupt discontinuation of iNO may precipitate V/Q mismatch, pulmonary hypertension, and hemodynamic compromise. iNO must be steadily tapered with concurrent clinical and hemodynamic evaluation to safely identify the patient's response to weaning iNO therapy. The effective dose of iNO may depend on the degree of reversible pulmonary arterial hypertension, the extent of V/Q mismatching, and the concurrent level of alveolar recruitment. Clinically, iNO doses between 5 and 20 ppm should produce a clinically apparent response in oxygenation and/or pulmonary vascular resistance. Continuous iNO >40 ppm does not produce greater benefit; rather it can produce increased measured levels of methemoglobin and nitrogen dioxide. In patients with hypoxemic respiratory failure, alveolar derecruitment has been associated with a poor response to iNO therapy at recommended doses. In patients with pulmonary hypertension, a decrease in pulmonary vascular resistance by 30% during a trial of 10 ppm iNO for 10 mins has been predictive of patients likely to derive a clinical response to oral agents. The effect of iNO administration on pain crises and acute chest syndrome in patients with sickle cell anemia is the subject of current clinical trials.

TABLE 14.2

FRACTION OF INSPIRED OXYGEN PROVIDED BY VARIOUS DELIVERY SYSTEMS

Delivery system	F_{IO_2} delivery	Flow required
Nasal cannula	24%–50%	<6 L
Face mask	<60%	6–10 L
Venturi mask	<60%	Variable
Partial rebreather	<60%	15 L
Nonrebreather	~100%	15 L

HELIUM OXYGEN MIXTURES (HELIOX)

Due to its low density, heliox can significantly decrease respiratory distress and work of breathing, and may improve the deposition of bronchodilator therapy to obstructed lower airways. Heliox provides a rapidly acting inhaled therapy for use that may afford the patient greater comfort and improved gas exchange while awaiting the therapeutic onset of slower definitive medical therapies (i.e., corticosteroids). Helium is an odorless, tasteless, noncombustible gas. Helium (0.179 micropoise) is approximately one-seventh the density of air (1.293 micropoise) and oxygen (1.429 micropoise). The density of heliox is dependent on the relative percentage of helium compared to oxygen. The higher the concentration of helium, the lower the concentration of oxygen and the lower the total density of the inhaled gas. Premixed helium-oxygen mixtures provide 20% oxygen (80:20 mixture), 30% oxygen (70:30 mixture), or 40% oxygen (60:40 mixture). Gas flow at high velocity through a relatively small cross-sectional area (e.g., gas flow within the upper airway or through partially obstructed air passages) is typically turbulent, whereas gas flow across a large cross-sectional area (e.g., in the lung periphery) is typically laminar. The lower density of heliox as compared to oxygen-enriched air improves gas flow through high-resistance airways with turbulent gas flow. Turbulent gas flow is mathematically defined by the Bernoulli principle. As gas flow becomes less turbulent in the affected airways, flow velocity is reduced, and the flow pattern may transition from turbulent to more laminar. This transitional zone is represented by the Reynolds number (Re). A lower Re number indicates gas flow with greater laminar flow characteristics. The low density of heliox allows greater gas flow through airways with high resistance and will decrease the Re number in airways with transitional gas flow pattern to generate more laminar flow of gas delivery to the distal airways. Furthermore, carbon dioxide diffuses 4 times as rapidly in heliox mixtures as in air or oxygen gas alone, which may contribute to the tendency for heliox to rapidly improve ventilation and to reduce patients' work of breathing. Administration with a tight-fitting mask is appropriate, while administration via nasal cannula or loose-fitting mask is ineffective. An oxygen analyzer should be placed in line with the patient inspiratory limb when administering heliox to ensure a known fractional percent of oxygen is being supplied to the patient. Heliox delivery through mechanical ventilators may also be effective to reduce air trapping and airways resistance in partially obstructed airways. Most mechanical ventilators can be adapted to administer heliox, but calibration is required. Ventilators are designed and calibrated for a mixture of oxygen and air; thus, adding heliox gas, which is of a different density, viscosity, and thermal conductivity, can affect both the delivered and measured tidal volumes. Unless appropriately calibrated for heliox use, diagnostic equipment, flow meters, gas blenders, and monitoring devices will report falsely low flow and tidal volume readings. For every 10 L/min flow of an 80:20 heliox mixture that is set, 18 L/min is actually delivered. Helium must always be administered with oxygen. Al-

though tanks of 100% helium are available, an interruption in O_2 delivery could result in the accidental administration of pure helium, which could be fatal. The higher the fraction of inspired oxygen required, the lower the helium concentration and the lower the therapeutic benefit derived. However, even those patients with high oxygen requirements (FIO_2 0.80 or greater) may have improved gas exchange with heliox allowing for reduced oxygen therapy. A brief (minutes) therapeutic trial can quickly assess for a clinical response, either by the patient's subjective report or based upon serial examination of respiratory effort, quality of air entry, and gas exchange. Clinically, it is appropriate to forewarn the patient that during heliox use, their voice may become high-pitched and their ability to generate an effective cough will be reduced.

INHALED BRONCHODILATOR THERAPY

Lower-airway respiratory disease is often accompanied by bronchoconstriction, inflammatory cell activation, mucosal edema formation, and inspissated secretions. Inhaled bronchodilator therapy is provided to relieve lower-airway bronchoconstriction, reduce airway resistance, and improve V/Q matching. Inhaled bronchodilators are often given in combination with other pharmacologic agents, including anti-inflammatory agents, decongestants, mucolytic agents, and pulmonary vasodilators, to reverse multiple processes limiting effective gas exchange. Inhaled bronchodilator therapy may include the use of beta-adrenergic receptor agonists (e.g., albuterol, metaproterenol, pirbuterol, levalbuterol, fenoterol, and salbutamol) and/or anticholinergic receptor blockade (e.g.. ipratropium bromide) Although systemic uptake of inhaled agents is negligible, clinically notable side effects may result due to receptor binding at nonpulmonary sites and nonselective receptor binding (e.g., vasodilation, decreased systemic vascular resistance, tremors, decreased insulin release, widened pulse pressure, hyperglycemia, hypokalemia, elevation of creatine phosphokinase and lactate dehydrogenase, tachycardia, palpitations, and/or arrhythmias). The R-isomer of albuterol, levalbuterol, may be associated with a lower incidence of side effects, toxicity, and tolerance.

Three principal types of devices are used to generate therapeutic aerosols: nebulizers, metered-dose inhalers (MDIs), and dry-powder inhalers (DPIs). All 3 types of devices may be equally effective for aerosol administration to the spontaneously breathing patient, but the dry-powder inhalers are ineffective devices for use in mechanically ventilated patients.

Nebulizers create an aerosol that can be effectively delivered to the distal airways by creating particle sizes between 1 and 5 μm. Particles that are too large (>10 μm) are deposited primarily in the oropharynx, and particles that are too small (<1 μm) are not effectively inhaled. Three variables affect nebulizer output: initial fill volume (volume of medication and sterile diluent), nebulization time, and gas flow rate. An increase in any one of these variables increases the effective delivery of inhaled medication. Inhaled aerosols can be effectively administered to the infant and pediatric patient using a face mask or a mouthpiece. A mouthpiece may be preferred as it can be used to direct aerosol therapy to the mouth of the younger patient. A MDI consists of drug suspended in a mixture of propellants, surfactants, preservatives, flavoring agents, and dispersal agents within a pressurized canister. To improve effective delivery for the pediatric patient, a spacer or valved holding chamber is commonly used. The MDI is actuated once, every 15–20 secs, into the accessory device to reduce the need to coordinate with inspiration. A spacer device is an open-ended tube or bag that allows the MDI plume to expand and the propellant to evaporate. DPIs are breath-actuated, thus delivering medication only upon inhalation. This reduces the problem of coordinating inspiration with actuation. However, release of the drug requires high inspiratory flow rates >50 L/min. This limits use in the younger patient <6 years of age and in the neuromuscularly weak patient.

Inhaled bronchodilators may be effectively administered and equally therapeutic in the mechanically ventilated patient using a nebulizer or MDI. To increase the effective drug delivery during mechanical ventilation, attention to several aspects of delivery is required: (a) location of delivery within the ventilator circuit, (b) humidity within the circuit, and (c) ventilator flow **(Table 14.3)**. Relative advantages of using an MDI versus a continuous nebulizer treatment for the intubated patient include less personnel time required for administration, lack of need to disconnect ventilator circuit (when an in-line MDI chamber is used), and no need to alter ventilator settings during administration.

NITROGEN (HYPOXIC GAS) AND CARBON DIOXIDE ADMINISTRATION

ICUs that manage patients with single-ventricle congenital heart disease may at times use supplemental nitrogen gas (forming a hypoxic gas mixture) or exogenous carbon dioxide administration to increase pulmonary vascular resistance (PVR) in an

---

TABLE 14.3

RECOMMENDED TECHNIQUES FOR METERED-DOSE INHALER AND NEBULIZER USE DURING MECHANICAL VENTILATION

Metered-dose inhaler
Agitate MDI and warm to hand temperature
Place MDI adaptor into inspiratory limb of circuit (10–18 cm from the Y-piece connector)

- Attach MDI to adaptor in ventilator circuit (chamber-style is best)
- Actuate ≥4 puffs at beginning of inspiratory cycle
- Cycle each actuation with a spontaneous or ventilator inspiratory cycle
- Wait ≥5 sec between actuations
- Assess patient response

Nebulizer
Establish dose to be administered
Place drug in nebulizer reservoir; fill with normal saline to ≥4 mL
Place nebulizer in inspiratory circuit ≥10 cm from the patient Y-piece connector
Initiate driving gas flow of oxygen ≥6 L/min; ≥12 L/min when heliox is used
Turn off flow by or continuous flow during nebulization
Continue nebulization treatment until sputtering occurs indicating end of treatment
Remove nebulizer and return ventilator to previous settings
Assure no leak in circuit
Assess patient response

Adapted with permission from James B Fink, MS, RRT.

---

effort to control the ratio of pulmonary (Q_p) to systemic (Q_s) blood flow. A patent ductus arteriosus in these patients is vital to either systemic or pulmonary blood flow based on the underlying structural cardiac defect. In the care of some patients with ductal-dependent single-ventricle congenital heart disease, excessive pulmonary blood flow may lead to clinically significant systemic hypoperfusion. With single-ventricle physiology, cardiac output is distributed based on the relative vascular resistances between the pulmonary and systemic vascular resistance (SVR) circulation. The ideal balance of these two circulations is reflected by an oxygenation saturation of ~80%.

Caution must be advised when delivering hypoxic gas mixtures to mechanically ventilated patients. Hypoxic gas mixtures are obtained by nitrogen dilution—the addition of low-flow nitrogen into the ventilator circuit. The F_{IO_2} control knob is no longer a control of administered O_2 but rather a control of either air or nitrogen. Therefore, if this knob is inadvertently turned (in either direction), the delivered concentration of hypoxic gas mixture may be significantly altered. It is impossible to deliver a hypoxic gas mixture via a ventilator and not defeat a safety mechanism. The oxygen analyzer alarm limits must be reset or turned off during hypoxic gas administration. Furthermore, commercially available O_2 analyzers do not accurately monitor these lower O_2 concentrations.

Pulmonary vascular resistance (PVR) is affected by alveolar O_2 tension, capillary CO_2 tension, and blood pH. Exogenous CO_2 may provide a dose-dependent increase in PVR. Some patients may respond to an elevated Pa_{CO_2} of 45–50 mm Hg, whereas in other patients, levels as high as 80–95 mm Hg Pa_{CO_2} may be required. As the Pa_{CO_2} tension increases, the resultant blood pH may fall, and acidemia may occur. Treatment of acidemia with buffering agents such as bicarbonate or THAM (tromethamine), especially in patients with underlying cardiac dysfunction, seems commonplace in many ICUs. Exogenous CO_2 may be administered into the ventilator outflow port and measured by a capnometer in the inspiratory limb of the ventilator circuit. Increased Pa_{CO_2} and acidemic pH are potent stimulators of respiration. Therefore, during exogenous CO_2 administration, minute ventilation must be maintained constant with the administration of sufficient sedation and, if necessary, neuromuscular blockade. Decreases in the ventilator set tidal volume and respiratory rate to achieve hypoventilation may have similar results as exogenous carbon dioxide administration, but if ventilator settings are decreased significantly, arterial desaturation may result secondary to the loss of lung volume. The therapeutic range of exogenous CO_2 is 1%–4% (8–30 mm Hg).

Caution must always be advised with any inhaled medical therapy that requires the alteration of or impairs safety features. Although hypoxic gas mixtures and CO_2 administration may achieve a similar degree of balance between the pulmonary and system blood flow, exogenous CO_2 gas therapy may do so without the need to defeat important safety controls. These therapies require technical skill and a thorough understanding of the underlying physiology to ensure appropriate use and patient safety.

INHALATIONAL ANESTHETICS

Inhalational anesthetics have been administered in the critical care unit to aid in the treatment of medically refractory bronchospasm (isoflurane, desflurane), for refractory pain (isoflurane, nitrous oxide), for treatment of status epilepticus, and for sedation

TABLE 14.4

COMPARISON OF ANESTHETIC POTENCY FOR THE INHALATIONAL ANESTHETICS USED IN THE PICU

Anesthetic agent	MAC (%)
Isoflurane	1.2
Desflurane	6.0
Nitrous Oxide	105.0[a]

MAC, minimum alveolar concentration; MAC (%), concentration of inhaled agent required to prevent movement in response to surgical stimuli in 50% of patients.
[a] Hyperbaric conditions are required to reach 1 MAC.

(isoflurane, desflurane). These agents provide an appealing alternative to more traditional intravenous therapies provided in the ICU because they provide (a) the rapid onset and titration of therapeutic effects, (b) a low side effect profile, (c) limited metabolism that is independent of renal or hepatic function, (d) the relief of bronchospasm, and (e) the potential to provide adequate sedation yet preserve spontaneous respiratory effort. The end-tidal alveolar gas concentration is continuously monitored to determine the median alveolar concentration (MAC; **Table 14.4**) of the volatile agent administered to the patient. For each inhaled anesthetic agent, 1 MAC refers to the concentration required to prevent movement in 50% of patients in response to surgical stimuli. MAC-hours references the patient's level of anesthetic exposure in hours.

Isoflurane induces rapid anesthetic induction and recovery and has been used to treat pain, sedation, and severe bronchospasm in cases refractory to conventional medical therapies. Isoflurane dosing in the ICU setting is initiated at 0.5% and titrated to clinical effect up to 2%. Dose-dependent side effects include systemic vasodilation, increased sympathetic stimuli resulting in increased cardiac output, skin flushing, and tachycardia. Isoflurane increases cerebral blood flow and may raise intracranial pressure, but it reduces cerebral oxygen consumption. Isoflurane is also a potent coronary vasodilator resulting in improved coronary blood flow and decreased myocardial oxygen consumption.

Use of inhalation anesthetics within the ICU requires proper facilities, personnel training, and equipment to facilitate a safe environment for patients and staff. To safely administer isoflurane outside the operative setting, specialized equipment for monitoring and scavenging the volatile anesthetic are needed. For delivery, an anesthesia machine or adaptation of the ICU ventilator is required. Active scavenging systems and appropriate turnover of ambient air is required to protect patients and staff from inadvertent exposure. The scavenging system should collect all exhaled gases, including ventilator exhaust, gas emitted around an endotracheal tube leak, gases emitted when the ventilator circuit is disconnected, and any gas collected within the anesthesia bag during manual ventilation. Continuous infrared monitoring equipment for both the inspired and expired concentrations of the inhalational agent is necessary. The high and low concentration alarms are set within a narrow range to immediately detect variation from desired settings. Prolonged administration may be associated with an abstinence syndrome. Symptoms, which are reversible, include agitation, choreoathetoid movements, hypertension, tachycardia, diaphoresis, and diarrhea. The abstinence syndrome may be prevented or treated with the gradual withdrawal of the inhalation agent or use of intravenous sedation as the agent is withdrawn. Fluoride ion nephrotoxicity is also associated with prolonged isoflurane exposure. Nephrotoxicity has been reported with serum fluoride levels 50 μm. Continuous temperature monitoring as well as carbon dioxide measurements are necessary to detect the rare but treatable onset of malignant hyperthermia. Dantrolene sodium should be readily available for any patient receiving inhaled isoflurane.

NITROUS OXIDE

Nitrous oxide is a relatively weak anesthetic agent, producing analgesia at low concentrations (20%) and requiring near-toxic concentrations to produce deep sedation. Concentrations between 20% and 80% produce analgesia and dose-dependent levels of sedation. Nitrous oxide must always be administered with oxygen and cannot be administered above concentrations of 80% due to the limitation imposed on fractional percentage of oxygen supplied. Nitrous oxide is eliminated via the lungs with metabolism that is independent of renal or hepatic function. Dose-dependent side effects include increased respiratory rate and depressed tidal volume, generally with minimal resultant effects on minute ventilation and carbon dioxide tension. Nitrous oxide increases cerebral blood flow and intracranial pressure, but these effects may be abolished when coadministered with IV sedation or narcotics. Nitrous oxide can be effectively delivered via nasal cannula, face mask, or non-rebreather. Safe handling practices must be followed when using nitrous oxide as both nitrous oxide and oxygen gases support combustion. Flow meters ordinarily calibrated for the administration of oxygen and nitrogen require calibration for the delivery of nitrous oxide. Nitrous oxide is contraindicated for any patient with pathologic air-filled cavities and with an increased risk or prior history of pulmonary hypertension. Nitrous oxide administration may result in expansion of an existing pneumothorax, pulmonary bullae, intracranial air, vascular air embolus, bowel obstruction, or intraocular air bubble. Nitrous oxide administration may cause megaloblastic anemia and a peripheral neuropathy secondary to vitamin B_{12} deficiency.

CHAPTER 15 ■ EXTRACORPOREAL LIFE SUPPORT

STEVEN A. CONRAD • HEIDI J. DALTON

The Extracorporeal Life Support Organization (Ann Arbor, MI) is a consortium of healthcare centers that use extracorporeal circulation for support of severe cardiopulmonary failure. These centers contribute detailed data into a registry on each extracorporeal life support (ECLS) case performed. The registry currently has data on >32,000 cases performed in 145 centers.

The components of an ECLS circuit, although based on the traditional cardiopulmonary bypass circuit, have been developed or adapted for long-term support (**Fig. 15.1**). Vascular cannulas are placed for blood drainage and reinfusion. A small drainage reservoir (bladder) helps to ensure continuous availability of blood for the pump. A roller-head or centrifugal pump provides the blood flow through the circuit. An artificial lung (membrane oxygenator) provides gas exchange, and a heat exchanger maintains a controlled temperature of reinfused blood. Other circuit components allow for infusion of medications, incorporation of a hemofilter for fluid control, and blood gas, flow, and pressure monitoring

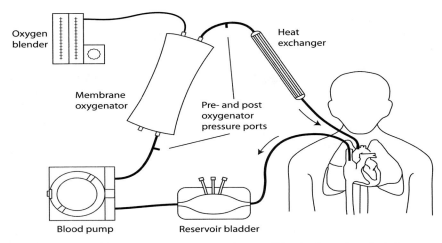

FIGURE 15.1. Components of a typical extracorporeal circuit. The circuit consists of a drainage reservoir (bladder), blood pump, membrane lung, heat exchanger, and connecting tubing. Blood is drained from the right atrium and returned to the arterial system via the carotid into the proximal aorta.

systems. Extracorporeal support requires blood flows equal to the cardiac output (for venoarterial support), and sometimes higher (100–120 mL/kg/min) for venovenous or hybrid support. Cannulas of sufficient sizes to support this level of flow are necessary. Most cannulas are constructed of polyurethane and may include wire reinforcement to prevent kinking.

Traditional cannulation employs two single-lumen cannulas, one for venous drainage and a second for return to the venous or arterial circulation. Single-lumen cannulas are used for all modes of support. The cannula size chosen is dictated by both the size and flow requirements of the patient as well as the size of the vessel(s) available for cannulation. Neonates have vessels that range from ~8–10 French (fr) (carotid artery) to 12–15 fr (internal jugular vein), whereas adolescents can accommodate up to 20 fr arterial and 24 fr venous (and larger). Double-lumen cannulas have been developed specifically for venovenous ECLS (Origen Biomedical, Austin TX; **Fig. 15.2**). Placed through the internal jugular, these cannulas have two drainage ports located at both atriocaval junctions and a reinfusion port between these two directed toward the tricuspid valve.

Two types of blood pumps are currently used for extracorporeal membrane oxygenation (ECMO) and are the same pumps used for cardiopulmonary bypass. The most popular is the *roller pump*, a positive-displacement pump in which a rotating roller head squeezes a length of blood tubing against a backing plate as the roller head rotates (**Fig. 15.3**). This pump is used with gravity drainage, so an assist reservoir

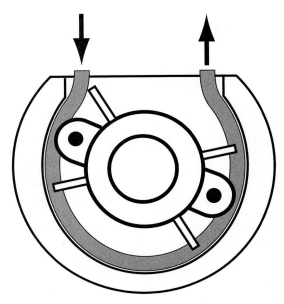

FIGURE 15.3. Roller pump used in extracorporeal circulation. The pump functions by having the rotor pinch and nearly occlude the raceway tubing against a backing plate, and the rotation forces blood through the tubing. The blood flow rate is linearly related to the size of the tubing and the rotational speed of the rotor.

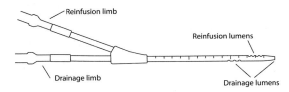

FIGURE 15.2. Double-lumen cannula for single-vessel (right internal jugular) access for venovenous extracorporeal life support.

(bladder) is required at the pump inlet to maintain a continuous supply of blood to the pump, since inlet occlusion can result in large negative pressures. In the event of outlet tubing obstruction, the pump can generate pressures high enough to cause tubing rupture, requiring continuous monitoring of circuit pressures. The *centrifugal pump* is a nonocclusive pump that generates flow via a spinning rotor with vanes . The device generates an active suction at the pump inlet. Occlusion of the inlet or outlet will result in only modest negative inlet or positive outlet pressures. Although this pump is safer from mechanical complications, hemolysis can develop rapidly in the case of tubing obstruction and is the most common complication of the use of a centrifugal pump.

Roller pump systems require a continuous availability of blood at the inlet to avoid development of large negative pressures and hemolysis. This is ensured by placing a small assist reservoir, or bladder, just before the pump inlet. Gravity assist is achieved by placing the reservoir and pump ~100 cm below the level of the cannula, providing a hydrostatic siphon for drainage and maintaining a positive pressure at the pump inlet. The reservoir also buffers against fluctuations in drainage. If drainage decreases, for example due to hypovolemia, the reservoir will begin to empty, signaling the need for correction of the reason for poor drainage. Most roller pump systems have the capability of servoregulation. A switch situated in the reservoir holder opens when the bladder empties, turning off the pump and allowing time for filling of the reservoir. With the pump off, the bladder refills, and the pump resumes operation.

The membrane lung, commonly called a membrane oxygenator, provides gas exchange between the blood and the atmosphere. Although called an oxygenator, it is more appropriately called an artificial lung, since it transports carbon dioxide as well as oxygen.

The spiral-wound solid silicone sheet membrane lung has been used in the majority of ECMO cases since its inception. Sizes range from 0.6 to 4.5 M^2. The larger devices have an integrated heat exchanger. Microporous hollow fiber devices, most commonly used for cardiopulmonary bypass, are increasing in popularity for ECMO because of their improved gas exchange performance and low resistance to blood flow. After several hours of contact with plasma, however, leakage of plasma ensues, and gas exchange is impaired.

SUPPORT MODES

As ECMO has evolved from cardiopulmonary bypass (e.g., venoarterial bypass with intrathoracic vas-

cular cannulation), the initial application mode of ECMO was also venoarterial. While venoarterial support remains important, especially with cardiac dysfunction, venovenous support has begun to supplant the traditional venoarterial mode, primarily for respiratory failure. A hybrid support mode combining features of venoarterial and venovenous has been described. More recently, pumpless arteriovenous support ($AVCO_2R$) has been shown to be clinically feasible for management of hypercarbic states. Each of these modes has particular advantages and disadvantages for different clinical situations (**Table 15.1**).

Venoarterial (VA) support is based on cardiopulmonary bypass, in which blood is drained from the right atrium via the central venous system and returned to the proximal arterial system. Both ventricles and the intervening pulmonary system are bypassed. In most cases, partial support is achieved, with some residual pulmonary blood flow present. Both cardiac and pulmonary support are provided with this mode. Cannulation is usually performed by surgical access to the right internal jugular vein for right atrial drainage and to the right carotid artery for return to the aortic root. This mode provides the highest levels of systemic arterial saturation but may be associated with lower coronary oxygen saturation when bypass is partial, since native cardiac output may be directed toward the coronary ostia. The gas exchange advantages of VA support are offset by a higher potential for complications such as cerebral embolism, the reduction in pulmonary blood flow, and the loss of the right carotid circulation from ligation.

In place of the cervical approach, cannulation may be made through the femoral vessels. This approach lends itself to percutaneous cannulation. Flow returning to the femoral artery will predominantly perfuse the lower half of the body, although retrograde flow up the aortic arch will also occur. The extent of retrograde flow is often dependent on the adequacy of native cardiac output, with more flow reaching the upper aorta under conditions of poor intrinsic cardiac function. With good cardiac function, the heart and brain predominantly receive blood from the native cardiopulmonary system. Thus, in patients with severe pulmonary failure and good cardiac function, desaturated blood may perfuse the brain and heart. Venous saturation entering the right heart is often elevated in this mode by the mixing of the lower body arterialized blood returned from the ECLS circuit with intrinsic venous blood—thus adequate oxygenation to the native cardiopulmonary circuit can be obtained.

Venovenous (VV) ECLS can effectively support pediatric patients with respiratory failure and

TABLE 15.1

COMPARISON OF CARDIOPULMONARY BYPASS AND DIFFERENT MODES OF EXTRACORPOREAL LIFE SUPPORT

	CPB	VA ECMO	VV ECMO	VVA	AVCO$_2$R
Setting	Cardiac surgery	Prolonged support	Prolonged support	Prolonged support	ER or ICU support
Support	Total cardiac and pulmonary	Cardiac and pulmonary	Pulmonary	Cardiac and pulmonary	Pulmonary
Cannulation	Intrathoracic (surgical)	Extrathoracic (surgical)	Extrathoracic (percutaneous)	Extrathoracic (percutaneous)	Extrathoracic (percutaneous)
Blood pump	Roller or centrifugal	Roller or centrifugal	Roller or centrifugal	Roller or centrifugal	None (pumpless)
ECMO blood flow (fraction of CO)	Total (100%)	Subtotal (70%–90%)	Subtotal	Subtotal (1/3 arterial, 2/3 venous)	Low (10%–20%)
Pulmonary flow	None	Low	Unchanged	Moderate decrease	Unchanged
Length of support	Hours	Days to weeks	Days to weeks	Days to weeks	Days
Anticoagulation	ACT >400	ACT 180–200	ACT 180–200	ACT 180–200	ACT 200–220
Reservoir	Large	Small or none[a]	Small or none[a]	Small or none[a]	None

CPB, cardiopulmonary bypass; VA ECMO, venoarterial extracorporeal membrane oxygenation; VV ECMO, venovenous extracorporeal membrane oxygenation; VVA, venovenoarterial; AVCO$_2$R, arteriovenous support

[a] Reservoir used for roller pump, optional for centrifugal pump.

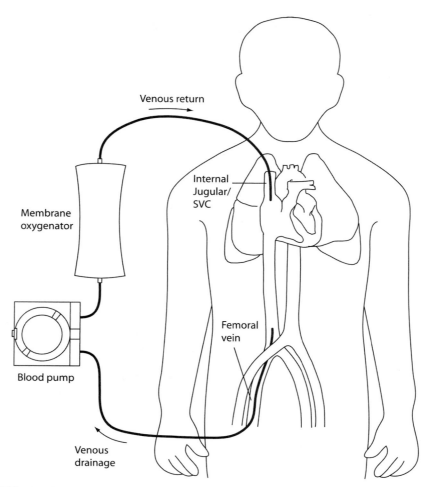

FIGURE 15.4. Venovenous mode of extracorporeal life support. Blood is drained from the inferior vena cava and returned to the proximal superior vena cava or right atrium.

is rapidly becoming the preferred mode for management of severe respiratory failure in children. This mode provides pre-pulmonary oxygenation by draining blood from the central venous circulation and returning it back into the venous circulation (**Fig. 15.4**). The reinfused blood elevates mixed venous saturation, diminishes the effect of intrapulmonary shunt, and delivers blood with a higher saturation to the coronary arteries. There is no direct cardiac support, though myocardial function commonly improves, often considerably, by elevation of myocardial oxygenation and reduction in intrathoracic pressures. VV support may be successfully applied even in the presence of inotrope dependence. An attractive aspect of VV support is the ability to cannulate the veins percutaneously, avoiding surgical vascular access and largely eliminating bleeding from the vascular access site. The carotid artery and jugular are spared from ligation, and venous return through

the jugular can be maintained. CNS complications are potentially lower with VV support, and this may be related to the less invasive nature of the vascular access technique. Cannulation is typically carried out through the right internal jugular vein and the right common femoral vein. The more recent development of double-lumen cannula for patients up to 10 kg has allowed even simpler access, requiring only a single cannulation through the internal jugular vein. Recirculation, in which some of the return flow into the venous system is directed back into the drainage cannula, is present to a variable degree and reduces overall gas transfer. Venous drainage may be obtained from the internal jugular and returned to the femoral sites or the direction of flow may be reversed (drainage from femoral with return to the jugular). Draining from the femoral veins has the advantage of reduced recirculation; however, usually less venous flow can be obtained than if drainage is via the jugular cannula. The use of a three-cannula approach can minimize recirculation even further.

The venovenoarterial (VVA) mode is a recently introduced hybrid mode that combines VV support for pulmonary failure and partial venoarterial support with the advantage of percutaneous cannulation. The typical circuit consists of a drainage cannula in the right femoral vein and two return cannulae connected via a Y-connection, one in the right internal jugular vein and the second in a femoral artery. Blood flow between the two return limbs is controlled to achieve ~30% flow into the arterial system by restricting the flow to the venous cannula. VVA support is ideally suited for larger pediatric patients requiring partial cardiac support in addition to pulmonary support.

In pumpless arteriovenous (AV) support of gas exchange, the arterial-venous pressure gradient drives flow through a membrane lung without the need for a pump. Since arterial blood is usually well oxygenated, oxygen transfer is limited, but carbon dioxide is readily removed. The applications of AV carbon dioxide removal ($AVCO_2R$) are identical to those of $ECCO_2R$ but without the need for an extracorporeal pump (i.e., reduction in mechanical ventilatory support and control of hypercapnia).

CANNULATION TECHNIQUES

The trend in vascular cannulation is toward percutaneous or modified percutaneous techniques, as this approach is more rapid, associated with less bleeding complications, and decannulation is simplified. The dual lumen catheter by Origen Biomedical (Austin, TX) is available in 12-, 15-, and 18-fr sizes and is suitable for neonates and infants up to ~10–12 kg. This cannula has both drainage and reinfusion lumens. This catheter is placed by percutaneous puncture of the right internal jugular, optimally under ultrasound guidance, using the Seldinger technique. A guidewire exchange system is available, in which the initial puncture is made with a small needle and guidewire (0.018 in), followed by an exchange for a larger wire (0.035 in) suitable for dilation and advancement of the cannula. VV cannulation in children >10–12 kg is accomplished by use of single-lumen cannulas in the femoral and right internal jugular veins. The internal jugular is large enough to accommodate a single reinfusion cannula (18–24 fr, depending on size). In larger children, a single femoral drainage cannula is usually suitable. The femoral veins in smaller children are smaller in relation to body size, and two drainage cannulas may be employed if drainage from a single site is inadequate. Choice of cannula size is dictated by the required flow (50–100 mL/kg/min). A modified percutaneous technique for cannulation of the internal jugular vein in neonates uses a limited surgical exposure of the internal jugular with percutaneous cannulation under direct visualization of the vein. Percutaneous arterial cannulation is limited to the femoral artery in larger children. This vessel is usually too small to accommodate full VA support, so this approach is limited to the provision of partial support. In the presence of respiratory failure, hybrid VVA support may be a suitable option. AV support for carbon dioxide removal ($AVCO_2R$) requires lower blood flows than those required for oxygenation support, on the order of 15%–20% of the cardiac output. Percutaneous cannulation of the femoral vessels with a 10- to 12-fr arterial cannula and 14- to 16-fr venous cannula provides adequate flow (500–1000 mL/min) for complete carbon dioxide removal in hypercapnic states.

The open surgical technique remains the approach of choice today for VA support through the common carotid artery and internal jugular vein. A transverse incision is made above the right clavicle over the vessels, and dissection is carried out to expose the carotid sheath (**Fig. 15.5**). Surgical placement of a dual-lumen venous cannula for VV bypass is performed in a similar manner, although without the need for carotid ligation and arteriotomy.

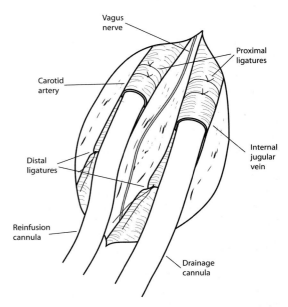

FIGURE 15.5. Open surgical approach to cervical cannulation. The carotid sheath is opened, the vessels exposed, and ligatures placed. An arteriotomy and venotomy provide access to the lumen for cannula insertion.

ECLS following failure to wean from cardiopulmonary bypass or sternotomy for resuscitation can be managed using the same cannulas placed for intraoperative support. These cannulas are placed into the right atrium and ascending aorta. The chest is incompletely closed, allowing the cannula to exit the wound and is dressed. If hemodynamic function improves in a short period of time, the patient can be weaned from support and decannulated in the operating room. If long-term support is deemed necessary, the patient can be converted to peripherally placed cannulas, as bleeding is less with this approach.

Termination of ECLS is followed by decannulation. If cardiopulmonary function is marginal after cessation of support, the decision may be made to maintain the cannulas in place for several hours or more. Provisions for maintaining anticoagulation and continuous flushing of the cannulas must be made.

DETERMINANTS OF ECLS CIRCUIT PERFORMANCE

The blood path in the extracorporeal circuit includes the vascular cannulas, circuit tubing, oxygenator, and heat exchanger. The point of greatest impedance to blood flow is in the vascular cannulas, in particular the venous drainage cannula, since it depends upon gravity drainage (roller pump) or a low level of suction (centrifugal pump). Optimization of conditions for venous drainage is essential, including selection of cannula size. The relationship between pressure and flow is nonlinear At lower blood flows, laminar flow predominates and is approximately described by the Hagen-Poiseuille equation, with flow (Q) directly related to pressure gradient (ΔP) and inversely related to catheter length (L):

$$\dot{Q} = \left(\frac{\pi r^4}{8\eta} \right) \bullet \frac{\Delta P}{L}$$

The catheter dimension with greatest influence on blood flow is the diameter; thus, the goal is to place the catheter with the largest diameter and shortest length as allowed by the venous anatomy. Blood delivered by the extracorporeal circuit must be fully saturated with oxygen by the membrane oxygenator in order to have maximal achievable oxygen delivery. A membrane oxygenator can fully saturate blood only up to a certain flow, above which saturation falls off and total oxygen delivery reaches a plateau. Gas transfer by the membrane oxygenator is determined by several factors. The membrane surface area, membrane diffusion coefficient, and thickness of the blood film in the oxygenator are determined by the manufacturer. The partial pressure gradient between the

blood and gas phases is in part governed by blood and sweep gas flows. The choice of the membrane oxygenator is usually made on selecting a sufficiently large surface area device to accommodate the calculated blood flow (50–100 mL/kg/min). Recirculation, in which some of the blood reinfused into the patient from the circuit is diverted back into the drainage cannula rather than continue into the pulmonary circulation, is unavoidable in VV ECLS.

CLINICAL APPLICATIONS AND SELECTION OF PATIENTS

Hypoxemic Respiratory Failure

Respiratory failure due to persistent pulmonary hypertension and meconium aspiration is replaced by pulmonary infection, pulmonary aspiration, systemic sepsis, the acute respiratory distress syndrome (ARDS) and others. These conditions present with features of their adult counterpart of ARDS rather than persistent pulmonary hypertension of the newborn and are frequently accompanied by extrapulmonary organ system involvement. The selection of patients for ECLS is founded in a set of criteria that have evolved over time and have historically predicted a high mortality (**Table 15.2**). The

---

TABLE 15.2

CRITERIA USED IN SELECTION OF PATIENTS FOR ECLS FOR PULMONARY SUPPORT IN HYPOXEMIC RESPIRATORY FAILURE

Severe, potentially reversible acute respiratory failure
Lack of response to conventional support measures[a]
Severe hypoxemia, e.g.:
  PaO_2 / FiO_2 <100
  Oxygenation Index (OI) >40
  Qs/Qt >0.5
Elevated inflation pressures, e.g.:
  MAP >20 on conventional ventilation, >25 on HFOV
  Persistent air leak or interstitial air
  Cardiovascular depression with shock (pH <7.25)
Lack of irreversible ventilator-induced lung injury, e.g.:
  Duration of mechanical ventilation <7 days

ECLS, extracorporeal life support; HFOV, high-frequency oscillatory ventilation; MAP, mean airway pressure
[a] Conventional support may include measures such as high-frequency oscillatory ventilation (HFOV), inhaled nitric oxide, prone positioning, surfactant, or others.

avoidance of ventilator-induced lung injury is a major goal of ECLS; thus, patients requiring excessive inflation pressures, even in the absence of life-threatening hypoxemia, should be considered for extracorporeal support. This is particularly important if lactic acidosis and shock result from high levels of ventilatory support. The presence of barotrauma (radiographic evidence of pneumomediastinum or pulmonary interstitial air, persistent air leak) should lead to consideration of ECLS, especially if it is progressive and uncontrollable. VV support is the preferred ECLS mode for hypoxemic respiratory failure. The presence of shock despite inotropes would be best supported with the VA approach.

Hypercapnic Respiratory Failure

Severe hypercapnia with respiratory acidosis, in particular severe asthma, is effectively managed by VV extracorporeal support. Since carbon dioxide is more effectively exchanged in the membrane lung than is oxygen, blood flows lower than that required for oxygenation are effective in control of hypercapnia. Other advantages of extracorporeal support of severe asthma is ability to perform bronchoscopy. An alternative to VV extracorporeal CO_2 removal is pumpless AV CO_2 removal (AVCO$_2$R). Percutaneous cannulation of the femoral artery and vein can be rapidly performed, and crystalloid priming of the circuit is simple. AVCO$_2$R can normalize pH and PCO$_2$, even in severe asthma. Decannulation is simple, since the small size of the arterial cannula permits hemostasis through direct pressure alone.

Acute Myocardial Dysfunction

ECLS has been a primary mode of support for pediatric patients with circulatory failure from acute myocardial dysfunction and accounts for the indication for support in over half of all pediatric ECLS cases beyond the neonatal period. Prolonged low cardiac output and shock in the face of appropriate fluid management and pharmacologic support can result in neurologic injury and other organ dysfunction and should be avoided by early consideration of ECLS. VA support is the mode of choice since it provides cardiopulmonary bypass and maintains systemic circulatory flow at normal levels. In the face of severe myocardial dysfunction, in which the ventricle cannot empty against the afterload associated with ECLS-maintained arterial pressure, persistent elevation of end-diastolic pressure can result in pulmonary hypertension, pulmonary edema, pulmonary hemorrhage, and impairment of myocardial recovery. When

required, the left heart can be decompressed via atrial septostomy, which can be performed in the cardiac catheterization suite or at the bedside. Nonsurgical causes of severe myocardial dysfunction are also supported with ECLS. Cardiomyopathies unrelated to cardiac surgery differ from the postoperative causes of myocardial dysfunction in that recovery may take place after prolonged support. Acute myocarditis can follow a rapidly progressive course and result in death in a majority of cases. VA ECLS can be used to bridge to transplantation.

Weaning from VA extracorporeal support is initiated when signs of ventricular recovery are noted. An early manifestation of recovery is improvement in pulsatility as evidenced by an increase in pulse pressure. Echocardiography permits serial noninvasive assessment of ventricular contractility and can assess the response to changes in ventricular loading associated with reduction in flow. Once ventricular recovery begins, the extracorporeal flow is gradually reduced, and the patient is assessed clinically for adequacy of perfusion. Measurements of blood gases, mixed venous oxygen saturation, and cardiac function by echocardiography ensure that native cardiac function is adequate.

Extracorporeal Cardiopulmonary Resuscitation

Recognition of the poor rate of recovery from cardiac arrest following external chest compression, particularly after prolonged efforts, has led to the expanded use of rapid-deployment ECLS. Also termed *extracorporeal cardiopulmonary resuscitation* or *resuscitation extracorporeal membrane oxygenation*, this technique involves the rapid institution of ECLS during cardiac arrest via percutaneous cannulation of the femoral vessels and a pre-primed or rapidly primed ECLS circuit.

Physiology of ECLS

Systemic blood flow during VA ECLS is the sum of native cardiac output and blood flow through the circuit. As circuit blood flow is raised, less venous return is available to the native heart. As the proportion of systemic flow provided by the nonpulsatile blood pump increases, stroke volume diminishes and is recognized as a diminishing pulse pressure on the arterial waveform. In severe cardiac dysfunction, systemic blood flow may be provided totally by the extracorporeal circuit. During total bypass, the left ventricle still receives some blood flow, mostly from the

Thebesian veins (in the myocardial wall) and deep bronchial veins and possibly intermittent flow across the pulmonary circulation. Nonpulsatile flow has potentially deleterious effects, including, increased peripheral vascular resistance and reduced renal and cerebral perfusion. Systemic oxygen delivery during ECLS is dependent on the mode of support and the degree of native lung function. During VA ECLS, in which native pulmonary blood flow is parallel to the circuit flow, oxygen delivery is the sum of that provided by fully saturated blood from the extracorporeal circuit mixed with that provided by the native lungs. With total bypass, systemic oxygen delivery is provided totally by the circuit, and is equal to the product of the pump flow and the oxygen content of fully saturated blood. With partial bypass, blood from the lungs is often poorly saturated due to pulmonary dysfunction and, therefore, functions as a shunt, decreasing the total oxygen content relative to the amount of native pulmonary blood flow. In VV support, the circuit and the native pulmonary circulation are in series, and the effects of oxygen content provided by the pump and that provided by the native lungs is additive. The resulting oxygen delivery is the incremental oxygen content added to the true mixed venous oxygen saturation by the circuit and the lungs. AV ECLS does not provide any significant degree of oxygen delivery, since the blood provided to the membrane already contains arterial levels of oxygen. Even under profound hypoxemic conditions, the small fraction of blood through the circuit (20% of cardiac output or less) would not contribute substantially to overall oxygen delivery. It is therefore most applicable to hypercapnic states without significant hypoxemia.

The mechanical pumping of blood and resulting high flow through a system that is recognized to produce high shear rates results in injury to erythrocytes, platelets, and plasma proteins. The extracorporeal circuit represents a large, non-endothelial contact surface that is known to induce profound effects on the coagulation system. Heparin is not an ideal anticoagulant but remains a drug of choice for numerous reasons, including the great degree of experience with its use. The extracorporeal circuit also induces a systemic inflammatory response. Activation of macrophages and other immune system–related cells results in the production of proximal proinflammatory mediators.

PRINCIPLES OF MANAGEMENT

The extracorporeal circuit volume is large relative to the patient's blood volume, mandating that the circuit be primed with a solution containing normal electrolyte concentration and acceptable acid-base status, oncotic pressure, and hemoglobin concentration. Priming begins with balanced electrolyte solution (such as Normosol or PlasmaLyte). Packed red blood cells and concentrated albumin are added, and heparin is administered (1–2 U/mL of prime). Preparation of the patient prior to cannulation includes adequate sedation and analgesia. Baseline measurement of activated coagulation time (ACT) is made prior to heparin administration. If percutaneous cannulation is chosen, ultrasonographic measurement of vessel size and patency may be performed and may also be used to guide needle insertion. Neuromuscular blockers are administered just prior to cannulation to prevent inspiratory efforts during cannula insertion that can result in a large air embolism. An initial bolus of heparin (50–100 U/kg) is administered just prior to cannulation. After vascular access is achieved, the primed circuit is connected and flow initiated a low flow rate, incrementally to the target rate over several minutes. Infants require 100–200 mL/kg/min. VV support targets the higher end of the range owing to recirculation. Pediatric patients require ~100 mL/kg/min, and adolescents require 50–100 mL/kg/min.

The goal for ventilator management is to provide a protective ventilation strategy: to maintain alveolar distention, avoid overdistension and atelectasis, minimize cyclic shear stress associated with tidal ventilation, and reduce exposure to elevated concentrations of oxygen. High-frequency oscillation with a mean airway pressure sufficient to minimize atelectasis is more commonly practiced in smaller children. In larger children, high-frequency oscillation or use of pressure-limited ventilation, elevated levels of positive end-expiratory pressure (PEEP) (10–20 cm H_2O), low respiratory rate (6–10/min), and small tidal volumes (4–6 mL/kg) will meet these goals. An appropriate level of PEEP can be obtained by recording a bedside slow dynamic pressure-volume curve and examining the inflection points on the inspiratory and expiratory curves.

The requirement for vasoactive agents is almost universal in patients about to undergo extracorporeal support. Patients with severe acute respiratory failure also have some degree of myocardial dysfunction. Right ventricular dysfunction due to acute pulmonary hypertension, myocardial depression from systemic inflammation, and altered ventricular filling due to high ventilation requirements are major contributors to myocardial dysfunction.

Provision of sedation and analgesia for patients receiving ECLS is accomplished with benzodiazepines (midazolam or lorazepam) and opioid analgesics (morphine or fentanyl). Dosing requirements may be elevated, as drugs may be adsorbed by the circuit, tolerance can develop, and hemofiltration can remove administered drugs. A major trend in extracorporeal support is to minimize sedation and allow spontaneous breathing and even interaction with staff. Use of minimal doses of benzodiazepines and narcotics can be supplemented by other agents. Atypical antipsychotic agents are effective in reducing agitation and delirium without sedation, and dexmedetomidine provides sedation from which the patient can be easily aroused. Propofol is a short-acting agent that is easily titratable; however, it cannot be used with microporous hollow fiber oxygenators. The lipid component can decrease surface tension at the pores of the membrane, leading to plasma leakage.

A goal of extracorporeal support is to provide sufficient blood flow to meet metabolic demands and avoid tissue hypoxia, yet not provide excessive flow. Mixed venous oxygen saturation (SvO_2) in the normal range of 70%–75% is the usual goal, and flow is adjusted accordingly. In VA mode, blood in the drainage limb of the circuit represents true SvO_2, allowing for continuous monitoring during support. Arterial blood during VA support should have normal oxygen saturation (>95%) and carbon dioxide tension and reflects the mixing of blood resulting from native cardiac output and that due to extracorporeal support. Assessment is more difficult during VV support. Measurement of true SvO_2 is precluded during this mode, since blood in the pulmonary artery is a mixture of blood returning from the tissues and the oxygenated blood provided by the circuit. Arterial saturation is then the result of oxygen transfer through the native lungs added to pulmonary artery saturation. In severe lung dysfunction, not uncommon during the initial phase of ECLS, the lungs may not transfer oxygen, and arterial saturation equals that of the pulmonary artery. VV support cannot provide full saturation of the venous blood as a result of incomplete drainage and recirculation; thus, arterial saturation during this mode of support is typically 85%–90%. These levels are well-tolerated if cardiac output is maintained. Assessing adequacy of support therefore depends on other assessments, such as resolution of lactic acidosis and clinical indices of perfusion. A technique to estimate true SvO_2 if a pulmonary artery catheter is in place during VV support is to temporarily interrupt support. Within a few seconds, the blood supplied by the circuit will have passed the pulmonary artery, and SvO_2 measured at this time will be close to true SvO_2.

Maintenance of normal intravascular volume is critical during ECLS, since adequate venous return is necessary to maintain pump flow. Insufficient volume can be detected by poor filling of the bladder and downregulation of the pump. In centrifugal pump systems without a bladder, blood flow variation at a constant pump speed heralds inadequate venous return and mandates prompt correction to avoid hemolysis. Volume can be replaced with crystalloid, colloid, or blood products. If blood products are needed, they are the first choice. Since patients on ECLS have a capillary leak syndrome, use of colloids, maintenance of colloid oncotic pressure (e.g., total protein >5.5), and minimization of crystalloid administration are commonly practiced. Excess interstitial edema leads to organ dysfunction, contributing to worsening pulmonary, cardiac, gastrointestinal, and renal function. Diuretics (intermittent or continuous infusion) are the first choice in reducing interstitial edema, but if response to diuretics is inadequate, hemofiltration can be easily incorporated into the ECLS circuit. Low oncotic pressure (total protein <5.5 g/dL) is corrected with fresh-frozen plasma (if also indicated for coagulation management) or concentrated albumin infusion (1–2 g/kg). The ECLS circuit is procoagulant, requiring continuous administration of a systemic anticoagulant. Inadequate anticoagulation leads to clot formation in the circuit, which cannot only affect circuit performance but accelerate platelet deposition and induce systemic fibrinolysis. By far the largest experience has been with heparin, and it remains the initial drug of choice. The level of anticoagulation is measured with a bedside assessment of ACT. Maintaining an ACT between 180 and 200 secs seems to best balance the risk of bleeding complications and circuit clotting. Platelet consumption is ongoing during ECLS support, and daily transfusions are not uncommon during the early phase of support. A platelet count of 80,000–100,000 is maintained during the initial phase of support and during management of bleeding complications, but lower values may be accepted once transfusion requirements have stabilized and bleeding is not problematic. Red blood cell transfusions are often required, especially in the presence of overt bleeding. Even in the absence of bleeding, transfusion requirements are above normal, as red blood cell lifespan is shortened. The target hemoglobin is 11–13 g/dL.

It is well established that enteral nutrition has substantial benefits over intravenous nutrition in critically ill patients and is the preferred route of administration. Parenteral nutrition has given way to enteral nutrition as the route of choice, which is well tolerated in adults and neonates on ECLS. The absence of bowel sounds does not predict intolerance and should not be used as a reason to withhold feeding. Postpyloric feeding may be better tolerated than gastric, but the addition of promotility agents such as erythromycin allows successful gastric feeding in the majority of patients. Contraindications to the enteral route include mechanical obstruction, ischemic bowel, and recent bowel resection. Intravenous nutritional support is used when the enteral route is contraindicated or to supplement it when full support cannot be achieved by the enteral route alone.

Following sufficient recovery of organ function to enable termination of extracorporeal support, the transition from ECLS (weaning) is initiated. In VA support, the extracorporeal flow rate can be gradually reduced at intervals with serial assessment of perfusion, myocardial function, and blood gases until a terminal flow of 5–10 mL/kg, or ~10% of full support. The response to cardiac loading is assessed with serial echocardiography. Ventilator settings are increased to compensate but only to levels considered safe (e.g., PIP ≤30 cm H_2O; FIO_2 ≤40%; PEEP ≤10 cm H_2O; and rate <30). In VV support, weaning is simpler since no cardiac support is being provided. Flow is decreased to reduce the amount of extracorporeal oxygen delivery as ventilator settings are increased. It had once been common practice to terminate support in apparently refractory cases if organ function had not returned after a period of time (~2–3 weeks) under the assumption that organ damage was irreversible by this time. Recent experience, however, indicates that organ function can recover after extended periods of time, and support for 2–3 mos or more with recovery are no longer uncommon. The decision to withdraw support is therefore an individualized one that includes underlying diagnosis, extent of organ dysfunction, complications, and perhaps further diagnostic tests to establish irreversibility.

COMPLICATIONS

The procedure of cannulation entails placement of a large vascular cannula, imposing the risk of injury to the vessel or failure to complete cannulation. Bleeding complications are among the most common problems associated with ECLS. Bleeding can occur at surgical (including cannulation) sites but can also be unrelated to procedures or trauma. Bleeding can be life-threatening, such as with intracranial hemorrhage. The initial approach to bleeding management is to identify causes that are surgically correctable, such as a bleeding vessel at a cannulation site. If no such treatable cause is found, the platelet count is increased, and the level of anticoagulation is decreased. An ACT of 160–180 secs, and perhaps 140–160, may be required for a period of time. If bleeding continues despite these efforts, aminocaproic acid can help control bleeding on ECLS by inhibiting thrombolysis. A loading dose of 100 mg/kg is given, followed by a continuous infusion of 25–50 mg/kg. Due to its tendency to induce thrombosis and cause clotting in circuits, aprotinin is now becoming a preferred agent. It is administered in a loading dose of 10,000 KIU/kg, followed by a continuous infusion of 2500 KIU/kg/hr. The loading dose can be added to the circuit prime in patients with bleeding complications prior to initiation of ECLS or in those with a high risk of bleeding. Recombinant factor VII can control bleeding on ECLS. Life-threatening or uncontrollable bleeding may require the discontinuation of ECLS. Heparin-induced thrombocytopenia due to heparin-associated antibodies (Type II HIT) is an uncommon but potentially life-threatening complication of heparin use. A precipitous fall in platelet count 5 days or after initiation of heparin in the presence of thrombotic complications mandates discontinuation of heparin and substitution of an alternative anticoagulant. Argatroban is a direct thrombin inhibitor that is gaining acceptance as the alternative to heparin and can be titrated with the ACT. Type I HIT may occur during ECLS but is unlikely to be distinguished from circuit-related thrombocytopenia.

Infections related to ECLS are uncommon but represent an additional morbidity that can impact outcome. Strict aseptic technique during placement and ongoing catheter care are essential. Limitation of other, non-ECLS vascular catheters is also important in reducing infection risk. Sepsis was once considered a contraindication to ECLS, but now it is not uncommon to support patients with sepsis-induced cardiopulmonary dysfunction. Hemodynamic support guidelines for pediatric septic shock include ECLS as a modality that may improve outcome.

CHAPTER 16 ■ RENAL REPLACEMENT THERAPIES

WARWICK W. BUTT • PETER W. SKIPPEN • PHILLIPPE JOUVET

The indications for, and the types of, renal replacement therapies (RRT) are summarized in **Table 16.1** and **Table 16.2**. Renal clearance is a quantitative measure of the rate of removal of a substance by the kidneys from the blood. It is expressed in terms of the volume of blood that could be completely cleared of a substance in 1 min and is expressed as "mL/min." Clearance is often standardized by adjusting for body surface area, and the units are described as "mL/min/m^2." Dialysis represents the process of exchange between two fluids (water and solute) across a semipermeable membrane. Usually, the fluids are blood and dialysis fluid.

PERITONEAL DIALYSIS

Fluid removal follows an osmotic gradient and is, therefore, more dependent on the concentration of the dialysis solution itself than on the peritoneal membrane. The peritoneal membrane is relatively impermeable to protein unless diseases, such as sepsis, systemic inflammatory response syndrome, cardiopulmonary bypass (CPB), pancreatitis, or shock, have caused a marked increase in capillary permeability. Clearance achieved by peritoneal dialysis (PD) depends on the size of the molecule (smaller molecules are cleared more quickly), the dialysis fluid osmolality (the higher the glucose concentration, the more rapid the fluid removal), the dwell time (most fluid removal occurs within the first 60 mins, because the concentration gradients change the most during this period), and the volume of dialysis fluid (the larger the volume, the greater the clearance because more fluid is in contact with the peritoneal membrane and its large surface area). Fluid removal also depends on the retention effect of lymphatic drainage on fluid being removed from the peritoneum and returned to the vascular compartment. Contraindications to PD include a defect in peritoneal membrane, abdominal sepsis with adhesions, and necrotizing enterocolitis.

Similar to other methods of RRT, PD can be associated with *fluid and electrolyte abnormalities*, in particular, potassium, sodium and, in small infants, lactate. Significant potential also exists for fluid imbalance, with too much or too little fluid being removed. Overall fluid balance, central filling pressures, and electrolyte balance of patients who receive PD must be closely monitored to avoid complications. *Peritonitis* is an uncommon complication that is mainly related to poor aseptic insertion or poor aseptic handling of the circuit and stopcocks. Diagnosis of peritonitis is confirmed if the dialysate is cloudy, if the white blood cell count is <100/mm^3, and if <50% of the cells are polymorphonuclear cells. Early empiric therapy with intraperitoneal cefazolin and gentamicin is commenced. A single IV dose of vancomycin may also be given if the patient is clinically unstable. Evidence of a pneumoperitoneum is also found in some patients with PD. Bowel perforation at the time of insertion is rare but is always a potential concern. Poor flow into the peritoneum can occur from kinking of the catheter, crystallization around the catheter instillation/drainage holes, or infection. *Hernias* (inguinal) due to increased intraabdominal pressure can occur, and the development of scrotal fluid (hydrocele) is common in the neonate. *Peritoneal fluid eosinophilia* may occur due to a reaction to the plastic tubing and may also be seen in fungal infection.

The choice of PD solution depends on the amount of fluid to be removed, the age of the patient, and whether metabolic acidosis is present. Instillation of 10–20 mL/kg normally provides good clearance and minimal risk of intra-abdominal hypertension. Increased volume of dialysate to 30–40 mL/kg gives a better clearance of solutes but an increased likelihood of intra-abdominal hypertension or respiratory embarrassment. PD is the commonest form of RRT in neonates and small children after bypass. PD continues to be effective even in low–cardiac output states, in hypotension conditions, and in infants with vasoconstrictors. However, as PD volumes increase or muscle relaxants are ceased and abdominal muscle tone increases, the potential increases for impairment of ventilation, gas exchange, and decreased cardiac performance.

CONTINUOUS RENAL REPLACEMENT THERAPY

CRRT can, over time, be equivalent in efficiency to intermittent hemodialysis and has the benefit of more hemodynamic stability. CRRT is effective,

TABLE 16.1

INDICATIONS FOR RENAL REPLACEMENT THERAPY

Renal
Oliguria (unresponsive to diuretics and/or fluid challenge)
Anuria (nonobstructive)
Metabolic acidosis (<7.1)
Hyperkalemia
pH <7.1
K^+ >6
Azotemia
Uremia symptoms (encephalopathy, myopathy, pericarditis, bleeding)
Hyperphosphatemia

Nonrenal
Fluid overload (pulmonary or cerebral edema)
Anticipated large transfusion in trauma or coagulopathy
Inborn errors of metabolism
Sepsis
Post-cardiopulmonary bypass systemic inflammatory response syndrome
Pancreatitis
Drug Overdose

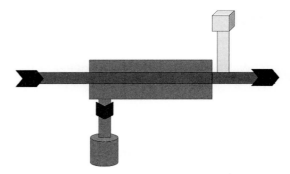

FIGURE 16.1. Continuous arteriovenous hemofiltration.

managing acute renal failure (ARF) by removing nitrogenous waste products and restoring acid-base balance, maintaining fluid balance while allowing nutrition or blood products to be given safely, purifying blood in conditions such as sepsis or metabolic disorders (e.g., hyperammonemia), and clearing ingested drugs or toxins.

Continuous arteriovenous hemofiltration (CAVH) provides a potential volume load to the heart in small infants that may not be well tolerated. In this mode, blood flows from artery to vein, and filtrate production depends on the patient's blood pressure, the filter surface area, and the height of the collecting system below the filter (**Fig. 16.1**). Continuous venovenous hemofiltration (CVVH) may be performed with a double-lumen catheter, which contains both a drainage and return lumen that is placed in a central vein. Clearance and fluid balance goals are chosen by the staff, and the

particularly in newborns with inborn errors of metabolism in whom very large volumes of ultrafiltrate and solute removal could be achieved. The goals of CRRT for the intensivist include restoring fluid and electrolyte balance, improving lung function by decreasing lung water and capillary permeability, improving hemodynamics by removing inflammatory mediators or bacterial toxins,

TABLE 16.2

SPECIFICS OF THE THREE TECHNIQUES OF RENAL REPLACEMENT THERAPIES IN THE PICU

	PD	HDi	CRRT
Method specificities			
Vascular access (ECC)	No	Yes	Yes
Complex method with specific expertise	Low	High	Moderate
Systemic anticoagulation	No	Frequent	Frequent
Dialysis dose			
Efficacy to remove a toxin	Moderate	High	High
Fluid balance	Moderate	Moderate	High
Clinical situation indication			
Hemodynamic instability	Yes	No	Yes
Intracranial Hypertension	Yes	±	Yes
ARDS	±	Yes	Yes
Abdominal surgery	±	Yes	Yes

PD, peritoneal dialysis; HDi, intermittent hemodialysis; CRRT, continuous renal replacement therapies; ECC, extracorporeal circulation; ARDS, acute respiratory distress syndrome

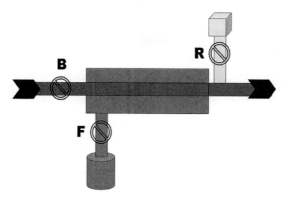

FIGURE 16.2. Continuous venovenous hemofiltration (postfilter replacement).

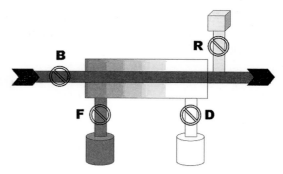

FIGURE 16.4. CVVHDF (post–filter replacement).

parameters are set on the dialysis machine as shown below (**Fig. 16.2**):

Choose filtrate rate: F = UFR = GFR (clearance of solute)

Choose fluid removal rate: F – RF

If no dialysis to be done concurrently: D = 0

Where:

$$F = \text{filtration rate}$$
$$UFR = \text{ultrafiltration rate}$$
$$GFR = \text{glomerular filtration rate}$$
$$RF = \text{Replacement fluid}$$
$$D = \text{dialysate flow rate}$$

Slow continuous ultrafiltration (SCUF) uses a low volume of filtrate with no replacement solution and is useful in removing small amounts of fluid (**Fig. 16.3**). Ideally, this can be done by using arterial drainage and venous return, which can eliminate the need for a pump.

Continuous venovenous hemodialysis (CVVHD) is illustrated in **Figure 16.4**, where:

D: dialysate flow rate (clearance)

Choose fluid removal rate: F – D

No replacement fluid: RF = 0

In continuous venovenous hemodiafiltration (CVVHDF), both solute clearance and fluid balance goals are chosen by staff and then set on dialysis machine (**Fig. 16.4**), where:

Determine replacement fluid rate, then

F – D – RF = fluid balance

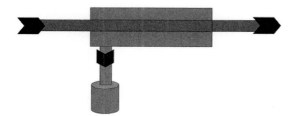

FIGURE 16.3. Slow continuous ultrafiltration (SCUF).

Where:

$$D = \text{dialysate flow (clearance)}$$
$$F – D = \text{filtration rate (clearance)}$$
$$RF = \text{replacement fluid}$$

In CAVH, Δp is the difference between the filter inlet and filter outlet pressure. In CVVH, desired blood flow is set on the dialysis machine. Lower blood flow across the filter can result in a higher tendency for clotting to occur. Transmembrane pressure (TMP) is the major force that acts on water and solute clearance outside the microtubule. Fluid moves through the microtubule into the external chamber of the filter, where it is removed as ultrafiltrate. The amount of ultrafiltrate obtained varies with the surface area, length and type of material from which the filter is made, and the patient's blood viscosity.

Substances are removed from the blood via 2 mechanisms: the passing of *solute* through the filter or *adsorption* to the surface of the plastic tubing and the filter itself. The substances that are removed by the filter vary, depending on the type of filter used and the modality of filtration. Examples of solutes removed are shown in **Table 16.3**. The sieving coefficient is the concentration of a substance in the filtrate divided by the concentration of the same substance in the plasma. Many small molecules have a sieving coefficient of ~1. Significant convective clearance occurs of "middle" molecules, including cytokines, complement, tumor necrosis factor, IL-1, IL-6, and IL-8, prostaglandin, myocardial depressant factor, interferon, and even Gram-positive bacterial exotoxins.

Differences in solute clearance between CVVH, CVVHD, and CVVHDF are shown in **Table 16.4**. Differences between type of dialysis and clearance were greater with larger molecules. It is clear that proteins (especially fibrinogen and albumin) and cytokines (such as TNF and IL) are adsorbed to the plastic surface of the circuit. Recommended CVVH catheters for children of different sizes and ages are listed in **Table 16.5**.

TABLE 16.3

SIEVING COEFFICIENTS FOR CLEARANCE OF VARIOUS SOLUTES

Solute	Sieving coefficient
CO_2	1.124
BUN	1.048
Chloride	1.046
Phosphorus	1.044
Glucose	1.043
Creatinine	1.020
Uric acid	1.016
Sodium	0.993
Potassium	0.985
Magnesium	0.879
Creatine phosphokinase	0.676
Calcium	0.637
Total bilirubin	0.030
Direct bilirubin	0.030
Total proteins	0.021
Albumin	0.008

BUN, blood urea nitrogen

TABLE 16.5

SUGGESTED SIZES OF CATHETERS FOR USE IN CONTINUOUS VENOVENOUS HEMOFILTRATION

Patient size	Catheter size and manufacturer
Neonate	Single-lumen 5 fr (Cook) Dual-lumen 7.0 fr (Cook/MedComp)
3–6 kg	Dual-lumen 7.0 fr (Cook/MedComp) Triple-lumen 7.0 fr (MedComp)
6–30 kg	Dual-lumen 8.0 fr (Arrow, Kendall)
>15 kg	Dual-lumen 9.0 fr (Arrow, Kendall)
>30 kg	Dual-lumen 10.0 fr (Arrow, Kendall) Triple-lumen 12.5 fr (Arrow, Kendall)

fr, French.

The key elements to the filter used for dialysis are:

- *Size:* The larger the surface area, the higher the filtration fraction and the less the hemoconcentration that occurs within the filter. Larger filters, however, have larger priming volumes and slower blood flow within the filter.
- *Type of membrane:* Filters may be composed of microtubules or a plate membrane.

The use of extracorporeal circulation and the infusion of solute with high flow create a substantial heat loss. The same solutions are used for dialysate and replacement fluids in CRRT. Commercial solutions usually include sodium, buffer, calcium, and magnesium, with concentrations similar to plasma. When prolonged CRRT is required, glucose and phosphorus should be present in the solution to limit deple-

tion in the patient The advantages of replacement fluid placement prior to the filter (predilution) are (a) increased urea clearance as diffusion of red cell urea into the plasma occurs and (b) a slight increase in filter survival due to hemodilution of blood and clotting factors.

Many strategies are used to prevent clotting in the extracorporeal circuits of RRT. Many factors lead to clotting within the circuit, including kinking of catheters; high circuit resistance; obstruction to inflow (blood drainage from patient) of catheter (often by side-hole occlusion by the vessel wall); slow blood flow or stasis; high blood viscosity due to high hematocrit, high plasma proteins, or from hemoconcentration due to excess fluid filtration; fibrinstrand formation from binding to the plastic surface of tubing or the filter; circulating procoagulants (particularly in sepsis or systemic inflammatory response syndrome); and inadequate anticoagulation. Examples of a CVVHDF circuit with various anticoagulation options are shown in **Figure 16.5**. Anticoagulant strategies include heparin prefilter and

TABLE 16.4

MEAN SOLUTE EFFLUENT: PLASMA RATIO (SD) FOR EACH TECHNIQUE

Solute	CVVH	CVVHD	CVVHDF	ANOVA
Urea	0.957 (0.038)	0.876 (0.109)	0.754 (0.123)	$p = 0.002$
Creatinine	0.942 (0.050)	0.934 (0.056)	0.814 (0.057)	$p = 0.002$
All amino acids	0.996 (0.344)	0.904 (0.196)	0.778 (0.180)	$p < 0.001$
Vancomycin	0.739 (0.082)	0.643 (0.063)	0.509 (0.081)	$p < 0.001$
Phenytoin	0.302 (0.028)	0.297 (0.036)	0.265 (0.035)	$p = 0.067$

SD, standard deviation; CVVH, continuous venovenous hemofiltration; CVVHD, continuous venovenous hemodialysis; CVVHDF, continuous venovenous hemofiltration; ANOVA, analysis of variance

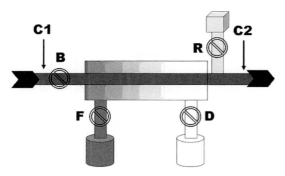

FIGURE 16.5. Continuous venovenous hemodiafiltration (CVVHDF) (post–filter replacement) with different anticoagulation options: C1 options: heparin, citrate, prostacyclin; C2 options: heparin, Ca^{2+}, protamine, nothing.

citrate prefilter and calcium postfilter. The easiest form of anticoagulation is a simple heparin infusion with regular monitoring of bedside activated coagulation times (ACTs) and daily laboratory coagulation tests. In situations of marked coagulopathy, such as sepsis, severe brain injury, trauma, liver failure, or active bleeding, it is logical to use regional anticoagulation, whereby the circuit is anticoagulated but the effect is reversed prior to blood return to the patient. Complications of extracorporeal therapy include:

- *Access*: To avoid limb ischemia and arterial bleeding complications, arterial access is not commonly used.
- *Infection*: Infection is usually related to catheter insertion sites.
- *Technical*: Equipment may malfunction.
- *Clotting of blood vessel or membrane filter*: Clotting is often related to the size of the catheter in relation to the size of the vessel.
- *Bleeding*: Patient bleeding may occur, but the degree of anticoagulation used for the dialysis circuit is fairly low or regional to minimize bleeding risk.
- *Embolism*: Although uncommon, embolization of air clots or debris returning from the circuit can occur.

HEMODIALYSIS

Hemodialysis (HD) is the extracorporeal exchange of fluid and solute that occurs across an artificial semipermeable membrane between blood and dialysis fluid that are moving in opposite (countercurrent) directions. HD uses dialyzers with larger surface area, higher blood flow rates, and higher dialysis flow rates than CRRT. Thus, HD is much more efficient at removing solute than CRRT. However, the intermittent nature of the technique (sessions usually last 4–6 hrs and are often repeated 3 times per week) lends

itself to being used in stable children with chronic renal failure or ARF due to renal disease (such as hemolytic-uremic syndrome or glomerulonephritis). HD can be used in children in the PICU for indications of both renal failure and nonrenal failure. It can also be used in hemodynamically stable children with hyperammonemia, inborn errors of metabolism, and drug overdoses in which rapid substance removal may be desirable. Increasing flow rates will increase solute transfer (increased blood flow brings more concentrated solute, while increased dialysate flow maintains low solute levels, thereby maintaining the concentration gradient); thus, small-molecule clearance is flow-dependent. Large molecules do not diffuse as easily and, therefore, are not flow-dependent, but they are dependent on physical characteristics (thickness, surface area, and type) of the plastic that constitutes the membrane dialyzer.

A large range of commercially available dialyzer membranes is used, and they have a number of features in common: small priming volume, biocompatibility (with minimal cytokine release), known sieving and filtration coefficients, known and consistent relationships between solute clearance and blood and dialysate flows, and low pressure drop across the membrane. Two types of dialyzers are available: *hollow fiber* (capillary), which is used in most major centers, and *plate dialyzers*.

In older children, the circuit is usually primed with saline or albumin. In children who weigh <10 kg, in children in whom the priming volume is <10%–15% of estimated patient blood volume, or in patients who are hemodynamically compromised, it is common practice to use a blood prime similar to that often used with CRRT. Hematocrit of the priming fluid should be <40%.

Heparin is the main method of anticoagulation. Other types of anticoagulation include enoxaparin, prostacyclin infusion, or regional anticoagulation with heparin/protamine or citrate/calcium. Monitoring of the level of anticoagulation with bedside testing of ACT is essential, with a goal level 1.5–2 times normal, depending on the patient's diagnosis, clinical condition, and risk for bleeding. When bleeding is a concern, regional anticoagulation with citrate can be given as in CRRT, with a target ionized calcium of 0.3 pre-dialyzer. To prevent systemic hypocalcemia, a calcium infusion is administered to maintain the patient's ionized calcium level at <0.9–1.2.

Multiple complications are associated with HD. *Disequilibrium syndrome* occurs when the patients' plasma becomes hypotonic relative to their brain cells and water enters the brain. Initial symptoms include nausea, headache, dizziness, and vomiting but can rapidly progress to seizures or coma. Children most at risk are those with high serum sodium or urea and those in whom very rapid HD is performed. When disequilibrium syndrome is recognized or in high-risk patients, an attempt should be made to have slow changes of solute occur by using low blood flow rates to decrease the rate of clearance. Mannitol at doses of 0.5–1.0 g/kg may also be helpful. *Hemolysis* can occur during dialysis from use of dialysate solution that is hypotonic, hyperthermic, hyponatremic, or contaminated with formaldehyde, bleach, copper, or nitrates. *Anaphylaxis reactions* still occur, albeit much less frequently than with the older styles of cellulose/cuprophane membranes. *Bacteremia/infection* can occur with poor aseptic technique. *Air embolus* is also possible, as is a blood or dialysate leak. *Hypothermia/hyperthermia* can occur if heaters/temperature baths malfunction. *Dosage* adjustment of drugs, both due to renal failure and removal of drug by HD, is essential. *Recirculation* can occur because of high blood flows and, in small children especially, the proximity of the 2 ends (the drainage and reinfusion holes) of the catheters.

When choosing the correct form of RRT, PD is used in small infants (<10 kg) after cardiac surgery and in those patients with early-onset chronic renal failure. CRRT tends to be used in the very sick or unstable patient with multiorgan failure, while HDi tends to be used in patients with ARF due to renal disease. In neonates and small infants with inborn errors of metabolism, all forms of extracorporeal RRT (CVVH, CVVHD, and CVVHDF) have been used, with rapid decrease in branched chain amino acids, keto-acids, lactate, and ammonia, resulting in minimizing cerebral injury.

CPB presents a unique situation in which it is known beforehand that a patient will suffer a significant insult that leads to a systemic inflammatory response with a marked cytokine response. Much effort is directed toward limiting this response with the use of pre-insult corticosteroids, heparin-bonded circuits, albumin-priming of circuits, and modified ultrafiltration at the end of CPB.

CHAPTER 17 ■ BLOOD PRODUCTS IN THE PICU

JACQUES LACROIX • NAOMI LUBAN • EDWARD C. C. WONG

RED BLOOD CELL TRANSFUSION

The concept of "permissive anemia" has become more popular because the safety of RBC transfusion has been questioned, at least in part due to the increased awareness among the general public regarding the risk of contracting viral diseases, especially human immunodeficiency virus and hepatitis. Less well recognized is the fact that transfusion of RBCs can modulate the inflammatory process, which may increase the risk or extent of multiple organ dysfunction syndrome (MODS).

Tissue hypoxia from low DO_2 may be due to a low Hb concentration (anemic hypoxia), cardiac output (stagnant hypoxia), or Hb saturation (hypoxic hypoxia). Anemia is defined as Hb concentrations below the "normal" range for age. Causes include repetitive phlebotomy losses, hemorrhage, intraoperative blood loss, chronic anemia (frequent in patients with cancer), and congenital anemia (e.g., sickle cell disease and thalassemia).

In critically ill patients, 2 phenomena may be present. First, the stress encountered by patients due to their disease frequently increases VO_2; this can upregulate the DO_2/VO_2 curve. Second, the critical threshold may be increased, which may explain why pathologic oxygen supply dependence is reported in selected patients, especially those with severe sepsis and septic shock. When the metabolic rate of a critically ill patient is increased, more nutrients and oxygen are necessary to meet energy requirements and a higher DO_2 may be required.

The formula for CaO_2 (arterial O_2 content) is:

$$(SaO_2 \times Hb \times 1.34) + (0.003 \times PaO_2)$$

where

Hb concentration is expressed in grams per deciliter

PaO_2 is expressed in millimeters of mercury (mm Hg)

Oxygen Kinetics

In healthy patients, DO_2 exceeds resting oxygen requirements, but despite significant reserves, safety margins may rapidly disappear during critical illness. Some investigators have shown that patients with sepsis do indeed have some DO_2/VO_2 dependence, which has led some to hypothesize that disease processes, such as sepsis, induce tissue hypoxia by producing an abnormally elevated anaerobic threshold. The resultant tissue hypoxia eventually contributes to the evolution of irreversible and often fatal MODS.

RBC transfusion may cause gut ischemia among septic adults, even if it increases DO_2. However, it remains unclear how transfused RBCs influence DO_2 in the microcirculation due to the difficulty in obtaining in situ measurements of blood viscosity, microcirculatory flow, and VO_2. Capillaries collapse if the hematocrit is too low, and RBC transfusion may be viewed "as a means of restoring blood viscosity." Conversely, capillary resistance to blood flow increases rapidly if the hematocrit level increases >0.45, which may result in microcirculatory stasis and impaired DO_2 to the tissues. Other authors have suggested that hematocrit has limited effects on microcirculatory flow. Characteristically, older RBC units have lower levels of 2,3-DPG, which alters Hb's affinity for O_2. Low levels of 2,3-DPG produce a left shift in the oxyhemoglobin-dissociation curve that may impede O_2 availability to the tissues, even if the DO_2 is increased. In addition, storage decreases RBC membrane deformability through alterations in cell membrane characteristics, which may influence end-capillary oxygen diffusion. Hemolysis does occur in packed RBC units over time; the amount of free Hb may increase from 0.5 mg/dL in a 1-day-old RBC unit to 250 mg/dL in a 25-day-old unit.

Transfusions of packed RBCs decrease the number of rejection episodes and improve renal and cardiac allograft survival. Many proinflammatory molecules are detected in RBC units, including cytokines, complement activators, O_2 free radicals, histamine, lysophosphatidylcholine species, and other bioreactive substances that may initiate, maintain, or enhance an inflammatory process. Giving an RBC transfusion to a critically ill patient with systemic inflammatory response syndrome may stimulate their inflammatory syndrome, which may result in the development of MODS (second-hit theory of MODS). The inflammatory risks of RBC transfusion decrease significantly if the packed RBC units are prestorage-leukocyte depleted.

Complications of Red Blood Cell Transfusion

Even though blood products are safer than in the past, RBC transfusion can cause many adverse events (**Tables 17.1–17.3**), which can be classified as early adverse reactions and delayed complications.

By definition, transfusion-related acute lung injury (TRALI) is pulmonary edema occurring during or within 6 hrs after the end of a transfusion. The European Haemovigilance Network has identified the following diagnostic criteria: (a) acute onset of respiratory distress during or within 6 hrs after the end of a transfusion; (b) no sign of circulatory overload; and (c) radiographic evidence of bilateral pulmonary infiltrates. A Canadian Consensus Conference held in 2004 added 2 criteria: (a) evidence of acute lung injury as defined by intensivists and (b) no preexisting acute lung injury or presence of risk factors for same. The latter criterion is a problem in critically ill recipients of blood products because a TRALI, a transfusion-associated circulatory overload, and an acute lung injury may coexist in the same patient. Most episodes of TRALI resolve within 48 hrs, which contrasts with cases of acute lung injury that are not transfusion-related.

More than 25% of deaths attributable to RBC transfusion are caused by blood-group incompatibility. The most significant risk of death from blood transfusion is from ABO mismatch, resulting in hemolysis (1/60,000) and death (1/600,000). In most instances, mismatch occurs when a patient receives blood prepared for another patient. Such errors occur more often in an emergency setting and can be avoided with careful identification of patient and donor unit.

Citrate anticoagulant can cause acidemia; however, if the liver is able to metabolize the citrate, a metabolic alkalosis develops. Citrate toxicity results if the capacity of the liver to metabolize citrate is overwhelmed, which occurs when >3 mL/kg/min of packed RBC or >1 mL/kg/min of whole blood or plasma are administered; severe hypocalcemia can ensue.

All RBC units contain potassium, which increases during refrigerated storage: potassium levels of 5 mmol/L after 1 day of storage, 22 mmol/L after 15 days, and >35 mmol/L after 25 days have been reported. Red cells stored in additive solutions have less potassium than those stored in citrate-monobasic sodium phosphate-dextrose (CPD) or CPD-adenine (CPDA-1). Irradiation further increases the concentration of potassium in the unit. To avoid hyperkalemia, transfusing at a rate of <0.3 mL/kg/min of RBCs is advised.

TABLE 17.1

INCIDENCE OF BLOOD PRODUCT TRANSFUSION-RELATED ADVERSE EVENTS

Serious adverse events	
Respiratory system	
Transfusion-related acute lung injury	1:20,000–1:5000 (5%–10% fatal)
Cardiovascular system	
Fluid overload	1:700–1:15,000
Hypotension[a]	1/102,000
Hematologic system	
ABO-incompatible transfusion	1:38,000
Death due to ABO-incompatible transfusion	1:1.8 million
Acute hemolytic transfusion reaction	1:12,000
Delayed hemolytic transfusion reaction	1:4000–1:12,000
Post-transfusion purpura	1:143,000–1:294,000
Mistransfusion	1:14,000–1:19,000
Other	
Anaphylaxis	1:1600 (platelets)
	1:23,000 (red blood cells)
Graft-versus-host disease	1:1 million (Canada)
Less serious adverse events	
Febrile nonhemolytic transfusion reaction	1:500
Allergic (urticaria)	1:250

[a]Hypotension can be caused by allergic or hemolytic reactions, septicemia, citrate toxicity, reaction to leukocyte reduction filters, etc. Such reactions have been reported with packed RBC units, plasma, platelets, and albumin. From Gauvin F, Toledano B, Hume HA, et al. Hypotensive reactions associated with platelet transfusion through leucocyte reduction filters. *J Intensive Care Med* 2000;14:329–32.

Massive transfusion is defined as the administration of >1 blood volume within a 24-hr period. Serious acute complications of massive transfusion include fluid overload, coagulopathy, thrombocytopenia, acidosis, hyperkalemia, and hypocalcemia.

The coagulopathy and thrombocytopenia observed after massive transfusion are attributed to hemodilution, hypothermia, administration of blood products with a prolonged duration of storage, and disseminated intravascular coagulation. Transfusion-related coagulopathy can be diagnosed if at least one of the following criteria is observed during or shortly after a massive transfusion: INR (international normalized ratio) of >2.0, activated partial

TABLE 17.2

DEFINITION OF SOME TRANSFUSION-RELATED ADVERSE EVENTS

Febrile nonhemolytic transfusion reaction. A in temperature ≥1°C that cannot be explained by the patient's clinical condition (i.e., other causes of fever must be excluded). A febrile nonhemolytic transfusion reaction may be accompanied by dyspnea and/or anxiety. Some of the following symptoms can also be present: rigors, dyspnea, tachycardia, or headache.

Hemolytic transfusion reaction (manifestations may range from mild to fatal). Hemoglobinuria or hemoglobinemia (measured as plasma free hemoglobin above the normal range) with at least one of the following symptoms/signs: fever, dyspnea, hypotension and/or tachycardia, anxiety/agitation, pain.

Major allergic and anaphylactic reaction (may be fatal). At least one of the following symptoms/signs must be present: cardiac arrest; generalized allergic reaction or anaphylactic reaction; angio-edema (facial and/or laryngeal); upper airway obstruction; dyspnea, wheezing; hypotension, shock; precordial pain or chest tightness; cardiac arrhythmia; loss of consciousness.

Circulatory overload (transfusion-related cardiac overload, TACO). Fluid overload with at least one of the following criteria: dyspnea or cyanosis; pulmonary edema de novo, tachycardia de novo, or hypertension.

Coagulopathy. At least one of the following criteria: INR >2.0; aPTT >60 secs; positive assay for fibrin-split products; D-dimers >0.5 mg/mL.

INR, international normalized ratio; aPTT, activated partial thromboplastin time.

TABLE 17.3

ESTIMATED RISK OF INFECTIONS FROM BLOOD PRODUCTS TRANSFUSION

Infectious agent	United States	Other countries
HIV (with NAT)	1:2.1 million (repeat donors) 1:1 million (first-time donors)	1:4.7 million (Canada)
HCV (with NAT) 1000	1:1.9 million (repeat donors) 1:791,000 (first-time donors)	1:2.8 million (Canada)
HTLV	1:641,000	1:1.9 million (Canada)
Hepatitis B virus	1:30,000–250,000	1:82,000 (Canada) 1:470,000 (France)
Hepatitis A virus	1:10 million	
Malaria	1:4 million	
Chagas disease	Extremely low	
Cytomegalovirus[a]	Unknown	
West Nile virus	Unknown	
Bacterial contamination		
Platelets[c]	1:1000–1:3000	1:14,000–1:38,000 (France)
Platelet fatality[b]	1:140,000	1:172,000 (France)
RBCs	1:500,000	1:66,000 (New Zealand)
RBC fatality	1:8 million	1:1 million (France)

HIV, human immunodeficiency virus; NAT, nucleic acid test; HCV, hepatitis C virus; HTLV, human T-lymphocyte viruses; RBC, red blood cell.
[a]The risk to contract cytomegalovirus from manufactured plasma derived products is theoretical if blood product is heat inactivated.
[b]Without pretransfusion culture of component.
Based on residual risk calculations published by Canadian Blood Bank Services and Héma-Québec (Infectious Diseases and Immunization Committee, Canadian Paediatric Society. Transfusion and risk of infection in Canada: Update 2006. *Paediatr Child Health* 2006;11:158–62).

thromboplastin time of >60 secs, positive assay for fibrin-split products, or D-dimers of >0.5 mg/mL.

In healthy animals undergoing acute hemodilution, evidence of heart dysfunction appears once the Hb concentration drops below 3.3–4 g/dL. However, animals with 50%–80% coronary artery stenosis can show evidence of ischemic insult to the heart with an Hb concentration as high as 7–10 g/dL. There may be some benefit in keeping the Hb concentration of hospitalized children above 5.0 g/dL. While RBC transfusion does not increase SaO_2 or PaO_2, it does increase the Hb concentration, which should improve arterial O_2 content. The efficacy of RBC transfusion to improve DO_2 is clear, but its usefulness is questionable. In 1995, the Blood Management Practice Guidelines Conference recommended a threshold of 7 g/dL if no cardiopulmonary disease is present; it also recommended a transfusion threshold of 10 g/dL in the perioperative period. The guidelines emphasized that the decision to administer RBC should be based on sound clinical judgment rather than on a Hb value. In practice, the consensus is that an RBC transfusion must be given to critically ill children if their Hb concentration drops below 5 g/dL. It is probably appropriate to use a higher threshold and to increase the Hb through transfusion in those children who are unstable; however, no consensus defines the threshold. The optimal Hb concentration may be even higher in cases of cyanotic congenital cardiomyopathy than in other kinds of congenital heart disease: thresholds as high as 13 and even 16 g/dL are recommended in some textbooks. Maintenance of a higher Hb concentration may be an advantage in traumatic brain injury. Some evidence suggests that transfusion is appropriate for critically ill children with congenital anemia (e.g., sickle cell disease), with acute chest syndrome, or in advance of an operative procedure.

All blood components must be administered through a macroaggregate particulate filter (170–260 μm), and the transfusion must be completed within 4 hrs of the time of release from the blood bank. "Third-generation" leukoreduction filters are used for WBC reduction of both RBC and platelet products. Benefits include reduced risk of CMV transmission, human leukocyte antigen (HLA) alloimmunization, and febrile nonhemolytic transfusion reactions. Solutions that can be coadministered with RBCs include normal saline (0.9% USP) and, under rare circumstances, 5% albumin, ABO-compatible plasma, or plasma protein fraction. Hypotonic or hypertonic saline, lactated Ringer solution, 5% dextrose, and medications must not be administered with blood or blood components, to avoid hemolysis and loss of anticoagulation and to distinguish transfusion-mediated reactions from reactions mediated by other causes. RBCs and whole blood can be safely warmed to 37°C, but not more than 42°C, using specifically designed devices.

Whole Blood

The standard single unit of whole blood contains 450 mL of collected blood into 63 mL of anticoagulant-preservative solution. The hematocrit is usually between 36% and 44%, and the whole-blood unit must be stored at 1°C–6°C. Depending on the anticoagulant-preservative solution, the shelf life will range between 21 and 35 days. However, after 24 hrs of storage, few functional platelets or granulocytes remain, and amounts of factors V and VIII are significantly decreased. Whole blood units, when available, may be used in patients who are actively bleeding, with massive volume loss (>25%), and who need both oxygen-carrying capacity and blood volume expansion.

Red Blood Cells

Units prepared in CPD are ~250 mL in volume, with a hematocrit of 70%–80% and a 21-day shelf life when they are stored at 1°C–6°C. Units prepared in CPDA-1 have a 35-day shelf life, with a similar volume and hematocrit as CPD-prepared units. Additive solutions, such as AS-1 (Adsol: dextrose, adenine, mannitol, sodium chloride), AS-3 (Nutricel: dextrose, adenine, monobasic sodium phosphate, sodium chloride), and AS-5 (Optisol: dextrose, adenine, mannitol, sodium chloride), are available to extend the shelf life further—up to 42 days at 1°C–6°C. Units prepared with 100 mL of additive solution are ~350 mL in volume, with a hematocrit of 50%–60%. They have essentially no plasma, and they flow rapidly. 1 unit of RBCs in an average-sized adult will usually raise the Hb concentration by 1 g/dL and the hematocrit by 3%–4%. In pediatric patients, a volume of 10 mL/kg (with an adjusted hematocrit of 80%) can be anticipated to raise the Hb concentration by 3 g/dL. For additive units (which have an adjusted hematocrit of 65%), a volume of 10 mL/kg

can be expected to result in less than a 3-g/dL increment.

Leukocyte-reduced Red Blood Cellss

One unit of RBCs contains ~10^8 white blood cells, which is approximately a log less than that contained in whole-blood units. Current prestorage third-generation leukocyte reduction filters can provide a 3-log, or 99.9%, reduction of WBC content to <5 × 10^6 WBCs and, with some filters, <1 × 10^6 per product. Leukocyte-reduced RBCs are indicated (a) for patients with repeated febrile, nonhemolytic transfusion reactions to cellular blood components or (b) to minimize alloimmunization to foreign HLA antigens.

Washed Red Blood Cells

RBC washing involves the use of sterile saline to remove the plasma that remains in an RBC unit. The procedure removes >98% of the plasma, including plasma proteins, microaggregates, and cytokines, as well as up to 20% of the RBCs. The procedure takes 1–2 hrs with an automated cell washer, and resultant product (~180 mL) is suspended in sterile saline to a hematocrit of 70%–80%. This product is indicated for severe, recurrent allergic reaction to blood components not prevented by premedication with one or more antihistamines. This component has a shelf life of only 24 hrs at 1°C–6°C. Washed RBCs are not a substitute for leukocyte reduction because washing reduces the WBC content by only 1 log.

Frozen Deglycerolized Red Blood Cells

A freezing process that involves a high glycerol concentration is used by blood centers for long-term storage (up to 10 years at −65°C or colder temperatures) of RBC units with rare phenotypes. Preparation requires thawing and deglycerolization using serial saline-glucose solutions. The final hematocrit is between 55% and 70%, with a 94%–99% reduction of WBC content and at least 80% of the original red cell mass remaining.

Prescription of Red Blood Cell Transfusion

Proper selection of RBCs and platelets by group and type of the donor and recipient is detailed in **Table 17.4.**

TABLE 17.4

COMPATIBILITY OF BLOOD PRODUCTS

If patient's blood type is:	O positive 37.4%ᵃ	O negative 6.6%	A positive 35.7%	A negative 6.3%	B positive 8.5%	B negative 1.5%	AB positive 3.4%	AB negative 0.6
These blood types will be compatible as packed red blood cells								
O positive	X	X						
O negative		X						
A positive	X	X	X	X				
A negative		X		X				
B positive	X	X			X	X		
B negative		X				X		
AB positive	X	X	X	X	X	X	X	X
AB negative		X		X		X		X
These blood types will be compatible as whole blood								
O positive	X	X						
O negative		X						
A positive			X	X				
A negative				X				
B positive					X	X		
B negative						X		
AB positive							X	X
AB negative								X
These blood types will be compatible as fresh frozen plasma								
O positive	X	X	X	X	X	X	X	X
O negative	X	X	X	X	X	X	X	X
A positive			X	X			X	X
A negative			X	X			X	X
B positive					X	X	X	X
B negative					X	X	X	X
AB positive							X	X
AB negative							X	X
These blood types are the first choice as platelets[b]								
O positive	X	X	X	X	X	X	X	X
O negative		X		X		X		X
A positive			X	X			X	X
A negative				X				X
B positive					X	X	X	X
B negative						X		X
AB positive							X	X
AB negative								X

[a] Proportion (%) of general population with this blood type.
[b] If the first choice is unavailable, other blood types may be used after volume reduction. Rh-negative patients may receive Rh-positive platelets in special situations with approval of the medical director.

In determining transfusion volumes:

$$\text{Volume (mL)} = [(\text{Hb}_{\text{targeted}} - \text{Hb}_{\text{observed}}) \times \text{blood volume}]/\text{Hb}_{\text{RBC unit}}$$

where
   $\text{Hb}_{\text{targeted}}$ is the Hb concentration targeted posttransfusion (for example, 10 g/dL)
   $\text{Hb}_{\text{observed}}$ is the most recently measured Hb concentration of the patient (g/dL)

Blood volume is expressed in milliliters
$\text{Hb}_{\text{RBC unit}}$ is the average Hb concentration in the packed RBC units (g/dL) prepared by the transfusion service
Blood volume is expressed in liters per kilogram (0.08 L/kg if child is <2 years old and 0.07 L/kg if child is 2–14 years old)

Older children of specific weight who are healthy can give their own blood, called *autologous donation*. RBC substitutes would be useful if available and effective. The response of critically ill patients to iron and erythropoietin is slow.

PLASMA

One unit of plasma is the quantity of plasma obtained from 1 unit of whole blood; plasmapheresis of a single donor can yield 500–800 mL. A typical whole-blood unit contains between 180 and 300 mL of anticoagulated plasma. Solvent/detergent plasma consists of a pool of 2500 plasma units that have been further processed to remove viral contaminants in a volume of 200 mL. One milliliter of plasma contains ~1 unit of each of the coagulation factors, as well as a concentration of complement, trace elements, and other plasma proteins. Labile coagulation factors, such as factors V and VIII, are unstable in plasma stored for prolonged periods at $1°C$–$6°C$, which explains why plasma is usually stored frozen at or below $-18°C$. FFP also contains significant amounts of glucose (535 mg/dL), sodium (172 mEq/L), potassium (15 mEq/L), and proteins (5.5 g/dL with 60% albumin). Plasma is used in the PICU to treat disseminated intravascular coagulation, to restore the blood concentration of deficient coagulation factors associated with massive transfusion or some diseases, or for rapid reversal of the Warfarin effect. Fresh frozen plasma (FFP) is sometimes used for isolated congenital coagulation factor deficiencies; recombinant or plasma-derived, pooled and virally inactivated factor concentrates are preferred when clinically indicated. Plasma can be required in patients who received massive transfusion of packed RBC units or whole blood. However, dilution of coagulation factors rarely appears before the patient receives >1.5 times his or her blood volume. Some surgeons request that plasma be administered once the patient receives 100% of his or her blood volume replaced by RBCs and if clinical evidence of oozing or microvascular bleeding is present. Plasma is used as a treatment measure of symptomatic thrombotic thrombocytopenic purpura and its related clinical entities, hemolytic uremic syndrome, and hemolysis, elevated liver enzymes, and low platelet syndrome. Plasma is also used as replacement fluid in some plasma exchanges performed by apheresis. Plasma is not recommended as a volume expander; crystalloids, synthetic colloids, or purified human albumin solutions are preferred.

Compatibility testing is not required before plasma transfusion, unless large volumes are given. FFP must be ABO compatible with the recipient's RBCs; AB plasma can be administered in severe and acute situations. Plasma dosing is calculated at 10–20 mL/kg, followed by repeat laboratory evaluation using a coagulation profile. In some cases, multiple repeat doses are necessary. FFP can be warmed in 7 mins using a microwave oven; however, only ovens specifically constructed for this task can be used, as standard microwaves will destroy the function of several coagulation factors. Thawed plasma must be used within 4 hrs of release to be used as FFP. A macroaggregate filter must be used. The effectiveness of FFP is often judged by cessation of bleeding, as the normalization of a coagulation profile may not always be seen. Additional plasma may be administered if the INR is higher than 2.5; the blood level of coagulation factors V, VIII, or IX is lower than 0.2–0.3 U/mL; or the fibrinogen level is <75 mg/dL (0.75 g/L).

PLATELETS

A platelet concentrate can be prepared from a single donor (apheresis procedure) or from a single whole-blood collection. A platelet concentrate from a single-donor apheresis procedure is the equivalent of 6–10 platelets derived from whole-blood donations. Non-leukoreduced platelets have $\sim 10^6$–10^8 leukocytes per unit. However, once leukoreduced, using current leukoreduction filters, $<5 \times 10^6$ leukocytes (and often $<1 \times 10^6$ leukocytes) per unit are present. Both apheresis and whole-blood–derived platelets contain substantial amounts of plasma, requiring the use of ABO-compatible platelets unless the plasma is substantially removed. However, platelet plasma is not an adequate source of coagulation factors, as factors such as factors V and VIII markedly decrease during platelet storage. Typical red cell content is substantially less with apheresis platelets (typically much less than 0.005 mL of RBCs per unit) than with whole-blood–derived platelet concentrates, which can contain on average ~ 0.5 mL of RBCs. The volume of a whole-blood–derived platelet concentrate is 50–70 mL while that of an apheresis platelet concentrate ranges from 200 to 300 mL. There are $\sim 5.5 \times 10^{10}$ platelets per whole-blood–derived unit (also called an "equivalent unit," or EU).

Thrombocytopenia and/or qualitative platelet defects increase the risk of bleeding, due to impairment in the ability to form a platelet plug. Platelet concentrates are given to patients at risk of bleeding in order to increase their platelet count or to supply them with more functional platelets.

Thrombocytopenia is defined by a platelet count of $<150,000/mm^3$ (150×10^9/L). High platelet consumption is frequently caused in the PICU by nonimmune-mediated mechanisms, such as disseminated intravascular coagulation, splenomegaly, and sepsis, and by immune-mediated mechanisms, as seen with alloimmunization in patients undergoing chemotherapy who have received numerous blood products, patients with autoimmune thrombocytopenia purpura, and patients who develop heparin-induced thrombocytopenia or other drug-induced antiplatelet antibodies. Decreased bone marrow platelet production can result from medications (most notably chemotherapy), sepsis, and viral infections, the latter of which can result in bone marrow histiocytic hyperplasia with hemophagocytosis (acquired hemophagocytosis syndrome).

Treatment of qualitative platelet function defects requires platelet transfusion in addition to the administration of certain drugs, such as antifibrinolytic agents (e.g., epsilon aminocaproic acid), and the use of cryoprecipitate to treat the platelet function defect associated with uremia. The risk of pulmonary hemorrhage is significant in mechanically ventilated patients if the platelet count is $<50,000/mm^3$, and most intensivists will prescribe a platelet transfusion in such an instance. A platelet transfusion must also be considered if the platelet count of a patient with an active hemorrhage is $<50,000-100,000/mm^3$. Transfusion to keep the platelet level above a threshold of $100,000/mm^3$ is recommended in the presence of an active intracranial hemorrhage or if extracorporeal membrane oxygenation is underway. It is also appropriate to consider a platelet transfusion even when the platelet count is higher than $100,000/mm^3$ if bleeding is active and severe or if bleeding is associated with a qualitative platelet defect. The administration of a large amount of crystalloids, packed RBCs, and/or whole blood (>1 blood volume), such as seen in surgical patients or in massive transfusion for trauma patients, can dilute the platelet count.

Platelet transfusion should not be used for the treatment of idiopathic thrombocytopenic purpura, except in the presence of intracerebral or life-threatening bleeding. Platelets are contraindicated in cases of thrombotic thrombocytopenic purpura and heparin-induced thrombocytopenia because of increased thrombotic risk. Alternatives to platelet transfusion, such as DDAVP [1-deamino(8-*d*-arginine) vasopressin] or antifibrinolytic agents, the use of steroids, plasmapheresis, and avoidance of heparin, when relevant, should be considered as first-line therapies.

It is prudent to use ABO-matched platelets. The use of ABO-incompatible platelets requires that the transfusion service remove a substantial amount of incompatible plasma. This additional procedure decreases the platelet content by 15%–20%, shortens the storage time to 4 hrs, and delays platelet release by ~1 hr. Administering 5–10 mL/kg of platelet concentrate (either whole-blood–derived or apheresis platelets) to infants who weigh <10 kg and administering 1 whole-blood–derived unit per 10 kg of weight (i.e., 1 unit for an 11–20-kg child, 2 units for a 21–30-kg child, etc.), or ~5 mL/kg if using apheresis or prepooled platelets, in older children who weigh >10 kg, should increase the platelet count by $50,000/mm^3$. Under certain circumstances, patients with renal failure may require volume-reduced platelets. From a regulatory perspective, platelet concentrates must be used within 4 hrs after release by the blood bank. Platelets should be transfused using a standard blood filter (pore size, 170–260 μm). If a single, whole-blood–derived platelet concentrate is given, an 80-μm filter may be used to avoid wastage. Leukoreduction cannot substitute for irradiation to eliminate the risk of transfusion-associated graft-versus-host disease (GVHD), which is associated with 90% mortality despite treatment. Patients most at risk for transfusion associated GVHD include patients with congenital cellular immunodeficiency, patients undergoing stem cell or solid-organ transplantation or chemotherapy, and patients receiving HLA-matched products or directed donations from blood relatives.

GRANULOCYTES

The degree of neutropenia as the result of chemotherapy correlates with the risk of infection. As a result, it has been hypothesized that the transfusion of granulocytes would benefit patients who are neutropenic for a protracted period. Granulocyte transfusions should be considered in severely neutropenic patients with bacterial sepsis or fungal infections when antimicrobial or antifungal therapy appears to be ineffective and bone marrow recovery is expected to be delayed as long as 2–3 weeks.

Because of the extremely high granulocyte count within a granulocyte product, granulocyte metabolic activity can rapidly deplete glucose, produce lactic acid, and increase cell death. This fact is accentuated because of the requirement to store granulocytes at room temperature, as cold storage inactivates neutrophils. From a regulatory standpoint, granulocytes must be transfused within 24 hrs; some even recommend transfusion as soon as possible. Granulocytes should be transfused over 1–2 hrs via a standard blood (150–200 μm) filter, with intermittent agitation of the unit to avoid settling of the granulocytes. Transfusion of granulocytes is frequently accompanied by fever, chills, and allergic reactions and should be discontinued in the case of severe pulmonary reaction. Granulocyte transfusion given at the same time as amphotericin is associated with severe pulmonary reactions.

LIMITING BLOOD PRODUCT UTILIZATION

The concept of bloodless medicine refers to all of the strategies that can be used to provide medical care without allogeneic blood transfusion, including blood conservation. Bloodless medicine strategy often begins before surgery by collecting autologous donation. Prescribing erythropoietin and iron supplements before a surgery can help to optimize the preoperative Hb level. Technology like acute normovolemic hemodilution, autologous blood cell salvage, intraoperative autotransfusion, and deliberate hypotension can also be considered. "Permissive anemia" is advocated by some experts. Phlebotomy remains a significant cause of blood loss, which can be decreased by limiting the number of blood tests and the volume of blood required. Days to weeks of therapy are necessary for erythropoietin and iron to effectively increase the Hb concentration in healthy patients; the response of critically ill patients to erythropoietin is blunted.

CHAPTER 18 ■ PLASMAPHERESIS AND TRANSFUSION THERAPY

PETER W. SKIPPEN • NIRANJAN "TEX" KISSOON • CARON STRAHLENDORF • WARWICK W. BUTT

Apheresis techniques involve an extracorporeal circuit whereby blood is removed from the patient, separated into its various components that are then modified by interaction with either a centrifuge or a filter, and then returned to the patient. The technique used in individual patients depends on the particular blood element targeted for removal and/or replacement—either plasma or cellular (**Fig. 18.1**). Plasmapheresis and therapeutic plasma exchange techniques are used interchangeably and have the same meaning. These procedures remove large particles (up to 3,000,000 Daltons), as compared with hemofiltration (up to 50,000 Daltons).

The centrifugal force generated separates the blood into a packed red blood cell layer, a plasma layer, and a buffy coat in between, according to their specific gravity (**Fig. 18.2**). The heavier red cells move to the outer wall, while the lighter plasma moves to the inside wall of the separation chamber. Therapeutic exchanges of cellular components or plasma involve both removal of the targeted component and replacement with donor cells, plasma, or albumin. Apheresis using a semipermeable filter membrane separates plasma from the whole blood based upon differences in solute size. The filter membrane is composed of porous, hollow fibers that are encased in a plastic cylinder. The pores are large enough to allow passage of all blood elements except the cellular components. The principle mechanisms that determine clearance are filter surface area, filter flow, transmembrane pressure, and the sieving coefficients of molecules cleared. Disadvantages of membrane separation techniques over centrifugation are the need for central venous access to generate adequate blood flow and the fact that membrane separation is limited to removal and replacement of the plasma component only. An advantage of membrane filtration is that it can be performed at the bedside using special filters and the same machines that are used for renal replacement therapy. It can also be combined with renal replacement therapy as an adjunct technique. In this age of improved automation, manual exchange transfusion is rarely performed, but it remains the preferred method in the neonatal period.

Molecular size is a more important factor affecting removal rates, as it determines access of the molecule to the intravascular space for removal by apheresis. For example, albumin, IgG, IgA, and C3 complement are distributed similarly between the intravascular and extravascular space, whereas >75% of IgM and fibrinogen are retained within the intravascular space. As a result of these distributions, the proportion of these molecules removed from the intravascular compartment may be substantially different from that of the total body. Based on one compartment modeling, a single-volume plasma exchange (~40 mL/kg) using a continuous pheresis method will remove ~63% of the IgM and IgG from the intravascular compartment. The whole-body IgM and IgG levels, however,

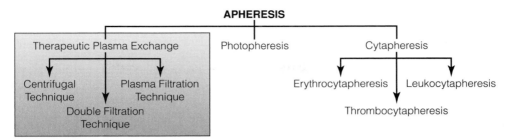

FIGURE 18.1. Apheresis refers to procedures that involve removing whole blood and separating it into its various components. Different techniques of apheresis exist. Blood components can be separated into various subunits based upon therapeutic indications, and the remaining blood components are returned to the patient's bloodstream.

will only be reduced by 47% and 28%, respectively. If the exchange volume is increased to 1.5 times the estimated plasma volume, the IgM and IgG levels in plasma will fall even more (by 78%), while the whole-body IgM and IgG levels will fall by 59% and 35%, respectively.

The effects of repeated procedures on serum and total-body levels of targeted substances can be predicted based on an approximate 48-hr period for complete equilibration to occur between the intravascular and extravascular spaces. For example, a goal of reduction in whole-body immunoglobulins by 85%–90% would require 4 single-volume plasma exchanges to deplete whole-body IgM and 6–7 exchanges to reduce IgG by a similar percentage. Increasing the exchange volume to 1.5 volume exchanges would reduce the number of total procedures required to only 3–5 to obtain similar removal of IgM and IgG.

In contrast to solute removal, removal of cells with apheresis is less efficient because of sequestration, which occurs in the liver and spleen, and adherence of cells to the vascular endothelium. Total circulating blood volume, rates of cell production, and release from extravascular sites also affect the amount of cellular depletion that can be obtained with apheresis. Because of these considerations, somewhat larger exchange volumes may be required to achieve clinically significant reductions in cell components. Modern cell separators are efficient in cellular depletions but require at least $2\times$ total blood volume exchanges for significant reductions to occur.

VASCULAR ACCESS

Like other hemofiltration procedures, adequate vascular access is a prerequisite to accommodate the high flow rates required to process between 1 and 2 blood volumes over the course of a few hours. Access flows of only 35–50 mL/min are required for centrifugal exchange, allowing the use of large-bore peripheral catheters, while membrane techniques require blood flow rates >100 mL/min, which necessitates central venous access. For patients who require hemapoietic progenitor stem cell collection, a temporary dialysis catheter is attached to a cell separator to collect the desired number of CD34+ cells.

ANTICOAGULATION

To maintain patency of the extracorporeal circuit, some form of anticoagulation must be used. As apheresis in the ICU patient is often used in the sickest patients with the highest bleeding risk, anticoagulation techniques that are regional in the apheresis circuit or that do not exert systemic anticoagulation are desired. A buffered citrate solution added to the patient's blood as it is withdrawn has become a common anticoagulant used for centrifugation

Centrifugal Separation of Blood Components

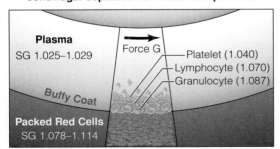

FIGURE 18.2. The mechanism of separation of blood components by centripetal force based upon specific gravity of the different blood elements in the separation chamber. The heaviest blood components are separated along the outside wall of the spinning channel. Plasma is the lightest component and locates along the inside wall of the separation channel.

apheresis procedures. Citrate acts by chelating the ionized calcium in the extracorporeal circuit without inducing a systemic anticoagulant effect in the patient. Higher blood flows require higher citrate flows. Modern apheresis instruments automatically adjust citrate flow rates, depending upon the blood flow rate into the extracorporeal circuit. Regional anticoagulation is achieved with circuit iCa^{2+} levels between 0.3 and 0.4 mmol/L. Citrate has a half-life of 30 mins and is readily metabolized. A calcium bolus may be required to prevent or treat the clinical signs of hypocalcemia due to citrate toxicity. Alkalosis may also be encountered, depending on the duration of the exchange and the total volume of citrate solution infused.

MAINTENANCE OF INTRAVASCULAR VOLUME

The ability of the critically ill child to compensate for acute volume or hemodilution changes depends upon the patient's cardiac, pulmonary, and renal functions. Any combination of crystalloid, albumin, fresh frozen plasma or IV immunoglobulin (IVIG) can be prescribed as replacement solutions to replace the plasma that is removed and discarded with the procedure, tailored to a specific child's other clinical issues (e.g., liver failure or severe sepsis). The extracorporeal volume is dependent on the type of equipment and the technique (intermittent vs. continuous), and the type of procedure (e.g., leukapheresis vs. plasmapheresis).

The separation chambers in centrifugal apheresis instruments vary widely in their requirement for specific volumes of packed cells to establish and maintain separation gradients. A red cell deficit occurs (dependent upon the equipment chosen and procedure performed) as the centrifuge chamber is filled at the start of the apheresis procedure. Total blood volume and red cell volume must be calculated according to the patient age, gender, and body habitus. If the extracorporeal volume is >15% of the patient's total estimated blood volume, priming of the apheresis machine with packed red cells should be considered. In practice, to minimize the impact of the circuit extracorporeal volume on patients who weigh <25 kg, an allogeneic blood prime that is discarded at the end of the procedure is usually performed. An alternate technique involves using a blood prime when the desired red blood cell depletion exceeds 30% of the original circulating red cell volume. In larger patients or in those in whom some degree of hemodilution is likely to be well tolerated, isotonic crystalloid or colloid can be infused during the initiation of the procedure to maintain cardiovascular stability until the separation chamber is filled.

Complications related to apheresis are most commonly due to difficulties with vascular access or related to the procedure itself. Protein-bound drugs, such as acetylsalicylic acid, tobramycin, phenytoin, and β blockers, may also be removed.

INDICATIONS

Most indications for apheresis fall within 4 main categories of disease: neurologic, hematologic/oncologic, autoimmune/rheumatic, and renal/metabolic. An additional ill-defined group includes sepsis syndrome and multiorgan failure with thrombocytopenia. Evidence-based indications and guidelines for apheresis have been published by the American Society for Apheresis and endorsed by the American Association of Blood Banks. Current recommendations reveal few well-established indications and few with category I evidence (**Tables 18.1–18.3**). Acute inflammatory demyelinating polyradiculopathy (AIDP), commonly referred to as Guillain-Barré syndrome, is the best-studied condition for which plasmapheresis is recommended. For all other category I indications, including thrombotic thrombocytopenic purpura (TTP), studies have been nonrandomized or case series. Emergency indications for apheresis relevant to the PICU include posttransfusion purpura and bleeding, TTP, red cell exchange for acute chest syndrome in sickle cell anemia, and pulmonary or central nervous system complications of hyperleukocytosis associated with acute leukemia.

HYPERVISCOSITY SYNDROMES

Leukapheresis, or therapeutic depletion of leukocytes, is used for hyperleukocytosis associated with leukemia. Extreme leukocytosis can cause sludging in the small vessels in the brain, leading to cerebral vascular hemorrhage. More commonly, pulmonary leukocytosis can result in respiratory compromise. Moreover, hyperleukocytosis is associated with early morbidity and mortality. Decreasing WBC loads to safe levels can be achieved easily with plasma exchange, evidenced by the effect of 2 leukophoretic exchanges.

Exchange transfusion or erythrocytapheresis has been recommended for neonatal polycythemia. A recent systematic review found no long-term neurodevelopmental benefit from partial exchange in polycythemic infants, and there was a relative risk of development of necrotizing enterocolitis of 8.68 in

GUIDELINES FOR APHERESIS: CATEGORY I

Disease	Procedure
Antiglomerular basement membrane antibody disease	Plasmapheresis
Thrombotic thrombocytopenic purpura	Plasmapheresis
Hyperleukocytosis	Leukapheresis
Sickle cell disease	Erythrocytapheresis
Thrombocytosis	Plateletpheresis
Posttransfusion purpura	Plasmapheresis
Guillain-Barré syndrome	Plasmapheresis
Chronic inflammatory demyelinating polyradiculoneuropathy	Plasmapheresis
Myasthenia crisis	Plasmapheresis
Demyelinating polyneuropathy with IgG and IgA	Plasmapheresis

Category I: Apheresis is standard and acceptable either as primary treatment or primary line adjunctive based on randomized, controlled trials or broad noncontroversial evidence.
Adapted from criteria endorsed by the American Association of Blood Banks (Smith JW, Weinstein R, Hillyer KL for the AABB Hemapheresis Committee. *Transfusion* 2003;43:820–2) and American Society of Apheresis (MacLeod BC. *J Clin Apheresis* 2000;15:1–5).

patients who received partial exchange (95% confidence interval, 1.06–71.1).

Uncontrolled thrombocytosis associated with myeloproliferative disorders may result in either severe thrombosis or hemorrhage. However, these conditions are rare in children. Platelet depletion (plateletpheresis) aims to reduce the platelet count to the near normal range (<600,000/mcL).

Exchange transfusion has been used in sickle cell disease for the treatment of stroke, severe intrahepatic cholestasis, prevention of sickling, and in bilateral retinal artery occlusion. The role of exchange transfusion in sickle cell crisis and in acute chest syndrome is well established. Evidence has shown that double-volume exchange transfusion lowers blood viscosity, relieves vaso-occlusion, and improves tissue oxygen delivery. The pre- and post-HbS quantification is helpful and may be a useful end point to determine transfusion requirements. Improvement in tissue oxygen delivery could also be used as a

GUIDELINES FOR APHERESIS: CATEGORY II

Disease	Procedure
Rapidly progressive glomerulonephritis	Plasmapheresis
Acute renal failure post transplant	Plasmapheresis
Cryoglobulinemia (adults)	Plasmapheresis
Idiopathic thrombocytopenic purpura (refractory)	Immunoabsorption
Polycythemia vera or erythrocytosis	Erythrocytapheresis
Hyperviscosity (monoclonal IgM, IgA, IgG)	Erythrocytapheresis
Coagulation factor inhibitors	Plasmapheresis
Demyelinating polyneuropathy with IgM	Plasmapheresis/immunoabsorption
Lambert-Eaton myasthenia syndrome	Plasmapheresis
Inflammatory bowel disease[a]	Plasmapheresis
Hypercholesterolemia[b]	Leukocyte pheresis
	Low density lipoprotein apheresis

Category II: Evidence is generally supportive or adjunctive based on randomized, controlled trials or case studies.
[a] Data from Sawada K, Kusugami K, Suzuki Y. Leukocytapheresis in ulcerative colitis: Results of a multicentre double-blind prospective case-control study with sham apheresis as a placebo treatment. *Am J Gastroenterol* 2005;100:1362–9.
[b] Data from Ziajka P. Role of low-density lipoprotein apheresis. *Am J Cardiol* 2005;96(4):67–9.
Adapted from criteria endorsed by the American Association of Blood Banks (Smith JW, Weinstein R, Hillyer KL for the AABB Hemapheresis Committee. *Transfusion* 2003;43:820–2) and American Society of Apheresis (MacLeod BC. *J Clin Apheresis* 2000;15:1–5).

TABLE 18.3

GUIDELINES FOR APHERESIS: CATEGORY III

Disease	Procedure
Hemolytic uremic syndrome	Plasmapheresis
Systemic lupus erythematosus	Plasmapheresis
Vasculitis	Erythrocytapheresis
Malaria or babesiosis	Plasmapheresis
Multiple sclerosis (acute, fulminant) (adults)	Plasmapheresis
Drug overdose and poisoning	Plasmapheresis
Acute hepatic failure	Plasmapheresis
Acute disseminated encephalomyelitis[a]	Plasmapheresis

Category III: Apheresis not indicated but reasonable as salvage therapy after failure of conventional therapy and lack of other options.

[a] Data from Khurana DS, Melvin JJ, Kothore SV. Acute disseminate encephalomyelitis in children: Discordant neurologic and neuroimaging abnormalities and response to plasmapheresis. *Pediatrics* 2005; 116:431–6.

Adapted from criteria endorsed by the American Association of Blood Banks (Smith JW, Weinstein R, Hillyer KL for the AABB Hemapheresis Committee. *Transfusion* 2003;43:820–2) and American Society of Apheresis (MacLeod BC. *J Clin Apheresis* 2000;15:1–5).

reasonable end point for titrating exchange transfusion in sickle cell disease.

The Centers for Disease Control recommends plasma exchange for *Plasmodium falciparum* infection when parasitemia is ≥10%, though exchange transfusion in malaria has yielded mixed results. The intent of transfusion in malaria is to reduce parasitic load and inflammatory mediators.

Plasma therapies are also being applied to thrombotic disorders, the best known of which is TTP, which involves an acquired autoantibody-mediated severe deficiency of ADAMTS 13 (a disintegrin and metalloprotease with thrombospondin type 1 motif), a plasma metalloprotease that is responsible for cleaving large von Willebrand factor multimers. Plasma exchange allows replacement of the deficient factor with fresh frozen plasma. Mortality for this condition has decreased from 90% to <10% following the introduction of plasma exchange as a therapy. Posttransfusion purpura is a rare bleeding disorder of platelet alloimmunization. It appears with sudden onset of severe thrombocytopenia, and purpura and is often associated with life-threatening hemorrhage. No single modality has proven effective alone, but plasmapheresis has been effective after failure of corticosteroids and IVIG.

Sepsis is one of the leading causes of death in children. Clinical derangements are thought to be due to the action of inflammatory and anti-inflammatory mediators. The inhibition or removal of these mediators by plasmapheresis is thought to be of possible benefit. Apheresis in sepsis fails to demonstrate an improvement in outcome because many studies have small numbers of patients and historical controls.

Plasma exchange may be of benefit for poisoning with drugs with high protein binding and low volume of distribution. It has been used effectively in vancomycin toxicity, theophylline poisoning, neonatal lead poisoning in combination with chelation, and isobutyl nitrate-induced methemoglobinemia.

SECTION I ■ RESPIRATORY DISEASE

CHAPTER 19 ■ THE MOLECULAR BIOLOGY OF ACUTE LUNG INJURY

TODD CARPENTER • R. BLAINE EASLEY • KURT R. STENMARK

The central derangement in acute lung injury (ALI) is the disruption of the alveolar-capillary barrier, which allows protein-rich plasma components to cross into the airspaces (**Fig. 19.1**). As the illness progresses, the disease enters a fibroproliferative phase in which lung compliance improves but lung function remains poor as a result of progressive scarring and thickening of the lung interstitium. Ultimately, many patients recover lung function completely or nearly so, but substantial numbers of survivors have long-lasting pulmonary function deficits.

Normal mechanisms of ventilation and perfusion matching are impaired in ALI, and the resultant maldistribution in pulmonary blood flow and increase in intrapulmonary shunting contributes to the severe systemic hypoxemia in these patients. Increased pulmonary pressure is a common feature of ALI and correlates with worse outcome. Increased microvascular pressure can occur as a result of increased blood flow through a given vascular segment due to uneven arterial vasoconstriction or as a result of elevated pulmonary venous resistance. Increased microvascular pressure, in turn, can lead to microfractures of the capillary endothelium and even of the epithelium, which cause increased permeability. While elevated pulmonary vascular pressures are rarely severe enough to cause overt right heart failure, changes in vascular tone may contribute substantially to edema formation.

Nitric oxide (NO) is a signaling molecule with profound effects in the lung. Its best-known function is as a vasodilator, though it has also been implicated in immune modulation, epithelial function, and control of endothelial permeability. NO acts in vascular smooth muscle by stimulating soluble guanylate cyclase to produce cyclic guanosine monophosphate (cGMP). cGMP activates a family of cGMP-dependent protein kinases that reduce intracellular calcium levels and reduce calcium sensitization by activating myosin phosphatase. The net effect of these events is to reduce myosin light-chain (MLC) phosphorylation and reduce vascular smooth muscle contraction. In addition to these effects on vascular tone, NO also appears to regulate endothelial permeability, though it has been reported to both increase and decrease lung microvascular permeability. NO is produced by a family of NO synthases (NOS). Endothelial NOS (eNOS) is constitutively expressed by endothelial cells, and neuronal NOS (nNOS) is expressed in neurons. Inducible NOS (iNOS) can be expressed as a response to inflammation or injury, in particular by lung macrophages and neutrophils in the setting of lung injury. The role of hypoxia in the control of pulmonary vascular tone is also pertinent to a discussion of ALI. Regional hypoxia is a characteristic of injured tissues and may be particularly evident in areas of dependent collapse in the injured lung, in which blood flow is reduced.

Once plasma fluids have breached the endothelial barrier, they must cross the epithelial barrier to reach the alveolar airspace. By most estimates, the permeability of the epithelial barrier is approximately tenfold lower than that of the endothelial barrier, suggesting that the epithelium is the greater barrier to edema formation. Direct epithelial cell death, as a result of bacterial or viral infection or direct injury by inhaled toxins, can alter permeability, as can mechanical injury to the epithelium from ventilator-induced lung injury. Airway lipopolysaccharide, presumably acting via Toll-like receptors, increases

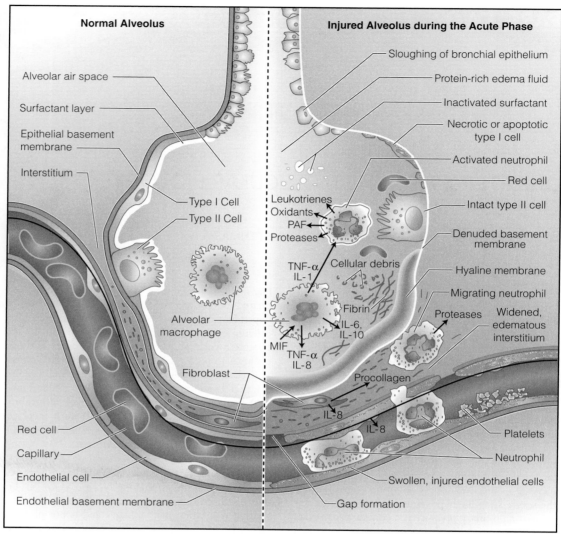

FIGURE 19.1. Cellular and molecular mechanisms of acute lung injury. Changes that occur as part of the early acute phase of lung injury are visible on the right half of the diagram in comparison to the left, including disruption of the endothelial and epithelial barriers, alveolar flooding, and influx of activated inflammatory cells into the alveolus and interstitium of the lung. Adapted from Ware LB, Matthay MA. The acute respiratory distress syndrome. *N Engl J Med* 2000;342(18):1334–49.

epithelial permeability via a mechanism that involves neutrophil influx and can be partially blocked by NO. For edema fluid to result in alveolar flooding, the movement of fluid into the airspaces must overwhelm these innate alveolar fluid clearance mechanisms (**Fig. 19.2**). ENaC subunit expression is downregulated by cytokines, such as TNF-α and IL-1β, and by infection with *Pseudomonas aeruginosa* bacteria.

The loss of surfactant activity from epithelial cell death or dysfunction and direct surfactant inactivation by plasma proteins flooding the alveolus

are prime characteristics of ALI. Pulmonary surfactant reduces surface tension in the air-liquid interface, facilitates the stability of the expanded alveolus, and is essential for normal lung function. In addition to its biomechanical properties, surfactant has been shown to contribute to the host's innate defense system and possess anti-inflammatory properties. The composition of surfactant is similar among various species and consists of ~90% lipids and 10% surfactant-related proteins. The lipid portion of surfactant contains 90% phospholipid, 75% of which is

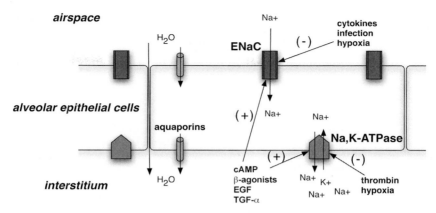

FIGURE 19.2. Molecular mechanisms regulating alveolar liquid clearance. Basolateral Na,K-ATPases (*pentagons*) pump sodium out the epithelial cell and into the interstitium, creating a gradient for sodium movement out of the airspaces via apical epithelial sodium channels, (ENaC) (*rectangles*). Water follows this gradient out of the airspaces via aquaporin channels (*cylinders*) and paracellular routes (*arrow*). Stimuli, including cytokines, thrombin, hypoxia, and β-agonists, can increase or decrease ENaC and Na,K-ATPase function. ENaC, epithelial sodium channels; cAMP, cyclic adenosine monophosphate; EGF, epidermal growth factor; TGF-α, transforming growth factor alpha.

phosphatidylcholine (PC). Approximately 40% of the PC exists in desaturated form as dipalmitoylphosphatidylcholine (DPPC), which is believed to be the main surface-tension–reducing component at the air-liquid interface. Surfactant proteins, especially SP-B and SP-C, play an important role in these processes. SP-A (32 kDa) and SP-D (43 kDa) are hydrophilic and belong to the collectin family. As collectins, their role appears predominantly related to host defense rather than to biophysical properties. Surfactant is synthesized in alveolar type II cells and secreted into the airspace via exocytosis. Within the airspace, alveolar surfactant exists as 2 structural forms (based on their buoyant density, composition, and function), designated as "large aggregates" and "small aggregates." Large aggregates are the heavier, surface-active components and contain the surfactant-associated proteins SP-A, SP-B, and SP-C. Small aggregates are lighter, vesicular forms that are not surface active. In normal lungs, both large and small aggregates are present in a consistent ratio. Deficiencies of either surfactant phospholipids or surfactant proteins are associated with impaired lung function, including poor compliance, atelectasis, inflammation, infection, and hypoxemia. Surfactant-associated protein concentrations are also decreased in Broncho Alveolar Lavage Fluid (BALF).

Mediators that initiate or maintain the injuries of ALI as well as providing crucial links to the immune system and coagulation system and to the process of angiogenesis are summarized in **Table 19.1**. A number of intracellular signaling pathways have been implicated in the development of ALI, one of the best described is the protein kinase C (PKC)

family of serine/threonine kinases. These molecules have been implicated in signal transduction pathways important to many cellular functions, including the control of endothelial permeability in the injured lung. Direct stimulation of PKC activity with diacylglycerol increases microvascular permeability, and PKC inhibitors reduce the increased lung vascular permeability caused by thrombin, vascular endothelial growth factor (VEGF), oxygen free radicals, TNF-α, and polymorphonuclear neutrophils (PMNs). PKC activation has been implicated in MLC phosphorylation in response to some agonists and in loosening of adherens junctions and focal adhesions in endothelial cells (**Fig. 19.3**).

Among the many transcription factors currently thought to be involved in ALI, hypoxia-inducible factor (HIF)-1, nuclear factor κB (NFκB), and SMAD transcription factors figure prominently. HIF-1 is a ubiquitously expressed protein the accumulation and activity of which in the nucleus are critical in cellular responses to hypoxia. The expression of many of the mediators involved in ALI (including VEGF and ET-1, among others) is controlled, at least in part, by HIF-1. NFκB is the most prominent transcriptional regulator of inflammatory responses and cytokine production and, thus, may control the amplifying effects of those mediators in ALI.

Cytokines may directly affect lung cells, promoting endothelial or epithelial injury or leading to fibroblast activation. They may also indirectly affect the injury process by recruiting circulating inflammatory or reparative cells. One of the most important cytokines in the lung is TGF-β, a well-described mediator of ALI. TGF-β is secreted by cells and stored

TABLE 19.1

KEY MOLECULAR MEDIATORS IMPLICATED IN ACUTE LUNG INJURY

Mediator	Source	Effects in ALI
Signaling molecules		
Protein kinase C (PKC)	Intracellular	Increases microvascular permeability
Transcription factors		
HIF-1	Intracellular	Upregulates hypoxia-responsive genes
NFκB	Intracellular	Regulates genes that control inflammatory responses
SMADs	Intracellular	Downstream of TGF-β; regulate genes that control endothelial and epithelial permeability, fibrosis
Cytokines		
TGF-β	Secreted by many cells	Increases endothelial and epithelial permeability; stimulates extracellular matrix production and fibrosis
TNF-α	Activated macrophages	Increases endothelial permeability
IL-1β	Activated macrophages	Increases endothelial permeability; amplifies immune responses; promotes epithelial repair
IL-6	Macrophages, endothelial cells, fibroblasts	Activates PKC, increases endothelial permeability
IL-10	Macrophages, lymphocytes	Inhibits cytokine production
HMGB1	Injured cells	Increases cytokine production
MIF-1	Macrophages, epithelial cells	Increases TNF-α, TLR-4 expression
Chemokines		
IL-8	Alveolar macrophages	Neutrophil recruitment
GRO	Alveolar macrophages	Neutrophil recruitment
ENA-78	Alveolar macrophages	Neutrophil recruitment
Angiogenic mediators		
VEGF	Epithelial cells, macrophages, smooth muscle	Increases endothelial permeability; involved in airway and vascular development and repair
Ang1	Vascular smooth muscle, endothelial cells	Reduces vascular permeability, decreases IL-8 expression
Ang2	Endothelial cells	Increases vascular permeability
Other mediators		
Thrombin	Cleavage of prothrombin	Increases endothelial permeability; activates TGF-β
S1P	Platelets	Reduces endothelial permeability
TGF-α		Promotes epithelial repair
KGF	Fibroblasts	Promotes alveolar epithelial proliferation
HGF	Fibroblasts	Promotes alveolar epithelial proliferation

in a latent form in the extracellular matrix. When enzymatically released from the latent form, active TGF-β binds to its receptors on the cell surface, phosphorylating and activating SMAD family transcription factors, which then move into the nucleus and regulate the transcription of many other genes. TGF-β is nearly ubiquitously expressed and causes a plethora of conflicting effects. In the setting of ALI, however, TGF-β1 directly increases the permeability of cultured endothelial monolayers through mechanisms that appear to involve SMAD phosphorylation, activation of RhoA and p38 mitogen-activated pro-

tein kinase (MAPK), and the disruption of adherens junctions. TGF-β activation increases both endothelial and epithelial permeability, which is one of many steps in the initiation and propagation of ALI.

One of the key physiologic triggers of ALI is sepsis, and many of the cytokines involved in systemic inflammatory responses to sepsis have also been implicated in ALI. For example, TNF-α and IL-1β are cytokines predominantly produced by activated macrophages, and both are key elements of the systemic response to sepsis. TNF-α stimulation triggers the upregulation of adhesion molecules in

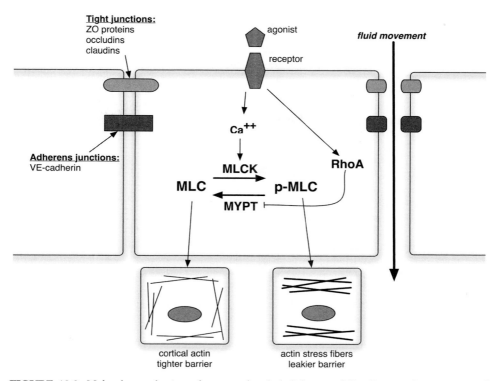

FIGURE 19.3. Molecular mechanisms that control endothelial permeability. Intact tight junctions and adherens junctions provide a barrier to paracellular fluid movement in unperturbed monolayers (*left side of figure*). Agonist stimulation leads to activation of MLCK via calcium influx and to suppression of myosin phosphatase activity via RhoA activation, with the net result of rearrangement of the actin cytoskeleton and increased actin-myosin interactions, leading to endothelial cell contraction. Combined with additional mechanisms that lead to the breakdown of intercellular junctions (tight junctions, adherens junctions), these changes cause endothelial cells to contract away from each other, allowing paracellular fluid flux (*right side of figure*). ZO, zonula occludens; VE-cadherin, vascular/endothelial-cadherin; MLCK, myosin light-chain kinase; MLC, myosin light chain; p-MLC, phosphorylated myosin light-chain; MYPT, myosin phosphatase target subunit.

human lung microvascular endothelial cells, which may lead to greater PMN attachment, cytoskeletal changes, and endothelial gap formation, which are mediated by activation of p38 MAPK, PKC isoforms, and RhoA. TNF-α has also been shown to induce the nitration of actin in endothelial cells, which may also cause endothelial barrier dysfunction in ALI. IL-1β has also been identified as a primary cytokine involved in the acute-phase inflammatory cascade in ALI. IL-1ra completely inhibits binding of IL-1 to its primary cell-surface signaling receptor, IL-1R1. Strong correlations exist between measures of IL-1β activity and clinical lung injury severity and outcome in patients with acute respiratory distress syndrome (ARDS). BALF IL-1 has a role in maintaining the inflammatory state in ARDS. IL-6 is consistently elevated in BALF and plasma from patients with ALI, and it increases endothelial permeability through activation of PKC. IL-10 is a potent anti-inflammatory cytokine

identified in ARDS, and higher levels in BALF are associated with improved survival. IL-10 inhibits cytokine production by macrophages and is closely related to TNF-α expression. IL-10 also downregulates human leukocyte antigen HLA-DR expression on monocytes from patients with septic shock and may play a role in modulating the host response to infections. A unique protein apparently involved in ALI is high-mobility group box 1 (HMGB1), which is a nuclear DNA-binding protein that is released from injured or necrotic cells and is a proinflammatory cytokine. Macrophage migration inhibitory factor (MIF) is produced by alveolar macrophages and bronchial epithelial cells, and MIF and TNF-α each promote and reinforce the other's production. MIF potentiates the effects of endotoxin and Gram-positive bacterial products; it also regulates macrophage responses to endotoxin through its regulatory effect on Toll-like receptor-4 expression.

High numbers of PMNs in BALF, as well as their persistence after the first week of ARDS, are associated with increased mortality, particularly in sepsis. PMNs must be recruited from the bloodstream to gain access to the alveolar space and airways. The ELR+ CXC chemokines IL-8, ENA-78, growth-related oncogene (GRO), and granulocyte chemotactic peptide (GCP)-2 are all produced by human alveolar macrophages. IL-8, ENA-78, and GRO are present in biologically significant concentrations in BALF in ARDS, and their concentrations correlate with PMN concentrations. Although GRO and ENA-78 concentrations are higher than IL-8 concentrations, IL-8 appears to be responsible for the majority of the PMN chemoattractant activity in human ARDS BALF.

The close linkage between coagulation and inflammation, particularly in the setting of sepsis, has recently become clear. Proinflammatory cytokines activate the coagulation system, primarily via the upregulation of tissue factor expression on endothelial and inflammatory cells and subsequent activation of the extrinsic clotting cascade. The generation of thrombin via this mechanism leads to increased inflammation and cytokine release. Similar mechanisms are active in the alveoli in ALI or pneumonia, and these could contribute to the pathogenesis of lung injury.

Many of the mediators involved in the formation of new blood vessels (angiogenesis) are activated by injury, and many of those mediators increase vascular permeability both in the lung and in other vascular beds. Three major families of molecules have been implicated in angiogenesis: the VEGFs, the angiopoietins, and the ephrins. While a role for the ephrins in regulating postnatal pulmonary vascular permeability remains speculative, solid evidence implicates both VEGF and angiopoietin family members in that process. VEGF is produced and secreted by many cell types in the lung, including alveolar epithelial cells, vascular smooth muscle cells, microvascular endothelial cells, and lung fibroblasts. Inflammatory cells, such as neutrophils and monocytes, can also produce VEGF, as can stimulated alveolar macrophages. VEGF in the normal lung is highly compartmentalized, with alveolar levels far exceeding plasma levels. This alveolar reservoir of VEGF may play a role in promoting epithelial integrity under normal conditions and may affect endothelial permeability if the epithelium is damaged, allowing the highly concentrated alveolar VEGF to reach the endothelial layer. VEGF expression in the lung is strongly upregulated by hypoxia and by numerous cytokines and inflammatory mediators associated with ALI, including TNF-α, TGF-β, IL-6, and ET. VEGF exerts its effects via several receptors, the 2 best characterized of which are VEGFR1 (also known as flt-1) and VEGFR2 (also known as flk-1). These receptors are tyrosine kinases, able to initiate downstream phosphorylation cascades that activate numerous intracellular signaling molecules. Both VEGFR1 and VEGFR2 are expressed on pulmonary vascular endothelial cells and on airway and alveolar epithelial cells. The angiopoietin family consists of several known ligands, the most important of which appear to be angiopoietin-1 (Ang1) and angiopoietin-2 (Ang2), and 2 receptors, TIE-1 and TIE-2. Postnatally, Ang1 stimulation reduces vascular permeability and improves integrity of the vascular barrier, reduces PMN adhesion to the endothelium, and reduces endothelial IL-8 production.

Sphingosine-1-phosphate (S1P) is a lipid mediator released from activated platelets that, in contrast to the mediators discussed above, exerts a protective effect on the lung endothelial barrier. S1P binds to a class of G-protein-coupled receptors known as Edg receptors. The net effect of activation of Edg receptors in the endothelium is to activate Rac-1, leading to the rearrangement of actin into a cortical pattern, which results in reduced permeability and to the assembly of focal adhesions and cadherins junctions.

FIBROPROLIFERATIVE PHASE OF ACUTE RESPIRATORY DISTRESS SYNDROME

The pathophysiology of ARDS consists of overlapping acute inflammatory and delayed "repair/ fibrotic" phases. Loss of alveolar capillary barrier function occurs early in ARDS and allows influx of proteinaceous fluid, blood, and inflammatory cells into the alveoli. Activation of the coagulation system and complement and the release of cytokines amplify the inflammatory response and contribute to further injury. It is now appreciated that overlapping with this acute exudative phase (rather than following it, as was previously thought) is a process of repair, markers of which have been identified as early as a few hours into the course of disease. This phase or process is characterized by the presence of intra-alveolar mesenchymal cells/fibroblasts, type II cell hyperproliferation, and extracellular matrix turnover. In many cases of ALI, the process of repair proceeds normally, with complete resolution of inflammation and fibrosis and a reestablishment of normal alveolar architecture. Clinically, the result of this fibroproliferative phase of ALI is a restrictive ventilatory defect and evidence of impaired alveolar membrane function, characterized by a prolonged reduction in the diffusing capacity for carbon monoxide.

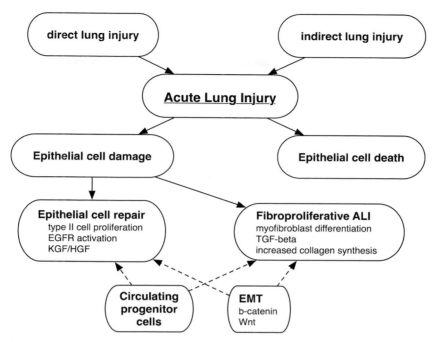

FIGURE 19.4. Fibroproliferation in lung injury. Direct and indirect triggers of acute lung injury lead to epithelial cell damage and death. Recovery from epithelial damage can proceed to normal regulated repair mechanisms or to dysregulated mechanisms of fibroproliferation. Circulating progenitor cells and epithelial-mesenchymal transitions (EMT) may contribute to both repair and fibroproliferation. EGFR, epidermal growth factor receptor; TGF-β, transforming growth factor-β; KGF, keratinocyte growth factor; HGF, hepatocyte growth factor.

Restoration of the normal air space architecture requires reconstitution of the denuded type I alveolar epithelial cells that have undergone apoptotic and necrotic death during the exudative phase of ALI. Regeneration of type II epithelial cells, in coordination with extracellular matrix turnover, is important in reestablishing surfactant production and ion transport, functions essential for maintaining open and dry alveoli. Proliferation of alveolar type II cells becomes significant 1–2 days after initiation of the injury.

Either during or following the acute inflammatory response to injury, interstitial fibroblasts migrate into the alveolar clot/coagulum, characterizing the beginning of the fibroproliferative phase of ALI (**Fig. 19.4**). The interstitial fibroblasts, either during or following migration, differentiate into myofibroblasts, which contain abundant α-smooth–muscle actin and vinculin. This much more "metabolically active" fibroblast proliferates in its new location and exhibits upregulated expression of important integrin receptors, including the fibronectin receptor $\alpha5\beta1$, CD44, and the receptor for hyaluronic acid–mediated motility, probably allowing for increased motility and specific interactions with the newly evolving microenvironment. Fibroproliferation is also seen in the microcirculation of the lung. In the airspace, fibroproliferation leads to shunt; in the microcirculation, it contributes to narrowing of the cross-sectional area, which contributes to pulmonary hypertension.

In addition to its likely roles in the acute phase of ALI, gTGF-β also has an important role in the fibroproliferative responses observed in ALI. TGF-β is a major regulator of gene expression, particularly of extracellular matrix molecules, in mesenchymal cells and lung fibroblasts. It is a potent inducer of collagen synthesis, has the ability to directly cause differentiation of fibroblasts into myofibroblasts, and inhibits collagenase production.

Corticosteroids may modulate the late fibroproliferative stage of lung injury. It has been demonstrated that dexamethasone can inhibit macrophage secretion of IL-1 but, in fact, it has very little effect on TGF-β1 secretion. Thus, it is possible that the variable efficacy of corticosteroid therapy in patients in the late stages of ALI is attributable to this divergence of effects, with corticosteroids causing a reduction in cytokine release but having little effect on TGF-β production by alveolar macrophages.

CHAPTER 20 ■ RESPIRATORY PHYSIOLOGY

FRANK L. POWELL • GREGORY P. HELDT • GABRIEL G. HADDAD

PULMONARY GAS EXCHANGE

Pulmonary gas exchange describes the process of O_2 uptake and CO_2 elimination by the lungs to supply the metabolic demands of the body. Normal oxygen values are shown in **Figure 20.1** as partial pressures (PO_2). The PO_2 decreases at every step, and this is called the "*oxygen cascade.*" A standard set of symbols developed for quantitative descriptions of respiratory physiology are summarized in **Table 20.1**. The alveolar-arterial PO_2 difference (**Fig. 20.1**) is caused by *gas exchange limitations*.

The Blood-Oxygen Equilibrium Curve

The blood-O_2 equilibrium curves (O_2 dissociation curves) quantify O_2 carriage in blood as graphs of concentration versus partial pressure. It is necessary to consider both partial pressure and concentration because partial pressure gradients drive diffusive gas transport in lungs and tissues, but concentration differences determine convective gas transport rates in lungs and the circulation. The concentration of a dissolved gas in a liquid is directly and linearly proportional to its partial pressure according to Henry's law ($C = \alpha P$, where α = solubility). Normal O_2 concentration in arterial blood (CaO_2) is ~20 mL/dL. (The usual units for O_2 and CO_2 concentration in blood are mL/dL, also called volume %; 1 mL/dL ≈0.45 mmol/L.) However, only 0.3 mL/dL is physically dissolved gas; normal arterial PO_2 (PaO_2) is 100 mm Hg, and the physical solubility of O_2 in blood is 0.003 mL/(dL × mm Hg) at 37°C. If arterial blood contained only dissolved O_2, cardiac output would have to be 100 L/min to deliver enough O_2 to the tissues for a normal adult metabolic rate of 300 mL O_2/min!

Hemoglobin

Hemoglobin (Hb) consists of 4 polypeptide chains, each with a heme (iron-containing) protein that can bind O_2 with iron in the ferrous (Fe^{2+}) form. Methemoglobin results when iron is in the ferric form (Fe^{3+}) and cannot bind O_2. Small amounts of methemoglobin normally occur in blood and slightly reduce the amount of O_2 that can be bound to Hb. One gram of pure adult Hb can bind 1.39 mL of O_2 when fully saturated, but methemoglobin reduces this value to 1.34–1.36. The O_2-equilibrium curve is S-shaped, or

sigmoidal (**Fig. 20.2**). The P_{50} quantifies the affinity of Hb for O_2. The 3 most important physiologic variables that can modulate P_{50} are pH, PCO_2, and temperature.

Changes in Hb concentration, [Hb], will change the maximum height of the concentration curve, according to the relationship between O_2 cap and [Hb]. Mean corpuscular Hb concentration (MCHC) quantifies [Hb] in RBCs and hematocrit (Hcrit) quantifies the percentage of blood volume that is RBCs. Typical adult values of MCHC = 0.33, Hcrit = 45%, and [Hb] = 15 g/dL are used for **Figure 20.2**, which shows normal CaO_2 = 20 L/dL and that CaO_2 = 15 mL/dL in mixed venous blood ($C\bar{v}O_2$).

Carbon monoxide (CO) is a deadly gas that also modulates the Hb-O_2 dissociation curve The affinity of Hb for CO is 240 times greater than it is for O_2, so even very small amounts of CO greatly reduce the capacity for Hb to bind O_2 (i.e., O_2 cap). CO is particularly dangerous because it is colorless and odorless. Hyperbaric O_2 exposure is used to treat CO poisoning because only very high PO_2 levels are effective at competing with CO for Hb-binding sites and driving CO out of the blood.

Oxygen Transport in Fetal Blood

Fetal Hb has a P_{50} of 20 torr, compared to 26 torr for adults, thus facilitating O_2 transfer to the fetus in the placenta (**Fig. 20.3**). Fetal Hb (HbF) is gradually replaced by adult hemoglobin in the first year. O_2 delivery across the placenta is limited by blood flow and PO_2 levels in the mother and fetus, but not by diffusion. For example, decreasing maternal PaO_2 <70 torr can reduce placental O_2 transfer. Increasing maternal PaO_2 to 600 torr, with oxygen breathing can increase fetal umbilical O_2 tensions by 3–5 torr, which can be important if the fetus is suffering any hypoxic stress.

Carbon Dioxide in Blood

Blood holds more CO_2 than O_2, in part, because CO_2 is carried by blood in 3 forms: physically dissolved CO_2 (0.067 mL/(dL mm Hg)), carbamino compounds, and bicarbonate ion (HCO_3^-), which is the most important form of CO_2 carriage in blood. CO_2 combines with water to form carbonic acid, and

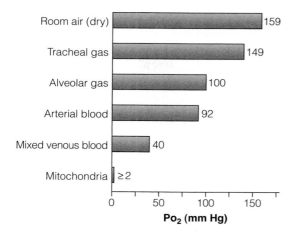

FIGURE 20.1. The "oxygen cascade" in a healthy subject breathing room air at sea level shows the pattern of P_{O_2} decrease between the different steps of O_2 transport, as described in the text. The difference between alveolar and arterial P_{O_2} occurs because of pulmonary gas exchange limitations. Adapted from Powell FL. Pulmonary gas exchange. In: Johnson LR, ed. *Essential Medical Physiology*, 3rd ed. Boston: Elsevier Academic Press, 2003.

this dissociates to HCO_3^- and H^+:

$$CO_2 + H_2O \leftrightarrow H_2CO_3 \leftrightarrow HCO_3^- + H^+$$

Carbonic anhydrase is the enzyme that catalyzes this reaction. Carbonic anhydrase occurs mainly in red blood cells.

The Haldane effect promotes unloading of CO_2 in the lungs when blood is oxygenated and CO_2 loading in the blood when O_2 is released to tissues.

Alveolar Ventilation and Alveolar P_{O_2}

Ventilation is the first step in the O_2 cascade, and the level of alveolar ventilation ($\dot{V}_A$) is the most important factor determining arterial O_2 for any given $P_{I_{O_2}}$ and level of O_2 demand ($\dot{V}_{O_2}$) in healthy lungs.

$$\dot{V}_E = f_R V_T$$

All of the tidal volume is not effective for gas exchange because the lung consists of a conducting zone, which does not exchange gas, and a respiratory zone, in which all gas exchange occurs. The gas volume of the conducting zone equals the *anatomic dead space*. The respiratory zone comprises the rest of the lung. A normal adult will have a total lung capacity (TLC) of 6 L but an anatomic dead space of only 175 mL (~1 mL/pound of body weight). $\dot{V}_A$ is the difference between total ventilation and dead space ventilation, and it is the effective conductance for pulmonary gas exchange. $\dot{V}_A$ can be determined using the *Fick principle*, which is a physiologic version of the principle

TABLE 20.1

SYMBOLS IN RESPIRATORY PHYSIOLOGY

Primary variables (and units)

C	Concentration or content (mL/dL or mmol/L)
D	Diffusing capacity (mL_{O_2} /(min × mm Hg)
F	Fractional concentration in dry gas (dimensionless)
P	Gas pressure or partial pressure (mm Hg or cm H_2O)
$\dot{Q}$	Blood flow or perfusion (L/min)
R	Respiratory exchange ratio (dimensionless)
RQ	Respiratory quotient (dimensionless)
T	Temperature (°C)
V	Gas volume (L or mL)
$\dot{V}$	Ventilation (L/min)

Modifying symbols

A	Alveolar gas
B	Barometric
D	Dead space gas
E	Expired gas
$\bar{E}$	Mixed-expired gas
I	Inspired gas
L	Lung or transpulmonary
T	Tidal gas
aw	Airway
w	Chest wall
es	Esophageal
pl	Intrapleural
rs	Transrespiratory system (total system)
a	Arterial blood
b	Blood (general)
c	Capillary blood
c′	End-capillary blood
t	Tissue
v	Venous blood
$\bar{v}$	Mixed-venous blood

Examples

$P_{A_{O_2}}$ = Partial pressure of O_2 in alveolar gas
Pa_{O_2} = Partial pressure of O_2 in arterial blood
$F\bar{E}_{CO_2}$ = Fraction of CO_2 in dry mixed, expired gas
$\dot{V}_{O_2}$ = O_2 consumption per unit time
$\dot{V}_A$ = Ventilation of the alveoli per unit time

of conservation of mass that describes gas transport by convection or bulk flow of air or blood. The Fick principle states that the amount of gas consumed or produced by an organ is the difference between the amount of the substance that enters the organ and the amount that leaves the organ. The alveolar ventilation equation shows how $\dot{V}_A$ and Pa_{CO_2} (or Pa_{CO_2}) are inversely related for any given metabolic rate. $\dot{V}_A$ is reduced from total ventilation by the amount of the dead space: Physiologic dead space can be calculated as:

$$V_D/V_T = (Pa_{CO_2} - P\bar{E}_{CO_2})/Pa_{CO_2}$$

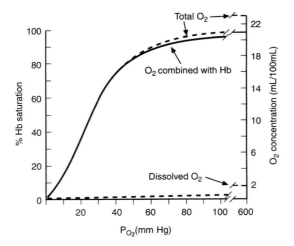

FIGURE 20.2. Standard human O_2-blood equilibrium (or dissociation) curve at pH = 7.4, PCO_2 = 40 mm Hg, and 37°C. Left ordinate shows O_2 saturation of hemoglobin (Hb) available for O_2 binding; right ordinate shows absolute O_2 concentration in blood. Most O_2 is bound to hemoglobin, and dissolved O_2 contributes very little to total O_2 concentration. From Powell FL. Oxygen and CO_2 transport in the blood. In: Johnson LR, ed. *Essential Medical Physiology*, 3rd ed. Boston: Elsevier Academic Press, 2003, with permission.

where $P\overline{E}CO_2$ = *mixed-expired* PCO_2 that is measured by collecting all expired gas in a bag or a spirometer and includes gas exhaled from the alveoli *and* dead space. In practice, arterial PCO_2 is substituted for alveolar PCO_2 because it is easily measured.

Alveolar PO_2 (PAO_2) can be predicted from the *alveolar gas equation*:

$$PAO_2 = PIO_2 (PACO_2 R)$$

where PIO_2 is inspired PO_2
  $PACO_2$ is alveolar PCO_2
  R is the respiratory exchange ratio

In practice, arterial PCO_2 is substituted for alveolar PCO_2 because $PaCO_2 = PACO_2$ in normal lungs and arterial samples are easily obtained. The alveolar gas equation is valid only if inspired PCO_2 = 0. The *respiratory quotient* (RQ), is the ratio of CO_2 production to O_2 consumption in metabolizing tissues.

$$RQ = \dot{V}CO_2 / \dot{V}O_2$$

RQ averages 0.8 on a normal, but it can range from 0.67 (fats) to 1 (carbohydrates). Substituting normal adult values in the alveolar gas equation predicts that PAO_2 = 100 mm Hg in breathing room air (PAO_2 = 150 – 40/0.8). Increases in $\dot{V}A$ (hyperventilation) increase PAO_2 by decreasing $PACO_2$, whereas decreases in $\dot{V}A$ (hypoventilation) decrease PAO_2.

Diffusion of O_2 from alveoli to pulmonary capillary blood is the next step in the O_2 cascade after alveolar ventilation. It is important to note that blood leaving the pulmonary capillaries is in equilibrium with alveolar gas in healthy lungs under normal resting conditions. Hence, the small decreases between PAO_2 and PaO_2 shown in **Figure 20.1** are not caused by diffusion but by ventilation-perfusion mismatching in healthy lungs under normal conditions.

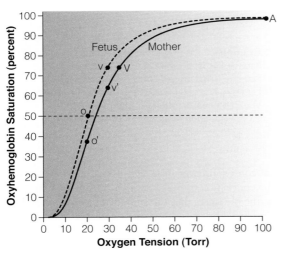

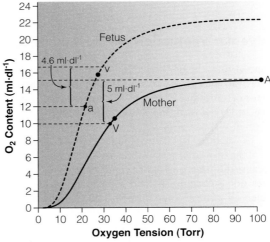

FIGURE 20.3. Oxygen-hemoglobin equilibrium curves for maternal and fetal hemoglobin. **A:** When PO_2 equilibrates between the fetal and maternal circulations, O_2 saturation is increased by 10% or more because of the lower P_{50} in fetal hemoglobin. **B:** Higher O_2 capacity of fetal compared to maternal blood further increases the amount of O_2 in blood for a given PO_2 and saturation. A = maternal arterial, V, maternal venous; a′, umbilical (maternal) arterial; v′, umbilical (maternal) venous; a, fetal arterial; v, fetal venous. Adapted from Powell FL. Pulmonary Gas Exchange. In: Johnson LR, ed. *Essential Medical Physiology*, 3rd ed. Boston: Elsevier Academic Press, 2003.

O_2 moves from the alveoli to pulmonary capillary blood barrier according to Fick's first law of diffusion:

$$\dot{V}O_2 = PO_2 \times DO_2$$

where:

PO_2 is the average PO_{2g} gradient across the blood-gas barrier.

DO_2 is a "diffusing capacity" for O_2 across the barrier.

DO_2 depends on both the molecular properties of the gasand the geometric properties of that membrane:

$$DO_2 = (\text{solubility}/MW)O_2 \bullet \text{area/thickness})_{\text{membrane}}$$

After O_2 diffuses into red blood cells, the finite rate of reaction between O_2 and Hb offers an additional "resistance" to O_2 uptake. Alveolar PO_2 is constant everywhere outside the capillary because diffusion is rapid in the gas phase. Any O_2 moving into the blood is instantly replaced by diffusive mixing in the small alveolar spaces. Hence, the gradient for O_2 diffusion changes along the length of the capillary, and the PO_2 value used in Fick's law is an average value, corresponding to the mean partial pressure gradient operating over the entire length of the pulmonary capillary.

The average capillary transit time of 0.75 seconds for adults is calculated from a cardiac output of 6 L/min and capillary volume of 75 mL (time = volume/flow rate). Note that diffusion equilibrium normally occurs between blood and gas in only 0.25 sec, providing a threefold safety factor. However, if DLO_2 is decreased sufficiently with lung disease, capillary PO_2 may not equilibrate with PAO_2 during the transit time. Only two conditions lead to diffusion limitation for O_2 in healthy adults. First, elite athletes at maximal exercise, with very high O_2 consumption and cardiac outputs, can have transit times that are too short for O_2 diffusion equilibrium. Second, normal adults exercising at altitude may not achieve diffusion equilibrium because transit time *and* PAO_2 decrease. Transit time will decrease with elevated cardiac output during exercise, but capillary volume recruitment and distension can preserve enough time for O_2 diffusion equilibrium to occur *if* PAO_2 is normal. At an altitude of 3050 m (10,000 feet), the barometric pressure is only 523 mm Hg and PIO_2 is 100 mm Hg [0.21 (523–47) mm Hg]. In a normal individual doing mild exercise at this altitude, PAO_2 is measured to be $\sim$55 mm Hg. The PO_2 gradient at the beginning of the capillary decreases from 70 mm Hg with mild exercise at sea level (100–30 mm Hg) to 31 mm Hg (55–24 mm Hg) at altitude.

Diffusion-limited and Perfusion-limited Gases

The anesthetic gas nitrous oxide (N_2O) achieves equilibrium rapidly, whereas CO never comes close to diffusion equilibrium. The uptake of a gas that achieves diffusion equilibrium depends on the magnitude of pulmonary blood flow. For example, N_2O diffuses rapidly from the alveoli to capillary blood; therefore, the only way to increase its uptake is to increase the amount of blood flowing through the alveolar capillaries. N_2O is an example of a *perfusion-limited gas*. Changes in the diffusing capacity have no effect on the uptake of a perfusion-limited gas or its partial pressure in the blood and body. All anesthetic and "inert" gases that do not react chemically with blood are perfusion-limited. Under normal resting conditions, O_2 is also a perfusion limited gas. The uptake of a gas that does not achieve diffusion equilibrium could obviously increase if the diffusing capacity increased. CO is an example of such a *diffusion-limited gas*. As Hb has a very high affinity for CO, the effective solubility of CO in blood is large. Therefore, increases in the CO concentration in blood are not effective at increasing partial pressure of carbon monoxide (PCO), which keeps blood PCO lower than alveolar PCO and results in a large disequilibrium and diffusion limitation. In practice, the only diffusion-limited gases are CO and O_2 under hypoxic conditions.All other gases are perfusion limited, including O_2 under normoxic conditions in healthy lungs.

The four kinds of pulmonary gas exchange limitations are (a) hypoventilation, (b) diffusion limitations, (c) pulmonary blood-flow shunts, and (d) mismatching of ventilation and blood flow in different parts of the lung.

Hypoventilation is the only pulmonary gas exchange limitation that does not increase the alveolar-arterial PO_2 difference. The magnitude of hypoxemia caused by hypoventilation is predicted by the alveolar gas equation:

$$PAO_2 = PIO_2 - (PACO_2/R)$$

Abnormal respiratory mechanics, such as increased airway resistance or decreased compliance with lung disease, may limit the effectiveness of the respiratory muscles in generating $\dot{V}A$. The ventilatory control system may be abnormal in terms of sensing PaO_2 and $PaCO_2$ changes and sending neural signals to the respiratory muscles to increase ventilation.

Shunt is defined as deoxygenated venous blood flow that enters the arterial circulation without going through ventilated alveoli in the pulmonary circulation. This kind of shunt is also called right-to-left

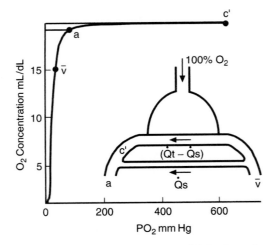

FIGURE 20.4. Two-compartment model for shunt flow ($\dot{Q}s$) and effective pulmonary blood flow ($\dot{Q}t-\dot{Q}s$). O_2-blood equilibrium curve illustrates how small shunt flows of mixed-venous blood ($\bar{v}$) significantly decrease PO_2 in arterial blood (a) relative to PO_2 in end-capillary blood leaving the alveoli (c'). From Powell FL. Pulmonary gas exchange. In: Johnson LR, ed. *Essential Medical Physiology*, 3rd ed. London: Elsevier/Academic Press, 2003, with permission.

shunt, to distinguish it from left-to-right shunt, which shunts systemic arterial blood into pulmonary artery flow with some congenital heart defects. Right-to-left shunt decreases PaO_2 by diluting end-capillary blood with deoxygenated venous blood. The effect of shunt on PaO_2 is illustrated in **Figure 20.4.** Alveolar and end-capillary PaO_2 are predicted to be >600 mm Hg during pure O_2 breathing. However, shunt significantly decreases PaO_2. Persistent hypoxemia during 100% O_2 breathing indicates a shunt if all of the alveoli are effectively ventilated with 100% O_2. If PaO_2 can be increased above 150 mm Hg during O_2 breathing, and cardiac output is normal, then 1% shunt increases the alveolar-arterial PO_2 difference ~20 mm Hg. In healthy adults, shunt during O_2 breathing averages <5% of cardiac output, including (a) venous blood from the *bronchial circulation* that drains directly into the pulmonary veins and (b) venous blood from the coronary circulation that enters the left ventricle through the Thebesian veins. If shunt is calculated during room air breathing, it is called *venous admixture*. Venous admixture is larger than the shunt during O_2 breathing because it is an "as if" shunt, which includes the effects of low PO_2 from poorly ventilated alveoli. Venous admixture occurs even in healthy lungs with ventilation-perfusion mismatching.

Mismatching of ventilation and blood flow in different parts of the lung is the most common cause of alveolar-arterial PO_2 differences in health and disease.

PAO_2 increases with $\dot{V}A$ according to the alveolar ventilation and alveolar gas equations. $\dot{V}A/\dot{Q}$ adds the concept of blood flow. The effect of $\dot{V}A/\dot{Q}$ on PAO_2 can be understood by thinking of $\dot{V}A$ as bringing O_2 into the alveoli and thinking of $\dot{Q}$ as taking it away. If $\dot{Q}$ suddenly increases and removes more O_2 from the alveoli (recall that O_2 is normally a perfusion-limited gas), then PAO_2 will decrease. However, if $\dot{V}A$ increases O_2 delivery to match increased O_2 removal (returning the $\dot{V}A/\dot{Q}$ ratio to normal), then PAO_2 will return to normal. Decreasing $\dot{V}A/\dot{Q}$ has the opposite effect and decreases PAO_2.

The O_2-CO_2 diagram shows the effects of changing $\dot{V}A/\dot{Q}$ in an ideal lung, modeled as a single alveolus in a steady state, with no shunts or diffusion limitations (**Fig. 20.5**). As $\dot{V}A/\dot{Q}$ is the alveolar ventilation-perfusion ratio, dead space is not a factor. The "$\dot{V}A/\dot{Q}$ line" on the CO_2-O_2 diagram shows all of the possible PCO_2-PO_2 combinations that could occur in this ideal lung, with $\dot{V}A/\dot{Q}$ ratios ranging from 0 to infinity.

Regional differences in alveolar ventilation occur because of the mechanical properties of the lung. In upright adults, gravity tends to distort the lung, and alveoli in the apex are more expanded than those in the base of the lung, resulting in basal alveoli operating on a steeper part of the lung's compliance curve, so that $\dot{V}A$ is greater at the bottom than at the top of the lung. $\dot{V}A$ per unit lung volume differs by a factor of 2.5 between the top and bottom of the upright adult lung (**Fig. 20.6**). $\dot{V}A/\dot{Q}$ heterogeneity increases the measured alveolar-arterial PO_2 difference without increasing alveolar-arterial PO_2 difference in any single gas exchange unit (see **Fig. 20.7**). 100% O_2 breathing will eliminate hypoxemia from $\dot{V}A/\dot{Q}$ heterogeneity if all of the alveoli equilibrate with inspired PO_2. With pure O_2 breathing, only O_2 and CO_2 (plus water vapor) are in the alveolar gas and PAO_2 is at least 600 mm Hg in all alveoli. O_2 breathing improves hypoxemia from $\dot{V}A/\dot{Q}$ heterogeneity but not nearly as quickly as it does with a pure diffusion limitation (which requires <1 min). If shunt is present, 100% O_2 breathing will never resolve the hypoxemia or decrease the alveolar-arterial PO_2 difference.

Other clinical measures of $\dot{V}A/\dot{Q}$ heterogeneity include physiologic shunt and dead space. Low $\dot{V}A/\dot{Q}$ gas exchange units and shunt have similar effects on PaO_2. Therefore, physiologic shunt (or venous admixture) can be used to quantify $\dot{V}A/\dot{Q}$ heterogeneity.

Carbon Dioxide Exchange

Hypoventilation has almost the same effect on both O_2 and CO_2. Differences between decreases in PaO_2 and increases in $PaCO_2$ with hypoventilation are

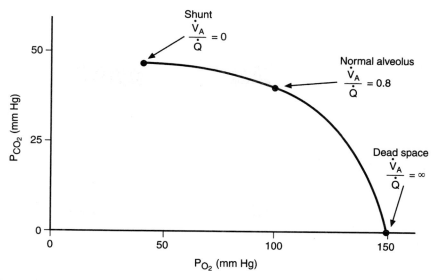

FIGURE 20.5. O_2-CO_2 diagram. The ventilation-perfusion curve describes all possible P_{O_2}-P_{CO_2} combinations in the alveoli (in an ideal lung ($P_{AO_2} = P_{aO_2}$)). Mixed-venous values occur in alveoli with no ventilation (shunt) and inspired values occur in alveoli with no perfusion (dead space). From Powell FL. Pulmonary gas exchange. In: Johnson LR, ed. *Essential Medical Physiology*, 3rd ed. London: Elsevier/Academic Press, 2003, with permission.

explained by the effect of the normal respiratory quetient (RQ) in the alveolar gas equation. The effects of shunts and ventilation-perfusion mismatching on P_{aCO_2} are similar and relatively small for two reasons: (a) P_{aCO_2} changes little when shunt or low $\dot{V}_A/\dot{Q}$ units increase CO_2 concentration because the CO_2-blood equilibrium curve is so steep, and (b) the linearity of the physiologic CO_2 dissociation curve means that increases in CO_2 concentration are offset by increasing $\dot{V}_A$, which decreases P_{aCO_2}. Normal ventilatory control will increase the overall $\dot{V}$ as necessary to restore P_{aCO_2} toward normal. In fact, some patients with shunts and low $\dot{V}_A/\dot{Q}$ units may actually have decreased P_{aCO_2} if hypoxemia is severe enough to override the normal control of P_{aCO_2}.

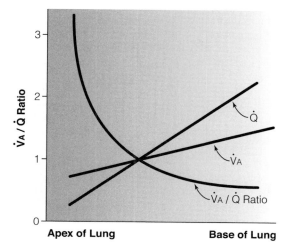

FIGURE 20.6. Gravity results in regional differences in alveolar ventilation ($\dot{V}_A$) and blood flow between the apex and base of adult lungs (as described in the text), which causes the $\dot{V}_A/\dot{Q}$ ratio to decrease ~2.5-fold from the top to the bottom of the lung. Adapted from West J, *Ventilation/Blood Flow and Gas Exchange*, 5th ed. Boston: Blackwell Scientific Pubs., 1990.

Cardiovascular and Tissue Oxygen Transport

The mitochondria are the ultimate site of O_2 consumption and CO_2 production. O_2 delivery is the product of cardiac output and arterial O_2 concentration ($\dot{Q}C_{aO_2}$). The tissues will extract enough O_2 to meet their needs as long as O_2 supply is sufficient. Hence, O_2 supply and demand determine venous O_2 levels. These factors are related by the Fick principle, which describes O_2 transport by the cardiovascular system as:

$$\dot{V}_{O_2} = \dot{Q}\,(C_{aO_2} - C\bar{v}_{O_2})$$

where $\dot{V}_{O_2}$ is O_2 consumption, $\dot{Q}$ is cardiac output, and the last term is the arterial-venous O_2 concentration difference. This equation can be used to calculate cardiac output from measurements of $\dot{V}_{O_2}$ and blood O_2 concentrations. The arterial-venous O_2 concentration difference can be predicted from

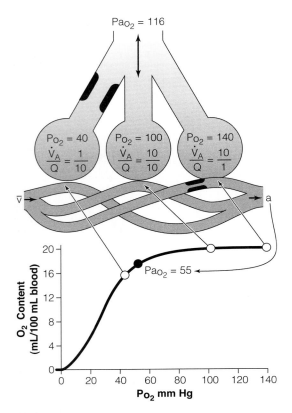

FIGURE 20.7. A three-compartment model showing how $\dot{V}_A/\dot{Q}$ differences between lung units can increase the difference between mixed-alveolar Po_2 ($P_{AO_2} = 116$ mm Hg) and mixed-arterial Po_2 ($Pa_{O_2} = 55$ mm Hg). Inspired Po_2 is assumed normal (150 mm Hg). Alveolar Po_2 in any individual unit is assumed equal to the Po_2 in end-capillary blood from that unit (*open circles on O_2 dissociation curve in lower panel*). However, Po_2 in mixed arterial blood is weighted toward Po_2 in the low $\dot{V}_A/\dot{Q}$ units, and Po_2 in mixed alveolar gas is weighted toward Po_2 in the high $\dot{V}_A/\dot{Q}$ units. The shape of the O_2 dissociation curve also contributes to the large alveolar-arterial Po_2 difference as described in the text. Adapted from West J, *Ventilation/Blood Flow and Gas Exchange*, 5th ed. Boston: Blackwell Scientific Pubs., 1990.

adult resting values for O_2 consumption ($\dot{V}O_2 = 300$ mL/min) and cardiac output ($\dot{Q} = 6$ L/min): (300 mL of O_2/min)/(6000 mL of blood/min) = 5 mL O_2/dL blood. If the normal value for $CaO_2 = 20$ mL of O_2/dL of blood, $C\bar{v}O_2 = 15$ mL/dL. The O_2-blood equilibrium curve is used to convert $C\bar{v}O_2$ (15 mL/dL) to mixed-venous O_2 saturation (75%) and $P\bar{v}O_2$ (40 mm Hg). Changes in $\dot{V}O_2$ can be achieved by increasing cardiac output ("flow reserve") and/or increasing the arterial-venous O_2 difference.

The main difference between O_2 diffusion in tissue and in the lung is that diffusion pathways are much longer in tissue. Tissue capillaries may be 50 μm apart, so that the distance from the capillary to

mitochondria can be 50 times longer than the thickness of the blood-gas barrier (<0.5 μm). Long diffusion distances can lead to significant Po_2 gradients in tissues.

LUNG MECHANICS, RESPIRATORY, AND AIRWAY MUSCLES

Pressure-Flow Relationships in the Respiratory System

The sum of the forces that make the lungs collapse is referred to as the *elastic recoil* and is reflected in the amount of pressure that must be applied across the lungs to produce both the end-expiratory lung volume and changes in the lung volume with breathing. During mechanical ventilation, this pressure is predominantly the pressure applied to the endotracheal tube. The respiratory muscles contract, and the pleural pressure (Ppl) decreases during inspiration from a negative value at end-expiration, which reflects the elastic recoil of the lungs. The transpulmonary pressure (Ptp), or the difference between the airway pressure (Paw) and Ppl, also decreases, which produces the inspiratory flow. The elastic recoil of the lungs increases linearly with lung volume. The main elastic elements of the lung are collagen and elastin.

In the first approximation, the PV relationship of an air-liquid interface can be modeled with a bubble on the end of a blow-tube, by the law of La Place (**Fig. 20.8**):

$$P = 2 \times \text{surface tension}/r$$

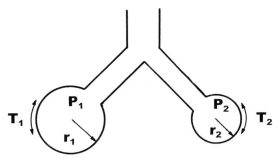

FIGURE 20.8. The distension pressure of two theoretical alveoli connected by a single airway is related by the law of La Place. In the larger alveolus, $P_1 = 2 \times \text{tension}_1/r_1$, and in the smaller alveolus, $P_2 = 2 \times \text{tension}_2/r_2$. If $\text{tension}_1 = \text{tension}_2$, the distending pressure of the smaller alveolus will be greater and will collapse into the larger alveolus. Alternatively, a greater pressure will be required to recruit the smaller alveolus, leading to overdistension and barotrauma to the larger alveolus.

where   P = the pressure applied, is the surface tension of the air-liquid interface
r = the radius of the bubble

The two theoretical alveoli presented in **Figure 20.8** have unequal radii. If the surface tension were the same in both alveoli, the alveolus with the smaller diameter would collapse into the larger one, as the pressure exerted by the surface-tension forces would be greater by this law.

The fact that the pulmonary surfactant decreases on compression overcomes this problem and makes lung inflation more homogeneous. Surfactant replacement therapy is a well-established therapy for premature infants with respiratory distress syndrome. The surfactant is manufactured from the washings or homogenates of animal lungs and processed for separation of surfactant lipids and surfactant-associated proteins. The primary synthetic surfactant, Exosurf, is not as effective as natural surfactants and has fallen out of common clinical usage. Therapy is most effective if given either prophylactically at birth or within the first 2 hrs after birth. Infants treated with surfactant have rapidly decreased oxygen and ventilatory requirements and can be weaned from mechanical ventilation more quickly. The use of prenatal steroids accelerates the appearance of endogenous surfactant and makes extremely premature infants more responsive to replacement therapy.

Flow Limitation

The second element in the mechanics of breathing concerns where and how airflow limitation occurs. In purely elastic systems, the energy put into the system that causes deformation is released back to the system when the deformation is relieved. In purely resistive systems, the energy put into the system during deformation is lost, usually in the form of heat. This dissipation of energy in the lungs occurs both in the airways and the tissue. The pulmonary resistance is usually thought to be that of the airways during spontaneous breathing, as most pathological states involve bronchoconstriction. Nevertheless, tissue resistive forces can more than equal those of the airways under certain pathologic states.

Airway resistance is usually modeled by the aerodynamics of flow through tubes. Flow through the airways is driven by a pressure drop between the alveoli and the atmosphere—or the endotracheal tube in the case of ventilated patients. The decrease in the pressure in the direction of the gas flow represents a dissipation of the kinetic energy of the gas. The rate of this dissipation depends on the conditions of flow. In laminar flow, the gas has a precisely ordered velocity profile, with the flow in the center being the

greatest, decreasing to zero at the walls. A boundary layer of very low flow forms at the walls. Laminar flow was first described by Poiseuille and theoretically has the least possible pressure drop or energy dissipation for a given flow and tube diameter:

$$Resistance = 8 \times viscosity \times length/\pi * radius^4$$

The resistance is dependent on the viscosity of the gas and is inversely proportional to the fourth power of the radius. This is an important consideration in endotracheal tubes of very small radius, as in the premature infant (<3.5 mm internal diameter).

A balance exists between the inertia of the gas and the viscous drag, which is expressed by the Reynolds number. This dimensionless number is proportional to the product of the gas density, the flow rate, and the diameter of the tube. When the Reynolds number is greater than ~2300, the inertial forces are greater than the viscous forces, and laminar flow cannot be established. Rather than moving in smooth lines straight down the tube, the gas is turbulent. The axial movement of the gas increases the pressure against the walls, and energy is dissipated at a greater rate than during laminar flow. During laminar flow, the pressure drop is proportional to the flow rate. During turbulent flow, the pressure drop is proportional to the square of the flow rate.

During inspiration (**Fig. 20.9A–C**), Ppl becomes more negative, the elastic recoil pressure increases, and the airways are supported by the negative

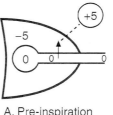

A. Pre-inspiration

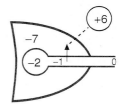

B. During inspiration

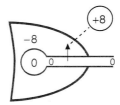

C. End-inspiration

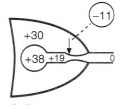

D. Forced expiration

FIGURE 20.9. Dynamic compression of the airways during forced expiration, caused by negative transmural airway pressure (D) beyond the equal pressure point. See text for details. From Powell FL. Mechanics of breathing. In: Johnson LR, ed. *Essential Medical Physiology*, 3rd ed. London: Elsevier/Academic Press, 2003, with permission.

pressure. During forced expiration, the Ppl adds to the elastic recoil pressure, producing the positive alveolar pressure to generate expiratory flow. When gas moves from the distal airways to the central airways, it is accelerated, as the cross-sectional area of the airways decreases rapidly. This acceleration requires a pressure drop down the airway in addition to viscous losses. At the point at which the expiratory flow equals that of the wave speed, the transmural pressure becomes negative, and a choke point is established, called the *equal pressure point* (**Fig. 20.9D**). Flow is then limited by the downstream segment and is independent of the expiratory effort. The higher the flow, the greater the pressure required. Therefore, the transmural pressure primarily reflects the elastic recoil pressure of the lung, because the lung parenchyma is closely linked mechanically to the peribronchiolar space. Thus, at high lung volume, when recoil pressure is greatest, the flow limitation is in the second and third generation of bronchi. At lower lung volumes, flow decreases, and the sites of flow limitation move peripherally. The P_{rs} is a mixture of laminar and turbulent flow. Flow in the large airways is turbulent, and the resistance in this flow regime is density dependent. In cases of extreme large airway obstruction, the resistance can be reduced by reducing the density of the gas with the use of a mixture of helium and oxygen (Heliox). This reduction may help to relieve obstruction such that intubation of the patient is avoided. The primary limitation is the oxygen requirement of the patient that dilutes the helium in the mixture.

The compliance represents the elastic recoil of the lung, determined by the tissue elastic and surface tension forces. The resistance consists of the dissipative forces of the airways and tissue.

Clinical Implications

The act of cyclic recruitment (popping open) and de-recruitment represents a resistive loss. By the same mechanism, recruitment and de-recruitment would involve changes in the elastance. Both the patency of the alveolar ducts and stability of the alveoli are greatly under the influence of surfactant.

PULMONARY CIRCULATION

Because the amount of blood pumped by the right and left ventricles is equal and because the pulmonary and systemic circulations are in series, adult lungs receive the same amount of blood flow as the rest of the body, placing the lung in a unique position to process blood. Many of the structure-function relationships in the

pulmonary circulation are explained by the fact that the lungs must handle high rates of blood flow.

Pulmonary Vascular Pressures

The pressures in the adult pulmonary circulation are generally lower than in the systemic circulation. For example, pulmonary artery pressure (systolic/diastolic) averages 25/8 mm Hg versus 120/80 mm Hg for the systemic arteries. Pressures at the end of the systemic circulation in the right atrium average 2 mm Hg, compared to 5 mm Hg in the left atrium, which collects pulmonary venous return. The pulmonary circulation is "pressure-passive" (i.e., it can accommodate large changes in flow with little changes in pressure). This is important, as the pulmonary circulation must receive the entire cardiac output (under normal circumstances), and minimizing the work of perfusing the lungs and allowing systemic venous return to pass to the systemic ventricle at low pressure decreases the overall circulatory work.

Mean pulmonary artery pressure can increase to >35 mm Hg during exercise, and pulmonary venous pressure can exceed 25 mm Hg in patients with congestive heart failure. Pressures in the pulmonary circulation also vary with normal breathing and especially with artificial ventilation because the heart is surrounded by the intrapleural space, in which pressure decreases during normal inspiration and increases during normal expiration. During positive-pressure artificial ventilation, alveolar and intrapleural pressures may increase considerably during inflation, leading to large increases in pulmonary circulatory pressures. When alveolar and arterial pressures both increase, pulmonary vascular resistance may increase. Similarly, positive end-expiratory pressure during artificial ventilation may increase pulmonary circulatory pressures and resistance in some circumstances, but not all, depending on the initial lung volume.

Pulmonary Vascular Resistance

The hydraulic analogy of Ohm's law can be used to define the relationship between pulmonary vascular pressure, flow, and resistance:

$$P = \dot{Q} \times PVR$$

where:

P is the pressure gradient between the inlet and outlet of a vessel (in mm Hg or cm H_2O)
$\dot{Q}$ is blood flow (L/min)
PVR is pulmonary vascular resistance.

PVR is by definition the resistance for both lungs; in adults, it is ~1.7 (mm Hg × min)/L for a normal cardiac output of 6 L/min, with an average pressure drop of 10 mm Hg from the pulmonary artery to left atrium. The dimensions of pulmonary vessels are strongly influenced by several external forces, unlike the situation for rigid pipes in a plumbing system or even in systemic arteries.

Increasing transmural pressure can affect capillary dimensions by two mechanisms: recruitment and distention. At very low pressures, some capillaries may be closed, and increasing pressure will open them by recruitment. At higher pressures, capillaries are already open, but they may be distended or stretched by increased transmural pressure. Together, recruitment and distention increase the effective size of the pulmonary capillaries and reduce PVR.

Fetal and Perinatal Pulmonary Circulation

The anatomy of the pulmonary circulation in the fetus differs from the adult because the placenta is the primary gas-exchange organ in utero (**Fig. 20.10**). Fetal blood flows into the placenta through the umbilical arteries. Oxygen diffuses from the maternal circulation into the fetus. Diffusion is relatively inefficient in the placenta compared to the lungs, but oxygen transfer is enhanced by the high oxygen affinity of fetal, compared to adult, hemoglobin. The end result is a maximum PO_2 of 30 torr in the fetal circulation in blood leaving the placenta and entering the inferior vena cava. Some of the oxygenated blood in the inferior vena cava flows directly from the right into the left atrium via the foramen ovale, which is a normal connection between the right and left atria in the fetus. Hence, blood leaving the left ventricle in the aorta has a relatively high PO_2, diluted only by other systemic venous blood in the inferior vena cava to ~25 torr. The rest of the blood returning from the inferior vena cava mixes with blood returning from the superior vena cava in the right atrium, reducing the PO_2 to 19 torr in the right ventricle.

Blood is pumped from the right ventricle into the pulmonary artery, but only 10% flows into the lungs; the remainder goes into the aorta via the ductus arteriosis, which is a shunt vessel normally present in the fetus. The small pulmonary blood flow is important for the normal development of the lungs and the surfactant system. The ductus arteriosis joins the aorta distal to the carotid and coronary arteries. This anatomy maximizes the PO_2 in blood that perfuses the brain and heart because PO_2 is greater in the left ventricle than in the right ventricle (**Fig. 20.10**). It is important to note that the output of the left ventricle is only approximately half that of the right ventricle in the fetus, in contrast to being equal in adults,

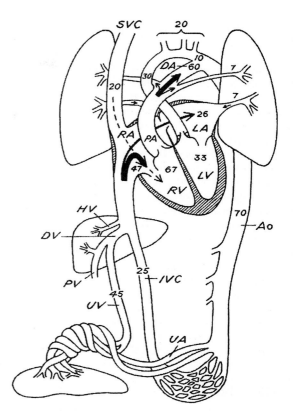

FIGURE 20.10. Schematic representation of human fetal circulation. Numbers refer to blood flow in mL/min through the main vascular channels. SVC, superior vena cava; DA, ductus arteriosus; RA, right atrium; PA, pulmonary artery; LA, left atrium; RV, right ventricle, LV, left ventricle; Ao, aorta; HV, hepatic vein; DV, ductus venosus; PV, portal vein ; UV, umbilical vein; IVC, inferior vena cava; UA, umbilical artery. Adapted from Comroe, JH. *Physiology of Respiration*, Chicago: Year Book Medical Publishers, 1965.

because the ductus arteriosis shunts blood from the pulmonary to systemic circulations.

The pressures in the fetal pulmonary circulation are high relative to adults because of the connection between the pulmonary arteries and the ductus arteriosis, which comes from the left ventricle, as well as high pulmonary vascular resistance in the fetal lung. Hypoxic pulmonary vasoconstriction helps to keep the pulmonary vascular resistance high in the fetus. At birth at term, the first few breaths expand the lungs, filling them with a relatively high oxygen tension, which makes several dramatic changes in the physiology. Hypoxic pulmonary vasoconstriction is reduced, and the pulmonary capillaries are stretched, opening them so that pulmonary blood flow greatly increases. The infant breathes deeply and rapidly, lowering the PCO_2 and raising the pH, which enhances the effects of decreased hypoxic pulmonary vasoconstriction.

With the increase in pulmonary blood flow upon air breathing at birth, left atrial pressure increases, thus closing the flap-like foramen ovale. This closure is also aided by the decrease in right atrial pressure as the umbilical blood flow decreases. Flow through the ductus arteriosis decreases as resistance to pulmonary blood flow decreases and the ductus constricts in response to increased PO_2 and circulating prostaglandin PGE_2.

This transition takes place in three stages. The first, which reduces the PVR to ~50% of the fetal level, occurs with the first few effective breaths. The second stage can take up to ~1 hr, during which time the ductus arteriosus constricts, and relief of the hypoxic pulmonary vasoconstriction is stabilized. During this stage, the systemic circulation is influenced by right-to-left shunting at the level of both the ductus arteriosus and the foramen ovale; the peripheral circulation can be sluggish, and some degree of peripheral cyanosis can occur. During this stage, the PVR is reduced by ~75% of the fetal level. This third stage takes several hours to several days, during which complete relaxation of the hypoxic vasoconstriction and remodeling of the vascular smooth muscle occur.

Distribution of Pulmonary Blood Flow

The zone model for pulmonary blood flow developed by West is illustrated in **Figure 20.11**. This model conceptually divides the lung into three zones to explain how gravity affects blood flow up the lung through alveolar vessels at different heights. The effect of mechanical ventilation on lung zones should be considered. Clearly, elevating alveolar pressure will convert some zone 2 lung to zone 1 and some zone 3 lung to zone 2. Thus, the effect of mechanical ventilation could be to create more alveolar dead space (zone 1) and improve V/Q matching in zone 2.

Hypoxic Pulmonary Vasoconstriction

Hypoxic pulmonary vasoconstriction is a direct response of vascular smooth muscle in pulmonary arterioles to decreased alveolar PO_2. Hypoxic pulmonary vasoconstriction can be reduced by low concentrations of inhaled nitric oxide (20 ppm nitric oxide) in humans. Nitric oxide also relaxes systemic vessels through a cyclic guanosine monophosphate (cGMP) pathway. A direct vasoconstrictor response to local alveolar PO_2 allows blood flow to be selectively diverted away from poorly ventilated regions of the lung. Hence, hypoxic pulmonary vasoconstriction is important for matching unequal distributions of ventilation and blood flow throughout the lungs. This response might be more important during the transition in the circulatory pattern at birth. Hypoxic pulmonary vasoconstriction reduces blood flow through the fetal lung when it is not ventilated. This response is greatest in the fetus and serves an essential function in utero, where its absence leads to hydrops, hypoxia, and fetal demise.

Blood pH has an effect even at high PO_2; therefore, the increase in pH with the onset of air breathing will also reduce pulmonary vascular resistance as PO_2 increases with air breathing in the newborn.

Lung Fluid Balance

Starling's law states that the net fluid flux across the capillary depends on a balance of hydrostatic forces (P) and colloid osmotic (or oncotic) forces (π):

$$\text{Net fluid flux} = K_{fc}[(Pc - Pi) - \sigma(\pi c - \pi i)]$$

where K_{fc} is a filtration coefficient that depends on the total surface area of the capillary and the number and size of pores in the capillary. Hydrostatic pressure in the capillary (Pc) tends to move fluid out, and interstitial pressure (Pi) tends to move fluid into the capillary. Conversely, capillary osmotic pressure (πc) tends to hold fluid in the capillary, and interstitial osmotic pressure (πi) tends to draw fluid out of the capillary. The osmotic reflection coefficient (σ) describes the effectiveness of osmotic pressure at moving.

Normally, the balance of forces results in net filtration, or the movement of a few milliliters per hour of fluid out of the capillaries in adults.

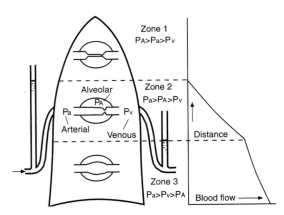

FIGURE 20.11. West's zone model for pulmonary blood flow predicts increasing blood flow down the lung because of the effects of gravity on pressures, as explained in the text. Pa, arterial pressure; PA, alveolar pressure; Pv, venous pressure. From Powell FL. Structure and function of the respiratory system. In: Johnson LR, ed. *Essential Medical Physiology*, 3rd ed. London: Elsevier/Academic Press, 2003, with permission.

Normal Pc $\approx$ 10 mm Hg, and normal Pi in the lungs is subatmospheric, so that a positive hydrostatic force moves fluid out of the capillaries. The interstitial space around alveolar capillaries is not compliant, and filtration in this region tends to increase local interstitial pressure. When this normal balance of forces is disturbed, filtration can exceed the capacity of reabsorption and lymphatic drainage, and fluid accumulates in the interstitium. Edema is the accumulation of excess filtrate outside the capillaries. Pulmonary edema fluid accumulates first in the peribronchiolar and perivascular spaces; this is called *interstitial edema*. Interstitial edema can alter local ventilation and perfusion and make gas exchange inefficient by decreasing compliance, increasing the work of breathing, and ultimately leading to loss of lung volume. As interstitial fluid accumulates, it can enter into the alveolus causing alveolar edema.

RESPIRATORY CONTROL

The overall aim of the respiratory feedback loop is to keep blood gases in a normal range with the least possible energy expenditure and O_2 consumption. The afferent limb consists of receptors that send information to a central controller. For example, the carotid bodies inform the central controller of the O_2 level. Both airway and carotid body sensors compare actual and baseline, or programmed, "set" signals to generate error signals. The carotid sinus nerve fibers, which carry impulses generated by the carotid glomus cells, synapse in the medulla oblongata. The efferent limb is the part of the feedback loop that is responsible for the execution of the decision made centrally (i.e., the respiratory muscles and their innervation) after integrating afferent signals. Among many muscles of respiration, the external intercostal and diaphragm muscles are the major muscles.

If presented with a number of neurophysiologic signals (representing options about various needs), the central controller can enhance or reduce the response to certain stimuli at the expense of others. Therefore, a hierarchy is used by brainstem networks in determining the response of the respiratory system at any one time. Temporal and spatial summation of excitatory and inhibitory postsynaptic potentials will be critical in deciding the behavior of these neurons. In addition, their cellular and membrane properties will indeed affect their output. Changes in the state of consciousness modulate the ability of the brainstem to respond to afferent stimuli. Age is very important, as the response of the brainstem to stimuli varies with maturation and cortical input to brainstem structures.

In addition to chemoreceptors, powerful mechanoreceptors in the lungs and chest wall function to preserve lung volume. Nowhere is this more evident than in the newborn, in whom the respiratory muscles are weak, whose lung mechanics are deranged, and whose oxygenation depends on maintenance of the FRC. The mechanoreceptors function to prolong inspiratory effort, shorten the expiratory time, and cause dynamic gas trapping. This tachypnea is commonly seen even in infants with normal gas exchange on mechanical ventilation. The mechanoreceptors are incorporated in the control of the airway muscles as well. Infants have expiratory grunting that can augment the expiratory transpulmonary pressure by several centimeters of H_2O to significantly increase their FRC.

A multitude of afferent messages converge on the brainstem. Chemoreceptors and mechanoreceptors in the larynx and upper airways sense stretch, temperature, and chemical changes over the mucosa and relay this information to the brainstem. Afferent impulses from these areas travel through the superior laryngeal nerve and vagus. Changes in O_2 or CO_2 tensions are sensed at the carotid and aortic bodies, and afferent impulses travel through the carotid and aortic sinus nerves. Thermal or metabolic changes are sensed by skin or mucosal receptors or by hypothalamic neurons and are carried through spinal tracts to the brainstem. Afferent information is not a prerequisite for the generation and maintenance of respiration. When the brainstem and spinal cord are removed from the body and maintained in vitro, rhythmic phrenic activity can be detected for hours. Among the many types of afferent information that affect the respiratory output of the central nervous system (CNS), CO_2 and O_2 are some of the most potent. If "afferent" is considered to be any information that converges on the brainstem respiratory network, CO_2 is certainly an important and powerful stimulus to respiration, even though it is sensed mostly in the CNS itself. Almost any change in CO_2 induces a change in ventilation and vice versa (for any given metabolic rate). Premature infants and full-term newborns have a reduced response to CO_2 for several days (or weeks) in early life, from a complex integration of changes in neural control (maturation of the CNS or peripheral nerves) and respiratory mechanics (chest-wall mechanics and/or respiratory muscles). In comparison to the adult, peripheral chemoreceptors assume a greater role in the newborn period.

The carotid bodies discharge and have an effect on ventilation when the PaO_2 reaches <55–60 torr. In general, other tissues react to such levels of PaO_2 but in very different ways. The effect on most tissues, however, is that they develop remarkable dysfunction when PaO_2 is <35–40 torr.

CHAPTER 21 ■ RESPIRATORY MONITORING

IRA M. CHEIFETZ • SHEKHAR T. VENKATARAMAN • DONNA S. HAMEL

It is a concerning phenomenon of modern intensive care that physical examination, and especially the stethoscope, are used with decreasing frequency. Clinical scoring systems have been developed to evaluate the clinical parameters of skin color, nasal flaring, retractions, accessory muscle use, and the presence and severity of an abnormal sound (e.g., rales, wheeze, or stridor). Scoring systems generally demonstrate that the more pronounced the abnormality, the worse the prognosis. Impedance pneumography is the method used most often for spontaneously breathing children to quantitate respiratory rate. Respiratory pauses last <5 secs and occur in children who are <3 months of age. Pauses occur in groups of 3 or more, are separated by <20 secs, and generally resolve by 6 months of age without medical intervention. A National Institutes of Health Conference consensus statement on infantile apnea defined apnea as cessation of breathing for >20 secs or any respiratory pause associated with bradycardia, pallor, or cyanosis.

ASSESSMENT OF GAS EXCHANGE

The primary functions of the cardiorespiratory system are to provide adequate O_2 to the tissues and to eliminate CO_2 (**Fig. 21.1**). Monitoring of oxygenation includes an assessment of O_2 transfer in the lungs, O_2 transport to the tissues and organs by the circulatory system (O_2 delivery, DO_2), and O_2 transfer to and utilization by the tissues (**Fig. 21.2**). Elimination of CO_2 similarly involves CO_2 production by the tissues, transfer of CO_2 from the tissues to venous blood, transport of CO_2 by the circulatory system to the lungs, and elimination of CO_2 by alveolar ventilation in the exhaled gas (**Fig. 21.2**).

Indices used to assess the lung as an oxygenator are (a) arterial O_2 tension (PaO_2); (b) arterial blood oxygen saturation (SaO_2); (c) intrapulmonary shunt fraction (Qs/Qt); (d) alveolar-to-arterial O_2 tension difference ($PA–aO_2$); (e) arterial-to-alveolar oxygen tension ratio (PaO_2/PAO_2); and (f) arterial-to-fraction of inspired O_2 ratio (PaO_2/F_iO_2). PaO_2, represents the net effect of O_2 exchange in the lung. At sea level, the normal PaO_2 in a newborn infant is between 40 and 70 mm Hg when breathing room air. With increasing age, the PaO_2 increases until it reaches an adult value of 90–120 mm Hg.

Hypoxemia is defined as a PaO_2 lower than the acceptable range for age, whereas hypoxia is inadequate tissue oxygenation.

Qs/Qt is defined as the fraction of right ventricular output that enters the left ventricle without oxygen transfer. In the absence of intracardiac shunts, Qs/Qt is calculated by the formula:

$$Qs/Qt = (Cc'O_2 − CaO_2)/(Cc'O_2 − CvO_2)$$

where:
$Cc'O_2$ = oxygen content of the pulmonary venous blood, assuming the lung to be a perfect oxygenator
CaO_2 = arterial oxygen content
CvO_2 = the mixed venous oxygen content

Oxygen content of whole blood is calculated as ($Hb × 1.34 × SO_2/100$) + ($0.003 × PaO_2$.

If the lung were a perfect oxygenator, pulmonary venous O_2 would be identical to the alveolar PO_2 (PAO_2), and if the right ventricular output traverses the ideal lung, PaO_2 would be the same as pulmonary venous O_2. PAO_2 is calculated from the simplified alveolar gas equation,

$$PAO_2 = (P_B − PH_2O) × FiO_2 − PaCO_2/RQ$$

where P_B = barometric pressure
PH_2O = partial pressure of water vapor (47 mm Hg when fully saturated with H_2O)
RQ = respiratory quotient (CO_2 production/O_2 consumption)

Oxygen consumption ($\dot{V}O_2$) is the amount of O_2 that is utilized by the body in a minute and can be measured by analyzing the inspired and expired gases using a Douglas bag or calculated using the Fick equation, where $\dot{V}O_2 = CI(CaO_2 − CvO_2)$. Fever, thyrotoxicosis, and increased catecholamine release or administration increase the metabolic rate and increase $\dot{V}O_2$. Hypothermia and hypothyroidism tend to decrease $\dot{V}O_2$. Measurement of $\dot{V}O_2$ may be important in critically ill patients, especially those with moderately severe cardiorespiratory dysfunction. Under normal conditions, $\dot{V}O_2$ is independent of $\dot{D}O_2$. In some critically ill patients, $\dot{V}O_2$ becomes $\dot{D}O_2$ dependent. If clinically possible, $\dot{D}O_2$ should be increased until $\dot{V}O_2$ is no longer $\dot{D}O_2$ dependent.

Mixed venous oxygen saturation (SvO_2) is commonly used as a measure of the balance between O_2 demand and supply. A low SvO_2 usually signifies that

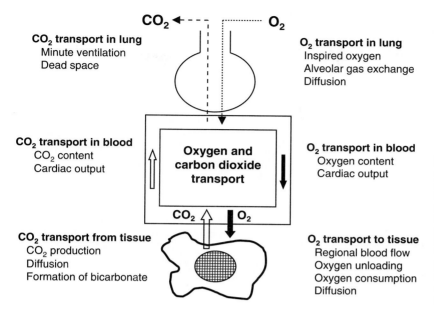

CO₂ transport in lung
Minute ventilation
Dead space

O₂ transport in lung
Inspired oxygen
Alveolar gas exchange
Diffusion

CO₂ transport in blood
CO₂ content
Cardiac output

Oxygen and carbon dioxide transport

O₂ transport in blood
Oxygen content
Cardiac output

FIGURE 21.1. Physiology of oxygenation and ventilation. The primary functions of the cardiorespiratory system are to provide adequate oxygen to the tissues and to eliminate carbon dioxide via the lungs. This gas transfer process involves an elaborate interaction between the lungs, circulatory system, and the tissues throughout the body.

CO₂ transport from tissue
CO₂ production
Diffusion
Formation of bicarbonate

O₂ transport to tissue
Regional blood flow
Oxygen unloading
Oxygen consumption
Diffusion

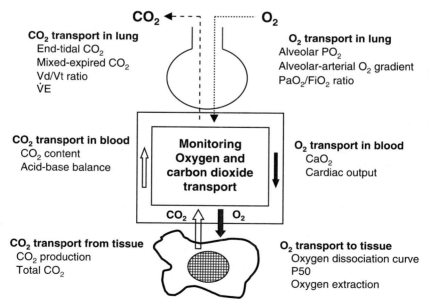

CO₂ transport in lung
End-tidal CO₂
Mixed-expired CO₂
Vd/Vt ratio
V̇E

O₂ transport in lung
Alveolar PO₂
Alveolar-arterial O₂ gradient
PaO₂/FiO₂ ratio

CO₂ transport in blood
CO₂ content
Acid-base balance

Monitoring Oxygen and carbon dioxide transport

O₂ transport in blood
CaO₂
Cardiac output

CO₂ transport from tissue
CO₂ production
Total CO₂

O₂ transport to tissue
Oxygen dissociation curve
P50
Oxygen extraction

FIGURE 21.2. Variables associated with cardiorespiratory monitoring at each point in the transport of oxygen and carbon dioxide. Monitoring of oxygenation includes an assessment of O_2 transfer in the lungs, O_2 transport to the tissues and organs by the circulatory system (i.e., oxygen delivery), and O_2 transfer to and utilization by the tissues. Elimination of CO_2 similarly involves CO_2 production by the tissues, transfer of CO_2 from the tissues to venous blood, transport of CO_2 by the circulatory system to the lungs, and elimination of CO_2 by alveolar ventilation in the exhaled gas. CO_2, carbon dioxide; E_TCO_2, end-tidal carbon dioxide; Vd/Vt ratio, dead space-to-tidal volume ratio; $\dot{V}_E$, expired minute volume; HCO_3, bicarbonate; Hb, hemoglobin; PaO_2, alveolar partial pressure of oxygen; $PA-aO_2$, alveolar-to-arterial O_2 tension difference; PaO_2, arterial partial pressure of oxygen; FiO_2, fraction of inspired oxygen; CaO_2, arterial oxygen content; SaO_2, arterial oxygen saturation.

TABLE 21.1

COMMON CLINICAL CONDITIONS ASSOCIATED WITH CHANGES IN MIXED VENOUS OXYGEN SATURATION

Reduction in SvO_2
↓Oxygen delivery
   ↓cardiac output
   ↓arterial oxygen saturation
   ↓hemoglobin concentration
↑Oxygen Consumption

Increase in SvO_2
↑Oxygen delivery
↓Oxygen consumption
   ↓oxygen extraction
Left-to-right intracardiac shunt
Sepsis

SvO_2, venous oxygen saturation

$\dot{D}O_2$ is significantly decreased and the body is extracting more O_2 from the blood. A high SvO_2 is usually seen in hypothermia due to decreased O_2 demand and in brain death, as the brain usually constitutes a major site of the total body O_2 consumption. The normal saturation of the Hb in the pulmonary artery is ~78% in the normal person (range, 73%–85%). Causes of changes in SvO_2 are listed in **Table 21.1**.

PULSE OXIMETRY

The arterial oxygen saturation of Hb (SaO_2) is the percent oxyhemoglobin in the arterial blood. The oxygen-dissociation curve describes the avidity with which oxygen binds to Hb. Acidemia, hypercarbia, increased temperature, and increased red-cell 2,3-diphosphoglycerate (2,3-DPG) level shift the curve to the right.

Pulse oximetry estimates arterial oxygen saturation by measuring the absorption of light in tissues. As pulse oximetry assesses whether oxygen is attached to Hb or is not, the relevant solutes are reduced Hb and oxyhemoglobin and their respective absorption characteristics. Wavelengths of 660 nm (red) and 940 nm (infrared) are used because the absorption characteristics of these 2 hemoglobins are significantly different at these 2 wavelengths. When light passes through a pulsating vascular bed, the transmitted light has nonpulsatile and pulsatile components. The nonpulsatile component is assumed to represent light transmitted through the tissues, capillaries, and veins. The pulsatile component is assumed to represent light transmitted through the arterial bed. By using the 2 wavelengths of light, the pulse oximeter

determines "functional saturation."

$$Functional\ SpO_2 = HbO_2/(HbO_2 + Hb)$$
$$where\ HbO_2 = oxygenated\ Hb$$
$$Hb = nonoxygenated\ Hb$$

Functional SpO_2 is contrasted with the fractional SpO_2 measured by co-oximetry on most blood gas analyzers, which provides the ratio of oxygenated Hb to the sum of *all hemoglobin types*, including carboxyhemoglobin (COHb) and methemoglobin (MetHb), which do not carry oxygen:

Fractional

$$SpO_2 = O_2\ Hb/(HbO_2 + Hb + COHb + MetHb)$$

The disadvantage of the determination of functional saturation is that other, possibly clinically significant Hb species, such as carboxyhemoglobin and methemoglobin, will be missed. This shortcoming can be overcome in ambiguous clinical situations by using periodic co-oximetry that uses 4–6 wavelengths to determine the fractional saturation. Factors that affect the performance of pulse oximeters include artifacts introduced by patient motion, poor peripheral perfusion, and false alarms (**Table 21.2**). Carboxyhemoglobin is interpreted as oxyhemoglobin by the photo detector of the 2-light-source photo oximeter. Thus, functional SpO_2 overestimates the true HbO_2, but fractional SpO_2 decreases dramatically. Methemoglobin absorbs light significantly at both the 660-nm and the 940-nm wavelengths, thereby confusing the oximeter photo detector into believing that both oxyhemoglobin and reduced Hb are increased. The microprocessor-driven algorithm results in the R/IR approaching unity and an SpO_2 of ~85% on the calibration curve. Methylene blue has a maximum absorbance at 668 nm. The oximeter interprets this extra absorbance as reduced Hb and, therefore, a lower SpO_2. Clinically, this is seen as a sudden (<30 secs) drop in saturation when methylene blue is injected for therapeutic or diagnostic purposes. This effect generally is limited to ~2 mins.

TABLE 21.2

FACTORS THAT CONTRIBUTE TO POTENTIAL INACCURACY OF PULSE OXIMETRY

Poor cardiac output/low perfusion states
Motion artifact
Increased venous pulsations
Optical interference from environment
Dyshemoglobinemias: carbon monoxide,
   methemoglobinemia, fetal hemoglobin
Dyes and pigments: methylene blue, indocyanine green

TRANSCUTANEOUS MEASUREMENT OF GAS TENSION

Monitors measure the PO_2 and CO_2 electrochemically. Electrodes are attached to the skin by adhesive patches to well-perfused, non-bony surfaces. The abdomen, inner thigh, lower back, and chest are desirable sites in neonates, as are the chest, abdomen, and lower back in larger children and adults. Perhaps the greatest benefit of this technology is continuous monitoring and trending that reduce the frequency of blood gas measurement and, hence, potentially decrease blood transfusions in neonates and infants.

Oxygen tension decreases linearly along the skin capillaries due to O_2 consumption in the dermis, which results in an arteriovenous difference in PO_2. Most transcutaneous monitors incorporate a heating element maintained at $42°C$–$44°C$. The heating of the skin increases blood flow and arterializes the blood in the capillaries underneath the electrode. The correlation between $P_{Tc}O_2$ and PaO_2 is excellent only when the blood pressure is within normal limits and peripheral circulation is normal. In circumstances wherein peripheral circulation is affected by hypotension, acidosis or drugs, the correlation becomes poor (**Table 21.3**). In critically ill newborns with mild circulatory failure, $P_{Tc}O_2$ can still reflect PaO_2, provided maximal hyperemia can be achieved. With moderate to severe circulatory failure, $P_{Tc}O_2$ no longer correlates with PaO_2. In these patients, $P_{Tc}O_2$ reflects skin perfusion more than PaO_2. The efficacy of various therapeutic maneuvers can be evaluated by their ability to restore the relationship between $P_{Tc}O_2$ and PaO_2. Advantages and disadvantages of $P_{Tc}O_2$ monitoring are summarized in **Table 21.4**.

TABLE 21.3

CONDITIONS ASSOCIATED WITH POOR CORRELATION BETWEEN $P_{Tc}O_2$ AND PaO_2

1. Shock	BP <2 Standard deviations below mean for age
2. Acidosis	pH <7.1
3. Hypothermia	Temperature <35°C
4. Following cardiac surgery	Probably due to 1, 2, and 3
5. Skin edema	Severe
6. Cyanotic heart disease	PaO_2 <30 mm Hg
7. Tolazoline infusion	Probably related to shunting in the skin blood vessels

$P_{Tc}O_2$, transcutaneous partial pressure of carbon dioxide; PaO_2, arterial oxygen tension.

TABLE 21.4

ADVANTAGES AND DISADVANTAGES OF $P_{Tc}O_2$ MONITORING

Advantages
Provides a reliably accurate measure of PaO_2 continuously and noninvasively
Accurate over a wide range of PaO_2 values
Very useful in neonates to maintain PaO_2 within a narrow range
Provides a trend of PaO_2 over time
Can detect variability and large changes in PaO_2 when SaO_2 is >95%
Provides a measure of circulatory dysfunction when $P_{Tc}O_2$ is <PaO_2

Disadvantages
Requires frequent calibration
Requires frequent site changes due to the possibility of local burns on the skin
Requires a warm-up time of 10 mins
Underestimates PaO_2 in hyperoxic range (>150 mm Hg)
Overestimates PaO_2 in hypoxic range (<50 mm Hg)
ess useful with increasing age

$P_{Tc}O_2$, transcutaneous partial pressure of carbon dioxide; PaO_2, arterial oxygen tension; SaO_2, arterial blood oxygen saturation.

Capnography

The normal E_TCO_2 in healthy subjects is <5 mm Hg different than the $PaCO_2$, representing normal anatomic dead space of the upper airway. Clinical conditions associated with alterations in E_TCO_2 are shown in **Table 21.5**. The phasic changes in CO_2 concentration that occur during the respiratory cycle are demonstrated in **Figure 21.3**.

Practical uses of E_TCO_2 monitoring in the ICU include adequacy of alveolar ventilation during mechanical ventilation, respiratory-rate monitoring, patient-ventilator system function, and endotracheal tube (ETT) patency and positioning. While the validation of ETT placement in the trachea is improved with E_TCO_2 monitoring, limitations do exist. False-positive readings (i.e., the monitor displays an end-tidal CO_2 value when the ETT is not in the trachea) may occur following prolonged bag-valve-mask ventilation prior to intubation, following ingestion of antacids or carbonated beverages, or when the tip of the ETT is in the pharynx. False-negative readings (i.e., no end-tidal CO_2 value is displayed when, in fact, the ETT is in trachea) may occur if the patient has severe airway obstruction, poor cardiac output, pulmonary emboli, or pulmonary hypertension. Capnography can be used to great advantage in mechanically ventilated patients if the waveform is

TABLE 21.5

CLINICAL CONDITIONS ASSOCIATED WITH ALTERATIONS IN E_TCO_2

Increases in E_TCO_2
Increased pulmonary capillary blood flow
Increased cardiac output
Hypoventilation
Increased carbon dioxide production
Sudden release of a tourniquet
Sodium bicarbonate administration

Decreases in E_TCO_2
Decreased pulmonary capillary blood flow
    Pulmonary hypertension
    Pulmonary embolus (thrombus or air)
Decreased cardiac output
Hyperventilation
Ventilator circuit leak
Obstructed endotracheal tube
Decreased carbon dioxide production

Absent E_TCO_2
Esophageal intubation
Ventilator disconnect

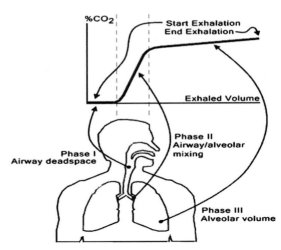

FIGURE 21.4. Volumetric capnogram. The initial portion of the volumetric capnogram (phase 1) represents the quantity of carbon dioxide eliminated from the large airways. Phase 2 is the transitional zone, which represents ventilation from both small and large airways. The third phase of the capnogram represents carbon dioxide elimination from the alveoli and, thus, the quantity of gas involved with alveolar ventilation. Figure Courtesy of Respironics, Inc., and its affiliates, Wallingford, Connecticut.

displayed and analyzed along with the numeric data. Mechanical failures can be detected, the adequacy of respiratory support can be analyzed, and changes can be made in the mode of ventilation to maximize the efficiency of ventilation, decrease the patient's work of breathing (WOB), and improve patient ventilator synchrony.

Volumetric capnography provides a measurement of CO_2 production (VCO_2) and enables calculation of alveolar minute ventilation and the ratio of volume of dead space (Vd) and tidal volume (VT), V_d/VT. The

net volume of CO_2 eliminated through the lungs each minute (VCO_2) varies depending on CO_2 production, ventilation, circulation/perfusion and, to a lesser degree, diffusion. The single-breath CO_2 waveform consists of 3 phases (**Fig. 21.4**). When weaning from mechanical ventilation, it is important to ensure that the volume of gas delivered actually participates in gas exchange (i.e., effective ventilation). Volumetric capnography provides clinicians with a continuous numerical representation of effective ventilation.

Responses to changes in ventilatory strategies and cardiac function can be detected with both time-based and volume-based (i.e., volumetric) capnography. Many conditions, such as pulmonary embolism, pulmonary hypertension, air embolism, and severe cardiac dysfunction increase dead-space ventilation, impair gas exchange, and cause a significant decrease in the expired CO_2 concentration.

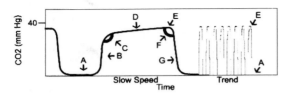

FIGURE 21.3. Normal features of a capnogram. (**A**) Baseline, represents the beginning of expiration and should start at zero. (**B**) The transitional part of the curve represents mixing of dead space and alveolar gas. (**C**) The alpha angle represents the change to alveolar gas. (**D**) The alveolar part of the curve represents the plateau average alveolar gas concentration. (**E**) The end-tidal carbon dioxide value. (**F**) The beta angle represents the change to the inspiratory part of the cycle. (**G**) The inspiration part of the curve shows a rapid decrease in carbon dioxide concentration. From Thompson JE, Jaffe MB. Capnographic waveforms in the mechanically ventilated patient. *Respiratory Care* 2005;50(1):100–9, with permission.

Monitoring Respiratory Mechanics

In a relaxed patient during mechanical ventilation, measurements of respiratory mechanics can be obtained by rapid airway occlusion during constant-flow inflation, when the proximal airway pressure increases as the lung is inflated to a maximal pressure (P_{max}). Rapid airway occlusion at end-inspiration results in an immediate drop in both airway pressure and transpulmonary pressure (Ptp) from P_{max},

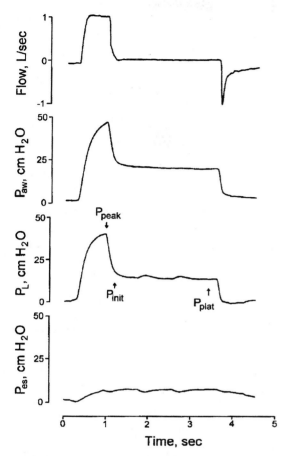

FIGURE 21.5. Flow (inspiration upward), airway pressure (P_{aw}), transpulmonary pressure (P_L), and esophageal pressure (P_{es}) tracings in a representative patient during passive ventilation. An end-inspiratory occlusion produced a rapid decline in both P_{aw} and P_{tp} from a peak value to a lower initial value, followed by gradual decrease until a plateau is achieved. From Jubran A, Tobin MJ. Passive mechanics of lung and chest wall in patients who failed and succeeded in trials of weaning. *Am J Resp Crit Care Med* 1997;155:916–21, with permission.

followed by a gradual decrease until a plateau (P_{plat}) is achieved after 3–5 secs (**Fig. 21.5**). The pressure drop from P_{max} can be partitioned into an initial almost linear drop followed by a slower, multi-exponential decrease to P_{plat}. P_{plat}, Ptp, and esophageal pressure (P_{es}) represent the static recoil pressure of the total respiratory system, lung, and chest wall, respectively.

Compliance is defined as a change in volume divided by a change in transmural pressure. *Elastance* is the reciprocal of compliance. Lung compliance is defined as the change in lung volume divided by the transalveolar pressure, which is equal to the difference between the alveolar pressure (P_{alv}) at the end of inflation and the pleural pressure (P_{pl} or P_{es}). At the bedside, the P_{plat} can be substituted for P_{alv} and tidal volume can be substituted for a change in lung volume (C_{lung}):

$$C_{lung} = VT/(P_{plat} - P_{es})$$

C_{lung} is also called *static lung compliance* (C_{stat}). Since esophageal pressure is often not measured in children, C_{lung} can be calculated by

$$C_{lung} = VT_{(effective)}/(P_{plat} - PEEP)$$

where $VT_{(effective)}$ is the tidal volume delivered to the patient (usually measured at the hub of the ETT or estimated by subtracting the compressible volume lost in the circuit from the ventilator-delivered tidal volume).

Dynamic compliance (C_{dyn}) is defined as the change in volume divided by the change in airway pressure from end expiration to end-inspiration during a mechanical breath. It is commonly calculated by dividing the VT by the difference between P_{max} and end-expiratory pressure.

$$C_{dyn} = VT/(P_{max} - PEEP)$$

In patients without $PEEP_i$, the end-expiratory pressure to be used is the set PEEP. In patients with $PEEP_i$, the end-expiratory pressure to be used for the calculation of C_{dyn} is $PEEP_i$.

A calculated VT represents the ventilator-determined VT minus the volume "lost" due to the distensibility (compliance) of the ventilator circuit. It should be noted that the calculated values can differ from those measured at the ETT. Additionally, it is preferable to index tidal volumes to body weight to be able to compare across patient populations.

The static recoil pressure of the respiratory system at end expiration may be elevated in patients who receive mechanical ventilation, especially in those who have lower-airway disease and obstruction. With lower-airway obstruction, inspiration may begin before exhalation is complete, thus resulting in an end-expiratory alveolar pressure that remains elevated above the proximal airway pressure. This positive recoil pressure, or static $PEEP_i$, can be quantified in relaxed patients by using an end-expiratory hold maneuver on a mechanical ventilator immediately before the onset of the next breath. Patients who are spontaneously breathing may need to overcome $PEEP_i$ to trigger a ventilator. Thus, $PEEP_i$ increases WOB and can contribute to muscle fatigue. Excessive $PEEP_i$ may also result in poor triggering because the patient is unable to generate the necessary negative pressure in the central airway. This problem can be largely overcome by flow triggering.

The inspiratory phase of the PV curve consists of 3 sections. As the lung is inflated from low lung volumes, the initial lung compliance is low. Then, as airway pressure is increased, lung compliance improves,

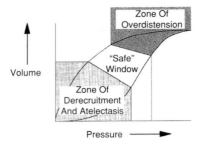

FIGURE 21.6. Pressure-volume curve. The inspiratory phase of the pressure-volume curve consists of 3 sections. As the lung is inflated from an initial low lung volume, the lung compliance is low. As airway pressure is increased, lung compliance improves, which continues until the lung is fully inflated. Inflating the lung further results in a reduction in the lung compliance at the end of inflation as the lung overdistends. The goal is to ventilate in the "safe window." From: Froese AB. High-frequency oscillatory ventilation for adult respiratory distress syndrome: Let's get it right this time! *Crit Care Med* 1997; 25(6):906–8, with permission.

which continues until the lung is fully inflated. Inflating the lung further results in a reduction in the lung compliance at the end of inflation (**Fig. 21.6**). The junction between the first and second portion of the curve is called the *lower inflection point*. The junction of the second and third portions of the curve is called the *upper inflection point*. In patients with acute lung injury, some investigators have recommended that PEEP should be set at a pressure slightly above the lower inflection point on a static PV curve.

WOB can be measured using esophageal manometry and measurement of tidal volume during spontaneous breathing. *Work* is defined as *force multiplied by displacement*. WOB can be estimated by integrating pressure and volume of a spontaneous breath.

Airway scalars are the most commonly reported waveforms. Scalars are composed of 3 distinct waveforms: flow, pressure, and volume (y-axis) plotted against time (x-axis). Convention dictates that, in these waveforms, positive values correspond to inspiration events and negative values correspond to expiration. Comparison of all 3 waveforms simultaneously facilitates analysis of the patient-ventilator interface. Patient-ventilator dys-synchrony becomes evident when the timing and magnitude of flow, pressure, and volume are disproportionate or delayed. Additionally, each of these parameters (flow, pressure, and volume) can be plotted against each other. PV and flow-volume loops can be particularly helpful in assessing alterations in resistance, compliance, WOB, pulmonary overdistension, and premature termination of exhalation.

A typical airway graphic during time-cycled, volume-limited ventilation is displayed in **Figure 21.7**. An inspiratory pause has been set and is represented by the lengthened T_i and the period of zero flow prior to exhalation. The plateau pressure corresponds to this zero-flow period during inspiration. The flow returns to zero during expiration, indicating the completion of exhalation. A typical airway graphic during pressure-limited ventilation with a variable, decelerating inspiratory flow pattern (i.e., pressure control) is displayed in **Figure 21.8**. PV and flow-volume loops provide insight into the patient's pathophysiology and the response to therapeutic interventions. PV loops depict pressure on the horizontal axis and volume on the vertical axis.

The typical PV and flow-volume loops during volume-limited ventilation are displayed in **Figure 21.9**. As the ventilator delivers gas to the patient, airway pressure increases from the set PEEP level until the set VT is reached and inspiration is terminated.

Note in **Figure 21.9** and **Figure 21.10** that only a small amount of volume is delivered during the initial phase of inspiration. As the inspiratory pressure

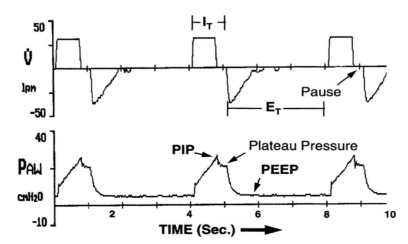

FIGURE 21.7. Normal scalar display of flow versus time and airway pressure versus time for volume-limited ventilation. Paw, airway pressure; PIP, peak inspiratory pressure; PEEP, positive end-expiratory pressure. Figure courtesy of VIASYS Healthcare Inc., Yorba Linda, CA.

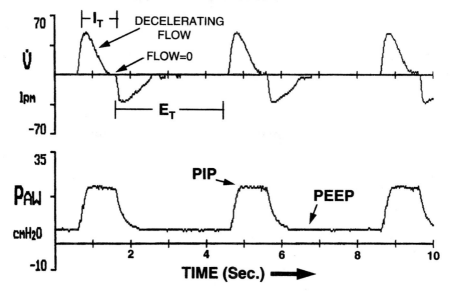

FIGURE 21.8. Normal scalar display of flow versus time and airway pressure versus time for pressure-limited ventilation. Figure courtesy of VIASYS Healthcare, Inc., Yorba Linda, CA.

increases, the critical opening pressure is achieved, and the tidal volume is delivered. Hysteresis, which is a nonlinear change in the PV relationship over time, is present during both inspiration and expiration. Acute respiratory distress syndrome (ARDS) reduces pulmonary compliance (compare **Fig. 21.9** with **Fig. 21.10**). The evaluation of inspiratory and expiratory flow patterns can provide important information as to the presence of increased inspiratory or expiratory resistance (**Fig. 21.11**). In patients with elevated resistance, the response of these abnormalities to various interventions, including suctioning, altering the inspiratory time, and/or bronchodilator therapy, can then be assessed.

Pressure-Volume and Flow-Volume Loops in Pressure-limited Ventilation

The decelerating flow pattern of pressure-control ventilation results in a more rapid rise in airway pressure during the initial phase of inspiration than does a traditional, volume-limited breath. The

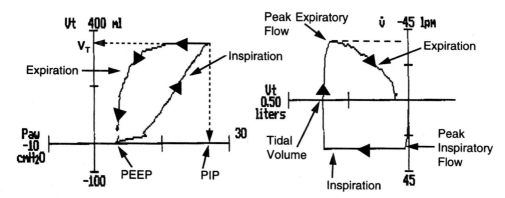

FIGURE 21.9. The pressure-volume graphic displays tidal volume on the vertical axis and airway pressure on the horizontal axis. The flow-volume graphic displays flow on the vertical axis and tidal volume on the horizontal axis. Note that in this flow-volume loop, the delivered inspiratory flow is represented during traditional volume-limited ventilation below the baseline as a square wave. Figure courtesy of VIASYS Healthcare, Inc., Yorba Linda, CA.

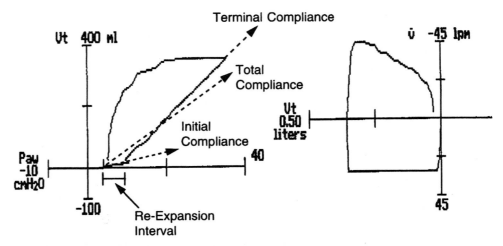

FIGURE 21.10. Pressure/volume and flow/volume loops for volume-limited ventilation during adult respiratory distress syndrome. Figure courtesy of VIASYS Healthcare, Inc., Yorba Linda, CA.

corresponding PV loop is demonstrated in **Figure 21.12**. During the initial phase of inspiration, the airway pressures are higher for a given VT, and the PV loop demonstrates an initial "scooping." Though the initial airway pressures are higher for a given VT, the VT is delivered at a lower PIP, peak inspiratory pressure (PIP), and dynamic compliance improves in this setting. This increase in dynamic compliance is demonstrated by the increased slope of the inspiratory loop (line connecting PEEP with PIP). The

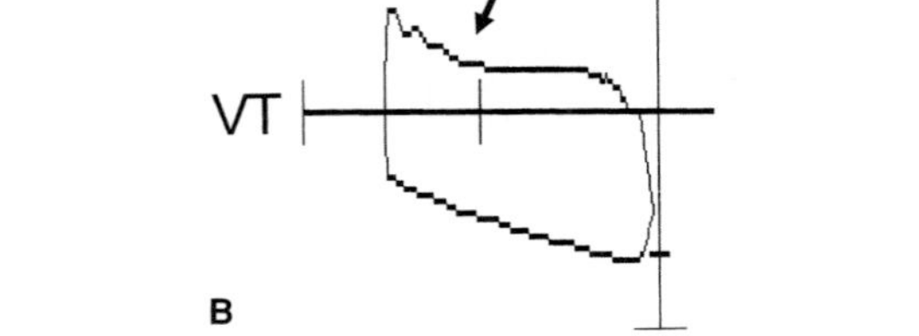

decelerating, variable inspiratory flow of pressure-control ventilation is higher than the fixed, constant flow of volume-limited ventilation. Thus, the peak inspiratory flow generated may better match the inspiratory demands of the patient.

Excessive levels of PEEP cause detrimental effects on cardiorespiratory function. These effects include (a) a reduction of venous return and cardiac output secondary to increased intrathoracic pressure and (b) overdistension of compliant lung units with redistribution of blood flow to the less compliant lung units. To optimize PEEP using graphics, the level of PEEP is increased gradually until the best balance is achieved in the following variables: the lowest PIP to deliver the desired VT, the highest compliance, and the best O_2 delivery (requires a determination/estimate of cardiac output and a measurement of arterial oxygenation).

Dynamic Hyperexpansion/Intrinsic Positive End-expiratory Pressure

The square-wave, constant-flow pattern during inspiration is demonstrated in **Figure 21.13**, as in **Figure 21.14**. The respiratory rate and T_i have been increased, resulting in a dramatic increase in mean airway pressure. With inadequate time to complete exhalation before the next breath is initiated, dynamic hyperexpansion or "gas trapping" occurs. Dynamic hyperexpansion occurs with premature termination of exhalation. Prolongation of the T_i may be beneficial in certain clinical conditions (i.e., ARDS) by decreasing PIP and increasing mean airway pressure, which would be expected to improve oxygenation.

FIGURE 21.11. Increased expiratory resistance. In the top panel, airway flow (V) is displayed over time. As noted by the arrows, exhalation is significantly prolonged, representing an increased expiratory resistance. In the bottom panel, airway flow is graphed on the vertical axis and tidal volume (VT) on the horizontal axis. The arrow again indicates that increased expiratory flow as the expiratory flow rate is greatly reduced early in exhalation.

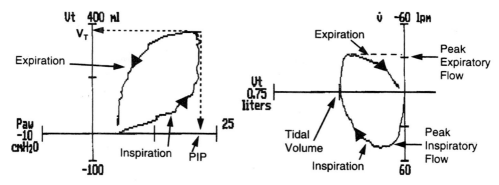

FIGURE 21.12. Normal pressure/volume and flow/volume loops for pressure-limited ventilation. VT, tidal volume. Figure courtesy of VIASYS Healthcare, Inc., Yorba Linda, CA.

Dynamic hyperexpansion may result in $PEEP_i$, which elevates the baseline airway pressure (externally applied PEEP + $PEEP_i$). However, $PEEP_i$ is relatively uncontrolled as compared to set PEEP, which can be more reliably titrated to achieve the desired oxygenation and ventilation end points. The increase in the baseline airway pressure secondary to $PEEP_i$ results in an increase in PIP that is required to maintain the set VT during volume-limited ventilation, or it results in a decrease in VT during pressure-limited ventilation (i.e., set total PIP).

Patient-Ventilator Dys-synchrony: Inaccurate Sensing of Patient Effort

Patient effort decreases airway pressure (arrows 1–3 in **Fig. 21.14**) and/or flow from baseline. Decreased airway pressure or flow (depending on the ventilator settings chosen) should result in an assisted mechanical breath in supported ventilation modes. However, with inadequate trigger sensitivity (**Fig. 21.14**), the ventilator is unable to determine that a patient effort has occurred (patient breaths 1–3). During patient

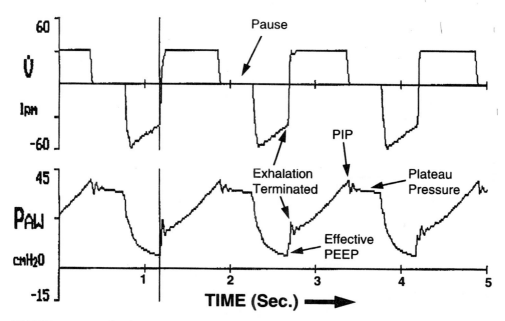

FIGURE 21.13. Scalar display of flow versus time and airway pressure versus time for volume-limited ventilation during adult respiratory distress syndrome. Premature termination of exhalation, which results in dynamic hyperexpansion (gas tapping), is shown. Figure courtesy of VIASYS Healthcare, Inc., Yorba Linda, CA.

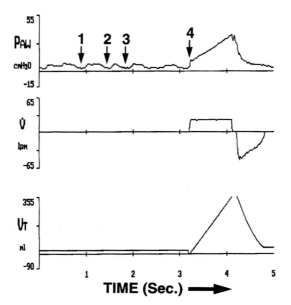

FIGURE 21.14. Scalar display of flow versus time, airway pressure versus time, and tidal volume versus time, representing patient-ventilator dyssynchrony to inadequate sensing of the patient effort. Figure courtesy of VIASYS Healthcare, Inc., Yorba Linda, CA.

breath 4, the ventilator delivers the preset VT at the preset rate without regard to patient effort. Inadequate sensing of patient effort leads to tachypnea, increased WOB, patient-ventilator dys-synchrony, and patient discomfort ("fighting the ventilator"). To improve patient-ventilator synchrony in conditions when the patient effort is not appropriately sensed, trigger sensitivity must be improved. Flow triggering is generally more sensitive than pressure triggering, as a small change in flow requires less inspiratory effort than a change in pressure. Dys-synchrony

may also occur when an air leak leads to the loss of PEEP, resulting in excessive ventilator triggering. This reduction in airway pressure or flow may be misinterpreted by the ventilator as a patient effort and results in a mechanical breath being triggered. This abnormality, commonly referred to as *autocycling*, may lead to frequent ventilator triggering without patient effort.

Patient-Ventilator Dys-synchrony: Inadequate Ventilatory Support

Figure 21.15 reveals a patient effort that results in a decrease in airway pressure (arrows 1 and 2) and triggering of a mechanical breath. However, the constant inspiratory flow of the delivered mechanical breath is inadequate to meet the patient's inspiratory demands. The patient is not satiated by the constant inspiratory flow of the mechanical breath and, as a result, attempts to initiate a spontaneous breath during the mechanical breath (arrow 3), causing a transient reduction of airway pressure, which is signified by a decrease in the airway pressure tracing during inspiration (flow dys-synchrony). Inadequate ventilatory support to meet the patient's inspiratory needs leads to tachypnea, increased WOB, and patient discomfort ("fighting the ventilator"). In volume-limited ventilation, a reduction of the inspiratory airway pressure as a result of a patient effort (arrow 3) during the mechanical breath may result in an increase in peak inspiratory pressure (arrow 4) being required to achieve the set VT. A variable flow mode may better meet the inspiratory demands of the patient. Such modes include pressure-support ventilation, pressure-assist/control ventilation, and pressure-regulated volume control. When increasing the flow rate or changing the inspiratory flow pattern is unsuccessful, inadequate

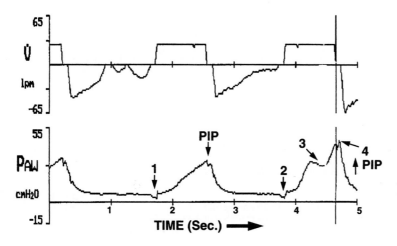

FIGURE 21.15. Scalar display of flow versus time and airway pressure versus time, representing patient-ventilatory dyssynchrony secondary to inadequate ventilatory support. Figure courtesy of VIASYS Healthcare, Inc., Yorba Linda, CA.

ventilatory support should be considered as the cause of the patient-ventilator dys-synchrony.

ESOPHAGEAL AND GASTRIC MANOMETRY

Esophageal manometry and gastric manometry are invasive methods by which to assess pressures generated during breathing. Esophageal manometry requires placement of an air-filled balloon attached to a catheter or a fluid-filled catheter in the lower third of the esophagus.

Transdiaphragmatic pressure (P_{di}) is defined as the difference between intrathoracic and abdominal pressures. It is usually calculated as the difference between P_{es} and gastric pressure (P_{ga}).

Diaphragmatic ultrasonography and fluoroscopy can be useful tools in detecting and diagnosing diaphragmatic paresis and paralysis. Diaphragmatic paresis and paralysis can occur from injury to the phrenic nerve or diaphragmatic muscle weakness. Diaphragmatic paresis is diagnosed by the reduction in excursion of the diaphragm during spontaneous breathing. Unilateral diaphragmatic paralysis can result in paradoxic movement of the diaphragm, when during inspiration, the normal diaphragm moves downward and the paralyzed diaphragm moves upward. It is important that testing be performed without positive pressure applied to the airway.

The pressure generated after the onset of inspiratory effort against an occluded airway in the first 100 msec ($P_{0.1}$) provides a measure of respiratory drive. In adults, $P_{0.1}$ can be used to predict weaning outcome. For extubated children, $P_{0.1}$ can be measured by placing a tight-fitting mask over the face and attaching a one-way valve that allows exhalation but not inspiration. Factors that influence the measurement of $P_{0.1}$ include chest-wall distortion (a problem in young children with compliant chest walls), alteration in expiratory lung volume, time constant of the respiratory system, expiratory muscle activity (such as in lower airway obstruction), shape of the driving pressure wave, and pressure-flow phase lags. An easier index to measure is the mean inspiratory flow (derived by dividing the VT by the T_i), which can be determined in intubated patients by measuring spontaneous VT and T_i using a pneumotachometer attached to the ETT without applying positive pressure to the airway. It can also be measured using respiratory inductive plethysmography, as previously described.

CHAPTER 22 ■ STATUS ASTHMATICUS

MICHAEL T. BIGHAM • RICHARD J. BRILLI

Status asthmaticus is defined as severe asthma that fails to respond to inhaled beta-agonists, oral or intravenous steroids and oxygen; and requires admission to the hospital for treatment. The majority of asthma related deaths in children occur as a result of respiratory failure or cardiopulmonary arrest that occurs prior to obtaining medical care. Asthma is an inflammatory disease characterized by air flow obstruction due to airway hyper-responsiveness and bronchospasm and airway inflammation with mucosal edema and mucous plugging of the small airways. The autonomic nervous system also contributes to bronchoconstriction through parasympathetic activation of M3 receptors by acetylcholine and excitatory non-adrenergic, non-cholinergic pathways mediated by tachykinins. Asthma is associated with air trapping with each breath and lung hyperinflation (**Fig. 22.1**). With higher end expiratory lung volumes, coupled with bronchospasm leading to increased airway resistance and reduced expiratory flow, expiration becomes an active, rather than passive process. Diaphragmatic flattening from hyperinflation causes additional mechanical disadvantages. Both forced expiratory volume and forced vital capacity are decreased in status asthmaticus as a result of high airway resistance. Total lung volumes are increased because of increased FRC.

Gas exchange abnormalities in status asthmaticus are due to ventilation/perfusion (V/Q) mismatch, including increased intrapulmonary shunt (atelectasis) and increased dead space (airway over-distension) resulting from small airway obstruction due to mucous plugging, edema, and bronchoconstriction. Typically this initially manifests as hypoxemia and hypocarbia. Atelectasis from small airway obstruction causes areas of decreased ventilation, but adequate pulmonary

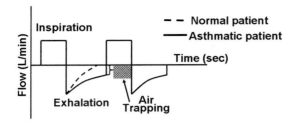

FIGURE 22.1. Flow-time waveform showing persistence of air flow at end expiration and air-trapping as a result.

blood flow and the resultant shunt leads to arterial hypoxemia. Dynamic hyperinflation in severe asthma can stretch the pulmonary vasculature, increasing pulmonary vascular resistance and increasing right ventricular after-load compromising right ventricular function. During the large negative intrathoracic pressure observed during inspiration, left ventricular after-load is increased, and systolic blood pressure decreases during inspiration. Exaggerated variation in systolic blood pressure associated with intrathoracic pressure variation during inspiration is termed *pulsus paradoxus* (**Fig. 22.2**). Systolic blood pressure decreases of >10–15 torr is associated with declining respiratory function in children with status asthmaticus.

PRINCIPLES OF CLINICAL MANAGEMENT

Four disparate clinical entities must be distinguished when the wheezing patient is first evaluated. These include asthma, pneumonia, foreign body aspiration, and congestive heart failure. Other diagnostic considerations in the differential diagnosis of wheezing can be divided into upper and lower airway diseases. Upper airway obstruction, while usually presenting with stridor, can also present with wheezing. Diagnostic considerations include fixed anatomic lesions such as vocal cord paralysis, anatomic webs,

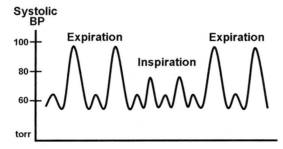

FIGURE 22.2. Pulsus paradoxus in status asthmaticus

and airway hemangiomas or dynamic airway obstruction such as laryngeal, tracheal, or bronchomalacia. Congenital anomalies such as complete tracheal rings and bronchial slings may also present with wheezing. Lower airway diseases that should be considered, besides infection and congestive heart failure, include cystic fibrosis and alpha₁ anti-trypsin deficiency. Children with status asthmaticus typically present with respiratory distress, cough, and wheezing that has progressed over 1–2 days. Allergen exposure or upper respiratory tract infection are often triggers for the onset of illness and frequently are identified by the child or family as inciting events. In contrast, foreign body aspiration will usually present with an abrupt onset of clinical symptoms. The presence of fever suggests lower respiratory infection, though asthma and pneumonia can both be present at the same time. When time permits, it is important to determine the presence of high risk factors for asthma severity and fatality, including previous severe sudden deterioration, past ICU admissions, and previous respiratory failure with the need for mechanical ventilation.

The use of the "rapid 30-second cardiopulmonary assessment" as described by the American Heart Association will allow quick determination of general appearance, airway patency, effectiveness of respiratory effort, and adequacy of circulation. Children with severe status asthmaticus often appear lethargic or diaphoretic, are unable to phonate, and have severe retractions with paradoxical thoracoabdominal breathing. Poor air movement found on chest auscultation is an ominous sign of impending respiratory or cardiopulmonary failure. Asymmetric wheezing may imply unilateral atelectasis, pneumothorax, or foreign body. Expiratory wheezing alone is found in mild-to-moderate illness, whereas both expiratory and inspiratory wheezing are present in moderate-to-severe status asthmaticus. The "silent chest" is an ominous sign and may indicate either pneumothorax or the complete absence of air flow due to severe airway obstruction and imminent respiratory failure. Hypoxemia as estimated by measured pulse oximetry is another sign of asthma severity. There are several clinical asthma scores that have been used to objectively assess the severity of status asthmaticus. The Becker asthma score (**Table 22.1**), modified by DiGiulio, determines severity by rating the acuity of four clinical characteristics: respiratory rate, wheezing, I/E ratio, and accessory muscle use and has the advantage of not requiring a PaO_2 measurement that is used in the Wood/Downes score. A Becker score >4 is considered moderate status asthmaticus. Children with scores ≥7 should be admitted to the ICU. Serial measurements allow an objective determination of disease progression, though there is often significant interobserver variability in assigning clinical scores.

TABLE 22.1

BECKER PULMONARY INDEX SCORE FOR ASTHMA

Score	Respiratory rate	Wheezing	I/E Ratio	Accessory muscle use
0	<30	None	1:1.5	None
1	30–40	Terminal expiration	1:2.0	One site
2	41–50	Entire expiration	1:3.0	Two sites
3	>50	Inspiration and entire expiration	>1:3.0	Three sites or neck strap muscle use

Laboratory tests commonly obtained in children with status asthmaticus include arterial or venous blood gas determination, complete blood count, and a basic metabolic panel. For spontaneously breathing children with status asthmaticus, clinical interventions should be primarily based upon the physical examination and not upon blood gas determinations. Typically early in the course of severe asthma, arterial hypoxemia and hypocarbia are found as a result of V/Q mismatch and hyperventilation. As the air trapping worsens and Vd/Vt increase, hypocarbia may be replaced by normal or elevated $PaCO_2$. Normal $PaCO_2$ in a tachypneic, hyperventilating child with status asthmaticus warrants close clinical observation and may be a sign of early respiratory muscle fatigue. Lactic acidosis is often present in status asthmaticus and, rarely, can suggest poor perfusion from impaired cardiac function associated with increased ventricular afterload caused by negative intrathoracic pressures (up to −60 to 100 cmH_2O). The presence of leukocytosis on complete blood count may suggest respiratory infection as the source of wheezing, though it can also represent a stress response to steroid administration or response to beta-agonist therapy. The WBC count in conjunction with chest radiography and the presence or absence of fever will help determine the need for antibiotic therapy. A basic metabolic panel may be useful to assess the degree of dehydration and the level of electrolyte disturbance. Hypokalemia may result from intracellular potassium shifts from exposure to beta-agonist therapy in children with status asthmaticus. Determining serum magnesium values may be important because the correction of relative hypomagnesemia in status asthmaticus may improve outcome.

A chest radiograph is not required at the time of hospital admission for all spontaneously breathing children with status asthmaticus; however, all children with first time wheezing or patients requiring ICU admission should receive a chest radiograph. Clinically relevant findings such as evidence of an infectious infiltrate, pneumothorax, cardiomegaly, pulmonary edema, or even unsuspected chest masses may be identified.

Children seen in emergency departments with mild-to-moderate status asthmaticus require inpatient care and are usually treated with oxygen, inhaled bronchodilators, and systemic corticosteroids. Clinical parameters that suggest the need for ICU admission include past ICU admissions, a history of rapid clinical deterioration, severe distress (inspiratory and expiratory wheezing, limited air entry, air hunger, and inability to phonate) despite initial bronchodilator therapy, or those with a Becker asthma score ≥7. Other indications for ICU admission include the child's sense of impending clinical doom, altered mental status, respiratory arrest, and a rising $PaCO_2$ coupled with clinical signs of fatigue.

Children admitted to the ICU require intravenous access, continuous cardiorespiratory monitoring, and continuous pulse oximetry. For spontaneously breathing children in the ICU, frequent blood gas monitoring is not required. Such children can usually be managed with close clinical observation without indwelling arterial or central venous catheters. For children requiring mechanical ventilation, a Foley catheter and arterial and central venous access will be required.

Critically ill children with status asthmaticus are often dehydrated as a result of decreased oral intake prior to admission and increased insensible fluid losses from increased minute ventilation. Providing appropriate fluid resuscitation and ongoing maintenance fluid is essential; however, overhydration should be avoided because these children are at risk for pulmonary edema due to microvascular permeability, increased left ventricular after-load, and alveolar fluid migration associated with the inflammatory lung process in asthma.

Most children with severe status asthmaticus will have some degree of mucous plugging, atelectasis, ventilation perfusion mismatch, and hypoxemia. In those lung segments with atelectasis, compensatory hypoxic pulmonary vasoconstriction is often present. Treatment with inhaled beta-agonists may induce generalized pulmonary vasodilatation and as a result exacerbate ventilation perfusion mismatch and worsen hypoxemia. Oxygen should be a part of the management for *all* children with status asthmaticus.

The overriding physiologic derangement in asthma is airway inflammation, and corticosteroids are a mainstay in the management of both acute and chronic asthma. Systemically administered corticosteroids reduce asthma hospitalization rates and hospital length of stay. Inhaled corticosteroids are of no clinical benefit in the treatment of status asthmaticus. Methylprednisolone is the most common agent used in the ICU and is preferred because of its limited mineralocorticoid effects. The initial dose is 2 mg/kg followed by 0.5–1 mg/kg/dose administered intravenously every 6 hrs. Other agents that are sometimes used include dexamethasone and hydrocortisone. Systemic corticosteroids begin to exert their effect in 1–3 hours and reach maximal effect in 4–8 hrs. Treatment duration depends upon the severity of illness but generally continues until the asthma exacerbation is resolved. Side effects often observed in the critically ill child include hyperglycemia, hypertension, and occasionally agitation related to steroid-induced psychosis. Prolonged steroid use may cause hypothalamic-pituitary-adrenal axis suppression, osteoporosis, myopathy, and weakness. The incidence of myopathy and weakness is increased when neuromuscular blocking agents are concomitantly administered in the mechanically ventilated asthmatic patient.

Beta-agonists as sympathomimetic agents cause direct bronchial smooth muscle relaxation and are key components of acute and chronic asthma therapy. In the treatment of status asthmaticus, inhaled beta-agonists are a bridge to support ventilation and oxygenation until the anti-inflammatory effects of corticosteroids take effect. Albuterol for inhalation is available in two forms: albuterol (salbutamol) and levalbuterol. Albuterol is a racemic mixture of two equal parts of mirror-image forms: R- and S-enantiomers. The R-enantiomer is the pharmacologically active enantiomer. The S-enantiomer is considered pharmacologically inactive, has a longer elimination half-life, and may contribute to airway irritation as a spasmogen. Levalbuterol consists solely of the R-enantiomer of albuterol, and some have suggested that levalbuterol has improved efficacy with fewer adverse effects when compared to racemic albuterol. The two primary delivery mechanisms are via small volume nebulizer and metered dose inhaler (MDI), usually with a vehicle delivery device (i.e., spacer). Breath-actuated inhaled beta-agonist delivery devices are another relatively new delivery method. Intermittent MDI dosing is infrequently used in the critically ill child with status asthmaticus. With continuous inhalation, patients have more rapid clinical improvement than with intermittent administration.

The usual dose of continuous albuterol nebulization is 0.15–0.5 mg/kg/hr or 10–20 mg/hr. During weaning from continuous albuterol inhalation, some practitioners transition children to intermittent albuterol MDI treatments—usually 4–8 puffs per dose with each puff delivering 90 mcg.

Untoward side effects of continuous albuterol nebulization include sinus tachycardia, palpitations, hypertension, diastolic hypotension, ventricular cardiac dysrhythmias, hyperactivity, tremors, and nausea with vomiting, hypokalemia, and hyperglycemia. Periodic serum potassium levels should be monitored during inhaled beta-agonist treatment.

Intravenous and subcutaneous administration of beta-agonists is most beneficial in children with severe status asthmaticus and limited respiratory air flow where distribution of inhaled medications may be significantly reduced. Nonselective beta-agonists such as ephedrine, epinephrine, and isoproterenol are rarely used because of their high side effect profile and the availability of more selective intravenous or subcutaneous agents.

Terbutaline has largely supplanted the use of epinephrine for subcutaneous administration. Subcutaneous administration of beta-agonists is primarily used for children with no intravenous access and as a rapidly available adjunct to inhaled beta-agonists. Subcutaneous dosing for terbutaline is 0.01 mg/kg/dose with a maximum dose of 0.3 mg. The dose may be repeated every 15–20 mins for up to 3 doses. Intravenous terbutaline therapy starts with a loading dose of 10 mcg/kg over 10 mins followed by continuous infusion at 0.1–10 mcg/kg/min. Side effects of subcutaneous or intravenously administered terbutaline are similar to those of inhaled beta-agonists. Some have suggested that the risk of myocardial ischemia is increased with the administration of relatively selective intravenous beta-agonists. It is often valuable to prospectively monitor cardiac-specific enzymes (CPK or troponin) in children who are receiving intravenously administered beta-agonists, including terbutaline.

For children hospitalized on the general care ward with status asthmaticus, theophylline adds little to oxygen, intermittent inhaled beta-agonist bronchodilators, and corticosteroids. For the critically ill asthmatic child, theophylline added to a regimen, including inhaled and/or intravenous beta agonists, inhaled ipratropium bromide, and corticosteroids, significantly improved clinical asthma score over time but did not reduce ICU length of stay. Theophylline therapy may be helpful in those critically ill children who are not responsive to steroids, inhaled and intravenous beta-agonists, and oxygen. Theophylline is administered by continuous intravenous infusion following a loading dose of 5–7 mg/kg infused over

20 mins. In general, a loading dose of 1 mg/kg will raise the serum theophylline level by 2 mcg/mL. For maximum therapeutic benefit, the goal serum theophylline level is 10–20 mcg/mL. Serum theophylline levels should be measured 1–2 hrs after the loading dose is completed. The continuous infusion should begin immediately after the bolus at a rate of 0.5–0.9 mg/kg/hr. The infusion should be adjusted to maintain levels as noted previously. Theophylline clearance is reduced in infants and adolescents. In these age groups, the usual dose for continuous infusion is closer to 0.5 mg/kg/hr. Serum levels >20 mcg/mL are associated with adverse effects that include nausea, jitters or restlessness, tachycardia (racing heart), and overall irritability. Serum levels >35 mcg/mL have been associated with seizures and cardiac dysrhythmias.

Ipratropium bromide is the most frequently used agent to provide anticholinergic effects in the treatment of status asthmaticus. Ipratropium promotes bronchodilation without inhibiting mucociliary clearance as occurs with atropine. Ipratropium bromide can be delivered either by aerosol or MDI. Initial dose range is 125–500 mcg (if nebulized) or 4–8 puffs (if via MDI) administered every 20 mins for up to 3 doses. Subsequent recommended dosing interval is every 4–6 hrs. Adverse effects of ipratropium are few because it has poor systemic absorption. The most common untoward effects are dry mouth, bitter taste, flushing, tachycardia, and dizziness.

The value of magnesium administration in the treatment of status asthmaticus remains controversial. The usual dose of magnesium is 25–50 mg/kg/dose over 30 mins administered every 4 hrs. Magnesium can be given by continuous infusion at a rate of 10–20 mg/kg/hr. With either dosing regimen, some have suggested a target magnesium level of 4 mg/dL to achieve maximal effect. Side effects of magnesium administration include hypotension, central nervous system depression, muscle weakness, and flushing, though in the studies previously mentioned there were no reported significant untoward effects. Severe complications such as cardiac arrhythmia, including complete heart block, respiratory failure due to severe muscle weakness, and sudden cardiopulmonary arrest, may occur in the setting of very high serum magnesium levels (usually >10–12 mg/dL). Serum magnesium levels should be regularly monitored.

Helium is a biologically inert, low density gas that, when administered by inhalation in a mixture with oxygen, reduces air flow resistance in small airways by reducing turbulent flow and enhancing laminar gas flow. These characteristics may also enhance particle deposition of aerosolized medications in distal lung segments. In aggregate, these characteristics make administration of a mixture of helium and oxygen (80% helium/20% oxygen: heliox) an attractive therapeutic option in the management of status asthmaticus, wherein turbulent air flow and high airway resistance are common. The use of heliox is sometimes limited by the degree of hypoxemia in the patient. If substantial supplemental oxygen is added to the two available mixtures of helium/oxygen (80/20 and 70/30), the salutary effect of low density gas administration on reducing turbulent gas flow is lost.

Mortality rates in mechanically ventilated children with status asthmaticus increase as compared to those children who do not require mechanical ventilation. Noninvasive positive pressure ventilatory support is an alternative to conventional mechanical ventilation in these patients.

In status asthmaticus, tracheal intubation is indicated for children following cardiorespiratory arrest, those with refractory hypoxemia, or significant respiratory acidosis unresponsive to pharmacotherapy. Children requiring mechanical ventilation are at increased risk for pulmonary barotrauma, nosocomial infection, pulmonary edema, circulatory dysfunction, steroid and muscle relaxant–associated myopathy, and death (**Fig. 22.3**).

Tracheal intubation of the asthmatic child with respiratory failure is oftentimes associated with hypotension because many patients have relative hypovolemia, which may be exacerbated by reduced preload as positive-pressure ventilation is initiated and by reduced vascular tone induced by anesthetic agents used for tracheal intubation. Histamine-producing agents such as morphine or atracurium must be

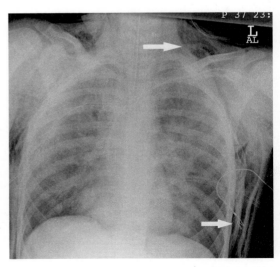

FIGURE 22.3. Significant barotrauma with bilateral pneumothoraces requiring chest tubes and large amount of subcutaneous air (*arrows*).

avoided. Ketamine is an excellent anesthetic agent for induction because of its relatively long half-life, its bronchodilating properties, and its relative preservation of hemodynamic stability. A cuffed endotracheal tube with the largest diameter appropriate for age should be used, as high ventilatory pressures are typical when treating mechanically ventilated children in status asthmaticus.

Ventilatory support in status asthmaticus should maintain adequate oxygenation, allow for permissive hypercarbia (moderate respiratory acidosis), and adjust minute ventilation (peak pressure, tidal volume, and rate) to maintain an arterial pH >7.2. Ventilator management strategies should attempt to minimize dynamic hyperinflation and air trapping (**Fig. 22.1**). This can usually be accomplished by employing slow ventilator rates with prolonged expiratory phase, minimal end-expiratory pressure, and short inspiratory time. Volume-control ventilation with constant or accelerating flow waveforms will provide stable tidal volumes from breath to breath but in the setting of dynamic airway resistance may result in high peak airway pressures, uneven distribution of tidal breaths, and increased risk for pulmonary barotrauma. Pressure-control ventilation with decelerating flow pattern results in lower peak pressure, higher mean airway pressure, and better distribution of gas into high-resistance long time constant airways. In pressure-control mode with pre-set peak inspiratory pressure, rapidly changing airway resistance can result in significant variation in delivered tidal volume and result in increased risk of pulmonary barotrauma if airway resistance changes abruptly. Pressure-regulated volume control is a relatively new mode of mechanical ventilation. There is limited experience with this mode of ventilation in patients with asthma; however, the decelerating flow pattern combined with the option to independently adjust pressure with a pre-set tidal volume is appealing to enhance gas distribution and minimize risk of barotrauma.

The use of positive end-expiratory pressure (PEEP) is controversial. Most authors suggest minimal PEEP because most patients with status asthmaticus already have increased FRC. High PEEP is likely to further increase FRC and exacerbate hyperinflation. Others argue that these patients have dynamic collapse of small airways during forced exhalation and PEEP may stent small airways open at the end of expiration and facilitate full expiration. Review of graphically displayed flow-time curves will demonstrate whether expiratory flow is completed prior to the next breath (**Fig. 22.1**). Adjustments can then be made to the ventilator rate, inspiratory time, expiratory time, or PEEP to facilitate full expiration between breaths.

The use of high-frequency ventilation has been described in a few case reports, though this mode of ventilation requires careful attention to the amplitude settings of the oscillator to avoid further hyperinflation. Some authors have suggested using pressure support ventilation without any pre-set rate and allow the patient to breathe spontaneously. This strategy avoids complications associated with continuous or frequent use of muscle relaxants. It has the further advantage of allowing the child to maintain forced exhalation while receiving support for inspiration. Tracheal gas insufflation has also been used to facilitate expiratory gas flow and reduce severe hypercarbia. Careful attention to secretion accumulation around the insufflation tube is necessary to avoid the development of tracheal tube mucous plugging.

Tracheal extubation should occur as soon as possible. Rapid weaning from the ventilator should take place—"Declare them well and pull the tube." The presence of the breathing tube, especially in awake children, may irritate the airway and stimulate further bronchospasm. Decreasing peak inspiratory pressure, adequate air movement by auscultation, and graphic evidence of full expiration of inspired tidal volume are sufficient criteria for tracheal extubation, even if expiratory wheezing is still present on clinical exam.

Chest physiotherapy (CPT) may augment airway clearance and encourage resolution of mucous plugging. This therapy should only be considered in children with clear segmental or lobar atelectasis. In all other populations of children with status asthmaticus, CPT has no therapeutic benefit. Some suggest that CPT is irritating to the severe asthmatic and may actually worsen clinical symptoms. CPT is not recommended as part of routine management in the critically ill patient with status asthmaticus.

Most asthma exacerbations are associated with or triggered by viral infections and not bacterial infections. For this reason, empiric antibiotic treatment for children with status asthmaticus is not indicated. Lower respiratory tract bacterial infections do occur in children with status asthmaticus. The most commonly identified organisms are *Mycoplasma pneumoniae* and *Chlamydia*. When findings on chest radiograph, leukocytosis, and fever suggest pneumonia, appropriate antibiotics should be administered, especially targeted at the organisms previously noted. Sinusitis is a common nonpulmonary infection found in children with status asthmaticus. When there is no evidence of bacterial pneumonia and high fever and peripheral blood leukocytosis are present, the diagnosis of sinusitis should be considered and, if found, antibacterial therapy should be instituted.

Sedation of the unintubated asthmatic is generally not indicated. Some children who are excessively anxious and who are not hypoxemic or hypercarbic as a cause for their anxiety may benefit from sedation. This should occur only in the closely monitored setting of the ICU. Ketamine is an excellent choice because it provides excellent sedation and bronchodilation with minimal risk of respiratory depression. Mechanically ventilated children require sedation and often muscle relaxants to prevent ventilator patient asynchrony and to reduce the risk of sudden cough–induced pulmonary barotrauma. Ketamine by continuous infusion is the first choice for sedation, usually combined with intermittent or continuous administration of benzodiazepines. Usual ketamine dosing is 1 mg/kg/hr and adjusted to achieve sufficient sedation. Increased respiratory secretions occur with ketamine administration; however, these side effects are usually manageable. When opiates are used, fentanyl is preferred because morphine causes histamine release, which may exacerbate bronchospasm. Neuromuscu-

lar blocking agents are frequently required to facilitate mechanical ventilatory support. Vecuronium is a commonly used agent. The starting dose is 0.1 mg/kg/hr, which should be titrated to train-of-four monitoring—usually 1–2 twitches. Drug holidays can be used to reduce the risk of overdose, prolonged paresis, and myopathy that is sometimes observed in children who receive continuous infusions of the non-depolarizing neuromuscular blocking agents. Inhaled general anesthetics have bronchodilating properties that have proven beneficial in the management of the intubated asthmatic. Hypotension and cardiac dysrhythmias are associated with the use of these agents and are more likely to occur in hypoxemic children.

When maximal medical therapy is failing, extracorporeal membrane oxygenation support should be considered. There are a number of case reports, all demonstrating high survival rates, even in a patient population that is gravely ill.

CHAPTER 23 ■ NEONATAL RESPIRATORY FAILURE

ELISABETH L. RAAB • LISA K. KELLY • PHILIPPE S. FRIEDLICH • RANGASAMY RAMANATHAN • ISTVAN SERI

Respiratory distress syndrome (RDS) due to surfactant deficiency is a significant life-threatening condition that is seen primarily in preterm infants. Under the influence of SP-A, which is co-secreted along with the lamellar bodies from type II pneumocytes, tubular myelin unravels to form mono- and multilayers of phospholipids rich in SP-B and SP-C. Surfactant therapy has decreased the mortality and incidence of pneumothorax in infants with RDS. Bronchopulmonary dysplasia (BPD) is defined clinically as the need for supplemental oxygen or mechanical ventilatory support at 36 weeks postmenstrual age.

Continuous positive airway pressure (CPAP) initiated in the delivery room stabilizes the alveoli, decreases the upper-airway resistance, and promotes the release of preformed surfactant from type II pneumocytes. The care provided in the delivery room and over the course of the first 12–24 postnatal hours is believed to have a large impact on the outcome of the extremely-low-birth-weight neonate. *Early rescue*

surfactant therapy given within 30–120 mins of age has been shown to be better than *delayed rescue therapy* by decreasing the need for additional doses of surfactant and allowing faster weaning of supplemental oxygen. Natural, modified surfactant preparations are summarized in **Table 23.1**. Among natural surfactants, poractant alfa may be associated with better clinical outcomes in preterm infants with RDS. It is recommended that saturations be kept in the high 90s once an infant's corrected gestational age reaches the late preterm range. Permissive hypercapnia involves allowing CO_2 levels in the blood to rise >40 mmHg to minimize the pressures (and volumes) required for ventilation and thereby potentially reduce the lung injury. Though procedures differ, CO_2 levels of 45–55 mmHg are generally accepted, with some centers allowing higher CO_2 levels without changing ventilatory management. Many neonatologists are now attempting to avoid intubation and mechanical ventilation altogether using CPAP delivered via nasal prongs.

TABLE 23.1

COMPOSITION AND DOSING OF NATURAL SURFACTANT PREPARATIONS COMMONLY USED IN PRETERM INFANTS WITH RESPIRATORY DISTRESS SYNDROME

Surfactant	Preparation, composition	Phospholipids (%)	Plasmalogen (mol %)	SP-B(mg/mMol PL)	SP-C	DPPC (mg/mL)	Dose (mL/kg)
Survanta	Minced bovine lung extract/ DPPC + palmitic acid + tripalmitin added	84	1.5	0–1.3	1–20	25	4
Infasurf	Bovine lung lavage/DPPC, cholesterol	95	NA	5.4	8.1	35	3
Curosurf	Minced porcine lung extract/ DPPC, polar lipids	99	3.8	2–3.7	5–11.6	80	1.25[a]

PL, phospholipid; SP-B, surfactant protein B; SP-C, surfactant protein C; DPPC, dipalmitoyl phosphatidylcholine
[a] Initial dose, 2.5 mL/kg.

BRONCHOPULMONARY DYSPLASIA

The pathologic description of BPD is divided into 4 distinct stages. Stage 1 describes the early findings of hyaline membrane disease, today referred to as RDS. Stage 2 occurs between days 4 and 10 of progression of the disease and is characterized by atelectasis, alternating with areas of emphysema, and increasing opacifications with air bronchograms on chest x-ray. In stage 3, typically present on days 11–30, permanent features of the disease appear, including bronchial and bronchiolar hyperplasia and cystic changes that were visible radiographically. The final stage (stage 4), presenting after the first postnatal month, is characterized by the pathologic findings of extensive fibrosis and destruction of the airways and alveoli. At this last stage, radiographic findings consist of fibrosis and areas of both consolidation and overinflation. In comparison to this "classic" form of BPD, the "new BPD" shows more uniform lung inflation and only minimal fibrosis. The risk factors for BPD include prematurity, intrauterine growth retardation, a family history of lung disease, inflammation triggered by mechanical ventilation–associated barotrauma and volutrauma, free oxygen radicals, increased pulmonary blood flow, and systemic or pulmonary infections.

The American Academy of Pediatrics currently recommends that neonatologists counsel parents about the risks and benefits of dexamethasone prior to initiating treatment. No evidence suggests that dexamethasone (or hydrocortisone) administration to prevent or treat BPD in very-low-birth-weight VLBW neonates improves pulmonary outcomes, and corticosteroid administration in general has significant side effects, including the occurrence of spontaneous intestinal perforation and poor neurodevelopmental outcome. Routine use of steroids must be discouraged, and their use should be restricted to brief administration of lower doses in patients with life-threatening respiratory failure despite optimum ventilatory and critical care support. The management and treatment of infants at risk of developing BPD should be directed toward (a) minimizing ventilatory support and alveolar overdistension, (b) supporting and maintaining functional residual capacity with optimal positive end-expiratory pressure, (c) optimizing growth, and (d) judiciously using diuretics and bronchodilators. These goals can be achieved in part by employing optimal alveolar recruitment strategies to prevent atelectasis and sustain functional residual capacity, allowing as much as possible for synchrony between the infant and ventilation, and by embracing moderate permissive hypercapnia. In addition to carefully applying ventilation strategies, it is important to determine an appropriate target for the oxygen saturation in preterm infants. It should be emphasized that in utero, the fetus is exposed to a PO_2 in the range of 25–30 mmHg and an oxygen saturation of between 60% and 80%. The optimization of growth and nutrition is essential to achieve early successful extubation. Vitamin A has been shown to decrease the incidence of BPD in clinical trials.

Transient Tachypnea of the Newborn

TTN is due to a delay in the cessation of production and ensuing clearance of fetal lung fluid. Infants born by elective cesarean section (i.e., cesarean section without labor) are at higher risk for developing TTN. Clinically, TTN presents with increased work of breathing, respiratory distress, hypoxemia, and CO^2 retention. The differential diagnosis includes sepsis, pneumonia, RDS, pulmonary hypertension, congenital lung malformation, and congenital heart disease. Early treatment is focused on supportive care with careful oxygen administration and positive pressure as needed, radiographs to rule out lung malformations, antibiotics while the infant is evaluated for sepsis, and an echocardiogram if indicated. TTN is by definition a transient disease, and though the infants may appear clinically sick with moderate respiratory failure initially, they typically improve significantly within 8–24 hrs. The initial chest x-ray findings of pulmonary edema, air bronchograms, and hyperexpansion also resolve within the same time frame, making x-rays an effective way to differentiate TTN from neonatal pneumonia, as the x-ray findings in pneumonia will persist beyond the first 24–48 hrs.

Persistent Pulmonary Hypertension of the Newborn

Persistent pulmonary hypertension of the newborn (PPHN) is a clinical syndrome of failure of pulmonary vascular transition to extrauterine life that results in increased pulmonary pressures, hypoxemia, and respiratory distress. The most common precipitating diseases are meconium aspiration syndrome, sepsis/pneumonia, perinatal depression/acidosis, abnormal pulmonary vascular development, pulmonary hypoplasia, and idiopathic "black lung" PPHN. Regardless of the etiology, hypoxemic respiratory failure in these infants is evident from birth or shortly thereafter, often with progressive cardiovascular compromise. The differential diagnosis includes congenital heart disease, sepsis/pneumonia, polycythemia, perinatal depression, and metabolic disease.

Initial treatment of PPHN includes correction of metabolic derangements, such as hypothermia, hypoglycemia, hypocalcemia, anemia, polycythemia, and hypovolemia. The use of alkalinizing agents is controversial, and induced alkalosis has been linked with adverse outcomes; however, correction of metabolic acidosis to physiologic pH is standard therapy. The appropriate use of vasopressor/inotropes (dopamine or epinephrine), inotropes (dobutamine), and lusitropes (milrinone) to support systemic perfu-sion (cardiac output) and myocardial function without inducing unwanted increases in the pulmonary vascular resistance (PVR) is important. The historic practice of using vasopressors/inotropes to drive the blood pressure to supraphysiologic levels to "force" blood through the lungs cannot be recommended, as increased PVR may occur. Monitoring of the preductal (right arm or right side of the face) and postductal (lower extremity) saturations can provide a reasonable estimation of ductal level shunting and severity of PPHN, assuming the ductus arteriosus is patent.

The goal of mechanical ventilation is to achieve "optimal" lung volume and recruitment (9–10 ribs) through the use of conventional or high-frequency oscillatory ventilation (HFOV) and to establish normal $PaCO_2$ levels and normal oxygenation. Failure to achieve lung recruitment at or above functional residual capacity contributes to hypoxemia and high PVR. Conversely, hyperexpansion, particularly with the constant distending pressure of HFOV may also worsen pulmonary hypertension by causing compression of capillaries and small arterioles and decreased cardiac output by interfering with venous return to the heart. iNO has been shown to improve oxygenation and decrease the need for extracorporeal membrane oxygenation (ECMO) in term infants with hypoxemic respiratory failure and an oxygenation index of >25 when started at 20 ppm. Surfactant is beneficial in improving compliance and oxygenation in infants with specific diseases. ECMO remains the final rescue therapy for infants with PPHN.

Meconium Aspiration Syndrome

Infants pass meconium in utero in response to stressful stimuli. A small subset of these infants who develop severe hypoxemia and acidosis and start gasping (second phase of apnea) will then aspirate the meconium-stained amniotic fluid (MSAF) into their airway, creating the scenario that can lead to meconium aspiration syndrome(MAS). MAS occurs when an infant born through MSAF develops a subsequent pneumonitis, leading to respiratory distress and PPHN.

The guidelines of the Neonatal Resuscitation Program no longer recommend the routine suctioning of the oropharynx of infants born through MSAF at the perineum (prior to delivery of the infant's body). However, the Neonatal Resuscitation Program does continue to recommend that nonvigorous infants born through MSAF be intubated and undergo tracheal suctioning by the neonatal team. In addition, it is no longer recommended to intubate and suction vigorous infants. Initial management of MAS includes supportive therapy, including intubation, cardiovascular support, analgesia, and antibiotics. The evidence at this time does not support the routine use of steroids in MAS. Surfactant replacement therapy improves lung compliance and oxygenation in infants with MAS and decreases the need for ECMO. iNO, is recommended for infants who do not respond to the above therapies (further discussed in the section on PPHN).

Congenital Diaphragmatic Hernia

CDH occurs owing to a failure of closure of the pleuroperitoneal folds resulting in a posterolateral diaphragmatic defect (Bochadalek hernia). The defect is most often on the left side. CDH is almost universally associated with lung hypoplasia primarily on the ipsilateral side; however, the contralateral side is typically hypoplastic as well.

When the presence of a CDH is known antenatally, the delivery room management focuses on immediate intubation, as bag-and-mask ventilation should be avoided to minimize distension of the stomach and the proximal intestine that would result in further compromise in lung expansion and cardiac filling. The stomach should immediately be decompressed with a sump tube. Many centers will routinely paralyze and sedate the infants to prevent them from swallowing air and to limit activity during the initial stabilization. On physical exam, breath sounds may be absent on the left side of the chest, the heart sounds may be shifted to the right, and the abdomen tends to be scaphoid owing to some of the abdominal organs shifting to the thorax. It may be difficult to effectively ventilate and resuscitate the patient. A chest x-ray confirms the diagnosis: Bowel loops are seen in the chest.

One of the major problems in CDH is pulmonary hypoplasia; therefore, it makes physiologic sense to avoid barotrauma, limit peak inspiratory pressures to 24–26 cm H_2O, allow spontaneous ventilation, and adopt the strategy of permissive hypercarbia. It is well known that infants with CDH have a high incidence of pulmonary hypertension; however, it is important to remember that the pulmonary vasculature in these patients is developmentally abnormal and hypoplastic; therefore, aggressive ventilator goals are likely to increase ventilator-induced injury rather than acutely lower the pulmonary pressures. iNO is effective in infants with hypoxemic respiratory failure without CDH; however, its role in CDH is less clear. Late pulmonary hypertension remains a significant problem in the CDH population. Researchers are investigating the role of pulmonary vasodilators such as sildenafil, inhaled prostacyclin, and chronic iNO therapy.

Congenital Cystic Adenomatoid Malformation

Clinically, infants with congenital cystic adenomatoid malformation (CCAM) present with a spectrum of illness, from severe respiratory failure to asymptomatic. The severity of respiratory compromise cannot always be predicted. Resection is recommended in all cases owing to the high likelihood of chronic infections in the lesion and the possibility of malignant transformation.

Pulmonary Sequestration

Pulmonary sequestration is another cystic lesion of the lung, differentiated from CCAM by the origin of its blood supply, which is systemic rather than pulmonary. Sequestrations can be intrapulmonary or extrapulmonary. Sequestrations present a risk for recurrent infections—historically, this was the typical way sequestrations came to medical attention prior to routine prenatal ultrasonography. Resection of the lesion is recommended in the first year of life, though timing depends on the case.

Pulmonary Hypoplasia

Pulmonary hypoplasia represents a broad spectrum of anatomic malformations ranging from total bronchial agenesis to mild parenchymal hypoplasia and may be either primary or secondary to other lesions. Primary pulmonary hypoplasia is typically unilateral and not associated with other malformations.

Oligohydramnios is associated with either renal disease in the neonate or chronic amniotic fluid leak. Fetal urine output becomes the primary source of amniotic fluid after 20–22 wks of gestation; before then, amniotic fluid is primarily produced by the placenta. Infants with bilateral renal agenesis, bilateral dysplastic kidneys, or obstructive uropathies have severe oligohydramnios owing to the lack of fetal urine output. Oligohydramnios related to amniotic fluid leak appears to have a slightly different pathophysiology, and the degree of pulmonary hypoplasia is very difficult to assess antenatally. Management is focused on limiting barotrauma while assessing the degree of lung hypoplasia and associated anomalies.

Air-leak Syndrome

Air-leak syndromes represent one of the most serious complications of assisted ventilation in the neonate. Air leaks begin with rupture of alveoli or distal airways and are associated with high ventilator pressures and severe lung disease. They can occur suddenly, often complicate the treatment of RDS, and may be life threatening if not rapidly identified and addressed.

Pulmonary Interstitial Emphysema

Pulmonary interstitial emphysema (PIE) results from overdistension of distal airways and usually occurs in the tiniest, most immature babies. The ruptured airways provide a pathway for leakage of air into the connective tissues that leads to the clinically observed findings of PIE on x-ray. As air moves within the connective tissues, it can further track toward the hilum of the lung. PIE increases the volume of gas within the lung parenchyma, thereby decreasing lung compliance and increasing airway resistance. An increased need for ventilation typically occurs as the result of increased respiratory dead space and reduced minute ventilation. Hypoxemia results from the reduction in alveolar ventilation and from intrapulmonary shunting. Death may occur owing to inadequate ventilation and oxygenation. PIE is diagnosed radiographically based on the characteristic linear and cyst-like radiolucencies that reflect the accumulation of interstitial air. PIE may involve a single lobe, one lung, or both lungs. The linear radiolucencies are coarse and rarely appear to branch. They must be differentiated from the smooth, branching, perihilar air bronchograms often seen with RDS. The cyst-like radiolucencies of PIE take the appearance of small bubbles, typically vary in size from 0.5 to 4 mm in diameter and are often present in large numbers.

No precise treatment for PIE exists. When PIE is unilateral, it is often suggested that the infant be positioned with the affected side down. When PIE is bilateral or extensive, an attempt can be made to decompress the air leaks by using a short inspiratory time, low inflation pressures, and small tidal volumes. One drawback to this approach is that it is often difficult to achieve optimal or even adequate oxygenation and ventilation while allowing for the collapse of the PIE-affected areas of lung. HFOV may allow for adequate ventilation and oxygenation in infants with PIE at lower peak and mean airway pressures than with conventional ventilation.

Pneumomediastinum and Pneumothorax

The diagnosis of pneumothorax and/or pneumomediastinum is easily confirmed by clinical examination and chest x-ray. Isolated pneumomediastinum is often asymptomatic or associated with mild respiratory symptoms. With a pneumothorax, infants are usually symptomatic with signs of respiratory distress (tachypnea, retractions, grunting, flaring), cyanosis, and poor perfusion. Bedside evaluation may reveal tachycardia with a narrow pulse pressure. It is important to note that differential breath sounds are an unreliable marker for the diagnosis of pneumothorax in infants. An acute clinical deterioration in a mechanically ventilated infant should prompt an urgent search for the possibility of an air leak.

Transillumination of the chest can sometimes be used to make the diagnosis of an air leak, but if time allows, the diagnosis should be confirmed by chest x-ray. Nitrogen washout is a therapy used for stable, minimally symptomatic non-mechanically ventilated neonates with air leak. The infant is placed on 100% inspired oxygen, typically delivered via an oxyhood, and monitored closely for resolution of the air leak. However, owing to the toxicity associated with the use of 100% oxygen, the risks of using the nitrogen washout technique may outweigh the risks associated with chest tube placement, especially in the unstable preterm infant, in whom recurrence of the pneumothorax is likely. Tube thoracostomy is indicated in neonates with cardiorespiratory compromise or those receiving mechanical ventilation. Needle aspiration may be useful for acute relief of a tension pneumothorax but should usually be followed by chest tube placement to allow for continued evacuation of the air leak while the lung tissue is healing. The chest tube is typically connected to 10–20 cm of negative water pressure and drainage and radiographs are monitored to determine the timing of resolution of the air leak and readiness for removal of the tube.

Pulmonary Hemorrhage

Pulmonary hemorrhage has been associated with a wide range of predisposing conditions, including prematurity, mechanical ventilation, sepsis, PDA, and asphyxia. Pulmonary hemorrhage reflects hemorrhagic pulmonary edema in most cases. An association exists between pulmonary hemorrhage and surfactant administration, especially in the presence of a PDA. The earliest clinical sign of pulmonary hemorrhage is usually the detection of blood-tinged secretions from the endotracheal tube. Chest x-ray may reveal fluffy infiltrates consistent with pulmonary edema, and the infant's respiratory status often deteriorates.

Treatment of pulmonary hemorrhage involves clearing the airway to prevent frank obstruction from the hemorrhagic fluid and adjusting support to provide adequate oxygenation and ventilation. However, every effort should be made to avoid unnecessary suctioning of the trachea, which may only exacerbate the bleeding. Increasing the mean airway pressure, typically achieved by increasing positive end-expiratory pressure, helps to prevent the continued flow of blood into the trachea. Blood tests for the presence of coagulopathy or new-onset infection, as well as to monitor the hematocrit are indicated. In most cases, packed RBC transfusion is unnecessary, and the additional volume only worsens the pulmonary edema. Therefore, volume administration in hypotensive neonates with pulmonary hemorrhage must be avoided, at least in the period immediately following the development of the hemorrhage.

Pulmonary Edema

Left atrial pressure may be elevated as a result of volume overload, presence of a PDA with left-to-right shunting, or obstruction to outflow due to congenital heart disease and abnormal anatomy, which leads to pulmonary edema. During the early postnatal period, pulmonary edema is associated with both PDA and RDS. Pulmonary edema complicates the respiratory management of the neonate. Every effort should be made to optimize nutrition and minimize barotrauma and excessive supplemental oxygen exposure during the patient's course. One must maintain a high degree of suspicion for persistent patency or reopening of the ductus arteriosus in VLBW neonates during the first days and weeks after delivery. Diuretics are frequently used as therapy for pulmonary edema to improve oxygenation and ventilation. Furosemide is typically used as the first-line agent of choice, but Diuril and Aldactone are frequently preferred for the management of the chronic phase of BPD, especially in the outpatient setting, to minimize the requirement for potassium and chloride supplementation, reduce the need for outpatient blood work to monitor electrolyte values, and decrease the risk of sensorineural hearing loss associated with chronic furosemide administration.

Airway Injury

Prolonged intubation carries the risk for significant upper-airway complications. For instance, marked stridor following extubation or a history of repeated failure to successfully extubate an infant may be due to airway injury secondary to long-term intubation. Injury can occur as a result of irritation from the endotracheal tube over time or from focal damage at the time of intubation and can range from edema, ulcerations, and granulations to vocal cord paralysis or subglottic stenosis. Endotracheal tubes should be upsized only if a leak around the endotracheal tube is compromising adequate ventilation and if the larger tube passes easily through the subglottis. A brief course of periextubation dexamethasone may decrease postextubation stridor in preterm neonates who are at high risk for subglottic edema. Nebulized

racemic epinephrine may also help reduce stridor in the acute setting after extubations, though it carries the risk of rebound edema formation once the medication is discontinued. The initial evaluation is at the bedside by flexible bronchoscopy, but rigid laryngoscopy in the operating room is often indicated to more completely visualize the extent and location of injury to the airway. Even when numerous extubation attempts have failed, extubation is sometimes successful when reattempted, after allowing time for growth and healing, and if CPAP, nasal, or nasopharyngeal intermittent assisted ventilation is used after extubation. Surgical options include an anterior cricoid split or tracheostomy.

Congenital Pneumonia

Congenital pneumonia frequently coexists with sepsis and is a significant source of morbidity and mortality in neonates. Infection is typically acquired when organisms ascend into the uterine cavity, either during or prior to labor, and come into contact with the fetus. Consequently, prolonged rupture of membranes is a significant risk factor for neonatal sepsis.

Group B *Streptococcus* (GBS) is the most common pathogen that causes early-onset neonatal pneumonia in the US. It is currently recommended that colonized women and those with other risk factors for neonatal sepsis be given intrapartum antibiotic therapy beginning at least 4 hrs prior to delivery. Other organisms that may cause pneumonia in the neonate include Gram-negative organisms, particularly *Escherichia coli*, group D *Streptococcus*, *Listeria*, pneumococci, *Staphylococcus* species, and fungus. *Chlamydia*, though acquired congenitally, typically presents as pneumonia at several weeks of age rather than in the immediate postnatal period. Interest has been renewed in the possibility that peripartum transmission of ureaplasma urealyticum to the respiratory tract of the preterm neonate may contribute to the development of severe respiratory failure and/or BPD. Though more typically a cause of late-onset pneumonia in neonates, viruses (herpes simplex virus, enterovirus, and adenovirus, in particular) can also cause congenital pneumonia and may have a severe and sometimes fatal course.

Neonates may present with respiratory distress at birth (or shortly after birth) for a wide range of reasons unrelated to infection. Tachypnea, retractions, grunting, and cyanosis can all result from processes as varied as transient tachypnea of the newborn, respiratory distress syndrome, CDH, pneumothorax, and polycythemia. In addition, neonates with pneumonia can present without focal respiratory signs, demonstrating only temperature instability (typically hypothermia), glucose instability, or jaundice. Fever and cough, frequent findings in older patients, are uncommon in newborns with bacterial pneumonia.

Numerous WBCs on the aspirate may signal the presence of infection, and growth of an isolated organism when present can guide therapy. Blood cultures should be sent to evaluate for bacteremia and can help determine appropriate coverage when culture growth is observed. A chest x-ray is indicated to evaluate for infiltrates, although it is often difficult to differentiate an infiltrate from atelectasis, RDS, retained lung fluid, and the edema seen with certain cardiac anomalies; serial radiograms may be useful in differentiating the various processes. Appearance of an infiltrate may lag behind the onset of clinical symptoms by 24–48 hrs. *Staphylococcus aureus* pneumonia is classically associated with empyema and pneumatocele formation. A decreased or elevated WBC count and/or a predominance of immature WBC forms are suggestive of infection. Though nonspecific, an elevated c-reactive protein indicates the presence of an infectious or inflammatory process.

It is standard for antibiotic therapy to be started prior to the determination of a definitive diagnosis of pneumonia in the neonate. Treatment is usually begun as soon as respiratory symptoms develop or troubling lab findings are identified in an infant at risk for sepsis. Typical treatment pending identification of the pathogen is broad spectrum, consisting of a penicillin in addition to an aminoglycoside. Coverage should be narrowed if the causative organism is identified. Ten days of IV ampicillin and gentamicin is probably the most widely accepted treatment, but treatment duration varies. Given the high incidence of coexisting bacteremia, many neonatologists would treat a documented Gram-negative pneumonia for a minimum of 14 days and rule out the possibility of meningitic involvement.

Nosocomial Pneumonia

Nosocomial pneumonia is defined by the CDC in patients who are <1 year of age at the appearance of a new or progressive infiltrate on chest x-ray, increased respiratory secretions or a change in sputum character, and isolation of the pathogen from a tracheal aspirate, bronchial washing, or biopsy specimen. Mechanical ventilation presents a risk because the respiratory tract, given time, will become colonized with bacteria, typically Gram-negative bacilli (*Pseudomonas aeruginosa*, *Klebsiella pneumoniae*, *E. coli*) or *Staphylococcus* species. Fungus, typically *Candida*, can also colonize the neonatal respiratory tract and

potentially cause pneumonia and/or systemic disease. Viruses, particularly respiratory syncytial virus, may also cause nosocomial pneumonia in NICU patients.

Nosocomial pneumonia should, in most cases, manifest itself with a clinical deterioration in the patient's respiratory status. The chest x-ray may show a focal infiltrate, but it is often difficult to clearly detect an infiltrate, as many preterm infants have significant radiographic findings of lung disease at baseline and frequently develop areas of atelectasis. A tracheal aspirate should be sent for Gram stain and culture, but it is important to realize that most ventilated patients will have colonization of the respiratory tract with bacteria and will subsequently have growth of bacteria when tracheal aspirate cultures are sent. It is important to critically analyze tracheal aspirate results in an attempt to differentiate colonization from infection and determine the need for antibiotic therapy. The presence of many or a moderate amount of WBCs has been used as an indicator of the presence of infection. In addition, growth of a single or predominant organism that is a known pathogen may be helpful. Growth of mixed flora and the presence of only a few WBCs are more consistent with colonization. Respiratory secretions can be sent for viral testing when a viral etiology is suspected.

Given that the pathogens responsible for nosocomial infections differ somewhat from those responsible for early-onset infections, the antibiotics administered for nosocomial pneumonia prior to identification of the responsible organism vary from those used for early-onset infection. Vancomycin is often used in combination with an aminoglycoside as the regimen of choice for a suspected nosocomial infection in the NICU. Vancomycin is used to optimally cover *Staphylococcus* species, particularly *S. epidermidis*, which is frequently oxacillin-resistant and a common cause of infection in NICU patients. Some centers choose to treat neonates who develop nosocomial infections with double Gram-negative antibiotic coverage while awaiting culture results, the theory being that Gram-negative organisms typically cause more aggressive disease, and vancomycin can always be added if clinical deterioration continues or significant growth of *S. epidermidis* from the cultures is seen. Sometimes, antibiotic therapy is directed at the bacteria that are known colonizers in the infant based on growth seen on prior bacterial cultures and/or based on the pattern of unit-specific cultures and resistance panels.

CHAPTER 24 ■ BRONCHIOLITIS AND PNEUMONIA

WERTHER BRUNOW DE CARVALHO • CíNTIA JOHNSTON
• MARCELO CUNIO MACHADO FONSECA

BRONCHIOLITIS

Acute bronchiolitis (AB) is generally self-limited, though in high-risk children (those who are premature or immunocompromised or those who suffer from bronchopulmonary dysplasia or congenital heart disease). AB can be associated with prolonged disease and a mortality rate as high as 30%. AB is a lower-respiratory-tract syndrome with acute onset. Typically, it begins with initial symptoms of an upper-airway viral infection, such as fever and coryza. Within 4–6 days, the lower-respiratory tract is involved, with clinical signs of cough, tachypnea, hyperinflation, chest retractions, widespread crackles, and wheezing. A wide range of agents (parainfluenza, adenovirus, influenza, *Mycoplasma pneumoniae*, rhinovirus, *Chlamydia pneumoniae*, human metapneumovirus [hMPV], and coronavirus) may cause AB; however, respiratory syncytial virus (RSV) (with its A and B subtypes), is by far the most frequently involved agent. Risk factors for clinical worsening of acute bronchiolitis are summarized in **Table 24.1**.

Influenza Virus

Though influenza infection is self-limited, it may cause complications, such as pneumonia, Reye syndrome, myositis, febrile convulsion, and acute encephalopathy. Hospitalization, increased disease severity, and complications are more frequent in children <2 years old and in those with risk factors (asthma or other chronic pulmonary disease, severe heart disease, immunocompromise, hemoglobinopathies, and diabetes mellitus).

Human Metapneumovirus

hMPV virus has universal distribution, especially during fall and winter seasons in temperate climates. It is associated with several clinical presentations, such as cold, AB, asthma exacerbation and airway-obstructive disease, pneumonia and, occasionally, severe infections in immunocompromised patients. Severe AB can be caused by combined infection with hMPV and RSV. The clinical syndrome of infected children ranges from mild respiratory symptoms to AB and pneumonia. The signs and symptoms of hMPV are fever (67%), cough (100%), rhinorrhea (92%), retractions (92%), wheezing (83%), vomiting (25%), and diarrhea (8%). Multiple reinfections of hMPV may occur in the same patient, particularly in the aged and immunocompromised.

Rhinovirus

Though the diseases caused by rhinovirus are not completely defined, its infection is the leading cause of asthma crisis in children and adults. It is still undetermined whether host factors such as innate immunologic response predispose to more severe disease and wheezing or whether repeated viral respiratory diseases cause wheezing due to airway and pulmonary lesions.

Coronavirus

A causal relationship between febrile respiratory disease and a new coronavirus (other than human coronavirus) was initially shown in China in 2003; this disease was named *acute respiratory syndrome*. Infants and young children were not detected as a risk group, and only a few cases were found in children <15 years old. In young children, signs of upper-airway infection are present; symptoms such as tremors, stiffness, and myalgia are usually not seen. Clinical manifestations are mild in young children when compared to adolescents and adults. Incubation time ranges from 2 to 7 days but may be >10 days, with fever higher than 38°C (100.4°F), dry cough, and dyspnea progressing to hypoxemia. Chest x-ray demonstrates early focal infiltration, progressing to generalization with interstitial infiltration in the majority of patients. Radiologic features are not distinct from bronchopneumonia caused by other pathogens. Laboratory changes include leukopenia or moderate lymphopenia with liver enzyme elevation.

TABLE 24.1

RISK FACTORS FOR CLINICAL WORSENING OF ACUTE BRONCHIOLITIS

Initial presentation	Tachypnea (RR >60–80 bpm or retractions)
	Hypoxia (SaO$_2$ 90%–95%)
	Feeding difficulty or dehydration
Age	Age <12 mos (the younger the child, larger the risk)
Comorbidities	Bronchopulmonary dysplasia
	Congenital heart disease
	Cystic fibrosis
	Immunodeficiency
Prematurity	Gestation age <36 weeks
Other	Malnutrition
	Poverty
	Overcrowding
	Parents and/or family members who smoke
	Genetic RSV infection predisposition

RR, respiratory rate; SaO$_2$, arterial oxygen saturation, RSV, respiratory syncytial virus.

TABLE 24.2

ADENOVIRUS CLINICAL SYNDROMES

System	Clinical manifestations
Respiratory	*Upper respiratory tract*
	Pharyngitis
	Coryza
	Lower respiratory tract
	Laryngotracheobronchitis
	Cough
	Acute bronchiolitis
	Pneumonia
Ocular	Conjunctivitis with respiratory disease
	Acute follicular conjunctivitis
	Epidemic keratoconjunctivitis
	Pharyngoconjunctival fever
Gastrointestinal	Diarrhea
	Immunocompromised host hepatitis
Urinary	Hemorrhagic cystitis
Nervous	Aseptic meningitis
	Meningoencephalitis, encephalitis
	Myelitis, acute flaccid palsy
	Myositis
Skin	Rash
Disseminated infections (immunocompromised newborns)	Multiple-organ failure

Adenovirus

Adenovirus is so named because it is frequently isolated from adenoid and other lymphatic tissues; 51 serotypes are currently identified. The incubation time ranges from 5 to 10 days. It is not common in the first 6 months of life, suggesting protection by maternal antibodies. Common symptoms are summarized in **Table 24.2**.

Parainfluenza

The seasonal pattern of types 1, 2, and 3 parainfluenza viruses is curiously interactive. Every second year, type-1 parainfluenza virus causes a defined epidemic, with a larger number of croup cases than AB. Type-2 parainfluenza virus epidemic is erratic and comes just after a type-1 epidemic; a type-3 parainfluenza virus epidemic occurs yearly (mostly in spring and summer) and has prolonged duration in relation to types 1 and 2. Parainfluenza viruses cause a disease similar to RSV with a lower hospitalization rate.

Respiratory Syncytial Virus

Mostly based on the surface of G glucoproteins, RSV is divided into 2 large groups: A (dominant strain) and B. This virus grows optimally in a pH of 7.5; although sensitive to temperature, in gloves contaminated with RSV-infected nasal secretions it is recovered more than 1 hr later. Owing to this stability, in a hospital setting RSV may be considered a nosocomial agent. One is exposed to RSV after contact with ocular or nasal secretion. Serum antibodies appear to offer some protection against RSV infection. High maternal antibody levels are associated with lower infection rates in infants. Prophylactic administration of antibodies has been effective in reducing, but not eliminating, severe RSV disease.

AB caused by RSV results from infection and inflammation of the respiratory mucosa. Symptoms of lower–respiratory tract obstruction are a consequence of the partial obstruction of the distal airways.

Clinical Manifestations

AB usually occurs in winter but can be observed in any season. Parents usually report that affected children attend daycare centers or had contact with people with cold symptoms. In the beginning of the disease, children have abundant rhinorrhea and typically a "tight" cough, along with poor food intake (4–6 days after symptoms start). The degree of fever in infants depends on the infecting organism. Infants with AB often have significant tachypnea, mild-to-moderate hypoxia, and signs of respiratory distress, such as nasal flaring and respiratory accessory muscle use. Physical examination frequently demonstrates audible wheezing, crackles or bronchi (apical ventilatory pattern), and a prolonged expiratory phase. Other common findings are conjunctivitis, acute otitis, and rhinitis. Many infants have a distended abdomen due to pulmonary hyperinflation.

A mild leukocytosis with a normal differential is frequently found in infants experiencing AB. Hypoxia is detected by pulse oximetry or arterial blood gases. CO_2 retention may be seen in severe cases. Virus-diagnosing test results may be used to limit inappropriate use of antibiotics. Chest x-rays often show nonspecific findings, including hyperinflation, gross infiltrates that are typically migratory and attributable to postobstructive atelectasis, and peribronchial filling. AB is not an alveolar space disease and, when a true alveolar infiltrate is seen, secondary bacterial pneumonia should be suspected. Wood-Downes score may be used to evaluate and grade AB severity (**Table 24.3**).

Treatment

An arterial saturation of <95% on pulse oximetry was the single best predictor of a more severe total disease course. Generally, a respiratory rate >80 bpm and hypoxia with SaO_2 <85% are predictors of the need for intensive care. Admission to the PICU is appropriate if clinical (progressive respiratory distress leading to respiratory fatigue, apnea episodes) and/or diagnostic signs (PO_2 <60 mm Hg; PCO_2 >50 mm Hg) of respiratory failure are noted despite administration of supplemental oxygen (40%–50% FIO_2).

Adequate hydration and oxygenation are the backbone of treatment of AB. Offering oral/enteral fluids or, when feeding is not tolerated, IV fluids and oxygen support is essential. Although hydration greatly varies among institutions, approximately half of uncomplicated bronchiolitis patients may require IV fluids. Supplemental oxygen, usually delivered via nasal prongs, is the single most useful therapy. SaO_2 should be kept above 92%. Careful monitoring, mainly among the more sick and high-risk children, is important, as more-aggressive ventilatory support may be required (mask, nasopharyngeal continuous positive airway pressure ventilation, or even endotracheal ventilation), and the timely introduction of ventilatory support is important to prevent further complications. β_2 agonist administration is almost a universal practice. If clinical improvement does not immediately occur or if worsening is observed after 60 mins of inhalation, β_2 agonists should be discontinued.

Results obtained with anticholinergics use (ipratropium bromide) are very limited. They were not superior to $\beta2$ agonists alone and did not improve the results when used in combination. Theophylline appears to be indicated for clinical apnea, but no studies have been conducted to evaluate this indication.

When compared to inhaled albuterol/fenoterol, epinephrine is more effective. A recent Cochrane review showed that epinephrine leads to small improvement on the clinical score but no change in the hospitalization rate. Racemic epinephrine 2.25% and L-epinephrine 0.1% are used at 0.1 mg/kg and 0.05 mg/kg, respectively, every 4 hrs. This treatment should be used only in the hospital setting with clinical, heart rate, and electrocardiographic monitoring. As a rebound effect may occur, the child should be

---

TABLE 24.3

WOOD-DOWNES SCORE

Score	Wheezing	Retraction	Respiratory rate	Heart rate	Ventilation	Cyanosis
0	No	No	<30	<120	Good Symmetrical	No
1	End expiratory	Subcostal/intercostal	31–45	>120	Regular Symmetrical	Yes
2	All expiration	Supraclavicular + nasal flaring	40–60		Very reduced	
3	inspiration and expiration	+ intercostal + suprasternal			Silent thorax	

The highest scores from each column are summed to attain the total severity score: 1–3, mild; 4–7, moderate; 8–14, severe.
Adapted from Wood DW, Downes JJ, Lecks HI, et al. A clinical scoring system for the diagnosis of respiratory failure. Preliminary report on childhood status asthmaticus. *Am J Dis Child* 1972;123(3):227–8, with permission.

observed for at least 1–2 hrs following cessation of treatment, and a decision to discharge prematurely should be avoided.

The use of inhaled and systemic steroids is also a controversial therapy, as these agents may produce little or no response at all. A Cochrane systematic review showed no benefit of systemic steroid use in the management of AB. Severely ill children who are receiving mechanical ventilation may benefit from steroid use; however, steroids do not prevent bronchospasm in patients following AB. DNase may also be effective in infections complicated by atelectasis, bronchial secretions, and mucous plugs that have high DNA concentration. The helium/oxygen mixture (heliox) reduces the work of breathing and expiratory wheezing in children with obstructive disease. Recommended techniques of respiratory physiotherapy for children with AB are based on positioning therapy, alveolar recruitment, expiratory airflow increase using hand-vibration, and airway aspiration. Extracorporeal membrane oxygenation is an option for severely ill children who cannot be supported by conventional mechanical ventilation due to their ventilation and cardiocirculatory condition. Nitric oxide used in the treatment of children severely infected with RSV improves oxygenation and respiratory-system resistance.

Conventional mechanical ventilation, using control-pressure ventilation mode, is indicated in those children with either obstructive or restrictive hypoxemic disease; however, a mixed mode (pressure regulated, volume controlled) can also be chosen. Due to the possibility of intrinsic positive end-expiratory pressure, efforts should be focused on maintaining a low RR (20 bpm) and an inspiratory:expiratory ratio of 1:3. Additionally, the initial positive end-expiratory pressure should be ~5 cm H_2O, with adjustments being made according to the degree of alveolar recruitment and clinical response. High-frequency oscillation ventilation is indicated for those patients whose condition continues to worsen despite conventional mechanical ventilation or for those with significant air leak (pneumothorax, interstitial emphysema, pneumopericardium).

Noninvasive positive-pressure ventilation use in AB children keeps airways open, improves respiratory flow, maintains functional residual capacity, improves pulmonary compliance, facilitates secretion mobilization, reduces work of breathing, improves gas exchange, and preserves surfactant synthesis and release. This therapy is indicated as first-choice ventilatory support in children who are experiencing apnea episodes and for preventing the use of invasive mechanical ventilation. This noninvasive support can be performed using continuous positive airway pressure or bilevel positive airway pressure ventilatory mode.

When continuous positive airway pressure is chosen, it is recommended to start with 4–6 cm H_2O; if bilevel positive airway pressure is chosen, it is recommended to begin with an inspiratory pressure of 8 cm H_2O and expiratory positive airway pressure of 4 cm H_2O.

Passive immunization against RSV may be made with monoclonal antibodies (palivizumab, approved by the US Food and Drug Administration in 1998). Once per month during the epidemic months, an intramuscular dose of 15 mg/kg should be administered.

PNEUMONIA

Pneumonia can be classified according to the anatomic location (lobar, lobular, alveolar, or interstitial), the location where it was acquired (community or nosocomial), or the causative organism. When a child presents with recurrent pneumonia, the possibility of an underlying disease (e.g., acquired or congenital lung anatomical abnormalities, immunodeficiency, prematurity, lung sequestration, tracheoesophageal fistula, foreign body, cystic fibrosis, heart failure, palatine cleft, bronchiectasis, ciliary dyskinesia, neutropenia and increased pulmonary blood flow) should be considered.

In children who are <1 year of age, viruses are the main pneumonia-causative pathogens. In the neonatal period, the most frequent pathogens are herpes simplex and cytomegalovirus. In children >6 months of age, RSV, influenza, parainfluenza, adenovirus, rhinovirus, coronavirus, measles, rubella, chickenpox, cytomegalovirus, and herpes are more frequent. In newborns and in infants <2 months old, the bacterial etiologies are more frequent: Group B Streptococci, Gram-negative bacilli (maternal genital tract or hospital flora), *Staphylococcus aureus*, *Chlamydia trachomatis*, and congenital syphilis (less frequently). From 2 months to 5 years of age, *Streptococcus pneumoniae*, type B *Haemophilus influenzae*, and *S. aureus* are frequently found. The prevalence of *Mycoplasma pneumoniae* increases in children >3 years, and the prevalence of *S. pneumoniae*, *M. pneumoniae*, type B Haemophilus influenza, and *Chlamydophila pneumoniae* increases in children ≥5 years of age. Pneumonias acquired after 48–72 hrs of hospitalization are considered nosocomial.

Aspiration Pneumonia

Children with obstructive lesions of the gastrointestinal tract, diseases with hypotonia, dysautonomia, compromised consciousness, or gastroesophageal reflux and/or swallowing incoordination can aspirate or regurgitate, which can cause chemical pneumonitis. Often, there is a time lapse between the aspiration and the signs/symptoms of pneumonia. Previously healthy, nonhospitalized, patients can be infected with agents of their own oral flora (predominantly anaerobes), and hospitalized patients can be colonized by Gram-negative bacteria. The usual signs and symptoms are fever, lethargy, poor appetite, pallor or cyanosis, toxemia, agitation, vomiting, and abdominal distension. Signs and symptoms of lung compromise are respiratory distress (nasal flaring, intercostal and subcostal retractions, thoracic pain). Tachypnea is the most sensitive parameter in children with pneumonia.

TABLE 24.4

LABORATORIAL TESTS FEATURES

Diagnostic Test	Characteristics
Blood count	Leukocytosis Leukopenia suggests a worse prognosis. Varied degrees of anemia
Erythrocyte sedimentation rate and reactive C protein	Nonspecific, used for follow-up control May be suggestive of bacterial etiology when very elevated.
Blood cultures	The ideal is to collect three samples before the beginning of the antibiotic therapy. High specificity Variable sensitivity depending on agent
Pleural fluid culture	Etiologic agent can be found in up to 60% of cases.
Tracheal aspirate culture	Intubated patients Growth $>10^5$–10^6 CFU/mL suggests infection.
Bronchoalveolar lavage culture (bronchoscopy)	High sensitivity and specificity Growth $>10^4$ CFU/mL indicates infection.
Culture of material obtained from aspirative puncture	Growth $>10^3$ CFU/mL indicates infection. Invasive method and therefore with restricted indications
Biopsies	Special restricted indications
Virus isolation and fibroblasts, HeLa, HEP2, and kidney monkey cells culture	Good positivity/high cost Used mainly during epidemic offspring investigations
Respiratory virus serologies	Blood samples in acute and convalescent phases Investigation of antibody elevation against a specific virus—useful as an epidemiologic instrument. Has no diagnostic usefulness in the acute phase because the serologic result will confirm the etiology only after the end of the acute phase.
Detection of bacterial antigens in corporal fluids	Urine and pleural fluid Reactions occur against *S. pneumoniae*, *H. influenzae*, group B streptococcus, and *N. meningitidis* serotypes A, B, C, Y and W135 In ~90% of the pneumonias due to *H. influenzae* with bacteremia blood or urine, samples are positive for group B streptococci; 5%–30% of the infections are due to *S. pneumoniae*.
Nasopharynx secretion sample Immunofluorescence	Detection of viral antigens Positivity up to 85% for RSV
Fast detection cryoagglutinins	The test is positive if defined micronodular agglutination occurs.
ELISA	For virus and bacteria
Complement fixation reaction	Performed for virus and *Mycoplasma pneumoniae* Retrospective diagnosis

CFU, colony-forming units; ELISA, enzyme-linked immunosorbent assay

TABLE 24.5

HOSPITAL ADMISSION CRITERIA

<3–6 mos
Acute respiratory failure (dyspnea, sustained tachypnea)
Toxemia/sepsis
Hemodynamic instability
Necessity for oxygen therapy
Domiciliary treatment failure
Extensive lung compromise
Immunosuppression, heart disease, or other serious
    underlying disease
Socioeconomic factors
Pneumonia complications

A diagnosis of pneumonia is possible in children who present with fever, cough, and tachypnea and have an infiltration on chest x-ray. However, several other diseases can have these signs and symptoms, such as AB, upper-airway infection, congestive heart failure, pulmonary embolism, thoracic tumors, or inflammatory diseases (systemic vasculitis). The radiologic pattern may suggest the disease etiology. The laboratory data are summarized in **Table 24.4**. Admission criteria are summarized in **Table 24.5**.

Therapy includes maintenance of nutritional state, fluid, electrolyte, and acid-base balance, and temperature; 30-degree head elevations, heated and humidified oxygen therapy, thinning of secretions, and physiotherapy. Initial antibiotic use is summarized in **Table 24.6**. Initial empiric therapy can be modified after the identification of the etiologic agent (**Table 24.7**).

Initial treatment of nosocomial pneumonia should cover Gram-negative and Gram-positive pathogens, using semisynthetic penicillin (oxacillin/cloxacillin) with third- or fourth-generation cephalosporins (ceftriaxone/ceftazidime or cefepime). In the presence of a high incidence of methicillin-resistant *S. aureus*, vancomycin, teicoplanin, or clindamycin should be administered with third- or fourth-generation cephalosporin. An optional treatment would be vancomycin with imipenem or meropenem. If risk factors exist for fungal infection, amphotericin B or fluconazole should be administered. If the patient has received a bone marrow graft or has lymphoma, leukemia, or acquired immunodeficiency syndrome, it is necessary to enhance the antibiotic spectrum for *Pneumocystis carinii*, adding trimethoprim-sulfamethoxazole or pentamidine.

Complications

Pneumonia with pleural effusion is defined by the presence of fluids in the pleural cavity and empyema

TABLE 24.6

EMPIRIC TREATMENT OF COMMUNITY-ACQUIRED PNEUMONIAS ACCORDING TO AGE

Age	Treatment
Newborns up to 2 mos	Possible infection due to Group B Streptococcus or Gram-negative bacilli: Ampicillin plus Gentamicin or ampicillin plus Amikacin If *Chlamydia trachomatis* infection is suspected: Erythromycin Suspicion of Herpes: Acyclovir Suspicion of CMV: Ganciclovir
Nonfebrile pneumonia up to 3 months	Probable infection due to *Chlamydia trachomatis*: Erythromycin
Nonfebrile pneumonia 3–4 mos to 5 yrs	Most frequent viral infections: Antivirals in special situations
2 mos to 5 yrs	Possible agents: *Streptococcus pneumoniae*, *Haemophilus influenzae*, and *Staphylococcus aureus*. Noncomplicated cases: oral amoxicillin, amoxicillin-clavulanate acid or cefuroxime, Moderate to serious infection: IV amoxicillin-clavulanate, cefuroxime, or oxacillin plus chloramphenicol or third-generation cephalosporin.
>5 yrs	*Mycoplasma pneumoniae* (frequent): macrolides (erythromycin, clarithromycin, azithromycin) Viral pneumonia is also possible Pneumonia and *H. influenzae*: non-complicated cases: amoxicillin-clavulanate or cefuroxime (orally). Complicated cases: erythromycin plus cefuroxime (IV) or third-generation cephalosporin.

TABLE 24.7

IDENTIFICATION OF THE ETIOLOGIC AGENT AND ANTIMICROBIALS

Agent	Antimicrobials
Chlamydia trachomatis	Erythromycin (40 mg/kg/day)
Chlamydia pneumoniae	Erythromycin (40 mg/kg/day)
Mycoplasma pneumoniae	Erythromycin (40 mg/kg/day)
Group B β hemolytic streptococcus	Ampicillin (100 mg/kg/day)
	plus gentamicin (5 mg/kg/day)
	OR
	plus amikacin (15 mg/kg/day)
Streptococcus pneumoniae	
Sensitive to penicillin	Crystalline penicillin (100,000–250,000 U/kg/day)
Intermediate sensitivity	Penicillin (200,000–250,000 U/kg/day)
Resistant to the penicillin	Cefotaxime (200 mg/kg/day) or Ceftriaxone (100 mg/kg/day)
Resistant to penicillin and	Vancomycin (40–60 mg/kg/day) + clindamycin (30–45
cephalosporins	mg/kg/day)–erythromycin (40 mg/kg/day) (follow antibiotic sensitivities)
Haemophilus influenzae	
β-lactamase negative	Ampicillin (100 mg/kg/day)
β-lactamase positive	Cefotaxime (200 mg/kg/day) or ceftriaxone (100 mg/kg/day)
Staphylococcus aureus	
methicillin sensitive	Oxacillin (200 mg/kg/day)
methicillin resistant	Vancomycin (40–60 mg/kg/day) or teicoplanin (10 mg/kg/day)
	plus clindamycin (30–35 mg/kg/day)).
Simian retrovirus, influenza b, parainfluenza	Ribavirin (15–20 mg/kg/day) (orally or IV) for immunocompromised patients, premature babies, those with chronic pulmonary diseases, congenital heart disease, or pulmonary hypertension, or critically ill patients
Influenza a and b	Amantadine 5 mg/kg/day (max. 150 mg/day)–from 1 yr to 9 yrs of age (PO)
	Amantadine 100 mg every 12 hrs–>9 yrs of age (PO)
	Zanamivir 10 mg every 12 hrs–>12 yrs of age (inhaled)
	Oseltamivir (Tamiflu) 45 mg PO BID × 10 days (>1 yo, 15–23 kg)
	Oseltamivir (Tamiflu) 60 mg PO BID × 10 days (>1 yo, 23–40 kg)
	Oseltamivir (Tamiflu) 75 mg PO BID × 10 days (adult dose, >40 kg)
Herpes simplex or zoster	Acyclovir (250 mg/m^2/8 hrs) (IV)
	(25–50 mg/kg/8 hrs)
	OR
	Foscarnet (60 mg/kg/8 hrs) (IV)
Cytomegalovirus	Ganciclovir 2,5 mg/kg/8 hrs initial (IV)
	5 mg/kg/12 hrs (2–3 wks) or foscarnet
Fungi	Amphotericin B (1 mg/kg/day)
	Liposomal amphotericin B (3 mg/kg/day) or fluconazole 6 mg/kg/day

when this fluid contains pus. Pleural effusions can occur associated with many etiologic agents, including *S. pneumoniae*, *S. aureus*, and *S. pyogenes*. Tuberculosis is also a frequent cause of pleural effusion, and it should be considered in the differential diagnosis of certain patients. Pleural effusions are classified as transudates and empyema, according to the laboratory analysis of the pleural fluid (**Table 24.8**). Additional data include a positive microbiologic study (Gram test, culture, or other diagnostic tests, such as polymerase chain reaction). All children with a diagnosis of pleural effusion should have a diagnostic

and sometimes therapeutic thoracentesis performed. Conservative treatment of pleural infection consists of isolated antibiotic therapy or antibiotic therapy and simple drainage. Most of the small parapneumonic effusions respond to antibiotic therapy without any additional intervention. However, the pleural effusions that increase volume and/or compromise breathing in an ill, feverish child must be drained. If the child has a significant pleural infection, a thoracostomy tube should be inserted. The initial empiric IV antibiotic therapy should cover *S. pneumoniae*. Broad-spectrum antibiotics are necessary for

TABLE 24.8

PLEURAL FLUID CHARACTERISTICS

	Transudate	Exudate
pH	>7.20	<7.20
Proteins (pleural fluid /serum level rate)	<0.5	0.5
LDH (pleural fluid/serum level rate)	<0.6	0.6
LDH (UI)	<200	200
Glucose (mg/dL)	>40	<40
Red cells (mm^3)	<5000	>5000
Leukocytes (mm^3)	<10,000 (PMN)	>10,000 (PMN)

LDH, lactate dehydrogenase; PMN, polymorphonuclear neutrophil

nosocomial infections, as well as those secondary to surgery, trauma, and aspiration. The antibiotic choice should be guided by the microbiologic results.

Intrapleural fibrinolytics may shorten length of hospital stay and are recommended by some for complicated parapneumonic effusions (loculated thick fluid) or empyema. Urokinase should be administered twice per day for 3 consecutive days: 10,000 units in 10 mL of normal saline for children <1 year of age and 40,000 units in 40 mL of nor-

mal saline in those ≥1 year old. Surgical treatment should be considered in patients who remain septic due to persistent pleural collection despite chest thoracostomy and antibiotic therapy. The 3 main surgical options are (a) video-assisted thoracic surgery; (b) mini-thoracotomy, which is similar to video-assisted thoracic surgery but is an open procedure; and (c) decortication, a more prolonged and complicated procedure. An organized empyema in a symptomatic child may require a thoracotomy and decortication.

CHAPTER 25 ■ ACUTE LUNG INJURY AND ACUTE RESPIRATORY DISTRESS SYNDROME

KATHLEEN M. VENTRE • JOHN H. ARNOLD

The American-European Consensus Conference suggested that the "adult" respiratory distress syndrome be renamed the "acute" respiratory distress syndrome (ARDS) to acknowledge the existence of this condition in children. The panel defined ARDS as acute, noncardiogenic pulmonary edema with bilateral pulmonary infiltrates on chest x-ray and a ratio of PaO$_2$ to FiO$_2$ of <200. Acute lung injury (ALI) was defined similarly but with a ratio of PaO$_2$ to FiO$_2$ of 200–300. ARDS develops following either "direct" or "indirect" lung injury. Pneumonia and pulmonary aspiration are among the most common conditions with the potential to inflict direct lung injury and ARDS, but traumatic pulmonary contusion, fat embolism, submersion injury, and inhalational injury are relatively common causes as well. The most common forms of indirect lung injury include systemic condi-

tions, such as sepsis, shock, exposure to cardiopulmonary bypass, and transfusion-related lung injury.

Regardless of the inciting factors, ARDS commonly progresses through stages defined by their associated clinical, radiographic, and histopathologic features. The first, or exudative, phase is characterized by the acute development of decreased pulmonary compliance and arterial hypoxemia. The alteration in pulmonary mechanics leads to tachypnea. Arterial blood gas analysis typically reveals hypocarbia at this stage. The chest x-ray usually reveals diffuse alveolar infiltrates from pulmonary edema. The proinflammatory events that occur during the exudative phase tend to create the setting for transition into the fibroproliferative stage of ARDS, during which an increased alveolar dead space fraction and refractory pulmonary hypertension may develop as a result of chronic inflammation and scarring of the alveolar-capillary unit. The fibroproliferative phase then gives way to a recovery phase, with restoration of the alveolar epithelial barrier, gradual improvement in pulmonary compliance, resolution of arterial hypoxemia, and eventual return to premorbid pulmonary function in many patients.

By definition, the edema in ARDS is not caused by cardiac failure but results from disruption of the structural components that regulate alveolar fluid balance under normal conditions. Normally, the pulmonary capillary endothelial cells are connected by tight junctions that allow some movement of fluid, but no movement of proteins or other solutes, into the interstitial space. The alveolar epithelium, conversely, normally is not permeable to fluid, proteins, or other solutes. The rate of fluid movement into the interstitium is governed by the net difference between hydrostatic pressure and osmotic pressure in the pulmonary capillaries, relative to the pulmonary interstitium. Generally, fluid movement across a semipermeable membrane, such as the pulmonary capillary endothelial layer, is characterized by the Starling formula:

$$Q = K_f[(P_c - P_{is}) - \sigma(\pi_{pl} - \pi_{is})]$$

where

Q = filtration rate across the semipermeable membrane

K_f = membrane filtration coefficient

P_c = capillary hydrostatic pressure

P_{is} = interstitial hydrostatic pressure

σ = membrane reflection coefficient

π_{pl} = plasma oncotic pressure

π_{is} = interstitial oncotic pressure

Injury to the pulmonary surfactant system is one of the more serious manifestations of damage to the alveolar epithelium and subsequent alveolar flooding. Surfactant is produced mainly by alveolar epithelial type II cells and contains phospholipid and protein components. Its major function is to promote alveolar and small airway stability by lowering surface tension, although its principal protein constituents also have an important role in facilitating clearance of infectious organisms. The Laplace equation illustrates the relationship between surface tension (T), cavity radius (r), and the pressure (P) required to maintain the patency of a spherical structure:

$$P = 2T/r$$

During inspiration, increasing transpulmonary pressure produces little change in lung volume until the patient reaches a lower inflection point on

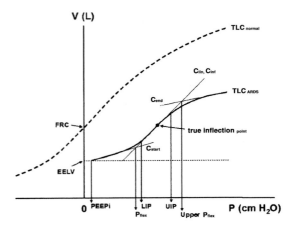

FIGURE 25.1. Volume-pressure curve in absence of disease (*dashed lines*) and in ARDS (*solid line*). Inspiratory curves are shown. Important transitions during lung inflation are indicated on the ARDS curve. Note that in ARDS, total lung capacity (TLC) is reduced, compared to TLC in the normal lung. In this example, a small amount of positive end-expiratory pressure (intrinsic PEEP, or PEEP$_i$) is present at EELV in the ARDS lung. EELV in the ARDS lung is below FRC. Compliance is indicated at various points as the slope of the volume-pressure curve. P$_{flex}$ is indicated on the curve as the intersection of the low-compliance portion of the curve obtained at low lung volume (C$_{start}$). Upper P$_{flex}$ is indicated at the transition between the nearly linear zone of maximal compliance (C$_{lin}$) and the zone of low compliance at high lung volume (C$_{end}$). The lower inflection point (LIP) and upper inflection point (UIP) are points at which the volume pressure curve begins to depart from C$_{lin}$ at the extremes of lung volume. The "true inflection point" marks the actual change in concavity of the volume-pressure curve. From Harris RS. Pressure-volume curves of the respiratory system. *Respir Care* 2005;50:78–98, with permission.

the inspiratory limb of the curve (lower P$_{flex}$) (**Fig. 25.1**). At that point, the change in lung volume produced by each upward increment of pressure (i.e., compliance) increases quickly, and then more slowly, until reaching an upper inflection point (upper P$_{flex}$) (**Fig. 25.1**) where compliance again decreases. The upward displacement of the expiratory limb relative to the inspiratory limb (**Fig. 25.2**) illustrates the difference in the transpulmonary pressures needed to maintain lung volume as the lung recoils and empties. This difference is potentiated by the properties of surfactant. In the injured lung, hysteresis is less pronounced, and the entire curve is displaced downward and rightward, reflecting the higher pressures required to achieve and maintain lung recruitment, and an overall decrease in lung compliance that is evident throughout the respiratory cycle (**Fig. 25.1,** **Fig. 25.2**).

The effect of alveolar and small-airways collapse on overall airway resistance can be explained by the

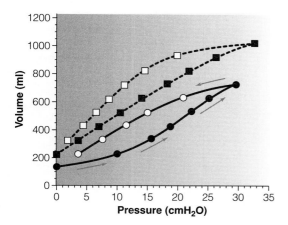

FIGURE 25.2. Pulmonary hysteresis. Volume–pressure relationships before and after lung injury. Inflation (*solid symbols*) and deflation (*open symbols*) volume-pressure data in a canine model before (*squares*) and 60 mins after (*circles*) oleic acid-induced acute lung injury. During inflation (expiration), higher lung volumes are maintained at lower transpulmonary pressures. Original experimental data are fitted with a sigmoidal equation to construct the curves ($R^2 > 0.9997$). Adapted from Venegas JG, Harris RS, Simon BA. A comprehensive equation for the pulmonary pressure-volume curve. *J Appl Physiol* 1998;84:389–95.

Hagen-Poiseuille equation describing laminar flow in straight circular tubes:

$$R = (8\eta l)/\pi r^4$$

where

    R = resistance to flow

    η = gas viscosity

    l = tube length

    r = airway radius

From this equation, it follows that a reduction in airway caliber, from peribronchiolar edema or outright airway collapse, produces a marked increase in airways resistance. Respiratory system resistance can be studied in vivo by plotting the decline in tracheal pressure following end-inspiratory airway occlusion until flow ceases and a plateau pressure is reached. Such techniques have suggested that increased total respiratory system resistance is observed in patients with ARDS as compared to controls, largely because of "mechanical unevenness" or instability of the respiratory system in this disease. In addition, there is a considerable contribution of abdominal distension to the alteration of respiratory system mechanics in patients with ALI and ARDS.

The permeability edema that is the defining feature of early ARDS sets the stage for reduced compliance and an end-expiratory lung volume (EELV) that decreases below functional residual capacity

(FRC) to a point approaching closing capacity, creating conditions that favor the development of regional atelectasis, intrapulmonary shunt, and alveolar hypoxia.

The fraction of pulmonary blood flow that ultimately enters the systemic circulation without being oxygenated is the "shunt fraction," or venous admixture. Shunted blood is low in oxygen and high in carbon dioxide, but intrapulmonary shunt does not tend to elevate systemic $PaCO_2$ because chemoreceptors sensitive to acute increases in $PaCO_2$ stimulate respiratory drive, eliminating CO_2 before an increase would be detectable by blood gas analysis.

In the upright human lung, spontaneous breathing creates a decreasing gradient of transpulmonary pressure from lung apex to lung base. In other words, the driving pressure for alveolar filling is greater in the (nondependent) apex than it is at the (dependent) lung base. Consequently, the less-distended, dependent alveoli are positioned on a more compliant portion of the volume-pressure curve, compared to the more distended nondependent alveoli (**Fig. 25.3**). Therefore, dependent alveoli collectively account for a greater portion of alveolar ventilation than do nondependent alveoli. "Physiologic shunt" fraction includes baseline $\dot{V}/\dot{Q}$ inequality, as well as blood from

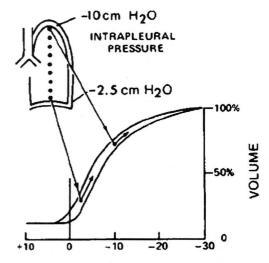

FIGURE 25.3. Regional differences in ventilation in the upright lung. The weight of the lung creates less negative intrapleural pressure at the lung base, while more negative intrapleural pressure is created at the apex. These differences translate into a decreasing transpulmonary pressure gradient in the dependent lung regions (see text). From West JB. Mechanics of breathing. In: *Respiratory Physiology: The Essentials*, 4th ed. Baltimore: Williams and Wilkins, 1990;87–113, with permission.

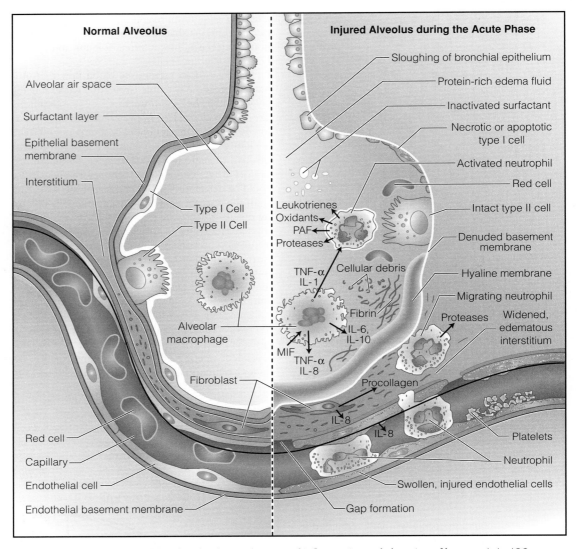

FIGURE 25.4. Cellular and molecular mechanisms of inflammation and alteration of hemostasis in ALI and ARDS. The normal alveolus is shown on the left, and the injured alveolus is shown on the right (see text). Adapted from Ware LB, Matthay MA: The acute respiratory distress syndrome. *N Engl J Med* 2000;342(18):1334–49.

the bronchial, pleural, and thebesian veins, which returns to the systemic circulation without passing through the pulmonary vascular bed. The influence of $\dot{V}/\dot{Q}$ imbalance on blood gas tensions is magnified in ALI and ARDS, in which consolidation and collapse of lung units are widespread and fluid-filled alveoli act as low $\dot{V}/\dot{Q}$ lung units with the potential to create detectable elevations in $PaCO_2$ and decreases in PaO_2.

Whether the individual patient with ALI and/or ARDS expresses, on balance, a predominantly procoagulant or anticoagulant phenotype seems likely to

be a function of the interaction between host genetics and the specific inciting factors that lead to disease development (**Fig 25.4**). Amplification of the immune response to lung injury is thus a product of redundancies and interactions among components of the innate immune system (cytokines), the complement system (C3a, C5a), products of membrane phospholipid metabolism (leukotrienes, PAF), and the coagulation cascade.

Pulmonary vascular resistance can be modified by lung volumes (**Fig 25.5**) as well as pharmacologic interventions.

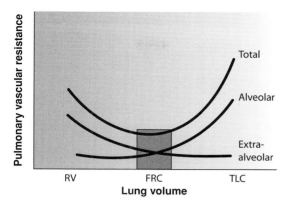

FIGURE 25.5. Effect of lung volume on pulmonary vascular resistance (PVR). "Optimal," or nadir PVR occurs at FRC. As lung volume increases toward total lung capacity (TLC), extra-alveolar resistance drops, while intra-alveolar vascular resistance escalates. As lung volume drops toward residual volume (RV), extra-alveolar vascular resistance increases as these vessels become tortuous, while alveolar hypoxia results in intra-alveolar vasoconstriction. The "Total," or net effect of these findings on overall PVR is represented by the uppermost curve. Adapted from Shekerdemian L, Bohn D. Cardiovascular effects of mechanical ventilation. *Arch Dis Child* 1999;80(5):475–80.

CLINICAL PRESENTATION

Diffuse alveolar disease that meets criteria for ALI and ARDS produces a predictable sequence of clinical changes. When fluid accumulation in the interstitial space exceeds the absorptive capacity of the pulmonary lymphatics, lung compliance declines and tachypnea ensues as the patient attempts to generate adequate minute ventilation in the face of lower tidal volumes. The eventual leakage of proteinaceous fluid into the alveolar spaces interferes with native surfactant function, creating conditions that favor regional atelectasis and small-airways closure, as well as a decrease in EELV to a point near or below closing capacity, especially in small infants and those with highly compliant chest walls (e.g., patients with neuromuscular disease). At this point, hypoxia rapidly worsens, and breathing becomes more labored in an effort to generate transpulmonary pressures sufficient to maintain alveolar patency. Hypocarbia is often present early in the disease process, when the patient first manifests tachypnea. However, as the work of breathing escalates, the $PaCO_2$ will further rise as respiratory muscle fatigue ensues. At this stage,

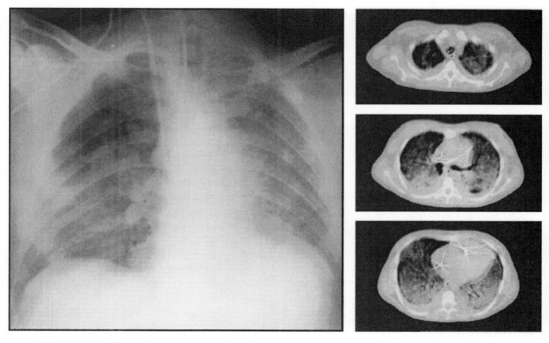

FIGURE 25.6. Nonuniform parenchymal involvement in acute respiratory distress syndrome (ARDS). AP chest x-ray and CT scans corresponding to lung apex, hilum, and base from a patient with sepsis and ARDS. Images are taken with the patient in supine position, at a positive end-expiratory pressure of 5 cm H_2O. The CT scans illustrate the influence of the gravitational axis on the pattern of alveolar consolidation in ARDS: Nondependent regions are aerated, while dependent regions remain consolidated. From Gattinoni L, Caironi P, Pelosi P, et al. What has computed tomography taught us about the acute respiratory distress syndrome? *Am J Respir Crit Care Med* 2001;164:1701–11, with permission.

TABLE 25.1

SUGGESTED THERAPY GUIDELINES FOR ALI/ARDS

	Pulmonary	Cardiovascular	Other
Resuscitation	Supplemental O_2 Early arterial access for disease identification (PaO_2/FiO_2, OI) and early implementation of therapy Consider early NPPV for alveolar recruitment in alert, cooperative patient[a] Endotracheal intubation and positive pressure ventilation for respiratory failure failing noninvasive therapy Titrate PEEP to achieve $FiO_2 \leq 0.5$–0.6/SpO_2 88%–95%. Limit tidal volume (6 mL/kg *ideal* body weight) and alveolar plateau pressure (≤ 30 cm H_2O).[b] Permissive hypercapnia unless contraindicated (coexistent increased intracranial pressure, etc.)	Crystalloid, colloid, or blood to optimize intravascular volume and support hemodynamics[c] Anticipate potentially adverse hemodynamic consequences of transition to positive pressure ventilation in setting of intravascular volume depletion Titrate supportive therapy to correct perfusion abnormalities and optimize urine output	Cultures Broad-spectrum antimicrobial agents Consider antifungal, antiviral, atypical agent coverage in immunocompromised population Consider early bronchoalveolar lavage in immunocompromised population
Escalation	Titrate PEEP upward if ongoing hypoxemia in setting of alveolar derecruitment Early transition to HFOV if high inflation pressures are necessary Consider prone positioning in selected cases Consider surfactant replacement in selected cases Consider NO in selected cases	Titrate fluid and vasoactive infusions to achieve age-appropriate blood pressure parameters and adequate end-organ function	Sedation/analgesia Neuromuscular blockade if necessary
Maintenance	Follow OI to track response to therapy Wean ventilator as allowable	Monitoring: CVP, serial clinical examination and review of organ function[d] Maintain euvolemia Diuretics	Nutrition: Implement enteral nutrition as early as feasible. Avoid excess glucose administration. Careful attention to nitrogen balance Neuromuscular blockade: Daily infusion interruption and discontinue as soon as feasible Sedation and analgesia: Daily infusion interruption and wean during plateau phase of illness
Advanced therapy	OI not improving on optimal ventilator strategy/HFOV: Consider ECMO	Consider early renal replacement therapy for persistent hypervolemia and oliguria despite diuretics	

OI, oxygenation index [100 × mean airway pressure × FiO_2]/PaO_2; NPPV, noninvasive positive pressure ventilation; PEEP, positive end-expiratory pressure HFOV, high-frequency oscillatory ventilation; CVP, central venous pressure; ECMO, extracorporeal membrane oxygenation.
[a]Early NPPV may avert need for intubation in certain immunocompromised patients.
[b]Optimal tidal volume and plateau pressure are not known, but use of 6 mL/kg has been associated with a 22% relative mortality benefit compared to 12 mL/kg. High tidal volumes are also associated with proinflammatory cytokine release.
[c]Optimal hemoglobin concentration is not known. In absence of cardiovascular disease, hemoglobin of 7–9 g/dL is probably adequate and may avert adverse effects of red cell transfusion.
[d]Current data suggest pulmonary artery catheter use in ALI/ARDS is not associated with improved outcomes and may be associated with increased incidence of catheter-related complications. CVP must be interpreted in context of surrounding compartment pressure (e.g., intrathoracic pressure for superior vena cava lines) and/or myocardial compliance. In absence of coexisting intracardiac shunt, mixed venous oxygen saturation may clarify adequacy of cardiac output.
Adapted from Fackler JC, Arnold JH, Nichols DG, et al. Acute respiratory distress syndrome. In: Rogers M, ed. *Textbook of Pediatric Intensive Care*, 3rd ed. Baltimore: Williams and Wilkins, 1996;197–233.

positive-pressure ventilation is required to open a sufficient number of atelectatic lung units for adequate gas exchange. On auscultation, the patient will typically demonstrate rales over areas of atelectasis or alveolar congestion and decreased air entry over areas that are largely consolidated. Occasionally, it is possible to appreciate wheezes over areas in which intermittent small-airways closure is occurring.

Imaging Studies

Clinical changes of early ALI and ARDS manifest on chest x-rays as diffuse alveolar infiltrates and air bronchograms that may be accompanied by pleural effusion and widespread atelectasis (**Fig. 25.6**). Areas of lung injury that are evolving into fibrosis may appear as prominent reticular opacities.

Principles of Clinical Management

The mainstay of therapy remains supportive care, of which a critically important component is the application of positive-pressure ventilation (**Table 25.1**).

CHAPTER 26 ■ CHRONIC RESPIRATORY FAILURE

THOMAS G. KEENS • SHEILA S. KUN • SALLY L. DAVIDSON WARD

Children treated in the PICU for acute respiratory failure (ARF) may emerge with chronic lung disease. A smaller proportion of survivors develops chronic respiratory failure (CRF), and may require long-term ventilatory support. Mechanical ventilation can now be performed in the home, with a relatively good quality of life for many children. The goals of ventilatory support in the home for children with CRF include (a) ensuring medical safety of the child, (b) preventing or minimizing complications, (c) optimizing the child's quality of life, (d) maximizing rehabilitative potential, and (e) reintegrating with the family.

RESPIRATORY SYSTEM IN CHILDREN

Ventilation varies with the state of the individual. It becomes less adequate during sleep, and it is less responsive to modulation by chemoreceptor input during active or rapid-eye-movement sleep. The diaphragm must perform most of the work of breathing. The factors that predispose to ventilatory muscle fatigue include hypoxia, hypercapnia, acidosis, malnutrition, hyperinflation, changes in pulmonary mechanics that cause increased work of breathing, and disuse. Underlying muscle pathology will further limit ventilatory muscle endurance. Acute respiratory failure is most commonly seen in children who experience the abrupt onset of a severe respiratory disorder, such as severe pneumonia or acute respiratory distress syndrome. This is accompanied by an increase in the respiratory load, which exceeds the ability of the child's physiology to continue performing that level of work. The ventilatory muscles fatigue while attempting to exert increased effort for breathing. Thus, the child breathes inadequately, which results in hypoxia, hypercapnia, and acidosis. Most children with acute respiratory failure can be weaned from mechanically assisted ventilation when the work of breathing decreases with recovery from the lung disease. Weaning is performed in such a way that the patient assumes increasing proportions of the work of breathing. CRF implies that a chronic, perhaps irreversible, underlying respiratory disorder is causing respiratory insufficiency that results in inadequate ventilation or hypoxia. The diagnosis of CRF is usually made once repeated attempts to wean from assisted ventilation have failed for at least 1 mo in a patient without superimposed acute respiratory disease or a patient who has a diagnosis with no prospect of being weaned from the ventilator (such as high spinal cord injury) Therapy should be directed toward (a) reducing the respiratory load, (b) improving ventilatory muscle power, and (c) increasing central respiratory drive as much as possible.

Reducing the respiratory load requires that pulmonary mechanics be optimized. Infection should be treated vigorously with appropriate antibiotics. Aggressive chest physiotherapy, with inhaled bronchodilators and anti-inflammatory agents, reduces atelectasis and pulmonary resistance by enhancing mucociliary activity and clearing secretions. In infants and young children, respiratory failure is often complicated by increased lung fluid, either interstitial or alveolar edema. Thus, diuretics may be helpful. Careful attention to electrolyte balance is required whenever diuretics are used.

Hypoxia, hypercapnia, and acidosis all decrease the efficiency of muscle energy production, predisposing to ventilatory muscle fatigue. Malnutrition decreases oxidative energy-producing enzymes in muscle. Hyperinflation places the diaphragm at a mechanical disadvantage. Pharmacologic neuromuscular blockade, sedation, and pain medications may also decrease ventilatory muscle function. Ventilator weaning techniques should be designed to improve ventilatory muscle power in an attempt to raise the child's fatigue threshold. The desired approach is similar to athletic training of any other skeletal muscle. Athletes train for performance by bursts of muscle activity (training stress) followed by rest periods. Sprint weaning is analogous to this form of athletic training, and ventilatory muscle training may result. Intermittent mandatory ventilation weaning imposes a gradually increasing functional demand on the ventilatory muscles, but it does not provide the alternating stress-and-rest training pattern. In a child with prolonged respiratory failure, sprint weaning, or sprinting, is instituted in the following way. Ventilator settings are adjusted to completely meet the child's ventilatory demands by the use of a physiologic ventilator rate for age and the attainment of normal noninvasive monitoring of gas exchange (SpO$_2$ ≥95% and end-tidal PCO$_2$ [P$_{ET}$CO$_2$] of 30–35 torr). The goal is to provide total ventilatory muscle rest. The patient is then removed from the ventilator for short periods of time during wakefulness ~4 times per day. In some cases, these initial sprints may last only 1–2 mins. The child is carefully monitored noninvasively during sprints to prevent hypoxia or hypercapnia, using pulse oximetry and P$_{ET}$CO$_2$ monitoring. Increased supplemental oxygen may be required during sprinting. Guidelines for terminating sprints, such as SpO$_2$ <95% or P$_{ET}$CO$_2$ >45–50 torr, should be provided as written orders. In addition, if the child develops signs of distress, tachypnea, retractions, diaphoresis, tachycardia, hypoxia, or hypercapnia, the sprint should be stopped. Note that the child with a respiratory control disorder may not exhibit these signs of distress. If the child develops signs of distress, tachypnea, retractions, hypoxia, or hypercapnia, the sprint is stopped. The length of each sprint is increased daily as tolerated. Initially, sprint-

ing should be performed only during wakefulness, as ventilatory muscle function and central respiratory drive are more intact during wakefulness than during sleep. Usually a child is weaned off the ventilator completely during wakefulness, before attempting to reduce sleeping ventilatory support. It is important to remember that sprint weaning requires that the child receive complete ventilatory support during rests.

Central respiratory drive can be inhibited by metabolic imbalance. Chronic metabolic alkalosis, for example, decreases central respiratory drive. Thus, electrolyte balance should be maintained, with careful attention to maintaining serum chloride concentrations >95 mEq/dl and avoiding alkalosis. Chronic hypoxia and/or hypercapnia may cause habituation of chemoreceptors, leading to a decrease in central respiratory center stimulation and decreased central respiratory drive. Although methylxanthines have been used to stimulate central respiratory drive by some clinicians, in general, pharmacologic respiratory stimulants are probably ineffective in the treatment of prolonged respiratory failure. This approach is summarized in **Table 26.1**.

Decision to Initiate Chronic Ventilatory Support

Ideally, the decision to initiate chronic ventilatory support in a patient may be made electively rather than nonelectively. Increasingly, the decision to initiate chronic ventilatory support is being made electively in order to preserve physiologic function and improve the quality of life. The most obvious example is the child with a progressive neuromuscular disorder, such as spinal muscular atrophy or muscular dystrophy. If the family opts for chronic ventilatory support, then noninvasive ventilatory support is usually initiated first, or a tracheostomy is performed and positive-pressure ventilation (PPV) is started electively before the patient develops major complications of CRF. Nocturnal ventilation allows ventilatory muscle rest and improves endurance for spontaneous breathing while awake; therefore, it is actually associated with an enhanced quality of life. Consensus has not been reached regarding the length of time that a child can remain intubated before airway damage from prolonged intubation occurs.

Candidates for Home Mechanical Ventilation

Children with CRF and relatively stable ventilator settings are candidates for home mechanical

TABLE 26.1

APPROACHES TO WEANING CHILDREN WITH PROLONGED RESPIRATORY FAILURE

Reduce the respiratory load

Relieve bronchospasm	Aerosolized bronchodilator
	Aerosolized corticosteroids or other anti-inflammatory agents
Remove excessive pulmonary secretions	Chest physiotherapy
	If ventilatory muscle weakness, consider cough-assist device
Reduce lung fluid and pulmonary edema	Diuretics with careful attention to electrolyte balance
Treat pulmonary infections	Antibiotics
	Consider aerosolized antibiotics for chronically colonized patients

Increase ventilatory muscle power

Increase ventilatory muscle strength	Eliminate or reduce hyperinflation
Increase ventilatory muscle endurance	Adequate oxygenation
	Avoid hypercapnia
	Avoid acidosis
	Achieve optimal nutrition
	Reduce respiratory load (as above)
Train ventilatory muscles to improve strength and endurance	Sprint weaning

Improve central respiratory drive

Avoid hypochloremic alkalosis	Maintain serum $Cl^- \geq 95$ mEq/dl
	Avoid chronic alkalosis
Reset chemoreceptors	Ventilate to adequate oxygenation ($SpO_2 \geq 95\%$) and ventilation ($P_{ET}CO_2 \leq 40$ torr)
Avoid respiratory depression	Reduce or avoid central nervous system–depressant medications

ventilation. The pulmonary component of the disorder is usually the most likely to provide instability. Therefore, the pulmonary disease must be such that the child does not require frequent adjustments in ventilator settings to maintain adequate gas exchange. Generally, the FIO_2 should be 40% or less. The requirement for peak inspiratory pressure (PIP) should be less than 40 cm H_2O. Although higher FIO_2 and PIP can be delivered by portable ventilators, patients requiring these settings may be too unstable to be successfully ventilated at home. Portable ventilators can now provide positive end-expiratory pressure and pressure support. Children with CRF fall into three basic diagnostic categories: ventilatory muscle weakness and neuromuscular diseases, central hypoventilation syndromes, and chronic pulmonary disease.

Ventilatory muscle weakness has three physiologic consequences. Inspiratory muscle weakness prevents children from inspiring deeply, resulting in atelectasis. Expiratory muscle weakness prevents effective coughing, resulting in decreased removal of pulmonary secretions and foreign material from the lungs, both of which increase the incidence and severity of pneumonia, which is the leading cause of

morbidity and mortality in children with neuromuscular disease. Two basic types of ventilatory muscle weakness are seen in neuromuscular disease: progressive and nonprogressive. In progressive neuromuscular disease, such as spinal muscular atrophy or muscular dystrophy, muscle weakness worsens with time, resulting in an inevitable and predictable development of CRF. In nonprogressive neuromuscular diseases, such as congenital myopathies, the muscle weakness per se does not progress. However, there may be a relative progression of impairment, because muscle strength cannot increase to overcome the increasing functional demands as the body grows. Many children with static neuromuscular disorders become nonambulatory and ventilator-dependent at or near puberty, because of the marked increase in body mass associated with the pubertal growth spurt. Often, children with chronically elevated $PCO_2 > 55–60$ torr due to ventilatory muscle weakness will develop progressive pulmonary hypertension. Although oxygen administration improves the PaO_2 and relieves hypoxia, this treatment alone is inadequate, as hypoventilation persists with resulting pulmonary hypertension. Thus, these children require home mechanical ventilation.

The cause of CRF in children with central hypoventilation syndrome is inadequate central respiratory drive, and the cause can be congenital or acquired. The congenital form may be idiopathic (congenital central hypoventilation syndrome or Ondine curse) or due to an identifiable brainstem lesion (Arnold Chiari malformation in myelomeningocele). Acquired forms of central hypoventilation syndrome may be due to brainstem trauma, tumor, hemorrhage, stroke, infection, and the like. In children with respiratory control disorders, usually little can be done to augment central respiratory drive. However, central respiratory drive can be further inhibited by metabolic imbalance, such as chronic metabolic alkalosis. Thus, serum chloride concentrations should be maintained at >95 mEq/dL, and alkalosis should be avoided. Pharmacologic respiratory stimulants are not helpful. Sedative medications and central nervous system depressants should be avoided, as these may cause apnea or hypoventilation. While central respiratory drive is impaired, the lungs and ventilatory muscles may be nearly normal, permitting reasonably stable ventilator settings to achieve adequate gas exchange.

Chronic pulmonary disease may increase the work of breathing to a level higher than can be sustained by the child. Often, the underlying lung disease is intrinsically unstable, requiring frequent adjustments in ventilator settings, but some children with chronic pulmonary disease will stabilize to the point where home mechanical ventilation is possible. No consensus has been reached on the P_{CO_2} level at which a child with chronic lung disease is considered to be in CRF, and to require chronic ventilatory support. However, in our experience, children with $P_{CO_2} \geq 60$ torr have a better clinical outcome if they use chronic ventilatory support to keep $P_{CO_2} \leq 45$ torr than if they remain with elevated P_{CO_2}. The improvement is seen primarily in improved growth, decreased hospitalization time, and avoidance of pulmonary hypertension. Many of these children will be able to wean from chronic ventilatory support with time. A common chronic lung disease for which home ventilation has been used in children is bronchopulmonary dysplasia. Newer, continuous-flow home ventilators have permitted successful home mechanical ventilation in children with restrictive lung disease, such as hypoplastic lungs from thoracic restriction (skeletal dysplasias) or interstitial lung diseases. Home mechanical ventilation has also been used in children with advanced obstructive lung disease, such as cystic fibrosis, as a bridge to lung transplantation. However, children with unstable lung disease, requirements for high oxygen and peak inspiratory pressures, or the need for frequent changes in ventilator settings are poor candidates for home mechanical ventilation.

Philosophy of Chronic Ventilatory Support

For most children on home mechanical ventilation, weaning is not a realistic goal in the short term. In order to optimize quality of life, these children must have energy available for other physical activities. Thus, ventilators are adjusted to completely meet their ventilatory demands, leaving much of their energy available for other activities. For children without significant lung disease, ventilators are adjusted to provide a $P_{ET}CO_2$ of 30–35 torr and a $SpO_2 \geq 95\%$. For children who do not require assisted ventilation while awake, ventilating to $P_{CO_2} \leq 35$ torr during sleep is associated with better spontaneous ventilation while awake. Optimal ventilation also avoids atelectasis and the development of coexisting lung disease. It has also been our experience that children who receive chronic ventilatory support actually have fewer complications and generally do better clinically, with some degree of hyperventilation during assisted ventilation. For the child who requires home mechanical ventilation, mobility and quality of life are maximized if the child can breathe unassisted for portions of the day. Even if a child cannot be weaned completely from assisted ventilation, nocturnal ventilation preserves waking quality of life and allows the ventilatory muscles a recovery period during the time when the patient is at highest risk for hypoventilation.

Modalities of Home Mechanical Ventilation

The ideal ventilators for home use are different from those used in hospitals for the treatment of acute respiratory failure. Because many children who require home mechanical ventilation do not have severe lung disease, a number of different techniques are available for providing chronic ventilatory support at home, including (a) portable positive-pressure ventilator via tracheostomy, (b) bi-level positive airway pressure ventilation via a mask or other interface, (c) negative-pressure chest shell (cuirass), wrap, or portable tank ventilator, or (d) diaphragm pacing.

Portable Positive-Pressure Ventilator via Tracheostomy

Portable PPV via tracheostomy is the most common method of providing assisted ventilation for infants and children in the home. Commercially available electronic PPVs have the capability for battery operation, are relatively portable, and maximize mobility. Portable PPVs are not as powerful, technologically sophisticated, or as versatile as hospital ventilators.

Consequently, when infants and children acquire a superimposed respiratory infection, portable ventilators may not be capable of adequately ventilating the child and hospitalization may be required. Most ventilator-assisted infants and small children are subject to frequent respiratory infections, which often require hospitalization and assisted ventilation with higher settings. A tracheostomy offers the advantage of providing ready access to the airway for hospital ventilators without the need for endotracheal intubation. For home mechanical ventilation, small, uncuffed tracheostomy tubes are preferred, as the work of breathing required to overcome the increased resistance is performed by the ventilator, not the child. The rationale for the small uncuffed tracheostomy tube is to (a) minimize the risk of tracheomalacia or tracheal mucosal damage, (b) allow a large expiratory leak so that the child may speak, and (c) provide a margin of safety because the child may still be able to ventilate around the tracheostomy tube. Further, the use of a one-way, positive-closure speaking valve enables the child to phonate from early childhood and thus to speak relatively normally in childhood and adolescence. Small, uncuffed tracheostomy tubes are associated with leaks, which can be large and variable, especially in small children. If the same PIP is achieved on each breath, the lungs are inflated to the same tidal volume, dependent on pulmonary mechanics, regardless of the amount of leak around the tracheostomy. Because of this, pressure ventilation is preferred, and it can be easily utilized on newer portable home ventilators with continuous flow. However, portable ventilators without continuous flow are volume-preset ventilators. A significant portion of the ventilator-delivered breath escapes in the leak around the uncuffed tracheostomy. The tracheostomy leak can be compensated for by using the ventilator in a pressure-limited modality (also known as pressure plateau ventilation) (**Fig. 26.1**). The remainder of the ventilator tidal volume is not delivered to the patient. It is important to note that the ventilator's high-pressure alarm, useful in detecting an occluded tracheostomy tube, will not function when pressure plateau is used. Thus, a back-up alarm, such as a pulse oximeter, is required. Pressure plateau ventilation is very successful in home ventilation of infants and small children. A second ventilator is required for those who require ventilatory support ≥20 hrs/day or who live a long distance from respiratory home care vendors who can provide emergency service in the event of malfunction.

Tracheostomy

A tracheostomy is performed when CRF is evident. After a tracheostomy is performed, it usually takes 7 days for the track to establish and mature. The first

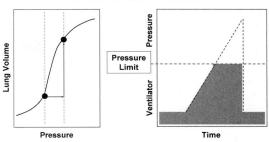

FIGURE 26.1. Pressure plateau ventilation. If the lungs are inflated to the same pressure on every breath, the same tidal volume will be achieved, according to the pressure-volume characteristics of the lungs (*left panel*). To establish pressure plateau ventilation on a volume preset ventilator without continuous flow (*right panel*), the pressure limit is set with a pressure pop-off valve to the desired peak inspiratory pressure. The ventilator-delivered tidal volume is set high to inflate the lungs and to compensate for the tracheostomy leak and compliance factors of the ventilator circuit. Even though the tracheostomy leak is variable, the lungs will be inflated to the same inspiratory pressure on each breath, ensuring a predictable tidal volume.

tracheostomy tube change is performed by an otolaryngologist to ensure that no complications arise with granulation tissue or false track and to document easy reinsertion. One of the most common complications for a child with a tracheostomy is mucous plugging. No standard scheduled time for suctioning is defined, as each child is different, and tracheal suctioning needs vary. Hence, vigilance for airway obstruction must be keen and constant. Mucous plugging is reportedly more prevalent at nighttime, when bedside observation is less rigorous. As the consequence of mucous plugging can be serious, caregivers should be trained to routinely triage a "breathing problem" by inspecting the airway for its patency. When in doubt, caregivers should suction and then change the entire tracheostomy tube. The weight of ventilator tubing pulling on the tracheostomy can cause erosion, laceration of the skin, and an exacerbation of granulation tissue growth. Bleeding from aggressive suctioning is another common problem, which uncommonly can lead to potential life-threatening bleeding in extreme situations. Granulation tissue forms from persistent irritation from suctioning and can obstruct the airway, compromising ventilation. Granulation tissue is an indication for bronchoscopy and possible laser removal. Tracheitis is a common complaint that requires medical attention. When systemic signs and symptoms of infection are not present, inhaled antibiotics are helpful to reduce upper respiratory infection and prevent pneumonia. If a tracheostomy tube is dislodged accidentally, an immediate replacement is recommended to ensure adequate ventilation and airway access. Tracheostomy stomas can shrink down and close in a very short time. A spare tracheostomy tube is necessary as a back-up at all times. While we advocate a small, uncuffed tracheostomy tube, some patients require a customized length or an extension from the stoma site. Newly developed types allow choices. A few children, especially the older ones, might need cuffed tubes to decrease the leak and allow better ventilation during sleep, when upper airway resistance decreases. Cuffed tubes, which are inflated during sleep, can almost always be deflated during wakefulness, permitting speech. Recommended cuffs can be tight to the shaft or with light, soft sleeves

Ventilator Circuits

A circuit is required to deliver air from a PPV to the patient. Gas from the ventilator goes through a heated humidification system. Ventilator gas must be humidified for infants and children. The desired temperature range is 26°–29°C (80°–85°F). Condenser humidifiers are not as effective for infants and small children as heated humidifiers, but they can be used for travel or for short periods of time. The circuit is usually connected to the tracheostomy with a swivel adapter. Dead space between the tracheostomy and exhalation valve should be minimized, to avoid elevated PCO_2. Two to three circuits are generally provided for home care, and they are changed each day. The circuit (tubing, valve, and cascade) not in use should be cleaned with mild soap and water, then rinsed in a disinfectant (such as 10% alkyl dimethylbenzol ammonium chloride), and dried.

Monitoring and Alarm Systems

Infants and children who require home mechanical ventilation have very little respiratory reserve. Caregivers should be trained to assess color change, chest excursion, respiratory distress, tachycardia, tachypnea, diaphoresis, edema, lethargy, and tolerance for spontaneous ventilation off the ventilator. Alarm systems are crucial, but they do not take the place of a trained and attentive caregiver. All PPVs have a low-pressure alarm that sounds in the event that a minimally acceptable pressure level is not being achieved. These alarms are important to detect a sudden disconnect of the ventilator from the tracheostomy or other very large leak in the circuit and are usually set to alarm if the maximal airway pressure achieved on a breath is less than the desired PIP minus 10 cm H_2O. However, if an infant or small child with a small tracheostomy is decannulated with the small tracheostomy still connected to the ventilator, sufficient resistance from the small tracheostomy tube

alone may keep the low pressure alarm from sounding. Ventilators also have high pressure alarms that sound if the pressure required to deliver a breath is too high. Very useful in detecting a plug or occlusion of the tracheostomy tube, these alarms are usually set to sound if the maximal airway pressure achieved on a breath is >10 cm H_2O above the desired PIP. As mentioned above, high pressure alarms will not sound if a ventilator is being used in a pressure plateau or pressure-controlled mode. Therefore, an additional monitoring system that is external to the ventilator and monitors the child directly is required. Currently, a pulse oximeter, which can alarm for low SpO_2 or low heart rate, is the recommended patient monitor. Alarms are usually set to sound for SpO_2 <85% or heart rate <60 bpm for ages 1–12 mos and 50 bpm for those >1 year of age. The pulse oximeter alarm should be used at all times during sleep and when a ventilator-dependent patient is not being observed. More sophisticated home ventilators have low- and high-minute ventilation alarms.

Bi-level Positive Airway Pressure Ventilation by Mask or Nasal Prongs

Noninvasive intermittent PPV is delivered via a nasal mask, nasal prongs, or face mask using a bi-level positive airway pressure ventilator. This technique is commonly used in older children but has also been used successfully in infants and small children. Bi-level ventilation can be used in children who require ventilatory support only during sleep and who have relatively mild intrinsic lung disease. Thus, bi-level ventilation is most frequently used in children with neuromuscular disorders and central hypoventilation syndromes. Bi-level ventilation has also been used for children with chronic lung disease who require ventilatory muscle rest. Bi-level ventilators are smaller, less expensive, and generally easier to use than conventional ventilators. Newer models have pressure and apnea alarms and adjustable rise times. Inspiratory positive airway pressure (IPAP) and expiratory positive airway pressure (EPAP) can be adjusted independently. The IPAP-to-EPAP difference is proportional to tidal volume. Tidal volume increases linearly, with IPAP-to-EPAP difference up to ~14 cm H_2O. Four modes of bi-level ventilation can be used: (a) continuous positive airway pressure, (b) spontaneous mode, which assists only generated breaths, (c) timed mode, which controls ventilation at a set rate, and (d) spontaneous/timed mode, which assists generated breaths as long as the patient breathes at least the set back-up rate and adds control breaths if the patient does not breathe at the minimum back-up rate. Only the spontaneous/timed and timed modes guarantee breath delivery and should be used in children with respiratory control disorders because these patients cannot be trusted to generate their own adequate respirations. Most side effects related to bi-level ventilation are minimal, such as rhinitis, aerophagia, conjunctival injection, and skin breakdown, most of which can be avoided by proper fitting of the mask. Noninvasive bi-level ventilation is not as powerful as PPV via tracheostomy. Thus, children may require intubation and more sophisticated ventilatory support during acute exacerbations, such as respiratory syncytial virus (RSV) infections, the risk of which is higher in young children.

Negative-Pressure Ventilation

Negative-pressure ventilators apply a negative pressure outside the chest and abdomen to generate inspiration. A chest shell ventilator uses a dome-shaped shell that is fitted over the anterior chest and abdomen. The negative-pressure wrap ventilator is a "jump suit" that fits snugly around the neck, wrists, and ankles to minimize leaks. A metal "cage" inside the jump suit creates a space where negative pressure can be generated during inspiration. A portable tank is a negative-pressure ventilator into which the child's torso is placed, with the head outside. Negative inspiratory pressure is generated inside the chest shell, wrap, or portable tank, which expands the chest and upper abdomen. The negative pressure is proportional to the tidal volume but may be limited by leaks around the chest shell or wrap. These ventilators can provide effective ventilation in children and adolescents, sometimes without a tracheostomy. However, with negative-pressure ventilation, synchronous activation of the upper-airway muscles does not occur as with spontaneous breathing. Thus, airway occlusion can occur when breaths are generated by a negative-pressure ventilator during sleep. Therefore, infants and young children may require a tracheostomy. In that the major potential benefit of negative-pressure ventilators is that a tracheostomy may not be needed in older children, this technique may offer little advantage over PPV in the infant or young child. Negative-pressure ventilators are not as portable as electronic positive-pressure ventilators, nor are they battery-operated. Negative-pressure ventilation may permit decannulation of a tracheostomy. Upper airway obstruction can be minimized by tonsillectomy and adenoidectomy. Reducing the inspiratory negative pressure and/or increasing the inspiratory time may also reduce obstructive apneas. Negative-pressure ventilation is not as powerful as PPV via tracheostomy. Thus, children

may require intubation and more sophisticated ventilatory support during acute exacerbations (e.g., RSV infections), the risk of which is higher in young children. The major benefit of negative-pressure ventilation is that a tracheostomy may not be required.

Diaphragm Pacing

Diaphragm pacing generates breathing using the child's own diaphragm as the respiratory pump. An antenna is taped on the skin over subcutaneously implanted receivers. The transmitter generates a train of pulses for each breath, and the receiver converts this energy to standard electrical current, which is directed to a phrenic nerve electrode by lead wires. The amount of electrical voltage is proportional to the diaphragmatic contraction, which generates tidal volume. In children, simultaneous bilateral diaphragm pacing is generally required to achieve optimal ventilation. Use of pacers requires that the phrenic nerves and the diaphragm function appropriately to enable effective ventilation. Therefore, ventilatory muscle myopathy and phrenic neuropathy are contraindications to pacer use. Obstructive apnea can be a complication of diaphragm pacing during sleep, because synchronous upper airway skeletal muscle contraction does not occur with inspiration. In general, diaphragm pacers can be used only up to ~14 hrs a day, and they cannot be used for 24 hrs continuously. Thus, patients who require ventilatory support 24 hrs/day should have an alternate form of ventilation for part of the day if pacers are used. The surgical technique is tricky, and use of the pacers once implanted requires a fair amount of experience. Therefore, diaphragm pacing should generally be performed in centers with experience in the technique. This technique may provide benefit to select groups of children with central hypoventilation syndrome or high cervical spinal cord injury.

HOSPITAL MANAGEMENT PRIOR TO DISCHARGE

Therapy for children who receive home mechanical ventilation should be directed toward relief of bronchospasm, clearance of pulmonary secretions, reduction in lung water, treatment of pulmonary infections, and prevention of aspiration. These children usually benefit from aerosolized bronchodilators followed by intensive pulmonary physiotherapy on a routine basis. Patients should receive the routine immunizations and annual split virion influenza vaccine. The patient's respiratory status must be stable on the child's home ventilator for at least

---

TABLE 26.2

NEEDS OF THE VENTILATOR-ASSISTED CHILD PRIOR TO HOSPITAL DISCHARGE

1. Medical stability of the child's condition, permitting relatively constant ventilator settings
2. Family commitment to care for the ventilator assisted child at home
3. Realistic assessment of the medical care requirements and arrangement for the family's ability to meet them, including in-home nursing assistance, if necessary
4. Thorough education of the family and other caregivers in technical aspects of medical care and equipment operation
5. Selection of a respiratory equipment vendor with ability to supply and service the desired equipment and 24-hr emergency availability
6. Selection of a local primary pediatrician to provide well child care, emergency care, and liaison with community resources
7. Informing of community emergency medical systems of the ventilator-assisted child and his/her needs
8. Notification of telephone and power companies to provide priority service in the event of interruption of service
9. Arrangement for routine and emergency transport from home to the medical center responsible for medical care
10. Arrangement for other medical, psychosocial, and developmental support, such as physical and occupational therapy, respite care, and school

1–2 weeks prior to discharge (**Table 26.2**). It is important to emphasize that settings on a home ventilator do not provide the same ventilation in the child as the same settings on a hospital ventilator. Therefore, the child must be tested on home equipment before discharge. Invariably, ventilator settings must be increased on the home ventilator to achieve the same level of gas exchange achieved on a hospital ventilator. In the hospital, it is important to use the actual ventilator and circuits that the child will use in the home. The equipment essential for home care of the ventilator-assisted child is listed in **Table 26.3**.

TABLE 26.3

HOME RESPIRATORY EQUIPMENT FOR HOME MECHANICAL VENTILATION (POSITIVE PRESSURE VENTILATOR VIA TRACHEOSTOMY)

1. Electronic portable positive pressure ventilator with:
   1 humidifier with humidifier jar
   1 heater and thermometer, water trap
   2 circuits with bleed-in adapter/connector
   Flex tubing
   Automobile cigarette lighter adaptor for car use, if available
2. Backup ventilator: Absolutely essential for patients who require $\geq$20 hrs/day of assisted ventilation or who are living long distances from medical and technical support
3. Deep-cycle marine gel battery with case and cables for operation of the ventilator and battery charger (unless built into the ventilator)
4. E-cylinder of oxygen with stand and regulator for emergency use
   Supplemental oxygen system, if necessary
5. Aerosol delivery system with:
   2 aerosol setups
   2 trach adapters
   2 22/15-cm connector/adapters
6. Portable suction machine with battery pack, connecting tubing, appropriately sized tracheal suction catheters, and tonsil fine-tip catheters
7. Resuscitation bag with appropriately sized mask
8. Pulse oximeter as an alarm system (alarm settings: SpO_2 <85%; low heart rate <60 bpm age 1–12 mos, <50 bpm age $\geq$1 yr); high heart rate off)
9. Other essential accessories:
   Tracheostomy tube holder
   Artificial nose (HMV = head moisture exchanger)
   In-line speaking valve
   Bacterial filter

TABLE 26.4

MANAGEMENT OF COMPLICATIONS OF HOME MECHANICAL VENTILATION

Medical problem	Management
Hypoxia	Evaluate oxygenation by noninvasive monitoring. If SpO_2 is <95%, add supplemental oxygen or increase ventilatory support.
Hypoventilation	Evaluate ventilator settings by noninvasive monitoring. If $P_{ET}CO_2$ is >35 torr, increase ventilatory support.
Chronic lung disease	Have a high index of suspicion. The diagnosis of chronic lung disease is often missed in ventilator-assisted children. Treatment includes bronchodilators (aerosolized and/or systemic), pulmonary physiotherapy, and diuretics.
Pulmonary hypertension	Ensure adequate oxygenation and ventilation. Periodically monitor electrocardiogram and echocardiogram for signs of pulmonary hypertension.
Pulmonary infections	Complete immunizations, including influenza A/B split virion vaccine. Treat respiratory infections aggressively with antibiotics and chest physiotherapy.
Growth delay	Ensure adequate caloric quantity and quality. Growth delay is a complication of chronic hypoxia or hypercapnia. Assess oxygenation and ventilation.

Service contracts for the maintenance of the ventilator and other respiratory equipment must be arranged. A backup ventilator and other essential equipment should be provided to all families, but *must* be provided for children who are ventilator-dependent ≥20 hrs/day or when they live long distances from medical or technical assistance. A resuscitation bag is necessary for resuscitation and to permit manual ventilation in the event of power failure or ventilator malfunction. The physical environment of the home should be evaluated for adequacy of space, grounded electrical outlets, and wiring. Prior to discharge from the hospital, the family must become familiar with all aspects of their child's care. Children who are ventilator assisted in the home must be closely linked to a medical center capable of providing the subspecialty care required. The local telephone and utility companies must be notified in writing of the patient's location and condition. In the event of a power outage or other interruption of service, the home ventilator patient should be given priority for restoration of service.

HOME MANAGEMENT OF THE VENTILATOR-ASSISTED CHILD

Following any change in the respiratory system (severe infection, hospitalization, etc.), settings should be checked and readjusted. These evaluations are usually performed by polysomnography, and it is important to monitor $P_{ET}CO_2$ as an indication of the adequacy of ventilation. Sleep studies during daytime naps may also be adequate for the evaluation of ventilator settings if the child's clinical course is reasonably stable. Supplemental oxygen may be required during spontaneous breathing and/or during mechanically assisted ventilation. Oxygen requirements must be assessed at regular intervals using noninvasive monitoring of oxygenation. Because home mechanical ventilation may not completely meet the ventilatory requirements at all times, even the most successfully managed patients may be exposed to periods of alveolar hypoxia and hypoventilation (**Table 26.4**). Thus, all ventilator-assisted children are at risk for development of pulmonary hypertension and cor pulmonale. The usual clinical findings of right-heart failure may not be present until late in the course. Echocardiography may be a more sensitive method for following right-heart function. When signs of pulmonary hypertension are discovered, it should be assumed that the level of mechanical ventilation is inadequate until proven otherwise. Common childhood illnesses pose a unique threat to the ventilator-assisted child. Placement of a ventilator-assisted child in the school system poses unique challenges to the teachers and the school district. Whenever possible, it is desirable to educate a ventilator-assisted child in as normal a school setting as possible. When the discharge team works closely with school district personnel, the optimal educational setting for the child can often be arranged. Educating school officials about the true nature of the child's disorder often eases fear and facilitates school placement and acceptance. Obviously, some children are better served in special schools, but this is usually dependent on disease involvement in bodily systems other than the respiratory system. Even with sophisticated management at home, venti-lator assisted children may succumb to a catastrophe stemming from a simple problem, such as a disconnected ventilator or plugged tracheostomy, emphasizing the need for compulsive care. However, home ventilator equipment failure is uncommon, occurring only approximately once every 1.3 patient-years.

CHAPTER 27 ■ SLEEP AND BREATHING

SALLY L. DAVIDSON WARD • THOMAS G. KEENS

Sleep-related breathing disorders (SRBD) may be severe enough to warrant admission to the PICU for management, or these patients may require PICU monitoring following surgical therapy. In addition, previously unrecognized SRBD may complicate the course of PICU patients admitted for other reasons. Breathing is under both voluntary and involuntary control during wakefulness. Chemoreceptor activity ensures that minute ventilation is appropriately matched to metabolic needs, whereas voluntary control of ventilation allows the integrated performance of complex behavioral activities. The ventilatory responses to hypoxemia and hypercapnia, both potent stimuli of chemoreceptor activity during wakefulness, are blunted during sleep. Important respiratory reflexes, such as coughing and swallowing, are also inhibited by sleep. The changes in lung volume that occur with moving from the upright to supine position reduce the caudal traction on the upper airway, thus increasing airway collapsibility. Rapid eye movement (REM) accounts for ~20% of normal sleep time in adults and children and 50% of sleep time in newborn infants.

OBSTRUCTIVE SLEEP APNEA SYNDROME

The most common form of sleep-disordered breathing in childhood is obstructive sleep apnea syndrome (OSAS). Obstructive sleep apnea (OSA) is defined as an absence of airflow at the nose and mouth despite continued respiratory efforts. Discrete events that are partial in nature (i.e., reduced but not absent airflow) are termed *obstructive hypopneas* and are often accompanied by hypoxemia, hypercapnia, and sleep disruption. Central apnea can be differentiated from obstructive apneas by monitors (**Fig. 27.1**). The patency of the upper airway during sleep is determined by the bony and soft tissue anatomy of the airway and the upper airway muscle tone. The latter is influenced both by state (wakefulness vs. sleep; and REM vs. non-REM sleep) and by neural and chemical controls. A number of conditions predispose to OSAS; the most common are listed in **Table 27.1**. These etiologies have the feature of an anatomically or functionally narrowed upper airway in common. With the onset of the obesity epidemic in children, the landscape of sleep-disordered breathing has changed dramatically, with many children and adolescents now at risk for severe obesity related OSAS. Complications of OSAS include systemic and pulmonary hypertension, failure to thrive, nocturnal enuresis, and worsening of parasomnias, such as sleepwalking. Because neither history nor physical exam is sufficient to firmly establish the diagnosis of OSAS, a polysomnogram (PSG; sleep study) is required to reliably make the diagnosis. Normative PSG values have been established for children and are quite different from those used in adults, as shown in **Table 27.2**. The importance of using age-appropriate normative values is illustrated by the fact that normal children have only 1–2 obstructive apneas or hypopneas per hour of sleep, whereas adults may have as many as 5 obstructive events per hour of sleep and still be considered normal.

Some patients are at higher risk for postoperative complications and require a higher level of care, often in the PICU for intensive cardiorespiratory monitoring. Complications of adenotonsillectomy (T&A) include postoperative bleeding, upper airway obstruction secondary to airway edema, pulmonary edema, and respiratory failure. Diagnostic groups at the highest risk for postoperative complications are listed in **Table 27.3**. A preoperative review of the history and the PSG can identify which patients can be scheduled for same-day surgery and those who

Central Apnea

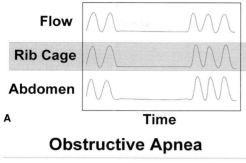

Obstructive Apnea

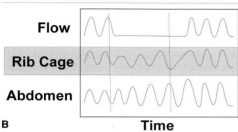

FIGURE 27.1. Home monitor detection of central and obstructive apnea. Home monitors detect breathing by chest wall motion (transthoracic impedance). Therefore, they can detect central apneas (**A**) because there is no chest wall movement (*gray area*). However, they cannot detect obstructive apneas (**B**) because there is chest wall movement (*gray area*).

will require postoperative care in the PICU. Increasingly, children with morbid obesity are presenting with OSAS. Unlike the majority of children with OSAS, respiratory control can be altered with resetting of chemoreceptor function, resulting in daytime hypoventilation. In this instance, ventilation may be dependent on hypoxic drive, requiring that oxygen be used judiciously and necessitating close monitoring, both preoperatively and postoperatively.

Therapy to support children with respiratory compromise following T&A or other airway surgery can include prolonged intubation or a nasopharyngeal airway. The use of noninvasive ventilation,

---

TABLE 27.1

CONDITIONS THAT PREDISPOSE TO OBSTRUCTIVE SLEEP APNEA SYNDROME IN CHILDREN

Adenotonsillar hypertrophy
Obesity
Craniofacial abnormalities
Down syndrome
Sickle cell disease
Cerebral palsy

---

either continuous or bi-level positive airway pressure, is attractive, as it avoids intubation and can often be performed in a pediatric unit after the patient is stable. However, some practitioners have questioned the safety of positive airway pressure in the immediate postoperative period, with concerns regarding subcutaneous emphysema dissecting at the surgical site, bleeding, or uncomfortable drying of the upper airway.

Most children with OSAS will be treated with T&A as first-line therapy, even if other anatomic or functional abnormalities are likely contributing to the upper airway obstruction. However, some will undergo a more extensive procedure, uvulopalatopharyngoplasty, which includes removal not only of the tonsils but the tonsillar pillars and uvula as well. This procedure is most often reserved for patients with cerebral palsy or Down syndrome, who have a high probability for residual obstruction following T&A alone. Mandibular distraction osteogenesis is being used with increasing frequency for infants and children with syndromes that include microagnathia. Pierre Robin syndrome, Treacher-Collins syndrome, and conditions that include hemifacial microsomia are examples. Treatment of OSAS in patients with Beckwith-Wiedemann (and occasionally Down syndrome) may require tongue reduction surgery. As a whole, the group of children who require complex surgical treatment for OSAS tend to have more severe sleep-disordered breathing and other risk factors for postoperative difficulties. Thus, they should be observed for a period of time in the PICU and may require several days of intubation following surgery.

Occasionally, the initial presentation of patients with OSAS will be as acute respiratory failure. This is less common in the current era, when the recognition of sleep-disordered breathing has increased, and the literature contains little evidence to guide treatment. These patients may be otherwise normal or have one of the risk factors listed in **Table 27.3**. Unlike the majority of patients with OSAS, they may have experienced long-term hypercapnia with resulting blunting of their respiratory drive, necessitating extreme caution in the use of supplemental oxygen. Pulmonary hypertension with right heart failure and pulmonary edema is often present, which will require treatment with diuretics and cardiology evaluation. Long-standing upper airway obstruction may have prevented adequate clearance of pulmonary secretions, and treatment with antibiotics may be indicated. Systemic steroids can be administered to acutely decrease the size of adenoidal and tonsillar tissue.

The stress of surgery has important effects on sleep architecture that can result in sleep

TABLE 27.2

NORMAL VALUES FOR PEDIATRIC POLYSOMNOGRAPHY

	Normal	Abnormal
Apnea hypopnea index (events/hr)	<1	>1
Maximal end-tidal P_{CO_2} ($P_{ET}CO_2$; torr)	≤53	>54
Duration of hypoventilation ($P_{ET}CO_2$ >45 torr; % of total sleep time)	≤45%	>46%
Minimal S_pO_2 (%)	92%	<91%
Fall in S_pO_2 (%)	≤8%	>9%

Data from McNamara F, Sullivan CE. Obstructive sleep apnea in infants: Relation to family history of sudden infant death syndrome, apparent life-threatening events, and obstructive sleep apnea. *J Pediatr* 2000;136:318–23.

fragmentation and deprivation and REM sleep reduction. REM sleep may be inhibited on the first postoperative night, but REM sleep rebounds on the second or third night.

Perioperative use of positive airway pressure therapy has been reported to reduce complications in adult patients with OSAS. Certainly, if this therapy has been used at home, arrangements must be made to continue it after surgery. Although patients with untreated OSAS may benefit from positive-pressure support after surgery, pressure titration and adaptation of the patient to the mask interface may be difficult when the child is recovering from surgery. Judicious use of narcotics in pain management, avoiding or minimizing sedation, and careful respiratory monitoring with frequent assessment of airway status are required with OSAS.

SUDDEN INFANT DEATH SYNDROME

Sudden infant death syndrome (SIDS) is defined as the sudden, unexpected death (apparently occurring

TABLE 27.3

CONDITIONS WITH A HIGHER RISK OF COMPLICATIONS FOLLOWING ADENOTONSILLECTOMY

Age <3 yrs
Severe OSAS (profound hypoxemia, AHI >10, significant hypoventilation)
Morbid obesity
Neuromuscular disease
Pulmonary hypertension
Down syndrome
Craniofacial anomalies

OSAS, obstructive sleep apnea syndrome; AHI, apnea hypopnea index

during sleep) of an infant <1 year of age that remains unexplained after a thorough investigation, including performance of a complete autopsy and review of the circumstances of death and the clinical history. The typical clinical scenario is that parents or caregivers place their apparently healthy baby down to sleep for an overnight sleeping period or a daytime nap. They return some time later to find that their baby has died. In some cases, the parents or caregivers have been within hearing distance of the baby, and they have returned within 30 mins of putting their baby down, to find that the baby has died during that short period of time. Yet, no sounds suggested that struggling occurred. Thus, SIDS appears to occur swiftly and silently. In a very small percentage of babies, resuscitation successfully retrieves a heartbeat, though spontaneous ventilation does not return, and the infant is transported to a PICU on life support. These babies should be evaluated for disorders that can cause rapid death, including sepsis, trauma (particularly head trauma), cardiac lesions (serious arrhythmias or anomalous coronary arteries), metabolic disorders, and respiratory disorders, (pneumonia or craniofacial abnormalities predisposing to obstructive sleep apnea syndrome). If child abuse or neglect is suspected, the intensivist should notify appropriate legal authorities. All states in the US and most Western countries require a thorough postmortem investigation, including an autopsy, to determine the cause of death of babies who die suddenly outside of a hospital. By definition, the autopsy does not reveal an identifiable cause of death in SIDS babies.

Usually, the "SIDS" event is accompanied by such severe hypoxemia that organs are not useful for transplantation. Infrequently, however, a baby who is diagnosed with brain death but has a heartbeat on life support may be a suitable organ donor. If the intensivist believes that organs may be suitable for transplantation, permission of the medical examiner is usually required before organs can be harvested.

The most important aspect of the intensivist's care of such SIDS infants is to provide the surviving family members with information about SIDS and resources for support. If the infant does not have evidence of trauma or another cause of death, SIDS is most likely to emerge as the cause of death after the postmortem evaluation. When speaking with the parents, the intensivist can indicate that it appears to have been a SIDS death, although further investigations and autopsy are needed to confirm. As an authority in healthcare, the intensivist can emphasize to parents that SIDS is a natural cause of death. Based on our current knowledge, SIDS parents do nothing to cause the death, and they could not have done anything to prevent it. SIDS parent support groups are the single best resource for SIDS parents; group participants are available 24 hrs/day to speak with newly bereaved SIDS parents and to provide comfort and support. In the US, the national SIDS parent support organization is First Candle/SIDS Alliance. In the UK, the support organization is called the Foundation for the Study of Infant Deaths, and in Canada, it is the Canadian Foundation for the Study of Infant Deaths.

By definition, SIDS occurs in the first year of life. It is most common between 2 and 4 months of age. It is less common in the first month of life. Sleeping environment plays an important role in SIDS. Sleeping in the prone position, on soft bedding, with soft items in the bed, overheating, and possibly bed sharing are all associated with an increased risk for SIDS. The SIDS rate has fallen dramatically since 1992 due to the "Back to Sleep" campaign, which seeks to educate parents regarding safe infant sleep practices.

APPARENT LIFE-THREATENING EVENTS

An apparent life-threatening event (ALTE) is defined as an event that is frightening to the observer, in which the infant is observed to have color change (cyanosis or pallor), tone change (limpness, rarely stiffness), apnea, and in which vigorous stimulation, mouth-to-mouth breathing, or resuscitation are required to revive the infant. In most cases, observers feared that the infant was in the process of dying. Sometimes, infants appear to respond quickly, and they may appear entirely normal when medically examined at a later time. Other infants require intensive intervention or resuscitation, and they may still exhibit signs of a serious hypoxic event several minutes later. It is this latter group, with persistent cardiorespiratory instability, who will usually be admitted to a PICU for observation and treatment. The presence of laboratory evidence for severe hypoxia (acidosis or elevated lactate, liver enzymes, or urinary hypoxanthines) can contribute to the assessment of the severity of the event. In order for a diagnosis of ALTE to be made, most clinicians require that significant intervention was necessary to revive the baby.

Clinically, infants who present with an ALTE are of concern because it has been believed that ALTEs are associated with an increased risk for SIDS. However, no scientific evidence supports this belief. The most important difference between ALTE and SIDS is that ALTE babies survive their episodes, while SIDS babies die. SIDS babies usually die from only one event. ALTE babies often have survived one or more events, even before treatment.

Principles of Management

Infants who experienced an ALTE and are being admitted to a PICU have evidence of ongoing cardiorespiratory instability, metabolic acidosis (presumably from a prolonged hypoxic event), or evidence of some other potentially life-threatening condition. Arterial blood gas, blood sugar, and chest x-ray are first-line diagnostic procedures. If the infant appears to be septic, a diagnostic evaluation for sepsis will be necessary, including a lumbar puncture. A list of possible etiologies for ALTE and appropriate diagnostic testing is shown in **Table 27.4**. Sleep studies are frequently used to evaluate infants with ALTE. They are extremely useful in diagnosing sleep-disordered breathing, which may have contributed to or caused an ALTE, such as OSAS, hypoxia due to chronic lung disease, or central hypoventilation syndromes. The most common causes of ALTE are shown in **Figure 27.2**.

The medical management of the ALTE infant in the PICU is primarily directed toward stabilizing the cardiorespiratory status of the infant following the ALTE event. Once this is achieved, a diagnostic evaluation, directed by the history and physical examination, is performed. If an identifiable cause explains the ALTE, the treatment should be directed toward that diagnosis

If a treatable cause for the ALTE cannot be found and if the original event was of sufficient severity to be of concern about the sequelae of subsequent events, most clinicians will manage these patients with home apnea-bradycardia monitoring. Home apnea-bradycardia monitors alert parents and caregivers to prolonged central apneic pauses and/or bradycardias by sounding an alarm (usually 90 dB). Then, trained caregivers must respond to evaluate the event and revive the infant if necessary.

TABLE 27.4

DIAGNOSTIC EVALUATION FOR APPARENT LIFE-THREATENING EVENT INFANTS

Potential diagnosis/etiology	Diagnostic tests
Infection Sepsis Asphyxia	Complete blood count Arterial blood gas (pH)
Hypocalcemia Electrolyte Imbalance Dehydration	Serum electrolytes Serum calcium BUN, creatinine
Hypoglycemia	Blood sugar
Sepsis	Blood, urine, cerebrospinal fluid cultures
Pneumonia Chronic lung disease Congenital heart disease Cardiomyopathy	Chest x-ray Electrocardiogram Echocardiogram
Cardiac arrhythmia Prolonged QT interval syndrome	Electrocardiogram 24-hr Holter monitoring
Trauma Child abuse	Skeletal series Skull x-ray Head CT scan
Seizures	Electroencephalogram
Gastro-esophageal reflux disease	Barium swallow Gastric scintiscan, esophageal pH monitoring
Sleep-disordered breathing Obstructive sleep apnea Central hypoventilation syndrome	Overnight polysomnography
Upper airway obstruction Craniofacial abnormality Congenital airway anomaly	Laryngoscopy Bronchoscopy
Inborn errors of metabolism	Serum ammonia level Urine organic acids Plasma amino acids
Arnold Chiari type I or II	MRI
Drug ingestion Toxic exposure	Serum and urine toxicology

BUN, blood urea nitrogen

Sleep in the PICU

Addressing the impact of sleep deprivation on healthcare providers is one of the most important aims of improving healthcare safety. Sleep deprivation also affects patients, particularly in the PICU setting. Inadequate sleep can cause neurocognitive and psychological deficits. Sleep deprivation is a physiologic stressor and can affect autonomic, immunologic, metabolic, and hormonal function. Sleep in critically ill patients is characterized by an abnormal distribution; with sleep times scattered throughout a 24-hr period rather than consolidated at night. Thus total sleep time may not be affected, but because sleep is fragmented, its restorative properties may be lacking. The arrangement of sleep stages is also affected with an increase in "light sleep" (stage 1) and decreased time in deeper sleep (stages 2, 3, 4, and REM). Sleep in the ICU is disrupted by frequent arousals and awakenings. Noise and light levels are high in the PICU and are not conducive to sleep. Poor synchrony between the patient and the ventilator, intubation, the ventilator mode, intermittent suctioning, and an inability to communicate all may contribute to sleep disruption. The medications used

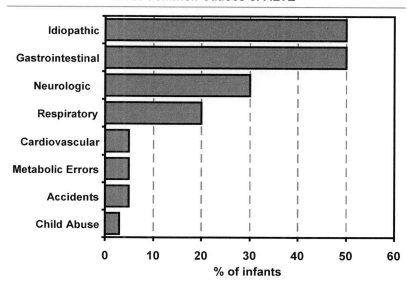

FIGURE 27.2. The most common causes of apparent life-threatening event (ALTE). The approximate proportion of infants (X-axis) who have ALTE that is caused by the listed categories. Modified from the data summary in Krimsky WR, Leiter JC. Respiratory control during sleep. In: Lee-Chiong T, ed. *Sleep: A Comprehensive Handbook.* Hoboken, NJ: John Wiley and Sons, Inc., 2006:663–7.

in the PICU often impact sleep, both during use and after discontinuation. Benzodiazepines and opioids cause REM suppression; consequently, a REM rebound effect follows discontinuation, which can result in nightmares or disturbing dreams. Sleep deprivation results in a number of neurologic and behavioral complications. Reduced vigilance and reaction time are the impairments most relevant for sleep deprivation in healthcare providers. Mood alterations (irritability) and organic brain dysfunction (delusions and hallucinations) are probably more important. Delirium can occur in the PICU setting,

and it has serious negative prognostic implications. Sleep deprivation in critically ill patients may impair immunologic function. Sleep loss affects the secretion of hormones that can play a role in the body's response to stress, including increases in cortisol, norepinephrine, and thyroid hormone. Critical illness can also alter these same hormones. Both sleep deprivation and critical illness cause insulin resistance that can be clinically significant. Controlling light exposure with open blinds during the day and decreased light at night has also been recommended.

CHAPTER 28 ■ ACUTE NEUROMUSCULAR DISEASE

SUNIT SINGHI • ALKA KHADWAL • ARUN BANSAL

Neuromuscular diseases (NMDs) can be classified according to the site of primary pathology: brain, spinal cord, peripheral nerve, neuromuscular junction, or the skeletal muscle (**Table 28.1**).

The lungs and surrounding chest-wall muscles form the ventilatory apparatus, which is similar in function to a pump. The integrity of this "respiratory pump" and the central control from brain and nerves is essential for maintaining normal breathing. The primary muscle of breathing is the diaphragm. The accessory muscles of breathing are located in the neck and the upper chest wall and include the sternocleidomastoid, trapezius, intercostal, and rhomboid muscles. Inspiration is an active process during which an increase in intrathoracic volume is produced by chest and lung expansion, resulting from contraction that causes a downward movement of the diaphragm. The intercostal muscles stabilize the chest wall during changes in intrathoracic pressure. Expiration is a passive process during quiet breathing that results from elastic recoil of the lungs as the diaphragm relaxes to resume its resting configuration.

Brain and brainstem diseases cause respiratory depression characterized by central patterns of respiration, including hyperventilation; irregular and ataxic (or cluster) breathing; hiccups; hypopnea; and apnea. Bulbar involvement may cause impaired clearing of secretions and aspiration. Children unable to clear secretions are more prone to pulmonary infection, which can lead to further deterioration of the clinical condition. A combination of these abnormalities often contribute to ineffective gas exchange (**Fig. 28.1**).

EVALUATION OF RESPIRATORY DYSFUNCTION IN A PATIENT WITH A NEUROMUSCULAR DISORDER

Monitoring of clinical parameters that indicate the severity and progression of weakness is summarized in **Table 28.2**. In many neuromuscular syndromes,

patients demonstrate a sign called *paradoxical breathing*. Early in the disease, weakness of the intercostal muscles is relatively greater than weakness of the diaphragm. The intercostal muscles usually stabilize the chest wall during inspiration. Paradoxical breathing occurs when, during inspiration, the chest wall is pulled inward due to weak intercostal muscles while the abdomen expands outward as the diaphragm contracts downward; this appears as a rocking motion of chest and abdomen. This pattern differs from normal inspiration in which diaphragm contraction results in abdominal expansion and intercostal contraction causes chest expansion (i.e., synchronized motion of the abdomen and chest).

A simple, single-breath counting test may be used at the bedside in older children and adolescents to assess severity and follow progression of weakness due to acute NMD. If the patient can count up to 10 in 1 breath, the forced vital capacity is likely to be at least 15–20 mL/kg. If he or she can count up to 25, the vital capacity is ~30–40 mL/kg. Monitoring the trend in single-breath counting may help to predict progression and the need for mechanical ventilation before actual respiratory failure.

A spirometric assessment can also be performed at the bedside in children >5 years to monitor both the severity of weakness and the progression of weakness using measurement of vital capacity and 2 clinically helpful respiratory pressures. A normal vital capacity is measured from maximum inspiration to maximum expiration (normal values range from 55 to 80 mL/kg). Maximum static respiratory pressures (i.e., maximum inspiratory pressure measured at residual volume; normal values are –100 to –120 cm H_2O for adult males and –80 to –100 cm H_2O for adult females) and maximum expiratory pressure (measured at total lung capacity, normal values 150–240 cm H_2O for adult males and 108–160 cm H_2O for adult females) are considered sensitive indicators of respiratory muscle strength. Both minimal values and changes in values have been associated with clinically significant deterioration, including an inability to cough and clear secretions, increased incidence

TABLE 28.1

ANATOMIC CLASSIFICATION AND EXAMPLES OF CONDITIONS WITH NEUROMUSCULAR WEAKNESS THAT REQUIRE PEDIATRIC INTENSIVE CARE

Brain
Intracranial hemorrhage
Hypoxic ischemic encephalopathy
Meningoencephalitis
Acute demyelinating encephalomyelitis

Spinal cord
Trauma
Epidural abscess
Myelitis
Acute poliomyelitis
Spinal muscular atrophy

Peripheral nerve
Guillain-Barré syndrome
Critical illness polyneuropathy
Toxic (lead, arsenic) neuropathy
Drug-induced neuropathy (e.g., vincristine)
Diphtheric polyneuropathy
Acute porphyria
Phrenic nerve injury—diaphragmatic paralysis

Neuromuscular junction
Myasthenia gravis and congenital myasthenic
   syndromes
Prolonged neuromuscular blockade
Antibiotic (aminoglycoside, d-penicillamine) therapy
Snake bite and scorpion sting
Organophosphorus poisoning
Botulism
Tick paralysis
Hypermagnesemia

Muscle
Critical illness myopathy
Hypokalemia
Muscular dystrophies
Congenital myopathies
Acute rhabdomyolysis
Inflammatory myopathies, (e.g., dermatomyositis)

of pulmonary infections, increased nighttime ventilatory insufficiency, hypercarbia, and need for ventilatory assistance. A 20/30/40 rule has been suggested for adult patients for minimal values that raise concern for respiratory failure. A vital capacity of ~20 mL/kg, a maximum inspiratory pressure less negative than −30 cm H_2O, or a maximum expiratory pressure of <40 cm H_2O are minimal values that raise concern for respiratory problems in adults with acute NMD. Also reported as concerning are values that fall by 50% from baseline or >30% in a 24-hr period.

On chest x-ray, an elevated hemidiaphragm, in fixed position during inspiration and expiration, suggests hemidiaphragm weakness or paralysis. A bell-shaped thoracic cage is indicative of intercostal muscle weakness or hypotonia. Nonspecific findings include patchy atelectasis or areas of consolidation in patients with aspiration or infection of the respiratory tract.

Intubation is considered (a) to protect the airway from severe aspiration because of oropharyngeal weakness; (b) to prevent respiratory failure from declining tidal volumes, hypoxemia despite supplemental oxygen, and hypercapnia; and if necessary, (c) to optimize pulmonary toilet.

If in doubt, *early assisted* ventilation should be the preferred treatment so as to ensure adequate minute ventilation. In severe cases, intubation and controlled mechanical ventilatory support are required. If the patient is able to generate some effort, synchronized intermittent mechanical ventilation, pressure-support ventilation, or a combination of both are appropriate modes for ventilation. *With synchronized intermittent mechanical ventilation, unassisted, spontaneous breathing may burden the accessory ventilatory muscles, but in pressure-support ventilation, inability to trigger breaths or unanticipated changes in lung compliance can result in insufficient ventilation. If fatigue, hypoxemia, or hypercapnia is encountered, the ventilatory support from either mode must be increased.*

Weaning from mechanical ventilation should be started when ventilatory muscle strength begins to return, provided the chest x-ray does not show atelectasis or infiltrates and the oxygenation is good. A vital capacity >10 mL/kg and a maximum inspiratory force of at least −20 cm H_2O are useful indicators of ability to wean. Weaning from synchronized intermittent mechanical ventilation can be accomplished by gradually reducing ventilation breaths or by increasing the duration of spontaneous breathing and time off of the ventilator. Weaning from pressure-support ventilation can be accomplished by gradually decreasing the inspiratory pressure support. During weaning, the patient should not be allowed to become significantly tachypneic, and end-tidal CO_2 should be monitored to confirm that PCO_2 is maintained within the normal range. Ventilatory support may be maintained at pre-weaning levels at night to provide rest. During sleep, some level of pressure support is usually required to prevent loss of lung volume and hypoxemia.

Generally, if a pressure support of 5 cm H_2O is well tolerated or the patient is maintaining minute ventilation without intermittent mechanical ventilation breaths, ventilation can be discontinued. A high-flow T-piece system with an end-expiratory pressure of 2.5–7.5 cm H_2O can be added to the endotracheal tube to prevent atelectasis during nonventilated periods. With increasing muscle strength, patients can

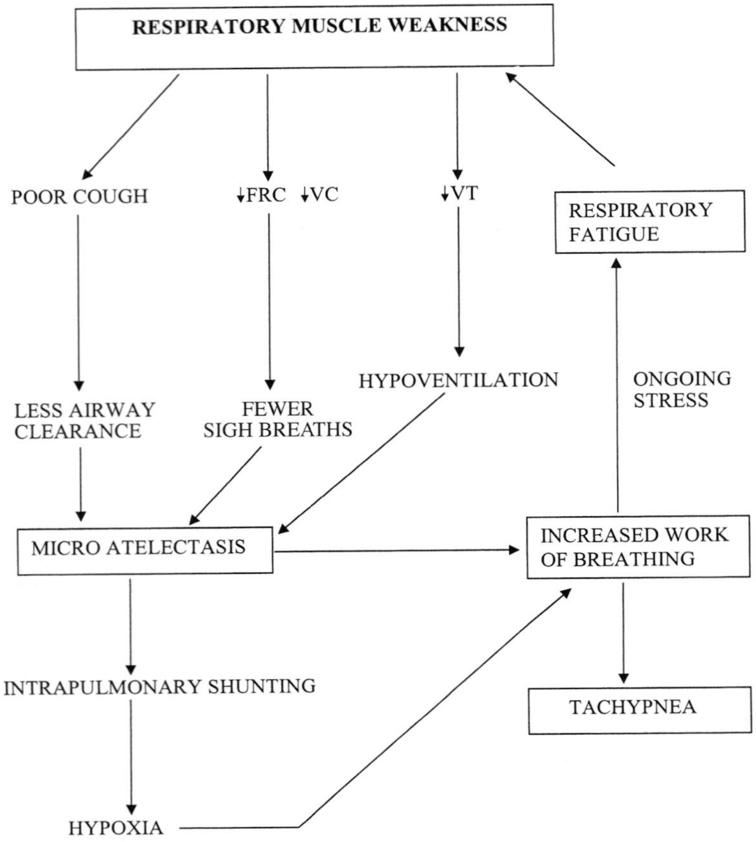

FIGURE 28.1. Pathophysiology of respiratory failure in neuromuscular disorders. FRC, functional residual capacity; VC, vital capacity; VT, tidal volume.

be kept off of the ventilator for increasing periods using either continuous positive airway pressure or a T-piece circuit. Before considering endotracheal tube extubation, clinical assessment of bulbar muscle weakness is very important, as upper-airway difficulties may compromise breathing after extubation.

Complications of mechanical ventilation depend on the duration of therapy. Nosocomial pneumonia and atelectasis are the most common complications. Long-term, invasive ventilation may result in tracheomalacia, tracheoesophageal fistula formation, or tracheal stenosis. Practicing sterile techniques during suctioning of the airway may decrease the incidence of nosocomial pneumonia.

Advantages of early tracheostomy include increased comfort, airway safety, and help in weaning from ventilation. No guidelines exist for tracheostomy in children with these disorders. Some disease-specific data suggest that children are less likely to require tracheostomy than are adults.

Patients on ventilators require special attention in preventing pressure sores and nerve compression by frequent and gentle posture changes, padding, and the use of air or water mattresses. A focus must also include prevention of deep vein thrombosis and

early enteral nutrition to prevent gastric mucosal atrophy and to reduce the incidence of nosocomial infection.

GUILLAIN-BARRÉ SYNDROME

Acute inflammatory demyelinating polyneuropathy, or Guillain-Barré syndrome (GBS), is an acute, autoimmune (often postinfectious), usually demyelinating disorder of the peripheral nervous system characterized by areflexic weakness of limbs. The Miller Fisher syndrome, a variant of GBS, is characterized by a triad of ophthalmoplegia, ataxia, and areflexia. A common initial symptom of GBS is paresthesia of the toes and fingers, followed by progressive weakness of the lower limbs and/or unsteadiness in gait. As the disease progresses over a period of a few hours to days and weeks, weakness of the upper limbs occurs, and cranial nerve palsies develop. This ascending weakness or paralysis is usually symmetric. Dysautonomia that presents as dizziness, sweating, and tachycardia may also occur. The hallmark of GBS on physical examination is ascending motor weakness, along with areflexia. Hyponatremia is common in GBS.

TABLE 28.2

CLINICAL AND LABORATORY PARAMETERS THAT ARE USEFUL IN ASSESSMENT OF ADEQUATE RESPIRATORY FUNCTION IN PATIENTS WITH NEUROMUSCULAR WEAKNESS

Clinical

Respiratory rate: Good index of response to hypoventilation caused by muscular weakness; tachypnea is the earliest response

Swallowing and handling of secretions

Quality of cough

Volume of speech

Single-breath count

Chest expansion

Presence of tachycardia/diaphoresis (nonspecific)

Use of accessory muscles

Orthopnea

Inward movement of abdomen during inspiration.

Breathing pattern alternates between accessory and major respiratory muscles, signifying weakness of major respiratory muscles

Change in status when sleeping: accessory muscle tone decreases

Rate of progression of generalized weakness

Laboratory

Vital capacity

Maximum inspiratory pressure

Maximum expiratory pressure

SaO_2, PaO_2, $PaCO_2$, pH

Chest x-ray

In its evolving phase, GBS must be differentiated from transverse myelitis, acute polyneuropathies caused by toxins/heavy metals, organophosphorus poisoning, tick paralysis, acute porphyria, diphtheria polyneuropathy, myelopathies (poliomyelitis and other enteroviral infections of anterior horn cell), myasthenia gravis, and electrolyte disturbances (especially hypokalemia). Asymmetric involvement, preserved or brisk reflexes, and extensor planter response should suggest a diagnosis other than GBS. If lumbar puncture is performed a week after onset of weakness, the CSF findings typically suggest demyelination (e.g., elevated protein >45 mg/dL) without cerebrospinal fluid pleocytosis (<10 cells/mm^3) (often referred to as albuminocytologic dissociation). Two weeks after of onset of symptoms, lumbosacral MRI with gadolinium contrast may reveal enhancement of the cauda equina nerve roots. Peripheral neurophysiology within the first week of symptom onset shows characteristic features of peripheral demyelination.

Children with GBS are at risk for life-threatening respiratory complications and autonomic disturbance. Endotracheal intubation may be required in children with GBS to protect the airway from aspiration, to overcome obstruction from loss of airway tone, or to facilitate supportive mechanical ventilation. Dysautonomia and potential for succinylcholine-induced hyperkalemia may increase the risks of endotracheal intubation in patients with GBS.

Independent predictors of the need for ventilation in adults with GBS were time from the onset of symptoms to admission of <7 days, inability to cough, inability to stand, inability to flex arms or head, increasing liver enzymes, and vital capacity <60% of predicted. Clinical signs that indicate the need for mechanical ventilation include ventilatory muscle insufficiency, an increasing oxygen requirement to maintain SpO2 >92%, or signs of alveolar hypoventilation (e.g., PCO_2 >50 torr). Other indications for initiating mechanical ventilation in GBS are forced vital capacity <15 mL/kg, rapid decline in vital capacity by 50% from baseline, and inability to generate a maximum negative inspiratory pressure of –20 cm H_2O.

Risk of dysautonomia is high in patients with respiratory failure, quadriplegia, or bulbar involvement. Transcutaneous cardiac pacing may be used for symptomatic bradycardia. Hypotension may be treated with volume repletion or, if refractory to fluids, a pure α agonist such as phenylephrine may be used to avoid potential arrhythmogenic effects from combined α and β agonists.

Constipation is common in patients with GBS as a result of adynamic ileus. Promotility drugs are contraindicated in patients with dysautonomia. Pain relief may be necessary, with acetaminophen usually the first choice. Opioids may be needed in addition, and carbamazepine or gabapentin may be used in case of neurogenic pain. The Cochrane Neuromuscular Group has concluded that steroids are not helpful but plasma exchange and IVIG (0.4 g/kg/day) are helpful in treating GBS.

MYASTHENIA GRAVIS

Myasthenia gravis (MG) is a disorder of the neuromuscular junction characterized by fluctuating weakness and fatigability of the voluntary skeletal muscles that result from autoimmune destruction of acetylcholine receptors (AchR).

Juvenile MG (JMG, autoimmune MG of childhood) has an age of onset between 3 months and 16 years, mostly before 3 years, and a clinical picture that is similar to MG in adults. Symptoms are least apparent on awakening, and they become more evident later in the day. Weakness may remain localized to the eye muscles or it may progress to be generalized. Ocular involvement is present in most children with JMG, taking the form of intermittent drooping of eyelids with a persistent upward gaze or double vision, especially while reading. This weakness is variable and often asymmetric. Weakness of respiratory muscles in combination with bulbar weakness warrants hospitalization for immediate evaluation and management.

On physical examination, findings are confined to the motor system, with no loss of sensation or coordination. Ptosis may be asymmetric, but extraocular muscle weakness is symmetric and fluctuating. Pupillary responses are not affected. Various maneuvers can be performed to unmask the underlying fatigability, including repetitive trips up and down the stairs, repetitive fun exercises in young children, and having the patient count to 100 or chew for 30 seconds, and may provide a rough assessment of fatigable weakness. An adaptation of a scale devised by Osserman is used commonly to grade strength and fatigability.

Transient neonatal MG presents shortly after birth. The features of transient neonatal MG may develop within a few hours of birth. Infants may show a range of symptoms from mild hypotonia to a generalized weakness, feeble cry, difficult feeding, ptosis, facial weakness, or life-threatening respiratory distress. Every newborn of myasthenic mothers should be observed during the neonatal period for signs of muscle weakness, respiratory failure, and any impairment of bulbar muscles. Treatment includes anticholinesterase and, if indicated, ventilatory support.

Congenital myasthenic syndromes present at birth with ptosis, ophthalmoparesis, dysphagia, dysarthria, poor feeding, weak cry, hypotonia, motor delay, respiratory distress, chronic respiratory and limb weakness, and arthrogryposis multiplex. Congenital MG must be differentiated from myopathies, muscular dystrophies, and JMG. Depending upon the defect, various treatment options are available, including pyridostigmine, 3,4-diaminopyridine, quinidine, and fluoxetine; however, immunotherapy has no role.

Myasthenic crisis and cholinergic crisis are two emergencies in MG associated with acute life-threatening respiratory failure. Myasthenic crisis is an acute exacerbation of the disease process that results in severe weakness from dysfunction of the neuromuscular junctions. Myasthenic crisis is characterized by respiratory failure due to weakness of either the upper-airway muscles or of the diaphragm and other respiratory muscles. This condition can be precipitated by respiratory infection, sepsis, aspiration, surgical procedures, rapid tapering of corticosteroid or immunotherapeutic drugs, initiation of corticosteroid therapy, and exposure to drugs.

Cholinergic crisis is severe weakness usually caused by an overtreatment with cholinergic medication, resulting in overstimulation and blockade of the already functionally compromised neuromuscular junction by acetylcholine. The muscarinic effects of cholinesterase inhibitors (CEIs) increase bronchopulmonary secretions, which can obstruct the airway and cause aspiration. Patients show features of cholinergic excess, including excessive salivation, excessive lacrimation, diarrhea, sweating, pupillary constriction, and possibly, muscle fasciculation.

Cholinergic crisis and myasthenic crisis may be difficult to distinguish. CEI treatment should be withheld initially to avoid contributing to cholinergic overload in cholinergic crisis. CEI treatment is potentially harmful in patients with myasthenic crisis if they have significant weakness, as it may cause increased secretions and thus hasten respiratory failure. Supportive care is generally required for both crises. CEI is withheld and atropine is used to treat cholinergic crisis. Removal of triggers and institution of plasmapheresis or administration of IVIG may be necessary to treat myasthenic crisis. Steroids, immunotherapy, and thymectomy are not immediately useful for myasthenic crises, as they may take weeks to be effective.

Tensilon is an IV cholinesterase-inhibiting agent with a rapid onset (30 secs) and a short duration (15 mins) of action. It acts by inhibiting the enzyme acetylcholinesterase, thereby allowing acetylcholine to diffuse widely throughout the synaptic cleft and to interact with AchRs, resulting in a larger and longer end-plate potential. Edrophonium is administered intravenously in incremental doses, beginning with 0.01 mg/kg up to a maximum of 0.1 mg/kg and observing for improvement in function. Bradycardia can be a significant side effect; therefore, patients should be on a cardiac monitor, and atropine should be available. Relative contraindications to this test are a history of bronchial asthma or cardiac dysrhythmias. Any group of muscles can be tested, but it is considered more sensitive and useful when improvement in ptosis and double vision are used as the diagnostic end points. Objective improvement in muscular strength is more important than the perception of improvement.

Some patients may not show a response to edrophonium, but they may show improvement to neostigmine or pyridostigmine. These agents have an onset of action 5–15 mins after intramuscular administration, and their effect may last for up to 4 hrs. This longer duration of action compared to edrophonium may make neostigmine and pyridostigmine more useful in the evaluation of children.

TABLE 28.3

PHARMACEUTICAL AGENTS WITH THE POTENTIAL TO AGGRAVATE MYASTHENIA GRAVIS

Antibiotics

Ampicillin, aminoglycosides (gentamicin, kanamycin, streptomycin, tobramycin), clindamycin, colistin, erythromycin, fluoroquinolones (e.g., ciprofloxacin, norfloxacin), lincomycin, neomycin, penicillin, polymyxin B, sulfonamides, tetracycline, trimethoprim-sulfamethoxazole, vancomycin

Anticonvulsants

Barbiturates, carbamazepine, gabapentin, phenytoin, trimethadione (no longer available in US)

Antirheumatic drugs

Chloroquine, penicillamine (could cause myasthenia gravis or elevation of antibodies)

Cardiovascular drugs

Bretylium, calcium-channel blockers (nifedipine, verapamil), lidocaine, oxprenolol, procainamide, propranolol and other β-blockers, quinidine

Psychotropic agents

Chlorpromazine, diazepam, lithium, promazine

Replacement hormones

Adrenocorticotropic hormone, corticosteroids, estrogens, oral contraceptives, thyroid hormones

Other drugs

Diuretics (lower serum potassium), interferon-α, iodinated radiographic contrast agents, muscle relaxants, magnesium, opioids, neuromuscular-blocking agents, quinine

Management in a PICU is indicated in patients with respiratory compromise or bulbar weakness and in those at risk for deterioration during initiation of therapy, myasthenic or cholinergic crisis, or perioperative management, including thymectomy. At the time of intubation, careful consideration should be given to the use of neuromuscular blocking agents because of prolonged and unpredictable duration. Resistance to the effects of succinylcholine is possible due to relative deficiency of AchRs, and higher doses may be needed to induce paralysis. Short-acting, nondepolarizing agents may be less likely to result in unwanted prolonged paralysis, but unexpected prolongation of any paralytic should be anticipated. Some medications exacerbate muscle weakness, and these should be avoided or stopped (**Table 28.3**).

In patients with moderately severe muscle weakness but no evidence of respiratory failure, it is reasonable to increase the dose of pyridostigmine every few days until a satisfactory response is apparent. In patients in acute respiratory failure, one approach is to gradually increase the dose of pyridostigmine while undertaking a course of plasma exchange. Side effects are related to increased peripheral cholinergic activity and include bronchospasm, excessive salivation, bradycardia, nausea, diarrhea, and miosis.

If no improvement in weakness is seen despite adequate CEI therapy, immunosuppressive drugs can be added. These include corticosteroids, azathioprine, cyclophosphamide, cyclosporine, and methotrexate.

These drugs suppress the immune system by inhibiting both cellular and humoral mechanisms and reducing the damage due to autoimmunity. Prednisolone, the most commonly used immunosuppressive agent, is added at a once-daily dose of 1.5–2 mg/kg in patients with moderate-to-severe disease that is refractory to CEIs. Plasmapheresis removes AchR antibodies from the circulation and has been advocated as an effective treatment for MG because it brings about improvement within a few days that lasts for several weeks. IV immunoglobin (IVIG) is considered to be as effective as plasmapheresis. With 2 g/kg given over 5 days (0.4 g/kg/day), 60%–70% of patients are expected to show response within days to weeks, and the response lasts up to 60 days. In patients with acute respiratory failure or who are in myasthenic crisis, IVIG is used if plasmapheresis is not available or cannot be done.

For patients with nonthymomatous autoimmune MG, thymectomy should be considered only as an option to increase the probability of remission or improvement. Patients selected for thymectomy should have pulmonary function testing, including vital capacity and maximum expiratory force, both before and after cholinergic inhibition. If the patient is already on CEIs and can tolerate withdrawal of drug for 6–8 hrs, preoperative low maximum expiratory force off of CEIs indicates the risk of postoperative respiratory complications. CEIs are discontinued on the morning of surgery to avoid interactions and side effects in the operating room. Atropine is recommended to reduce secretions, and in patients on corticosteroids, preoperative, stress-dose, hydrocortisone is used for 3 days postoperatively.

ACUTE INTERMITTENT PORPHYRIA

Acute intermittent porphyria (AIP) is characterized by an acute life-threatening attack of neurovisceral symptoms. Common to all acute porphyrias is overproduction and accumulation of 5-aminolevulinic acid (ALA) and porphobilinogen (PBG). The neurovisceral symptoms are due to the neurotoxic effect of PBG and ALA and interaction of ALA with GABA receptors. The classic features of acute porphyrias are abdominal pain, altered mental state, and peripheral neuropathy. Neurologic symptoms may involve both the central and peripheral nervous systems and include paresthesias, myalgias, paresis, neuropathy, seizures, and coma. Motor neuropathy of acute, severe attacks usually presents with paresis and muscle weakness at an early stage. The weakness begins proximally, in the arms rather than the legs. It is usually symmetric, resembling GBS, and can progress to quadriparesis and bulbar and respiratory muscle weakness. The deep-tendon reflexes may be lost. Hyponatremia frequently complicates the acute porphyrias and may precipitate seizures. Other electrolyte disturbances (e.g., hypokalemia, hypomagnesemia, hypochloremia) may also occur.

Four main categories of factors can either induce or worsen an attack of acute porphyria: medications, starvation, hormonal factors, and infection. The medications include anticonvulsants (i.e., barbiturates, phenytoin, carbamazepine, diazepam) and antibacterials (i.e., chloramphenicol, erythromycin, metronidazole, sulfonamides). The goals of treatment are to identify the triggering event, alleviate symptoms, and reverse ALA synthetase activity with medication. Dehydration, malnutrition, or infection should be managed. Morphine or other opiate analgesics can be used to control pain. Propranolol can be used for hypertension, and diazepam can be used to acutely treat seizures. Long-term seizure control can be achieved with valproate or clonazepam. Hyponatremia and hypomagnesemia should be corrected. Gastrointestinal symptoms can be treated with chlorpromazine or phenothiazine. Enzyme activity is reversed by administering 10% glucose and hemin infusion. These act by directly suppressing ALA synthetase activity. Hemin infusion is given in a dose of 3–4 mg/kg once daily for 4 days.

INTENSIVE CARE–ACQUIRED NEUROMUSCULAR DISORDERS (CRITICAL ILLNESS NEUROMUSCULAR ABNORMALITIES)

Critical illness neuromuscular abnormality (CINMA) is the term given to those NMDs that are acquired de novo during the treatment of critical illnesses other than primary neuromuscular condition. A number of factors increase the risk of CINMA, including sepsis, systemic inflammatory response, multiorgan failure, mechanical ventilation, corticosteroids, neuromuscular-blocking drugs, aminoglycosides, hyperosmolality, parenteral nutrition, and hyperglycemia.

Prolonged neuromuscular transmission blockade has been described in those who receive muscle relaxants for several days or weeks. These patients become ventilator-dependent and have persistent paralysis and areflexia long after the drug is discontinued. Renal failure or dysfunction is an important factor, as many commonly used neuromuscular blocking agents (NMBAs) have significant clearance via the kidney. Hypermagnesemia and metabolic acidosis are other risk factors in prolonging neuromuscular blockade.

Critical illness polyneuropathy (CIP) is characterized by acute, generalized neuropathy occurring after overwhelming sepsis and multiorgan dysfunction. Clinical signs usually develop 2–3 weeks after the onset of sepsis. Rapid development of flaccid quadriparesis or paraparesis with hyporeflexia/areflexia occurs. The problem is recognized when an obvious difficulty is encountered in weaning from mechanical ventilation. During recovery, some patients may complain of painful paresthesia and some may develop weakness after discharge. Loss of sensation in glove-and-stocking distribution is seen.

Terms used to describe critical illness myopathy (CIM) include acute quadriplegic myopathy, floppy-person syndrome, necrotizing myopathy of intensive care, thick-filament myopathy, and steroid-induced quadriparesis. Exposure to corticosteroids or NMBAs appears to be the major risk factor for developing CIM. Other risk factors include sepsis and multiorgan failure. Patients have flaccid tetraparesis or tetraplegia. Deep-tendon reflexes are either normal or diminished but usually are not completely lost. Sensation is preserved. Painful stimulation elicits facial grimacing without limb withdrawal, unlike the finding in CIP. Weaning from mechanical ventilation is difficult.

Nerve conduction studies and electromyography can be performed at the bedside. CNS and non-neurologic causes can be excluded, and the cause of weakness can be localized to either muscle or nerve in most cases.

No specific treatments have been recommended for CINMA. Early physiotherapy and good nutrition should help recovery. Studies have shown that glutamine, glutathione supplementation, and branched-chain amino acid supplementation are associated with improved survival and shorter ICU stay. Avoidance of prolonged immobilization and oversedation, strict glycemic control, and minimization of dosages and duration of corticosteroids and NMBAs can minimize the development of CINMA.

DIAPHRAGMATIC PALSY

Bilateral diaphragmatic palsy is usually due to systemic illnesses, while unilateral palsy is due to injury to phrenic nerve (cervical motor neurons C3–C5). The most common causes of unilateral diaphragmatic palsy in children are birth trauma (due to difficult or breech delivery), congenital diaphragmatic eventration, and cardiothoracic surgery. Children present with tachypnea, increasing need for oxygen, hypercapnia, atelectasis, pneumonia, and a mediastinal shift. Chest x-rays show an elevated affected hemidiaphragm. Fluoroscopy on sniffing is a traditional method of diagnosing diaphragmatic movements. The normal diaphragm descends during a sniff. In the presence of unilateral diaphragmatic palsy, the affected diaphragm ascends. Sonographic assessment of diaphragmatic motion can be used for diagnosis and to follow the progression of diaphragmatic function at the bedside. Management of eventration of the diaphragm secondary to phrenic nerve injury in the newborn period invariably requires surgery.

CHAPTER 29 ◼ CHRONIC NEUROMUSCULAR DISEASE

JONATHAN GILLIS • MONIQUE M. RYAN

Children with chronic neuromuscular diseases (CMDs) have recurrent admissions, and the duration of admission is longer than most other patients; as a result, they have a disproportionate impact on ICU resources. The children and their families become well known to the nursing and medical staff, with sometimes complex and difficult interactions. For the staff, these admissions often generate ethical discussions about the appropriate use of intensive care resources and quality-of-life outcomes. Unfortunately, however, there exists a large amount of misconception about these diseases, their morbidity and mortality, their natural history, and the quality-of-life outcome for these children.

CLINICAL PRESENTATION AND DIFFERENTIAL DIAGNOSIS

The presentation of these conditions relates largely to their pathophysiology (**Table 29.1**). Diagnosis is based on clinical findings, ancillary investigations such as the serum creatine kinase and neurophysiologic studies, and muscle and nerve biopsy. CMD can be usefully discussed under the headings of neuropathies, neuromuscular junction disorders, and muscle disorders. Children with CMD can present before a diagnosis is made or at different stages of their disease thereafter. An underlying diagnosis of a CMD should be suspected in all children in whom it is difficult to wean ventilation after an acute respiratory illness. Later presentations are (a) routine postoperative admissions, (b) acute respiratory compromise, and (c) possible terminal admissions. One of the main issues here is whether the acute episode is reversible (i.e., is there a good chance the child can over time revert to his or her previous function and level of respiratory support, or will the acute episode lead to increasing dependency and a need for increased respiratory support, or is the respiratory deterioration the natural progression of the disease and, if this is so, is this a terminal deterioration). Most presentations to the ICU, in children with CMDs, will be for the management of respiratory compromise because of intercurrent illness, surgery, or disease progression. The severity of pulmonary compromise in children

TABLE 29.1

CHRONIC NEUROMUSCULAR DISORDERS OF CHILDHOOD

	Etiology	Age of onset	Course
ANTERIOR HORN CELL			
Spinal muscular atrophy	Genetic (AR)	Variable (infancy-adulthood)	Progressive
Poliomyelitis	Infectious	Variable	Static
Acid maltase deficiency	Genetic (AR)	Variable (infancy-adulthood)	Progressive
PERIPHERAL NERVE			
Congenital hypomyelinating neuropathy	Sporadic/genetic (AD/AR)	Neonatal	Static
Déjérine-Sottas disease	Sporadic/genetic (AD/AR)	Infancy	Static
Charcot-Marie-Tooth disease	Genetic (AD, AR, XL)	Childhood	Slowly progressive
Chronic inflammatory demyelinating polyneuropathy	Autoimmune	Variable (childhood)	Relapsing-remitting or progressive
NEUROMUSCULAR DISORDERS			
Congenital myasthenic syndromes	Genetic (AR, AD)	Neonatal or infancy	Static
Myasthenia gravis	Autoimmune	Variable (childhood)	Relapsing-remitting
MYOPATHIES			
Congenital myopathies	Genetic (AR, AD, XL)	Variable (infancy-adulthood)	Static or slowly progressive
Congenital muscular dystrophies	Genetic (AR)	Infancy-childhood	Static or slowly progressive
Myotonic dystrophy	Genetic (AD)	Variable (neonatal-adulthood)	Static or slowly progressive
Duchenne and Becker muscular dystrophies	Genetic (XL)	Childhood	Progressive
Other muscular dystrophies	Genetic (AD, AR)	Variable (infancy-adulthood)	Progressive

AR, autosomal recessive; AD, autosomal dominant; XL, X-linked recessive

with neuromuscular disease depends on the pattern and severity of involvement of respiratory muscles, the development of secondary thoracic wall abnormalities, and resultant changes in lung compliance.

Inspiratory muscle weakness causes loss of the ability to take deep breaths, leading to collapse of peripheral airways. Respiratory muscle weakness may also cause an ineffective cough reflex. The cough reflex involves initial inhalation of gas (which is reduced by inspiratory weakness), closure of the glottis (which is impeded by bulbar muscle weakness), the generation of an expiratory force against a closed glottis (which is impeded by expiratory muscle weakness) and, finally, rapid expiratory flow once the glottis opens. Impairment of the cough reflex results in inability to clear secretions and the development of atelectasis. Superimposed upper–respiratory tract

infections increase the volume of secretions, leading to frequent and rapid development of pneumonia. Weakness of the bulbar musculature can lead to chronic aspiration, which may further impair respiratory function. The pattern of respiratory muscle weakness varies with the underlying disease. In normal children, the chest wall and abdomen expand out together during inspiration. In children with Duchenne muscular dystrophy (DMD) and congenital myopathies, weakness of the diaphragm develops at the same rate as weakness of the intercostal and abdominal muscles. This means that though these children may develop significant respiratory compromise, their pattern of breathing is normal. In such children, diaphragmatic weakness is frequently worse in the supine position (i.e., during sleep).

In contrast, in children with spinal muscular atrophy (SMA), the intercostal muscles are more affected than the diaphragm, and the work of breathing is done mainly by the downward descent of the diaphragm. This creates a negative intra-thoracic pressure. As the weak intercostal muscles cannot support the thoracic cage, there is an inward collapse of the chest and outward expansion of the abdomen during inspiration—"paradoxical respiration." This abnormal pattern of breathing can lead to secondary chest wall deformities with development of a bell-shaped chest and abnormalities in lung development. Atelectasis causes ventilation/perfusion mismatch, exacerbating abnormalities of gas exchange, which in combination with increased chest wall rigidity in older children increases the work of breathing, causing respiratory muscle fatigue. These problems may lead to chronic alveolar hypoventilation, the development of hypercarbia, and chronic respiratory failure. The initial manifestation of significant respiratory muscle weakness is that of excessive nocturnal apneas associated with desaturations, which are followed by the development of hypercapnic alveolar hypoventilation and, ultimately, daytime respiratory failure. Acute hypercapnic episodes during respiratory tract infections complicate the situation. Two types of respiratory failure (type 1 and type 2) are typically seen in children with neuromuscular disease. Type 1 respiratory failure refers to acute failure of oxygenation and occurs most frequently in the setting of acute pneumonia. It is characterized primarily by hypoxemia and a low-to-normal pCO_2 and is corrected by delivery of oxygen. Patients with respiratory muscle weakness and alveolar hypoventilation may also present with type 2 respiratory failure, which is characterized by hypoxemia and CO_2 retention. Patients with type 2 respiratory failure may adapt to chronic hypercapnia, relying on hypoxemia-responsive peripheral chemoreceptors to maintain respiratory drive. Administration of oxygen alone to patients suffering from type 2 respiratory failure may therefore lead to a decreased respiratory drive and respiratory depression. In addition to supplementary oxygen, these patients require ventilatory support in order to improve gas exchange. Positive-pressure ventilation acts primarily by improving lung expansion. Increased lung expansion improves alveolar gas exchange, decreases the work of breathing, and reduces respiratory muscle fatigue.

Factors leading to respiratory compromise in these children include recurrent aspiration secondary to oropharyngeal motor problems and gastroesophageal reflux; poor cough and limited ability to clear the airways, leading to further aspiration; and respiratory muscle weakness: "Intercostals are affected relatively early, causing paradoxical breathing (chest wall sucked in as abdomen goes out) and a bell-shaped chest. Diaphragm weakness occurs later and heralds the onset of respiratory failure. Hypoventilation tends to occur during sleep first, as weak intercostals become even more hypotonic during rapid-eye-movement sleep; respiratory drive is decreased, and upper airway obstruction may also occur." Kyphoscoliosis with resultant restrictive lung function, sleep apnea, bulbar palsy, and hypotonic pharyngeal muscles/airway cause hypoventilation and hypoxemia during sleep. This can further lead to pulmonary hypertension.

Intensive care admission is therefore usually against a background of increasing respiratory compromise. In most cases, the acute deterioration is due to intercurrent infection and/or aspiration. These children are particularly vulnerable to influenza and other viral infections. Sometimes the episode represents the inevitable progression of the underlying illness. On admission, the child's primary physician should be contacted, and the following information should be obtained from both the family and the physician: (a) What is the child's present level of respiratory and bulbar function? Inability to clear secretions can make noninvasive mask ventilation difficult to maintain, necessitating intubation; (b) What is the present level, if any, of respiratory support? (c) Have discussions occurred about prognosis and have previous decisions been made about the level of artificial ventilation to be offered? From this history, it should be possible to decide on a treatment plan, but in general reversibility should be assumed. Treatment should include physiotherapy, antibiotics, and respiratory support. Respiratory support may include noninvasive ventilation (NIV) via face or nasal mask. For those already receiving nocturnal NIV, an attempt should be made at first to increase pressures and provide oxygen with the same method of NIV. Those usually receiving continuous positive airway pressure (CPAP) often benefit from a 2–3-day period of bi-level mask ventilation. Many children respond easily to increasing support to 24 hrs/day for a number of days. Those not responding to an increase in NIV should be intubated. Many children can be successfully extubated even after prolonged periods of respiratory decompensation.

PRINCIPLES OF MANAGEMENT IN THE ICU

The overall objective of any admission to the PICU should be the discharge of the child in his or her previous respiratory state. Indeed, studies have shown that most children with neuromuscular disease admitted to PICU will recover and are discharged without the need for prolonged invasive ventilation. Many will, however, require continued noninvasive respiratory support. Indications for ongoing ventilatory support include CO_2 retention ($PaCO_2 > 50$ mm Hg), chronic hypoxia ($PaO_2 < 90$ mm Hg), vital capacity of <1 L, and recurrent pneumonia.

ICU admission requires a clear plan on ventilation weaning. The major obstacle to this is the lack of continuity in most PICU, and this problem should be confronted and attended to shortly after admission. Case management coordinates the multidisciplinary care, including physiotherapy, occupational therapy, social work, nursing staff, and numerous different medical specialists. Neurology and chronic ventilation teams need to be involved early in decision making. Almost all children can be extubated to noninvasive bilevel ventilation that should initially be provided for 24 hrs/day, then weaned to nocturnal ventilation. Depending on the individual child, bilevel ventilation can usually then be weaned to CPAP.

Delivery of Respiratory Support

NIV can be delivered by nasal mask, face mask, or mouthpiece interfaces and bilevel pressure-targeted ventilators. Most bilevel pressure-targeted ventilators include a CPAP mode in addition to spontaneous and timed bilevel support modes. In the CPAP mode, the ventilator delivers a flow of gas set at a constant positive pressure. CPAP is therefore not always helpful when the patient suffers from frequent central apneas and hypoventilation. Bilevel positive airway pressure ventilators also provide continuous positive airway pressure but allow independent control of expiratory and inspiratory muscles. NIV is contraindicated in patients with upper-airway obstruction and uncontrollable airway secretions. Severe swallowing impairment secondary to bulbar involvement is a relative contraindication to NIV. Complications of NIV include pneumothorax, facial irritation, gastric distension, and midface hypoplasia.

Bulbar Dysfunction

Neuromuscular disorders causing significant facial and bulbar weakness usually cause feeding difficulties in infancy and can lead to recurrent aspiration, dysarthria, poor articulation, and poor control of secretions in older children. In the ICU setting, poor control of oral secretions predisposes to recurrent aspiration and may slow extubation. Feeding problems in the newborn period often necessitate gavage feeds. Insertion of a gastrostomy tube, with or with-

out fundoplication, should be considered if problems persist after the first few months of life. Careful attention to nutrition is important, particularly during acute illnesses. Approaches to control excessive drooling include oral anticholinergic agents, such as glycopyrrolate, but such agents can increase the viscosity of secretions, resulting in atelectasis. More recently, salivary gland botulinum toxin injections have been trialed in some children with mixed results.

Orthopedic Complications

All children with chronic neuromuscular disorders can develop scoliosis and kyphosis. Progressive spinal deformity can lead to pain, loss of independent mobility, and difficulty in standing, sitting, or balancing. Respiratory function may be further compromised by the development of restrictive lung disease. Operative stabilization is often required to halt the progression of spinal deformity. Surgery is indicated if the curve is progressing, pulmonary function is impaired, and spinal fusion is unlikely to impair motor function. Many of these children are admitted to the PICU for postoperative care. Complications are more common in children with vital capacities <30%–40% predicted and those with spinal curves of >100 degrees. With appropriate perioperative care, however, even children with severe restrictive lung disease can have good outcomes following scoliosis surgery.

Cardiac Function

Cor pulmonale may be seen associated with advanced respiratory disease. Patients with these conditions should undergo annual cardiac review, including electrocardiography, echocardiography and, where relevant, Holter monitoring. Advanced DMD is commonly associated with cardiac conduction defects, resting tachycardia, and cardiomyopathy. Mitral valve prolapse and pulmonary hypertension may also occur. Myotonic muscular dystrophy is rarely associated with cardiomyopathy, but children with myotonic dystrophy commonly develop symptomatic or subclinical conduction disturbances, which may cause left ventricular dysfunction. Patients with myotonic dystrophy require monitoring of cardiac conduction and may require pacemaker placement.

Anaesthesia

In general, patients with congenital myopathies and muscular dystrophies tolerate surgical procedures and general anesthetics well, but there is the potential for decompensation of respiratory function and rapid loss of muscle conditioning. Children with myotonic dystrophy may be extremely sensitive to anesthetics and analgesic medications, especially barbiturates and opiates, with a tendency to postoperative apnea and excessive sedation. Paradoxical reactions to depolarizing muscle relaxants have also been reported. Close postoperative monitoring is recommended after general anesthesia, particularly in those with diminished respiratory reserve. Aggressive pulmonary physical therapy, assisted-cough device treatments, nasal bilevel positive airway pressure, and careful postoperative monitoring may be indicated. Malignant hyperthermia (MH) is an autosomal dominant pharmacogenetic disorder characterized by an increase in skeletal muscle metabolism in response to certain inhalation narcotics (particularly halothane) and depolarizing muscle relaxants (particularly succinylcholine). The triggering agent increases sarcoplasmic calcium concentrations, resulting in uncontrolled muscle contraction and hyperthermia, which may be fatal if untreated. Central core disease and minicore myopathy are associated with an increased risk of MH. Malignant hyperthermia has not been definitely associated with other congenital myopathies, although a single report describes three children with nemaline myopathy and increased body temperature with surgery. MH has, however, been reported in DMD and other less common muscular dystrophies. Because the underlying diagnosis is unknown in many patients undergoing muscle biopsy, MH precautions should be taken in all patients prior to definitive diagnosis. Triggering anesthetic agents should be avoided in susceptible individuals.

OUTCOME AND QUALITY OF LIFE IN CHILDREN VENTILATED FOR NEUROMUSCULAR DISEASE

It is a common, if unstated, concern of intensive care staff that, once intubated for an acute episode of respiratory compromise, children with neuromuscular disease will not be able to be extubated and weaned from full ventilation. This concern is not supported by the literature.

Specific Disorders

Spinal Muscular Atrophy

Type 1 (SMA 1) is a devastating disease of childhood caused by recessive mutations that result in a progressive motor neuronopathy. Four clinical subtypes

of SMA are defined on the basis of disease severity and progression. Infants with SMA 1 never sit unsupported, children with SMA type 2 sit but never stand, those with type 3 SMA are able to walk without assistance, and SMA type 4 is of adult onset. Children with SMA type 1 present in the first months of life with hypotonia and decreased spontaneous movement. Progressive weakness causes loss of antigravity strength and increasing difficulty in breathing and feeding. Without ventilatory support, death from chronic respiratory insufficiency before the age of two is virtually universal. Noninvasive ventilatory support, by nasal prongs or face mask has been variably successful in SMA 1. Prolonged survival into the second decade of life has been reported by a single American center, with other units reporting less success. With invasive ventilatory support (mechanical ventilation via tracheostomy), long-term survival in SMA 1 has been reported from a number of centers.

Congenital hypomyelinating neuropathy presents in the first few years of life with hypotonia, weakness, and absent deep-tendon reflexes, often in association with congenital or acquired joint contractures. These disorders are most often related to dominant or recessive mutations in genes for myelin proteins and represent an extreme of the Charcot-Marie-Tooth disease spectrum. Respiratory muscle involvement is variable.

Neuromuscular Junction Disorders

Congenital myasthenic syndromes (CMS) are genetic disorders of neuromuscular transmission characterized by fatigable weakness of the ocular, bulbar, and limb muscles presenting in the first months or years of life. Most are inherited in an autosomal recessive fashion. Physical findings may include ptosis, ophthalmoplegia, bulbar dysfunction, hypotonia, joint contractures, and depressed reflexes. Muscle weakness may be fatigable or fixed. Diagnosis is based on characteristic abnormalities on repetitive nerve stimulation with negative testing for antibodies to acetylcholine receptors. There may be some response to treatment with acetylcholinesterase inhibitors. Quinidine, fluoxetine, ephedrine, and 3,4 diaminopyridine, a potassium channel blocker, may be useful for specific CMS. Symptomatic management of episodic weakness should be focused on respiratory support and prevention of aspiration.

Myasthenia gravis (MG) is an autoimmune disorder characterized by fluctuating weakness and fatigue affecting the ocular, facial, bulbar, or limb muscles and caused by autoantibodies directed against neuromuscular junction acetylcholine receptors. Symptomatic treatment with acetylcholinesterase inhibitors ameliorates weakness in MG, while immunosuppressive therapies such as prednisone, azathioprine, mycophenolate mofetil, and thymectomy may induce temporary or permanent disease remission. Plasmapheresis and intravenous immunoglobulin are often effective in management of myasthenic crises, which may be precipitated by intercurrent illness or surgery. Children with acute exacerbations of facial, bulbar, and respiratory muscle weakness in MG are at risk of hypoventilation, respiratory failure, and aspiration and must be monitored very carefully. Serial measurements of vital capacity may prompt intubation and mechanical ventilation. A number of medications are known to affect neuromuscular transmission and should be avoided in children with MG. These include certain antibiotics (gentamicin, erythromycin, and ampicillin), antiarrhythmics, and phenytoin. Neuromuscular blocking agents should be administered with caution.

Muscle Disorders

The congenital myopathies are summarized in **Table 29.2**. All may be associated with early-onset generalized weakness, hypotonia and hyporeflexia, poor muscle bulk, dysmorphic features secondary to muscle weakness (pectus carinatum, scoliosis, foot deformities, a high arched palate and elongated facies), and a distinguishing but not necessarily specific morphological abnormality on muscle biopsy. Affected patients may present later in life with delayed motor milestones, frequent falls, or disease complications such as contractures, scoliosis, and respiratory insufficiency. Muscle weakness in the congenital myopathies is generally static or slowly progressive. Facial weakness is common. There may be distal as well as proximal weakness, which is often static or only very slowly progressive, although some children experience deterioration during the prepubertal period of rapid growth. The respiratory muscles are usually involved, but cardiac involvement is rare. Respiratory muscle involvement in the congenital myopathies is variable but generally parallels the extent of limb weakness. Some disorders (myotubular myopathy and nemaline myopathy) may present at birth with severe hypotonia and weakness, little spontaneous movement, and respiratory insufficiency. In infants with such severe muscle weakness, death from respiratory insufficiency, aspiration, or pneumonia is common during the first weeks or months of life. However, even severely hypotonic patients with minimal respiratory effort at birth have been known to survive, sometimes with little residual disability. With less severe myopathies, respiratory impairment may be apparent only at the time of intercurrent illness (aspiration or pneumonia) or with anesthesia. In-

creasing weakness of the axial musculature may cause spinal deformities, which can progress rapidly during periods of rapid skeletal growth, particularly adolescence. Paraspinal muscle rigidity and kyphoscoliosis frequently result in significant restriction of lung capacity and respiratory insufficiency, which may be rapidly progressive.

The congenital muscular dystrophies group of disorders includes the "pure" congenital muscular dystrophies (which affect only muscle) and those associated with structural abnormalities of the brain and eyes (**Table 29.3**). In contrast to the congenital myopathies, which relate to genetic abnormalities of the muscle contractile apparatus, the muscular dystrophies are generally caused by muscle membrane abnormalities. These conditions are associated with generalized weakness that is often progressive, a raised serum creatine kinase, and fibrotic (dystrophic) changes in muscle. Respiratory insufficiency is common and may be exacerbated by intercurrent illness or aspiration. Some of these diseases are associated with a characteristic pattern of axial weakness, spinal rigidity, and early respiratory insufficiency with relative sparing of the appendicular (limb) muscles. Such conditions may present with respiratory failure while affected children remain ambulant and relatively active.

Myotonic dystrophy is passed from the effected mother. Infants with congenital myotonic dystrophy present with congenital contractures, generalized hypotonia, and weakness. Facial weakness causes the characteristic tented upper lip and scaphoid temporal fossae. Swallowing difficulties are common, most children requiring gavage feeds. Respiratory insufficiency is common in children presenting in the first few weeks of life. Hemidiaphragmatic elevation (right more so than left) is common. Bulbar weakness predisposes to aspiration. Persistent pulmonary hypertension of neonate and central respiratory control failure may be exacerbated by prematurity and asphyxia. Around 50% of patients with congenital myotonic dystrophy require ventilation at birth. Older children with myotonic dystrophy remain at risk of aspiration pneumonitis and symptomatic respiratory insufficiency. Systemic manifestations of myotonic dystrophy include cardiac arrhythmias, gastrointestinal smooth-muscle involvement, diabetes mellitus, and learning difficulties. Anesthesia should be undertaken with a mind to these potential complications.

Duchenne and Becker muscular dystrophies are related muscle disorders caused by mutations in the gene for dystrophin. DMD affects 1 in 3,000 boys and is the most common muscular dystrophy of childhood. DMD usually presents between the age of 3 and 5 years with an abnormal ("waddling") gait and frequent falls. Progressive muscle weakness causes

TABLE 29.2

CONGENITAL MYOPATHIES

	Inheritance	Muscle biopsy findings	Natural history	Additional findings
Central core disease	AD	Type 1 fiber predominance Cores in type 1 muscle fibers	Muscle weakness static or slowly progressive Most patients remain ambulant	Scoliosis Congenital hip dislocation Predisposition to malignant hyperthermia
Nemaline myopathy	Variable: AD, AR, sporadic	Type 1 fiber predominance Nemaline bodies on trichrome stain	Muscle weakness static or slowly progressive Variable severity Respiratory insufficiency common Bulbar involvement common	Scoliosis Acquired joint contractures
Myotubular myopathy	X-linked	Central nuclei all muscle fibers	Severe congenital weakness Most ventilator-dependent Significant early mortality	Ptosis Ophthalmoplegia Macrocephaly Pyloric stenosis
Centronuclear myopathy	AD, AR	Central nuclei all muscle fibers	Variable weakness presenting in childhood or later Most patients remain ambulant	Ophthalmoplegia in some Respiratory insufficiency may present late
Minicore myopathy	AR	Type 1 fiber predominance Multiple small cores in type 1 muscle fibers	Moderately severe weakness Most are ambulant Respiratory insufficiency in those with spinal rigidity	Ophthalmoplegia in some Spinal rigidity Hand involvement Cardiomyopathy in minority
Congenital fiber-type disproportion	AD, AR, XL	Type 1 fiber predominance Type 1 fibers small	Variable weakness Respiratory insufficiency in some	Ophthalmoplegia in some Scoliosis common

AR, autosomal recessive; AD, autosomal dominant; XL, X-linked recessive

235

TABLE 29.3

CONGENITAL MUSCULAR DYSTROPHIES

Site of defect	Protein defect	Disorder/inheritance	Natural history	Additional findings
Extracellular matrix protein	Laminin α2 (merosin)	Merosin-deficient CMD (CMD type 1A) (AR)	Severe muscle weakness Respiratory insufficiency common	Leukodystrophy Demyelinating neuropathy
	Collagen VI	Ullrich (AD, AR) and Bethlem (AR) CMDs	Mild–moderate muscle weakness Respiratory insufficiency by late childhood-adolescence	Proximal joint contractures Distal hyperlaxity Follicular keratosis
Sarcolemmal proteins	Integrin α7 (AR)		Congenital muscular dystrophy	
Glycosyltransferase enzymes	Fukutin (AR)	Fukuyama CMD (AR) Walker-Warburg disease (AR)	Severe muscle weakness Early respiratory insufficiency	Cerebellar dysgenesis Cobblestone lissencephaly Severe mental retardation
	POMGnT1	Muscle-eye-brain disease (AR)	Severe muscle weakness Early respiratory insufficiency	Cerebellar dysgenesis Cobblestone lissencephaly Severe mental retardation
	POMT1	Walker-Warburg disease(AR) Limb-girdle MD with mental retardation (AR)	Severe muscle weakness Early respiratory insufficiency	Cerebellar dysgenesis Cobblestone lissencephaly Severe mental retardation
	Fukutin-related protein	CMD type 1C (AR) LGMD type 2I (AR)	Variable muscle weakness	Macroglossia Calf hypertrophy Cardiomyopathy
	ARGE	CMD type 1D (AR)	Moderately severe muscle weakness	Severe mental retardation Leukodystrophy
Endoplasmic reticulum protein	Selenoprotein 1 (*SEPN1*)	CMD with spinal rigidity (AR) Multiminicore disease (AR) Congenital fiber-type disproportion (AR)	Axial rigidity Axial weakness Respiratory insufficiency	Characteristic facies

AR, autosomal recessive; AD, autosomal dominant; XL, X-linked recessive; CMD, congenital muscular dystrophy; LGMD, limb-girdle muscular dystrophy loss of independent ambulation between the ages of 8 and 13 years in untreated boys. Becker muscular dystrophy presents later and is more slowly progressive. Loss of ambulation is followed by rapid progression of orthopedic abnormalities, such as scoliosis and contractures. Other findings in DMD include muscle pseudohypertrophy, which most commonly affects the calves, and cardiomyopathy. Diagnosis is based on characteristic clinical findings with marked elevation of the serum creatine kinase.

Limb-girdle muscular dystrophies present in adulthood. These relatively uncommon neuromuscular conditions are associated with characteristic patterns of muscle weakness preferentially affecting the pectoral and pelvic girdle muscles and generally sparing the face.

SECTION III ■ NEUROLOGIC DISEASE

CHAPTER 30 ■ DEVELOPMENTAL NEUROBIOLOGY, NEUROPHYSIOLOGY, AND THE PICU

LARRY W. JENKINS • PATRICK M. KOCHANEK

The emerging field of neurointensive care for infants and children is challenged with designing and implementing optimal therapies for complex insults, such as traumatic brain injury (TBI), asphyxial arrest, stroke, status epilepticus, and central nervous system (CNS) infections, for what is uniformly recognized as the most complex organ system—the CNS. The challenge is magnified in pediatrics by the need to accomplish this goal in a manner that is optimal, whether the patient is a newborn, infant, child, or adolescent.

Throughout the first month of human gestation, specific CNS regions, such as the forebrain, midbrain, and hindbrain, form due to neurogenesis and cellular migration (**Fig. 30.1**). Major CNS development milestones in gestational weeks are as follows: At 3–4 wks, the formation of the neural tube occurs; at 5–10 wks, the hemispheres form; at 8–18 wks, neuronal proliferation is ongoing; at 12–24 wks, neuronal migration proceeds; at 25+ wks, neuronal arborization, synaptogenesis, programmed neuronal death, and neural connectivity occur; and at 40+ wks, myelination is ongoing. Human brain size increases dramatically, beginning from early gestation and continuing for at least 2–3 postnatal years. CNS growth, based upon changes in gross brain size, peaks at ~4 months postnatally. However, specific brain regions have different growth time windows and periods of genetic and environmental vulnerabilities before and after birth. In general, the forebrain develops more slowly than the hindbrain, with the medial aspects of the hindbrain developing faster than the lateral. The neocortical and hippocampal structures grow mostly during the fetal period but do have some continuing neuronal and glial postnatal development. In contrast, the thalamus and hypothalamus develop during the early fetal and late embryonic periods, as does the mesencephalon. The pons and medulla of the hindbrain develop primarily during the embryonic period, which in humans encompasses weeks 3–7.5 of gestation.

The prenatal stage of brain development is characterized by rapid cell division under the control of the cell cycle and, in turn, numerous cell-signaling pathways, including at least 9 different growth factor cascades. Cells also must duplicate their organelles and cellular molecules to maintain their size; thus, growth processes must also be coordinated with cellular replication. It has been estimated that ~200,000 new neurons are produced each minute at between 8 and 18 wks of gestation. In contrast, it has been proposed that little neurogenesis occurs after birth, except in some select brain regions that continue into adulthood.

Neuronal cell type and number are regulated by apoptotic cell death during CNS development, which occurs in waves. Programmed cell death (PCD)

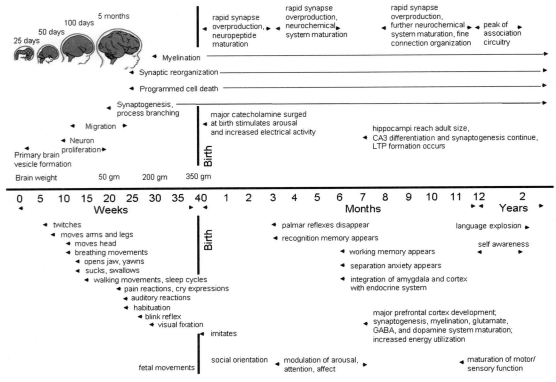

FIGURE 30.1. The key events of the human developmental timeline. The appearance of specific structural and functional developmental events is shown for the human fetus, infant, and young child up to 2 years of age. Modified from Lagercrantz H, Ringstedt T. Organization of the neuronal circuits in the central nervous system during development. *Acta Paediatr* 2001; 90:707–15; additional data from Levitt P. Structural and functional maturation of the developing primate brain. *J Pediatr* 2003; 143:S35–45, and from Herschkowitz N. Neurological bases of behavioral development in infancy. *Brain Dev* 2000; 22:411–16.

begins in zones of proliferation and recurs as CNS remodeling proceeds based upon the kind and number of connections made by each individual neuroblast and neuron. Furthermore, PCD persists postnatally due to continued CNS development. Two types of developmental PCD have been classified: (a) a proliferative apoptosis that affects morphogenetic processes involving neural precursor cells and postmitotic neuroblasts and (b) a neurotrophic-related apoptosis that affects postmitotic neurons that fail to establish appropriate synaptic connections. Apoptotic regulation of neurons that undergo PCD prior to developing synaptic contacts (proliferative apoptosis) has been proposed to differ from target-dependent neuronal death pathways (neurotrophic-related apoptosis). Proliferative neuronal apoptosis prevents premature and dysfunctional neurogenesis from occurring secondary to premature differentiation signals. Interference in normal developmental neuronal death cascades by environmental or genetic stress can result in a number of different pathologies. In contrast to the trophin-mediated signals that

promote growth and survival, extracellular signaling proteins exist that inhibit these processes. The Bcl-2 protein family, the adaptor protein Apaf1, and the cysteine-protease caspase family are the principal regulators of PCD. As many as 70% of developing neurons die via PCD during embryogenesis to eliminate excess cell numbers and to assist in neural tube closure. Due to the upregulation of PCD machinery during development, the developing CNS may be more prone to injury-related PCD than is the adult brain. An especially sensitive age for injury-induced CNS PCD would be in newborn infants in the PICU environment.

Neuronal migration occurs at between 12 and 24 gestational weeks in humans and is modulated by neurotransmitters, such as glutamate. Importantly, glutamate *N*-methyl-D-aspartate (NMDA) receptor antagonists can inhibit neuronal migration and affect developmental neuronal apoptosis, which may have important effects upon developing CNS recovery and plasticity. The developmental processes responsible for the progression of neural lineages from stem cells to progenitors to postmitotic precursors and, ultimately, to mature neurons are controlled by multiple pathways. Four primary types of signals guide axonal growth and target contact: chemoattractant, chemorepellent, contact attractive, and contact repellent.

Synaptogenesis is one of the most important developmental processes that occur during childhood and is an important potential mechanism of CNS injury and recovery in PICU-relevant injuries. Based upon nonhuman primate studies, a tentative timetable composed of 5 temporally distinct phases of synaptogenesis has been proposed for human development (**Fig. 30.1**). At ~6–8 wks of gestation, phase 1 of synaptogenesis is limited to the subplate. Beginning at ~12–17 wks of gestation, synaptogenesis phase 2 remains somewhat limited to the cortical plate with most new synapses on neuronal dendritic shafts. Phase 3 is more rapid and dynamic; with up to 40,000 new synapses made per second, it begins at ~20–24 weeks of gestation and lasts up to 8 months postnatally. Similarly, phase 4 has a high rate of synaptogenesis, lasting until puberty. The third and fourth phases are more influenced by use-dependent experience. Lastly, phase 5 levels of synaptogenesis persist throughout adulthood to age 70 but with significant synapse loss during this period as well.

Glia are not passive participants in CNS development; rather, they exert significant influence over neuronal development. Glia include astrocytes, oligodendrocytes, radial glia, and microglia. Astrocytic development occurs well after neuronal migration and differentiation, and oligodendrocytic development occurs after that of axogenesis. Astrocytes have a multitude of functions in the CNS aside from the structural support of neurons. These functions include K^+ buffering, H^+ and Ca^{2+} ion homeostasis, ammonia detoxification, free radical scavenging, metal sequestration, growth factor production, immune response participation, and neuronal metabolic support functions (pH regulation, neurotransmitter uptake, supply of glycogen and tricarboxylic acid cycle intermediates, and provision of neurotransmitter precursors). Astrocytes also participate in synaptogenesis and neurogenesis in CNS development as well as cognitive function. Protoplasmic astrocytes occur in gray matter and fibrous astrocytes in white matter. An important feature of astrocytes is the use of the energy-dependent Na^+ gradient to uptake glutamate and K^+ and to regulate H^+ ions. As a result, excessive release of glutamate, energy failure, neuronal depolarization, or tissue acidosis in brain injury result in astrocytic swelling in both the perivascular and perineuronal astrocytic compartments, which can increase diffusion distances in the brain for metabolic gases (O_2 and CO_2), substrates, and waste products. It

has been proposed that severe glial swelling may compress capillaries to reduce cerebral blood flow (CBF) and distort synaptic contacts, resulting in neuronal synaptic deafferentation. These changes can become important in a variety of CNS insults.

Microglia are CNS immune cells of myeloid origin that are similar to macrophages and represent 10% of the CNS cell populations in adults. They are normally in a resting state in normal brain, but with activation in response to infection or CNS injury, they morphologically (enlarge) and functionally change, resulting in the upregulation of cytokines and chemokines, as well as surface antigens. They have been implicated in the response to encephalitis, ischemia, TBI, and demyelinating diseases.

Oligodendrocytes produce myelin, modulate axonal function in the CNS, and are vulnerable to excitotoxic injury, decreased trophin levels, and oxidative stress conditions. Neurons and oligodendrocytes signal one another during myelination to modulate neurofilament spacing, phosphorylation, and axonal diameter. As myelination continues to occur until 10 years of age, injury to oligodendrocytes and altered myelination is an important consideration in the PICU in children who suffer brain injuries.

Myelination persists longer than most other CNS developmental processes, continuing through adolescence, making it, like synaptogenesis, another aspect of CNS development of special relevance to the PICU infant or child (**Fig. 30.1**). In fact, myelination continues in humans until ≥30 years of age, and new evidence suggests that myelination may even be an important mechanism of activity-dependent plasticity (defined as both short- and long-term changes in synaptic strength stimulated by altered neural electrical activity via altered synaptic protein levels, protein posttranslational modifications, and nerve conduction velocity).

NEUROTRANSMITTER AND NEUROTROPHIN DEVELOPMENT

The synapse serves as the anatomic substrate for information flow between neurons and the point at which the release and response to neurotransmitters predominantly occur within the nervous system. The release of neurotransmitters from within presynaptic vesicles occurs by fusion with the presynaptic plasma membrane due to electrical depolarization and the influx of Ca^{2+} into the presynaptic bouton, which contains synaptic vesicles (**Fig. 30.2**). Receptors in the postsynaptic membrane couple directly to ion channels or second messengers to mediate downstream effects. The removal of neurotransmitters that

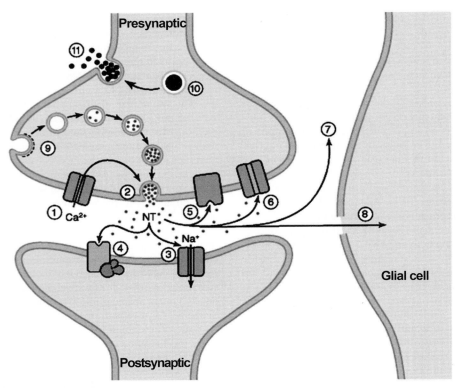

FIGURE 30.2. Schematic of a typical axodendritic synapse as seen at a dendritic spine. Calcium entry triggered by presynaptic terminal depolarization (1) induces neurotransmitter (NT)-containing synaptic vesicle exocytosis (2), which in turn, releases neurotransmitters into the synaptic cleft. NTs bind to their receptors at the postsynaptic density (concentration of postsynaptic proteins involved in synaptic function) of the postsynaptic membrane. These receptors modulate either ion channels (3) or on G proteins that stimulate second messenger production (4). Similar NT presynaptic receptors (5) are also activated, which can modulate subsequent NT presynaptic release. The uptake of many NTs occurs via a transport protein coupled to the sodium gradient at the presynaptic terminal (e.g., dopamine, norepinephrine, glutamate, and GABA) (6) or by degradation (acetylcholine) (7) or uptake by glia (glutamate) (8). Synaptic vesicle membranes are recycled by clathrin-mediated endocytosis (9). Large, dense core vesicles (10) that store protein and neuropeptides are released by repetitive stimulation at a more distant site from the postsynaptic density (11). From Holz RW, Fisher SK. *Basic Neurochemistry*, 6th ed. Philadelphia: Lippincott Williams & Wilkins, 1999, with permission.

have been released occurs by glial uptake, enzymatic degradation, or transport proteins coupled to the Na^+ gradient established by synaptic and glial sodium and potassium adenosine triphosphate translocase enzymes (Na^+-K^+ATPase). Neurotransmitter levels and receptor expression serve critical roles in synapse formation and in the circuitry and networks necessary for behavioral function in the immature and mature CNS. Furthermore, synaptic activity mediated by neurotransmitters is a requirement for the survival of developing synaptic contacts in the immature brain. It is well documented that neurotransmitters both mediate synaptic transmission and have trophic functions. Neurotransmitters and neuromodulators that have been shown to play important roles in development include glutamate, gamma-aminobutyric

acid (GABA), acetylcholine, catecholamines, serotonin, and opioids. The human developmental neurotransmitter timeline displays considerable regional and temporal variation for various transmitter systems. These variations come into play when considering age- and regional-dependent injury, manipulations of the transmitter systems, and the possible effects of the transmitter systems on recovery. Insults to the brain at vulnerable developmental periods can produce long-term structural and functional CNS changes.

Preterm fetuses and newborn infants appear to be at particularly critical periods of developmental neurotransmitter vulnerability. Before birth, the majority of neuromodulators and neurotransmitters increase during synaptogenesis. At birth, increased brain activity and a surge of catecholaminergic activity are associated with arousal. A decrease in adenosine occurs, along with a desensitization of adenosine receptors during the first postnatal days. In addition, periods of developmental "switches" in neurotransmitter function occur at birth, and sensitivity to glutamate toxicity may be especially high and vulnerable at this time.

Glutamate and GABA

Amino acids are the most abundant neurotransmitters in the CNS and have important functions in brain development regarding neural networks, CNS structure, and plasticity. Glutamatergic and GABAergic neurotransmission play major roles in brain development. In fact, many of the CNS behavioral and functional milestones during development can be correlated with the maturation of these systems and their receptors.

Glutamate Receptor Development

Almost half of the synapses of the forebrain are glutamatergic, and excessive glutamate synapse creation occurs during the most active period of synaptogenesis in the first 2 years of postnatal human brain development. Each of the 5 types of major glutamate receptors contains various subtypes. Three general types of glutamate ionotropic receptors exist that couple to Na^+ and Ca^{2+}: 4 alpha-amino-3-hydroxy-5-methyl-4-isoxazolepropionic acid (AMPA) receptor subtypes ($GluR_{1-4}$), 5 kainate receptor subtypes ($GluR_{5-7}$, KA_{1-2}), and 7 NMDA receptor subtypes (NR_{1-3B}). Eight G protein-coupled metabotropic glutamate receptors ($mGluR_{1-8}$) exist, which positively or negatively couple to phosphoinositide and cyclic nucleotide second messengers to varying degrees with pre- and postsynaptic and regional CNS distributions. AMPA receptors (which normally activate NMDA receptors) mature more slowly than do NMDA receptors; thus, the NMDA receptor must depend on other systems (the immature $GABA_A$ receptor) to help depolarize immature neurons and activate the NMDA-coupled calcium channel. Immature NMDA receptors, which contain higher levels of the NR2B subunit, are relatively more excitable during early phases of development to promote use-dependent plastic changes that are necessary for (a) normal development and (b) learning and memory. However, higher levels of NR2B make the brain more sensitive to excitotoxic insults, such as ischemia, TBI, and status epilepticus.

GABA and the GABA Switch

In addition to its neurotransmitter role on neuronal excitability, GABA has trophic actions upon synaptic and neuritic outgrowth, as well as neuronal viability during development. GABAergic inhibition of excitatory synaptic CNS activity occurs by neuronal hyperpolarization via postsynaptic $GABA_A$ (outward chloride channel) and $GABA_B$ (G protein-coupled inward potassium channel) receptors in the adult brain. The inhibitory actions of GABA are also mediated by a reduction of presynaptic excitatory neurotransmitter release via presynaptic $GABA_B$ receptors. In contrast, GABA is an excitatory neurotransmitter during prenatal development prior to birth in humans. The $GABA_A$ receptor binds barbiturates, benzodiazepines, and ethanol, which alter chloride (Cl^-) flux thorough the channel. Thus, GABA is mainly excitatory during the fetal period but becomes inhibitory around birth in humans. The so-called "GABA switch" marks the point at which GABA becomes a predominant inhibitory, rather than excitatory, neurotransmitter.

Adenosine

Adenosine is a neuronal, glial, and cerebrovascular transmitter that affects the excitability of neurons and the functional processes of oligodendrocyte progenitor proliferation and myelination during infancy and childhood. Four receptors—A_1, A_{2a}, A_{2b}, and A_3—have been identified with different regional and pre- and postsynaptic distributions. A1 receptors are inhibitory and provide a line of defense against developmental excitotoxic cascades and, along with GABA, may be the most important inhibitory neurotransmitter-receptor system in the brain. A_{2a} receptors modulate dopaminergic D_2 receptor function and are highly concentrated in the basal ganglia. Due to the importance of adenosine receptor modulation of neuronal excitability and developmental processes, this system may be an important therapeutic target in brain injury.

Acetylcholine

Acetylcholine is one of the major excitatory transmitter systems of the CNS and is important in cognition and attention, motor function, and pain. Five muscarinic receptor subtypes have been identified, with $M_{1,2,5}$ coupled primarily to phosphoinositide turnover and $M_{2,4}$ coupled to cyclic AMP production. As with many receptors, some receptor subtypes couple to more than one second messenger system.

Norepinephrine and Dopamine

Monaminergic neurons form during telencephalic vesicle formation, and catecholamines are thought to play a significant role in early development. Norepinephrine is important in cognitive function, anxiety, arousal, and attention and is necessary for normal brain development. Noradrenergic neurons appear at 5–6 weeks in humans, and adrenergic alpha$_2$ and beta$_1$ receptors predominate in the CNS. In addition, as stated above, a surge of catecholamine levels is associated with increased brain activity and arousal at birth (**Fig. 30.1**). Dopamine is also important in cognition, motor function, and addiction behavior. Five dopamine receptors have been identified (D$_1$–D$_5$), with the major CNS dopaminergic receptors being D$_1$ and D$_2$. Dopaminergic neurons begin to develop at 6–8 weeks in humans. D$_1$ receptors, in particular, are critical for working memory function during the first year of life (**Fig. 30.1**). The use of catecholamines for blood pressure support in the PICU in infants with immature or injury-altered blood-brain barrier (BBB) function warrants consideration due to the potent catecholinergic excitatory actions at birth, which in theory could be potentially excitotoxic at this critical developmental time.

Serotonin

Serotonin (5-HT) neurons have extensive contacts and synchronize complex motor and sensory information, and at least fifteen 5-HT receptors are identified. The 5-HT$_1$ receptors, in general, inhibit cyclic AMP formation and open K$^+$ channels, while 5-HT$_2$ receptors stimulate phosphoinositide second messengers, release intracellular calcium, and are generally excitatory. Serotonin also modulates developmental proliferation, differentiation, migration, and synaptogenesis. Aberrations in serotonin levels during development and early childhood result in CNS connectivity malformations and may contribute to later psychiatric disorders.

Neurotrophins

Growth factors, both intrinsic and extrinsic to the CNS, play a major role in normal brain function, developmental processes, and in the injury and repair process. Nerve growth factor (NGF), brain-derived neurotrophic factor (BDNF), and neurotrophins 3–5 (NT3, NT4/5) are diffusible peptides that compose the neurotrophin family of trophic factors in mammalian brain. Receptors for the neurotrophin peptides are the tropomyosin kinase receptors (TrkA,

TrkB, and TrkC) and the p75 neurotrophin receptor (p75 NTR), a member of the transforming growth factor receptor family. NTs are critical for neuronal survival, and the loss of NT activity after CNS injury can contribute to neuronal death and loss of function. NT precursors are called *proneurotrophins* and are cleaved by proteases to produce mature NTs. Proneurotrophins can also activate NT receptors and appear to be the preferred ligand for p75 NTR. ProNGF induces apoptosis via p75 NTR, and proNGF and NGF produce opposite responses—cell death and cell survival, respectively. NT receptors couple to a number of protein and lipid kinase intracellular pathways, such as the mitogen-activated proteins kinase, the phosphoinositide 3-kinase (PI3K), and the PKB pathways. The regional distribution of NGF is highest in regions innervated by the cholinergic system of the basal forebrain, such as the neocortex and the hippocampus. Lower but significant levels are also seen in other brain regions. BDNF has a wider distribution than NGF, having been detected in the hippocampus, amygdala, thalamus, neocortex, cerebellum, and other brain regions.

SYNAPTIC AND BEHAVIORAL DEVELOPMENT

Due to ongoing developmental synaptogenesis, connectivity, wiring, and myelination, an associated increase and development of CNS electrical activity occurs. A measurable electrical encephalogram (EEG) develops and matures with gestational and postnatal age. However, birth is the point of significantly increased neural activity due to the arousal effects of neurotransmitters, neuromodulators, and neurotrophins.

Primary behavioral and functional developments in the infant (**Fig. 30.1**) over the first 2 years include the following: (a) the cortical inhibition of brainstem reflexes due to maturation of GABA inhibition and myelination occurs postnatally at ~3 mos; excessive cortical inhibition of brainstem nuclei, such as respiratory centers, may increase the risk for the sudden infant death syndrome; (b) the development of recognition memory also takes place near the postnatal age of 3 mos, which requires adequate hippocampal and cortical visual development; (c) working memory (recent past memory that enables one to solve a current cognitive task) develops in the infant over the latter half of the first year; it is dependent upon prefrontal cortical function and is modulated by glutamate, GABA, and dopamine; and (d) between 7 and 10 mos, infant prefrontal cortices undergo dramatic maturation in synaptic density and neurotransmitter systems and have increased glucose utilization required for both growth and activity-dependent processes. Similarly, the hippocampus reaches adult size, and synaptogenesis, coupled with the maturation of neurotransmitter systems, makes LTP development possible. During this time of rapid growth and activity-dependent synaptogenesis and maturation, the infant brain is especially vulnerable to injury, resulting in either short- or long-term changes in behavioral function. For example, at 2 yrs of age, rapid language development and acquisition occur, which has been further linked to increased connections between prefrontal cortex and associational cortical regions with the limbic and motor systems. Significant synaptogenesis also occurs in many of these same brain regions.

ANTIOXIDANT DEVELOPMENT

Free radicals are molecules that contain one or more unpaired electrons, such as superoxide, peroxynitrite, and hydroxyl radicals. Enzymes and low-molecular-weight antioxidants are the major brain antioxidant defense systems. Major enzyme systems include peroxyredoxins, thioredoxins, superoxide dismutase, catalase, and peroxidases that vary in concentration depending on species and brain regions. Glutathione, vitamin E, ascorbate, and coenzyme Q are water- or lipid-soluble low-molecular-weight antioxidants. Oxidative stress, produce by abnormal free radical generation in the brain, is at least partially quenched by these defense systems. The levels of these antioxidant enzymes and molecules in the brain vary with developmental age. In general, lower levels occur during fetal development but increase at birth, as the transition from a low- to high-oxygen environment occurs. Based upon enzyme levels, catalase appears to be more of a contributor to antioxidant defenses in the immature brain, which may influence the choice of antioxidant interventions in the developing brain after injury.

CEREBROVASCULAR AND METABOLISM DEVELOPMENT AND FUNCTION

The CNS vascular system develops in 3 phases: vasculogenesis (formation of new blood vessels) angiogenesis (generation of new blood vessels from existing vessels), and barriergenesis.

Vascular reactivity of the cerebral circulation is an important neuroprotective mechanism whereby the CNS vessel diameter adjusts to physiologic changes (i.e., perfusion pressure, PaO$_2$, PaCO$_2$.) to regulate

CBF so that metabolic demands of the brain can be met. The ability of the cerebrovascular system to dilate or constrict has limits that are defined physiologically as the upper and lower limits of autoregulation. Impaired CBF autoregulation and vascular reactivity are considered potential candidates in the etiology of secondary injury across the spectrum of age. For example, loss of pressure autoregulation could underlie, in part, the marked vulnerability of the acutely injured brain in a child to otherwise tolerable hypotension. Similarly, it is believed to contribute to periventricular hemorrhagic venous infarction in preterm infants.

Pressure autoregulation is the major cerebrovascular response to acute changes in perfusion pressure that result, at the extreme range, in either hypotension with hypoperfusion and tissue ischemia or in hypertension and possible hyperemia and BBB disruption. Vascular tone in the cerebral circulation compensates for changes in cerebral perfusion pressure over a range of pressures to maintain CBF constant (between a cerebral perfusion pressure of ~40–160 mm Hg in adults) (**Fig. 30.3**). Cerebral perfusion pressure is equal to the difference between mean arterial pressure and intracranial pressure. Developmental studies of pressure autoregulation of CBF in newborns suggest a narrower perfusion pressure range, with a similar lower limit to that seen in adults—but an upper limit that is only ~90–100 mm Hg (**Fig. 30.4**).

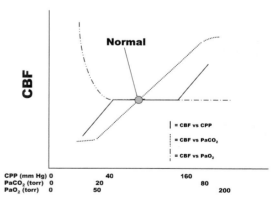

FIGURE 30.3. Relationships between cerebral blood flow (CBF) and cerebral perfusion pressure (CPP), PaCO$_2$, and PaO$_2$ across therapeutic ranges generally encountered in the PICU. These values are provided based on normative data from adults. Pressure autoregulation maintains CBF constant between a CPP of between ~40 mm Hg and 160 mm Hg. CBF is linearly related to PaCO2, with an ~4% change in CBF per torr change in PaCO$_2$ between ~20 torr and 80 torr. Below 20 torr, this curve dramatically flattens. Above ~80–100 torr, this relationship also more gradually flattens. The relationship between CBF and PaO$_2$ is relatively flat until a PaO$_2$ of ~50 mm Hg is reached, below which, a dramatic increase in CBF is observed.

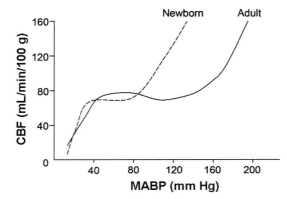

FIGURE 30.4. Comparison of the relative pressure: Cerebral blood flow (CBF) autoregulatory curves from studies of subhuman primate newborns and adults. In the adult, CBF is maintained relatively constant when arterial blood pressure is between 50 and 160 mm Hg, while in newborns, CBF is maintained over a narrower range due to a reduced upper limit of CBF autoregulation. CBF autoregulation of newborns makes them more vulnerable to hypertensive episodes. MABP, mean arterial blood pressure. From Hardy P, Varma DR, Chemtob S. Control of cerebral and ocular blood flow autoregulation in neonates. *Pediatr Clin North Am* 1997; 44:137–52, with permission.

The cerebrovascular response to changes in PaO_2 is mediated locally and results in vasodilation under reduced-oxygen conditions (hypoxic) and in vasoconstriction in high-oxygen conditions (hyperoxia) to maintain CBF constant over a range of pO_2 values (**Fig. 30.3**). This curve is relatively flat, except at reduced PaO_2 levels (less than ~50 torr), at which a steep rise in CBF curve occurs to maintain cerebral oxygen delivery.

The cerebrovascular response to changes in $PaCO_2$ is mediated locally by changes in perivascular pH. However, in contrast to changes in perfusion pressure and PaO_2, a nearly linear relationship between $PaCO_2$ and CBF exists between the range of $PaCO_2$ values of 20 torr and 80 torr, with an approximate 4% per mm Hg change in $PaCO_2$ (**Fig. 30.3**). At the ends of the spectrum (either hypocapnia or hypercapnia), the response is blunted, and these curves flatten. Consequently, vasodilation is seen with increasing arterial carbon dioxide concentration (hypercapnia), and vasoconstriction is seen with low arterial carbon dioxide concentration (hypocapnia). This vasoreactivity is the basis of hyperventilation-mediated reduction in CBF and the resultant reduction in cerebral blood volume that serves therapeutically to reduce intracranial hypertension. The CBF response to changes in $PaCO_2$ is generally related to the level of CBF at rest in a given brain region; thus, hyperventilation tends to equalize CBF throughout the brain. In addition, the CBF response

to changes in $PaCO_2$ is transient, lasting <24 hrs for a given change and is believed to be mediated by compensatory changes in brain interstitial bicarbonate concentration, which take time to manifest. When a hyperventilation-mediated reduction in $PaCO_2$ is used to reduce intracranial pressure, despite flattening of the CBF response to reduction in $PaCO_2$, relative ischemia has been suggested to occur, in part due to a reduction in CBF. Relative ischemia may also result from limited off-loading of oxygen from hemoglobin as the dissociation curve shifts to the left. CO_2 reactivity appears to be less vulnerable to injury than is pressure autoregulation. Altered CO_2 reactivity may suggest substantial damage to the brain region that is being assessed, and global loss of CO_2 reactivity is a concerning finding. Finally, CO_2 reactivity and pressure autoregulation are separate entities, as demonstrated by the fact that pressure autoregulation is maintained despite a new baseline CBF value when $PaCO_2$ is altered.

CEREBROVASCULAR REGULATION—DEVELOPMENTAL ISSUES

Given that the most dramatic change facing the developing child is birth, going from a relatively hypoxic to an oxygen-rich environment, it is intuitive that the cerebrovascular system would normally be ready to respond to such challenges. However, even in normal term infants, it appears that several days are required for such vascular responses to further mature. Experimental studies in piglets have shown that CO_2 reactivity and pressure autoregulation are present but poorly developed at birth; however, both autoregulation and CO_2 reactivity mature rapidly over the first postnatal days. Resting CBF levels also increase over the first few postnatal days, and studies in preterm human infants have confirmed that CBF increases over the first 3 postnatal days. Similarly, CO_2 reactivity increases from birth to early postnatal age, as do EEG amplitude and arterial blood pressure. However, during this postnatal period, CBF in infants is still lower than in adults. CBF further increases in children until 5–6 years of age, when it may be as much as 50%–85% higher than in adults, then decreases to adult levels by 15–19 years of age (**Fig. 30.5**). **Figure 30.5** shows the developmental changes in cerebral metabolism of glucose and CBF for both human and rat. The rat fuels a large percentage of cerebral metabolism during the synthetic work related to early postnatal developmental growth spurts by utilizing ketone oxidation due to the higher fat content of rodent maternal milk. In humans, CBF

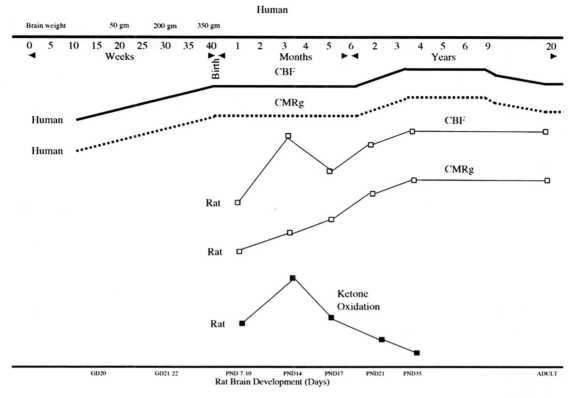

FIGURE 30.5. Developmental changes in cerebral metabolism of glucose (CMRg) and cerebral blood flow (CBF) for both human and rat. The rat fuels a large percentage of cerebral metabolism during the synthetic work related to early postnatal developmental growth spurts. In humans, peak CBF and CMRg occur between 3 and 9 years of age, corresponding to a very active growth period. GD, gestational day; PND, postnatal day. From Nehlig A. Cerebral energy metabolism, glucose transport and blood flow: Changes with maturation and adaptation to hypoglycaemia. *Diabetes Metab* 1997; 23:18–29, with permission.

parallels glucose metabolism, and peak CBF and glucose metabolism occur between 3 and 9 years of age, corresponding to a very active growth period. However, it has been estimated that human infants also may utilize up to 20% of their energy needs from ketones during the postnatal period, when nourishment is based primarily on maternal milk.

Cerebral Blood Flow—Metabolism Coupling

In adults, a tight coupling of CBF to brain metabolism normally occurs and is termed "flow-metabolism coupling," as described previously. It has been shown that CBF-metabolism coupling appears intact in normal newborn infants. The peak in cerebral glucose utilization during development correlates with the density of glucose transport proteins. Postnatal changes in regional CBF and cerebral metabolism occur in parallel in the human infant,

with the highest rates of local cerebral metabolic rate for glucose (LCMRg) and CBF occurring at between 3 and 9 years of age during the well-recognized period of rapid cognitive development (**Fig. 30.5**). Glucose is normally the lone cerebral substrate fueling active growth during this same period.

Cerebral Metabolism

Glucose serves as the major energy source for the developing brain. Glucose utilization through glycolytic and oxidative decarboxylation pathways parallels the energy demand of the developing brain. Consequently, LCMRg increases with developmental maturation and critical periods of growth and functional activity. Glucose entry into brain occurs via glucose transporter proteins (GLUTs). Of the 5 GLUTs (GLUT1–GLUT5), 2 (GLUT1 and 3) are located in the brain, with GLUT1 found in the BBB and choroid plexus and GLUT3 found in neurons. GLUT5 is located in activated brain microglia. GLUT expression in the developing brain is proportional to energy demand, increases during maturation, and is highest during peak synaptogenesis. Peak GLUT protein expression correlates with glutamate receptor maturity and learning and memory development in the developing CNS.

Germane to the PICU is the fact that cerebral energy metabolism and blood flow peak between 3 and 8 years of age in humans. Glucose utilization in 5-week-old infants in most brain regions is 71%–93% of that in the adult brain. LCMRg increases over the next 3 months, especially in the basal ganglia and parietal, temporal, and occipital cortices. Frontal cortex LCMRg further increases by 8 months—at which time cognitive function is rapidly developing. Adult levels of LCMRg are found by the time children are 2 years of age. LCMRg increases further until it reaches its highest levels, which are maintained until age 9 (**Fig. 30.5**). From this point forward, LCMRg declines until about age 20. Thus, the child's brain has considerable metabolic demand compared to adults.

In addition to the metabolism of glucose by the developing brain, the immature brain can utilize lactic acid, ketone bodies, and a large number of other metabolites, such as amino acids and free fatty acids. Monocarboxylate transporters for lactate and pyruvate develop over the midgestation period in the human brain, providing another significant energy source, using both extracellular lactate and pyruvate

as substrates. Lactate and pyruvate have also been shown to modulate the LTP and LTD that may be involved in synaptic plasticity critical to cognitive development at later stages of brain maturation. Due to the high fat ingestion of infants secondary to milk intake, more ketones are available in infant blood than in adult blood and can represent up to 20% of the carbon skeletons used in energy production in infants. The BBB is quite permeable to ketones, and coupled with enhanced developmental brain enzymatic activity for ketone use compared to adults, ketones play a more important role in bioenergetics of the immature CNS. CNS substrate use of ketones may also be linked to amino acid and lipid biosynthetic pathway precursors, which are subsequently used in developmental membrane and myelin formation. However, as has been shown in rats (**Fig. 30.5**), once the child is no longer dependent on maternal milk, the use of ketones as a metabolic fuel would decrease as well.

BLOOD-BRAIN BARRIER AND CHOROID PLEXUS DEVELOPMENT

Primary BBB functions serve to isolate brain blood compartments, provide selective transport of metabolites, ions, and molecules, and either metabolize or modify many blood- or brain-borne substances (**Fig. 30.6**). The BBB is impermeable to

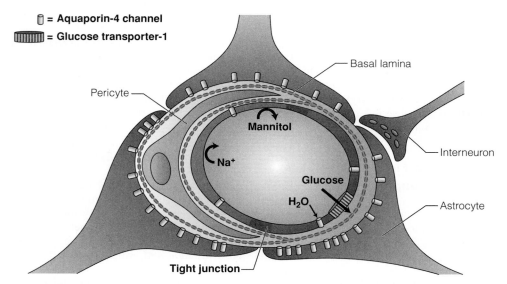

FIGURE 30.6. The structure of the mature blood-brain barrier (BBB) consists of endothelial cells connected by tight junctions, specialized supportive cells called pericytes, a basal lamina and perivascular astrocytic end feet. Modified from Abbott NJ, Ronnback L, Hansson E. Astrocyte–endothelial interactions at the blood-brain barrier. *Nat Rev Neurosci* 2006; 7:41–53.

hydrophilic molecules, ions, and proteins, while key metabolic substrates (e.g., glucose) enter via transport proteins (e.g., glucose transporter-1), and water passes through the BBB via aquaporin-4 channels. In addition, numerous metabolic barriers block the passage of molecules from blood to brain via the BBB, including P-glycoprotein (which involves energy-dependent movement of hydrophobic drugs out of the CNS) and enzymes (such as monoamine oxidase to metabolize catecholamines), which protect synaptic function.

The BBB is commonly thought to be "leaky" during fetal development and in the newborn infant. However, this issue remains a matter of debate (based upon experimental technical approaches), as evidence suggests that the fetal BBB is highly developed during the developmental period, including some mechanisms not found in the adult BBB. Tight junctions develop early during CNS maturation, and most proteins do not gain access to the extracellular compartment via the BBB during development. Cerebrospinal fluid (CSF) protein concentration is higher during early brain development and is thought to result from an immature choroid plexus; however, high CSF protein concentrations during development are not reflected in the extracellular space due to junctional complexes forming barriers at the CSF-brain interfaces that are not found in the adult brain. BBB permeability to ions and amino acids develops as transport systems mature in the brain; however, lipid insoluble molecules are more permeable in the immature brain than in the adult brain. The majority view suggests that fetal BBB permeability to macromolecules is similar to adults, but small molecules enter the fetal brain more readily than in the adult CNS. Ion permeability decreases just before birth in large animal experiments.

Small lipophilic molecules, such as CO_2, O_2, and ethanol, can readily pass through the BBB. However, the mature BBB is impermeable to many molecules and substances that are provided by cerebrovascular endothelial cell tight junctions, which form the complete zona occludens (**Fig. 30.6**). Small polar molecules needed for brain function, such as glucose and amino acids, are transported across the barrier by carrier proteins (e.g., GLUT-1 for glucose and the L-system carrier L1 for large neutral amino acids, such as leucine). Some small molecules and lipids are transported across the BBB by receptor-mediated endocytosis. The BBB is also able to remove hydrophobic molecules via p-glycoprotein—the energy-dependent, broad-spectrum efflux carrier, which plays a key role in BBB transport of a number of drugs. Finally, the cerebrovascular endothelial cells have an important metabolic function that is an integral component of the BBB. They contain

monoamine oxidase and can defend brain synaptic function against circulating catecholamines. Abbott and Romero have characterized the BBB as having important "static and dynamic properties." In addition, the barrier is surrounded by astrocyte foot processes, and these astrocytes can further modulate entry and egress of substances across the BBB via their possession of various channels and transporters (such as GLUTs previously discussed and the aquaporins discussed below) and through intracellular metabolism. A complete discussion of astrocyte metabolic function is beyond the scope of this chapter.

A number of specific proteins mediate barrier functions at tight junctions. Germane to pediatric critical care medicine, cerebrovascular tight junctions effectively prevent the movement of hydrophilic substances, such as cations (Na^+, K^+) and osmolar agents (e.g., mannitol), along with proteins, among other molecules (**Fig. 30.6**). Thus, the intact BBB is impermeable to salts and proteins, making osmolar gradients rather than oncotic gradients critical to water movement across the barrier and serving as the theoretical basis for the use of hypertonic saline and mannitol in the treatment of intracranial hypertension (discussed later in several chapters). Water movement across the BBB is mediated via special water channels, termed *aquaporins*. In the BBB and astrocyte foot processes, water movement is facilitated specifically by aquaporin-4 channels. These are in relatively low concentration in the vascular endothelial cells and in higher concentration in the astrocytes, which use them for their rapid astrocytic influx of water during uptake of potassium, glutamate, and other substances (**Fig. 30.6**). The role of the BBB and astrocytes in CNS injury is discussed in detail in Chapter 52, as it relates to excitotoxicity and cellular swelling.

CEREBROSPINAL FLUID DYNAMICS

Two pathways of CSF circulation have been proposed—a minor and a major pathway. While the details of CSF dynamics during development remain unclear, it is classically thought that they differ in the developing brain as compared to the adult. The major pathway of CSF absorption is via the arachnoid villi (arachnoid granulation) into the venous sinuses. The minor pathway includes drainage via ventricular ependyma, the interstitial and perivascular space, and perineural lymphatics. In adult humans, CSF production is ~500 ml/24 hrs, and the turnover may be 3–4 times a day. Interplay between the 2 drainage pathways maintains normal homeostasis and the neurochemical milieu in balance. The CSF circulation begins in development, with choroid plexus formation ~40–60 days of gestation, depending on the ventricle. The arachnoid granulation appears just before birth, and CSF reabsorption occurs at later ages.

The minor CSF pathway is the major route for CSF dynamics in the developing immature human brain, with arachnoid granulation function occurring in the late infant stages. Radiologic evidence for the arachnoid granulation as a gross structure occurs around age 7 and continues to develop until age 20.

CHAPTER 31 ◼ MOLECULAR BIOLOGY OF BRAIN INJURY

PATRICK M. KOCHANEK • HÜLYA BAYIR • LARRY W. JENKINS • ROBERT S.B. CLARK

Knowledge of the pathophysiology of central nervous system (CNS) injury, such as intracranial and cerebrovascular dynamics, has guided brain-oriented therapy. Most research on developmental brain injury suggests that, in many ways, the immature brain is more resistant to injury and more capable of recovery than is the adult brain as a result of enhanced plasticity (rewiring or repair). Ablative brain lesions in laboratory models, such as hemispherectomy in cats, demonstrate that the earlier the brain lesion occurs in development, the better the outcome. Some suggest possible critical windows in development represent periods of enhanced vulnerability of the brain to specific developmental processes. Some developmental aspects do predispose the immature brain to greater injury than the adult. However, outcome from out-of-hospital cardiac arrest is worse in children than in adults. The mechanism that underlies the cardiac arrest in children—asphyxia—is particularly injurious to the brain, compared to ventricular fibrillation. Similarly, reported outcomes in infants from severe traumatic brain injury (TBI) can be as bad as or worse than those in adults. This finding likely results from the contribution of inflicted childhood neurotrauma (child abuse) to severe TBI in infancy. Thus, although most data suggest that the developing brain exhibits both resistance and resilience to injury versus the adult, the mechanisms of injury are often severe in children.

SECONDARY INJURY

The essence of neurointensive care is the prevention of secondary injury. Two distinct types of secondary injury are frequently lumped into a single concept.

First, endogenous secondary injury cascades evolve in the minutes to days after the initial insult. Such processes as excitotoxicity, oxidative stress, and delayed neuronal death cascades, among others, kill neurons and injure other components of the CNS at varying rates. Emerging evidence supports the concept that these cascades can be abrogated in some cases, resulting in salvage of injured tissue and improved recovery of function. In contrast to the endogenous secondary injury cascades, a parallel form of secondary injury involves the occurrence of secondary insults in critically ill patients in the field, emergency room, or ICU that produce adverse consequences on a CNS with enhanced vulnerability after cardiac arrest, stroke, TBI, status epilepticus, or CNS infection. For example, hypoxemia, at a level tolerated by the normal brain, can have devastating effects after TBI.

Studies have begun to unravel the mechanisms producing secondary damage that are relevant to cardiac arrest, stroke, TBI, status epilepticus, CNS infection, and other insults. Five categories of mechanisms can be defined: those associated with (a) ischemia and energy failure and (b) excitotoxicity, both initiating cell death cascades; (c) inflammation; (d) direct tissue disruption; and (e) axonal injury. Within each category, a constellation of mediators of secondary damage is involved. The quantitative contribution of each mediator to outcome and the interplay between these mediators remains unclear and varies with the insult. A sixth component of the response to brain injury is the role of endogenous neuroprotectants, repair, and regeneration. The ultimate result of the primary injury that results from TBI, setting into motion these five cascade initiators, is summarized in **Figure 31.1.**

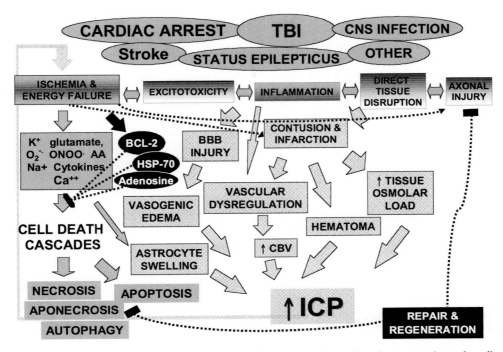

FIGURE 31.1. Secondary cascades triggered by the five initiators of secondary damage are shown for cell death cascades (*gray*), and for brain swelling-related process (*stippled gray*). In addition, a sixth category of endogenous neuroprotectants and repair and regeneration is initiated; the components of this cascade are shown in black. TBI, traumatic brain injury; $O_2^{\cdot-}$, superoxide anion; ONOO, peroxynitrite; AA, arachidonic acid; HSP-70, heat shock protein 70; CBV, cerebral blood volume; ICP, intracranial pressure.

Global Cerebral Ischemia

The brain is exquisitely vulnerable to ischemia, which represents a unifying mechanism involved in the evolution of secondary damage across CNS insults. When cerebral blood flow (CBF) globally ceases, such as in cardiac arrest, a stereotypic time course of events occurs that is initiated by acute cellular energy failure. Phosphocreatine is depleted in 1 min, and the adenylate energy charge is depleted in ~5 min. After this time, no useful energy can be made available to ATP-requiring reactions. Membrane failure follows, with loss of ionic gradients, increases in intracellular Ca^{2+} and Na^+, and a decrease in intracellular K^+. Free fatty acid release from the neuronal membrane also occurs, and electroencephalogram and evoked potentials fail. If energy failure is sustained beyond a critical period, an irreversible insult to neurons occurs and is believed to be manifest by acute necrotic death, with membrane failure, cellular sodium and calcium accumulation, cellular swelling, and acute failure of organelles, such as mitochondria. However, during complete global brain ischemia, assessment of brain tissue with light microscopy reveals no obvious pathologic derangement, and electron microscopy

reveals only chromatin clumping. The resultant damage to neurons, glia, and white matter does not manifest until reperfusion, suggesting a critical role for reperfusion in the evolution of secondary damage, as well as the intriguing possibility that even prolonged periods of ischemia might be survived with good outcome if the deleterious consequences of reperfusion could be eliminated. The duration of irreversibility for global cerebral ischemia in ventricular fibrillation cardiac arrest is believed to be between 5 and 10 min, although it can be modified by factors that include temperature, blood glucose concentration, and pH, among others.

Focal Cerebral Ischemia

Unlike global brain ischemia, focal ischemic insults (strokes) produce brain regions with different degrees of blood-flow reduction related to the vascular anatomy surrounding the area of occlusion. The typical result is an ischemic core, where flow reductions are profound, surrounded by penumbral brain regions that have less severe but still compromising CBF reductions. The most sensitive biochemical or molecular event to CBF reduction in the ischemic penumbra is protein synthesis, which is inhibited by ~50% at a CBF of 55 mL/100 g/min and generally fails below 35 mL/100 g/min. Other homeostatic processes that fail at decreasing CBF thresholds in focal ischemia include glucose utilization below 25 mL/100 g/min and ATP depletion, beginning at a CBF less than ~20 mL/100 g/min. Periinfarct depolarization waves occur at CBF of 50–70 mL/100 g/min and are postulated to contribute to damage in the penumbra by transiently increasing metabolic demands in this compromised zone. Electroencephalogram fails at a CBF below ~30 mL/100 g/min, hemiparesis is seen at CBF thresholds of ~23 mL/100 g/min, and anoxic depolarization occurs at CBF values between 15 and 20 mL/100 g/min, resulting in ionic failure. These CBF thresholds for failure of molecular and cellular homeostasis represent estimates for the adult brain. Corresponding ischemic threshold values in the developing brain are less well-established. If neuronal metabolic demands are increased (i.e., hyperthermia, seizures), the CBF threshold value that would trigger neuronal death could be higher, consistent with enhanced vulnerability.

Neuronal death can occur by multiple pathways, necrosis, programmed cell death (PCD) or apoptosis, and mixed phenotypes. Necrosis, which is characterized by denaturation and coagulation of cellular proteins, results from a progressive reduction in cellular ATP. Necrosis involves progressive derangements in energy and substrate metabolism that are followed by a series of morphologic alterations, including, swelling of cells and organelles, subsurface cellular blebbing, amorphous deposits in mitochondria, condensation of nuclear chromatin and, finally, breaks in plasma and organellar membranes. Mixed phenotypes of neuronal death exist that have features of both necrosis and apoptosis. The development of PCD involves new protein synthesis and the activation of endonucleases, with a characteristic cleavage of DNA into nucleosomal fragments of double-stranded DNA, called "DNA laddering." After cardiac arrest, stroke, TBI, epilepsy, and CNS infections, a continuum may exist in neurons from recovery to necrosis that depends on the severity and duration of the insult, the local milieu, and the given brain region.

Autophagy is a process that mediates normal turnover of cellular constituents, such as organelles and membranes in autophagic vacuoles. It is associated with cell death during starvation. However, after ischemia and TBI, disruption of this process may lead to "autophagic stress" or "macroautophagy," with accumulation of autophagic vacuoles resulting in cell death.

Three pathways are involved in cell death. First, Ca^{2+} activates several degradative enzymes (including calpain proteases and phospholipases) that modify mitochondrial proteins and lipids. Second, oxidative stress further modifies mitochondrial constituents. Finally, unchecked Ca^{2+} sequestration in mitochondria leads to mitochondrial permeability transition, which involves formation of a large conductance pore in the inner mitochondrial membrane and produces uncoupling of oxidative phosphorylation, osmotic swelling, release of matrix metabolites, and ultimately, physical rupture. These processes can lead to neuronal necrosis, apoptosis, or mixed cellular phenotypes.

Excitotoxicity is the process by which glutamate and other excitatory amino acids (EAAs) cause neuronal damage. Several cell injury mechanisms are linked to glutamate toxicity, which is also associated with neuronal damage in cardiac arrest, stroke, TBI, epilepsy, CNS infection, and hypoglycemia. Glutamate is the predominant excitatory neurotransmitter in the brain and acts through receptor types that are characterized according to specific EAA agonists. The 3 main glutamate receptors are the N-methyl-D-aspartate (NMDA), kainate, and α-amino-3-hydroxy-5-methyl-4-isoxazoleproprionic acid (AMPA) receptors (**Fig. 31.2**). Excitotoxic damage seems to be largely mediated by NMDA-receptor stimulation after stroke and TBI.

After cardiac arrest, stroke, and TBI and in CNS infection, a number of biochemical pathways contribute to a marked increase in free radical production. Oxidative stress-mediated injury is of heightened importance in CNS because of the high level of polyunsaturation of lipids, high metabolic rate, and the association between excitotoxicity and free radical production. Other sources of free radicals include cyclooxygenase-2, peroxidases (including myeloperoxidase and cytochrome-c), and both invading and resident inflammatory cells (**Fig. 31.3**).

Another important trigger for neuronal death is trophic factor withdrawal, and this process likely has relevance in the evolution of secondary damage after CNS insults in pediatric neurointensive care. Neurotrophins, such as nerve growth factor, brain-derived neurotrophic factor, and basic fibroblast growth factor, etc., are constitutively produced by neurons and glia, bind to receptors on target neurons, and are essential to survival and plasticity. Loss of trophic input to a target neuron via death of, or damage to, neuronal input from another brain region can trigger death of the target neurons.

In mature tissues, PCD requires initiation by either intracellular or extracellular signals. These signals have been characterized in vitro and are

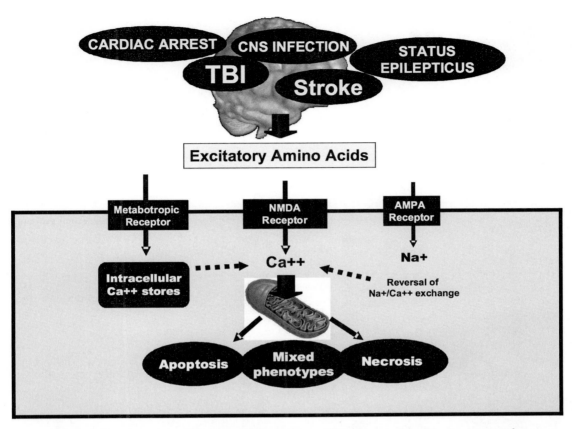

FIGURE 31.2. Receptors and key intracellular events resulting from excitotoxicity in neurons after PICU-relevant CNS insults. NMDA, *N*-methyl-D-aspartate; AMPA, α-amino-3-hydroxy-5-methyl-4-isoxazoleproprionic acid.

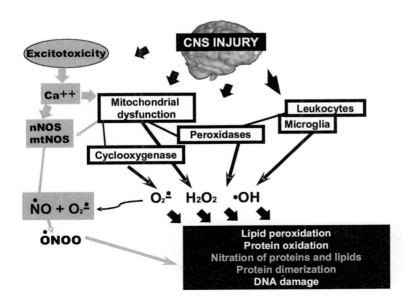

FIGURE 31.3. Pathways of oxidative and nitrative stress after CNS injury. Mitochondrial failure is a key participant with other pathways. Free radicals and other oxidants are generated, leading to lipid peroxidation, protein oxidation and dimerization, protein and lipid nitration, and DNA damage. mtNOS, mitochondrial nitric oxide synthase; n, neuronal; O_2^{-}, superoxide anion; ONOÖ, peroxynitrite; •OH, hydroxyl radical; H_2O_2, hydrogen peroxide.

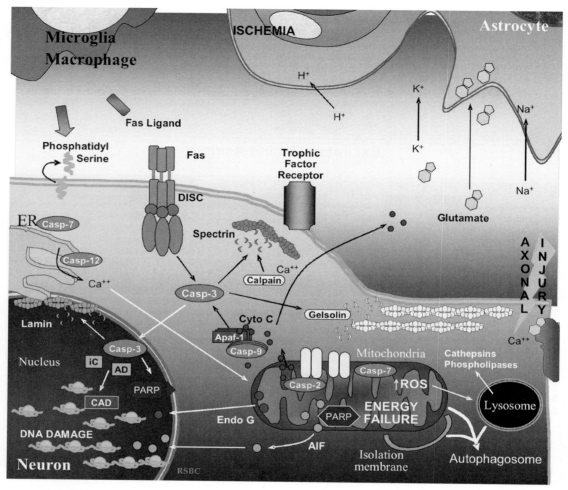

FIGURE 31.4. Neuronal death cascades resulting from necrosis, apoptosis [intrinsic, extrinsic, and apoptosis-inducing factor (AIF) pathways], and autophagy in CNS injury. ER, endoplasmic reticulum; Casp, caspase; CAD, caspase activated deoxyribonuclease; Endo G, endonuclease G; ROS, reactive oxygen species; PARP, poly (ADP ribose) polymerase.

becoming better characterized in vivo (**Fig. 31.4**). Intracellular signaling appears to be initiated in mitochondria, triggered by disturbances in cellular homeostasis, such as ATP depletion, oxidative stress, or calcium fluxes. Mitochondrial dysfunction leads to egress of cytochrome c from the inner mitochondrial membrane into the cytosol. Cytochrome-c release can be blocked by anti-apoptotic members of the bcl-2 family (bcl-2, bcl-xL, Mcl-1) and promoted by proapoptotic bcl-2 family members (bax, bad, bid). Cytochrome-c in the presence of dATP and a specific apoptotic-protease activating factor (Apaf-1) in cytosol activates the initiator cysteine protease caspase-9. Caspase-9 then activates the effector cysteine protease caspase-3, a key apoptosis effector that cleaves

cytoskeletal proteins, DNA repair proteins, and activators of endonucleases.

An additional intracellular cascade of PCD linked to mitochondrial injury is the apoptosis-inducing factor (AIF) pathway. This caspase-independent pathway is activated by mitochondrial permeability transition and results in the release of AIF from the mitochondrial membrane. AIF release leads to large-scale DNA fragmentation. Another intracellular pathway that can trigger apoptosis independent of mitochondrial failure is through synthesis of unique proapoptotic factors associated with endoplasmic reticulum (ER) stress. The aforementioned reduction in ER Ca^{2+} concentration that results from IP3-mediated Ca^{2+} release from the ER leads to induction of proteins such as CHOP in neurons, which mediate apoptosis.

Extracellular signaling of apoptosis occurs through the tumor necrosis factor (TNF) superfamily of cell surface death receptors, which include TNFR1 and Fas/Apo1/CD95. Receptor-ligand binding of TNFR1-TNFα or Fas-FasL promotes formation of a trimeric complex of TNF- or Fas-associated death domains, respectively. These death domains facilitate caspase recruitment.

Neurotrophic factors, neurotransmitters, cytokines, and reactive oxygen species (ROS) activate multiple upstream signaling pathways linked to either prosurvival or prodeath activities. These receptors couple to signal transduction pathways, involving interactions and cross-talk between multiple serine/threonine and tyrosine protein kinase cascades. Many kinases involved in the cell-death process are serine/threonine protein kinases. Important participants in the cell-death cascades include the mitogen-activated protein kinases.

The enzyme PARP plays a role in neuronal death in ischemia and TBI. PARP is found both in mitochondria and the nucleus and plays a homeostatic role in DNA repair in these 2 organelles. PARP, when activated by DNA damage, catalytically adds poly (ADP ribose) units onto proteins in mitochondria and the nucleus, such as histones, to help direct DNA repair enzymes to sites of damage. However, a deleterious consequence of PARP activation in CNS injury is the consumption of large quantities of NAD, thus depleting mitochondrial energy stores. This paradoxic consequence of PARP activation has been labeled the "PARP cell suicide theory" and leads to mitochondrial failure and cell death, either from overwhelming energy failure or delayed neuronal death through release of cytochrome-c and/or AIF.

Increases in intracellular Ca^{2+} in neurons activates calpain proteases, which sets into motion a cascade of protease activation that has been referred to as the "calpain-cathepsin cascade." Calpains (both mu and m isozymes) are located in dendritic regions and in axons and, when activated, cleave key cytoskeletal targets, such as spectrin, kinases, phosphatases, membrane receptors, and, importantly, lysosomes. Lysosomal rupture, believed to be mediated in part by calpains, leads to release of >80 hydrolytic enzymes, of which cathepsins B, D, H, and L are believed to play a role in executing neuronal death.

The endogenous retaliatory response to ischemic and excitotoxic insults are summarized in **Fig. 31.1**. Adenosine is an endogenous neuroprotectant produced in response to both ischemia and excitotoxicity. Adenosine antagonizes a number of events thought to mediate neuronal death. Breakdown of ATP leads to formation of adenosine, a purine nucleoside that decreases neuronal metabolism and increases CBF, among other mechanisms. Another endogenous neuroprotectant is HSP70, which is induced as part of the classic preconditioning response in brain. Bcl-2 is an important endogenous inhibitor of PCD in vitro. Several processes that result from injury may lead to substantial functional impairments without cell death. These include synaptic damage, disturbances in cell signaling and glial-neuronal cross talk, and alterations in neurotransmitter balance.

Brain Swelling

A unifying concept in brain injury is the occurrence of brain swelling. Cerebral swelling invariably develops, resulting from edema and/or increased cerebral blood volume (CBV), and can contribute to secondary ischemia from raised ICP, local compression, or the devastating consequences of herniation (**Fig. 31.5**).

Cellular swelling, a term that has supplanted the traditional "cytotoxic edema," occurs predominantly in astrocyte foot processes and is less representative of a "toxic" rather than a homeostatic or mediator-driven process. An additional molecular aspect of brain edema formation germane to astrocyte swelling is the role of endogenous water channels called *aquaporins*.

The blood–brain barrier (BBB) permeability, with resultant vasogenic edema, can also contribute to secondary brain swelling; this is particularly true in CNS infections, stroke and, to some extent, in TBI. This mechanism is likely of less importance after cardiac arrest. In acute bacterial meningitis, the acute inflammatory cascade also contributes to BBB damage and includes cytokine-mediated induction of leukocyte-adhesion molecules, neutrophil accumulation, and related oxidative injury to vascular endothelium. In addition, an important role for matrix metalloproteinases (MMPs) has also been reported in experimental meningitis. MMPs are endoproteases that can degrade the extracellular matrix.

A mechanism that appears to contribute greatly to the development of edema, particularly in TBI, is osmolar swelling in areas of contusion necrosis. Ironically, reconstitution of the injured BBB and/or development of an osmolar barrier around a necrotic focus may contribute to marked focal edema as the local osmolar load of the tissue increases, as macromolecules are degraded to constituents. This mechanism has been shown in adult TBI and likely represents one of the underpinnings for the beneficial

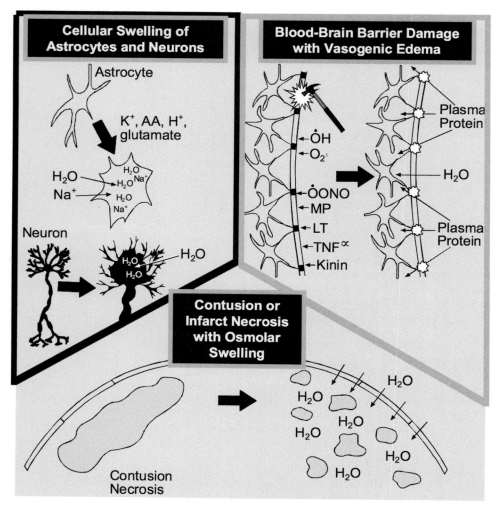

FIGURE 31.5. Three major mechanisms underlying the development of cerebral edema, including cellular swelling, blood-brain barrier injury with vasogenic edema, and osmolar swelling that develops in both contusions and infarcts. AA, arachidonic acid; O_2^{-}, superoxide anion; ONOÒ, peroxynitrite; •OH, hydroxyl radical; MP, metalloproteinase; LT, leukotriene; TNF-α, tumor necrosis factor α.

effects of osmolar therapy in the setting of cerebral contusion.

When an increase in CBV is seen after CNS injury, it may contribute to raised ICP and result from local increases in cerebral glycolysis "hyperglycolysis". In regions with increases in glutamate levels, such as in contusions, increased glycolysis is seen because astrocyte uptake of glutamate is coupled to glucose utilization. Hyperglycolysis may also mediate a coupled increase in CBF and CBV and resultant local brain swelling. As glutamate uptake by astrocytes is coupled to Na^+ and water uptake, local cellular swelling is also seen.

Regeneration and plasticity play important roles in mediating beneficial long-term effects on recov-

ery, and these responses are linked to inflammation. Macrophage infiltration and differentiation of endogenous microglia into resident macrophages may link inflammation and regeneration, with elaboration of a number of trophic factors (i.e., nerve growth factor among others). A link has been reported between IL-6 and nerve growth factor production.

It remains unclear whether anti-inflammatory therapies will improve outcome in clinical CNS injury. If inhibition of the inflammatory response is considered, exacerbation of infection risk must also be anticipated, and any deleterious consequences on the link between inflammation and regeneration must be addressed.

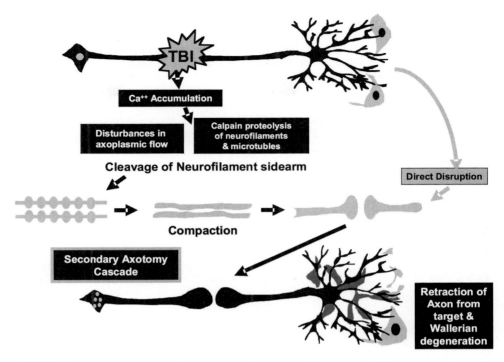

FIGURE 31.6. Cascades of axonal injury seen in either traumatic brain injury (TBI) or cerebral ischemia. Direct disruption of axons can occur in TBI, as shown on the right side of the figure. Believed to be more important, however, are two cascades of secondary axotomy related to either disturbances in axoplasmic flow or calcium-mediated proteolytic events, resulting in neurofilament compaction. These cascades may be responsive to some therapies, similar to those used to target neuronal death.

Axonal Injury

Axonal injury plays an important role in TBI, and perinatal brain injury and white matter injury may also be important in stroke. The most established type of white matter damage in PICU-relevant CNS insults is traumatic axonal injury (TAI). The classic view that TAI occurs due to immediate physical shearing is represented primarily in severe injury, in which frank axonal tears occur. However, recent experimental studies suggest that TAI occurs by a delayed process termed "secondary axotomy" (**Fig. 31.6**).

MECHANISMS OF ENHANCED VULNERABILITY OF INJURED BRAIN

The injured brain is extremely vulnerable to secondary physiologic derangements that occur in the field, emergency department, or ICU, and hypotension and hypoxemia have received the most investigation. Hypoxemia to PaO_2 levels between 40 and 50 mm Hg for periods as short at 30 min can exacerbate neuronal death. Increased metabolic demands early after CNS insults are substantial and result from both direct excitation of neurons, clinical or subclinical seizures, and increases in glucose utilization from glycolytic demands of astrocytes in EAA reuptake and mitochondrial dysfunction. The most likely candidate for enhanced vulnerability in this phase is concomitant brain swelling, which generally peaks between 24 and 72 hrs. Hypotension or hypoxemia, even within the autoregulatory range, results in compensatory vasodilation with an increase in CBV, further increasing ICP and potentially leading to a vicious cycle. Compromised CBF can also impair protein syntheses, as regeneration is beginning. Other mechanisms may also be important.

Hyperthermia-mediated exacerbation of secondary brain injury is marked at the time of injury but has been reported even days after experimental brain injury. Exacerbation of the inflammatory response may be involved. Heightened metabolic demands in injured brain with inability to compensate with an appropriate increase in CBF could also be occurring. These experimental findings have served to support the need for prevention of fever after cardiac arrest, stroke, and TBI, though this is less clear in CNS infections.

Vulnerability of the normal brain to hypoglycemia is well described in the classical experimental brain injury literature. It might be advisable to avoid tight glucose control in patients with brain injury, in favor of a more conservative approach. Although care must be taken to avoid hypoglycemia after CNS in-

sults, it is also well recognized that hyperglycemia can exacerbate CNS injury. The mechanisms involved in this exacerbation of ischemic brain injury by hyperglycemia include worsened brain swelling by lactate-mediated osmolar effects, along with greater local brain tissue acidosis with enhanced iron-catalyzed lipid peroxidation. It appears that before or after brain injury, marked hyperglycemia (>180 mg/dL) should be avoided or treated.

CHAPTER 32 ■ EVALUATION OF THE COMATOSE CHILD

NICHOLAS S. ABEND • SUDHA KILARU KESSLER • MARK A. HELFAER • DANIEL J. LICHT

Consciousness is a state of wakefulness and awareness of self and surroundings. Coma is a state of altered consciousness with loss of both wakefulness (arousal, vigilance) and awareness of the self and environment, and it is characterized by sustained, pathologic, eyes-closed, unarousable unresponsiveness. Sleep-wake cycles are absent. Coma is a type of transitory state that can evolve toward recovery of consciousness, a minimally conscious state, a vegetative state, or brain death. *Lethargy* is a state of reduced wakefulness with attention deficits. *Obtundation* is characterized by blunted alertness and diminished interaction with the environment. *Stupor* is a state of unresponsiveness with little or no spontaneous movement, resembling deep sleep but differing from coma because vigorous stimulation induces temporary arousal. A patient in a persistent vegetative state is awake but unaware and has sleep-wake cycles but no detectable cerebral cortical function. The eyes may be open without visual fixation or pursuit. Generally this state is not diagnosed until 1 month after coma onset. A patient in a minimally conscious state has severely altered consciousness with minimal but definite behavioral evidence of self or environmental awareness, such as following simple commands or making simple nonreflexive gestures. *Akinetic mutism* is a condition of extreme slowing or absence of bodily movement with loss of speech. Wakefulness and awareness are preserved, but cognition is slowed. Causes include extensive bihemispheric disease and lesions that involve the inferior frontal lobes bilaterally, the paramedian mesencephalic reticular formation, or the posterior diencephalon. The locked-in syndrome is a state of preserved consciousness

and cognition with complete paralysis of the voluntary motor system. Cortical function is intact, and electroencephalogram (EEG) patterns are normal. Locked-in syndrome may result from lesions of the corticospinal and corticobulbar pathways at or below the pons but may also arise with severe peripheral nervous system disease, such as Guillain-Barré syndrome, botulism, and critical illness polyneuropathy. Eye movements, most commonly vertical eye movements, may be preserved, allowing for some communication. Coma must also be distinguished from brain death, which is the permanent absence of all brain activity, including brainstem function. Delirium is an acute confusional state characterized by changes in level of consciousness, impaired attention, and a fluctuating course. It may occur with toxic-metabolic encephalopathy, focal lesions, or seizures.

The causes of coma are broad and are listed in **Table 32.1.** An algorithm for initial evaluation of coma is outlined in **Table 32.2.** Guidelines have been published online (www.nottingham.ac.uk/paediatric-guideline) by the Pediatric Accident and Emergency Research Group of the Royal College of Paediatrics and Child Health and the British Association for Emergency Medicine.

A detailed history may not always be available on initial evaluation of the comatose child, but historic information must be gathered as quickly as possible, as it may be crucial in identifying the cause of coma. The most widely used instrument is the Glasgow Coma Scale (GCS), which was initially developed to evaluate adults with head injury. Pediatric adaptations to the GCS, more developmentally appropriate for infants and children, include the

TABLE 32.1

ETIOLOGIES OF COMA

Trauma
Parenchymal injury
Intracranial hemorrhage
  Epidural hematoma
  Subdural hematoma
  Subarachnoid hemorrhage
  Intracerebral hematoma
Diffuse axonal injury

Nontraumatic causes
Toxic/metabolic
Hypoxic-ischemic encephalopathy
  Shock
  Cardiopulmonary arrest
  Near drowning
  Carbon monoxide poisoning
Toxins
  Medications: narcotics, sedatives, antiepileptics,
    antidepressants, analgesics, aspirin
  Environmental toxins: organophosphates, heavy metals,
    cyanide, mushroom poisoning
  Illicit substances: alcohol, heroin, amphetamines, cocain
Systemic metabolic disorders
  Substrate deficiencies
    Hypoglycemia
    Cofactors: thiamine, niacin, pyridoxine
  Electrolyte and acid-base imbalance: sodium, magnesium,
    calcium
  Diabetic ketoacidosis
  Thyroid/adrenal/other endocrine disorders
  Uremic coma
  Hepatic coma
  Reye syndrome
  Inborn errors of metabolism
    Urea cycle disorders
    Amino acidopathies
    Organic acidopathies
    Mitochondrial disorders
Infections/postinfectious/inflammatory
  Meningitis and encephalitis: bacterial, viral, rickettsial,
    fungal
  Acute demyelinating diseases
    Acute disseminated encephalomyelitis
    Multiple sclerosis
  Inflammatory/autoimmune
    Sarcoidosis
    Sjögren disease
    Lupus Cerebritis
Mass lesions
  Neoplasms
  Abscess, granuloma
  Hydrocephalus
Paroxysmal neurologic disorders
  Seizures/status epilepticus
  Acute confusional migraine
Vascular
  Intracranial hemorrhage
  Arterial infarcts
  Venous sinus thromboses
  Vasculitis

Pediatric Coma Scale, the Children's Coma Scale, and the Glasgow Coma Scale-Modified for Children (**Table 32.3**). Pupils (**Fig. 32.1** and **Table 32.4**) are examined first by observing the size of both pupils in dim light and then by assessing reactivity to a bright light shined in each eye. Asymmetric pupils are caused either by disruption of the oculomotor nerve (cranial nerve III) or impairment of sympathetic fibers (Horner syndrome). Because the oculomotor nerve innervates the pupil constrictors, oculomotor nerve impairment results in an abnormally dilated pupil. Oculomotor nerve palsy also results in ptosis and ophthalmoparesis and may be a sign of uncal herniation. Horner syndrome describes disruption of the sympathetic innervation to the face, characterized by mild ptosis over an abnormally small pupil (meiosis). In traumatic coma, Horner syndrome may be an important clue to dissection of the carotid artery, along which the sympathetic fibers travel, or an injury to the lower brachial plexus (C8–T1). Anisocoria (asymmetric pupils) is an important physical finding, and differentiating whether a pupil is abnormally large or abnormally small is crucial to identifying underlying pathology. In brief, in pupils that are more asymmetric in bright light, the pathology lies with the larger pupil and is likely the result of oculomotor palsy (cranial nerve III). Investigations to rule out uncal herniation or an aneurysm of the posterior communicating artery should follow. In pupils that are more asymmetric in darkness, the pathology lies with the smaller pupil. Investigation of the carotid artery, the low cervical–high thoracic spinal cord, or brachial plexus roots should follow to find causes of the Horner syndrome.

Abnormalities of eye position and motility may be signs of cortical, midbrain, or pontine dysfunction. Conjugate lateral eye deviation is caused by destructive lesions of the ipsilateral cortex or pons or by focal seizures in the contralateral hemisphere. Rarely thalamic lesions may cause "wrong-way eyes," in which the eyes deviate away from the side of the destructive lesion. Tonic down-gaze suggests dorsal midbrain compression. The complete dorsal midbrain syndrome of Parinaud includes pupillary light-near dissociation, lid-retraction, and convergence-retraction nystagmus.

Dysconjugate gaze suggests extraocular muscle weakness or, more commonly, abnormalities of the third, fourth, or sixth cranial nerves or nuclei. Unilateral or bilateral abducens nerve (cranial nerve VI) palsies are commonly seen in increased intracranial pressure (ICP), presumably because the nerve is stretched. This sign is therefore considered a "false localizing sign," as it suggests a focal brainstem lesion but, in fact, represents a more diffuse ICP change. An eye with oculomotor nerve (cranial nerve III) palsy

TABLE 32.2

INITIAL EVALUATION OF COMA

Airway, breathing, and circulation assessment and stabilization
Ensure adequate ventilation and oxygenation.
Blood pressure management depends on considerations regarding underlying coma etiology. If hypertensive encephalopathy or intracranial hemorrhage, lower blood pressure. If perfusion-dependent state, such as some strokes or elevated intracranial pressure, reducing blood pressure may reduce cerebral perfusion.

Draw blood for glucose, electrolytes, ammonia, arterial blood gas, liver and renal function tests, complete blood count, lactate, pyruvate, and toxicology screen.

Neurologic assessment
GCS score
Assess for evidence of raised intracranial pressure and herniation.
Assess for abnormalities that suggest focal neurologic disease.
Assess for history or signs of seizures.

Administer glucose IV (in an adult, thiamine should be given first)

If concern for infection delays lumbar puncture, broad-spectrum infection coverage should be provided (including bacterial, viral, and possibly fungal).

Give specific antidotes if toxic exposures are known.
For opiate overdose, administer naloxone.
For benzodiazepine overdose, consider administering flumazenil.
For anticholinergic overdose, consider administering physostigmine.

Identify and treat critical elevations in intracranial pressure.
Neutral head position, elevated head by 20 degrees, sedation
Hyperosmolar therapy with mannitol 0.25–1 g/kg or hypertonic saline
Hyperventilation as temporary measure
Consider intracranial monitoring.
Consider neurosurgical intervention.

Head CT

Treat seizures with IV anticonvulsants. Consider prophylactic anticonvulsants.

Investigate source of fever and use antipyretics and/or cooling devices to reduce cerebral metabolic demands.

Detailed history and examination

Consider lumbar puncture, EEG or extended long-term EEG monitoring, MRI, metabolic testing (amino acids, organic acids, acylcarnitine profile), autoimmune testing (ANA panel, antithyroid antibodies), thyroid testing (TSH, T3, T4).

is ptotic, depressed, and abducted and has a dilated pupil. As discussed below, oculomotor nerve palsy in a comatose patient suggests uncal herniation with midbrain compression and requires urgent intervention. Trochlear nerve (cranial nerve IV) palsy causes hypertropia in the affected eye.

Roving eye movements are seen in comatose patients with intact brainstem function. Their disappearance may signal the onset of brainstem dysfunction. Periodic alternating gaze (ping-pong gaze) describes conjugate horizontal eye movements back and forth, with a pause at each end. It may be seen with extensive bilateral hemispheric, basal ganglia, or thalamic-midbrain damage with an intact pons and is thought to result from disconnection of cortical influences on oculovestibular reflex generators. It has also been reported in reversible coma from monoamine oxidase and tricyclic antidepressant toxicity.

Oculocephalic and oculovestibular reflexes are useful for assessing the integrity of the midbrain and pons in a comatose patient without spontaneous eye movements. To test oculocephalic reflexes, the examiner holds the patient's eyelids open and quickly moves the head to one side. In a comatose patient with an intact brainstem, the eyes will move in the direction opposite the head motion. For example, if the head is moved to the right, the eyes will move conjugately to the left. After several seconds, the eyes may return to a neutral position. The head should be tested in both horizontal and vertical directions. Oculocephalic reflexes should not be tested if the patient

TABLE 32.3

GLASGOW COMA SCALE AND MODIFICATION FOR CHILDREN

Sign	Glasgow coma scale	Modification for children	Score
Eye opening	Spontaneous	Spontaneous	4
	To command	To sound	3
	To pain	To pain	2
	None	None	1
Verbal response	Oriented	Age-appropriate verbalization, orients to sound, fixes and follows, social smile	5
	Confused	Cries, but consolable	4
	Disoriented	Irritable, uncooperative, aware of environment	3
	Inappropriate words	Irritable, persistent cries, inconsistently consolable	
	Incomprehensible sounds	Inconsolable crying, unaware of environment or parents, restless, agitated	2
	None	None	1
Motor response	Obeys commands	Obeys commands, spontaneous movement	6
	Localizes pain	Localizes pain	5
	Withdraws	Withdraws	4
	Abnormal flexion to pain	Abnormal flexion to pain	3
	Abnormal extension	Abnormal extension	2
	None	None	1
Best total score			15

has sustained cervical spine trauma or if the spine has not been cleared.

The oculovestibular reflex, commonly referred to as cold calorics, tests the function above the pontomedullary junction. The child must have an open

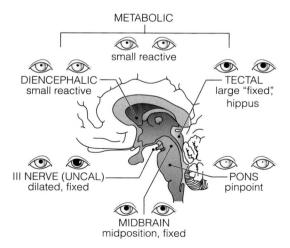

FIGURE 32.1. Pupils in comatose patients. Adapted from Plum F, Posner JB. *The Diagnosis of Stupor & Coma*, 3rd Ed. Philadelphia: F.A. Davis, 1982.

external auditory canal with an intact tympanic membrane (including the absence of pressure equalization tubes), and visual inspection of the canal is an important first step. With the head elevated at 30 degrees, up to 120 mg of ice water is introduced in the ear canal with a small catheter. A conscious patient would experience nystagmus with slow deviation of the eyes toward the irrigated ear and a fast corrective movement away from the ear (the mnemonic COWS, *cold opposite, warm same,* applies to the fast phase). In a comatose patient, the fast correction mediated by the cortex is not seen. Instead, the eyes will deviate slowly toward the irrigated ear and remain fixed there. If the brainstem vestibular nuclei (located at the pontomedullary junction) are impaired, no movement will be seen. In brain death, in which brainstem function is nonexistent, no eye movement is seen with both ears tested. Five minutes should be allowed before the second ear is tested to allow return of temperature equilibrium between the 2 ears. Vertical eye movements may be tested by simultaneously irrigating both auditory canals with cold water, producing downward deviation in the comatose patient. Warm water irrigation produces upward gaze.

The remaining brainstem reflexes provide information about the integrity of lower regions of the

TABLE 32.4

PUPIL ABNORMALITIES IN COMA

Etiology/localization	Pupil appearance
Metabolic	Small, reactive
Hypothalamic	Small, reactive
Tectal	Large, nonreactive, hippus
Pontine	Pinpoint
Midbrain	Mid-position, fixed
Oculomotor nerve, uncal herniation	Ipsilateral pupil dilated, fixed
Severe hypoxic-ischemic encephalopathy	Bilateral dilated, fixed
Opiate intoxication	Pinpoint
Anticholinergic poisoning	Dilated and fixed, unreactive to 1% pilocarpine

brainstem. The corneal reflex is tested by tactile stimulation of the cornea, which should elicit bilateral eyelid closure. The afferent (sensory) signal is carried by the trigeminal nerve (cranial nerve V), and the efferent (motor) pathway is carried by the facial nerve (cranial nerve VII). Completion of the reflex loop requires intact trigeminal and facial nerve nuclei in the mid- and lower pons. The cough reflex, which may be seen with stimulation of the carina when a patient is intubated or undergoes suctioning, is mediated by medullary cough centers; sensory and motor signals are carried by the glossopharyngeal (cranial nerve IX) and vagus (cranial nerve X) nerves. When the soft palate is stimulated, the gag reflex is elicited, manifested as elevation of the soft palate. As in the cough reflex, afferent and efferent signals are carried by the glossopharyngeal and vagus nerves, with processing in the medulla. Narcotics may suppress cough reflex, an important consideration for accurate assessment of brainstem function.

LABORATORY, IMAGING, AND ELECTROPHYSIOLOGIC INVESTIGATION

Investigation should continue with laboratory, neuroimaging, and electrophysiologic testing (**Table 32.5**). Once the patient has been stabilized and the etiology of coma remains unclear, a brain MRI may be performed for diagnostic and prognostic purposes.

INCREASED INTRACRANIAL PRESSURE

Causes of increased ICP in coma include intracranial hemorrhage, space-occupying lesions, and cerebral edema. Cerebral edema may be vasogenic, cellular, or osmolar. Cellular swelling is predominantly astrocyte swelling as a consequence of homeostatic processes to control excitotoxicity or acidosis with sodium and water accumulation. Osmolar swelling can also occur in necrotic foci such as infarcts or contusions. Herniation syndromes often herald impending catastrophic deterioration and death unless ICP is lowered by medical or surgical means. Initial management of critically raised ICP includes IV hyperosmolar therapy (mannitol or sodium) and hyperventilation to achieve a pCO_2 of 35 mm Hg. Further reduction in pCO_2 may be necessary to achieve rapid but temporary reductions in cerebral blood flow and this ICP, but excessive or prolonged hyperventilation may compromise cerebral perfusion, resulting in further hypoxic ischemic injury. These initial measures may provide only temporary reductions in ICP. Barbiturate coma or hypothermia may reduce cellular energy requirements and may thus help protect the brain during periods of hypoxia and ischemia. Similarly, providing adequate sedation and paralysis may further reduce energy demand and prevent spikes in ICP. Maintaining a neutral neck position and elevation of the head of the bed at 20–30 degrees may improve venous drainage. Surgical decompression may be required for more definitive therapy. Often a large craniectomy is performed with wide margins to allow space for brain expansion. If the margins are too small, fungating herniation may occur through the skull defect. Cushing triad (hypertension, bradycardia, and a change in respirations) may occur with any type of increased intracranial hypertension, and more specific signs of herniation depend on the location of the herniation syndrome. These are summarized in **Table 32.6**. While neuroimaging will demonstrate the exact nature of the herniation, waiting for and transport to neuroimaging may be detrimental, and medical interventions should be implemented emergently prior to neuroimaging.

TABLE 32.5

INVESTIGATION OF NONTRAUMATIC COMA IN PEDIATRICS

Investigations	Indication/clinical clues	Possible abnormality	Further investigation if abnormal	Possible diagnoses	Action
Dextrostix	All	Low	Blood glucose	Hypoglycemia secondary to:	IV dextrose
Blood glucose			Liver function tests	Fasting	Fluids/insulin
			Blood ammonia	Severe illness	
			Blood lactate	Reye syndrome	
			Blood and urine amino acids	Organic aciduria	
			Urine organic acids	Fatty-acid oxidation defect	
				Hemorrhagic shock and encephalopathy	
	Previous polydipsia/polyuria	High		Diabetic ketoacidosis	
Blood sodium	All	Low	Urinary sodium	Hypo/hypernatremia ± dehydration	Appropriate fluids
		High			
Blood urea	All	High	Blood creatinine	Dehydration	Rehydrate
			Blood film	Hemolytic-uremic syndrome	Dialysis, plasmapheresis
Aspartate transaminase	All	High	Blood ammonia	Reye Syndrome	
				Hypoxia-ischemia	
Blood Ammonia	All (unless cause known)	High	Blood orotic acid	Urea cycle defect	Sodium benzoate
			Urine organic acids	Organic acidemia	
Full blood count and film	All	Low Hb	Hb electrophoresis	Anemia	Transfusion
	Residence in endemic area	High WBC		Infection	3rd-generation cephalosporin
	Pica	Low platelets		DIC infection	Dialysis, plasmapheresis
		Sickle cells		Sickle cell disease	Quinine
		Burr cells		Hemolytic-uremic syndrome	Chelation
		Parasites on thick/thin films		Malaria	
		Basophilic stippling	Wrist x-ray—lead line	Lead encephalopathy	
Blood culture	All				Appropriate antibiotics
Stool culture	All	Shigella, enteroviruses			
Mycoplasma IgG, IgM	All (unless cause known)		Chest x-ray	Mycoplasma encephalitis	Erythromycin, ?prednisolone

(continued)

TABLE 32.5

INVESTIGATION OF NONTRAUMATIC COMA IN PEDIATRICS (CONTINUED)

Investigations	Indication/clinical clues	Possible abnormality	Further investigation if abnormal	Possible diagnoses	Action
Viral titers	Analyze if unexplained		Repeat at discharge		
Urine for toxin screen	Analyze if unexplained		Blood film—basophilic stippling, wrist x-ray—lead line	Poisoning	Antidote
Blood lead	Analyze if unexplained				Chelation
CT scan without contrast	All (after resuscitation, afebrile patients should ideally be transferred for CT scan to a unit with neurosurgical facilities)	Blood			
		Subdural	Skull x-ray/skeletal survey/clotting screen	Nonaccidental injury	Neurosurgical referral Child protection
		Extradural			Neurosurgical referral
		Intracerebral			Neurosurgical referral
		Space-occupying lesion		Tumor	
		Hydrocephalus Obstructive Communicating	CSF examination	?Space-occupying lesion ?Meningitis, especially tuberculous	Antituberculous cover Neurosurgical referral Neurosurgical referral
		Abscess	Culture aspirate Contrast CT/MRI		Neurosurgical referral Anaerobic cover
		Swelling Focal low density		Cerebral abscess, herpes simplex, stroke, ADEM	Mannitol 0.25 g/kg
		Abnormal basal ganglia	Plasma/CSF lactate, blood gas	Leigh syndrome, hypoxic-ischemic, striatal necrosis	
Lumbar puncture	In febrile patient if no clinical or radiologic evidence of raised ICP (delay and treat if doubt)				
Pressure measurement		High			Mannitol, ventilate
Microscopy		High WBC	CT	Meningitis/e encephalitis	3rd-generation cephalosporin, acyclovir
Gram stain, bacterial culture		High RBC	CT (traumatic tap should clear by third bottle)	Hemorrhage/encephalitis/ nonaccidental injury	Neurosurgical referral, acyclovir, child protection

Investigation				Diagnosis	Treatment
Glucose		Low		Tuberculous meningitis	Immediate and prolonged antitubercular therapy
Protein		High		Tuberculous meningitis	Immediate and prolonged antitubercular therapy
PCR for viruses, TB Prolonged search for acid-fast bacilli, culture for TB on Lowenstein-Jensen	Prodome >7 days, optic atrophy, focal signs, abnormal movements, CSF polymorphs <50%, hydrocephalus and/or basal enhancement on contrast CT			Tuberculous meningitis	Immediate and prolonged antitubercular therapy
Antibodies; (e.g., herpes simplex, mycoplasma)				Encephalitis	Acyclovir, erythromycin
Lactate	Abnormal breathing/eye movements, basal ganglia lucencies		Muscle biopsy	Leigh syndrome	
EEG	All, especially if ventilated or evidence of subtle seizures (nystagmus, tonic deviation of eyes, clonic jerking limbs)	Epileptiform discharges Asymmetrical foci of spikes or periodic lateralizing epileptiform discharges on slow background		Status epilepticus Herpes simplex encephalitis (many patients do not have characteristic EEG)	IV benzodiazepines, phenytoin, thiopentone High-dose IV acyclovir for 2 weeks
MRI	Unexplained encephalopathy	Frontotemporal abnormality Thalamic abnormality	CSF for herpes simplex, PCR CSF for EBV (arboviruses in endemic area)	Herpes simplex encephalitis	High-dose IV acyclovir for 2 weeks

hb, hemoglobin; WBC, white blood cell; CSF, cerebrospinal fluid; RBC, red blood cell; TB, tuberculosis; EEG, electroencephalogram; PCR, polymerase chain reaction; EBV, Epstein Barr virus
From Kirkham FJ. Non-traumatic coma in children. *Arch Dis Child* 2001; 85:303–12, with permission.

TABLE 32.6

HERNIATION SYNDROMES

Herniation syndrome	Location	Signs
Central herniation	Increased pressure in both cerebral hemispheres, causing downward displacement of the diencephalon through the tentorium, causing brainstem compression.	**Diencephalic stage:** withdraws to noxious stimuli, increased rigidity, or decorticate posturing; small, reactive pupils with preserved oculocephalic and oculovestibular reflexes; yawns, sighs, or Cheyne-Stokes breathing. **Midbrain-upper pons stage:** decerebrate posturing or no movement; mid-position pupils that may become irregular and unreactive; abnormal or absent oculocephalic and oculovestibular reflexes; hyperventilation. **Lower pons-medullary stage:** no spontaneous motor activity, but lower extremities may withdraw to plantar stimulation; mid-position fixed pupils; absent oculocephalic and oculovestibular reflexes; ataxic respirations. **Medullary stage:** generalized flaccidity; absent pupillary reflexes and ocular movements; slow irregular respirations, death.
Uncal herniation	Uncus of the temporal lobe is displaced medially over the free edge of the tentorium.	Ipsilateral third-nerve palsy (ptosis, pupil fixed and dilated, eye deviated down and out). Ipsilateral hemiparesis from compression of the contralateral cerebral peduncle (Kernohan notch). Other signs of brainstem dysfunction from ischemia secondary to compression of posterior cerebral artery.
Subfalcine (cingulate) herniation	Increased pressure in one cerebral hemisphere leads to herniation of cingulated gyrus underneath falx cerebri.	Compression of anterior cerebral artery leads to paraparesis.
Tonsillar herniation	Increased pressure in the posterior fossa leads to brainstem compression.	Loss of consciousness from compression of reticular activating system. Focal lower cranial nerve dysfunction. Respiratory and cardiovascular function can be significantly affected early with relative preservation of upper brainstem function, such as pupillary light reflexes and vertical eye movements.

SEIZURES

Subclinical seizures in critically ill patients may be an under-recognized phenomenon; therefore, the index of suspicion in a comatose child should be high. Likewise there are many issues that can modify the perceived prognosis of patients with brain injury leading to an inappropriately pessimistic outlook.

PHYSICAL EXAMINATION

Many patients with severe brain injury receive paralytic or sedative medications that can affect the physical examination. The effect of these agents must be carefully considered before interpreting the potential significance of a comatose child's physical examination. Children with hypoxic-ischemic

TABLE 32.7

GENERAL GUIDELINES FOR NEUROIMAGING IN THE INITIAL EVALUATION OF SELECT CAUSES OF COMA

	Head CT	Diffusion-weighted image	T2	T1	Echo gradient	Gadolinium contrast
Acute ischemia Minutes to hours	± (Usually normal)	Bright signal indicates restriction of water diffusion (cytotoxic edema)	Hyperintense signal after several hours	Variable	May demonstrate petechial hemorrhage	– early + late (increasing after 3 days)
Subacute ischemia 3 days to week	Hypodense (dark)	Restriction of water will fade at 7–10 days	Hyperintense	Variable, hyperintense in neonate	Petechial or hemorrhagic transformation	+ enhancement
Acute hemorrhage hour to days	Hyperdense (bright)	N/A	Very hypointense	Hypointense	Strongly positive	
Subacute hemorrhage First several days	Heterogeneous to hypodense	N/A	Very hyperintense	Very hyperintense	Strongly positive	
Infection	Hypodense/isodense	Restriction of water diffusion if abscess	Very hyperintense	Very hypointense	± petechial hemorrhage	+ enhancement

Intensity is relative to normal brain parenchyma (hypointense, dark relative to normal tissue; hyperintense, bright relative to normal tissue; isointense, same intensity of normal tissue).

encephalopathy (HIE) that the absence of spontaneous ventilation and absence of pupillary reflexes at 24 hrs after insult had 100% positive predictive value (PPV) of poor outcome. In children with coma due to multiple etiologies, the absence of motor response to pain on day 3 after injury had PPV for unfavorable outcome of 100%. Together, these studies suggest that if not confounded by medications, the neurologic examination is quite predictive when performed >24 hrs after the inciting event. Falsely pessimistic predictions can be limited by using SEP in conjunction with the physical exam.

EVOKED POTENTIALS

When a sensory stimulus is delivered to nerves, neural structures along the particular sensory pathway produce electrical signals that can be detected by electrodes. On initial testing, abnormal SEPs have a PPV for unfavorable outcome of 98% when absent bilaterally and PPV for favorable outcome of 91% when present. All patients with favorable outcomes despite absent SEPs had structural lesions, such as subdural effusions or brainstem hemorrhage. In children with only HIE in whom prognosis was unclear at 24 hrs after resuscitation, the finding of bilateral absent N20 waves on the SEP had 100% PPV for unfavorable outcome, with 63% sensitivity.

Brainstem auditory-evoked potentials (BAEP) use an auditory stimulus to evaluate brainstem but not cortical function. Thus, while they may be predictive of survival versus death, they lack utility in predicting neurocognitive outcome, which is based largely on cortical function.

Visual-evoked potentials (VEP) use a flickering light to activate the visual system. Bilaterally absent cortical somatosensory-evoked potential (SEP) responses are predictive of death or severe disability.

The role of BAEP and VEP is less clear. The role of SEP in children with traumatic brain injury (TBI) is less clear.

ELECTROENCEPHALOGRAM

The EEG is a good indicator of thalamocortical function, but the utility of a single EEG is limited by the lack of specificity of findings. For example, a burst suppression pattern, which refers to an EEG background exhibiting alternating periods of low- and high-amplitude activity, may be seen in hypoxic-ischemic encephalopathy, metabolic encephalopathy, or with sedating medications. Thus, serial EEG recordings combined with clinical information may be required for prognostic purposes. Mild slowing and rapid improvement of the EEG are associated with good outcome, while burst suppression, electrocerebral silence, and lack of reactivity are associated with poor outcome. Repeating the EEG to determine whether improvement occurs is important, as is ensuring that EEG changes are not pharmacologically induced or compromised by scalp edema or subdural collections. Prolonged EEG monitoring may be helpful to determine whether sleep-wake rhythms exist.

NEUROIMAGING

MRI, especially diffusion-weighted imaging, may be more sensitive to early HIE changes than is cranial CT (**Table 32.7**). Newer MR imaging techniques have been useful in predicting outcome after TBI. Susceptibility-weighted MR imaging detects hemorrhagic diffuse axonal injury particularly well. MRS determines metabolic ratios in specific brain regions. Fluid-attenuated inversion recovery is also helpful.

CHAPTER 33 ■ NEUROLOGIC MONITORING

BRAHM GOLDSTEIN • MATEO ABOY • ALAN GRAHAM

There is increasing evidence that there are tangible benefits from neurologic monitoring in a variety of PICU patients. Continuous electroencephalogram coupled with digital video monitoring for status epilepticus, diagnosing nonconvulsive seizures, and as part of a surgical approach for intractable seizures is routinely applied with good results Though sparse,

there are evidence-based data for intracranial pressure monitoring in patients with severe traumatic brain injury. And intra- and postoperative neurophysiologic monitoring of children undergoing repair of congenital cardiac disease with near infrared spectroscopy (NIRS) can improve outcomes. **Table 33.1** provides definitions for engineering terms.

TABLE 33.1

ENGINEERING TERMS AND DEFINITIONS

Aliasing—The apparent conversion of high-frequency signals to low-frequency signals owing to an insufficient sample rate.

Analog to digital (A/D) conversion—The electrical conversion of an analog signal (often a voltage) to a digital representation that enables manipulation and processing by computers.

Band-pass filter—A filter that eliminates low- and high-frequency components of a signal but retains an intermediate range.

Bandwidth—The range of frequencies spanned by a signal. When applied to band-pass filters, this describes the range of frequencies that are allowed to pass through the filter.

Capacitance—A measure of the ability of a circuit element to store electrical charge. Elements with a large capacitance dampen or resist rapid fluctuations in voltage.

Demodulation—The process of extracting an information-bearing signal from another signal. This is analogous to extracting a file of interest from a compressed or encrypted file.

Hertz (Hz)—A measure of frequency and equivalent to cycles per second (cps).

High-frequency noise—Many types of artifact in physiologic signals contain significant power at high frequencies. This noise is often emitted by medical equipment near the patient.

Highpass filter—A filter that eliminates low-frequency components of a signal but retains high-frequency components.

Inductance—A measure of the ability of a circuit element to store energy in a magnetic field. Elements with a large inductance dampen or resist rapid fluctuations in current.

Linear interpolation—The process of estimating a value of a signal or function between two intermediate values using a line between the two points.

Low-frequency noise—Some types of artifact in physiologic signals contain significant power at low frequencies. This noise is often caused by patient movement.

Lowpass filter—A filter that eliminates high-frequency components of a signal but retains low-frequency components.

Modulation—The process of embedding an information-bearing signal in another signal. This is analogous to creating an encrypted or compressed file that contains a file of interest.

Moving window—A technique for estimating an average quality of a signal continuously by averaging over a period of the preceding 3–5 secs. For example, the systolic blood pressure is usually calculated by averaging the systolic peaks over a moving window of 3–5 secs.

Nonlinear—Any system or device whose behavior is governed by a set of nonlinear equations. In general, these systems do not produce an output that is proportional to the input.

Signal power—The power contained in a signal is generally defined as the square of the signal. This is often averaged over a moving window to create a smoothly varying continuous estimate.

SCIENTIFIC FOUNDATIONS

General Engineering Aspects of ICU Monitoring

Medical instrumentation systems are often composed of sensors, signal conditioning hardware and software, output displays, and auxiliary signals. Sensors are used to convert a physical measure (i.e., a quantity, property, or condition of interest) into an electrical signal output. The sensors used for medical instrumentation purposes are designed to be minimally invasive and to respond to the source of energy present in the measure while excluding all the others as much as possible. Generally, the electrical signal produced by these sensors cannot be connected directly to the output display device. Signal conditioning and processing such as amplification and analog filtering are typically required. Additionally, the sensor outputs are analog signals and must be converted to digital form before they can be processed using more advanced digital signal processing techniques. Analog-to-digital conversion involves signal conditioning, anti-aliasing filtering, uniform sampling, and quantization. These filters are usually linear bandpass or highpass filters used to remove drift, prevent aliasing, and to reduce noise. These frequency-selective filters can distort the waveform morphology due to nonlinear phase in the passband or removal of signal frequencies.

To accurately represent the signal on patient monitor displays, the sampling rate must be high enough that a linear interpolation between the sample points results in a visually smooth and representative signal. To achieve this, the sampling rate should be at least 10× higher than the highest frequency component of the pre-filtered signal. For most physiologic signals that vary with the cardiac and respiratory cycles, a sampling rate of 100 Hertz (Hz) is sufficient. Due to the impulsive nature of the electrocardiographic wave (QRS) complex, electrocardiographic (ECG) signals have a higher bandwidth than most other physiologic signals encountered in the ICU and require a higher sampling rate of at least 250 Hz to accurately represent different segments of the ECG waveform. Electroencephalograms (EEG) also require a higher sampling rate, though this signal is infrequently displayed directly on ICU patient monitors.

Once the physiologic signals have been converted to digital form, more advanced algorithms are used to process these physiologic digital signals and extract clinical significant parameters. For instance, heart rate is estimated from the ECG signal using automatic QRS detection algorithms and diastolic and systolic pressures are obtained from pressure signals.

Patient monitors typically generate alarms *after* the alarm condition has persisted for several seconds. And the obverse is also true. After a successful resuscitation from cardiopulmonary arrest, the arterial oxygen saturation value will typically lag a few seconds after the patient's cyanosis has resolved.

Clinically Important Physiologic Systems and Signals

There are a limited number of physiological systems that may be monitored within the CNS. The EEG has been widely available for decades to record and quantitatively measure the brain's electrical activity. Intracranial pressure monitoring technology has also been available but now is almost always done with more accurate fiberoptic technology. However, the most recent advances have occurred in our ability to monitor cerebral blood flow, both on a global and a regional basis, using direct and indirect methods such as ultrasound, tissue oxygenation, jugular venous oxygenation, and local blood flow and oxygenation indices. "Multimodality neuromonitoring" refers to combinations of the above methods used simultaneously to provide a physiologic picture of CNS activity from the organ to tissue to the cellular level.

APPLICATION TO PEDIATRIC INTENSIVE CARE

Electroencephalogram

The EEG is electrical activity of the brain observed via scalp electrical potentials. The EEG's sources are neurons located predominantly in the outermost layers of the cerebral cortex. Thus, the EEG is a spatial phenomenon following the spatial topography of the cortex.

Continuous EEG

While a 1-hr EEG is often used in most clinical circumstances, the use of continuous 24-hr EEG or video EEG monitoring is becoming increasingly commonplace in most ICUs for various clinical indications, such as monitoring status epilepticus and therapeutically induced coma for refractory status epilepticus and traumatic brain injury. It has proven also useful in the surveillance of patients at risk for subclinical seizures and persistent nonconvulsive status epilepticus, metabolic encephalopathies, and neurologic conditions that limit a patient's ability to respond (brainstem injuries, severe peripheral neuropathic syndromes) The depth of impaired consciousness or coma can be immediately assessed, as can the degree to which ongoing electrographic seizures contribute to that state.

The most common pediatric EEG is a 20-lead EEG with continuous recording and simultaneous digital video recording with clinical annotations made by bedside observers, usually the PICU nurse or a parent. A variety of channel configurations (i.e., bipolar or reference montages) can be used depending on the area of interest. Additional electrodes may include eye leads to discern ocular movements, electromyography, ECG, and a measurement of respiratory frequency. A channel is simply a representation of the potential difference between two recording electrodes. Current digital EEG technology has been used for the past 10 years when increased computer power and storage capability resulted in the older, less flexible, and less information-rich analog pen-and-paper systems being phased out.

Current digital acquisition systems record continuous EEG data to computer hard drives (1–1.5 GB/24 hrs/patient). Systems can acquire 32, 64, 128, or more channels, with higher numbers used for large arrays of electrodes, usually in patients undergoing intracranial recording for epilepsy surgery (**Fig. 33.1, Fig. 33.2**). Most patients require 32 or fewer channels. Sampling rates vary from 60 Hz to 257 Hz. Data can be instantly remontaged to allow better

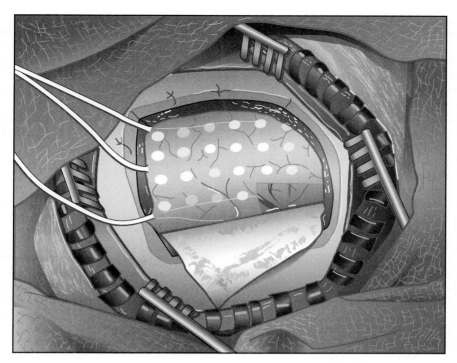

FIGURE 33.1. High-density subdural electrode grid placed intraoperatively over the frontotemporal region in a patient with intractable focal seizures.

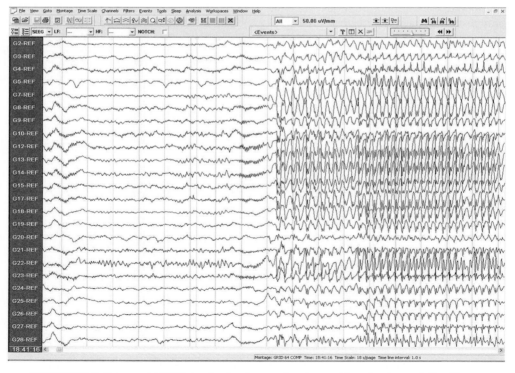

FIGURE 33.2. Intracranial EEG showing focal onset of a seizure with regional spread after 10 secs.

localization and interpretation of focal or generalized abnormalities.

A variety of software packages are available to interpret EEG data, often in real time. Specialized software can identify numerous epileptiform abnormalities and detect electrographic seizure activity. The parameters of these detection algorithms can be adjusted to increase yield and decrease false detections. Special software packages are available for the detection of neonatal seizures. Other packages can identify sleep stages. The systems can trigger alarms when a seizure or abnormality of interest is detected.

Most digital EEG monitoring systems can also acquire simultaneous digital video and audio signals. Temporal resolution is excellent, far surpassing analog video modalities. Data can be recorded from cart-mounted cameras and microphones in the patient room or remotely via wall- or ceiling-mounted devices. Digital video files can be large, and though file size can be decreased by reducing image resolution, video captures can occupy >12 GB/24 hrs/patient using MPEG-2. This can make storage and transmission of data across hospital networks expensive and difficult. Many programs can automatically prune files into time samples based on preselected criteria, saving only portions of every hour or time period as well as computer-detected abnormalities. Compression algorithms may also be of use in creating smaller files for storage, transmission, or review via cable linkage to main workstations in the neuroepileptologist's laboratory.

Newer technology includes various quantitative and graphic techniques, such as compressed spectral arrays and voltage maps that can transform the EEG signal using a range of frequency and amplitude modulations and can be easily derived from EEG data to aid in interpretation and source localization of abnormalities of interest. Recent advances in material sciences and in engineering have led to new dense-array EEGs that can be specifically designed for children and infants. The spatial information obtained from EEG data collected with standard electrode arrays is confounded by spatial aliasing error. However, a dense-array EEG allows sensors placed at >100 sample locations, making possible accurate measurement of the EEG as a time-varying, spatially distributed electrical potential. Advantages to dense-array EEGs are that the time for electrode placement and removal is minimal as the sensor net is just soaked in a solute bath, and the smell and potential skin irritation from collodion glue are eliminated.

Limitations of the continuous EEG monitoring primarily involve the level of expertise required for data interpretation. In many cases, ICU staff can be taught to identify seizures and patterns of interest, but full review and analysis usually require a neurophysiologist or neurologist. The time required for interpretation has been reduced by technologic advances in digital acquisition, spike- and seizure-detection algorithms, and networked systems, but remains significant. Automatic detection software remains error-prone. If full analysis is to be delayed, many of the benefits of anticipatory care may be lost. Lastly, the application and maintenance of electrodes usually require trained technologists, and prolonged electrode placement, usually with colloidon, can cause scalp breakdown.

Bispectral Index

The BIS monitor (BIS, Aspect Medical Systems, Natick, MA) (**Fig. 33.3**) integrates time domain, frequency domain, and higher-order spectral analysis of limited EEG signals to create a univariate descriptor of the level of sedation that is represented as a dimensionless number ranging from 0 to 100. The BIS monitor was developed with data from adults with the goal of decreasing the occurrence of awareness in operating room. The bispectrum evaluates the coherence of sinusoidal frequencies using phase and power information. In the awake individual, there are multiple independent CNS signal generators, and the resultant EEG is chaotic. As deeper sedation occurs, phase coupling of different frequencies is thought to indicate a common source unifying some EEG signals. As phase angles for sinusoidal frequencies become coupled, the higher biocoherence is demonstrated by a large spike on the bispectrum display. The sequential signal

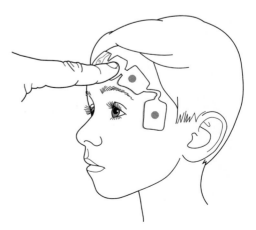

FIGURE 33.3. Illustration of BIS monitor leads placed over the forehead of a patient.

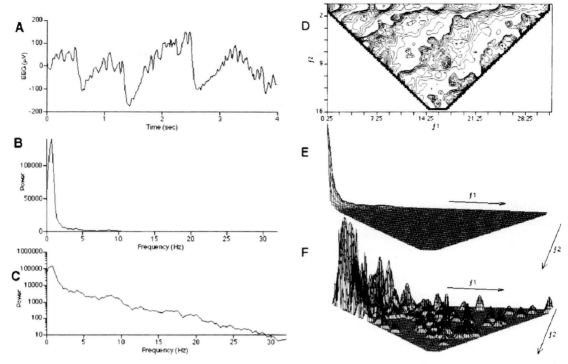

FIGURE 33.4. Examples of the processes of bispectral analysis. **A:** An epoch of raw EEG. **B:** The power spectrum after Fourier analysis of the epoch in part A. In this epoch, the large contribution from frequencies around 1 Hz overwhelms the contributions from higher frequencies. **C:** The same data as part B are plotted with a logarithmic power scale, allowing the contribution from faster waves to be identified despite the presence of large slow waves. **D:** After computing the complex spectrum for this epoch of data, the bispectrum may be calculated. **E:** The same bispectral data plotted in three-dimensional perspective. **F:** Bicoherence plot with phase coherence features visible in a wide distribution of frequency.

processing from raw EEG to bispectrum is demonstrated in **Figure 33.4**.

Evoked Potentials: Visual, Auditory, Somatosensory, and Motor

Vision, hearing, sensory, and motor functions may all be discretely monitored to assess peripheral and CNS damage in patients with suspected injury. The integrity of the complete neural pathways may be assessed with abnormalities assigned to specific levels or sites of injury. While these tests do not lend themselves for continuous monitoring in the PICU, one-time evaluations may prove useful for diagnostic or prognostic purposes.

Assessment of clinical conditions including level of sedation, vegetative states, brain death, peripheral nerve damage, and stroke may provide useful information. The main limitation is the limited clinical utility in an essentially one-time assessment of neural pathways versus continuous monitoring.

Intracranial Pressure

Raised intracranial pressure (ICP) is the most common cause of death in neurosurgical patients and it is extremely common in patients suffering from head injury. Elevated ICP following traumatic brain injury (TBI) often results in secondary injury due to decreased cerebral perfusion pressure (CPP). Therapeutic interventions aimed directly at controlling abnormally elevated ICP have resulted in improved survival and neurologic outcomes. In other brain injuries, such as hypoxic and ischemic injuries, monitoring of ICP has not been shown to improve outcome. The major aim of monitoring and managing elevated ICP is the prevention of cerebral ischemia. The most common methods of ICP monitoring use either an intraventricular catheter or an intraparenchymal catheter. Of these two, the intraventricular catheter is more frequently used, since it is a more direct method, is believed to provide more accurate measurements, and results in the most satisfactory waveforms for off-line analysis. Additionally, the intraventricular catheter allows for removal of small amounts of cerebral spinal fluid to reduce ICP and infusion of saline to determine the pressure-volume relationship of the brain, which can then be used to estimate cerebral compliance. From a safety point of view, intraventricular catheters present a risk of infection and are generally removed as soon as is practical.

Relatively recently, fiberoptic transducer-tipped catheters have been introduced into clinical practice and are the standard of care in most PICUs. These devices monitor the variations in the amount of light reflected from a pressure-sensitive diaphragm located at the catheter tip. The advantages include versatility (they can be placed into intraventricular, subarachnoid, or intraparenchymal regions), robustness to artifacts cased by patient movement or from fluid column sources, and ability to perform ventricular drainages and monitoring simultaneously. Some of the drawbacks include the need for dedicated equipment for waveform display as opposed to conventional ICP systems that use existing bedside monitoring devices.

Cerebral Perfusion Pressure

CPP is defined as the difference between the mean arterial pressure and the ICP. Because CPP drives the cerebral blood flow (CBF) and keeps oxygen and other essential nutrients flowing to the brain, it is believed to be necessary to maintain a certain CPP or else run the risk of cerebral ischemia. CPP is a continuous calculation derived from the time-averaged difference between two physiologic signals (CPP = MAP − ICP). In severe pediatric TBI, CPP should be kept at a minimum of 40 mm Hg while in adult TBI, CPP should be maintained >70 mm Hg.

Jugular Venous Bulb Oxygen Saturation

Jugular venous bulb saturation ($SjvO_2$) refers to the oxygen saturation of the venous blood in the jugular bulb, at the base of the skull. Placement of a fiberoptic $SjvO_2$ catheter allows for continuous monitoring.

The saturation normally ranges between 60% and 80%. The physiologic concept is that the difference between $SjvO_2$ and SaO_2 is an indirect measure of global CBF as the SO_2[a-v] is inversely proportional to the cerebral metabolic rate of oxygen. When CPP and CBF decrease, the brain has to extract the same amount of oxygen from a smaller amount of blood so the SjvO2 decreases. In general, $SjvO_2$ values <50% are indicative of cerebral ischemia.

Abnormalities that increase oxygen consumption (e.g., fever or seizures) or that decrease oxygen delivery (e.g., increased ICP, hypotension, hypoxemia, hypocapnia, or anemia) may decrease $SjvO_2$. Secondary insults may be identified with the $SjvO_2$ monitoring and contribute to the patient's neurologic injury.

Errors may be due to improper catheter placement, such as curling in the bulb or when the catheter tip is adjacent to the vessel wall, or with changes in head position. Accuracy of measurements of $SjvO_2$ is dependent upon precise in vivo calibration. Finally, while jugular venous bulb monitoring can be used to assess the adequacy of CPP and CBF, it measures only global but not regional ischemia.

Transcranial Doppler

Transcranial Doppler (TCD) allows for portable, invasive, and repeatable measures of regional CBF. Although not strictly a continuous signal in terms of 24-hr availability, a multidirectional ultrasound probe for simultaneous TCD of the middle cerebral artery, ophthalmic artery, and/or supratrochlear artery has been constructed. The middle cerebral artery is the most commonly studied in children.

Technical limitations of TCD include obtaining adequate ultrasound windows through the bony skull, assessment of only medium- to large-sized vessels, measurements that may vary between studies, lack of correlation with other indices of CBF, and that only CBF velocity is actually measured while flow is inferred.

Regional Brain Tissue Oxygenation Monitoring by NIRS

NIRS technology uses a modification of the Beer-Lambert Law, which describes the relationship between absorption of light and the concentration of intravascular chromophores such as deoxyhemoglobin (Hb), oxyhemoglobin (HbO_2), and the intracellular chromophore cytochrome aa_3. NIRS technology differs from pulse oximetry in that it does not require a pulse; therefore cerebral NIRS monitoring can be used during cardiopulmonary bypass.

The range of baseline cerebral oxygen saturation values is very wide. In healthy children, cerebral oxygen saturations are reported to be 68% ± 10% while in children with cyanotic heart disease baseline values range from 38% to 57%. Limitations of NIRS technology include varying ratios of brain and extracranial tissues between patients and that the DPF varies with age and pathologic state. Icteric patients have depressed cerebral rSO_2 values, presumably due to absorption of light by bilirubin. Ongoing blood loss is associated with a decrease in rSO_2 despite a stable SjO_2, which may indicate that a changing Hb level confounds cerebral oximetry measurement. Furthermore, the reproducibility of cerebral oxygenation measurements in infants is poor.

Laser-Doppler Cortical Flowmetry

Laser-Doppler cortical flowmetry (LDF) measures the frequency shift reflected off RBCs to calculate local CBF velocity. LDF measures blood flow velocity in the microvessels of a small volume of brain tissue rather than in a large artery such as with TCD. Flow is determined by calculating the velocity times the volume of tissue. A small optical fiber is placed in brain parenchyma through same site as the ICP monitor. Limitations of this technique include measurement reliability and movement of artifact.

Regional Brain Tissue O2 (Pti$_2$), C$_2$ (PtiCO$_2$) and pH

A tissue-monitoring catheter (0.5 mm diameter) may be placed alongside the ICP catheter in the frontal cortex to a 2–3-cm depth to measure regional brain tissue changes in O_2, CO_2, and pH. The technology uses fluorescent dyes that respond to O_2, CO_2, and

pH or can use a Clark electrode for PO_2 measurements. A temperature probe may be added to obtain continuous brain tissue temperature measurements. Limitations of this technology include measurements reflecting regional rather than global changes and a reported lack of correlation with other metabolic measures, such as $SjvO_2$.

Microdialysis

A microdialysis catheter may be inserted into brain tissue and connected to a microdialysis pump that delivers perfusion fluid that equilibrates with the extracellular brain tissue fluid through the dialysis membrane of the catheter. Changes in levels of glucose, lactate, pyruvate, and various amino acids in the interstitial fluid may be measured. Extracellular concentrations of lactate and glutamate concentrations are reported increased during episodes of jugular venous desaturation.

CHAPTER 34 ■ NEUROLOGIC IMAGING

DAVID JOSHUA MICHELSON • STEPHEN ASHWAL

COMPUTED TOMOGRAPHY

One major factor in favor of CT in comparison with MRI is that it can be quickly and easily obtained. Helical (spiral) scanners have shortened the acquisition times required for high-quality images. One of the drawbacks of CT is radiation exposure, particularly of concern for young patients and those who require repeated studies, given the known dose-related risk of radiation-associated disease and possible risk of developmental impairment. Considering this, alternative studies, such as ultrasound, MRI, or CT of lower-resolution (and thus lower radiation dose) may be preferable. Also, while the radiodense, iodinated contrast agents used in CT scanning are well tolerated by most children, acute allergic reactions can occur. Fatty tissue, water, and air appear dark, soft tissues appear as intermediate shades of gray, and mineralized bone, concentrated blood, iodinated contrast, and metallic objects appear bright. CT is limited by streaking artifacts in areas around metal prostheses, fragments (such as dental fillings or gun-

shot pellets), and dense bone (such as the temporal petrous bones in the posterior fossa). Areas of abnormal signal on CT can be characterized as hypodense, isodense, or hyperdense, relative to the normal neural tissue. The differential for hypodense parenchymal lesions includes edema, infarction, neoplasia, demyelination, inflammation, and cyst formation. Hyperdensity is found in areas of contrast enhancement, hemorrhage, calcification, and hypercellularity. Abnormal calcification can be seen with congenital or chronic infections, tumors and hamartomas, abnormal blood vessels, areas of ischemia, metabolic disorders, and endocrine disorders. Isodense lesions may be recognizable by their replacement of, or effect on, normal structures, unless they show abnormal contrast enhancement. CT angiography allows the vascular anatomy of the brain to be imaged fairly well by high-resolution CT scanning that is closely timed with an intravenous bolus of an iodinated contrast agent. Thinly cut source images can be reformatted into 2- and 3-dimensional images that are nearly as detailed as MR angiograms.

MAGNETIC RESONANCE IMAGING

MRI is the modality of choice when resolution of fine anatomic detail is desired. Moreover, this technology also offers several specialized sequences that highlight metabolic changes within the brain and are applicable to a wide variety of diagnostic situations. MRI is also the imaging test of choice for spinal cord injury when neurologic deficits are present, as CT images of the spine, while superior for visualizing fractures and dislocations, do not allow for assessment of the cord. MRI also allows for far more precise imaging of posterior fossa structures, as it is not subject to the artifact produced by the dense temporal petrous bones on CT. The principal drawback of MR imaging is the long acquisition time, which frequently necessitates procedural sedation. When intravenous propofol is used for sedation, concentrations of supplemental oxygen >60% can cause artifactual cerebrospinal fluid (CSF) hyperintensity within the sulci and cisterns that can be mistaken for subarachnoid hemorrhage. Another drawback of MRI is the incompatibility of ferromagnetic materials with the strong electromagnetic field within the imaging suite. Plastic and aluminum MR-compatible monitors are available, and ventilator-dependent patients can be ventilated manually, but patients with metallic bullet fragments or implants, including cardiac pacemakers and neurostimulators, may not be able to undergo MRI safely.

Conventional Anatomic Imaging

The shade of a an MR image is referred to as its *intensity*, which is determined by factors such as proton mobility (T1 relaxation) and local magnetic effects (T2 relaxation). Various sequences, such as spin echo, gradient-recalled echo, and fluid-attenuated inversion recovery (FLAIR), use programmed pulses of radiofrequencies and gradient magnetic fields to produce images that highlight T1 or T2 signal effects. On T1-weighted images, fat, methemoglobin, and gadolinium-containing contrast agents appear bright (or hyperintense), while CSF, muscle, deoxyhemoglobin, and hemosiderin, appear dark. On T2-weighted images, CSF, edema, extracellular methemoglobin, and areas of hypercellularity, infarction, and demyelination appear bright, while muscle, cortical bone, deoxyhemoglobin, and hemosiderin appear dark. Routine brain imaging begins with a sagittal T1-weighted sequence that serves as a localizer for subsequent sequences and allows evaluation of the corpus callosum, pituitary gland, cerebellar vermis, and other midline structures. In standard diffusion-weighted imaging (DWI), bright areas reflect decreased or restricted movement of water. DWI is particularly useful in the early evaluation of ischemia, as diffusion restriction becomes apparent within minutes after cytotoxic injury is sustained. DWI is also used in the evaluation of brain tumors, helping to distinguish cystic tumors from epidermoid tumors and recurrent tumors from areas of peritumoral edema. Diffusion restriction is also seen within cerebral abscesses and empyemas; this methodology is helpful when a suspected abscess cannot otherwise be distinguished radiologically from a tumor with central necrosis.

Other MR Technologies

Reconstructions of the arterial supply and venous drainage of the brain can be obtained from maximum intensity projections (MIP) that correlate with blood flow, rather than luminal diameter, and can exaggerate the true degree of vascular stenosis. As the process of generating MIP images is also prone to producing artifacts, any suspected abnormality should be confirmed in the source images. Spectroscopic imaging most often analyzes the signals generated by protons from a number of clinically important neuronal and glial metabolites, including N-acetyl aspartate, choline and phosphatidylcholine, creatine and phosphocreatine, myoinositol, and lactate. A number of MR methods have been developed for measuring cerebral perfusion. Applications for perfusion imaging include assessing the risk of ischemia in tissues with decreased perfusion, identifying the decreased perfusion in primary and secondary vasculopathies, and grading the vascularity of tumors. Deoxygenated blood and such blood breakdown products as hemosiderin are weakly paramagnetic, and the artifacts that they produce on particular MR sequences can be exploited in the evaluation of patients for vascular abnormalities and small hemorrhages. Gradient echo T2-weighted images have been used for this purpose for some time and are widely available, but they are not nearly as sensitive as susceptibility-weighted imaging that makes these same paramagnetic artifacts far more apparent.

SELECTED CLINICAL APPLICATIONS

Trauma

The initial workup of children with known or suspected head trauma will usually begin with a CT of the head and neck, looking for evidence of acute

THE EVOLVING APPEARANCE OF HEMORRHAGE ON CT AND MR IMAGING

Timing	Hyperacute (<1 day)	Acute (1–3 days)	Early subacute (3–7 days)	Late subacute (7–14 days)	Chronic (>14 days)
Blood product	OxyHb (intracellular)	DeoxyHb (intracellular)	MetHb (intracellular)	MetHb (extracellular)	Hemosiderin (extracellular)
CT image	Hyperdense	Hyperdense	Isodense	Isodense	Hypodense
MR image					
T1-weighted	Dark or gray	Dark or gray	Bright	Bright	Dark or gray
T2-weighted	Bright	Dark	Dark	Bright	Dark

Adapted from: Bradley WG Jr: MR appearance of hemorrhage in the brain. *Radiology* 1993; 189:15–2.

hemorrhage, fracture, or displacement of vertebrae out of their normal alignment. Young children who suffer traumatic brain injury are at particular risk of upper–cervical spine injury because of the relative weight of the cranium, weakness of the paraspinous muscles, elasticity and redundancy of the interspinous ligaments, and horizontal orientation of the incompletely ossified facet joints. Children <8 years of age have such mobility of their cervical spine as to have a normal atlantodental space as wide as 5 mm and anterior movement of C2 on C3 and of C3 on C4 of up to 4 mm. Alignment of the spinolaminar line is disrupted in true subluxation. Spinal MRI should be considered in children, even when no evidence of misalignment or fracture of the vertebrae is seen on plain imaging in a neutral position, as soft tissue and cord edema, ischemia, and hemorrhage may only be visible on spinal MRI. The tendency of children to develop soft-tissue and spinal cord injury without radiologic abnormality refers only to plain film and CT imaging. As children reach adolescence, they are increasingly likely to sustain bony injuries with spinal trauma, but less severe injuries can still occur without plain film evidence of fractures. Adolescents are also more likely than young children to present with lower cervical injuries and traumatic disc herniation. MRI of the brain provides greater sensitivity than CT for brainstem injury, edema and petechial hemorrhages from axonal shearing, small extra-axial fluid collections, and older blood products and is, therefore, the study of choice once a patient has been stabilized. Imaging may find traumatic hemorrhage that is parenchymal, due to contusion or axonal shearing, or extraparenchymal, with the development of an epidural or subdural hematoma. On CT, hemorrhages appear hyperdense in the first week, isodense to brain between 1 and 3 weeks, and increasingly hypodense thereafter. Contrast administration causes enhancement of the outline of the hematoma that becomes increasingly intense as the hemorrhage

organizes. On MRI, hyperacute blood is dark on T1-weighted images and bright on T2-weighted images, in contrast to acute blood, which is bright on T1-weighted images and dark on T2-weighted images. **Table 34.1** summarizes the evolution of the appearance of hemorrhage on CT and MRI. With layering of blood cells within a hematoma, the upper layer of fluid appears bright on T1- and T2-weighted images, while the bottom layer appears isodense to brain on T1-weighted images and dark on T2-weighted images. Finding signs of both old and new traumatic brain injury adds to the suspicion for nonaccidental trauma in infants. Subarachnoid hemorrhage due to trauma is most commonly seen layering along the falx cerebri in the posterior interhemispheric fissure or the tentorium cerebelli and is best detected in the acute stage by CT. Subacute hemorrhage can be detected by FLAIR sequences on MRI. Children may have normal-appearing CT and MRI in the first 12 hrs after even severe traumatic brain injury, with severe cerebral edema becoming evident thereafter. Diffusion-weighted MRI can show areas of restricted diffusion due to cytotoxic edema within hours of injury.

Hypoxic-Ischemic Injury

Infarction occurs in ~40% of children with cerebral sinovenous thrombosis, with accompanying hemorrhage in more than half of the patients. Presenting symptoms depend on the age of the child and the severity of the injury but range from signs of focal injury, such as neurologic deficits and seizures, to diffuse signs of increased intracranial pressure, such as altered level of consciousness, headache, and vomiting. Greater degrees of venous outflow reduction progressively cause vasogenic edema, infarction, and hemorrhage, all of which appear differently on neuroimaging. A CT scan may show areas of

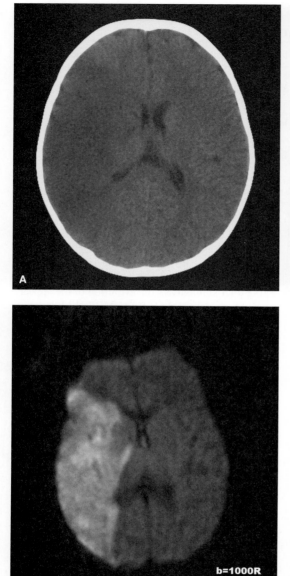

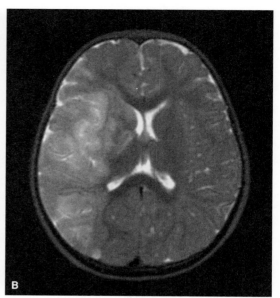

FIGURE 34.1. Two-year-old girl who awoke with left hemiparesis and right-gaze preference. (**A**) A wedge-shaped area of hypodensity is seen on axial CT. MRI shows (**B**) T2 hyperintensity and (**C**) corresponding diffusion restriction, indicative of an ischemic stroke in the distribution of the right middle cerebral artery.

subcortical white-matter hypodensity due to cerebral edema and areas of hyperdensity due to hemorrhage. Intravenous contrast is often necessary for detection of the venous thrombosis, with the flow of contrast around the thrombus described as the empty delta sign. MRI will show corresponding changes on routine T1- and T2-weighted images and is likely to visualize the thrombosis within the venous system, even without the use of contrast. MR venography can be useful when the diagnosis is suspected but uncertain. DWI may show reduced, normal, increased, or mixed water movement, depending on the relative contri-

butions of vasogenic and cytotoxic edema. Focal arterial infarction appears on CT as a wedge-shaped area of hypodensity that involves the cortex and white matter supplied by the occluded artery (**Fig. 34.1A**). MRI is even more sensitive than CT for the detection of ischemia-related cerebral edema (**Fig. 34.1B**), though both modalities may appear normal within the first 24 hrs after the appearance of clinical symptoms. DWI, conversely, can show restricted water movement from cytotoxic edema (**Fig. 34.1C**) in as little as 1 hr after injury. Angiography, using either CT or MR, can be used to assess the possibility

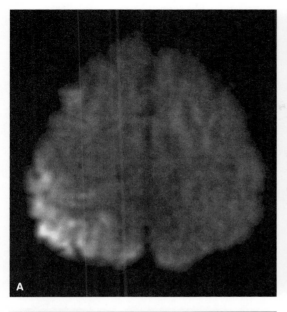

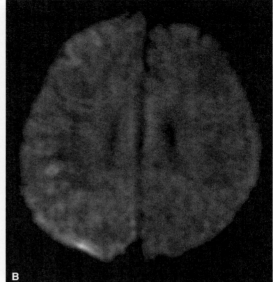

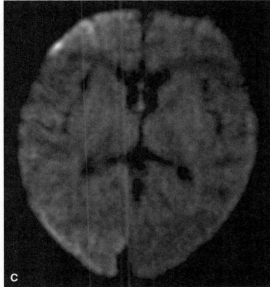

FIGURE 34.2. Thirteen-month-old boy presenting with pneumococcal meningitis and mild left-sided weakness. Diffusion-weighted image shows restriction within the interarterial or watershed regions of the right frontal and parietal cortex.

of medium-to-large vessel abnormalities, such as occlusion, thrombosis, dysplasia, or dissection. Neither method can exclude the type of small-vessel vasculopathy. Diffuse hypoxic-ischemic injury can result from cardiopulmonary arrest or from severe hypotension or hypoxia. The cortical areas supplied by branches of the carotid artery, especially the intervascular boundary zones, are vulnerable to ischemic injury, often resulting in a pattern referred to as a "watershed" distribution (**Fig. 34.2**). CT can be used for initial imaging of unstable patients, although scans within the first 24 hrs may be read as normal despite

the presence of severe global ischemia. Even the earliest appreciable changes, such as basal ganglia hypodensity and effacement of the perimesencephalic cisterns, may be very subtle. Later CT scans will show clearer evidence of cerebral edema, with decreased differentiation between cortex and white matter, effacement of sulci and cisterns, and hypodensity of deep and cortical gray matter. Particularly ominous for prognosis is the "reversal sign," with white matter appearing denser than cortex, which may be due to impaired venous drainage. Early changes of global ischemia can be as subtle on conventional MRI as they

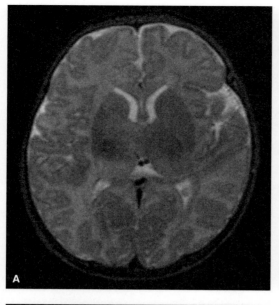

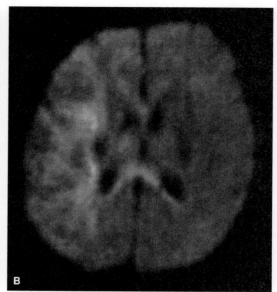

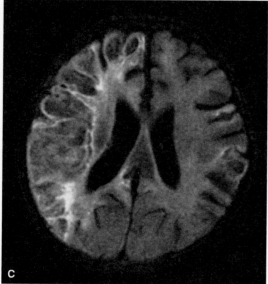

FIGURE 34.3. Ten-week-old girl who presented with focal seizures and hemiparesis due to herpes simplex virus meningoencephalitis. MRI done on admission shows (**A**) normal signal characteristics on T2-weighted images but (**B**) widespread right hemispheric diffusion restriction. MRI obtained 3 wks later shows (**C**) corresponding extensive right hemispheric encephalomalacia on axial FLAIR image.

are on CT, although early diffusion restriction can be seen in areas of infarction, and proton MR spectroscopy can show a rise in glutamate and glutamine, with or without the presence of lactate. However, very early DWI can significantly underestimate the complete extent of ischemic injury.

Meningitis

When CNS infection is clinically suspected and a lumbar puncture is being contemplated, it is common practice to first obtain a CT of the head to determine

whether a mass lesion is present that might predispose to cerebral herniation. CT may show meningeal contrast enhancement when meningitis is present, especially in its later stages, and is important for investigating possible sources of infection such as mastoiditis, sinusitis, and skull-based fractures. Complications of meningitis, such as ischemic stroke from vasculitis, obstructive and communicating hydrocephalus, and hemorrhage from venous thrombosis, are also evaluated well by contrast-enhanced CT. MRI is more likely to show meningeal contrast enhancement in uncomplicated meningitis but has also been shown to predict the diagnosis of tuberculous meningitis

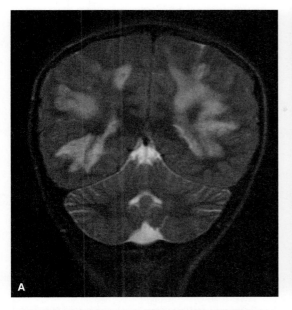

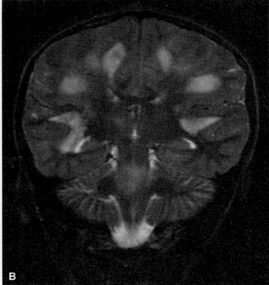

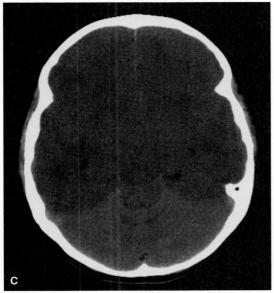

FIGURE 34.4. Seven-year-old girl who presented with hallucinations and obtundation due to acute disseminated encephalomyelitis. **A,B:** T2-weighted coronal MR images show diffuse T2 hyperintensity within the subcortical white matter, right thalamus, and pons. The patient deteriorated clinically despite aggressive immunomodulatory therapy. **C:** CT shows diffuse hypodensity of the supratentorial tissues with obliteration of the perimesencephalic cisterns. Autopsy showed diffuse cerebral edema and transtentorial herniation.

when the meninges appear bright on precontrast T1-weighted magnetization transfer images. MRI with DWI is superior to CT in demonstrating some infectious and vasculitic complications of meningitis, including encephalitis, cerebritis, abscess, empyema, ventriculitis, and ischemia.

Meningoencephalitis

CSF analysis is the principal method employed for diagnosing viral meningoencephalitis, but in children infected with the most common etiologic agent, herpes simplex virus (HSV) I, false negative polymerase chain reaction testing is not uncommon when done within the first 72 hrs of illness. MRI with DWI is highly sensitive for the detection of the cytotoxic edema and necrosis associated with this infection, and the presence and extent of such lesions is predictive of the long-term neurologic prognosis. **Figure 34.3** shows an infant with evolving necrosis from HSV encephalitis. Imaging findings in encephalitis due to other viral agents, including enteroviruses and arboviruses, are often nonspecific and may be limited to

TABLE 34.2

METABOLIC DISORDERS THAT PRODUCE GRAY MATTER IMAGING ABNORMALITIES

Cortical gray matter
  Neuronal ceroid lipofuscinoses
  Mucolipidosis I

Deep gray matter
  Striatal T2 hyperintensity
    Mitochondrial disorders (Leigh and MELAS syndromes)
    Juvenile Huntington disease
    Organic acidopathies
    Hypoxia-ischemia or hypoglycemia
  Globus pallidus T2 hypointensity
    Pantothenate kinase-associated neurodegeneration (PKAN)
    Oculodigital dental dysplasia
  Globus pallidus T2 hyperintensity
    Methylmalonic academia
    Toxins (carbon monoxide, manganese, cyanide)
    Kernicterus
    Succinate semialdehyde dehydrogenase deficiency
    Guanidoacetate methyltransferase deficiency
    Isovaleric academia

Adapted from Barkovich AJ. *Pediatric Neuroimaging*.
Philadelphia: Lippincott Wiliams & Wilkins, 2005.

TABLE 34.3

METABOLIC DISORDERS THAT PRODUCE WHITE MATTER IMAGING ABNORMALITIES

Subcortical white matter
  Megalencephalic leukoencephalopathy with subcortical cysts
  Alexander disease
  Galactosemia
  Salla disease
  4-Hydroxybutyric aciduria

Deep white matter
  Krabbe disease
  GM1 or GM2 gangliosidosis
  X-linked adrenoleukodystrophy
  Metachromatic leukodystrophy
  Phenylketonuria
  Maple syrup urine disease
  Lowe disease
  Sjögren-Larsson syndrome
  Hyperhomocysteinemia
  Radiation/chemotherapy
  Childhood ataxia with diffuse central nervous system hypomyelination
  Merosin-deficient congenital muscular dystrophy
  Dentatorubropallidoluysian atrophy

Lack of myelination
  Pelizaeus-Merzbacher disease
  Trichothiodystrophy
  18q- syndrome
  Salla disease

Nonspecific pattern of involvement
  Nonketotic hyperglycinemia
  Urea cycle disorders
  3-hydroxy-3-methylglutaryl-coenzyme A lyase deficiency
  Collagen vascular diseases
  Demyelinating diseases
  Viral infections

Adapted from Barkovich AJ. *Pediatric Neuroimaging*.
Philadelphia: Lippincott Wiliams & Wilkins, 2005.

subtle T2 hyperintensity within the cortical and subcortical gray matter. Ring-enhancing lesions should raise the possibility of unusual causes of meningoencephalitis, including fungi (cryptococcus, aspergillus, and candida), parasites (toxoplasmosis, cysticercosis, amoebae), and mycobacterium tuberculosis. The differential is expanded in patients who are immunocompromised.

Spinal Infections

Spinal CT with contrast enhancement has a higher detection rate for paraspinal infection than does plain x-ray, which may only detect bony erosion and vertebral destruction, but it is insufficiently sensitive to exclude the presence of an early discitis or epidural abscess and does not directly assess the integrity of the spinal cord. Given the urgency with which surgical intervention might be needed to avoid permanent spinal cord injury, MRI should be performed early in the evaluation of all patients with suspected spinal infections if no contraindication exists. In patients with spinal epidural abscesses that show no cord compression but have signs of severe neurologic impairment, neuroimaging can reveal cord ischemia due to vascular compression or thrombosis.

Postinfectious Encephalomyelitis

Inflammatory neuropathies with an autoimmune basis are thought to be triggered in most cases by infections, vaccinations, and traumatic injuries. Any portion of the central or peripheral nervous systems can be involved individually, as in such isolated syndromes as optic neuritis, acute cerebellar

TABLE 34.4

METABOLIC DISORDERS THAT PRODUCE GRAY AND WHITE MATTER IMAGING ABNORMALITIES

Cortical gray matter only

  Cortical dysgenesis
    Congenital CMV infection
    Congenital muscular dystrophy
    Peroxisomal disorders

  No cortical dysgenesis
    Mucopolysaccharidoses
    Lipid storage disorders

Deep gray matter

  Early thalamic involvement
    Krabbe disease
    GM1 or GM2 gangliosidosis
    Wilson disease
    Profound neonatal hypotensive encephalopathy

  Early globus pallidus involvement
    Canavan disease
    Kearn-Sayre syndrome
    Methylmalonic academia
    Toxins (carbon monoxide and cyanide)
    Maple syrup urine disease
    L-2-hydroxyglutaric aciduria
    Dentatorubropalliodoluysian atrophy
    Urea cycle disorders
    Cree leukoencephalopathy

  Early striatal involvement
    Mitochondrial disorders (Leigh and MELAS syndrome)
    Wilson disease
    Organic acidurias
    Molybdenum cofactor deficiency
    β-Ketothiolase deficiency
    Biotinidase deficiencies
    Hypoxia-ischemia or hypoglycemia
    Cockayne syndrome
    Toxins

Adapted from Barkovich AJ. *Pediatric Neuroimaging.* Philadelphia: Lippincott Wiliams & Wilkins, 2005.

ataxia, transverse myelitis, and Guillain-Barré syndrome. Alternatively, multiple areas of the nervous system can be involved at once with various manifestations of acute disseminated encephalomyelitis (ADEM). MRI is well suited for the detection of ADEM lesions within the brain and spinal cord, although patients may have severe optic neuritis without radiologic evidence of optic nerve involvement. The differential considered in some cases of ADEM includes atypical infection (e.g., cryptococcal meningitis), tumor (e.g., lymphoma), ischemic stroke, and recurrent demyelination from multiple sclerosis. MR spectroscopy and DWI may be particularly helpful in difficult cases in which biopsy would otherwise be considered necessary.). A fulminant case of ADEM is presented in **Figure 34.4A–C**.

Toxic Metabolic Injury

A wide variety of metabolic disorders, from inborn errors of metabolism and acquired endogenous or exogenous toxins can have similar, nonspecific patterns of injury on neuroimaging. From an imaging perspective, these patterns can be characterized by whether they affect gray matter, white matter, or both (**Tables 34.2–34.4**). Although CT is sometimes useful for the detection of the calcifications that can occur in these disorders, MRI is superior for identifying the pattern of injury and can, in some instances, provide a specific diagnosis, as with T2-weighted imaging in pantothenate kinase-associated neurodegeneration and with MR spectroscopy in leukodystrophies like Canavan disease. While nonspecific, detection of otherwise unexplained deep gray-matter lactate contributes to the diagnosis of mitochondrial disorders such as mitochondrial encephalopathy (MELAS syndrome).

CHAPTER 35 ■ HEAD AND SPINAL CORD TRAUMA

ROBERT C. TASKER

Mechanical forces at the time of accident (e.g., direct or contact force, acceleration and deceleration forces, and rotational or torsional forces) are responsible for primary injury. As a consequence of these forces, a variety of primary and secondary brain injuries occur. Inflicted traumatic brain injury (iTBI) includes one or more of the following features: shaking injury, cerebral lesions as a result of direct impact, compression, and penetrating injuries. Shaking injury is the most frequent form of iTBI in infants (birth to 12 mos). **Spinal cord injury** (SCI) in children involves bony fractures and dislocations of the pediatric spine. In general, head injuries conform to 1 of 3 types: the *blunt* head injury, the *sharp* head injury, or the *compression* injury.

TRAUMATIC BRAIN INJURY

A blunt injury occurs when the head comes into forcible contact with a flat, smooth surface. This injury can be caused by a fall when the head hits the ground or a blow to the head by a blunt object. The injury combinations that are likely to follow blunt head injury to the vault are summarized in **Table 35.1**. The area of impact and extent of skull distortion is small in sharp head injury. Laceration of the scalp, local depression or fragmentation of the skull, tearing of the dura, and bruising and laceration of the underlying brain may be seen. A compression or crush injury is unusual (**Table 35.2**). The approach to these patients are outlined in: Guidelines for the acute medical management of severe traumatic brain injury in infants, children, and adolescents.

HEMORRHAGE AND OTHER FOCAL BRAIN TISSUE EFFECTS

In infants, epidural hematomas (EDH) of venous or bony origin is found in the posterior fossa adjacent to the venous sinuses. These venous EDHs often have a delayed presentation because the infant has significant intracranial reserve from unfused sutures and open fontanelles. In older children, EDH arises from arterial bleeding. Patients may have a short, lucid interval after injury, but they will deteriorate rapidly with an increasing intracranial mass. Subdural hemorrhage (SDH) is a problem in children who suffer iTBI. It is the associated brain injuries that account for immediate unconsciousness at the time of accident and any focal neurologic deficits (e.g., hemiparesis, pupillary abnormalities, and seizures). Traumatic intraparenchymal hematomas, or contusions, are not common in children, but their frequency increases with age.

Diffuse Injury Involving Axons

Diffuse injury that involves axons results from shearing forces that act at interfaces of the brain with differing structural integrity, such as grey-white-matter boundaries. The neuronal axons that cross multiple brain regions are particularly vulnerable. Traumatic axonal injury (TAI) may vary from small foci of axonal injury to a more severe form of diffuse TAI, in which injury is widespread throughout the brain, including the brainstem. MRI is more sensitive to the white-matter changes usually seen with TAI. It is possible that iTBI contains an important component of both hypoxia-ischemia and axonal injury and that these factors likely vary with the spectrum of injury in this complex disorder.

Diffuse Swelling of the Cerebrum

During the early phase of posttraumatic coma in children, cerebral swelling develops and generally peaks between 24 and 72 hrs after injury. In some instances, specific focal injury may occur in combination with diffuse injury. Tissue herniation syndromes can exist despite normal global intracranial pressure (ICP) (**Table 35.3, Fig. 35.1**).

Posttraumatic Ischemia and Metabolism

Cerebral blood flow (CBF) is reduced, and secondary insults such as hypotension and hypoxemia have devastating effect. Brain swelling and any accompanying intracranial hypertension can contribute to this early secondary ischemia. Following early posttraumatic hypoperfusion, CBF may increase to levels greater

TABLE 35.1

FEATURES ASSOCIATED WITH VAULT FRACTURES IN BLUNT HEAD INJURY

Site of impact	Features associated with fracture lines
Mid-frontal	**Clinical** CSF rhinorrhea Meningitis, pneumocephalus Anosmia **Brain** General concussion Direct bruising of underlying cortex Laceration of subfrontal cortex **Hemorrhage** SAH, SDH
Lateral frontal or temporofrontal	**Clinical** CSF rhinorrhea and meningitis in anterior fractures Blindness in medial fractures EDH in posterior fractures **Brain** General concussion Motor aphasia from a blow to the left side **Hemorrhage** SAH, SDH, EDH
Lateral or temporoparietal	**Clinical** Movement of the brain is restricted by dural folds, but their sharp edges may cut into the brainstem If fracture lines involve the base of the skull 5th, 6th, 7th, and 8th cranial nerves may be involved, as well as the sella turcica Involvement of middle meningeal vessels with EDH Middle-ear involvement with CSF otorrhea and meningitis **Brain** Concussion is not that severe in general. Local contusions beneath impact may cause aphasia or contralateral weakness if the Rolandic fissure is involved **Hemorrhage** SAH is uncommon SDH follows small lacerations related to point of impact
Posterolateral or occipitoparietal	**Clinical** CSF otorrhea, meningitis, and hearing loss when the petrous temporal bone is involved **Brain** Concussion is severe. Distant injury with laceration of the frontal and temporal poles **Hemorrhage** EDH may occur in fractures in the middle fossa or posterior fossa High risk of tearing of vessels: SAH and SDH formation
Midline posterior or occipital	**Clinical** Often associated fracture of cervical spine Lower cranial nerve palsies **Brain** Concussion is severe Distant subfrontal or temporal contusions and laceration **Hemorrhage** Subfrontal or temporal SAH and SDH

CSF, cerebrospinal fluid; SAH, subarachnoid hemorrhage; SDH, subdural hemorrhage; EDH, extradural hemorrhage

TABLE 35.2

COMPRESSION FRACTURES

Type	Clinical problem

Side-to-side
Fracture passes through the middle fossa across the sella turcica to the opposite side
	Injuries include:
	    Anterior group of cranial nerves may be involved, in particular, 6th nerve
	    Internal carotid artery may be torn

Front-to-back
Wide fissures through the frontal sinus extending back through the cribriform and ethmoid regions
	Disruption of:
	    Frontal sinus
	    Cribriform plate
	    Roof of the orbit

TABLE 35.3

TYPES OF BRAIN TISSUE HERNIATION SYNDROMES

Syndrome	Mechanism	Clinical features
Foramen magnum	*Herniating tissue:* Downward mesial displacement of cerebellar hemispheres *Compression:* Unilateral or bilateral medulla by ventral parafolliculi or tonsillae through foramen magnum	Episodic tonic extension with opisthotonic posturing, leading to quadriparesis Changes in blood pressure, heart rate, and arrhythmias Ataxic breathing Small pupils and disturbance of conjugate gaze
Central tentorial	*Herniating tissue:* Downward displacement of one or both cerebral hemispheres *Compression:* Diencephalon and midbrain through tentorial notch	ICP is usually raised Bilateral decorticate or decerebrate posturing An "upward" form of this syndrome may occur if supratentorial ventricles are decompressed in the presence of cerebellar mass
Uncal (lateral transtentorial)	*Herniating tissue:* Medial temporal lobe (uncus and parahippocampal gyrus) forced into the incisura *Compression:* Midbrain and posterior cerebral artery	ICP is usually raised Contralateral hemiparesis Ipsilateral pupillary dilatation and ptosis Unilateral or bilateral occipital lobe infarction Obstructive hydrocephalus from compression of aqueduct or peri-mesencephalic cistern Regions of necrosis and hemorrhage in tegmentum, subthalamus, midbrain, and upper pons
Cingulate	*Herniating tissue:* Cingulate gyrus herniates under the anterior falx *Compression:* Anterior cerebral artery	Infarction of regional tissue seen on imaging Contralateral lower extremity paresis
ICP, intracranial pressure		

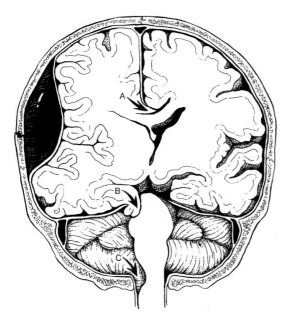

FIGURE 35.1. Herniation syndromes: (**A**) subfalcine and cingulate, (**B**) uncal, (**C**) foramen magnum (see **Table 56.3**). Subfalcine herniation occurs when one cerebral hemisphere is displaced under the falx cerebri across the midline (**A**). Uncal herniation refers to displacement of supratentorial structures inferiorly under the tentorium cerebelli, causing distortion and compression of the blood supply to infratentorial structures (**B**). Downward herniation of the cerebellum causes compression of the brainstem (**C**).

than metabolic demands, producing a state of relative hyperemia. Alternatively, a phase of increased cerebral metabolism of glucose may accompany posttraumatic hypoperfusion.

The brain tissue extracellular lactate-to-pyruvate ratio, obtained using cerebral microdialysis, has been considered a useful and sensitive marker of cerebral ischemia after TBI and subarachnoid hemorrhage. Ratio <20 suggests uncomplicated cerebral metabolism, and a rise in ratio is a sensitive indicator of a fall in brain tissue partial pressure of oxygen ($P_{bt}O_2$). In TBI, an increased ratio results from a 10- to 100-fold reduction in pyruvate concentration in association with a 2- to 5-fold increase in lactate concentration.

Hypothalamic-pituitary Injury

The pituitary gland and its anatomic attachment to hypothalamic structures are vulnerable to injury following TBI, even though they are protected by the bony sella turcica. In this instance, the pituitary stalk is at risk of trauma. In other forms of injury, the

reason for pituitary vulnerability may be vascular or ischemic, as tissue swelling and edema cause compression of the hypophysial blood vessels within the restrictive space of the sella turcica. In moderate or severe TBI, the frequency of hypopituitarism may be high.

TRAUMATIC SPINAL CORD INJURY

The features and variety of spinal cord syndromes that may occur in the setting of trauma are summarized in **Table 35.4**.

Spinal Cord Injury without Radiographic Abnormality

The anatomic characteristics of the younger child (i.e., lack of muscular development of the neck and the relatively large head size) also lead to the frequent occurrence of an entity known as "spinal cord injury without radiographic abnormality" (SCIWORA). That is, the elasticity of the immature spine may allow for significant distraction and flexion to injure the cord without resulting in either ligamentous or bone disruption and, hence, no apparent abnormalities on radiographic investigation. SCIWORA may occur in older children even though bone maturity is reached by age 9 years because ligamentous laxity continues into adolescence.

The possibility of SCIWORA should be considered in all pediatric TBI cases. The clinical features range from tingling dysesthesias or numbness to frank weakness or paralysis. MRI demonstrates 5 classes of post-SCIWORA cord findings: complete transection, major hemorrhage, minor hemorrhage, edema only, and normal.

Traumatic Atlanto-occipital Dislocation

Atlanto-occipital dislocation is defined as disruption of the supporting ligaments such that displacement occurs in either transverse or vertical direction. This lesion is rare in children and adolescents.

INITIAL CLINICAL ASSESSMENT

It is important to know the mechanism of injury in cases of TBI because this information will help in anticipating potential patterns of injury and problems (**Tables 35.1, 35.2.**).

TABLE 35.4

SPINAL CORD SYNDROMES IN TRAUMA

Syndrome	Mechanism	Findings
Complete cord transection	Trauma Secondary vascular	Loss of all motor function Loss of sensory function Above C_3—apnea and death
Brown-Sequard (cord hemisection)	Penetrating trauma	Ipsilateral loss of proprioception Ipsilateral loss of motor function Contralateral loss of pain and temperature sensation Suspended ipsilateral loss of all sensory modalities
Central cord	Neck hyperextension	Motor impairment greater in upper limbs than in lower limbs Suspended sensory loss in cervicothoracic dermatomes
Anterior cord	Hyperflexion Anterior spinal artery occlusion	Variable motor impairment Pain and temperature loss with sparing of proprioception
Conus medullaris	Direct trauma	Extension to lumbosacral roots may produce both upper and lower motor neuron signs Spastic paraparesis Sphincter dysfunction Lower sacral "saddle" sensory loss

Primary Survey

The primary survey is a rapid, abbreviated, initial physical examination that is aimed at identifying and treating quickly any life-threatening injuries. The identification and correction of airway obstruction, inadequate ventilation, and shock take priority over detailed neurologic assessment. The approach is outlined in the 2003 *Guidelines for the Acute Medical Management of Severe TBI in Infants, Children, and Adolescents* that were endorsed by the American Association for the Surgery of Trauma, the Child Neurology Society, the International Society for Pediatric Neurosurgery, the International Trauma Anesthesia and Critical Care Society, the Society of Critical Care Medicine, and the World Federation of Pediatric Intensive and Critical Care Societies.

Airway

The initial evaluation begins by demonstrating the presence of a patent, maintainable airway; the patient must be conscious, alert, and breathing spontaneously. The aim is to prevent hypoxia or hypercarbia, which may lead to secondary brain injury. The range of indications for endotracheal intubation is listed in **Table 35.5**. Beyond the prehospital setting, any children who are unable to open their eyes or

TABLE 35.5

INDICATIONS FOR INTUBATION IN THE HEAD-INJURED CHILD

Upper airway obstruction or loss of airway protective reflexes
  Loss of pharyngeal muscle activity and tone
  Inability to clear secretions
  Foreign body
  Direct trauma
  Seizures

Abnormal breathing due to
  Chest wall dysfunction
  Respiratory muscle dysfunction
  Pulmonary disease: aspiration, contusion, neurogenic
  Cervical spine injury

Apnea

Arterial partial pressure of carbon dioxide ($Paco_2$)
  Hypercarbia: $Paco_2$ >45 mm Hg
  Hypocapnia: spontaneous hyperventilation, causing $Paco_2$ <25 mm Hg

Pupils
  Anisocoria >1 mm

Glasgow Coma Scale (GCS) score
  GCS <9
  Fall in GCS score of >3, irrespective of initial GCS

verbalize must be considered candidates for intubation because of concerns about absent or impaired airway protective reflexes. Similarly, an unconscious patient must be assumed to have an obstructed airway that requires immediate evaluation. Intracranial hypertension with impending herniation may be inferred from the presence of dilated, unresponsive pupils or a triad of symptoms that includes systemic hypertension, bradycardia, and abnormal pattern of breathing.

The recommended route of airway control is orotracheal intubation; nasotracheal intubation should be avoided because of the possibility of fracture of the base of skull. Precautions to protect the cervical spine and minimize the rise in ICP associated with intubation should be undertaken. The patient's neck should be maintained in a neutral position, with axial traction applied by a person whose only role is to maintain the position of the neck. All trauma patients with supraclavicular injury should be assumed to have cranial and cervical spine injuries until proven otherwise.

Ventilation

In patients with SCI, the pattern of respiratory dysfunction depends on the level of injury (**Fig. 35.2**). Complete injury above C_3 causes respiratory arrest and death unless immediate ventilatory assistance is given. Injury at the C_3–C_5 level leads to respiratory failure, but the onset might be delayed. The *Guideline* for severe TBI is that supplemental oxygen, with 100%, should be provided in the resuscitation phase of care for all patients with moderate-to-severe TBI in order to prevent, and immediately correct, hypoxia that could cause secondary brain injury.

Circulation

After the airway and ventilation are confirmed as being adequate, the next step is assessment and optimization of the circulation. The injured brain is at risk for hypotension and inadequate perfusion. Neurogenic shock may be present in cases of SCI above T_4.

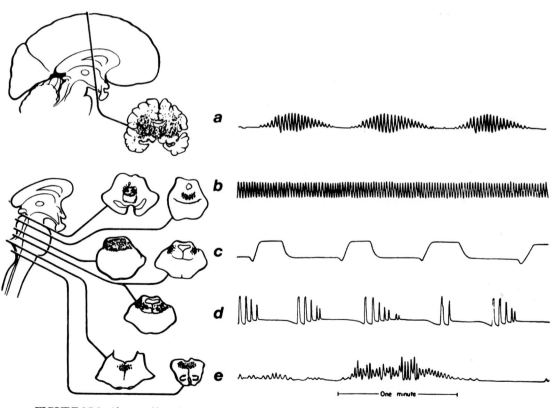

FIGURE 35.2. Abnormal breathing patterns due to lesions at different levels of the brain. Injury to different portions of the brain leads to distinctive abnormal breathing patterns that may help to localize the area of injury. A prolonged abnormal respiratory pattern may interfere with oxygenation and ventilation. From Mettler FA. *Neuroanatomy*. St. Louis: CV Mosby, 1948:816, with permission.

This hemodynamic syndrome reflects sympathetic denervation of the heart (T_1–T_4) and vasculature, with resulting decreased inotropism, chronotropism, and arterial and venous dilation. Initial treatment of hypovemia is with 20 mL/kg isotonic crystalloid (0.9% sodium chloride solution) administered as soon as vascular access is obtained. Hypotonic fluid should not be used in the initial resuscitation phase, and subsequent doses of fluid should be guided by serial assessment of blood pressure, perfusion, and hematocrit.

Neurology

The next step after adequate initial survey and stabilization is assessment of the neurologic examination. This process should be succinct and aimed primarily at diagnosing and treating life-threatening intracranial hypertension with imminent brain-tissue herniation (**Table 35.3**). A rapid assessment includes evaluation of the patient's pupillary size and its response to light, level of consciousness, and response in their extremities to a painful stimulus. The level of consciousness is graded using the Glasgow Coma Score (GCS). This descriptive scoring system evaluates performance in three areas: eye opening, which relates to the level of arousal; verbalization, which relates to content and mentation; and motor ability

(**Table 35.6**). The GCS score has not been validated in children, and in those <2 years of age, it is almost impossible to use.

SECONDARY SURVEY

The aim of the secondary survey is to identify all traumatic injuries and to begin to prioritize treatment. A thorough physical examination is required; the areas of this survey that are especially important in TBI are discussed below.

Head

Examination of the head entails careful inspection for surface depressions, swellings, lacerations, or ecchymoses that would indicate underlying injury. Evidence of base of skull fracture includes Battle sign (i.e., retro-auricular ecchymosis), raccoon eyes (i.e., periorbital ecchymosis), cerebrospinal fluid (CSF) otorrhea, CSF rhinorrhea, and hemotympanum. Evidence of facial fracture includes instability of facial bones and zygoma (i.e., Lefort fracture) and facial step-off abnormality (i.e., orbital rim fracture). If any lacerations are present, they should be explored with a gloved finger so that underlying open or depressed skull fracture or foreign material can be identified. In infants, the fontanelles and sutures should be

TABLE 35.6

GLASGOW COMA SCALE SCORE FOR CHILDREN AND INFANTS

Activity	Child response	Infant response	Score
Eye opening (E)	Spontaneous	Spontaneous	4
	To verbal stimuli	To verbal stimuli	3
	To pain	To pain	2
	None	None	1
Verbal (V)	Oriented	Coos and babbles	5
	Confused	Irritable cries	4
	Inappropriate words	Cries to pain	3
	Nonspecific sounds	Moans to pain	2
	None	None	1
Motor (M)	Follows commands	Normal spontaneous movement	6
	Localizes pain	Withdraws to touch	5
	Withdraws in response to pain	Withdraws to pain	4
	Flexion in response to pain	Abnormal flexion	3
	Extension in response to pain	Abnormal extension	2
	None	None	1

Total score: minimum, 1E + 1V + 1M = 3; maximum, 4E + 5V + 6M = 15 palpated. The tone of the fontanelle (i.e., bulging, soft, or sunken) is an indication of intracranial pressure ICP level. If possible, the head circumference should be measured and recorded.

Neck

Injury to the cervical spine must be assumed to have occurred in any head-injured patient until such time as neck soft tissue or bony injury has been ruled out. The neck should be immobilized in an appropriately sized collar, and manipulation should be kept to a minimum. If the collar is removed for any reason, the neck should be held in midline position and gentle axial traction should be applied by a single operator. Obvious deformity, swelling, or ecchymosis of the neck should be visible on inspection.

Thorax

The chest wall should be observed for the pattern and adequacy of ventilation. Specific patterns of breathing are seen with head injury and may have important localizing value (**Fig. 35.2**).

Neurology

Assessment of ocular signs and responses, the motor system, and functional integrity of the spine and spinal cord should be conducted. The American Spine Injury Association (ASIA) recommends use of the following scale of findings for the assessment of motor strength in SCI: 0, no contraction or movement; 1, minimal movement; 2, active movement but not against gravity; 3, active movement against gravity; 4, active movement against resistance; 5, active movement against full resistance. The motor level is defined as the lowest segment in which muscle strength is assessed as able to move and hold in an antigravity position (i.e., ≥3). The systematic examination required for formal assessment in SCI is best recorded using the ASIA charts. However, by way of summary, **Figure 35.3** and **Table 35.7** provide general criteria for determination of sensory and motor level. Flaccid areflexic paralysis and anesthesia to all modalities characterize *spinal shock*. SCI above the seventh thoracic vertebra may mask the tenderness normally associated with an intra-abdominal injury. Therefore, a high index of suspicion is needed in these patients to diagnose intra-abdominal bleeding.

INITIAL INVESTIGATIONS

The purpose of emergency laboratory and neuroradiologic investigations (along with the primary and secondary survey) in the child with TBI or SCI is to be able to respond to 4 key questions:

- Are there any systemic metabolic or acid-base derangements that require correction?
- Does this patient have intracranial pathology that requires emergency surgery?
- Does this patient have an unstable spine that needs fixation?
- Does this patient require full investigation for suspected nonaccidental head injury (NAHI) or shaken-baby syndrome?

Guidance can be found in reports from the American Academy of Pediatrics and the Royal College of Paediatrics and Child Health (**Table 35.8**).

Head CT

An unenhanced head CT scan is the test of choice for patients who have moderate-to-high risk of injury after head trauma, as it reveals both hemorrhage and bony injury. The indications for head CT include GCS ≤14, progressive headache, decline in level of consciousness, seizure, unreliable history, vomiting, amnesia, signs of skull fracture or facial injury, penetrating skull injury, suspected iTBI, or focal or abnormal neurology. The initial head CT should include visualization of the craniocervical junction so that atlanto-occipital dislocation, rotatory subluxation of C_1 on C_2, and other craniocervical disruptions can be evaluated. Patients with negative CT scans and mild neurologic disturbances, such as posttraumatic seizures, vomiting, headache, irritability or GCS score of 12–15, can be observed. Children with normal examination or minimal neurologic deficit and small EDH, SDH, or intraparenchymal hemorrhage may also be closely observed. In the child with lower GCS score, the absence of abnormalities on initial CT does not rule out ICP elevation. A skull x-ray is only helpful if head CT scan is not available.

Brain imaging provides some insight into the evolving mechanism of injury in the acute stage of iTBI. For example, patients with acute SDH (interhemispheric or convexity) can be categorized as those with diffuse cerebral hypoattenuation or those with focal cerebral hypoattenuation. Diffusion-weighted imaging and apparent diffusion coefficient maps—forms of MRI sensitive to ischemia and cytotoxic edema—can be used to reveal nonhemorrhagic infarction much earlier than CT, in fact within hours.

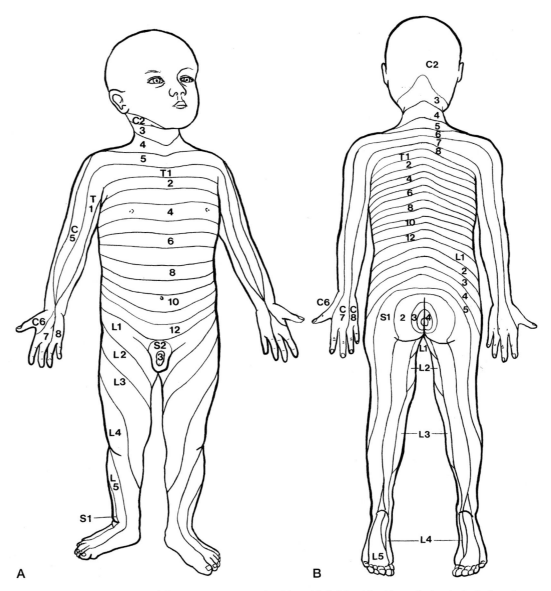

FIGURE 35.3. Segmental dermatomes are reproducible and helpful in identifying the level of spinal cord injury.

Spinal Imaging and Assessment of Stability

Imaging of the spine should be obtained in all patients with neck or back pain or tenderness, sensory or motor deficits, or an impaired level of consciousness or in those with painful, distracting injuries outside of the spine region. The goal of imaging is to rapidly identify injury of the spine that places neural tissue at risk. Spinal CT scan is indicated when the spine has not been visualized adequately on standard films or

if it appears abnormal. Spinal MRI is highly sensitive to changes in the spinal cord, hemorrhage, and ligamentous injury and is indicated in the presence of cord-related neurologic findings.

Spinal Stability

Spinal stability is defined as the capacity of the spine to withstand physiologic loading without neurologic injury, deformity, or pain. In practice, this state is

TABLE 35.7

NERVE ROOTS UNDERLYING MUSCLE FUNCTION AND REFLEXES

Nerve root	Muscles and function	Reflexes
C_4	Diaphragm Inspiration	
C_5	Deltoid Shoulder flexion Shoulder abduction	Biceps (C_5, C_6)
C_6	Biceps Elbow flexion	
C_7	Extensor carpi radialis Wrist extension	Triceps (C_7, C_8)
C_8	Flexor digitorum superficialis Finger flexion	
T_1	Interossei Finger abduction Finger adduction	
T_2–T_7	Intercostals Expiration Forced expiration	
T_8–T_{12}	Abdominals Expiration Trunk flexion	Superficial abdominals
L_2	Iliopsoas Hip flexion	Cremasteric (L_1, L_2)
L_3	Quadriceps Knee extension	Knee (L_3, L_4)
L_4	Tibialis anterior Foot dorsiflexion	
L_5	Extensor hallucis longus Great toe extension	Hamstring (L_5, S_1)
S_1	Gastrocnemius Foot plantar flexion	Ankle (S_1, S_2)
S_2–S_5	Anal sphincter Fecal continence	Bulbocavernosus (S_3, S_4) Anal wink (S_5)

predicted by clinical examination and imaging. For the thoracolumbar spine, instability is defined as injury to more than 2 CT-based "columns": the *anterior column*, which consists of the anterior longitudinal ligament and the anterior half of vertebral body or disc; the *middle column*, which consists of the posterior half of the body or disc and the posterior longitudinal ligament; and, the *posterior column*, which consists of the posterior arch and ligaments.

Clearance of the cervical spine as being stable is controversial. Some standards have been established for clearing the cervical spine in adults. Adults who are awake, alert, not intoxicated, and have no other distraction injuries, neck pain, or tenderness do not require any supplemental radiographic assessment to clear the cervical spine as being stable. These guidelines can be used in children older than 9 years. In children with significant TBI or significant neck pain, a reasonable practice is to maintain cervical spine immobilization until an MRI can be performed to ex-

clude ligamentous injury. However, there are no formal guidelines exist on this practice. In the conscious child, immobilization can be discontinued when the pain has resolved and flexion and extension radiographs reveal no apparent injury.

NEUROCRITICAL CARE MONITORING OF INTRACRANIAL PRESSURE

Traditionally, ICP monitoring is performed via a ventriculostomy. Newer technologies rely on fiberoptic monitoring, with the catheter sensor-tip placed in the brain parenchyma. The advantage of the ventriculostomy is that it enables CSF drainage as a treatment. However, it can be difficult to place and maintain function in the child with small, compressed, or distorted ventricles.

TABLE 35.8

ESSENTIAL BASELINE MEDICAL ASSESSMENT OF AN INFANT WITH SUBDURAL HEMORRHAGE AND SUSPECTED INFLICTED TRAUMATIC BRAIN INJURY

Assessment	Notes
Clinical history	Full case history Full documentation of all possible explanations for injury Identification of any previous concerns about unexplained injury Identification of relevant criminal record of care providers
Examination	Thorough general examination Documentation and clinical photographs of coexisting injury Head circumference, weight, and length plotted on centiles
Eyes	Ophthalmologist to examine both eyes through dilated pupils
Radiology	Initial cranial CT scan Repeat neuroimaging at 7 and 14 days Neuroradiologic report of all imaging Full skeletal survey; repeat at 10–14 days
Serology	Full blood count repeated over first 24–48 hrs Coagulation screen Urea and electrolytes, liver function tests, blood cultures
Follow-up investigations indicated by tests above	Exclude glutaric aciduria in cases with frontotemporal atrophy Lumbar puncture where meningitis is possible Save serum for viral serology

ICP AND CEREBRAL PERFUSION PRESSURE TARGET LEVELS

Normal ICP is usually <10 mm Hg in adults, varies between 3 and 7 mm Hg in younger children, and is <6 mm Hg in infants. In adults, the threshold for initiating treatment of intracranial hypertension is taken as 20–25 mm Hg. It is likely that the ICP threshold for poorer outcome is similar across all ages. Cerebral perfusion pressure (CPP) is calculated as the difference between the mean systemic arterial pressure and the mean ICP. The pediatric *Guideline* for severe TBI is that "CPP >40 mm Hg should be maintained." A modification of this recommendation is to titrate the CPP threshold according to age: thresholds of 40–50 mm Hg in infants and toddlers, 50–60 mm Hg in children, and >60 mm Hg in adolescents.

NEUROCRITICAL CARE TREATMENTS

After endotracheal intubation and insertion of an ICP monitor, the first step used to reduce ICP is to ensure adequate sedation, analgesia, and neuromuscular blockade by using standard dosing of agents chosen by the treating physician. Propofol should not be used in children with severe TBI. The other "first-tier" therapies include elevation of the head of the bed to 30 degrees and positioning of the head in the midline, ensuring no obstruction to cerebral venous return. If ICP remains elevated and a ventriculostomy tube is in place, CSF can be drained.

If ICP is still elevated after these initial measures, mannitol or hyperosmolar therapy using hypertonic saline can be instituted. Intermittent, IV infusions of mannitol, usually in the range of 0.25–0.5 g/kg, can be administered. Serum osmolality should be assessed before redosing and the mannitol infusion withheld if the serum osmolality is >320 mOsm/L, as dehydration induced by mannitol can precipitate renal failure. Some centers use furosemide as an adjunct to mannitol to potentiate its effects as a diuretic. A continuous infusion of 3% saline (between 0.1 and 1.0 mL/kg/hr administered on a sliding scale) is effective management of ICP. Infusions can be continued if serum osmolality is below 360 mOsm/L.

If the patient still continues to have raised ICP despite using all first-tier therapies, a number of "second-tier" therapies can be considered. If the basal cisterns are open on concurrent cranial CT scan and no significant mass or midline shift is

TABLE 35.9

PEDIATRIC INTENSITY LEVEL OF THERAPY (PILOT) SCALE

Variable	Score	Maximum score
Individual daily scored components are denoted 'a', 'b' or 'c' in the scoring section		
General (at any time in previous 24 hrs) Treatment of fever (>38.5°C) or spontaneous temperature (<34.5°C) Sedation (opiates, benzodiazepines: any dose) Neuromuscular blockade	1a 1b 2c	1a + 1b + 2c = 4
Ventilation (most frequently observed $Paco_2$ in 24 hrs) Intubated/normal ventilation ($PaCO_2$ 35.1–40 mm Hg) Mild hyperventilation ($PaCO_2$ 32–35 mm Hg) Aggressive hyperventilation ($PaCO_2$ <32 mm Hg)	1a 2a 4a	4
Osmolar therapy (total dose in 24 hrs) Mannitol ≤1 g/kg Mannitol 1.1–2 g/kg Mannitol >2 g/kg Hypertonic saline (any dose or rate, regardless of [Na])	1a 2a 3a 3b	3a + 3b = 6
Cerebrospinal fluid drainage (times in 24 hrs) 0–11 times 12–23 times ≥ 24times or continuous	1a 2a 3a	3
Barbiturates (total dose in 24 hrs; for score, 5 mg thiopental is equivalent to 1 mg pentobarbital) Pentobarbital ≤36 mg/kg Pentobarbital >36 mg/kg	3a 4a	4
Surgery (at any time in 24 hrs) Evacuation of hematoma Decompressive craniectomy	4a 5b	4a + 5b = 9
Other treatments (at any time in 24 hrs) Induced mild hypothermia (≥35°C–37°C) Induced moderate hypothermia (<35°C) Lumbar drain Induced hypertension (≥95th percentile for age)	2a 4a 2b 2c	4 + 2 + 2 = 8
Total possible score		4 + 4 + 6 + 3 + 4 + 9 + 8 = 38

Data from Shore PM, Hand LL, Roy L, et al. Reliability and validity of the pediatric intensity level of therapy (PILOT) scale: A measure of the use of intracranial pressure-directed therapies. *Crit Care Med* 2006; 34:1981–7.

present, a lumbar CSF drain can be considered by the neurosurgical staff. If the patient has no medical contraindications to using barbiturates, pentobarbital can be used to induce burst suppression and control elevated ICP by reducing cerebral metabolic activity. A commonly used protocol for pentobarbital is to use a loading dose of 10 mg/kg over 30 mins, followed by 5 mg/kg every hour for 3 doses, and then a maintenance infusion of 1 mg/kg/hr. The dose is titrated to the effect required (i.e., ICP control) while hypotension and unnecessary central nervous system depression are avoided. Alternatively, with ev-idence of brain swelling on CT scan, decompressive craniectomy can be considered. Other therapies that can be used as adjuncts to care include induced hypothermia (or at least maintenance of normothermia), controlled hyperventilation ($PaCO_2$ 30–35 mm Hg) in those with cerebral hyperemia, and controlled arterial hypertension. The Pediatric Intensity Level of Therapy scale assigns scores to a variety of first- and second-tier treatments used in ICP control (**Table 35.9**). The intensity of treatment in subgroups of patients and in different PICUs can be compared using this scale.

Spinal Cord Injury-directed Therapies

In adults, high-dose methylprednisolone became the standard of care in the management of nonpenetrating acute SCI. The Canadian Association of Emergency Physicians no longer recommends high-dose methylprednisolone as the standard of care. The Congress of Neurological Surgeons states that steroid therapy "should only be undertaken with the knowledge that evidence suggesting harmful effects is more consistent than any suggestion of clinical benefit." The American College of Surgeons has modified their Advanced Trauma Life Support guidelines to state that methylprednisolone is "*a* recommended treatment" rather than "*the* recommended treatment." If steroids are recommended, they should be initiated within 8 hrs of injury with the following protocol. Methylprednisolone 30 mg/kg bolus over 15 mins and an infusion of methylprednisolone at 5.4 mg/kg/hr for 23 hrs beginning 45 mins after the bolus, if the patient started therapy within 3 hrs of injury. If the patient starts treatment between 3 and 8 hrs after injury, the infusion can be continued for a total of 48 hrs.

Last, adults with SCI are at risk for deep vein thrombosis and venous thromboembolism. Current guidelines recommend that patients with SCI receive prophylaxis with low-molecular-weight heparin. Gastroparesis and paralytic ileus are also common, and treatment with prokinetics may be useful.

Seizures and Anticonvulsants

Seizures are the most common complication after a head injury. The standard definition for an early posttraumatic seizure is that it occurs within one week of trauma. In patients who are refractory to treatment, which appears to be quite common in iTBI, continuous infusion of midazolam can be utilized. The alternative is high-dose phenobarbitone or anesthesia with short-acting barbiturates. The main problems with barbiturates are the zero-order kinetics once treatment is prolonged and the inability to assess clinical neurology. In children, medications for seizure prophylaxis include phenytoin, phenobarbital, and carbamazepine.

Posttraumatic Meningitis and Fever

Posttraumatic meningitis is a risk of mid-frontal, lateral-frontal, or temporofrontal fractures and posterolateral fractures (**Table 35.1**). It is best treated after an infective organism is cultured so that the antibiotic can be tailored appropriately. Initial empiric therapy after culture should cover *Streptococcus* and *Staphylococcus*. Ceftriaxone with or without vancomycin, depending on the local incidence of resistant Gram-positive organisms, is a reasonable choice until the specific organism is cultured.

Fever may be the earliest sign of meningitis, but in severe TBI, this is not always the cause. Early hyperthermia (i.e., temperature $>38.5°C$) within the first 24 hrs of admission often occurs after TBI; this phenomenon appears to be a function of severity of injury and is to be expected in children with moderate degrees of subarachnoid hemorrhage. Generally, a rise in temperature of $>39°C$ demands investigation, and the presence of a compound fracture, either internal or external, should serve to focus attention immediately upon the possibility of meningitis. Extracranial causes of fever are also possible (e.g., chest infection, fat embolism, wound infection) and must be sought. Neurogenic hyperthermia may be due to primary brain lesions associated with TAI and dysautonomia with storming episodes. Another possibility is dehydration.

Fluids and Nutrition

It is clear that use of low-sodium-containing crystalloids is associated with mortality and morbidity in children. However, prolonged use of IV 0.9% sodium chloride will inevitably cause hyperchloremia and acidosis. IV saline-induced hyperchloremic acidosis causes reduced urine flow, confusion, and increased morbidity in adults who undergo major surgery. Glucose-containing IV solutions are not recommended in adults who have suffered TBI. In fact, the emphasis is on limiting glucose in the insulin-resistant critically ill and on controlling blood glucose within a tight range by using supplemental insulin. This so-called tight glycemic control with intensive insulin therapy appears to be associated with better ICP control in TBI. Until more is known about the relationship between blood glucose, brain glucose, and outcome, it is advisable to continue with one's current fluid strategy. An *option* that circumvents these issues is to initiate enteral nutritional support by 72 hrs after injury and aim for full nutritional replacement by day 7.

Hypothalamic-pituitary Dysfunction

In adults with moderate-to-severe TBI, the endocrine changes in the first few hours and days immediately after injury share similarities with the changes in hypothalamic-pituitary-endocrine dysfunction observed in other critically ill patients. In particular, low basal cortisol levels with subnormal cortisol responses to stress test have been observed. Posterior pituitary dysfunction that leads to abnormalities in water homeostasis and results in either cranial (central) diabetes insipidus or syndrome of inappropriate antidiuretic hormone (SIADH) secretion is also commonly observed in the acute period after TBI. In the majority of cases, perturbations in water balance are usually transitory and resolve within a few days or weeks of the event. SIADH is manifest as hyponatremia (serum sodium ≤130 mmol/L), which will exacerbate cerebral swelling, worsen ICP, and cause seizures. Cerebral salt wasting may also cause hyponatremia. SIADH is treated with volume restriction, and cerebral salt wasting is treated with volume and sodium repletion. The differentiation between these entities can be difficult to discern, but the single, clear, differentiating factor is the patient's volume state. Patients with high volume status have SIADH, while those with low intravascular volume have cerebral salt wasting. In that patients with SIADH tend to make smaller amounts of highly osmolar urine, careful documentation of urine volume and urinary sodium concentration may assist in the diagnosis. Mineralocorticoids also have a role in facilitating sodium retention.

In patients with acute-phase basal cortisol concentration between 200 and 400 nmol/L, we consider replacement therapy if the child has features that could be due to adrenal insufficiency (e.g., hypotension, hyponatremia, or hypoglycemia). Assessment of growth hormone, gonadal, and thyroid axes is not necessary in the acute phase because, in adults, no evidence suggests that acute phase replacement of these hormones in the deficient patient improves outcome.

CHAPTER 36 ■ STATUS EPILEPTICUS

KIMBERLY D. STATLER • COLIN B. VAN ORMAN

Status epilepticus (SE) is classically defined as seizure activity, either continuous or episodic without complete recovery of consciousness, lasting for ≥30 mins (**Table 36.1**). The evolution of SE can be conceptualized in stages: (a) premonitory or prodromal SE, characterized by an increasing frequency of serial seizures with recovery of consciousness between episodes; (b) incipient SE, defined as continuous or intermittent seizures lasting up to five minutes without full recovery of consciousness; (c) impending or early SE, marked by seizure activity persisting 5–30 mins; and (d) established SE, defined as seizures lasting >30 mins. When SE lasts >30–60 mins, subtle SE usually develops. Subtle SE is characterized by progressive electromechanical dissociation in which clinical signs diminish yet electroencephalographic (EEG) seizure activity persists. Finally, nonconvulsive SE (NCSE) refers to ongoing EEG seizure activity without associated clinical signs. An operational treatment definition advocates defining SE as seizure activity lasting >5 mins, given that prompt intervention is crucial.

GENERALIZED CONVULSIVE STATUS EPILEPTICUS

Generalized convulsive status epilepticus (GCSE) is characterized by tonic, clonic, or tonic-clonic seizure activity involving all extremities. In primary GCSE, seizure onset cannot be localized to one brain region by either clinical or EEG findings. In secondary GCSE, which is more common, seizures begin focally but spread to involve the entire brain. Focal motor SE, also called simple complex SE, somatomotor SE, or epilepsy partialis continua, is characterized by involvement of a single limb or side of the face. Focal motor SE is less common than GCSE and is frequently associated with focal brain pathology (**Table 36.2**). Myoclonic SE is characterized by irregular, asynchronous, small-amplitude, repetitive myoclonic jerking of the face or limbs. Myoclonic SE is more common in comatose patients and is associated with several specific conditions, particularly anoxia or cardiac arrest (**Table 36.3**).

NONCONVULSIVE STATUS EPILEPTICUS

NCSE is characterized by continuous nonmotor seizures and requires EEG confirmation for diagnosis. NCSE may occur in ambulatory or comatose patients. The most common type of NCSE in ambulatory children is absence SE, which is characterized by altered consciousness. NCSE in comatose patients may be difficult to diagnose and should be

TABLE 36.1

CLASSIFICATION OF STATUS EPILEPTICUS

Convulsive	Nonconvulsive
Generalized convulsive	Absence
Focal motor	Complex partial
Myoclonic	NCSE with Coma

NCSE, nonconvulsive status epilepticus

considered in any patient with prolonged obtundation after seizure cessation or with coma of unclear etiology.

REFRACTORY STATUS EPILEPTICUS

Refractory SE (RSE) is seizures that fail to remit despite treatment with adequate doses of two anticonvulsants.

NEONATAL STATUS EPILEPTICUS

SE presents differently in neonates than in older infants and children. Neonates are unlikely to demonstrate GCSE or continuous seizure activity; however, frequent, serial seizures without recovery of consciousness can occur and may involve rapid extensor or flexor posturing, tremor of extended extremities, apnea, eye deviation, or automatisms.

TABLE 36.2

COMMON ETIOLOGIES OF FOCAL MOTOR STATUS EPILEPTICUS

Brain tumor
  Astrocytoma
  Oligodendroglioma
  Glioblastoma
Infection
  Brain abscess
  Viral encephalitis
  Cysticercosis
  Tuberculosis
Vascular
  Cortical vein thrombosis
  Arteriovenous malformation
  Cerebrovascular accident
Trauma
  Posttraumatic cyst
  Chronic subdural hematoma
  Focal gliosis

TABLE 36.3

COMMON ETIOLOGIES OF MYOCLONIC STATUS EPILEPTICUS

Anoxic injury
  Cardiac arrest
  Cardiopulmonary bypass
  Carbon monoxide poisoning
  CO_2 narcosis
Infection
  Viral encephalitis
  Acute demyelinating encephalomyelitis
  Subacute sclerosing panencephalitis
  Opportunistic infection
Injury
  Heat stroke
  Lightning
  Intracranial hemorrhage
Metabolic
  Hepatic failure
  Renal failure
  Hypoglycemia
  Hyponatremia
  Nonketotic hyperglycemia
  Thiamine deficiency
Toxins
  Tricyclic antidepressants
  Anticonvulsants
  β-lactam antibiotics
  Opiates
  Lithium
  Heavy metal poisoning
Genetic/epilepsy syndromes
  Juvenile myoclonic epilepsy
  Lennox-Gastaut syndrome
  Absence epilepsy
  Degenerative myoclonus epilepsy
  Angelman syndrome

Conditions commonly associated with neonatal SE are presented in **Table 36.4**.

COMMON ETIOLOGIES

Though initial supportive and anticonvulsant therapies are similar regardless of cause, diagnostic tests and adjunctive treatments are guided by suspected etiology. The etiologies of SE are commonly classified as cryptogenic, remote symptomatic, febrile, acute symptomatic, or progressive encephalopathy (**Table 36.5**). Febrile or acute symptomatic etiologies are most common in younger children. Tapering or withdrawal of anticonvulsant medications is a common inciting event among older children. CNS infection, metabolic abnormalities, traumatic brain injury, and anoxic brain injury are the most common specific etiologies of acute symptomatic pediatric SE. Other common inciting events are listed in

TABLE 36.4

COMMON ETIOLOGIES OF NEONATAL STATUS EPILEPTICUS

Perinatal or acute insults
  Hypoxia-ischemia
  Intracranial hemorrhage
  Cerebral vascular accident
Infection
  Meningitis
  Encephalitis
  Abscess
Metabolic
  Hypoglycemia
  Hypocalcemia
  Hyponatremia
  Hypomagnesemia
  Bilirubin encephalopathy
Inborn errors of metabolism
  Phenylketonuria
  Nonketotic hyperglycemia
  Pyridoxine deficiency
  Histidinemia
  Hyperammonemia
  Homocitrullinemia
  Maple syrup urine disease
  Leucine-sensitive hypoglycemia
Toxins
  β-lactam antibiotics
  Anesthetics
  Drug withdrawal
  Heavy metal poisoning
Cerebral malformations
  Neuronal migration defect
  Neurocutaneous syndrome
Degenerative diseases
  Leigh's encephalopathy
  Leukodystrophies
  Alper's disease
  Sandhoff's disease
  Tay-Sachs disease
Benign familial syndromes
  Benign familial neonatal seizures
  Benign neonatal sleep myoclonus

Table 36.6. Meningitis is more frequent in infants. Anoxia is more common in children >5 years old. Hypoxic-ischemic injury is the most prevalent cause of neonatal SE in developed countries, but electrolyte abnormalities continue to be more common in developing regions.

Behavioral and Electroencephalographic Manifestations

The progression of both clinical and experimental CSE may be divided into five stages. The first stage is characterized by discrete seizures, which are typically focal with secondary generalization and manifest as generalized tonic-clonic convulsions. With time, the discrete seizures merge to produce an EEG pattern of asymmetric sharp and spike waves with waxing and waning amplitude accompanied by either generalized convulsions or serial tonic or clonic seizures involving one or more extremities. The third stage is characterized by continuous EEG seizure discharges and either clonic jerks or subtle clonic convulsive activity. In the fourth stage, flat periods of EEG activity interrupt continuous seizure discharges, and behavioral clonic convulsions may be overt, subtle, or absent. During the fifth stage, the EEG shows monomorphic repetitive sharp waves, called periodic epileptiform discharges, on a flat background, and accompanying motor manifestations are absent. In the immature (vs. the adult) brain, the EEG progression through all five stages is less consistent, and behavioral manifestations are less discrete. Treatment with anticonvulsants can interrupt both EEG and behavioral progression of SE.

Seizure Initiation and Progression

Seizure initiation and propagation involve a failure of gamma-aminobutyric-acid (GABA) mediated inhibition and/or an increase in glutamate-mediated excitation. A predominance of inhibition is required for seizure termination and may be achieved by augmenting inhibition or blocking excitation. Mechanisms implicated in seizure termination include a predominance of GABA activity, membrane stabilization by acidic extracellular pH, magnesium blockade of N-methyl-D-aspartate channels, activation of the Na^+/K^+-ATPase system, and activation of K^+ conductance to allow membrane repolarization. Adenosine, an endogenous neuroprotectant, is though to regulate basal neural inhibition and may also prove important for seizure termination. Treatment with adenosine antagonists, such as caffeine or aminophylline, is proconvulsive.

Cerebral Injury Induced by Status Epilepticus

Seizures lasting 30–60 mins are sufficient to cause neuronal injury. Importantly, both CSE and NCSE may be injurious, and both must be controlled as efficiently as possible. Neuronal injury induced by SE is predominantly due to prolonged seizure activity, not to systemic complications, such as hypoxia, hypoglycemia, or hyperthermia. In the presence of an accompanying acute neurologic insult, the seizure duration necessary to cause neuronal injury may be

TABLE 36.5

ETIOLOGIC CLASSIFICATION OF STATUS EPILEPTICUS

Etiology	Definition
Cryptogenic (idiopathic)	Status epilepticus in the absence of an acute precipitating CNS insult or metabolic dysfunction in a patient without a preexisting neurologic abnormality
Remote symptomatic	Status epilepticus in a patient with a known history of a neurologic insult associated with an increased risk of seizures (e.g., traumatic brain injury, stroke, static encephalopathy)
Febrile	Status epilepticus provoked solely by fever in a patient without a history of afebrile seizures
Acute symptomatic	Status epilepticus during an acute illness involving a known neurologic insult (e.g., meningitis, traumatic brain injury, hypoxia) or metabolic dysfunction (e.g., hypoglycemia, hypocalcemia, hyponatremia)
Progressive encephalopathy	Status epilepticus in a patient with a progressive neurologic disease (e.g., neurodegeneration, malignancies, neurocutaneous syndromes)

Adapted from Shinnar S, Pellock JM, Moshe SL, et al. In whom does status epilepticus occur: Age-related differences in children. *Epilepsia* 1997;38:907–14.

TABLE 36.6

POTENTIAL ETIOLOGIES OF ACUTE SYMPTOMATIC STATUS EPILEPTICUS

	Newborn	1–2 Months old	Infancy and childhood
Acute insult	Hypoxic-ischemic CNS infection Intracranial hemorrhage	CNS infection Subdural hematoma Anoxia VP shunt dysfunction	CNS infection Intracranial hemorrhage Anoxia VP shunt dysfunction
Genetic and metabolic	Hypoglycemia Hypernatremia Hyponatremia Hypocalcemia Hypomagnesemia Hyperbilirubinemia Organic acidemia Urea cycle defects 　Nonketotic hyperglycemia 　Congenital lactic acidosis Pyridoxine dependency	Hypoglycemia Hypernatremia Hyponatremia Hypocalcemia Organic acidemia Urea cycle defects Phenylketonuria Riley-Day syndrome	Hypoglycemia Hypernatremia Hyponatremia Hypocalcemia Lysosomal defects Urea cycle defects Uremia Hepatic failure
Malformation	Neuronal migration defect Chromosomal anomaly	Sturge-Weber syndrome Neurofibromatosis Tuberous sclerosis	
Other	Toxins Drugs Narcotic withdrawal	Cocaine toxicity Drugs Narcotic withdrawal	Febrile convulsion Drugs 　Tricyclic antidepressants 　Anticonvulsants 　Calcineurin inhibitors 　β-Lactam antibiotics 　Opiates Narcotic withdrawal

<30–60 mins. Seizures increase glucose metabolism and intracranial pressure, placing vulnerable cerebral tissue at greater risk for injury.

CLINICAL PRESENTATION AND DIFFERENTIAL DIAGNOSIS

Generalized Convulsive Status Epilepticus

Generalized convulsive status epilepticus (GCSE) may be tonic-clonic, clonic, or tonic in nature. GCSE often starts as increasing frequency of serial seizures with recovery of consciousness between episodes (premonitory SE), and prompt treatment during this stage may prevent progression. Serial seizures typically last 1–3 mins but tend to shorten as time elapses. Between seizures, patients are obtunded, showing autonomic signs such as salivation, bradypnea, cyanosis, and arterial hypotension. In some cases, cardiovascular collapse may occur. Neurologic examination may reveal abnormal cranial nerve function and unilateral or bilateral Babinski responses. Cerebrospinal fluid pleocytosis as a consequence of GCSE has been documented in all ages.

Clonic Status Epilepticus

Clonic SE may persist hours or even days, waxing and waning in intensity, and a persistent post-ictal hemiplegia is usually observed. The behavioral manifestations of clonic SE are variable. Seizures tend to be continuous and may be generalized, unilateral, or restricted to one limb or segment. Fluctuations between different patterns of involvement may occur during a single episode of clonic SE. Additionally, the rhythm of jerks is variable and may also fluctuate. Clonic seizures in young children are predominantly unilateral; however, they may shift from side to side.

Tonic SE is less common than tonic-clonic or clonic SE and occurs almost exclusively in children and adolescents with known epilepsy. Importantly, tonic SE has been precipitated by intravenous or oral benzodiazepine treatment of absence SE in children with Lennox-Gastaut syndrome. The duration of tonic SE may be much longer than that of other CSE types, persisting for several days. Serial tonic seizures are typical, and autonomic manifestations, particularly increased bronchial secretions, may be pronounced. Over time, behavioral manifestations become limited to slight eye deviation, respiratory irregularities and marked tracheobronchial obstruction due to hypersecretion. Consciousness is mod-

erately to severely impaired, and a post-ictal confusional state may persist for days. The initial behavioral manifestations of tonic SE may be attenuated or even subclinical. In these cases, polygraphic monitoring is necessary to demonstrate the tachycardia, altered respiratory rhythm, occasional hypertonus of the trunk or neck muscles, and EEG activity indicative of tonic SE.

Focal Motor Status Epilepticus

Focal motor SE may affect children with acute inciting insults (**Table 36.2**) or those with known epileptic disorders. Focal motor SE due to an acute illness, such as encephalitis, typically develops into secondary GCSE. Conversely, in children with epilepsy, focal motor SE tends to have a more restricted distribution and may be manifest only as jerking of the corner of the mouth or cheek, salivation, swallowing difficulties, and absent speech. Even with narrowly localized seizures, autonomic disturbances and some impairment of consciousness may be present. Children who clinically appear to be in focal motor SE may be treated despite a lack of seizure activity on EEG.

Myoclonic SE is characterized by the incessant repetition of massive myoclonic jerks. Acute hypoxic-ischemic encephalopathy is the most common cause of myoclonic SE among critically ill children. When associated with anoxic brain injury, myoclonic SE indicates severe diffuse brain damage and can be difficult to control. Myoclonic SE also occurs with metabolic insults, such as hypoglycemia, hepatic or renal failure, or heavy metal intoxication (**Table 36.3**). Physical trauma or inflammatory disease rarely causes myoclonic SE. Importantly, myoclonic SE may be induced by high doses of beta-lactam antibiotics, especially in patients with renal failure. Intrathecal administration of radiologic contrast agents is also associated with myoclonic SE, typically with a favorable prognosis. Finally, myoclonic SE also affects children with epilepsy and has been described with Angelman syndrome.

NCSE is defined as (a) prolonged (>30 mins) alteration of consciousness or complex partial seizures without full recovery of consciousness, (b) epileptiform changes on the EEG that are different from the pre-ictal state, and (c) prompt observable improvement in both the EEG and clinical state after administration of an intravenous antiepileptic medication. NCSE can present agitation and aggression, lethargy, confusion, delirium, fugue-like state, decreased speech, mutism, echolalia, blank staring with or without blinking, chewing and picking, tremulousness, subtle facial or limb myoclonus, rigidity, or waxy flexibility or vegetative features. NCSE is seen in children with epilepsy, such as Landau-Kleffner syndrome, and ring chromosome 20. Additionally, critically ill patients with unexplained coma or prolonged obtundation after CSE may have NCSE.

Absence NCSE

Generalized NCSE is widely known as absence SE, although it has also been called *petit mal status* and *spike-wave stupor*. Absence SE is characterized by a variable impairment of consciousness, ranging from mild slowing of higher cognitive functions to barely perceptible responsiveness. Complex automatisms may occur, and motor manifestations, including myoclonic twitches of the eyelids and facial muscles, bilateral or unilateral limb myoclonus and/or atonic phenomena producing falls, head nods, knee buckling or other alterations of posture, are seen in about half of the cases. Patients are totally or partially amnestic of these episodes. Of note, patients typically do not show the cycling in the clinical state that characterizes complex partial SE.

Complex partial SE is also known as psychomotor status, focal NCSE, temporolimbic SE, or localized NCSE. It occurs less commonly in children but can be seen in the course of focal epilepsies. Complex partial SE can present as frequently recurring partial seizures without full recovery of consciousness between seizures or continuous long-standing episodes of mental confusion and behavioral disturbance with or without automatisms. Complex partial SE is often marked by cyclic alterations between unresponsive staring and partial responsiveness with quasi-purposeful reactive automatisms.

RSE may occur with any classification or etiology of SE and is associated with greater morbidity and mortality than more responsive SE. Although RSE typically has motor manifestations, it may begin as NCSE. Even in patients who present with GCSE, RSE frequently becomes subtle or nonconvulsive (NCRSE). Patients with acute structural lesions are at higher risk for NCRSE, and a high degree of suspicion with continuous EEG monitoring is required for timely and accurate diagnosis. Additionally, continuous EEG monitoring is important to guide therapy in any patient with RSE.

Systemic Manifestations

GCSE can be divided into early and late phases. During early SE, compensatory mechanisms to attenuate seizure-associated injury are prominent. The transition from early to late SE occurs after ~30–45 mins of continuous seizure activity. Late SE is marked by failure of compensatory mechanisms and seizure associated injury. Additionally, once the transition from early to late SE has occurred, SE is more difficult to terminate.

During early SE, increased catecholamine levels result in tachycardia, hypertension, increased central venous pressures, and hyperglycemia. Cerebral blood flow increases in response to increased cerebral metabolic demands. Lactic acidosis commonly results from continued, rigorous muscle activity. Mild hypoxemia and modest hypercarbia may occur, but patients usually maintain sufficient oxygenation and ventilation if the airway remains patent. Other autonomic signs, including diaphoresis, hypersecretion, and mydriasis, are frequent. During late SE, compensatory reserves are exhausted and marked hyperthermia, hypotension, and hypoglycemia may occur. Cerebrovascular autoregulation is lost, and cerebral blood flow becomes pressure-dependent, making prompt correction of hypotension crucial. Cerebral edema may accompany late SE. Sustained motor convulsions may result in rhabdomyolysis and hyperkalemia. Hypoxia and hypercarbia are frequently more exaggerated during late SE. Respiratory compromise, associated with apnea or poor handling of secretions, is common. Pupillary and corneal reflexes may be absent in the ictal or post-ictal phases of both early and late SE. Rarely disseminated intravascular coagulation and multiorgan failure may be induced by SE itself or by the inciting cause. Myoglobinuria or dehydration and shock may lead to renal failure. Hepatic insufficiency or failure may result from the underlying cause of SE, as a side effect of anticonvulsant therapy, or from hyperpyrexia. Finally, emesis is common, and patients with SE are at high risk for aspiration.

Differential Diagnosis

CSE is usually easy to diagnose and not readily confused with other disorders in a nonparalyzed patient. However, pseudo-SE can be confused with CSE on occasion with disastrous results. Clinical signs suggestive of nonepileptic psychogenic seizures include motor movements that fluctuate in intensity, frequency, and/or distribution with lack of facial muscle involvement and pelvic thrusting. Vocalization, bizarre behavior, explosive emotional expression, and resistance to examination are common. Although urinary incontinence, tongue biting, and cyanosis can occur, they are less common than in CSE. In pseudostatus epilepticus, the EEG is often obscured by muscle and movement artifact, and no post-ictal EEG changes occur. A well-developed alpha rhythm can be discerned during brief moments of cessation of movement or on termination of pseudoseizures. In contrast, patients with CSE have both ictal and post-ictal EEG changes. Furthermore, the muscle artifact associated with pseudoseizures lacks the repetitive characteristics seen in true CSE. In contrast, the seizure behavior associated with NCSE is nonspecific and may produce diagnostic confusion. Two common conditions that may simulate the seizure behaviors of NCSE are post-ictal drowsiness and anticonvulsant-induced sedation. Continuous EEG recordings may be necessary to accurately distinguish these disorders. Toxic-metabolic (including drug intoxication and drug withdrawal) and infectious (including para-infectious and post-infectious) encephalopathies of numerous etiologies present with altered mental status and may be clinically indistinguishable from NCSE. Additionally, altered mental status mimicking NCSE can be caused by acute structural lesions, including traumatic brain injury, tumors, and stroke. Neuroimaging studies are helpful for differentiation of these etiologies. Finally, psychiatric disorders may need to be considered in patients with behavioral changes not associated with appropriate ictal and inter-ictal EEG changes.

PRINCIPLES OF CLINICAL MANAGEMENT

As with any critically ill child, the first priority of initial stabilization is to ensure airway patency and control. The patient should be positioned so that ongoing seizure activity will not cause physical harm. Nothing should be placed into the patient's mouth, due to the risk of aspiration. Supplemental oxygen should be provided and respiration assisted as needed. Precautions should be taken to prevent aspiration. In patients with hypoxia, hypoventilation, or a Glasgow Coma Score <8, rapid-sequence endotracheal intubation should be considered for airway protection and respiratory support. A short-acting barbiturate, such as thiopental, is commonly used, although dose-associated hypotension should be anticipated and avoided. Benzodiazepines or narcotics are also acceptable choices. If neuromuscular blockade is necessary to facilitate intubation, a short-acting, nondepolarizing agent such as rocuronium is preferable. In the absence of a known normal serum potassium level, succinylcholine should be avoided due to the risk of hyperkalemia associated with ongoing seizure activity. Repeated or continued neuromuscular blockade should also be avoided, as it may mask ongoing seizure activity. Reliable intravenous access should be established as soon as possible. If

placement of intravenous catheters is difficult or prolonged, an intraosseous catheter may be considered. Hypotension or dehydration should be treated with isotonic fluid resuscitation. Hypertension is common with ongoing seizure activity, and treatment should not be considered unless it persists after seizure activity has stopped. Hypoglycemia should be considered as an inciting event and a serum glucose level checked promptly. In the absence of rapid testing, empiric dextrose should be administered intravenously. Thiamine (50–100 mg IV) may be considered prior to dextrose administration in older children at risk of nutritional deficiencies. Electrolyte abnormalities, such as hyponatremia or hypocalcemia, should be evaluated. Due to the potential for exacerbating cerebral injury, significant hyperthermia (>40°C) should be treated with passive cooling. Precautions should be taken to prevent shivering associated with passive cooling. If neuromuscular blockade is required, continuous EEG monitoring is indicated to assess for ongoing seizure activity.

Diagnostic Tests

Swift cessation of seizures is crucial, and anticonvulsant therapy should not be delayed to facilitate diagnostic testing. All patients with SE should receive serum glucose and electrolyte testing. Further diagnostic tests are guided by probable or suspected etiology. Serum anticonvulsant medication levels should be measured in children on chronic therapy. Blood and urine specimens should be obtained for culture, especially in febrile children. Serum and urine toxicology screening tests should be sent in patients with possible ingestions. After the seizures have stopped, a head CT scan is appropriate in patients with new onset seizures or at risk for anatomic abnormalities, mass intracranial lesions. Once a mass intracranial lesion or cerebral edema has been excluded, lumbar puncture is indicated in patients at risk for meningitis or those with a new-onset seizure disorder. Due to the risk of downward herniation, lumbar puncture should be avoided in patients with evidence of increased intracranial pressure. Serum ammonia, lactate, and serum amino and urine organic acid levels should be checked in infants and children at risk for inborn errors of metabolism. More specific metabolic testing may be appropriate for certain patients and should be considered in consultation with a pediatric neurologist or geneticist.

Medications for Seizure Termination

Rapid cessation of SE is associated with improved response rates and clinical outcomes. Consequently,

TABLE 36.7

PREFERRED MEDICATIONS FOR CONVULSIVE STATUS EPILEPTICUS

	GCSE	Focal motor	Myoclonic	Neonatal
First-line	Lorazepam	Lorazepam	Lorazepam	Phenobarbital
Second-line	Fosphenytoin	Fosphenytoin	Fosphenytoin Valproate	Fosphenytoin Lorazepam

GCSE, generalized convulsive status epilepticus. Data from Wheless JW, Clarke DF, Carpenter D. Treatment of pediatric epilepsy: Expert opinion, 2005. *J Child Neurol* 2005; 20 Suppl 1:S1–56.

administration of anticonvulsants for SE should proceed along a defined timeline, with the goal of controlling SE within 30 mins of presentation. The progression of treatment includes administration of a first-line agent, administration of second-line agent, and initiation of pharmacologic coma for treatment of RSE. First- and second-line medications for SE are determined by SE classification (**Tables 36.7, Table 36.8**). Recommended medication doses are detailed in **Table 36.9**. IV administration of lorazepam is the first-line treatment for all types of convulsive SE except neonatal SE, for which it is a second-line agent. The peak effect of IV lorazepam occurs 15 mins after dosing and the duration is 3–6 hrs. If a single dose is not effective, a second dose is recommended before or concurrent with administration of a second-line agent. Both diazepam and midazolam may be administered IV as well. Given IV, both diazepam and midazolam have shorter durations than lorazepam (roughly 15–30 and 30–80 mins, respectively). Administration of diazepam per rectum (0.2–0.5 mg/kg) is acceptable for patients receiving prehospital care or in those without established IV access. Midazolam may be given via intramuscular (0.1–0.15 mg/kg; max 0.5 mg/kg), buccal (0.3 mg/kg), or intranasal (0.2–0.5 mg/kg; max 0.5 mg/kg) administration in patients without IV access.

Phenobarbital is the first-line agent for neonatal SE and a second-line agent for GCSE or complex partial SE. IV administration of phenobarbital results in an onset of action after roughly 5 mins and peak levels after 15 mins. Dose adjustment may be indicated in patients with severe renal or hepatic failure. Phenobarbital can cause dose-dependent respiratory and hemodynamic depression, and these potential side effects should be anticipated and avoided. Fosphenytoin is the second-line agent for GCSE, complex partial SE, and neonatal SE. Fosphenytoin is a pro-drug that is dephosphorylated to phenytoin. Fosphenytoin is dosed as phenytoin equivalents (PE units), and peak levels of phenytoin are achieved roughly 20 mins after intravenous dosing. Phenytoin is highly protein-bound, and in patients on chronic phenytoin therapy, fosphenytoin may displace phenytoin from albumin-binding sites and raise free phenytoin levels rapidly. Similarly, valproate may displace phenytoin from albumin-binding sites. Therapeutic total levels of roughly 20 mg/dl are typically targeted, although in patients with hypoalbuminemia or concurrent valproate therapy, total levels may underestimate free plasma concentrations. In these patients, free phenytoin levels should be followed. Valproate is the second-line agent for absence SE and may be useful as an adjunctive therapy for GCSE, complex partial SE, or myoclonic SE. Therapeutic valproate levels are 50–150 mcg/mL; both efficacy and toxicity may be increased at higher doses. Valproate is generally well tolerated but may rarely

TABLE 36.8

PREFERRED MEDICATIONS FOR NONCONVULSIVE STATUS EPILEPTICUS

	Absence	Complex partial	NCSE with coma
First-line	Lorazepam	Lorazepam	Lorazepam
Second-line	Valproate	Fosphenytoin	Fosphenytoin Pharmacologic coma

NCSE, nonconvulsive status epilepticus. Data from Wheless JW, Clarke DF, Carpenter D. Treatment of pediatric epilepsy: Expert opinion, 2005. *J Child Neurol* 2005; 20 Suppl 1:S1–56.

TABLE 36.9

MEDICATION DOSING FOR STATUS EPILEPTICUS

Medication	Dose	Delivery rate	Comments
Lorazepam	0.05–0.15 mg/kg/dose IV (max 4 mg)	2 mg/min	Repeat in 5 mins
Phenobarbital	15–20 mg/kg IV	60 mg/min	Repeat in 5 mg/kg dose PRN to ~40 mg/kg
Fosphenytoin	15–20 mg PE/kg IV	100 mg PE/min	
Valproate	15–20 mg/kg	20 mg/min	Repeat in 10 mg/kg/dose PRN to ~40 mg/kg

PE, phenytoin equivalents

cause hypotension during acute administration. Hepatotoxicity and hyperammonemia are associated with valproate use, and transaminase levels and liver function should be monitored during treatment. Additionally, valproate has been associated with thrombocytopenia and coagulation disorders, possibly due to decreased hepatic production of clotting factors, as well as pancreatitis.

Refractory Status Epilepticus

Due to the ongoing risk for seizure-induced cerebral injury and systemic complications, RSE, whether convulsive or nonconvulsive, should be treated urgently (**Table 36.10**). Pharmacologic coma is continued for 24 hrs after seizure control before tapering. If seizures recur on a reduced dose of medication, coma can be reinstated for an additional 24 hrs. Pharmacological coma is typically achieved using benzodiazepine or barbiturate infusions, guided by continuous EEG monitoring. The endpoint of

pharmacological coma may be either cessation of EEG seizure activity or burst suppression. The three most common therapies for RSE are midazolam, pentobarbital, and propofol. Midazolam infusion, the most common therapy, is associated with the longest duration of therapy, the highest incidence of breakthrough seizures, and the greatest number of changes in therapy due to lack of efficacy but the least hemodynamic compromise. Conversely, pentobarbital is associated with the shortest duration of therapy, the lowest incidence of breakthrough seizures, the least changes in therapy, and the most hypotension. Midazolam infusions of ~15 mcg/kg/min have been used to treat neonatal and pediatric RSE. In comparison, the mean effective infusion rate in adults was 8 mcg/kg/min. Barbiturate coma is a common therapy for RSE. Fluid resuscitation and low-dose vasopressor or inotropic support are frequently required due to the cardiovascular effects of high barbiturate doses. Although dosing is usually

TABLE 36.10

MEDICATION DOSING FOR REFRACTORY STATUS EPILEPTICUS

Medication	Dose	
	Loading	Infusion
Midazolam	0.2 mg/kg IV	0.05–2 mcg/kg/min[a]
Pentobarbital	10–15 mg/kg IV initially, then 2–5 mg/kg q5min to stop seizure	1–3 mg/kg/h
Thiopental	5 mg/kg IV initially then 1–2 mg/kg q5min to stop seizure	3–5 mg/kg/h
Propofol	2–5 mg/kg IV	25–65 mcg/kg/min
Valproate	40 mg/kg IV	3 mg/kg/min
Ketamine	1.5 mg/kg IV	0.01–0.05 mg/kg/h
Topiramate	25 mg/kg NGT	Increase by <25 mg/kg/d NGT every other day

[a]Higher infusion rates may be used, as delineated in the text. NGT, nasogastric tube

titrated to burst suppression, targeting cessation of EEG seizure activity may provide similar efficacy with fewer side effects. Pentobarbital and thiopental are the most commonly used barbiturates. Dosing for either agent is titrated to effect and higher infusion rates than those listed in **Table 36.10** are frequently necessary. Propofol, valproate, ketamine, topiramate, and volatile anesthetics have been used as adjunctive therapies for RSE. The use of prolonged propofol infusions for SE is associated with propofol infusion syndrome, which is characterized by metabolic acidosis, lipidemia, arrhythmias, and cardiovascular collapse. Risk factors for propofol infusion syndrome include lean body mass, high dose, and >24 hrs of administration. In response, propofol use for sustained sedation in children <16 years of age has been contraindicated in the US, Canada, and the European Union. If used, the infusion duration should be as short as possible, and the dose should not exceed 67 mcg/kg/min. During propofol therapy, patients should be closely monitored for the development of metabolic acidosis or lipidemia, and therapy should be stopped at the first indication of toxicity.

Valproate has been added as adjunctive therapy in adults and children with RSE. When administered as a continuous infusion, the mean efficacious dose is roughly 3 mg/kg/min. Of note, valproate may be particularly helpful in patients with myoclonic SE, absence SE, or Lennox-Gastaut syndrome. Ketamine has been used in clinical RSE. Ketamine may increase intracranial pressure and should not be administered in the absence of neuroimaging excluding mass intracranial lesions. Topiramate is typically used for chronic seizure control via nasogastric tube. Topiramate dosing is rapidly escalated to total doses of 300–1600 mg/day. High-dose topiramate is also efficacious for infantile spasms. Finally, volatile anesthetics, such as isoflurane, may be used to treat RSE.

Surgical Treatment Options

RSE that fails to respond to high-dose suppressive therapy is associated with high mortality and morbidity in children. Lobar resection or hemispherectomy can be considered in patients with discrete, localized seizure foci. Epilepsy syndromes commonly amenable to resection include hemimegalencephaly, Rasmussen's encephalitis, prenatal cerebral artery infarction, tuberous sclerosis, malformations of cortical development, and Sturge-Weber syndrome. Other surgical options may include multiple subpial transections, corpus callosotomy, and implantation of a vagal nerve stimulator.

CHAPTER 37 ■ CEREBROVASCULAR DISEASE AND STROKE

JOHN PAPPACHAN • FENELLA KIRKHAM

Acute focal signs in childhood can be symptomatic of a variety of pathologies (**Table 37.1**). The World Health Organization definition of stroke is "rapidly developing clinical signs of focal (or global) disturbance of cerebral function, with symptoms lasting 24 hrs or longer, or leading to death, with no apparent cause other than of vascular origin." Patients whose signs resolve within 24 hrs have transient ischemic attacks by definition, but many have recent cerebral infarction or hemorrhage on imaging.

Hemorrhagic stroke includes intracerebral hemorrhage (ICH) (**Fig. 37.1A**), most commonly due to arteriovenous malformation, and subarachnoid hemorrhage (SAH), often secondary to aneurysm, but sinovenous thrombosis may cause either. The most common predisposing conditions of stroke in childhood are heart disease and anemias, including sudden cardiac death (SCD). Other acquired conditions, such as leukemia and brain tumor; chromosomal disorders, including Down syndrome; and genetic disorders, such as neurofibromatosis, are also usually obvious at the time of presentation. Those previously well may have a history of trauma or recent infection (e.g., with *Varicella*; **Fig. 37.2A**), and investigation often reveals vasculopathy and/or hereditary coagulopathy. They may also have single-gene disorders with a highly significant predisposition to stroke, such as homocystinuria, Fabry disease, and Menkes disease. Hemorrhagic stroke and sinovenous thrombosis may also occur in the context of acquired illnesses.

TABLE 37.1

DIFFERENTIAL DIAGNOSIS IN CHILDREN WHO PRESENT WITH ACUTE FOCAL NEUROLOGIC DEFICIT

- **Primary hemorrhagic stroke ± mass effect**
- **Acute ischemic arterial stroke ± hemorrhage ± mass effect**
- **Acute venous stroke ± hemorrhage ± venous infarction ± mass effect**
- **Postictal** (As Todd paresis is of short duration, if persistent, neuroimaging is essential; children with prolonged seizures may develop permanent hemiparesis)
- **Hemiplegic migraine** (but diagnosis of exclusion, as migrainous symptoms are commonly seen in cerebrovascular disease, e.g., dissection)
- **Acute disseminated encephalomyelitis**
- **Brain tumor**
- **Nonaccidental injury** (subdural hematoma, strangulation with compression of internal carotid artery)
- **Encephalitis** (e.g., secondary to Herpes simplex; usually have seizures)
- **Rasmussen encephalitis**
- **Posterior leukoencephalopathy** (hypertension/hypotension or immunosuppression)
- **Unilateral hemispheric/focal cerebral edema** (e.g., secondary to metabolic)
- **Alternating hemiplegia**

Note: All stroke syndromes are potential neurosurgical emergencies and should always be discussed with a pediatric neurologist on presentation. Further management and any transfer must involve liaison with the nearest available PICU.

CONGENITAL HEART DISEASE

Cardiac embolism occurs, particularly at the time of interventions such as catheterization or surgery or secondary to infective endocarditis, but echocardiography often fails to reveal a source of clot; other pathophysiologies, including sinovenous thrombosis and primary cerebral arterial disease, should be excluded. In contrast to studies in young adults, previously undiagnosed cardiac disease, such as patent foramen ovale, is relatively uncommon, but otherwise asymptomatic abnormalities of the aortic valve are associated with primary cerebrovascular disease (CVD), such as cervicocephalic dissection and moyamoya.

Sickle Cell Disease

Most children with overt ischemic stroke have intracranial, large-vessel disease (**Fig. 37.2B**). Ischemic

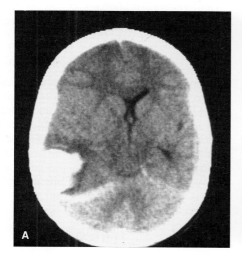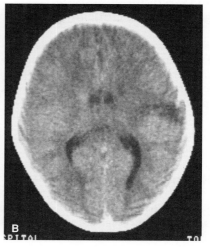

FIGURE 37.1. CT scans from children with hemorrhagic and ischemic (arterial and venous) stroke and its mimics. **A:** Spontaneous intracerebral hemorrhage with midline shift. **B:** Cortical ischemic stroke after minor head injury.

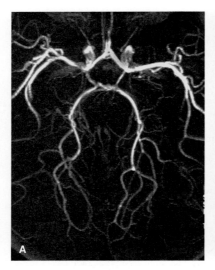
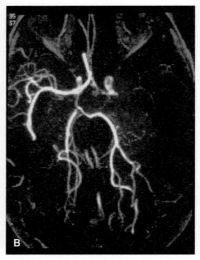

FIGURE 37.2. MRA from children with first and recurrent arterial ischemic stroke. **A:** "Transient" cerebral arteriopathy associated with basal ganglia infarct. **B:** Unilateral occlusion at the origin of the middle cerebral artery in sickle cell anemia with a large middle cerebral artery territory infarct.

stroke predominates in childhood, while the majority of adults have spontaneous ICH or SAH secondary to aneurysm, although hemorrhage secondary to hypertension and steroid use has been well documented in children, and sinovenous thrombosis and posterior leukoencephalopathy and watershed ischemia (**Fig. 37.3D**) have probably been previously underrecognized. The predisposition to large- and small-vessel disease, "silent" (covert) and clinical (overt) infarction, seizures, and cognitive deterioration may be in part related to genetic makeup but is probably also linked to environmental exposure (e.g., infection, poor nutrition, or hypoxemia).

Infection, Inflammation, and Immune Deficiency

Bacterial and tuberculous meningitis are well-recognized associations with stroke. Frank immunodeficiency, either inherited or acquired, also appears to be an occasional association. Recently, chickenpox within the previous year has been documented to be more common in otherwise cryptogenic stroke than in controls (**Fig. 37.2A**).

Hyperhomocysteinemia

Classic homocystinuria (deficiency of cystathionine β-synthase) has long been recognized as an important cause of arterial vascular disease and infarction. Apart from genetic predisposition, homocysteine levels are also influenced by the dietary intake of folate, vitamin B$_{12}$, and vitamin B$_6$. Supplementation may reduce homocysteine levels.

Hypertension

Hypertension is one of the most important risk factors for stroke in young adults and in the elderly but has largely been ignored in the pediatric literature.

Lipid Abnormalities

In a series of childhood stroke, 9% of those in whom random cholesterol was measured had high levels, while 31% had high triglyceride levels, and 22% had high lipoprotein (a), a risk factor for atherosclerosis in adults. In another series, apolipoprotein abnormalities were seen more commonly in association with childhood stroke. High lipoprotein (a) was a risk factor for recurrent stroke in German children with arterial ischemic stroke (AIS).

Disorders of Coagulation

Factor V Leiden (which is common in white populations and is the most common cause of activated protein C resistance) and the prothrombin 20210 mutation are important risk factors for venous thrombosis in adults and may be associated with neonatal and childhood sinovenous thrombosis and perhaps with AIS. A significant proportion of children with stroke have multiple prothrombotic disorders, and evidence exists for interaction between the factor V Leiden mutation and hyperhomocysteinemia.

Nitric Oxide

Nitric oxide is one of the most potent naturally occurring vasodilators and is a regulator of normal vascular tone, cell adhesion, and thrombosis, probably playing an important role in determining whether or

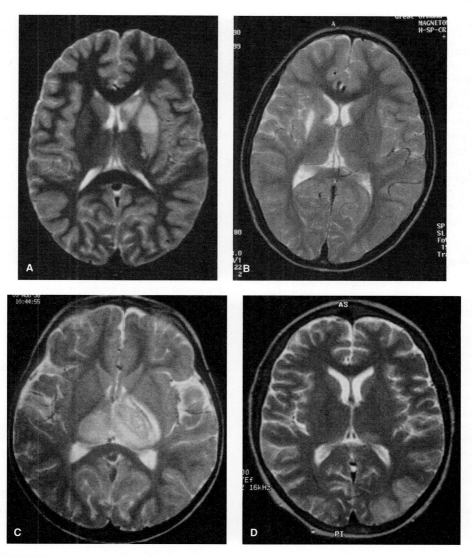

FIGURE 37.3. MRI scans from children with first and recurrent ischemic (arterial and venous) stroke and its mimics. **A:** Small infarct associated with middle cerebral artery stenosis. **B:** Deep white matter infarct in *Haemophilus influenzae* meningitis. **C:** Bilateral thalamic infarction in sinovenous thrombosis. **D:** Occipital edema in distribution compatible with reversible posterior leukoencephalopathy in sickle cell anemia and acute chest crisis.

not the endothelium is damaged (e.g., in SCD). A delicate balance exists between hypoxia-driven vaso-constriction and nitric oxide–driven vasodilatation in hypoxic conditions, and factors that affect nitric oxide biosynthesis may play a key role in the pathogenesis of vascular occlusion and stroke.

Arterial Disease

Up to 80% of children with AIS have abnormal conventional or magnetic angiographic studies (**Fig. 37.2**). A non-abrupt onset of stroke is characteristic of those with arteriopathy. Typical abnormalities include internal carotid artery (ICA) or vertebral dis-

section, stenosis or occlusion of the distal ICA or middle cerebral artery (MCA), moyamoya syndrome (bilateral severe stenosis or occlusion of the internal carotid arteries with collateral formation), and occasionally, rarer patterns such as small-vessel vasculitis.

Extracranial/Intracranial Dissection

Risk factors include minor trauma, infection migraine, hyperhomocysteinemia, and rare disorders such as fibromuscular dysplasia, Marfan or Ehlers-Danlos syndrome, and α-1 antitrypsin deficiency. Dissections are caused by blood penetrating and splitting the wall of an artery that supplies the brain. The origin of the dissection is likely to be a small intimal tear or primary intramural hemorrhage of the vasa vasorum. Arterial dissection results in an intramural hematoma and its variable extension along the course of that artery. The MRA is not usually diagnostic, but a lesion in the neck vessels may be suggested by reduced flow in the intracranial vessels. In many cases, the intramural hematoma may be demonstrated using fat-saturated T_1-weighted MRI of the neck, although conventional arteriography may sometimes be required to demonstrate the tapering partial occlusion of the artery ("rat's tail"). Head or neck trauma is a well-recognized cause of dissection, and it is worth noting that intraoral injuries can contuse the carotid artery in the peritonsillar area.

Other Intracranial Arteriopathies

Moyamoya derives from the Japanese word meaning "something hazy like a puff of smoke drifting in the air" and describes the appearance of the collaterals seen in association with bilateral severe stenosis or occlusion of the terminal ICAs in childhood. Moyamoya syndrome is associated with SCD, Down syndrome, Williams syndrome, neurofibromatosis, cranial irradiation, and arteriopathies, including fibromuscular dysplasia.

"Transient" cerebral arteriopathy may involve an inflammatory response to infections such as *Varicella*,*Borrelia*, or tonsillitis. Cerebral imaging (**Fig. 37.2A**) typically shows small subcortical infarcts located in the basal ganglia and internal capsule and, on conventional arteriography, multifocal lesions of the arterial wall are seen, with narrowing in the distal ICA, and the proximal anterior, middle, or posterior cerebral arteries.

Narrowing of the distal ICA and proximal MCA and anterior cerebral artery is also characteristic of SCD (**Fig. 37.2B**), although in these patients, gradual progression to occlusion commonly occurs with or without moyamoya collaterals.

Vascular Malformations

Arteriovenous malformations are defined by the presence of high-flow arteriovenous shunts through a nidus of abnormal thin-walled, coiled, and tortuous connections between feeding arteries and draining veins, without an intervening capillary network (**Fig. 37.4**). Capillary telangiectasias are collections of dilated ectatic capillaries with normal intervening neural tissue, without smooth muscle or elastic fibers; they are not commonly associated with ICH or SAH.

Cavernous angiomas (cavernomas) are vascular malformations that comprise thin-walled sinusoidal spaces lined with endothelial tissue and contain in-

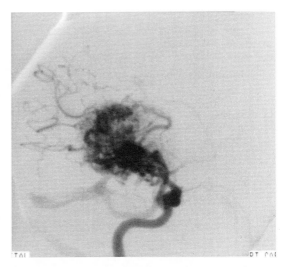

FIGURE 37.4. Conventional cerebral angiography showing arteriovenous malformation in an 11-year-old boy presenting with a spontaneous intracerebral hemorrhage.

travascular or intervascular calcifications, without any intervening parenchymal tissue. Cavernomas may present with symptoms related to frank ICH or with epilepsy, possibly secondary to intermittent leakage of blood around the cavernoma.

Sturge-Weber syndrome is a sporadic condition characterized by a venous angioma of the leptomeninges, a choroidal angioma, and a facial capillary hemangioma involving the periorbital area, forehead, or scalp that probably result from a failure of regression of a vascular plexus around the cephalic portion of the neural tube at between 6 and 9 wks of gestation. Epilepsy, hemiplegia, and learning disability, often progressive, are probably the result of an ischemic mechanism. The patient may be relatively well between episodes of status epilepticus or acute hemiparesis. Aspirin may reduce the frequency of stroke-like episodes. If intractable epilepsy cannot be controlled by medical means, hemispherectomy may be beneficial.

Vein of Galen malformation is an embryonic choroidal arteriovenous malformation. It can be diagnosed antenatally, has a male preponderance but no known genetic predisposition, and usually presents in the neonatal period as heart failure or, in older children with hydrocephalus, seizures, proptosis, or prominent scalp veins.

Aneurysms

Three fourths of patients with arterial aneurysms present with ICH. Approximately 10%–15% of arterial aneurysms are posttraumatic; a similar proportion are mycotic and are associated with infection (e.g., *Staphylococcus, Streptococcus,* Gram-negative organisms, and HIV). Mycotic aneurysms may also arise secondary to embolization of infective thrombi into the intracranial circulation in patients with subacute bacterial endocarditis. Other associations with arterial aneurysms in children are polycystic kidney disease, SCD, tuberous sclerosis, Marfan syndrome, Ehler-Danlos syndrome type IV, pseudoxanthoma elasticum, and hypertension, but no underlying systemic disorder is found in a substantial proportion.

Cerebral Sinovenous Thrombosis

The "deep venous system" includes the inferior sagittal sinus and the paired internal cerebral veins, which join to form the vein of Galen and the straight sinus, draining predominantly into the smaller caliber left lateral sinus and jugular vein. In neonates, pathogenesis of sinovenous thrombosis may be related to mechanical distortion of the cranial bones during birth. In older children, trauma, sepsis, and underlying illnesses such as malignancy or systemic inflammation play a larger role. Septic foci include the inner ear, mastoid, or air sinuses and lead to thrombophlebitic sinovenous thrombosis. Dehydration, anemia, and inherited prothrombotic disorders (congenital or acquired) are also recognized risk factors.

Venous Infarction

Cerebral infarction results when perfusion to the affected area of the brain is reduced to critical levels. In sinovenous thrombosis, "outflow" obstruction causes venous hypertension in the affected region of the brain, leading to focal cerebral edema (**Fig. 37.3C**). When tissue hydrostatic pressure exceeds arterial inflow pressure, infarction, which may be hemorrhagic, ensues.

Intracranial Hypertension

Sinovenous thrombosis leads to disruption of cerebrospinal fluid absorption within the superior sagittal sinus, resulting in diffuse cerebral swelling, communicating hydrocephalus, or pseudotumor cerebri (benign intracranial hypertension).

Posterior Circulation Arterial Stroke

Arterial disease in association with posterior circulation infarction in the cerebellum, brainstem and parieto-occipital lobes may require conventional angiography in the acute phase, as MRI and MRA commonly miss the diagnosis in the posterior circulation (**Fig. 37.5**). Etiologic factors include minor trauma, subluxation of the cervical spine at the

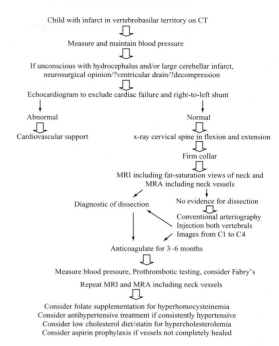

FIGURE 37.5. Algorithm for the management of posterior circulation stroke.

extremes of flexion and extension, chiropractic manipulation, frequent neck movements (e.g., secondary to athetoid cerebral palsy, hypertension, cardiac anomalies, and perhaps Fabry disease; **Fig. 37.5**). Some patients with conventional risk factors for stroke (hypertension, hypercholesterolemia, hyperhomocysteinemia) have vascular imaging compatible with early atheroma.

Reversible Posterior Leukoencephalopathy and Borderzone Ischemia

Reversible posterior leukoencephalopathy (RPLS) (**Fig. 37.3D**) is a cliniconeuroradiologic syndrome characterized by seizures, disorders of consciousness, altered mental status, visual abnormalities, and headaches, all of which are associated with predominantly posterior white matter abnormalities on CT and MRI examinations but without arterial or venous disease. RPLS is a relatively common stroke mimic and has been recognized in an increasing number of medical settings, including hypertensive encephalopathy, eclampsia, after acute chest crisis in SCD and immunosuppression. Acute hypotension in the context of poor cardiac function and/or anemia may also cause occipital infarction without vascular disease. As treatments are different, it is essential to distinguish RPLS from posterior circulation embolic stroke secondary to vertebrobasilar dissection; the latter typically presents "out of the blue," and is typically associated with infarction in the cerebellum and/or brainstem as well as the occipitoparietal cortex, but MR and conventional arteriography may be required to make a positive diagnosis. It is also important to exclude sinovenous thrombosis, particularly of the sagittal and straight sinuses, which may be associated with venous infarction in the parietal and occipital lobes as well as the thalami. Most patients make a full clinical and radiologic recovery after conservative measures, including slow reduction of blood pressure and maintenance of normal oxygenation.

Acute Disseminated Encephalomyelitis

MRI may reveal demyelination in children who present with acute focal neurologic signs. Evidence suggests that IV methylprednisolone reduces the duration of the illness and perhaps improves long-term outcome.

Metabolic Stroke

Diabetes and inborn errors of metabolism can cause acute focal neurologic symptoms and signs (metabolic stroke) due to either vascular injury or direct tissue injury, which may be permanent or transitory. Some organic acidemias, urea cycle disorders, and other inborn errors of metabolism can cause metabolic stroke. Mitochondrial disorders can cause stroke-like episodes (such as mitochondrial encephalopathy with lactic acidosis and stroke-like episodes). In the organic acidemias and urea cycle disorders, it is likely that accumulation of a toxic metabolite causes infarction of a selectively vulnerable area of the brain. By contrast, mitochondrial disorders are liable to cause infarction because of deficient energy supply and by the generation of oxygen free radicals. As arginine supplementation may be beneficial, it is important to exclude mitochondrial disorders.

CLINICAL PRESENTATION AND DIFFERENTIAL DIAGNOSIS

The important clinical clues for diagnosis are often (a) for symptomatic stroke, a preexisting diagnosis, and (b) for cryptogenic stroke, the trigger(s) (**Figs. 37.5, 37.6, 37.7, 37.8**). As a result of controlled trials of thrombolysis, increased awareness of the need for rapid assessment and appropriate management of

acute stroke in adults and the concept of "brain attack" have received widespread publicity. Thrombolysis must begin within 3 hrs; however, few children are triaged this quickly. The common clinical presentations are presented in **Table 37.1**. The importance of the recognition of these as a medical/surgical emergency cannot be overstated. Children may present with an immediate airway problem in coma, needing anesthesia and intubation for airway protection, with status epilepticus resistant to first-line therapy and requiring airway protection for second-line therapy (e.g., barbiturate coma) or with a reduced level of consciousness either requiring observation in the PICU or mandating airway protection for further investigation (**Fig. 37.9**).

PICU MANAGEMENT AND INVESTIGATION

The aim should be maintenance of oxygen saturation, cardiac output, systemic and cerebral perfusion pressure (CPP), normothermia, and careful avoidance of hypoglycemia and hyperglycemia. Blood should be taken for biochemical and hematologic analysis by the referring hospital (including a full coagulation profile and platelet count in case surgery or intracranial pressure (ICP) monitoring is required immediately after arrival at the tertiary center). The presence of shock should be treated aggressively to normalize perfusion and systemic hemodynamics. The primary goal should be optimization of intravascular volume, stroke volume, and perfusion pressure with the appropriate use of aggressive volume loading. Any total body water deficit should be estimated using standard algorithms and corrected over 24–48 hrs. IV maintenance fluids should be titrated to age and initial plasma sodium.

In any unconscious child with a stroke syndrome, it is reasonable to assume a degree of intracranial hypertension (assumed ICP of 20 mm Hg) and target a minimum mean arterial pressure of ICP + 50 mm Hg to achieve a satisfactory CPP (**Fig. 37.9**). After fluid administration, perfusion pressure augmentation should be achieved, if required, with the use of centrally administered noradrenaline. Hypertension should be assumed to be physiologic (reflecting disrupted cerebral autoregulation in response to intracranial hypertension) and not treated, at least initially. In consultation with the treating neurosurgeon, hypertension following ICH associated with an arterial/arteriovenous malformation may require treatment, as the risk of rebleeding must be balanced against the need to maintain CPP. Children who are not already intubated and whose level of

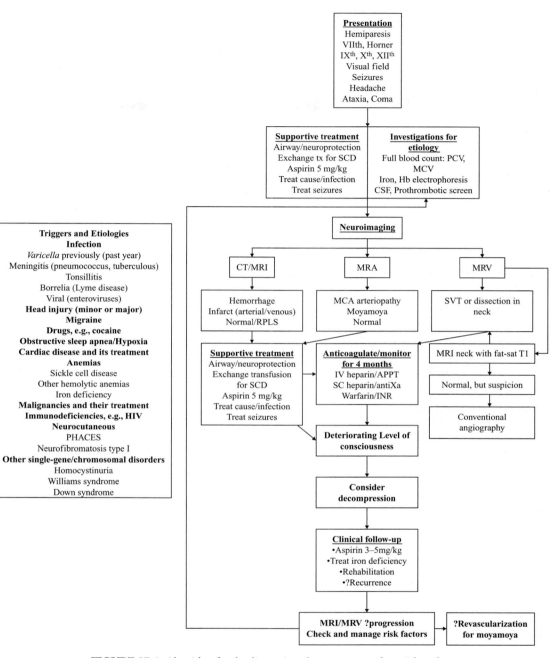

FIGURE 37.6. Algorithm for the diagnosis and management of arterial stroke.

consciousness deteriorates should be mechanically ventilated, and emergent neurosurgical consultation should be obtained in case they require drainage of a hematoma, ventriculostomy for hydrocephalus, or craniectomy for intractable intracranial hypertension. Seizures in the acute phase should be managed according to standard algorithms.

Neuroprotection—Controversies and Recommendations

Neonates, infants, and smaller children are at risk of hypoglycemia if isotonic glucose-free maintenance fluids are used prior to the successful initiation of

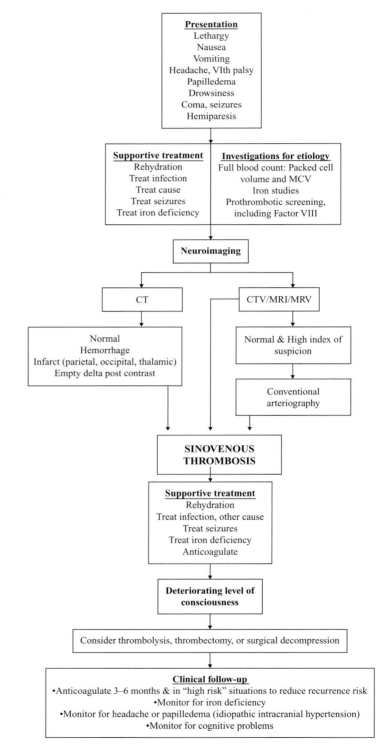

FIGURE 37.7. Algorithm for the management of sinovenous thrombosis.

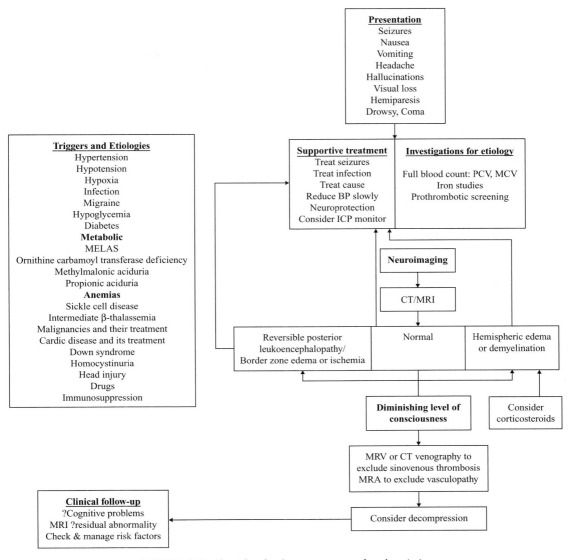

FIGURE 37.8. Algorithm for the management of stroke mimics.

enteral nutrition. We therefore recommend that this group of children receive isotonic normal saline with extra glucose added to achieve a final concentration of either 5% or 10%. For older children, glucose-free isotonic maintenance fluids using normal saline will normally suffice until enteral feeding is established. Enteral nutrition must be the gold standard, and perhaps more rigorous efforts should be made to establish post-pyloric feeding, either with radiologically (neonate, infant, and small child) or endoscopically (older child) placed nasogastric/orogastric jejunal feeding tubes. In the particular context of sinovenous thrombosis, when prothrombotic states and dehydration are common etiologic factors, it may even be necessary to rehydrate in addition to prescribing maintenance fluids.

We would recommend attention to normoglycemia; tight glycemic control to the degree used in the adult study cannot be recommended at this stage. A compromise might be to aim for blood glucose levels between 6 and 8.5 mmol/L and certainly to treat levels >10 mmol/L with a sliding scale of insulin. The pediatric population, especially neonates and infants, is at far greater risk than is the adult population of hypoglycemia, and an adequate glucose load of at least 4 mg/kg/hr of dextrose must accompany insulin infusions.

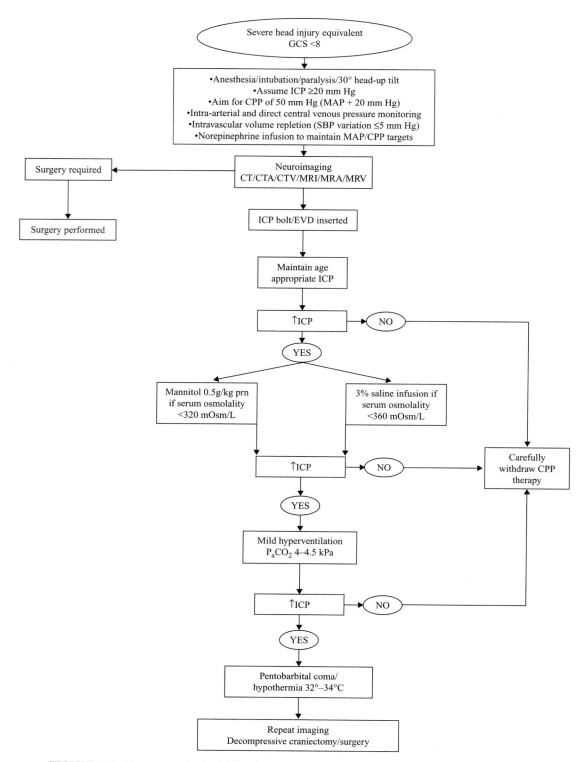

FIGURE 37.9. Neuroprotection in childhood stroke. EVD, external ventricular drain; CPP, cerebral perfusion pressure; CTA, computerized tomography-angiography; CTV, CT-venography; MRA, magnetic resonance angiography; MRV, magnetic resonance venography.

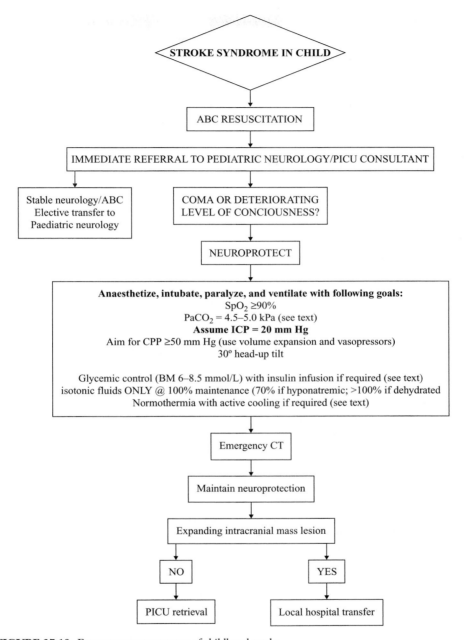

FIGURE 37.10. Emergency management of childhood stroke.

Medical management steps include maximizing sedation (including thiopentone to achieve burst suppression as analyzed by a bedside cerebral function monitor), paralysis, elevating the head of the bed (30 degrees), a loading dose (18 mg/kg) and subsequent maintenance dose of phenytoin, a hypertonic 3% saline infusion to achieve a plasma osmolality ≥320 mOsm/L, hyperventilation to a $PaCO_2$ of 30–37.5 mm Hg (4.0–5.0 kPa), and active cooling to between 32°C and 34°C (**Figs. 37.9**, **Fig. 37.10**). Chronic hyperventilation cannot be recommended, but acute hyperventilation in the context of imminent herniation does rapidly decrease ICP. If intracranial hypertension persists (despite maximal medical management and cerebrospinal fluid drainage via an external ventricular drain) or if clinical evidence exists of impending central or uncal transtentorial herniation, decompressive craniectomy and/or hypothermia can

TABLE 37.2

EMERGENCY IMAGING FOR CHILDHOOD STROKE

Magnetic resonance imaging (MRI) (including diffusion and perfusion), arteriography (MRA), venography (MRV)
Exclude hemorrhage
Define extent and territory of infarct
MRA to define vascular anatomy of circle of Willis and neck vessels
T_1-weighted spin echo of the neck with fat-saturation sequence to exclude dissection
MRV to exclude sinovenous thrombosis
Diffusion imaging to differentiate acute from chronic infarction
Perfusion imaging to demonstrate areas of tissue larger than demonstrated on diffusion imaging of abnormal cerebral blood flow, blood volume, and mean transit time

CT scan to exclude hemorrhage if MRI not available acutely

Conventional angiography if
Hemorrhage without coagulopathy and cause is not obvious on MRA or MRV
Ischemic stroke, MRA normal, and fat-saturated T1-weighted MRI of the neck does not demonstrate dissection

be considered. The indications for emergency neuroimaging are outlined in **Table 37.2.**

Sinovenous thrombosis may be accompanied by hemorrhagic or bland infarction—typically occipital, parietal, frontal, or thalamic (**Fig. 37.3C**); although often missed on CT, the occluded sinus may be seen on MRI or CT/MR venography. Importantly, most of the conditions that mimic ischemic stroke, such as acute disseminated encephalomyelitis, metabolic disease, and posterior leukoencephalopathy (**Fig. 37.3D**), may be recognized on MRI, which may mean that a child is not exposed to the unnecessary risks of antithrombotic therapy but receives the appropriate evidence-based management strategy for the condition.

Emergency electroencephalogram may be helpful in diagnosing hemiplegic migraine and electrical seizure activity in the unconscious patient. Epilepsy with postictal hemiparesis may be diagnosed on electroencephalogram. This study in hemiplegic migraine usually shows unilateral slow background activity, in addition to the evidence of edema on diffusion- or T_2-weighted MRI.

Specific Measures

Patients with hemorrhagic stroke require immediate transfer to a PICU with on-site neurosurgery in the event that craniectomy is required, but pediatric neurology and hematology consultations should also be obtained in view of the wide differential diagnosis. Hemorrhagic disease of the newborn should be treated with vitamin K, and disseminated intravascular coagulation should be treated with fresh frozen plasma or Beriplex (a prothrombin complex containing a concentrate of factors II, VII, IX, and X). Fresh platelet transfusion is required if the hemorrhage has occurred in the context of thrombocytopenia, and recombinant factor VIII is the treatment for hemophilia. The use of recombinant activated factor VII (rFVIIa) should be considered in hemorrhagic stroke with large clot volumes.

If an underlying arteriovenous malformation is present, the recurrence risk is 2%–3% per year for life if untreated, and a carefully considered decision regarding management (neurosurgery, neuroradiology with coils, or stereotactic radiotherapy) must be made once the patient has recovered from the acute phase. Although less common, aneurysms are associated with a significant rebleeding risk, particularly soon after presentation.

Ischemic Stroke

Some children with ischemic stroke (**Figs. 37.6, 37.7**) are candidates for emergency management of the stroke, such as exchange transfusion for patients with SCD or anticoagulation for venous sinus thrombosis. Ideally, neuroimaging to identify the pathology of the infarct and of the vascular disease should be performed either before or as therapy commences. The Seventh ACCP Conference on Antithrombotic and Thrombolytic Therapy developed guidelines for antithrombotic therapy in children, including those who had suffered an ischemic stroke. At about the same time, the Paediatric Stroke Working Group of the RCP produced guidelines that are available on the Internet (http://www.rcplondon.ac.uk/pubs/books/childstroke/childstroke_guidelines.pdf).

Stroke Due to Sickle Cell Disease

Children with SCD are at high risk for stroke. Hemoglobin and sickle hemoglobin percentages should be measured at presentation with any neurologic complication, and packed RBCs (20 mL/kg) should be cross-matched as quickly as possible. The accepted goal is to begin transfusion within 2–4 hrs of presentation, particularly if the deficit is persisting or progressing. If available, exchange (using a manual regime or an automated cell separator for erythrocytapheresis) transfusion is recommended rather than simple transfusion. Over the first 48 hrs, the goal is to reduce the hemoglobin S percentage to <20% and raise the hemoglobin to 10–11 g/dL, with a hematocrit of >30%. Blood should be leukocyte depleted and ABO, Rhesus D and K, Fy, Jk, and MNS red cell phenotype compatible with the recipient to minimize the risk of alloimmunization.

Thrombolysis with Tissue Plasminogen Activator

In adults with ischemic stroke, the main focus of recent studies has been in looking at the possibility of minimizing the effect of the initial stroke by promoting recanalization of the occluded artery using thrombolysis. After detailed counseling and consultation with the family, very occasionally, thrombolysis with IV tPA within 3 hrs or intra-arterial tPA within 6 hrs may be considered for MCA infarction, or intra-arterial tPA within 12 hrs may be considered for basilar artery occlusion.

Anticoagulation

The use of anticoagulation remains controversial. For AIS, the ACCP guidelines recommend anticoagulation with unfractionated or low-molecular-weight heparin for 5–7 days or until cardioembolic stroke and dissection are excluded, and they offer a practical regimen.

Antiplatelet Agents

The RCP guidelines suggest aspirin (5 mg/kg/day) be administered immediately following AIS, except in the presence of evidence of hemorrhage, followed by 1–5 mg/kg/day long term, whereas the ACCP guidelines recommend aspirin (2–5 mg/kg/day) once anticoagulation has been discontinued. The RCP guidelines suggest continuing aspirin at a dose of 1–5 mg/kg/day in children with cerebral arteriopathy other than dissection or moyamoya; however, if well tolerated, long-term, low-dose aspirin is probably a reasonable approach for all non-SCD children with AIS, in that though the risk of recurrence is greatest in the first year after stroke, risk is ongoing, even for those with cryptogenic stroke. In an attempt to produce a consistent approach, members of the International Paediatric Stroke Study have agreed to consistently use a dose of 3–5 mg/kg of aspirin as short- and long-term prophylaxis if they do not choose anticoagulation.

CHAPTER 38 ■ HYPOXIC-ISCHEMIC ENCEPHALOPATHY

ERICKA L. FINK • MIOARA D. MANOLE • ROBERT S.B. CLARK

Hypoxic-ischemic encephalopathy (HIE) can be defined as damage to cells in the brain due to hypoxia. Prolonged hypoxemia and ischemia lead to brain injury by triggering multiple pathologic cascades that can lead to cell death and loss of neurologic function. Interwoven with pathologic cascades are endogenous neuroprotective responses to minimize damage. HIE can result from global or focal disease. Global HIE can result from respiratory arrest, cardiac arrest, strangulation, poisoning or, rarely, other conditions such as sagittal sinus thrombosis or profound shock states. Final common pathways after critical global or focal ischemia include excitotoxicity from membrane failure with increased release and decreased reuptake of excitatory amino acids, such as glutamate and glycine, oxidative stress, mitochondrial dysfunction, energy failure, and initiation of cell death cascades (**Fig. 38.1**). Neuronal and glial cell death can result from necrotic, apoptotic, and autophagic pathways. *Necrosis* is a process characterized by immediate mitochondrial and energy failure, leading to cellular swelling, loss of membrane integrity, and a prominent inflammatory response in surrounding tissues. *Apoptosis* is an energy-requiring process that

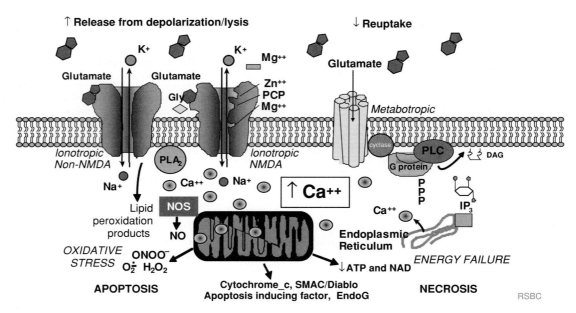

FIGURE 38.1. Cellular mechanisms resulting in cell death and hypoxic-ischemic encephalopathy. Prominent contributory mechanisms include excitotoxicity, disturbances in calcium homeostasis, oxidative stress, energy failure, and release of substances triggering cell-death pathways.

generally requires new protein synthesis. Enzymatic degradation of cytoskeletal proteins results in cell somal and nuclear shrinkage, and DNA is characteristically fragmented via endonucleases. In contrast to necrosis, apoptosis produces minimal inflammation. Autophagy is an adaptive response to starvation and results in autodigestion of cellular proteins and organelles to feed the cell.

CARDIAC ARREST

Asphyxial cardiac arrest, accounting for ~80%–90% of pediatric cardiac arrests, begins with respiratory failure followed by hypoxemia, hypercarbia and acidosis, hypotension, pulseless electrical activity, then ultimately asystole. The most common clinical entities associated with asphyxial cardiac arrest include sudden infant death syndrome, pneumonia, aspiration, and submersion injury. Cerebral blood flow (CBF) during and after cardiac arrest is phasic in nature. During cardiac arrest, global ischemia occurs, with no-flow or low-flow if cardiopulmonary resuscitation is being provided. CBF in the postarrest period can be divided into 4 phases : multifocal no reflow (Phase I), global hyperemia (Phase II), delayed hypoperfusion (Phase III), and restitution of normal blood flow (Phase IV). Data from adults who were resuscitated from cardiac arrest show that at 24 hrs after restoration of spontaneous circulation (ROSC), patients can have low, normal, or high CBF. "Luxury

perfusion syndrome" refers to a relative hyperemia in relationship to the brain's metabolic needs.

SYSTEMIC VARIABLES THAT AFFECT CBF AFTER CARDIAC ARREST

CBF is influenced by $PaCO_2$, PaO_2, blood pressure, and temperature. Low $PaCO_2$ produces vasoconstriction and decreased CBF, and higher $PaCO_2$ produces vasodilatation and increased CBF. Extreme hyperventilation and hypocarbia could exacerbate hypoperfusion and therefore should be avoided in the early postresuscitation period. Normocarbia and normoxia in patients during and after cardiac arrest should be the target CBF is maintained constant with the brain's ability for autoregulation over a range of cerebral perfusion pressure, ~50–150 mm Hg in adults. Adults resuscitated from cardiac arrest may have compromised autoregulation, with either absent autoregulation or increased lower limits of autoregulation (range, 80–120). Patients with higher mean arterial pressure in the first 2 hrs after cardiac arrest are more likely to have better outcomes. Hypothermia, now a class IIb recommendation from the American Heart Association (AHA) for postresuscitation treatment of cardiac arrest, typically decreases CBF, but this occurs via a coupled reduction in cerebral metabolism (**Tables 38.1, 38.2**).

TABLE 38.1

IMPORTANT CHANGES IN RECOMMENDATIONS FOR PEDIATRIC RESUSCITATION FROM
THE INTERNATIONAL LIAISON COMMITTEE ON RESUSCITATION CONSENSUS ON
SCIENCE, WITH TREATMENT RECOMMENDATIONS FOR PEDIATRIC AND NEONATAL
PATIENTS: PEDIATRIC BASIC AND ADVANCED LIFE SUPPORT

Recommendation change	Classification[a]
Recommended chest compression–ventilation ratio: For lone rescuers with victims of all ages: 30:2	IIa
For healthcare providers performing 2-rescuer CPR for infants and children: 15:2 (exception, 3:1 for neonates)	
Use of 1 shock followed by immediate CPR is recommended for each defibrillation attempt, instead of 3 stacked shocks	IIa
Biphasic shocks with an automated external defibrillator are acceptable for children >1 year of age. Attenuated shocks using child cables or activation of a key or switch are recommended in children <8 years old.	IIa
Routine use of high-dose IV epinephrine is no longer recommended.	III
Intravascular (IV and intraosseous) route of drug administration is preferred to the endotracheal route.	IIa
Cuffed endotracheal tubes can be used in infants and children provided correct tube size and cuff inflation pressure are used.	IIa
Exhaled CO_2 detection is recommended for confirmation of endotracheal tube placement.	I
Consider induced hypothermia for 12–24 hrs in patients who remain comatose following resuscitation.	IIb

[a] *Class I:* General agreement that a procedure or treatment is useful and effective.
Class II: Conflicting evidence or divergence of opinion exists.
Class IIa: Weight of evidence or opinion favors utility or efficacy of procedure or treatment. *Class IIb:* Weight of evidence or opinion is less well established.
Class III: Evidence or general agreement that the procedure or treatment is either not useful or not effective or, in some cases, may be harmful.
Increased emphasis on performing high-quality CPR: "*Push hard, push fast, minimize interruptions of chest compression; allow full chest recoil, and don't provide excessive ventilation.*"
Adapted from The International Liaison Committee on Resuscitation (ILCOR) Consensus on Science with Treatment Recommendations for Pediatric and Neonatal Patients: Pediatric basic and advanced life support. *Pediatrics* 2006; 117:e955–77.

Oxygen stores are depleted after ~20 secs, and loss of consciousness occurs. Glucose and ATP stores are depleted within 5 mins, whereupon the patient's brain crosses the threshold for cerebral ischemia. Following ROSC and reperfusion, typically a transient cerebral hyperemia occurs that lasts minutes and may be followed by global hypoperfusion. The duration and degree of postresuscitative hypoperfusion is proportional to the duration of the cardiac arrest, is related to ultimate severity of injury, and can last hours to several days; this period, during which the brain is at risk of secondary injury, may represent a therapeutic target.

Although all parenchymal cells in the brain are susceptible to hypoxia-ischemia, most attention has been directed toward neurons. Various neuronal populations are known to be selectively vulnerable to hypoxia-ischemia, including neurons within the CA1 region of the hippocampus, cerebral cortical layers 3 and 5, amygdaloid nucleus, basal ganglia, and cerebellar Purkinje cells, which have a predilection to undergo delayed neuronal death—even up to 5 days after injury.

CLINICAL ASPECTS OF HYPOXIC ISCHEMIC ENCEPHALOPATHY

The clinical goals for treating pediatric cardiac arrest are effective cardiopulmonary resuscitation (CPR), rapid ROSC, and prevention of secondary injury. Time to initiation and quality of CPR can strongly impact survival and neurologic outcome. Community education in bystander CPR may influence

TABLE 38.2

EVIDENCE IN SUPPORT OF THE USE OF THERAPEUTIC HYPOTHERMIA (32°–34°C FOR 12–24 HRS) IMMEDIATELY AFTER RESUSCITATION FROM CARDIAC ARREST

Evidence	Level[a]
Two prospective, randomized studies of adults with VF arrest (1,2)	1,2
Two prospective, randomized studies of newborns with birth asphyxia (3,4)	2
Numerous animal studies of both asphyxial and VF arrest (5)	6
Acceptable safety profiles in adults (1,2) and neonates (3,4) treated with hypothermia for up to 72 hrs	7

[a]*Level 1:* Randomized clinical trials or meta-analysis of multiple clinical trials with substantial treatment effects
Level 2: Randomized clinical trials with smaller or less significant treatment effects
Level 3: Prospective, controlled, nonrandomized cohort studies
Level 4: Historic, nonrandomized cohort or case-controlled studies
Level 5: Case series: patients compiled in serial fashion, control group lacking
Level 6: Animal or mechanical model studies
Level 7: Extrapolations from existing data collected for other purposes, theoretical analyses
Level 8: Rational conjecture (common sense); common practices accepted before evidence based guidelines

1. Mild therapeutic hypothermia to improve the neurologic outcome after cardiac arrest. *N Engl J Med* 2002;346: 549–56.
2. Bernard SA, Gray TW, Buist MD, et al. Treatment of comatose survivors of out-of-hospital cardiac arrest with induced hypothermia. *N Engl J Med* 2002;346:557–63.
3. Gluckman PD, Wyatt JS, Azzopardi D, et al. Selective head cooling with mild systemic hypothermia after neonatal encephalopathy: multicentre randomised trial. *Lancet* 2005;365:663–70.
4. Shankaran S, Laptook AR, Ehrenkranz RA, et al. Whole-body hypothermia for neonates with hypoxic-ischemic encephalopathy. *N Engl J Med* 2005;353:1574–84.
5. Tisherman SA, Sterz F. Therapeutic Hypothermia. In: Clark RSB, Carcillo JA, eds. *Molecular and Cellular Biology of Critical Care Medicine*, Vol. 4. New York: Springer, 2005.

Adapted from The International Liaison Committee on Resuscitation (ILCOR) Consensus on Science with Treatment Recommendations for Pediatric and Neonatal Patients: Pediatric basic and advanced life support. *Pediatrics* 2006;117:e955–77.

outcome after out-of-hospital arrests. Many hospitals have brought this concept to in-hospital cardiac arrest and organized dedicated rapid-response teams. The AHA provides pediatric advanced life-support guidelines, with supporting scientific review. Important new guidelines from the AHA are shown in **Table 38.1**. A treatment guideline algorithm based on the literature and protocols and practice at the Children's Hospital of Pittsburgh is provided in **Figure 38.2**. Patients remain at significant risk of secondary brain injury after ROSC from hypotension, hypoxemia, seizures, hypoglycemia, and hyperthermia.

PICU MANAGEMENT

PICU management of patients after cardiac arrest consists largely of supportive care and prevention of secondary insults. Monitoring of intracranial pressure (ICP), once a standard measurement after cardiac arrest, is no longer considered standard practice, largely because aggressively treating elevated ICP in children after submersion injury may increase the number of surviving patients with severe disability and vegetative state.

A head CT scan can be rapidly obtained but may often be normal. Findings of cerebral edema, loss of cortical gray- and white-matter density and interface, reversal sign, and/or cerebral swelling, indicate more severe injury and less favorable neurologic outcome. An initial CT may be helpful in situations in which the etiology of arrest is unclear or concomitant trauma may exist. Following cardiac arrest, serial head CT scans are indicated only if new or evolving pathology, such as hemorrhage, evolving mass lesion, or herniation, is suspected.

NEUROINTENSIVE CARE MONITORING

Currently, CBF can be measured using stable Xenon CT, positron-emission tomography, or perfusion MRI. Transcranial-Doppler ultrasonography is a noninvasive bedside method for estimating CBF and may be used to extrapolate effects of cerebral edema and ICP on CBF velocity. Transcranial-Doppler measures middle–cerebral artery blood-flow velocity as a surrogate for CBF but does not provide a

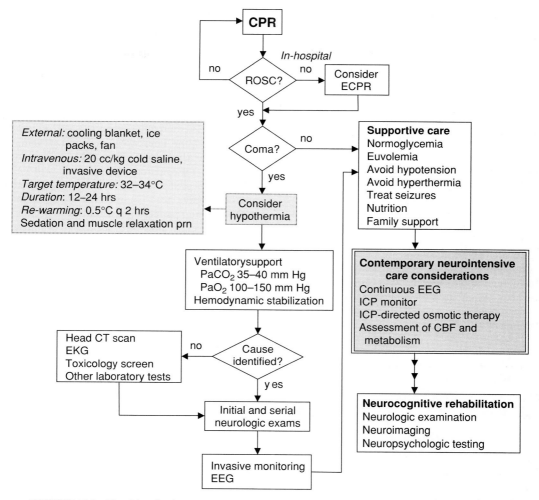

FIGURE 38.2. Algorithm for the management and treatment of post-circulatory arrest syndrome in infants and children. Guidelines based on medical literature and protocols and practice at the Children's Hospital of Pittsburgh. CPR, cardiopulmonary resuscitation; ROSC, return of spontaneous circulation; ECPR, extracorporeal cardiopulmonary resuscitation; EEG, electroencephalogram; ICP, intracranial pressure; CBF, cerebral blood flow; EKG, electrocardiogram.

direct measurement. Brain oxygenation can be measured using near-infrared spectroscopy. Brain oxygenation can also be determined invasively using a fiberoptic catheter placed into brain parenchyma to measure brain tissue oxygen partial pressure. Global cerebral metabolism can also be measured directly if a jugular bulb catheter is placed and CBF is measured simultaneously. Cross-brain extraction of oxygen—arteriovenous difference of oxygen content—and glucose—arteriovenous difference of glucose—can be used to calculate $CMRO_2$ and CMRGlu, respectively. Examining jugular venous bulb oxygen saturation ($SjVO_2$) as a reflection of cerebral metabolism also has potential utility, particularly if direct CBF measurements are not available and given that arterial oxygen saturations are typically at or near 100%. $SjVO_2$ is frequently employed to monitor patients with TBI, with normal values reported to be 55%–71% and values <50% considered the critical threshold for brain ischemia.

EEG is a noninvasive bedside method increasingly being used after HIE to diagnose and monitor response to treatment of nonclinical seizures. A newer indication is continuous monitoring during periods of muscle relaxation, especially during the induction of hypothermia, which is increasingly being used for postresuscitation therapy in cardiac arrest patients. EEG alone or in combination with other methods has been used to predict outcome after pediatric cardiac arrest. Presence of a discontinuous EEG and epileptiform spikes or discharges correlated with poor outcome. Somatosensory-evoked potentials use electrical stimulation of peripheral nerves and record the response of somatosensory pathways.

MR imaging provides detailed information about ischemic brain injury, is noninvasive, and does not use ionizing radiation. A scoring system validated in infants that combines MRI with neurologic examination has been used to predict outcome in HIE late after initial injury. MRI coupled with arterial spin labeling can be used to trace arterial and venous blood supply to the brain and quantify CBF and cerebral blood volume. Brain MR spectroscopy has been used experimentally to demonstrate the relationship of metabolites such as lactate, pyruvate, glutamate, N-acetylaspartate, and phosphocreatine to outcome in patients with HIE.

No single clinical, laboratory, or imaging test exists to detect occult or evolving brain injury or to predict neurologic outcome with certainty after cardiac arrest in children (or adults). Serum and urine biomarkers are surrogates of brain injury that present a promising approach to these problems (**Fig. 38.3**).

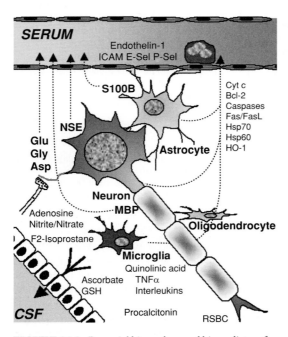

FIGURE 38.3. Potential biomarkers and biomediators for identifying and following brain injury, validating mechanisms of injury, and serving as targets for therapeutic drug monitoring.

THERAPIES THAT TARGET PREVENTION AND TREATMENT OF HYPOXIC-ISCHEMIC ENCEPHALOPATHY

Mild, induced hypothermia has come to the forefront as a promising strategy for improving survival and neurologic outcome after cardiac arrest in adult patients, but the benefits in pediatric patients remain to be determined. The AHA now endorses this therapy for comatose adult patients with VF- or VT-induced cardiac arrest. Whole-body hypothermia or selective head cooling is now also endorsed in the neonatal population for reduction of morbidity and mortality after birth asphyxia. Whole-body cooling may be the more effective modality, given that deeper brain structures are cooled as well as superficial brain structures, and selective head cooling may not be as effective outside the neonatal period. Extrapolating from these and an abundance of experimental studies that showed the efficacy of induced hypothermia with a good safety profile, the AHA recommends considering induced hypothermia (32°–34°C for 12–24 hrs) for comatose pediatric patients after cardiac arrest as a type IIb recommendation (**Table 38.2**). During induction of hypothermia, particular attention should be paid to electrolyte abnormalities, volume status, shivering, coagulopathy, dysrhythmias, and effects on drug metabolism. Previous concerns about the potential adverse effects of hypothermia on successful defibrillation/cardioversion appear unfounded. The multicentered clinical studies cited show that hypothermia is effective even when applied up to 6 hrs after cardiac arrest.

Certain centers with the capability to provide extracorporeal membrane oxygenation are now applying it as a rescue therapy for in-hospital pediatric cardiac arrest or imminent cardiac arrest (called extracorporeal cardiopulmonary resuscitation) and for patients with impending heart failure after cardiac surgery. Other "cutting-edge" strategies to improve outcomes after prolonged cardiac arrest are currently under investigation. These include high-volume, continuous, venovenous hemofiltration, thrombolytics, coenzyme Q with mild, induced hypothermia, and bicarbonate given during resuscitation. Failed clinical trials include magnesium with and without diazepam, calcium channel blockers, barbiturates, and corticosteroids.

CHAPTER 39 ■ METABOLIC ENCEPHALOPATHIES IN CHILDREN

PHILLIPE JOUVET • ANNE LORTIE • BRUNO MARANDA • ROBERT C. TASKER

Metabolic encephalopathies include a large variety of disorders divided into three groups according to their pathophysiology (**Table 39.1**).

ENCEPHALOPATHIES WITH ENDOGENOUS INTOXICATION

Encephalopathies with endogenous intoxication include liver failure and several inborn errors of metabolism (IEMs) in the catabolic pathway of amino acids may induce a metabolic encephalopathy by endogenous intoxication. In those diseases, intermediate products of amino acid catabolism are not detoxified by the liver (and/or the kidney), accumulate, and contribute to neurologic symptoms (**Fig. 39.1**). Cerebral edema is frequently associated mainly due to cytotoxic mechanisms. In that the encephalopathy is related to toxic metabolite accumulation, specific therapeutic strategies to decrease this accumulation are required to restore brain function.

Blood ammonia concentration $>300–500$ μmol/L is associated with severe CNS dysfunction, including cerebral edema and coma. Ammonia is mainly released by intestine and muscles. In the absence of a functional hepatic urea cycle that transforms ammonia into urea, the ammonia free base (NH_3) enters the brain through the blood-brain barrier. This barrier has a much lower permeability to NH_4^+, which implies that the diffusion of ammonia across the blood-brain barrier depends partly on the arterial blood pH. In the brain, ammonia is buffered by the formation of glutamine via astrocytic enzyme glutamine synthetase. As the enzyme functions are at near maximal capacity under normal physiologic conditions, hyperammonemia rapidly exceeds the brain capacity to synthesize glutamine and ammonia concentrations rise significantly. High ammonia levels in the brain may lead to cell swelling and cerebral edema through the following mechanisms: (a) glutamine accumulation, which induces astrocyte swelling and disturbed function, (b) increased cerebral blood flow, and (c) alterations of mitochondrial functions and consequent changes in cerebral energy metabolism, with reduction of brain ATP concentration. A number of human disorders are associated with hyperammonemia. IEMs with hyperammonemia include primary urea cycle enzyme defects and secondary inhibition of urea cycle by organic acidurias (propionic, methylmalonic aciduria) or fatty acid oxidation disorder (FAOD).

Reye syndrome is characterized by the combination of liver disease and metabolic encephalopathy. In 1980, the Centers for Disease Control defined Reye syndrome as an acute noninflammatory encephalopathy with microvesicular fatty metamorphosis of the liver confirmed by biopsy or autopsy and/or a threefold increase of transaminases and/or ammonia without cerebrospinal fluid pleocytosis and without reasonable explanation for the neurologic presentation of the hepatic abnormality.

Hepatic encephalopathy is characterized by cytotoxic brain edema, including brain astrocyte swelling. Mechanisms involved in hepatic encephalopathy include (a) synergetic effects of toxic accumulation, including ammonia, mercaptans, fatty acids, and phenol; (b) changes in the GABA-benzodiazepine system; (c) changes in blood-brain barrier; and (d) neurotransmission disturbances. Among the amino and organic acid disorders, those that most frequently cause patients to be admitted to the PICU for acute metabolic encephalopathy are maple-syrup-urine disease (MSUD), propionic acidurias, and methylmalonic acidurias. Damage caused by copper accumulation in the basal ganglia of the brain may be oxidative in nature. In one-third of cases, Wilson's disease is associated with initial neurologic presentation between 10 and 20 yrs of age.

ENCEPHALOPATHIES WITH ENERGY FAILURE

Any mechanism that causes reduction in brain energy supply may create an encephalopathy. It is the case in hypoxemia-ischemia, and it occurs when energy substrates are decreased for other reasons. Cerebral energy is supplied by mitochondria, and the principal energetic source is glucose (**Fig. 39.2**). As the encephalopathy is secondary to energy deprivation, specific therapeutic strategies that decrease cerebral energetic consumption and increase energy production, when possible, are required to restore brain function.

Under normal conditions, the human brain derives its energy from glucose metabolism. Glucose has to be transported across the blood-brain barrier

TABLE 39.1

CAUSES OF METABOLIC ENCEPHALOPATHIES CLASSIFIED ACCORDING TO THEIR PATHOPHYSIOLOGY

Endogenous intoxication
Hyperammonemia and liver diseases
   Urea cycle disorders
   Reye syndrome
   Hepatic encephalopathy
Organic acids disorders: MSUD, PA, MMA, IVA,
   3HiB-uria, GA type I
Ketolysis defect
Wilson disease

Energy failure
Hypoglycemia: hyperinsulinism, GSD
Mitochondrial defects: pyruvate dehydrogenase
   deficiency, pyruvate carboxylase deficiency,
   respiratory chain deficiency
Fatty acid oxidation disorders
Thiamine deficiency
Biotin-responsive basal ganglia disease

Water, electrolyte, and endocrine disturbances
Disorders of osmolality: Diabetic ketoacidosis and
   nonketotic hyperosmolar coma, hyponatremia,
   hypernatremia
Hypocalcemia
Hypercalcemia
Hypomagnesemia
Hypophosphatemia
Thyroid disorders
Intestinal diseases that induce encephalopathy
Burn encephalopathy

MSUD, maple syrup urine disease; PA, propionic aciduria;
MMA, methylmalonic aciduria; IVA, isovaleric aciduria;
3HiB-uria, 3 hydroxyisobutyric aciduria; GA type I, glutaric
aciduria type I; GSD, glycogen storage disorders

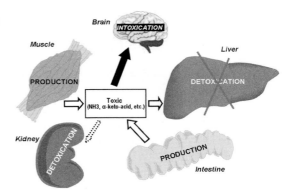

FIGURE 39.1. Endogenous intoxication model: nitrogen metabolism impairment due to liver failure or IEM on catabolic pathway of amino acids. The nitrogen essentially produced by intestine and muscle amino acid catabolism is not properly metabolized, resulting in toxic accumulation and brain damage. From D Rabier (Biochemical Laboratory, Necker Hospital, France), with permission.

via the GLUT1 glucose transporter. Mutations in this gene are associated with hypoglycorrhachia without hypoglycemia. Glycogen storage disease, hyperinsulinism, and FAOD may present with severe hypoglycemia. Under conditions of prolonged fasting, the brain can switch to lactate oxidation and increase ketone uptake to partially restore energy balance.

Primary mitochondrial energy metabolism defects include pyruvate dehydrogenase complex deficiency, tricarboxylic acid cycle deficiencies, and respiratory chain defects. All of these diseases may present with acute encephalopathy, which results from lack of energy production, despite normal brain oxygenation. FAODs comprise another group of diseases with impaired mitochondrial energy metabolism. However, encephalopathy observed in FAOD are not fully understood and may result from a multifactorial

insult, including one or more of the following mechanisms: (a) hypoglycemia concomitant with abnormally low ketones as fuel for the brain, (b) hyperammonemia, and (c) decrease in cerebral blood flow due to collapse.

Thiamine (vitamin B_1) plays an important role in several metabolic processes—in the decarboxylation of pyruvate and α-ketoglutarate (two steps of the tricarboxylic acid cycle), with magnesium as a cofactor, and in the conversion of 5-carbon to 6-carbon sugars by means of the enzyme transketolase. Thiamine deficiency, therefore, decreases energy available to the brain and increases the concentrations of several metabolites. Patients who receive total parenteral nutrition, chronic dialysis, or high carbohydrate diet during debilitating illness are at risk of thiamine deficiency, and Wernicke encephalopathy may be observed. In these settings, the features are highly variable and may manifest by sudden collapse and death or seizures or by the classic but extremely rare triad of ataxia, confusion, and ocular abnormalities.

ENCEPHALOPATHIES WITH ACUTE WATER, ELECTROLYTE, AND/OR ENDOCRINE DISTURBANCES

The osmolality of a solution is determined by the number of particles in the solution. Sodium salt, glucose, and urea are the primary osmoles of the extracellular space, potassium salts are the primary osmoles of the intracellular space, and plasma proteins

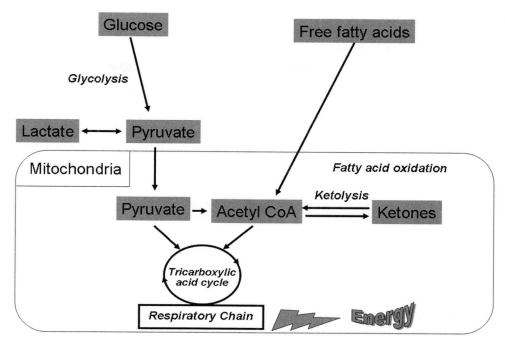

FIGURE 39.2. Energy failure model of metabolic encephalopathy. Hypoglycemia and any enzyme defect in mitochondria energy production may result in metabolic encephalopathy. The pathophysiology of metabolic encephalopathy by fatty acid oxidation defect is multifactorial.

are the primary osmoles of the intravascular space. Because cell membranes are permeable to water, an osmotic equilibrium is maintained (e.g., the volume of intracellular fluid is determined by osmolality of the extracellular space). Hypernatremia and hyperglycemia are the major causes of serum hyperosmolality, and hyponatremia is the major cause of hypoosmolality. Any modifications of brain water volume may result in acute encephalopathy.

Cerebral edema in diabetic ketoacidosis (DKA) typically occurs in the first 12 hrs after the onset of treatment but can be present before treatment initiation. Regardless of the final mechanism, treatment is focused upon vigorous hydration only as required to initially achieve hemodynamic stability with normal saline or Ringer's lactate and to subsequently complete volume repletion over a 48-hr period. In the presence of cerebral edema, the rate of fluid administration is reduced and mannitol (0.25–1 g/kg IV over 20 min) or hypertonic saline (NaCl 3%, 5–10 mL/kg over 30 min) may be given. Hyperosmolar hyperglycemic nonketotic coma is rare in childhood and shares similar pathogenesis with DKA without ketone body contribution.

Osmotic disequilibrium between a low osmolality plasma compartment and higher osmotic pressure within glial cells will result in astrocytic water accumulation and brain edema. Rapid decrease in sodium

concentration is much more likely to cause severe edema. Hyponatremia may result from water retention, sodium loss, or both. Water retention is often caused by inappropriate antidiuretic hormone secretion and sodium loss from renal disease, vomiting, and diarrhea. Both mechanisms of hyponatremia are worsened by infusion of hypotonic solutions. Conversely, a too-rapid correction of hyponatremia can induce a central pontine myelinolysis. This syndrome is characterized by confusion, cranial nerve dysfunction and, when the lesion is larger, by a "locked-in" syndrome and quadriparesis.

Hypernatremia is associated with cellular dehydration, which affects brain function. Because the brain can compensate for slow or chronic osmolality changes, acute changes should be treated acutely, and chronic changes should be treated slowly. Hypernatremia is usually caused by dehydration, in which water loss exceeds sodium loss or by overhydration with hypertonic saline solution.

Acute uremic encephalopathy is multifactorial and does not strictly correlate with concentrations of blood urea nitrogen alone. Hypertensive encephalopathy may be associated. The treatment is dialysis. However, dialysis encephalopathy is caused by the rapid shift of fluids and electrolytes between intracellular and extracellular spaces and may be associated with acute transitory neurologic disturbances which usually occur toward the end of dialysis or up to 24 hrs later.

Calcium is the major divalent cation in the extracellular fluid. It is an important regulator of cellular function and is essential for numerous cellular processes, especially neurotransmission. Severe hypocalcemia and hypercalcemia may both induce encephalopathy. Magnesium is the second most abundant intracellular cation in the body and is required for the maintenance of normal activities. It is a cofactor of numerous enzymes that play vital roles in energy metabolism. Hypomagnesemia (usually in association with other electrolyte abnormalities: hypocalcemia, etc.) and hypermagnesemia may both induce encephalopathy. Hypophosphatemia may also cause neurologic dysfunction.

Thyroid disorders, both hyperthyroidism (thyrotoxicosis) and hypothyroidism, affect the CNS and may lead to coma.

Intestinal invagination and abdominal surgery in children may be associated with depressed levels of consciousness. This type of presentation may be explained either by a possible endogenous opioid poisoning by massive secretion of endorphins during paroxysms of pain or by gastrointestinal release of neurotoxic vasoactive peptides and neuroactive gut hormones.

In burn encephalopathy, a few days after severe burn injury, awareness and responsiveness may decline without any neurologic findings in the physical exam. The mechanism is not known.

PRINCIPLES OF CLINICAL MANAGEMENT

The challenge of metabolic encephalopathies is to quickly diagnose treatable disorders to ensure prompt recovery. The diagnosis is suspected on the combination of clinical course and laboratory investigations. Metabolic encephalopathies must be considered in parallel with other common conditions, such as sepsis, anoxo-ischemic encephalopathy, encephalitis, exogenous intoxication, and brain tumors.

Metabolic encephalopathy may present within hours or days of progressive confusion, diverse motor and sensorial abnormalities and, rarely, hallucinations. A careful history may guide the diagnosis in some circumstances, such as a polyuropolydipsia syndrome that precedes the encephalopathy in diabetic ketoacidosis or an infusion of hypotonic solutions in the perioperative period in hyponatremia encephalopathy. In other circumstances, especially in the case of IEMs, the history is not obvious and requires specific details of the events that lead to

behavioral change. Drug exposure, personal history, and family history must be carefully determined and considered. Acute metabolic encephalopathy in treatable IEMs usually results from an increased protein catabolism and/or change in energy metabolism. The decompensation may occur at any age from the neonatal period to adulthood.

Endogenous intoxication and FAODs may decompensate with fasting, as protein catabolism is increased and free fatty acids are preferentially used as fuel. The decrease in consciousness turns into a vicious cycle in which the child cannot feed and worsens.

Both anesthesia and surgery induce protein catabolism and increase energy demand.

Infections increase protein catabolism and increase energy demand. The most typical cause of acute onset in infants is gastrointestinal infection, which combines the infectious effect on metabolism and a fasting state.

Endogenous intoxication and FAODs may decompensate with prolonged exercise, as it creates protein catabolism and increases free fatty acid use.

Valproic acid may decompensate urea cycle disorders and respiratory chain disorders by enzyme inhibition. Steroids and adrenocorticotropic hormone increase protein catabolism.

Protein intake is restricted in endogenous intoxication disorders. Noncompliance to the diet, typically seen surrounding the holidays, may lead to acute decompensation.

An IEM should be suspected when the following personal and/or familial history is found: (a) recurrent coma, (b) any unexplained death in the family or any neonatal death, even if it was attributed to another etiology (sepsis, anoxia, etc.), or (c) parent's consanguinity. Although most genetic disorders are hereditary and transmitted as recessive disorders, the majority of cases appear sporadically in developed countries because of small family sizes. Clinical manifestations are usually nonspecific, except for the following presentations. In the comatose state, characteristic changes in muscular tone and involuntary movements appear in some diseases. In MSUD, generalized hypertonic episodes with opisthotonos are frequent, and boxing or pedaling movements, as well as slow limb elevations, spontaneous or upon stimulation, are observed. In organic aciduria, axial hypotonia, and limb hypertonia with large amplitude tremors and myoclonic jerks, which are often mistaken for convulsions, are observed. Intracranial hypertension is a presenting symptom in metabolic encephalopathies. Focal signs can mimic a stroke in certain mitochondrial encephalopathies. Other patients with organic acidemias and urea cycle defects present with focal neurologic signs and cerebral edema. These patients

TABLE 39.2

LABORATORY INVESTIGATIONS IN METABOLIC ENCEPHALOPATHY

	Routine tests	Storage of samples and metabolic tests[a]
Urine	Smell (special odor) Look (special color) Acetone (Acetest) Ketoacids (DNPH)[b] pH Electrolytes (Na^+,K^+) Urea, creatinine	Fresh sample in the refrigerator, frozen sample at $-20°C$, for metabolic testing (AAC, OAC, orotic acid)
Blood	Electrolytes (Na^+, K^+, Cl^-, HCO_3^-) glucose, Ca^{2+}, Mg^{2+}, phosphate urea, creatinine Osmolality Blood gases Transaminases, bilirubin, γGT Ammonia Lactic acid Creatine kinase Blood cell count Prothrombin time	Plasma heparinized at $-20°C$ (5 ml); whole blood (10 ml) collected on EDTA at $-20°C$ (for molecular biology studies); plasma or blood on filter paper for acylcarnitine dosage; redox status if lactate >10 mmol/L (AAC, OAC, acylcarnitines)
Miscellaneous	CSF if no intracranial hypertension with concentration of lactate and pyruvate	CSF (1 mL) frozen for AAC *Other metabolic tests*: Skin biopsy for fibroblast culture; If death: liver and muscle biopsy

[a] Tests should be discussed with specialists in metabolic diseases.
[b] This test screens for the presence of alpha-keto acids, as occur in MSUD. It can be replaced by an amino acid chromatography, if available, in an emergency situation.
Adapted from Saudubray JM, Martin D, de Lonlay P, et al. Recognition and management of fatty acid oxidation defects: A series of 107 patients. *J Inherit Metab Dis* 1999;22:488–502.
DNPH, dinitrophenylhydrazine test; AAC, amino acid chromatography; OAC, organic acid chromatography; CSF, cerebrospinal fluid

can be mistakenly diagnosed as having cerebrovascular accident or cerebral tumor.

Hepatomegaly may be observed, especially in organic academia, FAOD, Wilson disease, hyperinsulinism, and glycogen storage diseases. An *abnormal urine or body odor* is present in some diseases in which volatile metabolites accumulate. In urine, an abnormal odor can be detected on a drying paper or by opening a container of urine that has been closed at room temperature for a few minutes. The three most important examples are fruity smell of ketoacid diabetic decompensation, maple syrup odor of MSUD, and sweaty feet odor of isovaleric acidemia. *Myoglobinuria* is an indicator of FAOD.

General supportive measures and laboratory investigations should be undertaken as soon as metabolic encephalopathy is suspected. The initial approach for investigations is outlined in **Table 39.2**. The systematic determination of plasma ammonia concentration is crucial when a metabolic encephalopathy is suspected because this is a life-threatening condition that necessitates urgent management. Venous blood should be collected in ammonia-free heparinized tubes, placed on ice at bedside, and transferred quickly to the laboratory, where the plasma should be separated immediately. IEMs are more difficult to diagnose, and the following biologic signs evoke such disorders (**Table 39.3**). Hyperammonemia with liver test abnormalities is seen in acute liver failure and Reye syndrome. Conditions that produce a Reye-like illness are detailed in **Table 39.4**.

Regardless of etiology, electroencephalogram during an acute encephalopathic process usually shows varying degrees of slow activity. The severity of slowing is usually well correlated with the severity of the encephalopathy. This slowing is not specific and only reflects cortical and subcortical dysfunctions. When evaluating a patient with consciousness fluctuation, it is essential to rapidly obtain a cerebral CT scan in order to eliminate underlying cerebral (such as stroke) or neurosurgical (such as hemorrhage)

TABLE 39.3

ALGORITHM FOR THE DIAGNOSIS OF IEM REVEALED BY AN ENCEPHALOPATHY

Clinical presentation	Predominant metabolic disturbance	Associated metabolic/ neurologic disturbance	Most frequent diagnoses (disorder/enzyme deficiency)	Differential diagnosis
Metabolic coma without focal neurologic signs	Metabolic acidosis	With ketosis	Organic aciduria (MMA, PA, IVA, GA I, MSUD) PC MCD Ketolysis Gluconeogenesis	Diabetes Exogenous intoxication Encephalitis
		Without ketosis	PDH Ketogenesis FAO FDP	
	Hyperammonemia	Normal glucose	Urea cycle defects	Reye syndrome Encephalitis Exogenous intoxication
	Hypoglycemia	Hypoglycemia	FAO HMG CoA lyase	
		With acidosis	Gluconeogenesis, MSUD, HMG CoA lyase FAO	
		Without acidosis	FAO Hyperinsulinism	
	Hyperlactatemia	Normal glucose	PC MCD Krebs cycle PDH Respiratory chain	
		Hypoglycemia	Gluconeogenesis FAO GSD	

Neurologic coma with focal signs, seizures, severe intracranial hypertension, strokes or stroke-like episodes	Biologic signs are variable, can be absent or moderate.			
		Cerebral edema	**MSUD** **OTC**	Cerebral tumor Migraine Encephalitis
		Hemiplegia or hemianopsia	**MSUD** **OTC** MMA PA PCK	
		Extrapyramidal signs	MMA GA I Wilson Homocystinuria	
		Caudate nucleus and putamen necrosis	**BBGD** **Urea cycle defect** MMA PA IVA	
		Stroke-like	Respiratory chain CDG **Thiamine responsive megaloblastic anemia**	Moya moya syndrome, Vascular hemiplegia Cerebral Thrombophlebitis Cerebral tumor

Treatable disorders appear in bold type.

MMA, methylmalonic academia; PA, propionic academia; IVA, isovaleric aciduria; GA I, glutaric aciduria type I; MSUD, maple syrup urine disease; PC, pyruvate carboxylase deficiency; PDH, pyruvate dehydrogenase; FAO, fatty acid oxidation; FDP, fructose-1,6-diphosphatase; HMG CoA lyase, 3-hydroxy-3-methylglutaryl coenzyme A lyase; GSD, glycogen storage disorders; OTC, ornithine transcarbamylase; PGK, phosphoglycerate kinase; BBGD, biotin-responsive basal ganglia disease; CDG, carbohydrate-deficient glycoprotein syndrome

Adapted from Saudubray JM, Martin D, de Lonlay P, et al. Recognition and management of fatty acid oxidation defects: A series of 107 patients. *J Inherit Metab Dis* 1999;22:488–502.

TABLE 39.4

CONDITIONS THAT PRODUCE A REYE SYNDROME–LIKE ILLNESS

Viral infection
Influenza A and B virus
Varicella zoster
Parainfluenza
Adenovirus
Coxsackie virus
Cytomegalovirus
Herpes simplex
Epstein Barr virus

Inborn errors of metabolism
Urea cycle defect
Organic acidemias
Fatty acid oxidation defects
Others: triple H syndrome (hyperammonemia, hyperornithinemia, homocitrullinuria), Biotinidase defect, HMG CoA lyase defect, FDP defect, fructosemia

Toxics and medications
Drugs: salicylates, valproic acid, antiemetics, paracetamol, outdated tetracycline, zidovudine
Toxics: aflatoxin, hypoglycin, ackee, pteridine, calcium hopantenate, isopropyl alcohol, methobromide, lead, margosa oil, diallyl acetate

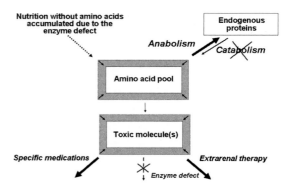

FIGURE 39.3. Schematic of the emergency treatment of errors of metabolism with endogenous intoxication.

conditions. If any clinical signs of intracranial hypertension are observed, a CT scan should be obtained after stabilization of the patient's condition (treatment of fluid and electrolyte imbalance, adequate oxygenation and perfusion, temperature control, etc.), MRI of the brain is much more precise than CT scan, and specific abnormalities can suggest diagnosis of certain pathologies, such as mitochondrial encephalopathies or biotin-responsive basal ganglia disease.

Intracranial pressure monitoring is not routinely performed in metabolic encephalopathy because of the potential rapid improvement with the correct treatment. However, in some circumstances, intracranial pressure monitoring may be helpful to maintain an adequate cerebral perfusion pressure. Using near-infrared spectroscopy to a continuously, directly, and noninvasively monitor cerebral oxygenation and cerebral blood volume may detect changes in cerebral hemodynamics in children with intracranial hypertension and may be helpful in the management of metabolic encephalopathy, especially if hemodynamics are not stable.

In the case of hyperammonemia or suspicion of mitochondrial disorder, seizure control is a priority but valproic acid is contraindicated. In endogenous intoxication, reduction of metabolic rate induced by hypothermia may decrease toxic production.

If an IEM is suspected, therapy must focus on treatable diseases. The first treatment is to infuse glucose (not protein or lipid) to limit protein catabolism (treatment of endogenous intoxication) and to bring enough energy through the glycolysis pathway (treatment of fatty acid oxidation and ketolysis defect). Concentrated solutions of glucose via a central line are necessary to achieve an ideal goal of 1000 kcal/m^2/day, which may require insulin infusion in case of hyperglycemia.

As soon as an endogenous intoxication is diagnosed, nutritional support should be discussed with the metabolism specialist and include the following (**Fig. 39.3**):

■ Promotion of protein anabolism: glucose and lipid without proteins preferably by enteral continuous feeding with a caloric intake of at least 1500 kcal/m^2/d. When the diagnosis is confirmed, special amino acid mixtures are used to supply nontoxic amino acids. For example, in MSUD, the enzyme defect involves the branched chain amino acids (leucine, valine, and isoleucine). The mixtures used are initially free of these three amino acids.
■ Avoidance of any factor that promotes protein catabolism, including steroid contraindication
■ Specific medications in some IEMs, such as ammonia removal drugs (**Table 39.5**)
■ Metabolite excretion: Small organic acids (methylmalonic, propionic, isovaleric, etc.) are excreted in urine, and hydration helps to decrease their concentration in blood and restore the acid-base balance.
■ Extrarenal therapy: When a high and/or prolonged toxic accumulation occurs, toxic removal

TABLE 39.5

SPECIFIC TREATMENTS OF IEMS

Drug	Effect	Indication(s)	Dose	Administration route
Sodium benzoate	Ammonia removal	NH_3 >200 mcmol/L	500 mg/kg/d	IV
Phenylbutyrate	Ammonia removal	NH_3 >200 mcmol/L	600 mg/kg/d	IV or PO
Arginine	Ammonia removal	NH_3 >200 mcmol/L	300 mg/kg/d	IVC
Carglumic acid	Ammonia removal	NAGS defect, MMA, PA, FAO, and NH_3 >200 mcmol/L	50 mg/kg/6 hrs	PO
Carnitine	Primary or secondary deficiency compensation	Organic aciduria Hyperlactacidemia FAOD	100 mg/kg/d	IVC or PO
Glycine	Increased urine	IVA	500 mg/kg/4 hrs	IVC or PO; removal of AIV
Vitamin B12	Enzyme cofactor	MMA	1–2 mg/d	IM
Metronidazole	Decreased toxin production by intestine bacteria	AMM, AP	20 mg/kg/d	PO
Biotin	PC cofactor	Hyperlactatemia	10–20 mg/d	IV or PO
Riboflavin	Acyls CoA cofactor dehydrogenase	FAOD	20–40 mg/d	IV or PO
Dichloroacetate or dichloropropionate	PDHk inhibitor	Hyperlactatemia >10 mmol/L	25 mg/kg/12 hrs	IV or PO

In suspected cases of IEM, the above specific treatments may be indicated in metabolic encephalopathy, after specialist consultation.
Some therapeutic are specific for toxic accumulation (i.e., hyperammonemia) and some are specific for a particular disease.
IV, intravenous; NAGS, N-acetylglutamate synthase; MMA, methylmalonic acidemia; PA, propionic acidemia; FAO, fatty acid oxidation defect; IVA, isovaleric acidemia; PC, pyruvate carboxylase; PDHk, pyruvate dehydrogenase kinase
Adapted from Jouvet P, Rustin P, Taylor DL, et al. Branched chain amino acids induce apoptosis in neural cells without mitochondrial membrane depolarization or cytochrome c release: implications for neurological impairment associated with maple syrup urine disease. *Mol Biol Cell* 2000;11:1919–32.

by dialysis is necessary to prevent further brain damage. The decision to dialyze is made with a multidisciplinary approach that involves intensivists, specialists in metabolic diseases, and nephrologists. The challenge is to quickly remove the toxins without worsening the cerebral edema by hemodynamic and/or osmotic shifts. The greater the cerebral edema, the higher the risk of cerebral herniation during therapy, especially in cases of hyperammonemia.

Treatment efficacy is evaluated on neurologic improvement, gastrointestinal tolerance that reflects calorie assimilation, toxic blood level decrease when measurable (amino acid chromatography in MSUD, pH in organic aciduria, ammonemia, etc.), negativation of urinary ketones if initially positive, and urea/creatinine urinary ratio decrease in MSUD and organic acid disorders, which reflects protein catabolism in the absence of renal failure and protein intake.

CHAPTER 40 ■ BRAIN DEATH

DANIEL L. LEVIN

DEFINITION OF DEATH

Recent History

Confusion and anxiety over the diagnosis of death has been attributed to the availability of recently developed technology and its introduction into the modern ICU. Patients who previously would have died with the loss of respiration, heartbeat, and consciousness can now be supported so that ventilation and heartbeat are maintained, even in patients with a persistent, dense coma and the loss of neurologic function clinically associated with death or brain death. Mollaret and Goulon in 1959 coined the term *coma depasse*, or a state beyond coma, to describe these patients. The importance of precisely defining death became more apparent in 1967 when, at Groote Schuur Hospital in Cape Town, Dr. Christiaan Barnard successfully transplanted the heart of Denise Ann Darvall, a young automobile crash victim, into Louis Washkansky, a man with terminal heart failure. Denise Ann Darvall was a brain-dead, beating-heart organ donor. According to Bernat, the analysis of death should proceed in three phases: (a) the definition of death that makes explicit the traditional implicit concept of death; (b) the measurable criterion of death that is both necessary and sufficient for death that can be employed in a death statute; and (c) devising and validating tests for death to show conclusively that the criterion has been fulfilled. According to Bernat, there are five assumptions to make concerning the definition of death: (a) Death is a non-technical word that is used broadly in common language and any definition should capture this common understanding as a univocal term; (b) death is primarily a biological phenomenon; (c) Death is irreversible; (d) death is understood as an event and not as a process; and (e) the event of death should be determinable by physicians (using tests to fulfill criteria) to have occurred at some specific time, at least in retrospect. Physicians should be able to distinguish a living organism from a dead one. In defense of the whole-brain concept as a criterion of death, Bernat and his colleagues define death as the permanent cessation of critical functions of the organism as a whole, not the whole organism. The pronouncement of death enables society to proceed in one or both of two directions. First, society can engage in death behavior. The grieving process can begin; religious rites, funer-

als, and burials can proceed; and the public can regard the person as a corpse. Legally, the pronouncement of death allows for the reading of wills, inheritance and distribution of property, payment of insurance, remarrying, succession and, if the criteria of brain death are fulfilled, proceeding with organ donation. In 1968, the Harvard criteria were established (**Table 40.1**). These criteria were followed by several other sets of criteria, each with their own variations. All of these criteria were based on the concept of whole-brain death, which included the brainstem, and not neocortical death, with all or part of the brainstem left intact. Thus, patients in a persistent vegetative state were excluded from these criteria.

These criteria applied mostly, though not exclusively, to adults, and the debate about whether they applied to children or infants (especially preterm infants) was put aside by the National Collaborative Study and the President's Commission (1981), which excluded from the criteria children <5 years of age. Since 1968, much discussion has focused on four areas: (a) Do the adult criteria apply to infants and children; (b) are ancillary tests necessary or even capable of establishing the criteria of brain death beyond the history, physical examination, and exclusion of confounding variables; (c) are there appropriate time intervals between triggering event(s), the physical examination of death, the ancillary tests, and the pronouncement of death; and (d) is the whole-brain death definition of death the only acceptable one, or are the exceptions to this criterion? The Special Task Force (1987) excluded infants of <1 wk from its guidelines for brain death in infants and children.

Ancillary Tests to Fulfill the Criteria of Brain Death

Though many authors believe that the clinical diagnosis of brain death based on history, physical examination, and an apnea test is sufficient, in some cases (e.g., barbiturate levels greater than the therapeutic range) one may wish to have ancillary tests available to speed up the ability to diagnose brain death. Other authors believe ancillary tests are needed to diagnose brain death and some have questioned the accuracy of apnea testing as well as the consistency of the application of the test. The British criteria do not recommend any confirmatory tests.

TABLE 40.1

HARVARD CRITERIA FOR BRAIN DEATH (1968)

1. Unresponsiveness, temperature >32.2°C
2. Absence of depressant drugs
3. No spontaneous movements
4. Apnea off respirator for 3 mins at room air
5. No reflexes including
    Decerebrate or decorticate posturing
    Pupils fixed and dilated
    Swallowing, vocalization
    Corneal and pharyngeal
    Stretch and deep-tendon reflexes
6. Isoelectric electroencephalogram
7. All of above should be repeated after 24 hrs

Currently, various tests are used to document brain death (**Table 40.2**). With the possible exception of a 4-vessel cerebral angiography test showing no cerebral blood flow, no test is absolutely confirmatory of brain death and can only be consistent with the diagnosis and, therefore, used to supplement the clinical impression, not to make the diagnosis. Frequently there are examples of disparities between the clinical examination and test results and among differing kinds of tests as well. In addition, there is disagreement in interpretations of the same test.

TABLE 40.2

ANCILLARY TESTS TO CONFIRM BRAIN DEATH

Test	Clinical Disparity
Electroencephalogram	Yes
Cerebral angiogram	Yes
Radionuclide angiogram	Yes
^{123}I-IMP and Tc-^{99}mHMPAO	Yes
Xenon CT	Yes
Brainstem-evoked responses (somatic, visual, auditory)	Yes
P-31 MRI, PET	Yes
Doppler sonography	Yes
Intracranial pressure monitoring	Yes
Endocrinologic function of the brain	Yes

For detailed list of references to these tests, see Farrell MM, Levin DL. Brain death in the pediatric patient: Historical, sociological, medical, religious, cultural, legal, and ethical considerations. *Crit Care Med* 1993;21:1951.
^{123}I-IMP, N-isoprpyl-(^{123}I) p-iodoamphetamine;
Tc-^{99}mHMPAO, technetium-^{99}m hexamethyl-propyleneamine oxime; PET, positron emission tomography

If one chooses to utilize ancillary tests to confirm the diagnosis of brain death, those tests available include all those examinations indicated in **Table 40.2**, although electroencephalography and radionuclide brain scanning are currently the two most frequently used tests.

Electroencephalography

The American Electroencephalographic Society's suggested guidelines for electroencephalography (EEG) are: The EEG must be performed over a 30-min period by a qualified technician, using a minimum of 8 scalp and ear reference electrodes with interelectrode distances of 10 cm; the machine sensitivity must be >2 μ/mm with electrode resistance between 100 and 10,000 ohms; the auditory and photic stimuli and reactivity to pain must be tested during the recording; and the electrocerebral inactivity cannot be determined using telephone electroencephalograms. Technically, the EEG may be difficult to perform on infants and small children, thus weighing against it as a confirmatory test of brain death. An isoelectric EEG, when performed on a premature infant or asphyxiated newborn, must be interpreted with extreme caution. Drug intoxication from barbiturates, diazepam, meprobamate, methaqualone, trichloroethylene, and succinylcholine may specifically cause electrocerebral inactivity.

Cerebral Arteriogram

Though the absence of cerebral blood flow on 4-vessel cerebral arteriography is irrefutable evidence of brain death, the converse is not true, and a patient can be brain-dead and have demonstrable flow. Nonfilling cerebral vessels on 2 aortocranial injections of contrast media 25 mins apart is required by the Swedish Criteria for brain death. Even with all the technical and logistic difficulties encountered in performing cerebral angiography, when the patient is in a barbiturate coma, only the arteriogram can be used to diagnose brainstem death without having to wait several days for the barbiturate levels to fall below the upper limit of therapeutic levels. Angiography will detect cerebral blood flow even though it may be suppressed by as much as 40% during barbiturate coma. In all other circumstances, however, examination remains the "gold standard" for the diagnosis of brain death.

Radionuclide Brain Scanning

Radionuclide brain scanning consists of intravenous injection of 99mTc pertechnetate, which passes through the cervical circulation into the intracranial vault. A tourniquet is placed around the patient's forehead to exclude detection of scalp circulation, and images are obtained with a portable gamma scintillation camera. Demonstration of the absence of intracranial circulation is confirmatory evidence of brain death. The presence of sagittal sinus activity in the absence of intracranial arterial circulation does not exclude the diagnosis of brain death. This technique has advantages of simplicity; however, its efficacy has not been proven in the premature infant and young child <2 mos of age. Another disadvantage of this technique is that cerebral blood flow in the premature infant may be only 12 mL/100 g/min, while the test assesses only flow to the cerebral hemispheres. In addition, the brainstem cannot be evaluated, and negative radioisotopic bolus study implies only that cerebral perfusion is <24% of the normal predicted blood flow. Therefore, neither the EEG nor the radionuclide scan can replace examination of the cranial reflexes. Radionuclide cerebral imaging is helpful only if it demonstrates the absence of flow.

Brainstem Auditory-evoked Potentials

Brainstem auditory evoked responses have been used to test the integrity of the anatomic pathway of hearing. This test can be performed at the bedside using portable equipment, where electrodes are placed over the mastoids and the vertex with sound delivered to each ear via headphones or tubal inserts. In normal individuals, waves I through V are visible. However, brain-dead patients demonstrate the absence of all waves, although the presence of wave I may not be incompatible with this diagnosis.

Time Intervals of Observation and Testing

The Task Force recommended observation periods according to age. For infants ranging in age from 7 days to 2 mos, it recommended 2 examinations and EEGs separated by at least 48 hrs. However, if 1 examination demonstrates the absence of flow on a radionuclide study, the second examination and EEG may be omitted. For infants >1 year of age, an observation period of at least 12 hrs in the presence of an irreversible cause is necessary. A longer period of 24 hrs may be required in certain instances (hypoxic-ischemic encephalopathy). As in the infants ranging in age between 7days and 2 months, however, if the EEG is isoelectric or the radionuclide study demonstrates no flow, the observation period may be shortened. The one major consideration with all these recommendations is that the physical examination must remain consistent with brain death throughout the observation.

CULTURAL, RELIGIOUS, AND LEGAL CONSIDERATIONS IN BRAIN DEATH

Cultural Consideration

In many societies, the concept of brain death is recognized, if not accepted in all, as a sufficient criterion of death for medical and legal purposes. Certainly it is not accepted as equivalent to the death of a person in all societies. Even when accepted medically and legally, it is not the most common mode of declaring death in Pediatric ICUs. Cultural differences certainly influence the acceptance of brain death as a criterion of death. These differences may be deep-seated and based in religion or societal norms but also may be as simple as practical consideration of availability of resources.

Legal Definitions

A statute was proposed in 1975 by the American Bar Association, and in 1981, the Uniform Determination of Death Act) was enacted and endorsed by both the American Bar Association and the American Medical Association. It states "An individual who has sustained either [1] irreversible cessation of circulatory and respiratory functions, or [2] irreversible cessation of all functions of the entire brain, including the brain stem, is dead. A determination must be made in accordance with accepted medical standards." Although brain death is not just a matter of facilitating organ transplantation, difficulties may arise without such legislation. Since the demand for organs far exceeds the supply, in 1968 the Uniform Anatomical Gift Act was enacted to help alleviate this problem. It recognized the legal status of donor cards, living wills, and the authority of the next of kin to make a donation on behalf of a loved one. The major limitation to widespread transplantation in the US is physician reluctance to discuss this issue with parents and next of kin. Many states now have a policy of "Required Request" that mandates inquiring regarding organ donation, regardless of the criteria used to define death. However, <5% of deaths meet brain-death criteria, and of those patients, <25% are possible organ donors.

ORGAN TRANSPLANTATION

Certainly according to most authors, the major purpose of having a concept of brain death as a criterion of death is for the practical issue of declaring a beating-heart, hemodynamically stable patient dead in order to procure whole organs for transplantation. The Pittsburgh protocol for allowing whole-organ donation from terminally ill patients who consent to have support withdrawn, wait 2–3 minutes for cessation of heartbeat, and be declared dead before having rapid organ procurement in an attempt to circumvent the tenants of the "dead-donor" rule (no patient should be harmed in order to procure organs for another). Although this protocol has recently gained substantial acceptance and endorsement from institutions and medical societies, there remains considerable debate about it on ethical grounds. There is an uneasy feeling that the patients were not truly dead in that they could possibly be revived if resuscitated.

Ethical Considerations

The patient must be declared dead prior to removal of organs, and it is never possible to allow some-

one to die in order that someone else may benefit from the use of their organs. Ethically, in terms of distribution of scarce resources, it is also wrong to maintain a brain-dead patient on a ventilator with no chance to benefit the patient. This approach is an abuse of bed space, economic resources, and the time of highly qualified personnel. There is an argument that a dead patient should remain on mechanical ventilation for the sake of the family, especially when events have progressed rapidly, in order to give the family time to accept the outcome. However, allowing the family a decent amount of time to adjust to the death poses many new problems. Usually this time period is adequate to talk to the family and await the arrival of other family members. Prolonged requests for delay may seem at first to have reasonable bases but alternatively may signal denial and bargaining. This course of action can result in situations in which mechanical support interferes with the delivery of healthcare to other patients and demoralizes the staff.

SECTION IV ■ CARDIAC DISEASE

CHAPTER 41 ■ CARDIAC ANATOMY

STEVEN M. SCHWARTZ • ZDENEK SLAVIK • SIEW YEN HO

SEGMENTAL APPROACH TO CONGENITAL HEART DISEASE

Two primary systems are currently in use for describing complex cardiac defects. Both of these systems are based on the principles that (a) specific cardiac chambers have unique, distinguishing characteristics that allow them to be clearly identified even when their right/left relationships to each other or connections to adjoining structures are altered or absent, and (b) that the precise nature of these relationships and connections should be carefully and fully described.

Atrial Situs

The terms "right" and "left" atria refer to specific, distinguishing morphologic characteristics of each

atrium, not to the side of the heart on which they are located or their accompanying venous or ventricular connections. Features that identify the *right* atrium include (a) a blunt atrial appendage with a wide connection to the smooth-walled part of the atrium, (b) the limbus of the fossa ovalis, and (c) remnants of the valves of the sinus venosus such as the Eustachian valve of the coronary sinus. The *left* atrium is characterized by (a) a hooked appendage with a narrower connection to the smooth-walled portion of the chamber, (b) the flap valve of the fossa ovalis, and (c) no remnants of venous valves. Venous connections are not used to designate the morphologic right and left atria, as these connections can be variable in congenital heart disease (i.e., total anomalous pulmonary venous return, unroofed coronary sinus, bilateral superior vena cava).

Once the morphology of the atria has been identified, the atrial arrangement, or situs, can be defined.

Atrial situs refers to the arrangement of the morphologic right and left atria within the heart. *Situs solitus* is the normal arrangement, wherein the right atrium is to the right and the left atrium is to the left. *Situs inversus* is the opposite arrangement; the right atrium is to the left, and the left atrium is to the right. *Atrial isomerism* is defined as the presence of two morphologically left or two morphologically right atria rather than one of each. Situs ambiguus refers to the situation in which separate right and left atria cannot be differentiated. Using this approach, anatomic variants that would be considered cases of atrial isomerism are more generally defined in terms of heterotaxy syndromes, and extracardiac abnormalities of laterality often coexist with the congenital heart disease. *Polysplenia syndrome* is thus often used to mean the same thing as left atrial isomerism, and *asplenia syndrome* is often used to describe the same atrial arrangement as right atrial isomerism.

The bronchi can be particularly helpful in identifying atrial situs because the right and left bronchi have characteristic features readily seen on chest x-ray, and bronchial situs almost always reflects atrial situs. Specifically, the right main stem bronchus is shorter, more vertically oriented, and located directly behind the mediastinal segment of the right pulmonary artery. The left main stem bronchus is longer and more horizontally oriented and below the left pulmonary artery. When the atria are inverted, the left-sided bronchus will usually have the orientation of a typical right bronchus and the left lung may contain 3 lobes. The right-sided bronchus will then have a typical left main stem bronchus anatomy. Isomeric arrangement of the atria usually is reflected by a bilaterally symmetrical bronchial arrangement of either a right or left type. In heterotaxy syndromes (atrial isomerism), abdominal structures in addition to the spleen can be abnormally distributed. Right atrial isomerism or asplenia can be thought of as bilateral right-sidedness and can be associated with a midline liver and intestinal malrotation. Left atrial isomerism, or polysplenia syndrome, can be thought of as bilateral left-sidedness and is also associated with an intestinal malrotation.

The finding of atrial isomerism is also typically accompanied by certain predictably associated intracardiac defects. Right atrial isomerism, or asplenia syndrome, usually includes anomalies of pulmonary venous return and atrioventricular canal-type defects, along with double-outlet right ventricle (DORV) or transposition, whereas left atrial isomerism tends to be more commonly associated with abnormalities of systemic venous connections, particularly interrupted inferior vena cava and DORV or normally related great arteries. Polysplenia can also be associated with atrioventricular canal defects and some abnormalities of pulmonary venous drainage but usually not to the degree that these are associated with asplenia.

The Atrial Septum

The atrial septum in its usual state contains a foramen ovale on the right side and the flap valve of the foramen on the left. The foramen, when patent, allows right-to-left shunting of blood when the right atrial pressure exceeds the left, but it is closed by the flap valve when left atrial pressure is higher. The foramen ovale is the remnant of the ostium secundum; therefore, atrial septal defects (ASDs) in this area are referred to as *secundum ASDs*. The foramen primum is the embryologic opening between the early atrial septum (septum primum) and the area where the endocardial cushions ultimately form.

Ventricular Morphology and Topology

As with the atria, the right and left ventricles are identified by certain constant morphologic patterns, not by their location within the heart or the body. The morphologic right ventricle is heavily trabeculated, contains the moderator band of the septum, and has septal attachments of the associated atrioventricular valve. The left ventricle is smooth walled, more bullet shaped, and has no septal attachments of the atrioventricular valve. When two distinct atrioventricular valves exist, the tricuspid valve is *always* associated with the morphologic right ventricle, and the mitral valve is *always* associated with the left ventricle.

The topology of the ventricles refers to the spatial anatomy of the ventricle with regard to the inflow and outflow. Determination of the "handedness" of a ventricle is made by considering the relationship of the inflow and outflow tracts of the ventricle when looking at the septal surface (**Fig. 41.1**). One can imagine placing the palm of the hand on the septal surface of the ventricle with the thumb extended toward the inflow and the fingers pointed toward the outflow. If this can be accomplished with the right hand, the ventricle is said to be "right-handed;" if it can be accomplished with the left hand, the ventricle is left-handed. In general, the right ventricle of a normal heart is said to have right-handed topology, and the left ventricle, left-handed topology.

Atrioventricular Connections, Junctions, and Alignments

Usually, two separate atrioventricular valves are present, one leading into each ventricle.

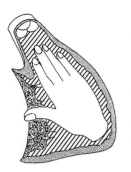 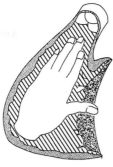

Right-Hand Topology   Left-Hand Topology

FIGURE 41.1. Ventricular topology is determined by imagining the palmer surface of the hand on the septal surface of the morphologically right ventricle, with the thumb pointing toward the inlet and the fingers pointing toward the outlet. Right-hand topology is present if this alignment can be accomplished with the right hand. Left-hand topology is present if this alignment requires use of the left hand. From Anderson RH. Nomenclature and classification: Sequential segmental analysis. In: Moller JH, Hoffman JIE, eds. *Pediatric Cardiovascular Medicine*. Philadelphia: Churchill Livingstone, 2000:263–74, with permission.

Furthermore, the right atrium usually opens into the morphologic right ventricle, and the left atrium opens into the left ventricle. The type of atrioventricular connection or alignment refers to the anatomic concordance or discordance of the atrium and ventricle. A normal heart has concordant atrial and ventricular connections, or alignments, in that the morphologic right atrium opens to the morphologic right ventricle and the left atrium opens to the morphologic left ventricle. A discordant connection or alignment is one in which the morphologic right atrium opens to the morphologic left ventricle and vice versa. When atrial isomerism is present or when both atria open into one ventricle, the relationship can be described as ambiguous and reference can be made to the topology of the ventricles or to the looping pattern.

When the heart has two atria, two atrioventricular valves, and two ventricles, the tricuspid valve is always associated with the morphologic right ventricle, and the mitral valve is always associated with the morphologic left ventricle. When one of the valves is atretic and/or the ventricle is hypoplastic, there are still considered to be two atrioventricular valves in terms of assignment of anatomic diagnosis (e.g., tricuspid atresia or hypoplastic left heart).

The nature of the atrioventricular connection can be further complicated when an inlet ventricular septal defect (VSD) is present. These types of VSDs often involve override or straddle of the atrioventricular valve. *Override* occurs when the annulus of the atrioventricular valve overrides the ventricular septum and thus allows the atrium associated with the overriding valve to empty into both ventricles. A *straddling atrioventricular valve* is one in which the chordal attachments of the valve cross the plane of the septum to attach to the contralateral ventricle.

Ventricular Arrangements

Topology is determined by imagining the palm of the hand on the septal surface of the morphologic right ventricle. If the right hand allows the thumb to point through the inlet while the fingers point at the outlet, the heart has right-hand topology. If this alignment of the thumb and fingers requires the left hand to be used, left-hand topology is present. When d-looping occurs, the embryologic ventricle ends up leftward of the bulbus cordis, thus placing the left ventricle to the left of the right ventricle. When looping occurs abnormally, with the apex of the loop to the left, the morphologic left ventricle ends up rightward of the morphologic right ventricle. This arrangement is referred to as a *levo* or *l-looped* heart.

The Ventricular Septum

The ventricular septum is normally composed of an *inlet portion* formed by endocardial cushion tissue, a *trabecular or muscular portion* that represents the muscular area between the ventricle and bulbus cordis after looping is completed (sometimes described as having sinus and trabecular portions), and the *outflow or conal portion* of the septum. Malalignment defects such as those that occur in tetralogy of Fallot or interrupted aortic arch are generally located in this area because they represent failure of proper alignment of the portions of the ventricular septum. The junction between all of these parts is the *membranous septum*, the most common site of VSDs.

The Great Arteries

The great arteries have relationships with the ventricles and with each other. The ventricular relationships are defined and determined by outflow tract anatomy and alignments. The relationship of one great artery to the other is considered in terms of anterior-posterior and left-right positioning. Normally, related great arteries occur when a heart has concordant ventriculo-arterial connections, with the aorta posterior and slightly rightward of the pulmonary artery. In ventriculo-arterial concordance, the aorta arises from the morphologic left ventricle, and the pulmonary artery arises from the morphologic right ventricle. Ventriculo-arterial discordance occurs when the aorta arises from the morphologic right ventricle and the pulmonary artery arises from the morphologic left ventricle. Concordance and discordance can thus be considered to be synonymous with normally related and transposed great arteries, respectively. With normally related vessels, the aorta is posterior to the pulmonary artery, and the relationship between them can be noted as *situs solitus* (s) when the aorta (aortic valve) is rightward of the pulmonary artery (pulmonary valve), or *situs inversus* (i) when the aorta is leftward of the pulmonary artery. In transposition, the aorta is generally anterior to the pulmonary artery, and the relationship can be described as *dextro* (d) when the aorta is rightward or *levo* (l) when the aorta is leftward.

SYSTEMIC AND PULMONARY VENOUS CONNECTIONS

The systemic and pulmonary venous connections are often abnormal in complex lesions. Abnormalities of systemic venous connections can include bilateral superior vena cava, left superior vena cava, or interrupted inferior vena cava. Furthermore, the site of major venous connections to the heart can be altered from normal such that a right-to-left shunt occurs. Pulmonary venous connections may be either partially or totally anomalous, returning to sites other than the left atrium. Usually, the important aspects of description include noting which pulmonary veins are anomalous and categorizing the connection as supracardiac, cardiac, or infracardiac.

CARDIAC POSITION

Chest x-ray is very helpful in making the diagnosis of an abnormally positioned heart, but a complete assessment usually requires echocardiography to identify the location of the cardiac apex. *Levocardia* is the normal positioning of the heart and describes a situation in which the heart is on the left side of the thorax; *dextrocardia* occurs when the heart is located predominantly in the right chest, and mesocardia is an intermediate situation with a more midline position.

CLINICAL EXAMPLES

Using the segmental approach to the description of cardiac anatomy, it can be seen that a normal heart has atrioventricular concordance, two atrioventricu-

lar connections, and ventriculo-arterial concordance. Alternatively, this anatomy can be referred to as *atrial situs solitus*, d-loop ventricles, and arterial situs solitus {S,D,S}. The most common form of transposition of the great arteries (d-TGA) has atrioventricular concordance and ventriculo-arterial discordance and can be referred to as atrial situs solitus, d-loop ventricles, and d-transposition of the great arteries {S,D,D}. A Taussig-Bing heart, which has a DORV, bilateral subarterial conus, and subpulmonary VSD (aorta completely committed to the right ventricle, pulmonary artery may override the septum) would be described as atrioventricular concordance, ventriculo-arterial discordance with double-outlet ventriculo-arterial connection—or as atrial situs solitus, d-loop, l-malposition of the aorta {S,D,L} with DORV and subpulmonary VSD.

Congenital Heart Defects with Left-to-Right Shunts

Ventricular Septal Defect

VSD is the most common congenital heart defect (30%). VSDs can be divided into *inlet*, *perimembranous*, *muscular*, and *outlet* (which may be subaortic, subpulmonic, or doubly committed) defects (**Fig. 41.2**). The high kinetic energy of the blood that reaches pulmonary circulation owing a large left-to-right shunt through VSD represents a risk for early onset of pulmonary vascular disease, and timely (<2 yrs of age) VSD closure is advocated. VSDs have a high rate of spontaneous closure, especially in isolated small defects (up to 90% by 6 yrs of age). They are frequently associated with other congenital heart defects (e.g., aortic coarctation), or the defect is part of a more complex congenital cardiac malformation (e.g., tetralogy of Fallot). Significant risk of infective endocarditis is associated with VSDs.

Atrial Septal Defects

Various parts of interatrial septum can be affected by defect and, according to their position, ASDs are divided into *secundum* (within oval fossa and around foramen ovale), *primum* (part of atrioventricular septal defect), and *sinus venosus* (superior or inferior adjacent to the orifice of the superior or inferior caval vein) (**Fig. 41.3**). The volume of left-to-right shunt depends on the size of the defect and the relative compliance of right and left ventricles. Large ASDs left untreated until adulthood are associated with risk of atrial dysrhythmias and pulmonary vascular disease. Paradoxical embolism may occur regardless of ASD size, but it is rare in children. Antibiotic prophylaxis for infective endocarditis (subacute bacterial

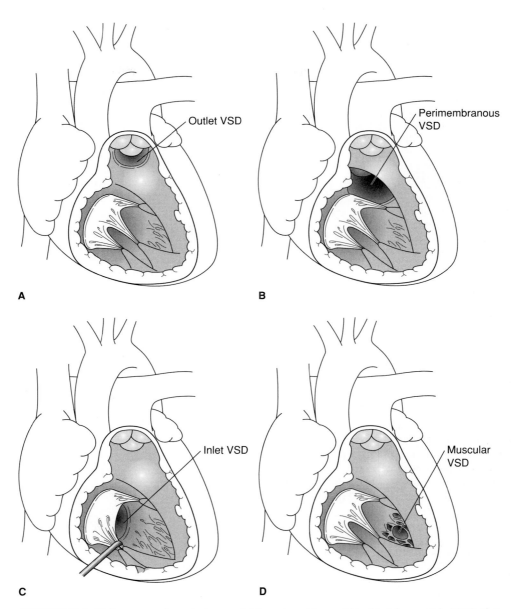

FIGURE 41.2. Various types of ventricular septal defects viewed from within the right ventricle. **(A)** Outlet, **(B)** perimembranous, **(C)** inlet, **(D)** muscular or trabecular.

endocarditis prophylaxis) is not required in isolated secundum ASDs or 6 mos after successful repair of an ASD.

Patent Ductus Arteriosus

The ductus arteriosus is part of the normal fetal circulation that joins the main pulmonary artery with the descending aorta. It allows for most of the blood that reaches the main pulmonary artery to bypass the lungs prenatally. The blood flow direction through the ductus arteriosus reverses postna-

tally, and the ductus arteriosus spontaneously closes in most neonates. Patency beyond 1 mo of age (3 mos in premature infants) is considered abnormal (**Fig. 41.4**). High rates of patency are common in preterm neonates. The patent ductus arterious (PDA) is the only source of pulmonary blood supply in some complex congenital heart defects (e.g., pulmonary valve atresia with intact ventricular septum), but it can be absent in others (e.g., most neonates with persistent truncus arteriosus) postnatally. Risk of pulmonary vascular disease is high in a large PDA left untreated

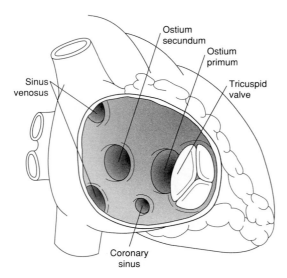

FIGURE 41.3. Various types of atrial septal defects (sinus venosus, ostium secundum, ostium primum) viewed through the right atrium. An unroofed coronary sinus may also act as an atrial septal defect.

into childhood. Subacute bacterial endocarditis prophylaxis is required prior to surgical correction.

Atrioventricular Septal Defects

The complete form of an atrioventricular septal defect (AVSD) is characterized by the absence of the interatrial septum primum and inlet part of the interventricular septum, with concomitant malformation of the common atrioventricular valve and a variable degree of valvar incompetence (**Fig. 41.5**). This

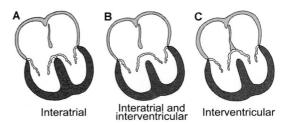

FIGURE 41.5. Atrioventricular septal defect (AVSD) due to deficiency between atrial and ventricular septal structures. (**A**) Shunting at atrial level (ostium primum ASD). (**B**) Shunting at both atrial and ventricular levels (complete AVSD). (**C**) Shunting at ventricular level only ("inlet VSD").

defect is often associated with Trisomy 21 and can lead to the early development of pulmonary vascular obstructive disease. A *partial form* affects either the interatrial or interventricular septum, with variable abnormality of the atrioventricular (AV) valve apparatus.

Truncus Arteriosus

Truncus arteriosus (TA) is a single arterial trunk that is guarded by a single truncal valve that arises from the heart to bifurcate into the ascending aorta and pulmonary arteries (type I) or to give rise to the branch pulmonary arteries at various locations (types II–IV) (**Fig. 41.6**). The truncal valve has a variable

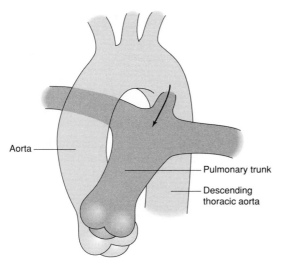

FIGURE 41.4. Patent ductus arteriosus (*arrow with left-to-right shunt*).

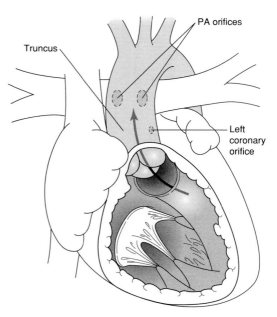

FIGURE 41.6. Truncus arteriosus type II. The relationship of the truncal artery (truncus) to the truncal valve, left coronary ostium, and ventricular septal defect (*arrow*) is shown.

number of cusps and overrides the ventricular septal defect, thereby receiving blood from both the left and right ventricle. Stenosis and/or incompetence of the truncal valve occurs. The origin of the pulmonary arteries from the persistent truncus varies resulting in the different subtypes of the lesion. TA has a strong association with chromosome 22q11 microdeletion (DiGeorge syndrome).

Aortopulmonary Window

Direct, side-by-side communication is present between the ascending aorta and the main pulmonary artery in the form of an oval opening. Separate aortic and pulmonary valves are found, distinguishing this lesion from TA. Free transmission of aortic blood pressure into pulmonary arteries represents a high risk of early onset of pulmonary vascular disease.

Partial or Total Anomalous Pulmonary Venous Connection

Abnormality in the pulmonary venous connections occurs when one (partial anomalous pulmonary venous connection) to all four (total APVC, TAPVC) pulmonary veins connect anomalously with the systemic venous system (inferior or superior vena cavae), right atrium, or coronary sinus. The partial variety, involving the right upper pulmonary vein connected with the superior vena cava, is often associated with a superior sinus venosus ASD. Depending on the insertion of the anomalous connection, total anomalous pulmonary venous connection (TAPVC) can be *supracardiac* (with pulmonary venous drainage into the innominate vein or superior vena cava), *intracardiac* (with pulmonary venous drainage into coronary sinus or right atrium), and *infracardiac* (with pulmonary venous drainage into hepatic or portal veins). Obstruction of the anomalous pulmonary venous connection (mainly in the supracardiac and infracardiac forms) results in profound cyanosis with severe pulmonary hypertension postnatally. Unobstructed TAPVC presents with signs and symptoms of mild cyanosis with congestive heart failure from the increased pulmonary blood flow.

Cyanotic Congenital Heart Defects

Tetralogy of Fallot

Tetralogy of Fallot is the most common cyanotic congenital heart defect, named for a combination of *VSD* with *overriding aorta*, *right ventricular outflow tract obstruction*, and *right ventricular hypertrophy* (**Fig. 41.7**). Interventricular septal malalignment

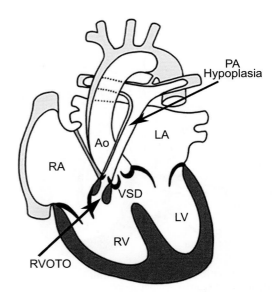

FIGURE 41.7. Tetralogy of Fallot. Ao, aorta; LA, left atrium; RA, right atrium; LV, left ventricle; RV, right ventricle; VSD, ventricular septal defect; RVOTO, right ventricular outflow tract obstruction; PA, pulmonary artery.

that involves superior and anterior shift of the outlet septum contributes to subvalvar pulmonary stenosis. Some degree of pulmonary annular and arterial hypoplasia is commonly present. Its severe form may involve pulmonary atresia and variable degrees of central pulmonary arterial hypoplasia, sometimes with additional aortopulmonary collateral arteries supplying different segments of the pulmonary circulation. AVSD, anomalous origin of the left anterior interventricular coronary artery from the right coronary artery, and/or right-sided aortic arch are the most common cardiac anomalies associated with tetralogy of Fallot. Chromosome 22q11 microdeletion (DiGeorge syndrome), is common.

Pulmonary Atresia with Intact Ventricular Septum

Pulmonary atresia with intact ventricular septum results in a spectrum of hypoplasia of the right ventricle and tricuspid valve (**Fig. 41.8**). The pulmonary arteries are usually of normal size due to blood flow from an obligate PDA, which arises from the aorta in a reverse angle. Coronary arterial fistulae connecting with the right ventricular cavity are present in up to one-third of all cases.

Transposition of Great Arteries

Ventriculo-arterial discordance leads to an aorta arising from the right ventricle and the pulmonary artery

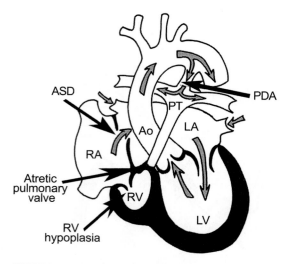

FIGURE 41.8. Pulmonary atresia with intact ventricular septum. ASD, atrial septum defect; Ao, aorta; PT, pulmonary trunk; PDA, patent ductus arteriosus; LA, left atrium; LV, left ventricle; RA, right atrium; RV, right ventricle.

arising from the left ventricle, which results in systemic and pulmonary blood flow configured in parallel circuits rather than in series (**Fig. 41.9**). Postnatal survival depends on mixing of blood between the systemic and pulmonary circulations, usually at the atrial and ductal levels. VSD and/or pulmonary stenosis are the most frequent associated cardiac defects. Coronary artery anomalies are common.

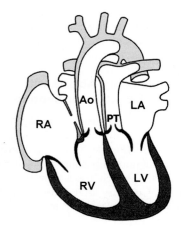

FIGURE 41.9. Transposition of the great arteries {S,D,D},with the pulmonary trunk arising from the left ventricle and the aorta arising from the right ventricle. RA, right atrium; Ao, aorta; PT, pulmonary trunk; LA, left atrium; RV, right ventricle; LV, left ventricle.

Obstructive Congenital Heart Defects

Pulmonary Valve Stenosis

A variable degree of commissural fusion between the valvar cusps is the most common cause of pulmonary stenosis. Tethering of the superior cusp edges and dysplasia of cusps themselves are less common varieties of stenosis. Mild, isolated stenosis rarely progresses. Severe forms of right ventricular hypertrophy may contribute to subvalvar stenosis. Supravalvar pulmonary stenosis that affects the main pulmonary artery or its branches may occur in isolation or in combination with valvar and subvalvar stenoses. This combination is seen as part of tetralogy of Fallot. ASDs and VSDs are the most common associated cardiac defects.

Aortic Valve Stenosis

Stenotic valves can be described as unicuspid, bicuspid, or tricuspid, depending on the number of functional commissures between valvar cusps. Unicuspid valves are usually most severely stenosed. Bicuspid valves, on the other hand, may present without stenosis in childhood.

Coarctation of the Aorta and Interruption of the Aortic Arch

In coarctation of the aorta, narrowing in the distal part of aortic arch around the aortic isthmus may be accompanied by variable degree and extent of aortic arch hypoplasia (**Fig. 41.10**). Aortic coarctation is closely associated with arterial ductal insertion into the aortic wall, and a discrete shelf inside the aortic lumen may become obvious only on ductal closure in some patients postnatally. Arterial ductal patency plays an important role in most cases with severe neonatal aortic coarctation, as it allows for blood flow to reach the lower part of the body. Collateral arteries that bridge the narrow aortic segment develop gradually during childhood in untreated patients. VSD, bicuspid aortic valve, and aortic and mitral valve stenoses are the most common associated anomalies.

In aortic arch interruption, a segment of the aortic arch is missing or replaced by a solid cord. Depending on the location of the missing aortic arch segment, the defect is categorized as type A, interruption distal to the left subclavian artery; type B (most common), interruption between the common carotid and left subclavian arteries; and type C, interruption between the two common carotid arteries. A PDA with right-to-left shunt is the only source of blood supply for body parts distal to the interruption. A VSD is the most common associated heart defect. Chromosome

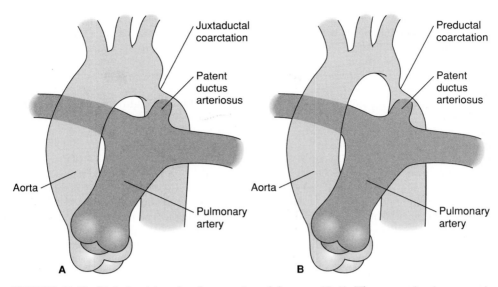

FIGURE 41.10. (A) Isolated juxtaductal coarctation of the aorta (CoA). The coarctation is most typically proximal to the patent ductus arteriosus (PDA) or ligamentum arteriosum. **(B)** Preductal coarctation associated with aortic arch hypoplasia.

22q11 microdeletion is strongly linked with type B interruption of the aortic arch.

Complex Congenital Heart Defects

Ebstein Anomaly of the Tricuspid Valve

Tricuspid valve malformation due to apical displacement of the septal and mural leaflet annular attachment is the leading underlying pathology of Ebstein anomaly. Annular attachment of the anterosuperior leaflet is usually normal. All leaflets of the valve may be larger or smaller than normal, contributing to the failure of all three leaflets to coapt successfully in ventricular systole. A variable degree of tricuspid valve incompetence is the most frequently encountered hemodynamic abnormality. Marked apical displacement of the tricuspid valve limits the size of the right ventricular cavity and may contribute to right ventricular outflow obstruction. An ASD is the most frequently associated anomaly. A wide spectrum of tricuspid valve malformations influences clinical presentation, from an asymptomatic child or adolescent presenting with supraventricular tachycardia or mild cyanosis (due to a right-to-left interatrial shunt) to a critically ill cyanotic neonate with severe obstruction to the right ventricular outflow and marked tricuspid regurgitation. Supraventricular tachycardia due to a manifest accessory connection (Wolff Parkinson White syndrome) can occur in utero, in infancy, in childhood, or in adolescence in patients with Ebstein anomaly.

Univentricular Hearts

A wide variety of congenital heart defects involves hypoplasia of one ventricle (right or left) and abnormality of the AV valves (tricuspid, mitral, or AVSD). The abnormality may be stenosis or atresia of the AV connection or both AV valves emptying into a

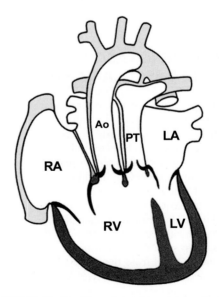

FIGURE 41.11. Double-outlet right ventricle with transposition physiology (aorta rightward and side-by-side with the pulmonary trunk). RA, right atrium; Ao, aorta; PT, pulmonary trunk; LA, left atrium; RV, right ventricle; LV, left ventricle.

dominant ventricle (i.e., double-inlet ventricle). A hypoplastic ventricle may communicate with the dominant ventricle through a VSD. Anomalies of systemic and pulmonary venous connections are common, as are anomalies of the ventriculo-arterial connections. The heterotaxy syndromes (asplenia/polysplenia) are strongly associated with these complex defects.

Hypoplastic Left-Heart Syndrome. This syndrome is a common form of univentricular heart with variable but mostly severe degrees of hypoplasia that affects the mitral valve, left ventricle, aortic valve, and aortic arch, including coarctation. The left ventricle is unable to support the systemic circulation postnatally. Systemic arterial blood flow and survival depend on a PDA with a right-to-left shunt. As pulmonary vascular resistance drops after birth, systemic perfusion (Qs) decreases due to excessive pulmonary (Qp) blood flow (an increased Qp:Qs ratio). The right ventricle must sustain both pulmonary and systemic circulations. If the ASD is markedly restrictive,

obstruction to pulmonary venous drainage occurs, which typically results in a very poor outcome. Anatomic anomalies of the CNS are common and should be investigated preoperatively, even in the absence of systemic hypoperfusion.

Double-Outlet Right Ventricle. In DORV, both aorta and pulmonary artery arise from the morphologic right ventricle. A semilunar valve is committed to a ventricle when $\geq 50\%$ of the valve arises from the ventricle. Thus, in DORV, the left ventricle ejects through a VSD into the semilunar valves (**Fig. 41.11**). The relative position of the VSD and the semilunar valves determines the distinctly divergent postnatal hemodynamics. A subaortic position of the VSD is more common and associated with pulmonary stenosis, which results in a tetralogy of a Fallot-like situation. When the VSD is in a subpulmonary position, a transposition-like physiology results, with the left ventricle ejecting blood through the VSD back into the pulmonary artery.

CHAPTER 42 ■ CARDIOVASCULAR PHYSIOLOGY

PETER OISHI • DAVID F. TEITEL • JULIEN I. HOFFMAN • JEFFREY R. FINEMAN

THE CARDIOVASCULAR CIRCUIT AND VASCULAR ANATOMY

Vessels are composed of concentric layers that include, from inside to out, the intima, media, and adventitia, although various vessel types can lack some layers. The innermost layer of the intima is the vascular endothelium, which is responsible for critical vascular metabolic processes. In addition, it functions as a barrier to the movement of fluid, gases, and solutes into the interstitial space with varying degrees of permeability. Capillaries are thin-walled vessels essentially lacking all but the endothelial cell layer, which makes them suitable for transporting and receiving substances to and from the tissues that they supply. Veins have the same basic layers as arteries but are less well organized and have thinner walls and larger luminal diameters as compared to arteries at similar locations in the circulation. In addition, many veins contain unidirectional valves, which prevent blood from moving backward away from the heart.

HEMODYNAMIC PRINCIPLES

At a constant flow, the velocity of blood through a vessel relates to the cross-sectional area of the vessel, by the equation:

$$v = Q/A$$

where

$$v = \text{velocity}, \ Q = \text{flow}, \text{ and } A = \text{the cross-sectional area}$$

Peak velocity occurs in the aorta and reaches its nadir in the capillary beds, which have tremendous cross-sectional areas. Velocity increases again as blood moves from the capillaries toward the central veins.

The relationship of pressure and flow to resistance can be understood by examining the hydraulic equivalent of Ohm's law:

$$R = (P_i - P_o)/Q$$

which states that the resistance to flow through a vessel is equivalent to the change in pressure across the vessel divided by the flow through the vessel. With rearrangement of Poiseuille's law to give the hydraulic resistance equation:

$$R = (P_i - P_o)/Q = 8\eta l/\pi r^4$$

Where P_i = inflow pressure, P_o = outflow pressure r = radius, η = viscosity, Q = flow and l = length. Resistance changes with the fourth power of the radius, so vascular contraction or relaxation has a profound impact on flow through a vessel.

A change in intravascular pressure results in a proportional change in intravascular volume. The incremental change in volume (ΔV) per unit change in pressure (ΔP) defines the compliance (C) of a vessel, as indicated by the equation:

$$C = \Delta V/\Delta P$$

INTERACTION OF THE CARDIAC PUMP AND THE VASCULATURE

Cardiac output is determined by heart rate, contractility, preload, and afterload. The vascular function curve describes how changes in cardiac output affect central venous pressure (CVP), or venous return. To understand this relationship, a conceptual model can be used to partition the circulation into components, including a pump, an arterial compartment with a given compliance (C_a), a resistor (which represents the resistance through the arterioles, capillaries, and venules), and a venous compartment with a given compliance (C_v). At some point, a maximal Q is achieved, whereby further reductions in the volume of blood in the venous compartment are not possible. Drawing blood from the venous compartment beyond this point would create a negative pressure within the venous compartment, which would tend to collapse the vessel walls. This point is termed the *critical closing pressure* (P_{cc}) and represents the lowest possible CVP and highest possible Q for any given blood volume. On the opposite extreme, when Q becomes zero, the system reaches a steady state, where pressures within the arterial and venous compartments are determined solely by compliance. In this situation, CVP would be at its maximum for any given blood volume.

The cardiac function curve is the reverse of the vascular function curve. That is, it examines how changes in CVP affect Q (**Fig. 42.1**). This relationship is based on Starling's law that describes increases in Q that result from increased stretch of the myocardium, which augments contractility. On the steep portion of the curve, increases in CVP, through

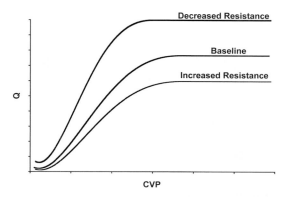

FIGURE 42.1. Cardiac function curves shown under conditions of varying degrees of systemic vascular resistance (afterload). The cardiac function curve describes how changes in central venous pressure (CVP) or venous return affect cardiac output (Q). On the steep portion of the curve, increases in CVP augment ventricular contractility. Increases in systemic vascular resistance (increased afterload) shift the curve downward, while decreases in systemic vascular resistance (decreased afterload) shift the curve upward.

increased venous return, distend the right ventricle (i.e., increase preload), which augments right ventricular contractility and flow through the pulmonary circuit. This then increases pulmonary venous return, which increases left ventricular preload and output. Though the cardiac function curve is directly related to CVP, it may also be affected by the other determinants of cardiac output, including afterload, contractility, and heart rate. For example, increases in systemic vascular resistance that increase afterload can result in a downward shift in the curve, while systemic vasodilation that decreases afterload will result in an upward shift in the curve (**Fig. 42.1**).

At any given time, the cardiovascular system operates at one theoretical point of intersection between the vascular and cardiac function curves. For example, if the pump suddenly ejected an increased volume of blood, volume and pressure would increase in the arterial compartment and decrease in the venous compartment. According to the cardiac function curve, subsequent ejection would decrease, as CVP was reduced. Over a short period of time, this decrease in Q would result in an increase in CVP in accordance with the vascular function curve, returning the system to the initial point of intersection. The superimposition of these curves in various physiologic states is useful, as it illustrates important interactions between cardiac output, preload, peripheral resistance (or afterload), and blood volume. For example, from **Figure 42.2**, it can be seen that alterations in vascular resistance affect both the vascular and cardiac function curves, whereas changes in blood volume only affect the vascular function curve.

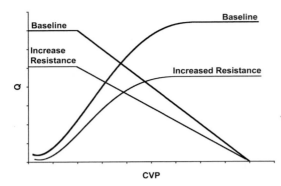

FIGURE 42.2. Effects of increased systemic vascular resistance on the vascular and cardiac function curves. Increased systemic vascular resistance (or afterload) shifts both curves downward, moving the operating state of the system that occurs at the point of intersection between the two curves downward. Increased systemic vascular resistance does not alter the vascular function curve at zero Q, as the CVP at this point is determined solely by the compliance of the venous compartment, at any given volume.

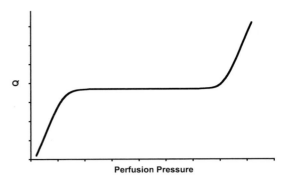

FIGURE 42.3. Autoregulation. Blood flow (Q) through most organs is maintained constant over a wide range of perfusion pressures. In general, decreases in perfusion pressure result in vasodilation, while increases in perfusion pressure result in vasoconstriction, thereby maintaining constant flow through alterations in vascular resistance. At the points of downward and upward inflection, maximal dilation or constriction have occurred, and constant blood flow can no longer be maintained in the face of decreased or increased perfusion pressures respectively.

REGULATION OF VASCULAR RESISTANCE

The main site of resistance within the circulation occurs at the level of the arterioles. However, larger arteries and veins of varying sizes also affect resistance and may become a primary site of resistance under various conditions. While a number of anatomic factors contribute to the resistance imposed by a vessel, smooth-muscle cell tone is the predominant regulating mechanism. Several mechanisms control the contractile state of vascular smooth muscle and, thus, vascular resistance, including neural control, hormonal control, endothelial derived factors, myogenic processes, and local metabolic products.

Blood flow to tissues remains relatively constant over a wide range of arterial blood pressures due to autoregulation (**Fig. 42.3**). Neural control of the circulation allows rapid regulation and provides simultaneous control of various regions within the circulation. Stretch receptors are found in the walls of the atria and ventricles. These stretch receptors provide feedback to the hypothalamus and inhibit secretion of antidiuretic hormone (vasopressin). Atrial stretch causes secretion of atrial natriuretic factor (ANF). Atrial stretch receptors are responsible for stimulation of increased heart rate by the Bainbridge reflex. Carotid baroreceptors are more important for control of sympathetic regulation of muscle blood flow, whereas cardiac receptors are more important in control of sympathetic regulation of kidney blood flow.

Two different types of sympathetic nerve fibers exist: vasoconstrictor and vasodilator. Sympathetic stimulation of the arterioles by vasoconstrictor fibers increases vascular resistance; these vessels are called *resistance vessels*. Sympathetic stimulation may also increase blood flow through activation of vasodilator fibers, which are primarily found in the vascular beds of skeletal muscle. The parasympathetic system primarily controls heart function and rate and has a very limited role in control of the peripheral circulation. The transmitter stored in nerve endings of the parasympathetic system is acetylcholine.

The vasculature in the peripheral circulation is responsive to various circulating substances, including catecholamines, angiotensin II, vasopressin, eicosanoids, nitric oxide (NO), neurokinins, and peptide hormones. Catecholamines are the hormones of the adrenergic system. Adrenergic receptors to catecholamines are present in the smooth muscle throughout the peripheral vascular system and can be categorized as α and β receptors. Stimulation of α receptors causes vascular smooth muscle to contract, causing vasoconstriction; stimulation of β receptors causes vascular smooth muscle to relax, causing vasodilation. These receptors are responsive to both endogenous catecholamines and sympathomimetic drugs. Norepinephrine, an α-adrenergic agonist, is secreted by the adrenal medulla and is carried by the bloodstream to receptors in the peripheral vasculature. Angiotensin II, a powerful vasoconstrictor, is produced by activation of the rennin-angiotensin-aldosterone system. The kidney secretes renin in response to decreased renal arterial pressure or a decrease in extracellular fluid volume. Renin, in turn, cleaves angiotensinogen to angiotensin I, which is then converted to angiotensin II by an angiotensin-converting enzyme found in lung and vascular endothelium. Angiotensin II has direct vasoconstrictor properties. Antidiuretic hormone is synthesized in the hypothalamus and secreted by the posterior pituitary. It is a very potent vasoconstrictor but plays a minimal role in regulation of the circulation under resting conditions.

Prostaglandins and other eicosanoids play a small role in regulation of flow in the systemic circulation. ANF is released from atrial myocytes of both atria and, in smaller amounts, from the ventricular myocytes. ANF is released in response to stretch of either atrium; increased circulating levels of ANF are detected when left atrial pressure is elevated, even when the right atrial pressure is normal. In the kidney, ANF decreases tubular reabsorption of sodium. In the circulatory system, ANF has vasodilator and cardioinhibitory effects. Circulating levels of ANF are increased in certain pathophysiologic conditions, such as congenital heart disease associated with elevated atrial pressures, congestive heart failure, valve disease, hypertension, coronary artery occlusion, and atrial arrhythmias. In addition, B-type natriuretic peptide has natriuretic, diuretic, and vasoactive properties.

The vascular endothelial cells are capable of producing a variety of vasoactive substances, which participate in the regulation of normal vascular tone. These substances, such as NO and ET-1, are capable of producing vascular relaxation and/or constriction, modulating the propensity of the blood to clot, and inducing and/or inhibiting smooth muscle migration and replication (**Fig. 42.4**). The vascular endothelium derived factors are used therapeutically, such as inhaled NO for pulmonary hypertension, L-arginine supplementation for coronary artery disease and the pulmonary vasculopathy of sickle cell disease, phosphodiesterase inhibitors (i.e., sildenafil) for pulmonary hypertensive disorders, endothelin-receptor antagonists for pulmonary hypertensive disorders and subarachnoid hemorrhage, and NO

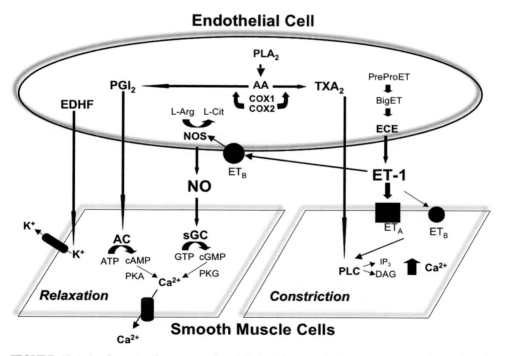

FIGURE 42.4. A schematic of some endothelial-derived factors, which may cause smooth muscle cell relaxation (**left**) and/or constriction (**right**). EDHF, endothelial derived hyperpolarizing factor; PGI_2, prostaglandin I_2; L-Arg, L-arginine; L-Cit, L-citrulline; PLA_2, phospholipase A_2; AA, arachidonic acid; COX1, cyclooxygenase-1; COX2, cyclooxygenase-2; TXA_2, thromboxane A_2; PrePro ET, PrePro endothelin; BigET, Big endothelin; NOS, nitric oxide synthase; ECE, endothelin-converting enzyme; ET_B, endothelin B receptor; NO, nitric oxide; ET-1, endothelin-1; K^+, potassium channels; AC, adenylate cyclase; sGC, soluble guanylate cyclase; ATP, adenosine-5′-triphosphate; cAMP, cyclic adenosine monophosphate; GTP, guanosine-5′-triphosphate; cGMP, cyclic guanosine-3′-5′ monophosphate; PKA, phosphokinase A; PKG, phosphokinase G; ET_A, endothelin A receptor; PLC, phospholipase C; IP_3, inositol triphosphate; DAG, diacylglycerol.

inhibitors for refractory hypotension secondary to sepsis and persistent patency of the ductus arteriosus.

NO is produced by NO synthase from L-arginine in the vascular endothelial cell. NO diffuses into the smooth-muscle cell and produces vascular relaxation by increasing concentrations of cGMP, via the activation of soluble guanylate cyclase (**Fig. 42.4**). NO is released in response to shear stress (flow) and the binding of certain endothelium-dependent vasodilators (such as acetylcholine, ATP, and bradykinin) to receptors on the endothelial cell.

ET-1 is produced by vascular endothelial cells and causes sustained hypertensive action. In fact, ET-1 is the most potent vasoconstricting agent discovered, with a potency 10 times that of angiotensin II (**Fig. 42.4**). The breakdown of phospholipids within vascular endothelial cells results in the production of the important byproducts of arachidonic acid, including PGI_2 and thromboxane (TXA_2). PGI_2 activates adenylate cyclase, resulting in increased cyclic AMP production and subsequent vasodilation, whereas TXA_2 results in vasoconstriction. Other prostaglandins and leukotrienes also have potent vasoactive properties.

In general, regional circulations regulate their flow so that they obtain required amounts of oxygen and nutrients, and all of the mechanisms described above may be invoked. However, an overriding principle exists wherein shear rate must be kept constant within narrow limits to avoid endothelial damage. Any increase in local organ flow is sensed by endothelial integrins that trigger a cascade of responses that culminate in release of NO. Tissues have the ability to regulate their own blood flow in response to changes in metabolic demands. Many tissues will release adenosine, a potent vasodilator, in response to increased metabolism or decreased oxygen tension. Other mediators include lactic acid, histamine, prostaglandin, ET-1, and NO.

REGULATION OF REGIONAL CIRCULATIONS

Fetal Circulation

The fetal ventricles primarily perform their postnatal functions as follows: The fetal right ventricle supplies the majority of its blood via the ductus arteriosus and descending aorta to the placenta for oxygen uptake, and the left ventricle supplies the majority of its blood via the ascending aorta to the heart and brain for oxygen delivery. So that the central venous circulation can facilitate these tasks, the least saturated venous blood must be directed to the right ventricle, and the most saturated blood must be directed to the left. Preferential streaming patterns among the various sources of venous return allow most of the poorly saturated blood from the upper body, myocardium, and lower body to reach the right ventricle and the more highly saturated umbilical venous return to reach the left ventricle.

Transition from the Fetal to the Postnatal Circulation

The changes in the central circulation at birth are primarily caused by external events rather than by primary changes in the circulation itself. Most important of these external events are the rapid and large decrease in pulmonary vascular resistance and the disruption of the umbilical-placental circulation. Abruptly at birth, the ductus arteriosus, until it closes in the first hours or days of life, changes from a right-to-left conduit of blood to the descending aorta, to a left-to-right conduit of blood to the lungs. The ductus venosus carries umbilical venous return primarily to the left heart. Although vasoactive processes are involved in the closure of the ductus arteriosus and may be involved in closure of the ductus venosus, closure of the foramen ovale at birth is entirely passive, secondary to alterations in the relative return of blood to the right and left atria.

Regulation of Prenatal and Postnatal Pulmonary Vascular Resistance and Pulmonary Blood Flow

Mechanical effects, state of oxygenation, and the production of vasoactive substances, regulate the tone of the fetal pulmonary circulation. The most prominent factor associated with high fetal pulmonary vascular resistance is the low blood O_2 tension (pulmonary arterial blood pO_2, 17–20 torr). NO appears to be especially important.

At birth, with initiation of pulmonary ventilation, pulmonary vascular resistance decreases rapidly and is associated with an 8–10-fold increase in pulmonary blood flow. By the first day of life, mean pulmonary arterial blood pressure is generally half systemic. After the initial abrupt decrease in pulmonary vascular resistance and pressure, a slow, progressive decrease follows, with adult levels reached after 2–6 weeks. The mechanisms that regulate the fall in pulmonary vascular resistance and increase in pulmonary blood flow after birth are in large part related to the increase in alveolar oxygen tension and the physical expansion of the lung. NO has been implicated as an important mediator of the decrease in pulmonary vascular resistance at birth that is associated with increased oxygenation.

The successful transition from the fetal to the postnatal pulmonary circulation is marked by the maintenance of the pulmonary vasculature in a dilated, low-resistance state. Two of the most important factors affecting pulmonary vascular resistance in the postnatal period are oxygen concentration and pH. Decreasing oxygen tension and decreases in pH elicit pulmonary vasoconstriction. This response to hypoxia is unique to the pulmonary vasculature; indeed, in most vascular beds (e.g., cerebral vasculature), hypoxia is a potent vasodilator.

Several other factors, unique to the lung, influence pulmonary blood flow in addition to pulmonary vascular tone. In a standing position, owing to gravity, mean pulmonary vascular pressures increase from the apex to the base of the lung, but alveolar pressure is relatively constant throughout the lung.

To characterize this relationship, West divided the lung into three theoretical zones that move down the lung from the apex to the base and are based on the relationship between pulmonary artery pressure (PAP), or inflow pressure, alveolar pressure (P_{av}), and pulmonary venous pressure (P_{ven}), or outflow pressure. In theory, no blood flows to zone I because P_{av} exceeds PAP, or $P_{av} > PAP > P_{ven}$. In this zone, intraalveolar vessels would be collapsed. Clinically, zone I conditions probably do not exist in a healthy lung, as pulmonary blood flow does occur at the apex. In zone II, PAP exceeds P_{av} and blood flow occurs independent of outflow pressures, or $PAP > P_{av} > P_{ven}$. In this zone, blood flow increases down the lung, as PAP, but not P_{av}, is influenced by gravity. In zone III, blood flow is dictated by the normal relationship of PAP to P_{ven}, or inflow pressure minus outflow pressure. In this zone, blood flow does not change dramatically down the lung as it does in zone II because gravity affects PAP and P_{ven} equally, or $PAP > P_{ven} > P_{av}$. Under normal conditions, pulmonary blood flow is largely determined by zone III conditions. However, with disease, less favorable conditions can predominate. Particularly pertinent to pediatric critical care are the effects of positive-pressure ventilation with high levels of peak end-expiratory pressure. Increased alveolar pressure may expand zone II and allow zone I conditions to be realized, resulting in mismatching of ventilation and perfusion and intrapulmonary shunting with hypoxia and hypercapnia.

Coronary Circulation

Blood flow to the myocardium is supplied by the right and left coronary arteries, which arise from the sinuses of Valsalva, just behind the right and left coronary cusps of the aortic valve. The right coronary artery supplies the right atrium and ventricle, while the left coronary artery, which divides into the left anterior descending artery and the circumflex artery, supplies the left atrium and ventricle. Venous return to the right atrium occurs principally through the coronary sinus, with a lesser portion returning through the anterior coronary veins. In addition, arteriosinusoidal, arterioluminal, and thebesian vessels connect the coronary arterial system to the cardiac chambers, forming an extensive plexus of subendocardial vessels.

Coronary blood flow is regulated by physical forces that are related to the anatomic position of the coronary vessels within and around the dynamic myocardium, metabolic factors that couple coronary blood flow to oxygen demand, and neural factors. If diastole is excessively shortened, such as with severe tachycardia and/or if perfusion pressure is decreased, subendocardial ischemia can occur. Conversely, flow within the coronary vessels that perfuse the right ventricular myocardium is normally maintained during systole and diastole because of the lower afterload induced by the pulmonary circulation that results in lower right ventricular intracavitary pressures. Perfusion of the hypertrophied right ventricle of severe pulmonic stenosis or tetralogy of Fallot would be expected to resemble that of the left ventricle.

Coronary blood flow is tightly coupled to the oxygen supply-to-oxygen demand ratio. Coronary blood flow increases when oxygen supply decreases and/or when oxygen demand increases. In this way, coronary blood flow is, in fact, linked to the overall oxygen needs of the body, as increases in cardiac output typically increase myocardial oxygen consumption. Likewise, when the body's metabolic needs decrease (e.g., during rest), myocardial oxygen consumption decreases, as does coronary blood flow. Under normal conditions, coronary blood flow is autoregulated such that if perfusion pressure is raised or lowered, there is a range over which almost no change in flow occurs; a rise in pressure evokes vasoconstriction, and a fall in pressure evokes vasodilatation. At perfusion pressures above some upper limit, flow increases, probably because the pressure overcomes the constriction. More importantly, at low perfusion pressures, flow decreases, indicating that the coronary vasculature is beginning to reach maximal vasodilatation and can no longer decrease resistance to compensate for the decreased perfusion pressure. A further decrease in perfusion pressure will cause ischemia. As sympathetic activation tends to increase myocardial oxygen consumption, in large part due to increases in contractility and heart rate, coronary blood flow increases in order to increase oxygen supply.

Right Ventricular Myocardial Blood Flow

Right ventricular myocardial blood flow follows the general principles of coronary blood flow, but differences exist that are related to the low right ventricular systolic pressure and to the fact that alterations in aortic pressure change coronary perfusing pressure without altering right ventricular pressure work. For example, if the normal right ventricle is acutely distended by pulmonary embolism, right ventricular failure will eventually occur; the increased wall stress increases oxygen consumption, but the raised systolic pressure reduces the coronary flow, so that when supply cannot match demand, right ventricular myocardial ischemia results. Raising aortic perfusing pressure mechanically or with α-adrenergic agonists increases right ventricular myocardial blood flow, relieves ischemia, and restores right ventricular function to normal. Improved coronary flow is not the only mechanism of this improvement; the increased left ventricular afterload moves the ventricular septum toward the right ventricle and im-

proves left ventricular performance. If right ventricular pressure is chronically elevated so that right ventricular hypertrophy occurs (as in pulmonic stenosis, many forms of cyanotic congenital heart disease, and some chronic lung diseases), right ventricular myocardial blood flow behaves in the same way as left ventricular blood flow, with one exception. If aortic pressure is lowered, left ventricular pressure also decreases, as does left ventricular work and oxygen consumption. However, in the right ventricle, the workload may not be reduced (if no ventricular septal defect is present) so that an imbalance between myocardial oxygen supply and demand may occur. The worst imbalance occurs when aortic systolic pressure is maintained but coronary perfusing pressure decreases, and this can occur in a child with tetralogy of Fallot who has an aortopulmonary anastomosis (e.g., Blalock-Taussig shunt) that is too large. The high aortic and left ventricular systolic pressures mandate an equally high right ventricular systolic pressure, but the low diastolic aortic pressure reduces coronary perfusion pressure in diastole and can cause both left and right ventricular ischemia and failure.

CHAPTER 43 ■ CARDIORESPIRATORY INTERACTIONS IN CHILDREN WITH HEART DISEASE

LARA SHEKERDEMIAN

Cardiorespiratory interactions describes the physiologic interrelationship between spontaneous or mechanical breathing and the cardiovascular system.

DETERMINANTS OF STROKE VOLUME: THE RIGHT HEART

Under most conditions, right ventricular (RV) stroke volume is primarily determined by RV filling (preload). Intrathoracic pressure is a key determinant of these conditions in health and in disease. Systemic venous return to the right heart is a passive phenomenon that relies on pressure gradients between the peripheral venous circulation, the extrathoracic great veins, and the right heart. At a very simplistic level, the circulation can be considered as

a "3-compartment model," consisting of the thorax, the abdomen, and the peripheries (**Fig. 43.1**). The peripheries are subject to a relatively constant pressure, which approximates atmospheric pressure. The extrathoracic great veins (in the abdomen) are subject to respiratory variations, largely due to diaphragmatic movement; and the intrathoracic veins and the right atrium are subject to pleural pressure.

During spontaneous inspiration, the pleural pressure becomes negative, and the mean right atrial pressure falls. Also during inspiration, the diaphragm descends, thus increasing the pressure to which the extrathoracic great veins are subject. Therefore, venous return from the abdominal compartment and from the peripheral circulation increases during inspiration, as the gradients increase in favor of blood flow to the thorax (**Fig. 43.1**). The increase in venous

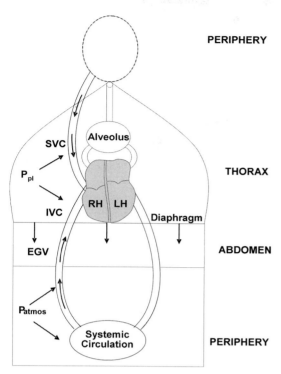

FIGURE 43.1. The "3-compartment" model of circulation. SVC, superior vena cava; IVC, inferior vena cava; EGV, extrathoracic great veins P$_{pl}$, pleural pressure; P$_{atmos}$, atmospheric pressure; RH, right heart; LH, left heart.

return as pleural pressure falls must not be limitless. A critical mean right atrial pressure below which no further increase in systemic venous return could occur exists at a mean right atrial pressure of between 0 and −5 mm Hg. At lower atrial pressures, the intrathoracic great veins tend to collapse, thus mechanically limiting central venous return and preventing right-heart volume overload. However, if, at a given pleural pressure, a bolus of fluid is given, the right atrial pressure and venous return (and therefore cardiac output) can be increased. Within normal physiologic boundaries, it is therefore the atrial pressure rather than pleural pressure that determines the *limits* of venous return.

During positive-pressure ventilation, the reverse occurs. As the intrathoracic pressure becomes increasingly positive, the right atrial pressure increases, and the venous pressure gradient is reduced between the peripheries, the extrathoracic great veins, and the right atrium. This reaction results in a fall in RV preload and can theoretically compromise the RV stroke volume, which may fall. However, in the intact circulation, the use of sensible ventilatory strategies, in tandem with intrinsic compensatory baroreceptor responses, largely mitigates against any overt clini-

cal manifestations of these adverse effects. At higher intrathoracic pressures, at which cardiac output may become compromised even in the healthy heart, colloid administration can help to restore RV preload and cardiac output.

INTRATHORACIC PRESSURE AND RIGHT VENTRICULAR AFTERLOAD

If venous return were the only determinant of cardiac output during positive ventilation, one would expect that, in the presence of normal myocardial function, volume expansion would preserve the cardiac output under conditions of increasing mean airway pressure; however, this is not always the case. Higher intrathoracic pressures and lung volumes directly influence pulmonary vascular resistance and RV afterload and, hence, RV function. Pulmonary interdependence describes the relationship between lung volumes (or alveolar distension) and the status of the pulmonary vessels (**Fig. 43.2**). As the lung volume is increased from residual volume to functional residual capacity, the extra-alveolar pulmonary parenchymal vessels increase in diameter and "straighten out"; thus, pulmonary vascular resistance falls. If a positive intrathoracic pressure is applied and lung volumes increase above functional residual capacity, the alveolar capillaries become stretched and their luminal diameter falls; thus, pulmonary vascular resistance increases. In practice, this phenomenon is observed at high levels of peak end-expiratory pressure (usually well above 10 cm H$_2$O). A fall in lung volume below functional residual capacity is associated with an elevation of

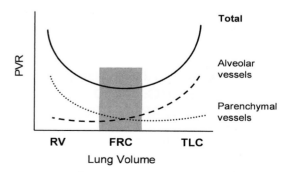

FIGURE 43.2. Lung volumes and pulmonary vascular resistance. Though lung volume has opposite effects on alveolar and parenchymal vessels, both types of vessels have the lowest pulmonary vascular resistance (PVR) at functional residual capacity (FRC). Hence, total PVR is lowest at FRC. RV, residual volume; TLC, total lung capacity.

pulmonary vascular resistance, and at low lung volumes, this may be further compounded by hypoxic pulmonary vasoconstriction (**Fig. 43.2**).

INTRATHORACIC PRESSURE AND THE LEFT VENTRICLE

Left ventricular (LV) stroke volume is determined by its contractility and the impedance to LV ejection or afterload. In a healthy individual, spontaneous and mechanical ventilation primarily influences the right heart. Left ventricular afterload is determined by its transmural pressure. Transmural pressure of an intrathoracic structure is the gradient "across" its wall and relates the measured pressure within the structure to the pressure surrounding it (the pleural pressure). An increased afterload can result from an increase in aortic (or arterial) blood pressure *or* from a fall in pleural pressure. During spontaneous inspiration, the intravascular aortic pressure may fall slightly, but the pleural pressure falls relatively more and becomes negative. Thus, the LV transmural pressure and afterload increase during spontaneous inspiration. In healthy individuals who are spontaneously breathing, respiration predominantly affects the right heart, and subtle changes in afterload of the LV do not adversely affect ventricular function.

However, the impact of changes in pleural pressure on the LV become much more significant if an exaggerated negative pleural pressure is applied. If healthy individuals perform a Mueller maneuver or an inspiratory threshold-loading maneuver, in which the pleural pressure falls to well below –20 cm H_2O, afterload increases significantly, and LV ejection fraction falls. This interaction can occur in otherwise healthy individuals with normal hearts—the "negative pressure pulmonary edema," which can occur during a severe asthma attack or with acute airway obstruction.

POSITIVE-PRESSURE VENTILATION AND LEFT VENTRICULAR AFTERLOAD

Positive-pressure ventilation reduces the transmural LV pressure and, therefore, lowers the LV afterload, which may result in increased LV stroke volume and a lower end-diastolic volume. Although in health, this cardiopulmonary interaction is of little clinical importance, it has important implications for the management of patients with acute and chronic heart failure.

CARDIORESPIRATORY INTERACTIONS IN CHILDREN WITH HEART DISEASE

Ventilation is a valuable though underutilized hemodynamic tool in pediatric cardiac intensive care. When used carefully and tailored according to a clinical situation, ventilation is often far more effective in manipulating the circulatory physiology than are cardiovascular pharmacologic agents (**Table 43.1**).

Cardiorespiratory Interactions during Resting Ventilation

Heart failure with *systolic* ventricular dysfunction is commonly encountered in the PICU. The term *heart failure* covers a broad clinical spectrum that includes the following:

■ Transient ventricular dysfunction after repair of congenital heart disease
■ Severe, acute decompensated heart failure secondary to myocarditis, sepsis, arrhythmia, or ischemia
■ Severe chronic (or acute-on-chronic) heart failure, secondary to dilated cardiomyopathy or congenital heart disease with systemic ventricular failure

Children with systolic heart failure are particularly susceptible to the interactions between spontaneous breathing and the heart for 3 main reasons:

■ LV afterload is elevated at baseline owing to activation of neurohumoral mechanisms, including the renin-angiotensin system and the intrinsic catecholamines.
■ The work of breathing is increased at baseline, compared to healthy individuals, and the negative inspiratory swings in pleural pressure are exaggerated owing to reduced lung compliance and increased lung water secondary to elevated left atrial pressures.
■ The right atrial pressure is increased, and cardiac output is reduced. The capacity of these patients to increase their cardiac output is greatly limited.

During spontaneous inspiration, the afterload on the LV and preload on the RV will further increase. Whereas these cardiorespiratory interactions are well tolerated (or are even desirable) under normal circumstances, they are exaggerated and can further exacerbate ventricular dysfunction in children with systolic heart failure. These interactions become even more pronounced with exertion, stress or agitation—circumstances in which either or both of the work of breathing and vascular tone are increased.

TABLE 43.1

BASIC CARDIORESPIRATORY INTERACTIONS IN CHILDREN WITH HEART DISEASE DURING SPONTANEOUS AND POSITIVE-PRESSURE VENTILATION

	Key issues	Spontaneous respiration	Positive pressure ventilation/CPAP	
Heart failure (acute or chronic)	Elevated LV afterload Systolic LV dysfunction	Increased work of breathing Exaggerated negative intrapleural pressure swings	Increased LV afterload	Reduced work of breathing Obliterated negative swings in pleural pressure	Reduced venous return Reduced LV afterload Improved LV function
Postoperative—tetralogy of Fallot	Good systolic function Diastolic RV dysfunction Preload-dependent	Increased RV preload Improved diastolic pulmonary artery flow	Improved cardiac output	Reduced RV preload Reduced diastolic pulmonary artery flow	Reduced cardiac output
Postoperative—Fontan/BCPS	Good systolic function Preload dependent Cardiac output depends on pulmonary blood flow.	Increased preload Negative intrathoracic pressure improves pulmonary blood flow.	Improved cardiac output	Reduced preload Reduced pulmonary blood flow	Reduced cardiac output
Duct-dependent systemic flow	Excessive pulmonary flow, leading to reduced systemic flow	Tachypnea and oversaturation are common. Limited control of pulmonary flow	Possible excessive pulmonary flow and reduced systemic cardiac output	Better control of pulmonary flow, pH, and pulmonary resistance	Improved systemic cardiac output

CPAP, continuous positive airway pressure; BCPS, bidirectional cavopulmonary shunt; LV, left ventricle; RV, right ventricle

Positive Pressure Ventilation in Heart Failure

Positive pressure ventilation produces beneficial cardiopulmonary interactions in children with acute or chronic heart failure, through a number of mechanisms. Positive pressure respiratory support facilitates the unloading of respiratory muscles, resulting in reduced respiratory effort and work of breathing. By increasing the mean airway pressure and reducing the work of breathing, positive pressure ventilation prevents the exaggerated negative inspiratory swings in spontaneously breathing patients with severe heart failure. A positive intrathoracic pressure lowers the pressure gradient between the thorax and the periphery and reduces the systemic venous return, resulting in reduced RV preload and RV end-systolic and end-diastolic volumes. Although this intervention may reduce stroke volume and cardiac output in the intact circulation, the reduced right-heart volume load in the failing heart results in improved cardiac performance and in better ventriculoventricular interactions.

Through its effects on intrathoracic pressure and work of breathing, positive pressure ventilation reduces the LV transmural pressure, thereby reducing the LV afterload, which improves LV stroke volume and ejection fraction. Patients with heart failure have elevated levels of endogenous catecholamines, increased myocardial oxygen consumption, and elevated cardiac sympathetic tone. These contribute to the elevated afterload and the increased stroke work of the impaired left ventricle. Positive intrathoracic pressure reduces the levels of norepinephrine in patients with chronic heart failure and reduces cardiac sympathetic tone and myocardial oxygen consumption.

The Treatment of Heart Failure with Positive Pressure Ventilation

Open cardiac surgery inevitably results in significant, albeit largely transient, myocardial injury owing to a number of intraoperative factors, including cardiopulmonary bypass, cross-clamp, temperature change, and cardiotomy. This injury is often associated with a degree of early postoperative systolic ventricular dysfunction. Most infants and children are intubated and ventilated with positive pressure ventilation when they are in the PICU early after open-heart surgery. Therefore, part of their "hemodynamic" support routinely includes positive pressure ventilation, which produces desirable effects on RV preload, LV afterload, and the work of breathing. Indeed, some neonates and younger infants will benefit from the continuing hemodynamic benefit of a period of continuous positive airway pressure (CPAP) immediately after endotracheal extubation.

Positive pressure ventilation is clearly beneficial for children with ventricular dysfunction, but in the nonsurgical setting, these are patients in whom the process of intubation may itself cause significant hemodynamic compromise. However, positive pressure ventilation does not necessarily require endotracheal intubation; it can safely and effectively be delivered to children of all ages via a face mask or a nasopharyngeal tube. Noninvasive positive pressure ventilation (CPAP or bilevel positive airway pressure), is now a mainstay of therapy in hospitalized adults with acute pulmonary edema secondary to decompensated heart failure. In these patients, noninvasive ventilation via CPAP or bilevel positive airway pressure results in symptomatic improvement, a reduced need for endotracheal intubation, and reduced early mortality. In adults with chronic congestive heart failure, CPAP improves cardiac volumes and LV ejection fraction. Long-term CPAP also improves functional status and quality of life in patients with end-stage heart failure.

Cardiorespiratory Interactions in Functionally Univentricular Circulation

The unifying feature of the preoperative and/or postoperative circulatory physiology of infants with functionally univentricular circulation is that the perfusion of the pulmonary and systemic (including coronary) circulations is from the output of a single (or functionally single) ventricle (**Table 43.2**). Thus, the relative delivery of the ventricular output to the systemic and pulmonary vascular beds depends on the relative resistances of the 2 circulations.

Infants with a critically obstructed systemic circulation, such as hypoplastic left-heart syndrome and its variants, have a duct-dependent systemic circulation at birth. Ductal patency requires pharmacologic treatment with prostaglandin. However, once the duct is wide open, the subsequent distribution of the cardiac output depends solely upon the resistance of the pulmonary and systemic circulations. If the systemic vasculature is constricted, blood preferentially flows to the lungs, compromising systemic and myocardial perfusion, clinically manifested as oversaturation, acidosis, end-organ dysfunction, and myocardial ischemia. Infants with

TABLE 43.2

NEWBORNS AND YOUNG INFANTS WITH FUNCTIONALLY UNIVENTRICULAR CIRCULATION: DIAGNOSTIC GROUPS

Diagnostic group	Preoperative physiology	Postoperative physiology
Hypoplastic left-heart syndrome (and variants)	Duct-dependent systemic circulation	Norwood-type operation
Interrupted aortic arch and ventricular septal defect	Duct-dependent systemic circulation	Biventricular circulation[a]
Truncus arteriosus	Single-outlet heart	Biventricular circulation[a]
Critically obstructed pulmonary circulation	Duct-dependent pulmonary circulation[a]	Neonatal systemic-pulmonary artery shunt

[a] Circulatory physiology, in which cardiopulmonary interactions do not fall within the scope of this chapter.

truncus arteriosus or hypoplastic left-heart syndrome are known to be the subgroup with congenital heart disease that is at greatest risk of neonatal necrotizing enterocolitis, which directly results from gut ischemia.

The pulmonary vasculature of neonates is highly sensitive to the vasodilating effects of inspired oxygen and alkalosis and to the constricting effects of carbon dioxide and acidosis. Routine resuscitation and early neonatal care of the infant with known or suspected duct-dependent systemic perfusion should include the avoidance, or cautious administration of, supplemental oxygen and the avoidance of significant alkalosis. In addition, pain and agitation should be avoided in all of these patients, so that sudden increases in systemic vascular resistance do not exacerbate systemic hypoperfusion.

Preoperative mechanical ventilation is commonly required in infants with functionally univentricular circulation, most frequently to optimize systemic perfusion. Ventilation can be used to control respiratory rate (and avoid respiratory alkalosis), to control the oxygen saturation, to optimize arterial carbon dioxide levels, to enable the administration of sedating agents, and to stabilize pulmonary vascular resistance.

In the early postoperative period following Norwood-type operations or placement of neonatal systemic-to-pulmonary artery shunts, ventilation should similarly be tailored to optimize systemic oxygen delivery, using the same basic principles. Optimal systemic oxygen delivery occurs when the pulmonary-to-systemic flow ratio (Qp/Qs) is ~1:1, corresponding to a systemic oxygen saturation of ~80%. The addition of 3% carbon dioxide to the ventilator circuit improves mixed venous saturation without changing systemic arterial saturation in both the preoperative and postoperative settings, suggest-

ing that supplemental carbon dioxide, but not nitrogen, improves systemic oxygen delivery in the functionally univentricular circulation.

Cardiorespiratory Interactions after the Fontan Operation

A low cardiac output state can complicate the early postoperative course of children after Fontan operations, only rarely due to systolic dysfunction of the systemic ventricle. The cause of this complication is much more commonly low output secondary to diastolic dysfunction or reduced pulmonary blood flow. Extubation undoubtedly results in a fall in central venous and, therefore, pulmonary artery pressures and an improvement in systemic cardiac output in Fontan patients.

Pulmonary blood flow is the key determinant of cardiac output in Fontan patients. In brief, the key elements of the Fontan circulation are that the systemic veins are in continuity with the pulmonary arteries, either through direct (cavopulmonary) anastomoses or via an atriopulmonary connection. The pulmonary venous return is to a pulmonary venous (left or common) atrium. In the absence of a subpulmonary pumping chamber, pulmonary blood flow is a passive phenomenon that is driven by a sufficient pressure difference across the lungs—or between the systemic veins and the pulmonary venous atrium. Negative-pressure ventilation using a cuirass device with a mean airway pressure of -6 to -9 cm H_2O may increase pulmonary blood flow.

Basic principles that should be followed in managing ventilation of children immediately after Fontan operations include (a) establishing spontaneous breathing early while intubated; (b) maintaining low peak end-expiratory pressure (3–5 cm H_2O);

(c) minimizing mean airway pressures; and (d) extubating early.

Cardiopulmonary Interactions after the Bidirectional Cavopulmonary Shunt

Pulmonary blood flow is the key determinant of systemic oxygen delivery in infants and children after a bidirectional cavopulmonary shunt (BCPS, or Glenn operation). Similar to Fontan patients, pulmonary blood flow in these patients is a passive phenomenon that depends on adequate venous return to a low-resistance pulmonary circulation. A unique feature of infants and children with a BCPS (but not of Fontan patients) is that pulmonary blood flow is entirely derived from upper-body (and cerebral) venous return. The systemic arterial oxygen saturations after a BCPS are highly indicative of pulmonary blood flow and systemic cardiac output. These patients are highly preload-dependent, and simple colloid or blood transfusion can produce improvements in arterial saturation. In patients who have undergone a BCPS, significant elevations of central venous (pulmonary artery) pressure, related to venous obstruction, pulmonary hypertension, or the use of excessively high airway pressures, result in venous congestion of the upper body, usually associated with systemic desaturation and signs of reduced systemic oxygen delivery. Similar to Fontan patients, extubation of infants and children after a BCPS is associated with hemodynamic improvement, with an increase in systemic cardiac output and a fall in pulmonary artery pressure.

Routine postoperative ventilatory practice after a BCPS should be tailored to optimizing systemic oxygen delivery and cerebral blood flow. On returning from the operating room, these patients should routinely be cared for with elevation of the upper body to assist systemic venous drainage, thereby encouraging pulmonary blood flow. In these patients, an increase in mean airway pressure reduces the pulmonary blood flow and, hence, systemic cardiac output. It is therefore standard practice to manage these infants similarly to the Fontan patient, using conservative airway pressures and aiming for early extubation. In ventilated patients with significant arterial hypoxemia early after a BCPS, a mild respiratory acidosis may result in improved oxygenation and systemic oxygen delivery. However, the strategy used to achieve this outcome is extremely important: Alveolar derecruitment is highly undesirable, as it is likely to complicate subsequent ventilatory weaning. Similar to infants with hypoplastic left-heart syndrome, therefore, a mild respiratory acidosis should be achieved through the addition of carbon dioxide to the inspired ventilator gases rather than by deliberate hypoventilation.

Cardiorespiratory Interactions in Patients with Diastolic Right Ventricular Dysfunction early after Tetralogy of Fallot Repair

A small subgroup of infants with a low cardiac output early after surgery, with elevated venous pressures and refractoriness to standard pharmacologic agents, systolic ventricular function is usually well preserved. Some of these patients have restrictive RV physiology early after tetralogy repair with a low cardiac output state. The hallmark of restrictive physiology is diastolic anterograde flow into the pulmonary artery, coincident with atrial systole. Although abnormal, this antegrade diastolic pulmonary arterial flow represents an important source of cardiac output and limits the duration of pulmonary regurgitation within the cardiac cycle. It would follow that a reduction in, or loss of, this flow could precipitate further clinical decline in some patients, or conversely, that augmentation of the flow could confer a hemodynamic benefit. The cardiac output of children with restrictive RV physiology after tetralogy of Fallot repair is highly sensitive to changes in intrathoracic pressure.

In children with restrictive physiology who are receiving positive pressure ventilation early after tetralogy repair, antegrade forward pulmonary artery flow is reduced during the inspiratory phase but is relatively preserved during expiration, suggesting that an increasingly positive intrathoracic pressure caused a significant reduction in pulmonary blood flow and, hence, cardiac output. Spontaneous inspiration augments diastolic pulmonary artery flow of infants with restrictive physiology. The principles of ventilatory management of children early after tetralogy repair should be similar to those in Fontan patients, with the use of conservative airway pressures and early establishment of spontaneous respiration. The first step in managing a child with a low cardiac output after tetralogy repair is to perform a detailed echocardiogram. If this test confirms restrictive physiology, the appropriate ventilatory strategies—use of conservative mean airway pressures and early establishment of spontaneous respiration—should be applied while minimizing the doses of inotropic agents.

Interestingly, restrictive RV physiology is not only an immediate postoperative phenomenon but affects a proportion of children and adults late after surgery. It is also likely that early restrictive physiology predicts its presence later in life, with identical associated cardiopulmonary interactions.

CHAPTER 44 ■ HEMODYNAMIC MONITORING

GILLIAN C. HALLEY • SHANE TIBBY

An ideal monitoring system would be noninvasive, safe, associated with no discomfort, and responsive to change in real time. The data collected would be reliable, accurate, repeatable, and continuously displayed, and the system would have the ability to store and retrieve information. As this ideal system does not yet exist, the potential benefits involved in monitoring patients must be balanced against the risks. As a general rule, the least invasive monitoring that is appropriate should always be used. The use of invasive monitoring should be reserved for those patients in whom it is essential for diagnosis, patient safety, or assessment of interventions or therapies.

PHYSICAL EXAMINATION

In the PICU, examination and reassessment are used to continuously monitor patients (**Table 44.1**).

ECG

A 12-lead electrocardiogram (ECG) is required to fully assess an abnormal rhythm, but much information can be gained from a 3-lead ECG (right arm, left arm, and indifferent leads). A rhythm strip from lead II is useful for displaying dysrhythmias. The CM5 configuration is able to detect 89% of ST segment changes due to left ventricular (LV) ischemia. In the CM5 configuration, the right-arm electrode is placed on the manubrium (*c*hest lead from *m*anubrium), and the left-arm electrode is on V5 position (5th interspace in left anterior axillary line). ECG interpretation can assist in the evaluation of heart rate and rhythm, ischemia, and conduction defects. Due to the relatively small stroke volume and the nature of the neonatal myocardium, changes in the heart rate of an infant will have a greater impact on cardiac output compared to an older child or adult. The ECG can be used as a trend monitor following cardiac surgery when changes in heart rate can assist in management decisions regarding intravascular volume requirements or choice of inotrope. Continuous bedside ECG monitoring can alert to the presence of myocardial ischemia (ST segment changes) or hyperkalemia (peaked T waves). The ECG is important in assessing whether a postoperative tachycardia is a sinus rhythm in origin. In this setting, p-wave identification may be aided by recording the ECG at a higher speed (50 mm/sec) or by utilizing surgically placed, temporary atrial pacing wires that can be attached to the ECG leads.

NONINVASIVE BLOOD PRESSURE MEASUREMENT

Systemic blood pressure (BP) is a fundamental cardiovascular parameter that varies with age, although the pressure obtained at any given time will also vary with the patient's underlying physiologic or pathophysiologic condition. Several methods of indirect arterial BP measurement have been developed, including the palpation method (Riva-Rocci), the auscultatory method (Korotkoff sounds), the oscillometric method, the rheographic method, the phase-shift method, and ultrasonic arterial wall motion detector. The cuff consists of an inflatable bladder within a restrictive cloth sheath and is connected to an inflation bulb that contains a control-release valve. In children, it is important that the center of the bladder (usually marked with an arrow) is placed directly over the artery. Turbulent blood flow, shock-wave formation, and instability of the arterial wall produce a series of audible frequencies (the Korotkoff sounds) as the external occluding pressure on a major artery is reduced (**Fig. 44.1**). Korotkoff sounds can be heard using a stethoscope or amplified using a Doppler device, which is particularly useful in infants and small children. The cuff is inflated above systolic BP (SBP) (the pulse is abolished) and then deflated slowly (~2–3 mm Hg/sec). When the cuff pressure is less than systolic, the arterial wall is partly open, and turbulent blood flow becomes audible. When cuff pressure is below diastolic blood pressure (DBP), the sounds muffle or disappear completely, as flow is no longer obstructed.

Phase I	systolic value, first sound
Phases II and III	sound character changes
Phase IV	sound becomes muffled
Phase V	sound becomes absent

DBP is recorded at Phase IV or V.

Automated BP devices such as Dinamap (*d*evice for *i*ndirect *n*oninvasive *m*ean *a*rterial *p*ressure) have

TABLE 44.1

CLINICAL MONITORING TOOLS FOR CARDIAC OUTPUT

Level of consciousness, activity, or agitation
State of hydration
Peripheral edema
Respiratory pattern
Peripheral perfusion/capillary refill time
Toe-core temperature gap
Heart rate and rhythm
Pulse characteristics
Urine output
Hepatomegaly
Jugular venous pressure
Pulmonary and cardiac auscultation

reduced the incidence of error associated with the manual technique of measurement. These devices employ the oscillometric method and can measure heart rate as well as SBP, DBP, and mean BP (MBP). The principal is that blood flow through a vessel produces oscillations of the arterial wall, and these are transmitted to an inflatable cuff. As the cuff pressure decreases, a characteristic change in the magnitude of oscillations occurs, which generates SBP, DBP, and MBP. SBP is recorded when a rapid increase occurs in oscillation amplitude, and at this point, arterial pres-

sure just exceeds cuff pressure. The mean pressure reading is taken at the maximum amplitude of oscillations during cuff deflation. The DBP coincides with a sudden decrease in oscillations.

One of the most important factors affecting the accuracy of measurement is the cuff size relative to the patient. A narrow cuff produces a higher pressure, and a wide cuff produces an artificially low pressure. The American Heart Association recommends that the width of the inflatable bladder be 40% of the mid-circumference of the limb and that the length should be twice the width. In children, the occluding bladder should be long enough to encircle the limb completely, as overlapping of the ends of the bladder in children does not appear to introduce an error in measurement. The accuracy of measurement is improved with slow cuff *deflation*, as this aids the detection of arterial pulsations. Rapid cuff *inflation* will help to avoid venous congestion. In shivering patients, muscle contraction around the artery lowers tissue compliance, which can raise the SBP artifactually ("pseudohypertension"). External pressure on the cuff or tubing can cause inaccurate reading. The accuracy is reduced in the presence of low cardiac output, significant hypotension, hypoperfusion, or vasoconstriction, dysrhythmias, or excessive body edema. The cuff pressure will tend to over-read in the presence of hypotension and under-read in the presence of is hypertension.

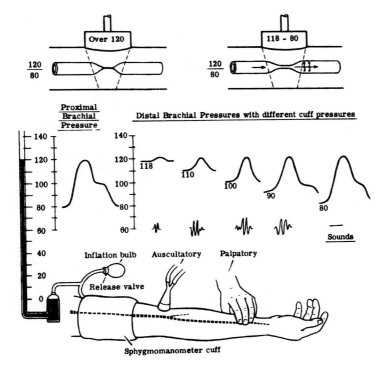

FIGURE 44.1. Method of obtaining blood pressure with a blood pressure cuff and Korotkoff sounds. From Abel FL, McCutcheon EP, *Cardiovascular function principles and applications.* Boston: Little Brown, 1979:231, with permission.

ARTERIAL BLOOD PRESSURE MONITORING

Pedal pressure is significantly higher than radial pressure in children. The equipment required for invasive BP monitoring includes an arterial cannula with a heparinized saline column and flushing device, a transducer, an amplifier, and an oscilloscope. A continuous column of fluid from the blood vessel lumen to the transducer diaphragm transmits variations in intraluminal pressure, causing changes in resistance and current that are converted into an electrical signal, which is amplified to display a waveform and digital pressure on the bedside monitor. The optimal dynamic response is achieved with a system that contains a liquid with low viscosity and minimal air bubble trapping in tubing that is short and wide with stiff walls. An optimal dynamic response results in one undershoot below baseline, followed by a much smaller overshoot above baseline, before returning to the underlying waveform (**Fig. 44.2**). In both underdamping and overdamping, the MBP is relatively unaffected.

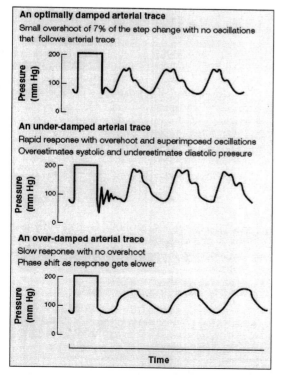

FIGURE 44.2. Quantification of the degree of damping via the fast-flush test. Reproduced from Anaesthesia UK Web site http://www.frca.co.uk/article.aspx?articleid=100382, with permission. Accessed 08/02/07.

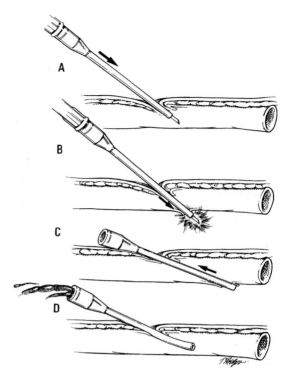

FIGURE 44.3. Radial artery cannulation. The catheter-over-needle unit is inserted into the artery (**A**). When arterial blood flow is seen in the needle hub, the catheter may be advanced over the needle into the artery. Another technique is to further advance the catheter and needle until blood flow ceases, thereby transfixing the artery (**B**), and to then remove the needle (**C**) and withdraw the catheter until blood flow is seen. The catheter is then advanced into the artery (**D**).

Cannulation can be performed by the transfixation method or the direct threading technique (**Fig. 44.3**). The risk of distal limb ischemia is increased in end arteries such as the brachial arteries that have a very poor collateral circulation. The radial artery is the most frequent site for cannulation, as this site is easy to access and has a low associated complication rate. Early cannulation of the umbilical artery may enable preservation of femoral vessels in the newborn who will need subsequent catheter or surgical procedures. However, the risk of infection and necrotizing enterocolitis must be considered in this population, and early removal of umbilical catheters is prudent.

In infants with patent ductus arteriosus, it is worth remembering that the right radial arterial blood represents blood oxygen saturation to the brain, as the right subclavian, right common, and left common carotid arteries originate from the aorta proximal to the duct. The left subclavian and descending aorta represent the postductal oxygen saturation, which is lower in the presence of a right-to-left shunt through the patent ductus arteriosus.

Collateral blood flow to the hand can be assessed by the Allen test prior to inserting the catheter, though the predictive value and benefit in children is questionable. Other sites of cannulation include ulnar, femoral, axillary, dorsalis pedis, and posterior tibial arteries. Catheterization of the femoral vein and artery in the same leg may increase the risk of limb ischemia, especially in low-flow states or when potent vasoconstrictors are used.

Vasospasm and thrombosis are the principal causes of arterial catheter failure. The addition of heparin (1 U/mL) and papaverine (a smooth muscle relaxant; 30 mg/250 mL) to the catheter infusion solution (0.9% or 0.45% NaCl) decreases the incidence of catheter failure. If arterial cannulation leads to thrombosis and early signs of circulatory compromise to an extremity, current guidelines recommend immediate catheter removal and systemic heparinization with unfractionated heparin. Thrombolytic therapy with tissue plasminogen activator may be added, if perfusion does not improve in 24 hrs. If all medical management fails, balloon thrombectomy via an arteriotomy can be employed to prevent limb loss.

Pulsus paradoxus is an exaggeration of the normal fall in SBP that occurs during the inspiratory phase of spontaneous breathing. During inspiration with spontaneous breathing, venous return to the right atrium and therefore right ventricular (RV) stroke volume increase, but venous return to the left atrium and LV stroke volume decrease. During positive-pressure breathing, pulsus paradoxus is reflected as an exaggerated SBP drop during the expiratory phase. Pulsus paradoxus is a classic sign of cardiac tamponade but can also be seen in constrictive pericarditis, early restrictive cardiomyopathy, or severe hyperinflation of the lungs, especially when combined with hypovolemia.

A common source of error is an inaccurate transducer level. Zero reference, or atmospheric pressure, must be set with the transducer at the same level as the chamber being measured—in this case, the heart. Recordings should be made with the child in the supine position and the transducer at the level of the mid-chest or mid-axillary line. If the transducer is set lower than the reference level, the pressure readings are falsely high, and if it is set higher than reference, the pressure is falsely low. Raising or lowering the system can introduce errors of 7.5 mm Hg for each 10 cm change in position. Regular zeroing is required to counteract baseline drift. Careful flushing of the catheter and pressure tubing to remove blood and air bubbles and choosing the shortest, stiffest, and largest catheter will minimize these errors.

TABLE 44.2

COMPLICATIONS OF INVASIVE BLOOD PRESSURE MONITORING

Bleeding
Thrombosis
Hematoma
Infection
Vascular compromise
Nerve damage
Accidental injection of air or thrombus
Digital necrosis
Arteriovenous fistulae
Carpal tunnel syndrome
Lymphatic damage

The risks of invasive arterial monitoring include bleeding, infection, vascular compromise, nerve damage, and accidental injection of hyperosmolar solutions (**Table 44.2**). Important additional risk factors for distal limb ischemia in children are critical illness, low cardiac output states, use of vasopressors, and large catheter size relative to the dimensions of the artery. In adults, it has been shown that the incidence of arterial occlusion (**Table 44.3**) increases linearly as the ratio of catheter outer diameter to vessel inner diameter increases, and this is even more important in children, in whom vessels are smaller; however, the catheter size cannot be reduced proportionally. Risk factors for catheter-related infection of arterial lines include the use of an arterial system that permits backflow of blood into the pressure tubing and the duration of catheterization. Care should be taken during flushing of arterial lines, particularly with axillary arterial catheters due to the risk of cerebral embolization of air or debris.

CENTRAL VENOUS PRESSURE MONITORING

Central venous cannulation allows secure IV access in critically ill children who may require large-volume fluid infusions or parenteral nutrition, and it is

---

TABLE 44.3

FACTORS THAT INCREASE THE RISK OF VASCULAR THROMBOSIS

Prolonged cannulation
Injection of hyperosmolar solutions
Underlying thrombogenic condition
Large catheter size
Multiple puncture attempts
Low flow states

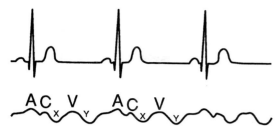

FIGURE 44.4. Central venous pressure trace with corresponding ECG. See text for explanation. From O'Rourke RA. The measurement of systemic blood pressure: Normal and abnormal pulsations of the arteries and veins. In: Hurst JW, ed. *The Heart.* New York: McGraw-Hill, 1990:159, with permission.

essential for the infusion of vasoactive drugs such as epinephrine and norepinephrine. A central venous catheter is not only essential for monitoring central venous pressure (CVP), which allows an indirect measurement of cardiac preload, but it provides access for blood sampling for measurement of mixed venous saturation. The monitoring of trends in mixed venous saturation enables trending of cardiac output in the absence of other continuous cardiac output devices.

The normal CVP trace has three positive waves (*a*, *c*, and *v*) and two negative waves (*x* and *y*). The *a* wave is caused by atrial contraction (after the P wave on the ECG), the *c* wave is caused by ventricular contraction against a closed tricuspid valve, and the *v* wave is caused by atrial filling. The x descent is due to the tricuspid valve being pulled away from the right atrium by the contracting ventricle, while the y descent occurs as the tricuspid valve opens and blood enters the ventricle (**Fig. 44.4**). The pattern of this waveform can change in pathologic conditions, as with the cannon *a* waves seen in complete heart block. In the presence of normal tricuspid valve function, the CVP is equal to the RV end-diastolic pressure, which is proportional to RV end-diastolic volume, which is the preload to the RV. The exact relationship between volume and pressure is compliance of the ventricle. It is important to avoid considering CVP purely as a reflection of "volume loading" of the ventricle, as ventricular compliance, afterload, and contractility will all affect the CVP. A change in CVP following a fluid challenge will depend on the state of venous filling and the compliance of venous capacitance vessels, as well as RV function and compliance. The CVP is measured using a catheter in a central vein with a reference point of the right atrium. Accurate zeroing is even more important than with the arterial system. The CVP will also vary with changes in intrapleural pressure that occur during spontaneous or positive-pressure breathing. The site of the

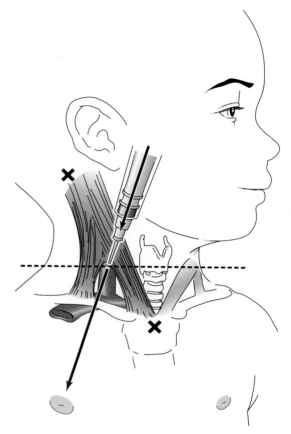

FIGURE 44.5. Internal jugular cannulation using the Seldinger technique. The head is turned to the opposite side, with needle puncture at the apex of the triangle formed by the heads of the sternocleidomastoid muscle (midway between the sternal notch and the mastoid process). The needle is aimed at the ipsilateral nipple. Adapted from Schleien CL. Cardiopulmonary resuscitation. In: Nichols DG, Yaster M, Lappe DG, et al., eds. *Golden Hour—The Handbook of Advanced Pediatric Life Support.* St Louis: Mosby—Year Book, 1991:124.

catheter will affect the absolute values obtained. Although trend monitoring from a non-central site (e.g., femoral venous catheter with a tip in the abdominal vena cava) is often used, elevated intrapleural pressures from high levels of positive-pressure ventilation can lead to significant differences between intrathoracic and intra-abdominal CVP measurements.

The Seldinger technique is used for catheter placement, and common sites include the internal jugular, subclavian, and femoral veins (**Fig. 44.5**). ECG monitoring is essential during central line placement because of the risk of inducing dysrhythmias when wires or catheters enter the heart. Careful positioning of the patient is important to the success of cannulation and to minimize the complications inherent in placement of a central venous catheter (**Table 44.2**). Ultrasonic guidance can be useful, though this is technically more difficult in the small patient. The risk of inadvertent arterial cannulation can be minimized by confirming three indicators of proper central venous placement in every patient: venous O_2 saturation, venous pressure waveform, and central vein location on x-ray.

Central venous catheters significantly increase the risk of infection in critically ill patients. They are also associated with long-term complications (**Table 44.2**) such as thrombosis (**Table 44.3**). Various strategies have been suggested to limit the associated morbidity, such as the use of heparin infusions or heparin-bonded catheters to reduce thrombosis risk, strategies to limit bacterial contamination with meticulous sterile techniques, antibiotic impregnated catheters, and smaller-diameter catheters.

LEFT ATRIAL PRESSURE MONITORING

The CVP estimates the LV end-diastolic pressure when cardiac and pulmonary functions are normal;

however, this does not commonly occur in the PICU. Therefore, a surgically placed left atrial catheter can be a very useful monitoring tool in the postoperative period, particularly when right atrial pressure is unlikely to reflect left atrial pressure, as in marked RV failure, pulmonary hypertension, and/or left failure. The most devastating complication of left atrial lines is the introduction of air embolism or thromboembolism, which may lead to stroke, myocardial infarction, or necrotizing enterocolitis. These risks are minimized by avoiding blood draws and flushes through the left atrial line. These lines should be removed as soon as possible after cardiac surgery (generally within 2 days).

CARDIAC OUTPUT MEASUREMENT

Cardiac output is the volume of blood ejected by the systemic ventricle each minute, typically measured in L/min. It is customary in pediatrics to index this measurement to body surface area (L/min/m^2), which results in a common reference range throughout infancy and childhood (**Table 44.4**). Once the decision

TABLE 44.4

COMMON HEMODYNAMIC VARIABLES

Parameter	Formula	Normal range	Units
Cardiac index	CI = CO/body surface area	3.5–5.5	L/min/m^2
Stroke index	SI = CI/heart rate	30–60	mL/m^2
Systemic vascular resistance index	SVRI = 79.9 × (MAP − CVP)/CI	800–1600	dyne-sec/cm^5/m^2
Pulmonary vascular resistance index	PVRI = 79.9 × (MPAP − LAP)/CI	80–240	dyne-sec/cm^5/m^2
Left ventricular stroke work index	LVSWI = SI × MAP × 0.0136	50–62 (adult)	g-m/m^2
Right ventricular stroke work index	RVSWI = SI × MAP × 0.0136	5.1–6.9 (adult)	g-m/m^2
Arterial oxygen content	CaO$_2$ = (1.34 × Hb × SaO$_2$) + (PaO$_2$ × 0.003)		mL/L
Oxygen delivery	DO$_2$ = CI × CaO$_2$	570–670	mL/min/m^2
Fick principle	CI = VO$_2$/(CaO$_2$ − CvO$_2$)	160–180 (infant VO$_2$)	mL/min/m^2
		100–130 (child VO$_2$)	mL/min/m^2
Mixed venous oxygen saturation		65%–75%	
Oxygen extraction ratio[a]	OER = (SaO$_2$ − SvO$_2$)/SaO$_2$	0.24–0.28	

CI, cardiac index; CO, cardiac output; SI, stroke index; SVRI, systemic vascular resistance index; MAP, mean systemic arterial pressure (mm Hg); CVP, central venous pressure (mm Hg); PVRI, pulmonary vascular resistance index; MPAP, mean pulmonary arterial pressure; LAP, left atrial pressure; LVSWI, left ventricular stroke work index; RVSWI, right ventricular stroke work index; CaO$_2$, arterial oxygen content; Hb, hemoglobin concentration (g/L); SaO$_2$, arterial oxygen saturation; PaO$_2$, partial pressure of dissolved oxygen; DO$_2$, oxygen delivery; VO$_2$, oxygen consumption; CvO$_2$, mixed venous oxygen content; OER, oxygen extraction ratio; SvO$_2$, mixed venous oxygen saturation.
[a]The equation given for OER is valid only if the contribution from dissolved oxygen is minimal. If this is not the case, oxygen content (CaO$_2$, CvO$_2$) must be substituted for saturation (SaO$_2$, SvO$_2$).

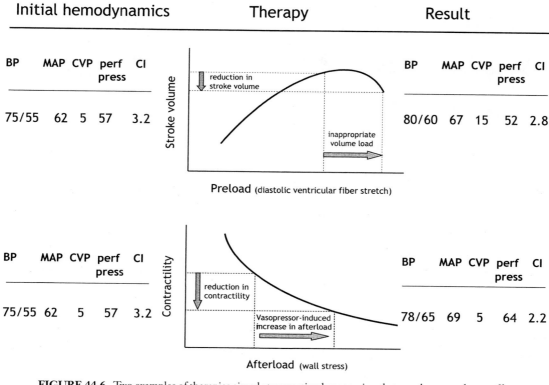

FIGURE 44.6. Two examples of therapies aimed at correcting hypotension that may have an adverse effect on cardiac output. In the top figure, an inappropriate volume load is given, resulting in an increase in blood pressure at the expense of a decrease in both cardiac output and perfusion pressure. In the bottom figure, the same initial hemodynamic profile is treated with vasoconstrictors, again increasing the mean blood pressure with a detrimental effect on cardiac output. BP, blood pressure; MAP, mean arterial blood pressure; CVP, central venous pressure; perf press, perfusion pressure (all mm Hg); CI, cardiac index (L/min/m²).

is made to measure cardiac output, a suggested checklist for its interpretation includes the following:

1. Is flow adequate for *this* patient at *this* time? Two common markers of adequacy of flow are blood lactate and mixed (or central) venous oxygen saturation.
2. How has the patient responded to the chosen therapy? An accurate measure of cardiac output and its associated determinants (preload, diastolic function, contractility, heart rate, afterload) may allow for an informed choice of therapy. Therapies instituted to correct hypotension are likely to have an affect on cardiac output, which may be detrimental despite correcting the BP (**Fig. 44.6**).

SPECIFIC TECHNIQUES

A valuable aspect of the Fick principle is that it allows cardiac output to be calculated separately for the systemic (Q_s) and pulmonary (Q_p) circulations. In the absence of an anatomic shunt, the cardiac output from both sides of the heart is essentially the same; thus $Q_p:Q_s = 1$ (ignoring the small amount of right-to-left shunt from thebesian and bronchial venous veins). However, in the presence of a shunt, the Fick equation can be rearranged to calculate the ratio of pulmonary-to-systemic blood flow ($Q_p:Q_s$).

$$Q_p = \frac{VO_2}{C_{pulm\,vein} - C_{pulm\,artery}}$$

$$Q_s = \frac{VO_2}{C_{aorta} - C_{mixed\,venous}}$$

$$Q_p:Q_s = \frac{C_{aorta} - C_{mixed\,venous}}{C_{pulm\,vein} - C_{pulm\,artery}}$$

$$\approx \frac{O_2\,sat_{aorta} - O_2\,sat_{mixed\,venous}}{O_2\,sat_{pulm\,vein} - O_2\,sat_{pulm\,artery}}$$

Care must be taken to sample at the correct anatomic site relative to the shunt. For example (**Fig. 44.7**), with a large atrial septal defect exhibiting a pure left-to-right shunt, systemic venous blood must be measured upstream to the atrium.

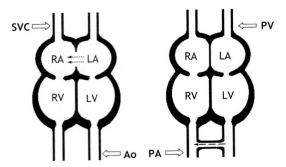

FIGURE 44.7. Calculation of pulmonary to systemic blood flow (Q_p:Q_s) in the setting of an anatomic shunt. The example on the left shows a large atrial septal defect with left-to-right shunt. In this setting, mixed venous blood should be sampled upstream of the shunt, for example, in the superior vena cava. On the right is a patent ductus arteriosus with pure left-to-right flow. Here, pulmonary artery blood should be sampled downstream of the shunt, to allow calculation of Q_p:Q_s. SVC, superior vena cava; RA, right atrium; LA, left atrium; RV, right ventricle; LV, left ventricle; Ao, aorta; PA, pulmonary artery; PV, pulmonary veins.

Oxygen content in the arterial and mixed venous blood is measured using co-oximetry (saturation) and a routine blood gas analyzer (PaO_2), via the formula:

$$O_2 \text{ content (mL } O_2 \text{ per liter of blood)} =$$
$$[1.34 \times \text{Hb (g/L)} \times \% \text{ saturation}/100] +$$
$$[PaO_2 \text{ (mm Hg)} \times 0.003]$$

where Hb = hemoglobin.

Cardiac output can be measured by multiple different techniques including thermodilution, carbon dioxide rebreathing, and dye dilution. All dilution techniques follow a similar principle. An indicator is injected into a central vein, and cardiac output is calculated by measuring the change in blood indicator concentration over time at a point downstream of the injection (**Table 44.5**). Calculation of the area under the curve is a fundamental challenge shared by all indicator methods, largely due to the problem of recirculation.

TABLE 44.5

DILUTION METHODS FOR DETERMINING CARDIAC OUTPUT

Method	Advantages	Disadvantages	Additional variables measured
Thermodilution: (pulmonary artery sampling)	Proven track record; semicontinuous mode available	Variations in cardiac output with respiratory cycle; difficult access in small patients; inaccurate at low flow; low but significant morbidity: infection, bleeding, catheter knotting	Pulmonary pressure; wedge pressure; mixed venous oxygen saturation
Thermodilution: transpulmonary (systemic artery sampling)	Easy access in small patients; repeatable; continuous if device is combined with arterial pulse contour method (combination commercially available)	Requires dedicated arterial line, safe length of insertion time unknown, frequent recalibration required if used in conjunction with pulse contour method	Intrathoracic blood volume (preload); cardiac function index (contractility); extravascular lung water; stroke volume variability (if used with pulse contour method)
Dye dilution	Accurate	Sequential measurements limited by dye clearance; commercial availability of dye and devices	
Lithium chloride dilution	Utilizes pre-existing central venous and arterial lines; continuous if device is combined with arterial pulse contour method (combination commercially available)	Sequential measurements limited by lithium clearance; theoretical risk of toxicity; requires blood sample with each measurement; unlicensed in <40kg; frequent recalibration required if used in conjunction with pulse contour method	Stroke volume variability (if used with pulse contour method)

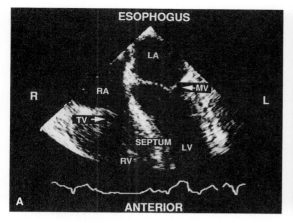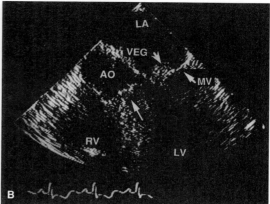

FIGURE 44.8. Two-dimensional transesophageal echocardiograms. (**A**) Four-chamber view showing left atrium (LA), right atrium (RA), right ventricle (RV), left ventricle (LV), with the septum and atrioventricular (AV) valves in the normal position. (**B**) Four-chamber view showing the aortic outflow (AO), LA, RV, and LV. In the center of the mitral valve (MV) is a highly echogenic vegetation (VEG). A subaortic membrane is also present (*arrow*).

Doppler ultrasound can be used as a stand-alone technique but is more commonly employed as an integral adjunct to bedside echocardiography. Echocardiography can provide a vast amount of functional and morphologic information in addition to cardiac output measurement, including indices of diastolic dysfunction, regional wall abnormalities, valve regurgitation, pericardial effusion, chamber dilatation, and cardiac chamber interdependence (**Fig. 44.8**).

MARKERS OF ADEQUACY OF FLOW

Mixed Venous Oxygen Saturation

The normal mixed venous oxygen saturation is ~73% (range, 65%–75%). The "typical" range for the arteriovenous oxygen saturation difference is 20%–33%, though this is highly variable and related to multiple factors. Because of the technical difficulties of measuring cardiac output in clinical practice, several measures of adequacy of organ flow and O_2 delivery are employed.

The oxygen extraction ratio can also be calculated as the following:

$$\text{oxygen extraction ratio} = (SaO_2 - SvO_2) / SaO_2$$

Normal values are between 0.24 and 0.28.

Blood Lactate

Hyperlactatemia can have multiple etiologies. A common cause, *tissue dysoxia*, whereby the cells can-

not utilize delivered oxygen, may be seen in states of mitochondrial dysfunction associated with sepsis, poisoning, and various inborn errors of metabolism. A second cause is accelerated aerobic glycolysis, in which lactate is generated predominantly from skeletal muscle.

Near Infrared Spectroscopy (Optical Monitoring Methods)

A variety of optical methods for measuring tissue perfusion are available, including laser Doppler flowmetry, near infrared spectroscopy (NIRS), orthogonal polarization spectral imaging, and the peripheral perfusion index. Among these techniques, NIRS has gained the most popularity. The commercially available NIRS device (INVOS System, Somanetics, Troy, MI) utilizes a sensor placed over the forehead to emit and detect the near-infrared light. The algorithm is weighted to sample venous blood predominantly. Hence, the numeric display reflects the venous O_2 saturation of the region of the brain being sampled (SrO_2 index). Generally, sensors are placed on each side of the forehead to reflect right and left cerebral cortical venous O_2 saturation. SrO_2 correlates well with jugular bulb O_2 saturation and moderately well with mixed venous O_2 saturation. The adequacy of regional cerebral perfusion should be investigated if the SrO_2 decreases 12–20 points from baseline, if SrO_2 is >30 points lower than the arterial O_2 saturation, or if the absolute SrO_2 index is <50 in a patient without an intracardiac shunt.

COMPONENTS OF CARDIAC OUTPUT

Five elements contribute to cardiac output: heart rate, preload, diastolic function, contractility, and afterload. Of these, only heart rate is measured routinely, which is complicated by the fact that these elements are interdependent, meaning that an apparent abnormality in one (or more) of these variables may actually be caused by an aberration in another (or several others). Rather than measuring preload, we are often more interested in addressing a related clinical question: "Will the patient respond to a fluid bolus by increasing stroke volume." Failure to do so can occur for three reasons: administration of inadequate volume, severely impaired contractility, and the patient is already functioning at the plateau of the Starling curve (**Fig. 44.6**).

Broadly speaking, measures of "preload" can be static or dynamic, with the latter more important in predicting fluid responsiveness. Two common static, pressure-based, measures of preload are CVP (or right atrial pressure) and pulmonary artery occlusion pressure (or left atrial pressure). Both are poor markers of volume status because many factors compromise the ability of a pressure measurement to act as a surrogate for volume status, including venous capacitance, cardiac chamber compliance, cardiac valve competence, pulmonary artery pressure, and the ability of the lung to function as a Starling resistor with positive-pressure ventilation. Nonetheless, CVP may be a reasonable trending measurement with a low value suggesting underfilling.

Diastolic Function

Diastolic function is crucial to maintaining an adequate cardiac output; yet, measurement of this entity remains challenging. Diastole is defined as the period from the end of aortic ejection (aortic valve closure) until the onset of ventricular tension that occurs with the following beat. It is an energy-consuming process, which is influenced by both active and passive mechanisms. Unfortunately, the ability to measure diastolic function at the bedside is limited in pediatric practice. The most common technique is Doppler echocardiography.

Contractility

Stroke work represents the area enclosed by the ventricular pressure-volume loop; however, this may be estimated by the product of stroke volume and arterial pressure measurements (**Table 44.4**). Although not a true measure of contractility, it allows some insight into cardiac reserve, namely, how stroke volume changes in the face of changing afterload.

The echocardiographic stress velocity index elaborates on the contractility-afterload relationship by plotting stress velocity (contractility) against end systolic wall stress (afterload). The slope of this relationship with changes in afterload helps to identify cardiac pathologies. The shortening fraction (SF), or percent change, in ventricular diameter is a convenient measure of global systolic function. Normal SF values are 29%–41%. SF is not a reliable measure of systolic function when ventricular geometry or regional wall motion is abnormal. Furthermore, SF is load-dependent. Therefore, even though intrinsic ventricular contractility is identical in two different patients, the patient with decreased preload will evidence lower SF. The ejection fraction (EF) provides similar information as the SF but uses the percent change in end-diastolic *volume*, such that:

$$EF = 100 \times (\text{end-diastolic volume} - \text{end-systolic } volume)/(end - diastolic\, volume)$$

The normal EF in children is 60% ± 7%.

Afterload

Afterload is the net force opposing LV fiber shortening during ventricular ejection and is quantified as LV wall stress. Wall stress is best measured at end systole and requires measurement of transmural ventricular pressure, LV end-systolic dimension, and wall thickness. The latter two variables are measured using echocardiography. Understanding wall stress allows for an appreciation of how factors that increase intrathoracic pressure, such as positive-pressure ventilation, result in a reduction in afterload.

CHAPTER 45A ▪ HEART FAILURE IN INFANTS AND CHILDREN: ETIOLOGY, PATHOPHYSIOLOGY, AND DIAGNOSIS OF HEART FAILURE

JEFFREY J. KIM • JOSEPH W. ROSSANO • DAVID P. NELSON • JACK F. PRICE • WILLIAM J. DREYER

PATHOPHYSIOLOGY

Heart failure is a constellation of structural and functional abnormalities, elevated filling pressures, neurohormonal activation, and signs or symptoms. Reference to acute decompensated heart failure (DHF) includes acute cardiovascular failure and shock, as well as the situation of exacerbated preexisting heart failure symptoms. The leading diagnosis that results in transplantation in pediatric patients is primary myocardial disorders, although palliated congenital heart disease is quickly becoming more frequent, emphasizing the evolving demographics of this patient population.

Heart Failure due to Structural Heart Disease

Symptomatic pulmonary overcirculation is a markedly different form of heart failure than the classic descriptions of congestive heart failure (CHF) described in adults. Ventricular systolic function is usually preserved in lesions that are associated with a large net left-to-right shunt, and low cardiac output is not a typical finding in this situation. However, if heart failure is thought of as a clinical syndrome characterized by elevated filling pressures, compensatory activation of the neurohormonal system, and progressive symptomatology, however pulmonary overcirculation certainly deserves to be recognized within the spectrum of heart failure. The sympathetic nervous system is activated, and plasma levels of norepinephrine increase, stimulating the renin-angiotensin-aldosterone system, causing peripheral vasoconstriction, and increasing the heart rate. Plasma levels of arginine vasopressin (antidiuretic hormone), a neurohormone that causes peripheral vasoconstriction and free water retention, are also increased in children with heart failure due to shunting lesions, as well as in situations of ventricular dysfunction. Natriuretic peptides are secreted by the atria and ventricles in response to myocardial stretch due to pressure or volume loads on the heart. Plasma levels of atrial natriuretic peptide and B-type natriuretic peptide (BNP) are elevated in children with congenital heart.

In acyanotic heart lesions such as ventricular septal defect and complete atrioventricular canal defect, signs and symptoms of heart failure usually develop during the first few weeks of life, after the pulmonary vascular resistance has fallen. Signs such as tachypnea, retractions, grunting, and diaphoresis with feeding usually herald this change in physiology. Other acyanotic lesions also associated with large left-to-right shunting include the patent ductus arteriosus, aortopulmonary window, and systemic arteriovenous malformations. These typical "runoff" lesions may manifest with signs of heart failure in the first few days (in premature infants) or weeks of life, with bounding pulses in addition to signs of respiratory compromise. If left uncorrected, over time, these defects can lead to pulmonary vascular disease.

Cyanotic cardiac defects can also be associated with pulmonary overcirculation and heart failure and include truncus arteriosus, total anomalous pulmonary venous connection, double outlet right ventricle (RV) without pulmonary valvar stenosis, and single ventricle lesions (both palliated and unpalliated) without obstructed pulmonary blood flow. In these lesions, an admixture of highly oxygen-saturated and less-saturated blood occurs at the atrial, ventricular, or great arterial level, and the mixed blood is then sent to the pulmonary and systemic circulations, preferring the path of least resistance. Chest x-ray may reveal increased pulmonary vascular markings despite low systemic arterial oxygen saturations. Classic signs of heart failure are also seen in infants with unrepaired or nonpalliated forms of cyanotic pulmonary overcirculation and include cardiomegaly, hepatomegaly, tachypnea, and poor weight gain.

Some forms of congenital heart disease can manifest with signs of heart failure in the early newborn period (first 3 days of life). Infants with critical aortic stenosis may present shortly after birth with shock or cyanosis. Critical coarctation of the aorta or interrupted aortic arch may also present in the first few days of life as the ductus arteriosus closes. These left-sided obstructive lesions often coexist, and the clinical spectrum can vary between an isolated bicuspid aortic valve with minimal obstruction to hypoplastic left heart syndrome. The RV will support the systemic circulation in the setting of a widely patent ductus arteriosus. When the ductus closes, however, the RV cannot adequately perfuse the systemic circulation, resulting in a profound metabolic acidosis and, if untreated, multiorgan system failure and death. Ventricular dysfunction caused by systemic hypertension can also lead to heart failure. In neuroblastoma, high levels of circulating catecholamines cause peripheral vasoconstriction and raise systemic vascular resistance. Patients with Wilms tumor may have high circulating levels of rennin, which also increases systemic vascular resistance.

Pulmonary valvular insufficiency that causes RV dysfunction or progressive heart failure is usually a result of previous surgery or catheter-based interventions on the pulmonary valve. Congenital forms of pulmonary insufficiency are also recognized, such as absent pulmonary valve syndrome. Most patients who undergo surgical correction of tetralogy of Fallot are left with some degree of pulmonary insufficiency. Acute and chronic aortic insufficiency can cause left ventricle (LV) dysfunction and heart failure. Dilation of the aortic root is a frequent cause of chronic aortic insufficiency and can be seen in patients with Marfan syndrome and other congenital conditions. Aortic root dilation has also been identified as a late finding following surgery for transposition of the great arteries and tetralogy of Fallot. Patients with a bicuspid aortic valve are also at risk for eventual aortic root dilation and concomitant aortic insufficiency.

Acute aortic insufficiency can also result from dissection of the aorta or rupture of a sinus of valsalva aneurysm, secondary to trauma or endocarditis. These patients are typically quite ill and may present in shock. In acute aortic insufficiency, aortic and LV pressures reach an equilibrium. LV dilation does not occur, and as the end-diastolic pressure acutely rises, pressure is transmitted back to the left atrium, leading to pulmonary edema (**Fig. 45A.1**). Immediate surgical intervention is necessary for survival. In moderate-to-severe chronic aortic insufficiency, the increased volume and pressure load on the LV can lead to ventricular hypertrophy and dilation. Over time, chamber dilation progresses, and myocardial dysfunction ensues with a decrease in LV ejection fraction. In decompensated chronic aortic insufficiency, patients develop symptoms of heart failure as elevated left heart pressures are transmitted to the pulmonary veins, causing congestion and exertional dyspnea.

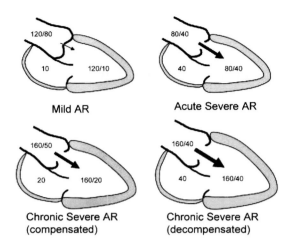

FIGURE 45A.1. Different stages of aortic regurgitation (AR). (**Top left**) In mild AR, LV size, function, and hemodynamics are normal. (**Top right**) In acute severe AR, there is equilibration of aortic and LV pressures (80/40 mm Hg in this example). Left atrial pressure is elevated, leading to pulmonary edema. (**Bottom left**) In chronic severe, compensated AR, the LV may begin to dilate, but LV ejection fraction is often maintained in the normal range by increased preload. Systolic arterial hypertension and a wide pulse pressure are present. However, LV filling pressures are normal or only slightly elevated, such that dyspnea is absent. (**Bottom right**) In decompensated chronic severe AR, the LV is dilated and hypertrophied, and LV function is often depressed as a result of afterload excess. Forward output is decreased, leading to fatigue and other low-output symptoms. Fibrosis and hypertrophy decrease LV compliance, leading to increased filling pressures and dyspnea. From Bekeredjian R, Grayburn PA. Valvular heart disease: Aortic regurgitation. *Circulation* 2005; 112:125–34, with permission.

Clinically significant tricuspid regurgitation is most often seen in patients with Ebstein anomaly, a congenital defect of the heart in which the annular attachments of the tricuspid valve are displaced toward the apex of the RV. The ventricle becomes divided into an "atrialized" inlet portion and functional apical and infundibular portions. Prograde pulmonary blood flow may be significantly compromised, and RV function may eventually deteriorate. Patients diagnosed in the newborn or infant period have the most severe form of the disease and develop signs of heart failure early on. Other causes of significant tricuspid regurgitation include endocarditis and tricuspid valvar dysplasia.

Mitral regurgitation is a common finding in pediatric heart failure, usually as a consequence of ventricular dysfunction and LV enlargement, rather than as an isolated cause of heart failure. In the setting of dilated cardiomyopathy (DCM) and heart failure, progressive chamber dilation causes the mitral valve annulus to stretch. The mitral valve leaflets fail to coapt, and regurgitation of blood into the left atrium results. Symptoms of pulmonary venous congestion develop as LV filling pressures increase. Isolated mitral valve disease can occur due to ischemia/infarction of a papillary muscle, trauma, or inflammatory disease processes; or it may be congenital in origin. When mitral regurgitation is not a result of DCM, the LV progressively dilates as a result of the volume load, and contractility is usually maintained or increased, as afterload is decreased. Eventually, as the regurgitant volume increases, LV function deteriorates and symptoms of heart failure ensue.

Right Heart Failure

Right heart failure in children is usually a result of a chronic volume and/or pressure overload on the RV, which often occurs in patients who have undergone surgery on the RV outflow tract (e.g., tetralogy of Fallot, truncus arteriosus, pulmonary atresia with ventricular septal defect, etc.) and are left with significant residual regurgitation or stenosis. RV dysplasia, an inherited cardiomyopathy characterized by RV dysfunction and dysrhythmias, is an uncommon form of right heart failure in children.

Low Cardiac Output Syndrome Following Cardiac Surgery

The transient drop in cardiac output after cardiac surgery has been referred to as *low cardiac output syndrome*. In the early postoperative period, this syndrome is due primarily to transient myocardial dysfunction, compounded by acute changes in myocardial loading conditions, including postoperative increases in systemic and/or pulmonary vascular resistance. Residual cardiac abnormalities, even if minor, may further aggravate an underlying low output state. Surgical repair of cardiac malformations exposes the myocardium to periods of ischemia, resulting in transient myocardial stunning or damage. Cardiopulmonary bypass, which activates the complement and inflammatory cascades, also contributes to myocardial injury, alterations in pulmonary and systemic vascular reactivity, and pulmonary dysfunction. In addition, some repairs require ventriculotomy, which further exacerbates myocardial dysfunction.

Heart failure alters the structure and function of the myocardium at both the molecular and cellular levels. In particular, calcium dysregulation can lead to maladaptive changes in the contractile apparatus as heart failure progresses. Also, disruption of sarcomeric proteins can threaten the structural integrity

of the myocardium. In the normal heart, cellular depolarization leads to voltage-gated Ca^{2+} influx into the myocyte cytoplasm, which in turn, triggers the release of Ca^{2+} stores from the sarcoplasmic reticulum via a receptor-mediated Ca^{2+} channel known as the ryanodine receptor channel. Dystrophin is a protein that has been strongly implicated in models of heart failure. In the stable myocyte, dystrophin and its associated complex connects the sarcomere to the sarcolemma/extracellular matrix and plays a key role in the transduction of physical force. Mechanical unloading of the heart with a ventricular assist device has subsequently been shown to lead to reverse remodeling.

Ventricular hypertrophy, an important part of myocardial remodeling, occurs in response to stimuli such as hemodynamic overload, mechanical stress, or disruption of myocyte structure and function. A major stimulus for myocardial remodeling and ventricular hypertrophy is mechanical stress secondary to hemodynamic overload. Exposure of cardiac myocytes to mechanical stress results in the activation of numerous molecular signaling cascades, as well as the reactivation of fetal gene programs, which leads to cellular growth, protein synthesis, and hypertrophic changes. This process is known as "mechano-transduction." Multiple signaling pathways have been implicated in the process of mechano-transduction, and they include humoral factors, G-protein-coupled receptors, changes in calcium signaling, and the activation of numerous kinases. The renin-angiotensin system is well documented to be activated in heart failure. Endothelin-1 is another vasoconstrictor peptide that is produced in increased amounts in the presence of hemodynamic overload and mechanical stretch, and it has been shown to be a potent inducer of cardiac hypertrophy, as evidenced by increased protein synthesis and cell size. Calcineurin, an intracellular Ca^{2+}-calmodulin-activated phosphatase, has been implicated in mechanisms of heart failure associated cardiac hypertrophy. High levels of circulating catechols (e.g., norepinephrine) have been shown to be directly toxic to myocardial cells via the induction of apoptosis, likely due to calcium overload. Natriuretic peptides are hormones that have been shown to act as a counter-regulatory system by providing beneficial effects such as vasodilation and natriuresis. Three distinct, major natriuretic peptides have been isolated and synthesized: atrial natriuretic peptide, BNP, and C-type natriuretic peptide. BNP is synthesized predominantly in the cardiac ventricles and is released in response to certain pathophysiologic states such as heart failure. BNP has physiologic counter-regulatory effects that ultimately lead to systemic vasodilation and natriuresis.

Inflammation in heart failure is a result of the coordinated activation of specific transcription factors in response to external stimuli (infection, oxidative stress, circulating neurohormones, etc.). The best understood of these transcription factors is NFκB. Once activated, the inflammatory cascade leads to the production of numerous proinflammatory and anti-inflammatory mediators. Tumor necrosis factor is produced endogenously by cardiac myocytes in response to stress or injury. Nitric oxide mediates improved relaxation, increased preload reserve, and decreased afterload, while detrimental effects include myocardial depression and β-adrenergic desensitization.

DECOMPENSATED HEART FAILURE

The clinical manifestations of decompensated heart failure (DHF) in children are somewhat dependent on the age at presentation. Therefore, the history and physical examination should be targeted for the appropriate clinical scenario. In neonates, common causes of DHF include perinatal asphyxia, toxemia, incessant tachyarrhythmias, neonatal myocarditis, severe anemia, or hyperviscosity syndrome. Certain types of CHD such as hypoplastic left heart syndrome with a severely restrictive atrial septum may manifest soon after birth as well but not usually as isolated heart failure. The history should include questions regarding prenatal course, birth history, potential perinatal insults, and family history. The physical exam, as expected, should evaluate for signs of left- or right-sided heart failure. In neonates, findings may include rapid, shallow breathing, dyspnea, wheezing, resting tachycardia, hepatomegaly, jugular venous distension, or hydrops. Cardiac evaluation should assess for gallops; a single, second heart sound; murmurs; and abnormal pulses.

Beyond the immediate perinatal period, DHF in infants can be broadly categorized into causes more likely to occur in the first few weeks of life and causes more likely to occur in the first few months of life. During the first weeks of life, CHD is dependent on ductal blood flow. Defects dependent on ductal flow for systemic perfusion (i.e., hypoplastic left heart syndrome, critical aortic stenosis, interrupted aortic arch, etc.) often present with increasing tachycardia, tachypnea, diminished pulses, and worsening perfusion. On the other hand, defects dependent on ductal flow for pulmonary circulation (i.e., critical pulmonary stenosis, pulmonary atresia, etc.) often present with progressive cyanosis. Again, assessment for cardiac murmurs; single, second heart sounds;

clicks; and pulses is critical. In this age group, evaluation of differential oxygen saturations (preductal and postductal) may also be of particular importance.

Lesions that present as DHF in infants beyond the first few weeks of life include those with increasing left-to-right shunting as pulmonary vascular resistance decreases. These shunting lesions include large ventricular septal defects, complete atrioventricular canal defects, aortopulmonary windows, truncus arteriosus, unobstructed total anomalous pulmonary venous return, and persistent patent ductus arteriosus, as covered previously. Of note, premature neonates with persistent patency of the ductus arteriosus may present earlier, particularly in infants who weigh <1500 g. Other important causes of DHF in infancy include primary myocardial diseases, myocarditis, and anomalous left coronary artery from the pulmonary artery (ALCAPA). In the pure sense, ALCAPA is a left-to-right shunting lesion that presents with heart failure secondary to LV ischemia, as flow in the left coronary system reverses with decreasing pulmonary vascular resistance (coronary steal). These infants may present with unique symptoms of intense irritability and angina, particularly during feeding.

Historic evaluation in all infants with suspected heart failure should include an accurate assessment of feeding (tachypnea with feeds, gagging, diaphoresis, time to complete feeding, etc.). It should also include an assessment of nutritional status and weight gain, as this may be the first manifestation of a failing heart. Along similar lines, physical examination in older infants should assess for cachexia and malnutrition, as well as the standard assessment for tachypnea, diaphoresis, and increased work of breathing. Precordial activity may be increased, and again, murmurs, gallops, or clicks may give important clues to etiology.

Older children are more likely to develop symptomatic heart failure from acquired or operated cardiac conditions, rather than newly recognized or unoperated CHD. Exceptions to this generalization include unrepaired large atrial septal defects, Ebstein anomaly of the tricuspid valve, or ventricular inversion. Patients with palliated CHD may develop DHF as a consequence of chronic pressure or volume overload. This population usually consists of patients with single-ventricle physiology, progressive valvular disease, or RV-dependent systemic circulations. As always, myocarditis or primary myocardial disorders can present at any age. Other potential etiologies of acquired heart failure in older children include rheumatic heart disease, hypothyroidism, or Kawasaki disease. The history in this age group should include questions regarding exercise capacity, easy fatigability, orthopnea, paroxysmal nocturnal dyspnea, and weight gain or weight loss. Physical examination should evaluate for resting tachycardia, tachypnea, hepatomegaly, jugular venous distension, ascites, edema, and diminished perfusion. Cardiac examination should focus on the presence of gallops, new murmurs, an RV impulse, and perfusion deficits. In all age groups, a directed history and physical examination can provide valuable clues into the presence and possible etiologies of impending DHF.

Cardiorenal Syndrome

Renal insufficiency commonly occurs in patients with DHF. The pathophysiologic process in which combined cardiac and renal dysfunction amplifies progression of end-organ damage has been termed the cardiorenal syndrome. The renal insufficiency that accompanies DHF is attributed to poor cardiac output and diminished renal perfusion.

Dysrhythmias in Acute Decompensated Heart Failure

Dysrhythmias can be the primary cause of ventricular dysfunction (tachycardia-induced cardiomyopathy), and patients with poor cardiac function are clearly prone to developing rhythm disturbances. Incessant atrial tachycardia, junctional tachycardia, accessory pathway-mediated tachycardia, and ventricular tachycardia have all been linked to the development of cardiomyopathy. Children with DCM are also more likely to develop secondary arrhythmias, which can be either atrial or ventricular in origin and may put these children at risk for sudden death.

Laboratory Evaluation of Decompensated Heart Failure

Classic findings on blood work include metabolic and respiratory acidemia due to poor tissue perfusion and pulmonary congestion, hyponatremia and hypochloremia due to free water retention, and elevated creatinine levels due to poor renal perfusion and compromised renal function. Measurement of serum BNP levels is clinically useful in differentiating pulmonary causes of dyspnea from cardiac causes of dyspnea. In children, BNP levels positively correlate with a clinical heart failure score and negatively correlate with ejection fraction.

An enlarged cardiac silhouette on chest x-ray due to cardiomegaly is frequently found. A cardiothoracic ratio of >0.55 in infants and >0.5 in children is the standard for cardiomegaly. The left lower lobe of the lung may also be collapsed due to compression of the left lower lobe bronchus. An electrocardiogram (ECG) can provide information regarding atrial enlargement, ventricular hypertrophy, strain, and changes in ST-segment or T-wave morphology. However, these changes are usually nonspecific, and their use in the diagnosis of heart failure is therefore limited. An exception to this may be in the cases of myocarditis, ALCAPA, or tachyarrhythmia-induced cardiomyopathy, in which pathognomonic ECG findings can sometimes be found. In patients with myocarditis, a pattern of myocardial infarction with wide Q waves and ST-segment changes may be seen.

The most precise way to quickly evaluate cardiac function and obtain a semiquantitative assessment of heart failure remains two-dimensional echocardiography. Although values vary with age, in general, normal values for shortening fraction range from 28% to 44%, while normal values for ejection fraction range from 56% to 78%. It is important to note that both of these classic measures of function are load dependent. Children with DCM have a dilated, dysfunctional LV on 2-dimensional and M-mode echocardiography. Segmental wall motion abnormalities are relatively common, but global hypokinesis is predominant. A pericardial effusion is frequently present. Doppler and color Doppler commonly demonstrate mitral regurgitation. Dilation of other chambers also may be seen. Cardiac output calculations may also be obtained and are frequently reduced. Coronary artery or structural abnormalities that could produce these features should be excluded. Improved techniques, particularly tissue Doppler imaging and myocardial velocity measurements, are being studied to better characterize tissue changes and monitor them over time.

In addition to providing an anatomic evaluation of the heart in failure, MRI can also provide accurate tissue characterization by measuring T1 and T2 relaxation times and spin densities. Relaxation time analysis provides a sensitive measure for acute myocarditis. Utilizing T1 spin-echo cine MR angiography and gadolinium-enhanced spin echo imaging, investigators demonstrated that focal myocardial enhancement combined with regional wall motion abnormalities strongly supported the diagnosis of myocarditis.

Cardiac catheterization is an invasive procedure with inherent risks and potential complications, which sometimes limits its application for diagnostic purposes. Catheterization can help in the hemodynamic assessment of patients by directly measuring LV end diastolic, pulmonary capillary wedge, pulmonary artery, and central venous pressures. Also, a cardiac catheterization with coronary artery angiography may be necessary to exclude coronary artery anomalies (both congenital and acquired).

CHAPTER 45B ■ HEART FAILURE IN INFANTS AND CHILDREN: CARDIOMYOPATHY

JOHN LYNN JEFFERIES • SUSAN W. DENFIELD • WILLIAM J. DREYER

Cardiomyopathies have been classified by the World Health Organization and the International Society and Federation of Cardiology task force into five forms according to phenotype. The first form is dilated cardiomyopathy (DCM), in which the left ventricle (LV) or both ventricles are enlarged and hypocontractile to variable degrees. In general, systolic dysfunction is the main clinical feature with resultant signs and symptoms of congestive heart failure (CHF). The second form is hypertrophic cardiomyopathy (HCM), also previously known as *idiopathic hypertrophic subaortic stenosis*, characterized by LV hypertrophy that may be asymmetric. Systolic function is usually preserved or hypercontractile, and symptoms may result from LV outflow tract obstruction, diastolic dysfunction, or arrhythmias resulting in sudden death. The third form is restrictive cardiomyopathy (RCM), which is recognized by markedly dilated atria with generally normal ventricular dimensions and systolic function. Diastolic filling is impaired, and symptoms result from pulmonary and right-sided systemic venous

TABLE 45B.1

SECONDARY CAUSES OF DILATED CARDIOMYOPATHIES

Infections	*Ischemia*
Viral	Hypoxia
Bacterial	Birth asphyxia
Fungal	Drowning
Protozoan (Chagas/toxoplasmosis)	Kawasaki disease
Rickettsial (Rocky Mountain spotted fever)	Coronary artery malformation
Spirochetal (Lyme disease)	Premature coronary artery disease
Arrhythmias	*Toxins*
Supraventricular tachycardia	Anthracyclines
Atrial flutter	Radiation
Ectopic atrial tachycardia	Other chemotherapeutic agents
Ventricular tachycardia	Sulfonamide sensitivity
Bradycardia	Penicillin sensitivity
	Iron (hemochromatosis)
Endocrine	Copper
Hyperthyroidism/hypothyroidism	
Excess catecholamines (pheochromocytoma or neuroblastoma)	*Systemic disorders*
Congenital adrenal hyperplasia	Systemic lupus erythematosus
	Juvenile rheumatoid arthritis
Metabolic diseases	Polyarteritis Nodosa
Disorders of glycogen metabolism	Kawasaki disease
Disorders of lipid metabolism	Osteogenesis imperfecta
Defects of B-oxidation enzymes	Peripartum cardiomyopathy
Carnitine deficiency syndromes	Hemolytic uremic syndrome
Fatty acid transport defects	Leukemia
	Amyloidosis
Nutritional deficiencies	Sarcoidosis
Protein: kwashiorkor	Reye syndrome
Thiamine: beriberi	
Vitamin E	
Selenium	
Phosphate	

Adapted from Denfield SW, Gajarski RJ, Towbin JA. Cardiomyopathies. In: Garson A, Bricker JT, Fisher DJ, et al., eds. *The Science and Practice of Pediatric Cardiology*, 2nd ed. Baltimore: Williams & Wilkins, 1998.

congestion. The fourth form is arrhythmogenic right ventricular dysplasia (ARVD) and is characterized by left-bundle-branch block, ventricular tachycardia, a dilated right ventricle (RV), and a dyskinetic RV outflow tract with replacement of myocardium by adipose tissue, beginning in the epicardium and extending to the endocardium. The above-mentioned organizations also recognize a fifth category of "other" cardiomyopathies. Left-ventricular noncompaction (LVNC) has gained considerable clinical attention as a "new" cardiomyopathy in this classification. In this form of cardiomyopathy, the LV wall is thickened with large spongiform trabeculations and the LV is typically hypocontractile.

DCM represents a heterogeneous group of myocardial disorders that result in ventricular dilation and impaired systolic contractile function in the absence of coronary artery disease, valvular abnormalities, and pericardial disease. Mitral regurgitation is common, as are ventricular arrhythmias, particularly ventricular tachycardia, torsade de pointes, and ventricular fibrillation. Impaired contractile function generally culminates with chamber enlargement. The regulation of normal contractile function necessary to maintain an appropriate cardiac output requires normal electrical conduction, normal intercellular and intracellular calcium signaling, appropriate energy production, sufficient force generation from the sarcomeric proteins, and adequate force trans-mission from the sarcomere through to the extracellular matrix via cytoskeletal proteins. Primary DCMs are disorders intrinsic to the myocardium that occur without a secondary cause and are presumably genetically transmitted diseases of one of the structural or regulatory proteins. Causes of secondary DCMs are summarized in **Table 45B.1**.

HCM is characterized by LV hypertrophy, a nondilated LV cavity, systolic hypercontractility, diastolic dysfunction, and, in ~20% of cases, obstruction to LV outflow (hypertrophic obstructive cardiomyopathy) secondary to mitral-septal contact during systole. HCM is recognized as the most common genetic cardiovascular disease and is the most common cause of sudden cardiac death in young healthy subjects in the US, particularly true with athletic activity, which accounts for approximately one-third of the deaths (**Fig. 45B.1**).

RCM is characterized by restrictive filling and reduced diastolic volume of either or both ventricles, with normal or near-normal systolic function and wall thicknesses. Increased interstitial fibrosis may be present. It may be idiopathic or associated with another disease. RCM has multiple causes (**Table 45B.2**). Mutations in desmin, Troponin I, and RSK2 have been reported in children with RCM. Diastolic function is primarily affected by ventricular compliance/stiffness and relaxation. In the normal heart, the phase of rapid or early filling occurs as the LV

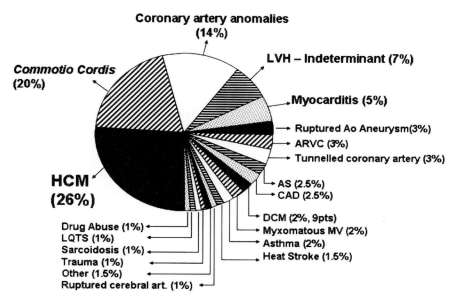

FIGURE 45B.1. Causes of sudden death in young competitive athletes, as reported to the Minneapolis Heart Institute Foundation national registry. Ao, aorta; art., artery; AS, aortic stenosis; CAD, coronary artery disease; DCM, dilated cardiomyopathy; LQTS, long-QT syndrome; LVH, LV hypertrophy; MV, mitral valve; and pts, patients. From Maron BJ, Pelliccia A. The heart of trained athletes: Cardiac remodeling and the risks of sports, including sudden death. *Circulation* 2006; 114:1633–44, with permission.

TABLE 45B.2

CAUSES OF RESTRICTIVE CARDIOMYOPATHIES IN CHILDREN AND ADULTS

Myocardial
Idiopathic
Familial
Scleroderma
Myocarditis
Cardiac transplantation
Pseudoxanthoma elasticum
Diabetic cardiomyopathy
Amyloidosis
Sarcoidosis
Gaucher disease
Hurler disease
Fatty infiltration
Hemochromatosis
Fabry disease
Glycogen storage diseases
Endomyocardial fibrosis
Hypereosinophilia syndrome (Löffler endocarditis)
Endocardial fibroelastosis
Carcinoid
Metastatic cancers
Radiation
Drugs
    Anthracyclines
    Serotonin
    Methysergide
    Ergotamine
    Mercurials
    Busulfan

pressure drops below that in the left atrium, just after the mitral valve opens. In the classic description of RCM, ventricular filling is completed in early diastole, with little or no filling in late diastole.

Arrhythmogenic RV cardiomyopathy (or dysplasia) is a form of cardiomyopathy that is characterized by fatty-fibrous replacement of the RV. This gradual process of replacement of normal myocardium with fatty and fibrous tissue predisposes patients to RV dysfunction and life-threatening ventricular arrhythmias. The ECG typically shows T-wave inversion in the precordial leads and a delayed S-wave upstroke. Echocardiography often shows dilation of the RV with segmental wall and/or global RV wall motion abnormalities. The RV outflow tract may be dilated, and an "echo-bright" moderator band and/or evidence of focal RV wall aneurysms may be seen. Cardiac MRI is now commonly used to further assess patients who are suspected of having ARVD. Cardiac MRI can be used to visualize fatty-fibrous replacement of the myocardium. Management of patients with ARVD may consist of antiarrhythmic agents, but the therapy with survival benefit appears to be implantation of an implantable cardioverter defibrillator.

LVNC is characterized by deep trabeculations in the LV endocardium. Typically, apical hypertrophy with variable systolic dysfunction is also seen. This disorder is also identified as fetal myocardium, noncompaction of the LV myocardium, and spongiform myocardium. The phenotypes display echocardiographic features that alternate between a DCM-like disorder and an HCM-like disorder, while others have primarily diastolic dysfunction. LVNC may be associated with systemic disorders such as Barth syndrome or mitochondrial or metabolic disorders. LVNC has also been associated with a variety of other diseases and syndromes, including Patau syndrome, Fabry disease, Melnick-Needles syndrome, and nail-patella syndrome. The diagnosis of LVNC is typically made by noninvasive methods, although LV angiography can also be used. Echocardiography is the most frequently noted modality. Other modalities such as cardiovascular MRI are becoming more widely used in the diagnosis of LVNC.

CHAPTER 45C ■ HEART FAILURE IN INFANTS AND CHILDREN: MYOCARDITIS

JOHN PHILIP BREINHOLT III • DAVID P. NELSON • JEFFREY A. TOWBIN

Active myocarditis is characterized by an inflammatory cellular infiltrate of the myocardium with necrosis and/or degeneration of adjacent myocytes. The etiologies are listed in **Table 45C.1**.

The pathogenesis of myocarditis involves direct invasion by the cardiotropic virus that leads to activation of an immune response and local inflammation. This activation induces production of B cells, which results in myocytolysis and further interstitial inflammation and production of anti-heart antibodies. A number of viruses have been implicated in the induction of apoptosis, including adenovirus, Epstein-Barr virus, and HIV.

In those cases in which resolution of cardiac dysfunction does not occur, chronic DCM results. Sudden cardiac death in infancy may result from myocardial inflammation.

TABLE 45C.1

CAUSES OF MYOCARDITIS

Viruses	Nonviral infectious pathogens	Noninfectious etiologies
Adenovirus	**Bacteria**	**Pharmaceuticals**
Arbovirus	*Borrelia burgdorferi*	Acetazolamide
Cytomegalovirus	*Brucella melitensis*	Amphotericin B
Enterovirus	*Chlamydia pneumoniae*	Anthracyclines
■ Coxsackie A and B	*Chlamydia psittaci*	Cephalosporins
■ Echovirus	Clostridium	Cocaine
■ Poliovirus	Klebsiella	Cyclophosphamide
Epstein-Barr virus	*Legionella pneumophila*	Digoxin
Hepatitis A and B	Leptospira	Diuretics
Herpes simplex virus	Meningococcus	Dobutamine
Human immunodeficiency virus	Mycobacteria	Indomethacin
Influenza A	*Mycoplasma pneumoniae*	Isoniazid
Measles	Salmonella	Methyldopa
Mumps	Streptococcus species	Neomercazole
Parvovirus B19	*Treponema pallidum*	Penicillin
Rabies	Tuberculosis	Phenylbutazone
Respiratory syncytial virus	Typhoid	Phenytoin
Rhinovirus	**Rickettsial**	Sulfonamides
Rubella	*Rickettsia rickettsii*	Tetracycline
Rubeola	*Rickettsia tsutsugamushi*	Tricyclic Antidepressants
Varicella	**Fungi and yeasts**	**Hypersensitivity/autoimmune**
Vaccinia virus	Actinomyces	Celiac disease
Toxins and other	Candida	Diabetes mellitus
Scorpion venom	Coccidiodes	Hashimoto thyroiditis
Diphtheria	Histoplasma	Mixed connective tissue disease
Smallpox vaccine	**Protozoa**	Myasthenia gravis
Cornstarch	*Entamoeba histolytica*	Pernicious anemia
Kawasaki disease	*Trypanosoma cruzi*	Rheumatoid arthritis
Sarcoidosis	*Toxoplasma gondii*	Rheumatic fever
Scleroderma	**Parasites**	Scleroderma
	Echinococcus granulosus	Systemic lupus erythematosus
	Hetereophyiasis	Takayasu arteritis
	Plasmodium falciparum	Thrombocytopenic purpura
	Schistosomes	Ulcerative colitis
	Taeniasis solium (Cysticercosis)	Wegener granulomatosis
	Toxocara canis	Whipple disease
	Trichinella spiralis	

CLINICAL MANIFESTATIONS OF MYOCARDITIS

In general, myocarditis should be considered in all children and adults with new-onset CHF in whom no other etiology is found. Any cause of acute circulatory failure may mimic myocarditis. The differential diagnoses of CHF based on age range are listed in **Table 45C.2**. In many cases, an antecedent, nonspecific flu-like illness or episode of gastroenteritis may precede the symptoms of CHF.

Distinct clinical presentations for myocarditis include acute, subacute, and fulminant forms of the disease. Patients with *acute and subacute myocarditis* present hemodynamically stable with no fever and requiring only low-dose inotropic support. *Subacute* presentation entails an indistinct onset of symptoms of heart failure that may have developed over weeks to months. Patients with *fulminant myocarditis* present with severe hemodynamic compromise with at least two of the following clinical features: fever, distinct onset of symptoms of heart failure (fatigue, dyspnea on exertion or at rest, acute-onset edema), and a history consistent with a viral illness within 2 wks of presentation. These patients are typically in extremis on presentation and often require high-dose inotrope

---

TABLE 45C.2

DIFFERENTIAL DIAGNOSIS OF MYOCARDITIS BY AGE

Newborn and infant
Sepsis
Hypoxia
Hypoglycemia
Hypocalcemia
Structural heart disease
Left atrial myxoma
Idiopathic dilated cardiomyopathy
Barth syndrome
Endocardial fibroelastosis
Pompe disease
Anomalous left coronary artery from the
    pulmonary artery
Cerebral arteriovenous malformation

Child
Idiopathic dilated cardiomyopathy
X-linked dilated cardiomyopathy
Autosomal-dominant dilated cardiomyopathy
Anomalous left coronary artery from the
    pulmonary artery
Endocardial fibroelastosis
Chronic tachyarrhythmia
Pericarditis

---

and/or mechanical support. One other subtype of the fulminant form of clinical phenotype is the patient who presents acutely—like the fulminant myocarditis patient, with symptoms of severe DHF—but additionally manifests an infarct pattern on ECG that mimics that seen in anomalous left coronary artery from the pulmonary artery, including deep Q waves in leads I and aVL, and V4 through V6. Endomyocardial biopsy typically reveals significant necrosis with severe cellular edema and cell breakdown and typically identifies a coxsackievirus as the viral etiology, or no virus identification is made.

Newborns or infants typically present with fever, irritability or listlessness, periodic episodes of pallor, tachypnea or respiratory distress, and diaphoresis. Poor appetite or vomiting is frequently seen. Sudden death may occur in this subgroup of children. On physical examination, pallor and mild cyanosis are commonly noted. The skin is usually cool and mottled, consistent with poor perfusion due to decreased cardiac output. Respirations are usually rapid and labored; grunting may be prominent, but rales are uncommon. The cardiovascular exam is consistent with CHF and includes resting tachycardia, a gallop rhythm, muffled heart sounds, and frequently a systolic regurgitant murmur due to mitral regurgitation. In some of these young children, particularly newborns, a tricuspid regurgitation murmur may also be identified. The pulses are usually thready, and hepatomegaly is usually obvious. Dysrhythmias (supraventricular or ventricular tachycardia) or atrioventricular block may also occur. It is important to remember that the younger the child, the more likely that intrauterine myocarditis has occurred and that the findings may be more associated with chronic disease than otherwise expected in acute disease.

Older children, adolescents, and adults commonly report a recent history of viral disease, generally 10–14 days prior to presentation. Initial symptoms include lethargy, low-grade fever, and pallor; the child usually has decreased appetite and often complains of abdominal pain. Diaphoresis, palpitations, rashes, exercise intolerance, and general malaise are common signs and symptoms. Later in the course of illness, respiratory symptoms become predominant. Physical exam findings are consistent with CHF. Unlike newborns, jugular venous distention and pulmonary rales may be found, and resting tachycardia is often prominent. Dysrhythmias, including atrial fibrillation, supraventricular tachycardia or ventricular tachycardia, and atrioventricular block, may occur. Syncope or sudden death may occur owing to cardiac collapse.

Appropriate diagnostic assessment includes chest x-ray, ECG, echocardiogram, and various laboratory studies.

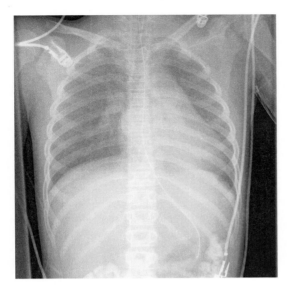

FIGURE 45C.1. Chest x-ray in a child with acute myocarditis. Presence of cardiomegaly and increased pulmonary vascular markings consistent with pulmonary edema.

As shown in **Figure 45C.1**, the chest x-ray on presentation usually demonstrates cardiomegaly with prominent pulmonary vascular markings that are suggestive of pulmonary edema, consistent with CHF. Comparisons over time may demonstrate significant improvement or normalization of the chest x-ray within a few months of presentation, suggesting a transient disease state (most typically, myocarditis).

Sinus tachycardia with low-voltage QRS complexes (<5 mm total amplitude in all limb leads) with or without low-voltage or inverted T waves are classically described. As shown in the example in **Figure 45C.2**, widened QRS complexes and ST-segment changes may be present. A pattern of myocardial infarction with wide Q waves (>35 msec) and ST-segment changes may also be seen in the fulminant necrotic presentation. Ventricular tachycardia, supraventricular tachycardia, atrial fibrillation, or atrioventricular block occurs in some children. A dilated and dysfunctional left ventricle consistent with DCM is seen on two-dimensional and M-mode echocardiography (i.e., left ventricle end-diastolic and end-systolic dimensions are increased; shortening and ejection fractions are decreased). Segmental wall motion abnormalities are relatively common, but global hypokinesis is predominant. Pericardial effusion frequently occurs. Doppler and

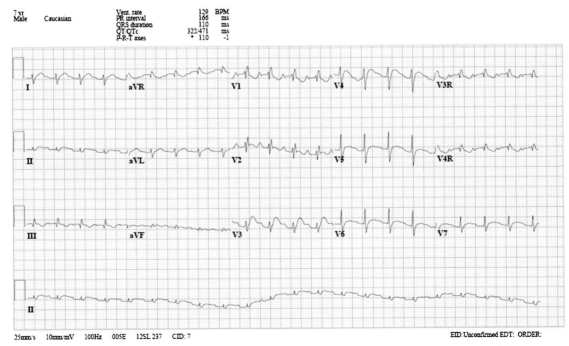

FIGURE 45C.2. Electrocardiogram in a case of myocarditis. Low-voltage QRS complexes with inverted T waves. Widened QRS complexes and ST-segment changes in the precordial leads consistent with ischemia noted throughout.

color-Doppler commonly demonstrate mitral regurgitation. Dilation of other chambers may also be seen. Cardiac output calculations may be obtained and are typically reduced. Coronary artery or structural abnormalities that could result in these features should be excluded.

Viral culture of peripheral specimens, such as blood, stool, or urine, is commonly performed but is unreliable at identifying the causative infection. A fourfold increase in antibody titer correlates with infection. However, these studies are nonspecific because prior infection with the causative virus is commonplace.

In adults who present with suspected myocarditis, serum cardiac biomarkers (e.g., creatine kinase, troponin I and T) are routinely measured. Creatine kinase and erythrocyte sedimentation rate have proven unhelpful, and troponin I and T have a low sensitivity.

In acute myocarditis, a right ventricular endomyocardial biopsy can be performed, and samples are evaluated histologically for inflammation. The inflammatory infiltrate is usually patchy and scattered within the ventricular myocardium. A mononuclear cell infiltrate is diagnostic of myocarditis, though this does not identify the etiology. The Dallas Criteria define myocarditis as "a process characterized by an inflammatory infiltrate of the myocardium with necrosis and/or degeneration of adjacent myocytes not typical of ischemic damage" due to coronary artery or other disease. The polymerase chain reaction amplification process, which identifies specific portions of a viral genome, is quite sensitive and specific.

CHAPTER 46A ■ TREATMENT OF HEART FAILURE IN INFANTS AND CHILDREN: MEDICAL MANAGEMENT

JOSEPH W. ROSSANO • JACK F. PRICE • DAVID P. NELSON

Heart failure is generally a chronic, progressive disorder, though certain types of cardiomyopathy such as left ventricular (LV) noncompaction can have an undulating phenotype, with periods of improvement and/or deterioration in function. Another exception is acute myocarditis, especially the fulminate form, in which patients often have a complete recovery of function. Guidelines for the management of chronic heart failure in adults and children have been published by the International Society of Heart and Lung Transplant, the American College of Cardiology, and the American Heart Association.

PHARMACOLOGIC AGENTS

Diuretics are recommended for patients with symptoms of heart failure and evidence of volume overload. Loop and thiazide diuretics remain the most commonly used diuretics. In adults, aldosterone antagonists such as spironolactone have been shown to improve mortality when added to standard heart failure management, though an increase in hyperkalemia may occur. Angiotensin-converting enzyme (ACE) inhibitors decrease the formation of angiotensin II, block the activation of the renin-angiotensin-aldosterone system (RAAS), and decrease adrenergic activity. Angiotensin-receptor blockers are primarily used in adults who are not tolerant of ACE inhibitors. Although they possess negative inotropic properties, the presumed benefit of β-blockers is inhibition of the effects of the sympathetic nervous system. Data on children have been extrapolated from adult studies, and the current recommendation of the International Society for Heart and Lung Transplantation is to use digoxin for symptomatic patients. Metoprolol may be used, as it has efficacy for heart failure and as an antiarrhythmic for arrhythmias where β blockers would be indicated (e.g., re-entrant tachycardia, ectopic focus tachycardia, rate control for atrial fibrillation). Amiodarone is an effective antiarrhythmic medication for a variety of arrhythmias. Patients with ventricular dysrhythmias and depressed LV function are at increased risk for sudden death, and consideration for implantable cardioverter-defibrillator (ICD) should be considered.

CARDIAC RESYNCHRONIZATION THERAPY

Restoration of ventricular synchrony with synchronized biventricular pacing is referred to as *cardiac resynchronization therapy* (CRT). When combined with an ICD, CRT may improve mortality. CRT may prove useful for pediatric and adult patients with congenital heart disease and an intraventricular conduction delay, as often seen in patients with tetralogy of Fallot or functionally univentricular hearts. The Heart Failure Society of America recommends that prophylactic ICD placement should be considered for patients with an ejection fraction ≤30% with mild-to-moderate heart failure symptoms. There are no current guidelines regarding pediatric patients.

ACUTE DECOMPENSATED HEART FAILURE

Heart failure is thought to occur after an index event produces an initial decline in heart function leading to compensatory mechanisms, including an activation of the sympathetic nervous system, salt and water preservation with activation of the RAAS, and production of inflammatory cytokines. A useful tool to help guide management of the patient with acute

decompensated heart failure is the rapid-assessment algorithm. Patients are characterized by the presence or absence of pulmonary or systemic congestion (i.e., elevated filling pressure) and the adequacy of perfusion. As shown in **Table 46A.1**, patients are classified according to signs of elevated filling pressures (wet or dry) and adequacy of perfusion (warm or cold). The goal is to maintain or transition a patient to the "warm and dry" category.

Patients with congestion but adequate perfusion likely comprise the largest group of patients with acute decompensated heart failure and the group that responds best to medial therapy. Diuresis, a critical component of the initial management of the patient with elevated filling pressures, may be the only therapy necessary to improve symptoms in the patient with adequate perfusion. β blockers and ACE inhibitors can generally be continued during hospitalization, but the negative inotropic effects of β blockers may necessitate discontinuation or dose reduction if perfusion is marginal. Some patients may not tolerate acute withdrawal from β blockade. Initiation of β blocker is usually contraindicated while the patient is in a decompensated state of heart failure. Delaying initiation of a β blocker until the patient has been transitioned back to the "warm and dry" state is generally advised.

Patients with congestion and poor perfusion require afterload reduction, as this is the more effective

TABLE 46A.1

PROFILE OF RESTING HEMODYNAMICS

	No congestion	Congestion
Adequate perfusion	"Warm and dry"	"Wet and warm"
	A	B
	Optimal profile: focus on prevention of disease progression and decompensation	Diuresis with continuation of standard therapy
Critical hypoperfusion	"Cold and dry"	"Wet and cold"
	L	C
	Limited further options for therapy	Diuresis and redesign of regimen with other standard therapies

Patients frequently progress from profile A to profile B or profile C. Profile "L" refers to patient's presenting with low output and no congestion. The letter L was chosen rather than the letter D to avoid the implication that this profile necessarily follows profile C or is a less desirable profile than C.
From Grady KL, Dracup K, Kennedy G, et al. Team management of patients with heart failure: A statement for healthcare professionals from The Cardiovascular Nursing Council of the American Heart Association. *Circulation* 2000; 102:2443–56, with permission.

way to increase cardiac output in the failing heart than "whipping" it with inotropic agents. Vasodilators and diuretics alone may be adequate therapy for many patients. Avoiding inotropic agents when possible appears to be beneficial. Nitroprusside is an effective vasodilator and has been used in the treatment of heart failure in adults for >3 decades. The drug has a rapid half-life and can be quickly up-titrated to effect. Blood pressure must be monitored, as hypotension can develop. Cyanide toxicity is an important potential side effect, especially with chronic use or renal impairment. The human recombinant B-type natriuretic peptide nesiritide has been shown to have positive lusitropic properties, promote vasodilation, improve natriuresis, and inhibit renin and aldosterone.

Inotropic agents may be required to improve perfusion in patients with acute decompensated heart failure. Many patients with significant ventricular dysfunction will remain compensated, do not need, and are potentially harmed by, inotropes. Traditional inotropic agents used for decompensated heart failure include dobutamine, dopamine, and milrinone. At low doses (2–5 mcg/kg/min), dopamine receptors in the renal, cerebral, coronary, mesenteric, and pulmonary vasculature are stimulated. Higher doses of dopamine stimulate β-adrenergic receptors, increasing contractility and heart rate. At higher doses (≥ 10 mcg/kg/min), significant α-adrenergic stimulation occurs, resulting in vasoconstriction and increased systemic vascular resistance (SVR) and pulmonary vascular resistance (PVR). The side-effect profile is similar to dobutamine, including the propensity for tachycardia, dysrhythmias, and increased myocardial oxygen consumption. Milrinone is a phosphodiesterase (PDE) inhibitor with inotropic, lusitropic, and vasodilatory properties. Levosimendan is a *calcium sensitizer* that increases inotropy and vasodilation. Traditional inotropic agents that increase intracellular calcium are associated with increased oxygen consumption, impaired myocardial relaxation, and dysrhythmias.

Patients with inadequate perfusion and normal filling pressures represent a tenuous patient population. Vasodilators may not be beneficial and can worsen perfusion in patients with marginal blood pressure. Inotropic agents are often needed. In the setting of significantly compromised perfusion or cardiogenic shock, additional or alternative agents such as calcium chloride (especially after bypass), epinephrine, or vasopressin may also be necessary. If perfusion can be improved by inotropic therapy, titration of vasodilation therapy may become feasible, but inotropic agents may not be sufficient to return the patient to an asymptomatic state.

Epinephrine, at higher doses, causes vasoconstriction and increased SVR. Although the increased SVR

and contractility may acutely improve perfusion, it may occur at the expense of increased myocardial oxygen consumption and myocardial work. High-dose catecholamines for inotropic support can promote tachycardia and proarrhythmic effects and increase myocardial oxygen consumption. The use of arginine vasopressin during and after cardiac arrest has been shown to improve return of spontaneous circulation and survival in some series.

In the setting of increased inotropic requirements for the failing myocardium, mechanical support should be considered to "rest the myocardium." In children, mechanical support in this setting has generally been used as a bridge to cardiac transplantation. In the setting of a potentially reversible process, such as myocarditis, mechanical support has been used as a bridge to recovery. As heroic efforts such as mechanical support may not be available, appropriate, or desirable in many patients, palliative care and withdrawal of support may be appropriate.

MEDICAL MANAGEMENT OF LOW CARDIAC OUTPUT AFTER CARDIAC SURGERY

Management of postoperative low cardiac output after cardiac surgery (LCOS) includes optimization of preload and afterload; prompt diagnosis of residual cardiac lesions; prevention of hypoxia, anemia, and acidosis; and administration of pharmacologic agents to improve myocardial contractile function. In addition, in low cardiac output associated with right heart failure, some children may benefit from creation or enlargement of an atrial-level shunt to allow right-to-left shunting. Fever in the setting of LCOS should be treated aggressively with anti-pyretic medication or surface cooling. A cooling blanket may be useful, but shivering should be avoided, as it may be associated with an increase in oxygen consumption. Total oxygen consumption can be decreased by the induction of heavy sedation, paralysis, or mild hypothermia that reduces the metabolic rate.

Causes of postoperative hypovolemia include bleeding, excessive ultrafiltration, and vasodilation from rewarming or afterload reduction. Cardiac tamponade impairs preload by altering diastolic compliance. Preload determination is predominantly a "trial and error" process. When atrial pressure is low, fluid administration augments end-diastolic volume and increases stroke volume. With successive fluid administration, however, increases in stroke volume become limited. A poorly compliant ventricle, such as with right ventricular (RV) dysfunction after tetralogy of Fallot repair, would be expected to have higher end-diastolic and, thus, right atrial pressures than a normal heart and may rely on higher filling pressures to generate adequate output. Patients with diastolic dysfunction may require more extensive postoperative volume administration to maintain preload and cardiac output. These patients will also benefit from lusitropic therapy intended to improve diastolic ventricular filling.

Sinus bradycardia, bundle-branch block, and atrioventricular block can occur after many cardiac surgical procedures; thus, temporary atrial and ventricular pacing wires are typically placed to facilitate pacing, if necessary. Dysrhythmias occur frequently in postoperative cardiac surgical patients and may require overdrive pacing, cardioversion, or pharmacologic intervention. Loss of atrioventricular synchrony can compromise preload, increase pulmonary congestion, and significantly diminish cardiac output; thus, maintenance of atrioventricular synchrony is essential (via pacing, if necessary). Junctional ectopic tachycardia (JET) is a common tachyarrhythmia that usually occurs in the first 48 hrs following surgery, especially after procedures involving closure of a ventricular septal defect and in younger patients. Recognition of JET and other dysrhythmias may be aided by careful surveillance of atrial pressure waveforms; loss of the distinct *a* and *v* waves, indicating loss of atrioventricular synchrony, is often the first indication of dysrhythmia and/or atrioventricular dyssynchrony. Hypomagnesemia may contribute to the onset of JET. If the hemodynamics allow it, an effort should be made to discontinue adrenergic agents, which contribute to the onset of JET and increase the JET rate. Pacing, either atrial (if atrioventricular conduction is preserved) or atrioventricular sequential, is the initial therapy of choice. If the junctional rate is too fast to allow pacing, the goal of pharmacologic therapy is to provide rate control to allow institution of atrial or dual-chamber pacing. While IV amiodarone is generally considered the drug of choice, induction of hypothermia and procainamide administration has also been shown to be effective.

Residual cardiac lesions in the postoperative patient can lead to LCOS and result in increased morbidity and mortality. As low cardiac output after pediatric heart surgery is often associated with some level of contractile dysfunction, inotropic support in the early postoperative period is usually necessary. At constant preload, increased contractility should increase stroke volume. In that stroke volume is not easily monitored, indirect measures of cardiac output (such as SVC saturation) or measures of end-organ perfusion (such as urine output) may be plotted against atrial pressure to attain a "modified" Starling relationship. Ionotropic support is often initiated with low-dose infusions of dopamine or dobu-

tamine (3–5 mcg/kg/min). The infusion rate is usually titrated to optimize systemic blood flow and pressure. High doses of dopamine are rarely used because of increasing vasoconstrictor and chronotropic effects. High-dose epinephrine (>0.1 mcg/kg/min) frequently results in tachycardia and systemic vasoconstriction. Epinephrine is often used in combination with IV vasodilators such as milrinone, sodium nitroprusside, and phenoxybenzamine to treat ventricular dysfunction and decrease systemic afterload. PDE inhibitors improve cardiac index by enhancing both systolic and diastolic function and by reducing SVR and PVR. For patients at high risk for LCOS, some centers prefer to load with milrinone during bypass to avoid potential hypotension associated with loading. The multicentered PRIMACORP study demonstrated that use of milrinone in children early after congenital heart surgery reduces the incidence of LCOS. Patients with renal insufficiency are at risk for toxicity due to excessive drug levels. Continuous infusion rates should thus be adjusted based on creatinine clearance to avoid excessive and prolonged vasodilation, especially in neonates.

Hypocalcemia occurs frequently in the postoperative period due to transfusion of citrate-treated blood and administration of loop diuretics. Ionized calcium, the physiologically active form of calcium, should be monitored frequently in the postoperative period, and normal or supernormal levels should be maintained with supplementation. Thyroid hormone therapy is a potential treatment for LCOS. Arginine vasopressin has been advocated as a therapeutic option for pediatric patients with refractory hypotension after surgery to improve systemic arterial blood pressure when conventional therapies fail. Low-dose corticosteroid administration has been suggested as an option for patients with refractory LCOS. Stress-dose hydrocortisone (50 mg/m^2/day) may help to reduce inotropic requirements in pediatric patients with LCOS that is refractory to conventional therapy.

Benefits of afterload reduction are particularly pronounced in neonatal hearts and in the setting of poor contractility. With neonatal hearts or impaired contractility, afterload reduction is particularly useful to augment stroke volume and overall cardiac output. As with inotropic agents, it is important to assess efficacy of these agents following initiation or dosage adjustment, as vasodilator agents also have unwanted side effects. The therapeutic goal of afterload reduction should be a greater stroke volume for a comparable preload. As phenoxybenzamine is a potent vasodilator with a very long half-life (>24 hrs), its use may be complicated by severe hypotension. For this reasons, many centers prefer to use sodium nitroprusside for afterload reduction and vasodilator therapy in patients with congenital heart disease. PDE inhibitors are useful in the postoperative pediatric cardiac surgical patient because enhanced inotropic and lusitropic effects are combined with systemic and pulmonary vasodilation. In patients who require high doses of adrenergic agents, it is especially important to use one or more vasodilator agents simultaneously.

Patients who undergo right heart procedures, including tetralogy of Fallot and Fontan procedures, often demonstrate restrictive physiology (diastolic RV dysfunction), characterized by antegrade diastolic pulmonary arterial flow coinciding with atrial systole. Children with acute RV restrictive physiology have a decreased cardiac index because the stiff RV has impaired diastolic filling. Alterations in ventricular compliance make patients with RV failure particularly sensitive to alterations in venous return caused by intrathoracic pressure changes. These patients benefit from ventilation strategies that minimize intrathoracic pressure. Patients with RV failure may benefit from manipulation of PVR to minimize RV afterload. PDE inhibitors are beneficial in these patients due to the combined lusitropic and pulmonary vasodilatory effects.

The ability to maintain a right-to-left shunt at the atrial level is beneficial in patients with RV dysfunction. In patients who undergo the modified Fontan procedure, fenestration between the Fontan pathway and atrium is beneficial. In patients who undergo tetralogy of Fallot repair, a right-to-left atrial shunt can be similarly facilitated by maintaining the patency of the foramen ovale or by creating a small fenestration in the atrial septum.

Ventilation Strategies in Patients with Ventricular Dysfunction

Tidal volumes should be maintained in the range of 8–10 mL/kg to avoid overdistension, which could increase PVR and RV afterload. Furthermore, evidence suggests that shorter inspiratory times may augment LV filling in patients with systemic ventricular dysfunction. Alterations in thoracic pressure may have opposing hemodynamic effects and systemic oxygen delivery should be monitored. Spontaneous inspiration enhances diastolic flow and, thus, overall cardiac output in these patients; therefore, early extubation can be beneficial. Due to the detrimental effects of positive-pressure ventilation on RV dynamics, alternative modes of ventilation such as negative-pressure or high-frequency jet ventilation have been studied. In postoperative Fontan patients, high-frequency jet ventilation decreased mean airway pressure,

reduced PVR, and increased cardiac index. Similarly, negative-pressure ventilation has been shown to augment cardiac output in patients with restrictive physiology after tetralogy of Fallot repair.

MEDICAL MANAGEMENT OF MYOCARDITIS

As it is more effective to reduce the work on the heart than to "whip a failing heart," afterload reduction is the cornerstone of therapy for patients with myocarditis and clinically significant contractile dysfunction. Sodium nitroprusside is often used alone or in conjunction with other inotropic agents. PDE inhibitors such as IV milrinone have been used to provide both inotropy and afterload reduction. In some circumstances, nesiritide may be beneficial. When chronic oral therapy is possible and hypotension is not present, an afterload-reducing drug such as captopril (0.3–3.0 mg/kg/day, divided every 8 hrs) or enalapril (0.2–0.4 mg/kg/day, divided every 12 hrs) may be used in addition to digoxin and diuretics. The addition of β blockers such as carvedilol or metoprolol also appears to enhance the normalization of cardiac function. Because catecholamines generally aggravate myocardial injury, use should be carefully assessed and doses should be minimized. Low-dose dopamine or dobutamine (<5 mcg/kg/min) may provide some assistance in the presence of decreased ventricular function, but greater doses or addition of more potent catecholamines such as epinephrine or norepinephrine should prompt consideration for mechanical support. Although the reduced use of high-dose catecholamines has reduced the frequency of dysrhythmias in these patients, they should be vigorously treated when they do occur. Complete atrioventricular block requires an immediate intravenous pacemaker. Mechanical support is provided for patients unresponsive to medical therapy. Transplantation becomes necessary in patients who do not acutely recover despite medical and mechanical support of the failed myocardium.

The use of immunosuppressive agents in suspected or proven viral myocarditis is controversial. The Myocarditis Treatment Trial demonstrated no improvement among patients treated with (a) azathioprine and prednisone versus (b) cyclosporine and prednisone, along with conventional medical therapy. Although immunosuppressive therapy has not been shown to be beneficial in most patients with histologically confirmed myocarditis, we advocate combined treatment with IV immunoglobulin and pulse-dose steroids for patients with the fulminant necrotic myocarditis phenotype of myocarditis. Due to anecdotal reports of benefit, patients with suspected fulminant necrotic myocarditis are treated with IV methylprednisolone (10 mg/kg body weight every 8 hrs for 3 total doses).

A frequently used but unproven therapeutic option for children with myocarditis is IV δ-globulin. Patients are typically treated with 1–2 doses of 1 g/kg of IV immunoglobulin. A prospective, randomized trial is pending.

MEDICAL MANAGEMENT OF CARDIOMYOPATHIES

Acute management of a child newly diagnosed with dilated cardiomyopathy (DCM) should include an effort to rule out myocarditis or surgically correctable causes (i.e., anomalous left coronary artery arising from the pulmonary artery, aortic arch obstruction). The risk of complications such as thromboembolic events or dysrhythmia should be minimized, and supportive care of heart failure symptoms should be provided. If an intramural thrombus is detected by echocardiography, systemic anticoagulation is indicated. Newly diagnosed patients should have inpatient telemetry and Holter monitoring performed. Electrolyte imbalances should be identified and corrected if present. If supraventricular or ventricular dysrhythmias are identified, they should be treated to improve an already diminished cardiac output. The choice of an antiarrhythmic agent should be balanced against its potential to further depress ventricular function. IV diuretics offer symptomatic relief from volume overload and venous congestion, as well as the administration of IV inotropes or PDE inhibitors to augment cardiac output. More recently, nesiritide, a recombinant form of B-type natriuretic peptide, has been useful in improving urine output and cardiac function. When the patients' acute decompensation has been controlled, however, the emphasis in treatment should shift to an oral regimen of ACE inhibitors, diuretics, and β blockers.

Therapy of hypertrophic cardiomyopathy is directed at reduction of symptoms, prevention of untoward complications, and prevention of sudden cardiac death, β blockers or nondihydropyridine calcium-channel blockers such as verapamil have been used. Both groups of drugs reduce the heart rate, which improves ventricular filling by prolonging diastole. Disopyramide, a type I antiarrhythmic drug, has also been used to reduce symptoms and outflow tract obstruction. At our institution, β blockers are used first line, with the addition of verapamil in patients with persistent symptoms and/or persistent severe LV outflow obstruction. Diuretics and ACE inhibitors rarely may have a role in some patients.

THERAPEUTIC STRATEGIES FOR RESTRICTIVE CARDIOMYOPATHY

No consistent approach to therapy has been established for restrictive cardiomyopathy in pediatric patients. A variety of medications have been administered in combinations, including digoxin, afterload-reducing agents, calcium-channel blockers, and β blockers. The role of ACE inhibitors and diuretics are controversial, and can be used in select patients. A variety of other therapies, such as implantable cardiac defibrillators (ICD) should be considered for patients with evidence of ischemia and ventricular dysrhythmias. Strenuous physical activity should be avoided. Management of patients with arrhythmogenic right ventricular dysplasia consists of antiarrhythmic agents, but the only therapy with survival benefit appears to be implantation of an ICD. In addition, therapies for heart failure may be instituted as the disease progresses toward a pattern similar to DCM. Cardiac transplantation is required in some cases.

The treatment of LV noncompaction is dependent on associated comorbidities. Patients with the hypertrophic phenotype with or without depressed systolic function or the dilated phenotype should be treated as outlined above. Aggressive anticoagulant therapy should be considered in cases of thrombus or systemic embolic events. In patients with associated mitochondrial myopathy, a combination of riboflavin, thiamine, coenzyme Q10, and carnitine may be considered. Serial Holter monitoring of patients with LV noncompaction should be considered, as these patients have an increased risk for dysrhythmias. Ventricular dysrhythmias have been associated with this condition and may prompt the placement of an ICD. Patients who are refractory to adequate medical therapy may require consideration for cardiac transplantation.

CHAPTER 46B ■ TREATMENT OF HEART FAILURE IN INFANTS AND CHILDREN: MECHANICAL SUPPORT

ANA LIA GRACIANO • JON N. MELIONES • KEITH C. KOCIS

EXTRACORPOREAL LIFE SUPPORT

Extracorporeal life support (ECLS) is the term used to describe prolonged extracorporeal partial CPB, achieved by extrathoracic (via the carotid/vena cava or femoral vessels) or transthoracic (via the open sternum) cannulation. ECLS is the preferred and most common technique used for short-term cardiac support (3–14 days) of the neonate, infant, child, and adolescent with refractory heart failure. *Cardiac ECLS* is provided with a system, consisting of a distensible venous drainage reservoir, a servoregulated roller pump, a membrane oxygenator in which gas exchange occurs, and a countercurrent heat exchanger to maintain blood temperature. Membrane oxygenators, which have greater longevity than do hollow-fiber oxygenators, are being used by most centers; however, hollow-fiber oxygenators are quickly and easily primed, making them very useful for rapid-deployment situations. Roller pumps are used by most of the ECLS centers, though centrifugal pumps are increasingly used. Centrifugal pumps have the advantage of maintaining venous inflow independent of gravity, which helps to maintain adequate venous return at higher flows. Crystalloid preprimed circuits are used at many large ECLS centers for rapid-deployment situations, while "dry circuits" can be rapidly primed on site while the patient is being cannulated. Patients are typically anticoagulated with heparin to prevent thrombosis within the circuit and prevent the development of thromboemboli.

ECLS for refractory cardiac failure should be used in patients in whom cardiac function is *reversible* and *expected* to recover within a short period of time (5–14 days). Pediatric cardiac patients considered for ECLS fall essentially into two groups: surgical (postoperative) and medical (i.e., myocarditis). All candidates have clear evidence of low cardiac output syndrome with or without shock (hypotension, elevated filling pressures, low mixed venous oxygen saturations, decreased urine output, elevated lactic acid) that is refractory to maximal "standard medical" support, including mechanical ventilation, vasoactive agents, analgesia, etc. In surgical patients, it is extremely important to exclude residual anatomic causes of postoperative myocardial dysfunction *before* considering ECLS.

Indications for Extracorporeal Life Support

Indications for ECLS in patients with single-ventricle physiology is controversial but may include dysrhythmia, low output, cardiac arrest, unbalanced circulation, and hypoxemia, Patients with the Sano shunt may require increased ECLS flows to maintain adequate Qp and systemic oxygen saturations. The use of ECLS for patients with single-ventricle physiology in the *preoperative* state remains dismal.

Extracorporeal cardiopulmonary resuscitation relates to ECLS after cardiac arrest. Recently, large centers have developed systems that allow rapid initiation of ECLS after cardiac arrest that does not quickly respond to conventional pediatric advanced life support therapy. These rapid deployment systems provide fast, reliable support in patients with acute, sometimes "unexpected," deterioration, leading to cardiac arrest. Preprimed circuits or modified, rapidly primed circuits are used with deployment and cannulation times of <1 hr.

Patients with *fulminant acute myocarditis* can have a rapidly progressive deterioration and fatal outcome if not managed aggressively with ECLS. Balloon atrial septostomy in these patients will decompress the left ventricle (LV) similar to LV vents in postoperative patients).

ECLS can be used as a bridge to heart transplantation.

Patient Management Issues for the Pediatric Cardiac Patient on Extracorporeal Life Support

Venoarterial ECLS provides biventricular and lung support for children with low cardiac output states and represents the preferred approach in most patients with ventricular dysfunction. Biventricular support is provided by draining blood from the right atrium into the ECLS circuit and returning it to the aorta, thus bypassing both ventricles and the lungs. Complete cardiac support *cannot* be provided while the patient is on venoarterial ECLS, as complete venous drainage of the heart by the venous cannula cannot be accomplished. Thus, some blood always remains (albeit small at high flows) that continues to circulate through the heart in a fashion dependent on the underlying anatomy of the patient.

Venovenous ECLS does not provide *direct* cardiac support; however, it can provide several indirect benefits to cardiac performance by perfusing the lungs and the coronary circulation with well-oxygenated, pH-balanced blood, without subjecting the patient to the risks of arterial cannulation. Patients *with reversible pulmonary artery hypertension* and secondary RV failure who do not respond to conventional therapies can sometimes be supported on venovenous ECLS, allowing pulsatile flow from the LV to the systemic circulation. This is not the case in instances of *irreversible* pulmonary vascular disease (i.e., Eisenmenger syndrome) with irreversible RV failure, in which case little improvement in hemodynamics is accomplished. Venovenous ECLS has several potential advantages over venoarterial ECLS, such as (a) not increasing LV afterload with the high-pressure aortic cannula in the aorta; (b) decreasing RV afterload with improvement in RV oxygen consumption (RV MVO$_2$); (c) improving the efficiency of LV filling, ejection, and function by decreasing RV overdistension and moving the interventricular septum into a more favorable position (interventricular dependence); and (d) improving regional oxygen delivery to the coronary circulation.

The three primary routes for arterial/venous access are transcervical (carotid artery/internal jugular vein), transthoracic (aorta, right atrium), and femoral (common femoral artery/vein). In small children, the transcervical approach is preferred, while femoral venoarterial cannulations can be used in older children in whom the risk of arterial ischemia is less. *Transthoracic cannulation* is the choice in patients who cannot be weaned from CPB in the operating room or in the immediate postoperative period. If the patient is placed on ECLS because of inability to wean from CPB, the cannulae placed in surgery are maintained. Although allowing for much greater venous return due to the size of the cannulae, the major disadvantages of this route include increased mediastinal bleeding, infection, and potential for cannulae dislodgment.

While on ECLS, coronary blood flow is nearly exclusively from the *non-bypassed blood* ejected from the systemic ventricle, except in unusual circumstances such as cardiac stun and aortic insufficiency. For this reason, lung rest strategies regularly employed in neonatal respiratory failure ECLS have the adverse effect of "hypoxemic and acidotic coronary perfusion." Currently, most centers maintain modest amounts of ventilatory support and oxygenation to the lungs while the patient is on ECLS to allow for improved myocardial oxygen delivery by improving the quality of the non-bypassed blood.

Cardiac stun refers to a transient state of profound myocardial dysfunction whereby the systemic ventricle is unable to generate sufficient pressure to open up the semilunar valve and eject blood into the aorta against the pressure generated by the ECLS aortic cannula. Cardiac stun is manifested by lack of pulsation in the aorta and resembles electromechanical dissociation. The heart is overdistended due to the lack of ejection, and coronary perfusion is extremely poor. It usually occurs within the first 6 hrs after initiation of flow and can last up to 2–3 days. In patients with poor LV function, left atrial decompression is required to prevent cardiac overdistension, mitral regurgitation, pulmonary edema or hemorrhage, and to improve coronary perfusion.

Assessing the hemodynamic state of a patient on ECLS is more complex due to the necessity to consider the individual contributions from the ECLS circuit and the patient's native cardiac output in individually or jointly providing the systemic and pulmonary blood flow. Mixed venous saturation is typically measured in the venous return of the circuit, with a goal of >75% in acyanotic patients. It must be remembered that if an LV vent is in place and ventilation is occurring with oxygen, there is a "left-to-right shunt," which will artificially increase the mixed venous saturation. In cyanotic patients, an arterial-to-venous SO$_2$ difference in saturations of 20%–25% is typically targeted. Lactate measurements can be helpful, although delay in clearance can occur after prolonged periods of extremely low cardiac output or cardiac arrest. Blood gases are obtained frequently to assess pH, PO$_2$, and PCO$_2$, which is necessary to adjust the ECLS circuit.

Large amounts of evaporative losses in the circuit and to the "exposed" patient occur, and capillary leak is common. Frequent blood draws for monitoring and bleeding require replacement of packed red blood cells. Coagulopathy is common, requiring replacement therapy. In addition, the systemic inflammatory response is highly activated, resulting in excess vasodilation. Systemic runoff with low diastolic (and, thus, mean) pressure can occur through either a BT shunt or systemic-to-pulmonary collaterals. Hypotension can occur as the result of mechanical problems with the circuit, such as inadequate venous drainage, cardiac tamponade, tension pneumo/hemo thorax.

Vasoactive agents usually used to manage hypertension include nitroprusside, nitroglycerin, phenoxybenzamine, nicardipine, and milrinone. Arterial pressure should be maintained at appropriate ranges for age. Factors that can lead to hypertension include hypervolemia, excessive inotropes, pain, agitation, hypothermia, and seizures.

Although inotropic agents are weaned rapidly after initiation of support, low-dose inotropes should be maintained to improve cardiac contractility and augment native cardiac output. These inotropes usually used include dopamine (3 mcg/kg/min), epinephrine (0.05 mcg/kg/min), milrinone (0.75 mcg/kg/min), and dobutamine (5 mcg/kg/min).

Due to extracorporeal circulation, anticoagulation is nearly always required, though a few centers have reported short-term success without anticoagulation with the use of heparin-bonded circuits. Heparin is almost exclusively used, although use of hirudin and argatroban (thrombin inhibitors) have been reported in those patients who develop heparin-induced thrombocytopenia. Aminocaproic acid (Amicar) and heparin-bonded circuits are used to reduce bleeding in postoperative patients. Use of aprotinin, a serine protease inhibitor, is controversial due to reports of excessive thrombosis. Typically, the degree of anticoagulation is followed closely with the activated clotting time (ACT) test, a gross aggregate measure of total clotting ability. Although ACT is typically maintained at between 180 and 200 secs when on full flow, it may be decreased to 160 secs when active bleeding is occurring. Platelets should be transfused to maintain platelet counts above 100,000/mm^3. Nonsurgical bleeding after cardiac surgery is usually related to heparin overdose, thrombocytopenia, and/or fibrinolysis. Clotting factors and fibrinogen levels must be maintained while the patient is on ECLS.

The overall goal is to ventilate the lungs while minimizing the negative effects of positive-pressure ventilation, such as barotrauma, volutrauma, and oxygen toxicity. Adequate ventilation is necessary to avoid atelectasis, decrease pulmonary vascular resistance, and optimize the quality of the blood perfusing the coronary circulation. Peak inspiratory pressures should be <30 cm H_2O, and positive end-expiratory pressures should be between 3 and 5 cm H_2O. Respiratory rates between 15 and 25 per minute are set, depending on the age of the patient. Chest x-rays are obtained to assess the adequacy of lung inflation, taking care to avoid over distension as well as collapse.

Most patients are managed with total parenteral nutrition, although trophic feeding can be started and advanced in select patients. Fluid balance is difficult to measure due to the large, insensible losses described above. Diuretics (furosemide) are commonly used as the patient weans from mechanical support. In anuric or oliguric patients, early placement of hemofilter into the ECLS circuit to provide continuous ultrafiltration, hemofiltration, or hemodialysis is recommended.

Adequate analgesia and sedation are essential for patients on ECLS. Morphine, fentanyl, and/or midazolam are usually used. Lorazepam can be used in intermittent doses, but infusions should not be used, as toxicity to propylene glycol has been reported. Neuromuscular blockade should be avoided, for it will limit clinical neurologic evaluation and induce muscle weakness. Daily head ultrasounds should be obtained in neonates and young infants to assess for bleeding in the central nervous system. If no evidence for intracranial bleeding is seen on the initial head ultrasounds, many centers defer further studies, unless a change in clinical status occurs. Daily surveillance cultures and broad-spectrum antibiotics are used in managing these patients.

Many sources of emboli can occur during ECLS, such as air, fibrin, platelets aggregates, and blood microemboli. Air emboli may originate from areas of low or negative pressure within the ECLS system. Both roller and centrifugal pumps generate negative pressure when venous inflow is obstructed; other sources of air embolism are cracks in the tubing and loose stopcocks. Massive air embolism can be fatal. Thrombi during ECLS form in areas of cavitation, turbulence, stagnant flow, and connector seams. Thrombosis within the ECLS system is more common during periods of low flow, when heparin infusions are decreased, or during platelet transfusions.

Weaning Strategies from Extracorporeal Life Support

The ideal duration of cardiac support on ECLS is between 3 and 7 days, although ECLS data suggest that cardiac recovery may take as long as 2 wks. If prolonged support is needed, patients should be converted to a ventricular assist device (VAD). As patients recover cardiac function and native cardiac output improves, ECLS flows can begin to be decreased. During this period, inotropic support may need to be increased but not to high levels. Afterload reduction and improved contractility can be provided by a variety of agents but, most commonly, milrinone. The amount of time that the patient is clamped off of the ECLS circuit (with cannulae being flashed so as to prevent thrombosis) is variable. Typically, the decision of the team to decannulate is made after an hour of relative hemodynamic stability. Echocardiographic assessment, either through the transthoracic or transesophageal route, is mandatory during these final weaning stages.

VENTRICULAR ASSIST DEVICES

Support for pediatric patients with body surface area of <0.7 m² is not possible with the devices designed for adults. Patients who have right, left, or biventricular dysfunction with adequate ability to oxygenate through their own lungs are ideally managed with a VAD. Long-term support (>30 days) is much more attainable and successful with a VAD than with ECLS. Cannulation differs depending on whether the device is being placed to support, right (RVAD), left (LVAD), or biventricular (BiVAD) function. These devices are powered pneumatically, electrically (including portable battery packs), or magnetically.

Indications for placement on a VAD are the same as for ECLS—typically, failure to wean from CPB but without the need for an oxygenator. Flows are maintained at 150 mL/kg/min. Anticoagulation is maintained with heparin infusions, with goal ACTs between 140 and 160 secs. Heparin-bonded circuits are being used at many centers. Plasma free hemoglobin should be <60 mg/dL and should be measured daily and, if values are higher (indicating high degree of hemolysis), pump replacement should be considered.

Other Forms of Mechanical Cardiac Support

The intra-aortic balloon pump (IABP) has a balloon (0.75–10 mL) mounted on a 4 or 5 F catheter that inflates during diastole in the aorta to provide coronary blood flow augmentation and then deflates before cardiac ejection. A few implantable, total artificial hearts (AbioCor™ and Jarvik 7) have been developed and are beginning to be used in adults.

CHAPTER 46C ■ TREATMENT OF HEART FAILURE IN INFANTS AND CHILDREN: CARDIAC TRANSPLANTATION

STEVEN A. WEBBER

Transplantation of the heart is generally considered to be indicated when expected survival is <2 years and/or when the patient has an unacceptable quality of life. The indications for heart transplantation in children were summarized in a 1999 report from the Pediatric Committee of the American Society of Transplantation and in a more report from 2007. Perhaps the most controversial indication for heart transplantation is hypoplastic left heart syndrome and related pathologies in the newborn. Relative and/or absolute contraindications include chronic infection with either hepatitis B or C, or HIV; prior nonadherence with medical therapy; recent or current treatment of malignancy with inadequate follow-up to ensure likely cure; active acute viral, fungal or bacterial infections; elevated and fixed pulmonary vascular resistance (PVR) above 10 IU; inadequate intraparenchymal pulmonary vascular bed; diffuse pulmonary vein stenosis; and major extracardiac disease felt to be nonreversible with heart transplantation (i.e., severe systemic myopathy). Inevitably, some centers consider specific contraindications absolute, whereas others may feel they are relative. A typical evaluation protocol is shown in **Table 46C.1**.

PREOPERATIVE EVALUATION OF THE PROPOSED RECIPIENT

The most complex anatomy may be transplanted, provided the lung vasculature is adequately developed and PVR is acceptable. Anatomic points of most interest to the surgeon include abnormalities of cardiac and visceral situs (especially anomalies of the systemic and pulmonary venous return) and the size and anatomy of the main and branch pulmonary arteries (including the presence of stenoses, distortions, and nonconfluence). Intracardiac anatomy is less important, as the bulk of the cardiac mass will be explanted. In general, children with indexed PVR (PVRI) ≤6 IU are considered low risk for acute donor right heart

TABLE 46C.1

EVALUATION OF CANDIDATES FOR HEART TRANSPLANTATION

History and physical examination

Required consultations
  Pediatric cardiologist, congenital cardiovascular surgeon, cardiac anesthesiologist, infectious disease specialist,
    psychiatrist or psychologist, transplant coordinator, social worker

Additional consultations (as required)
  Neonatology, genetics, neurology, dental, oncology, immunology, nephrology, nutritional services,
    physical/occupational therapy, developmental pediatrics, hospital finance

Cardiac diagnostic studies
  Chest radiograph, electrocardiogram, echocardiogram, cardiac catheterization
  In selected patients: exercise test, ventilation-perfusion scan, chest CT or MRI, pulmonary function tests

Blood type (ABO), anti-HLA antibody screen, complete blood count and white cell differential, platelet count,
    coagulation screen, blood urea nitrogen, serum creatinine, glucose, calcium, magnesium, liver function tests, lipid
    profile, brain natriuretic peptide.

Serologic screening for antibodies to the following pathogens: cytomegalovirus; Epstein-Barr; herpes simplex virus;
    varicella-zoster virus; HIV; hepatitis A, B, C, D, and measles; antibodies to *Toxoplasma gondii*

PPD/Mantoux tuberculosis test placement

Update immunizations, including hepatitis B, pneumococcal and influenza (in season)

---

failure. If resistance is between 6 and 10 IU, the risks are higher, but transplantation is still generally not considered to be contraindicated. A PVRI >10 IU is usually considered a contraindication to isolated heart transplantation, unless a major fall is achieved (to well below 10 IU) with pulmonary vasodilator therapy (100% O_2 and/or nitric oxide). In borderline cases, restudy of hemodynamics after several days of inotropic and vasodilator therapy may be necessary.

The laboratory tests that should be conducted in a transplant candidate are summarized in **Table 46C.1**. Blood typing is necessary to ensure ABO compatibility with the transplanted organ, though infants and young children with absent or low anti-A and anti-B isohemagglutinin titers may be safely transplanted across traditional ABO barriers. Evaluation for the presence of preformed anti-HLA antibodies ("sensitized") is performed using panel-reactive antibody and solid-phase assays. Infectious disease evaluation includes serologic testing for cytomegalovirus (CMV), Epstein-Barr virus (EBV), varicella, herpes simplex virus, *Toxoplasma gondii*, HIV, measles and hepatitis viruses A, B, C, and D. Serologic status for these agents may guide prophylaxis as well as the diagnostic evaluation of posttransplantation fever.

Each candidate is evaluated by a multidisciplinary team that includes the transplant cardiologist and surgeon, social worker, transplant coordinator, and infectious disease expert. A screening psychiatric/psychologic examination of the patient and the family is also very important. Additional consultations may be required from specialist services such as hematology-oncology (when the patient has a past history of malignancy), child development, genetics, neurology, and feeding/nutritional specialists. Patients with Fontan circulation require evaluation of the liver for evidence of cirrhosis and may require formal hepatology consultation.

PREOPERATIVE EVALUATION OF THE PROPOSED DONOR

Evaluation of the proposed donor is summarized in **Table 46C.2**.

IMMEDIATE POSTOPERATIVE MANAGEMENT FOLLOWING HEART TRANSPLANTATION

Most heart transplant recipients will benefit from low-dose inotropic support in the immediate postoperative period, though often this is only required for 2–3 days. Low-dose dobutamine and isoproterenol are common choices. The latter is sometimes recommended because of its combined properties of chronotropy, inotropy, and pulmonary

TABLE 46C.2

EVALUATION OF THE CARDIAC DONOR

History
  Donor age, height, weight, and gender
  Cause of brain death
  History of cardiac arrest and length of resuscitation
  Evidence of chest trauma
  History of IV drug usage
  Past history of cardiovascular disease
  Distance from transplant center
  History of malignancy

Cardiovascular status
  Heart rate, blood pressure, central venous pressure
  Fluid balance
  Blood gas
  Types and doses of IV inotropes
  Inotropic support increasing or decreasing

Cardiovascular testing
  Electrocardiogram
  Chest radiograph
  Echocardiogram
  Cardiac enzymes

Other testing
  Infectious disease screen: CMV, EBV, *Toxoplasma gondii*, HIV-1, HIV-2, HTLV-1, HTLV-2, RPR, hepatitis B and C
  All culture results since admission to ICU

vasodilatation. The addition of a combined vasodilator/inotropic agent such as milrinone is logical in the presence of low cardiac output and evidence of high systemic vascular resistance.

In contrast to the nontransplant cardiac surgical patient, systemic hypertension is common. Many factors contribute to this, including vigorous function of an oversized donor organ and use of high dose corticosteroids. It is not unusual to observe quite severe systolic hypertension within 24 hrs of a successful transplant procedure. Treatment with a variety of IV vasodilators, including β blockers, is necessary.

PVR is a risk factor for acute right ventricular failure. Nitric oxide is begun in the operating room and is used to wean from cardiopulmonary bypass. Acidosis must be avoided, and high levels of inspired oxygen are provided. Generous sedation is provided in the early postoperative period. If necessary, prostaglandin E_1 can also be used. The right heart may require significant inotropic support, and sometimes epinephrine may be required in addition to milrinone and dobutamine. If right ventricular dysfunction persists with poor cardiac output despite this level of support, then mechanical assistance should be provided.

The most common postoperative rhythm abnormality (other than sinus tachycardia) is sinus bradycardia, with or without an atrial or junctional escape rhythm. The denervated sinus node responds appropriately to exogenous chronotropic agents, and isoproterenol is useful in this respect. A simpler approach is atrial pacing, and all transplant recipients should have temporary pacing wires placed in the operating room. Ventricular ectopy and nonsustained ventricular tachycardia may occur in the first week or two after transplantation but rarely requires treatment.

Primary Graft Failure

The term *primary graft failure* is often reserved for the finding of acute left ventricular or biventricular failure not due to elevated PVR. Poor donor selection, prolonged ischemic time, poor preservation technique, and hyperacute rejection should all be considered. The latter is extremely rare with routine recipient pretransplant screening for anti-HLA antibodies. When primary graft failure occurs, recovery is frequently possible if the circulation can be supported, which is usually achieved with extracorporeal membrane oxygenation.

Respiratory Support

Early extubation should be the goal. The patient who has required prolonged preoperative mechanical ventilation will usually need more prolonged ventilatory support postoperatively, as retraining of respiratory muscles will be required. Infants with long-standing cardiomegaly will often have significant tracheobronchomalacia, and persistent or recurrent pulmonary atelectasis is not unusual.

Renal Function

The combination of chronic heart failure, cardiopulmonary bypass, and use of cyclosporine or tacrolimus all contribute to postoperative renal dysfunction, which is exacerbated with a low postoperative cardiac output state. Oliguria is common. Persistent oliguria is managed with loop diuretics and low-dose dopamine (e.g., 3–5 mcg/kg/min). Low output is managed with inotropic agents. Administration of a continuous furosemide infusion (up to 6 mg/kg/day) may be helpful. These maneuvers are usually successful in stimulating an adequate urine output (>1 mL/kg/hr). In some cases, particularly in neonates and infants, IV prostaglandin E_1 may also provide a diuretic effect. When urine output remains low, it may be necessary to decrease or hold calcineurin inhibitors (tacrolimus or cyclosporine), which can be facilitated by the use of IV induction agents as part of the early immunosuppressive regimen.

Gastrointestinal Considerations

Gastrointestinal complications are quite common early after pediatric heart transplantation. All patients should receive intravenous and, subsequently, oral H_2 antagonists to decrease the risk of stress ulcers in the early postoperative period. These are usually continued until corticosteroids have been weaned to low doses or discontinued. The nasogastric tube is removed as soon as the patient is extubated and able to take oral feeds and medications. Attention is paid to providing optimal calories without use of excessive volumes, as most patients will tend to retain fluid in the early postoperative period. Pancreatitis is not uncommon following transplantation and should be sought in the presence of abdominal pain or unexplained feeding intolerance. Immunosuppressive regimens that avoid the use of azathioprine and corticosteroids may reduce this complication. Symptoms of gastrointestinal perforation may be subtle in small children on immunosuppressive medications, especially if corticosteroids are being used. Many children with chronic heart failure have gastroesophageal reflux disease; this should be aggressively managed but with knowledge that many drug interactions occur between immunosuppressant medications and drugs used for gastroesophageal reflux disease, including antacids, antihistamines, and prokinetic agents.

Infectious Precautions

During the first week after transplantation, invasive lines and drains are removed as soon as possible. A short course of antibiotics (e.g., 72 hrs) is given as prophylaxis against mediastinal and wound infection. Usually, a first-generation cephalosporin will suffice. Broader staphylococcal coverage (i.e., vancomycin) is given if the patient has had a prolonged ICU stay and has long-standing vascular catheters in place. Such lines are usually replaced in the operating room. Patients colonized with methicillin-resistant *Staphylococcus aureus* are also covered with vancomycin. Oral nystatin is started in the ICU, along with ganciclovir, if recipient or donor is seropositive for CMV. Patients at high risk for yeast infections (e.g., patients on pretransplant extracorporeal membrane oxygenation) are frequently given prophylaxis with fluconazole. However, it should be noted that all "azole" antifungals have a profound effect on calcineurin-inhibitor metabolism (via the cytochrome P450 system). A marked reduction in tacrolimus or cyclosporine dosing (50%–90% reduction) is required during concomitant use of an azole antifungal agent. Initiation of prophylaxis against *Pneumocystis carinii* can follow closer to the time of hospital discharge.

Immunosuppression and Early Acute Rejection

High-dose IV methylprednisolone (e.g., 15–20 mg/kg) is given in the operating room. A tapering course of corticosteroids is usually given over the next 1–2 weeks, with the majority of centers discharging patients on maintenance corticosteroid therapy. However, steroid-free immunosuppressive regimens are increasingly being used in pediatric practice. Cyclosporine or tacrolimus is commenced generally within 24–48 hrs of surgery once good urine output has been established. Both agents can be given intravenously or enterally. If anti–T-cell induction therapy is used (most commonly, polyclonal rabbit antithymocyte globulin; less often with an IL-2 receptor antagonist), then there is less urgency to introduce a calcineurin inhibitor in the immediate (first 1–2 days) posttransplant period. The principals of maintenance therapy are summarized in **Table 46C.3**.

Rejection is generally delayed with use of induction therapy. Pallor, increasing tachycardia, abdominal pain, gallop rhythm, and oliguria all are suggestive of severe rejection. Ideally, rejection is identified by echocardiography and/or surveillance biopsy before such signs develop. The electrocardiogram may show reduced precordial voltages. If evidence of new graft dysfunction is unequivocal, empiric treatment of bolus intravenous corticosteroids is given. Endocardial muscle biopsy generally shows lymphocytic infiltrates (predominantly T cells) with varying degrees of edema and myocyte dama.

MEDIUM-TERM AND LATE COMPLICATIONS

Patients remain at risk for acute rejection indefinitely. Systolic dysfunction is associated with acute rejection, and rapid deterioration is common, even when the patient appears well. Thus, it is prudent to admit all patients with acute graft failure to the ICU for initiation of therapy. If systolic failure is more

TABLE 46C.3

POTENTIAL COMBINATIONS OF MAINTENANCE IMMUNOSUPPRESSIVE DRUGS USED IN PEDIATRIC HEART TRANSPLANTATION

Number of agents	Potential combinations	Comments
Monotherapy	Tacrolimus or cyclosporine	Monotherapy rarely used with cyclosporine.
Dual therapy	Tacrolimus or cyclosporine *with* azathioprine *OR* mycophenolate mofetil *OR* sirolimus/everolimus or corticosteroids	Little experience with the mTOR (target of rapamycin) inhibitors sirolimus and everolimus in children. Steroid avoidance increasingly common in pediatric heart transplantation.
Triple therapy	Tacrolimus or cyclosporine *with* corticosteroids *with* azathioprine *OR* mycophenolate mofetil *OR* sirolimus/everolimus	In triple therapy regimens, mycophenolate mofetil is being used with increasing frequency in lieu of azathioprine.

than mild, IV milrinone should be initiated, and the patient should be monitored for dysrhythmias. Unless graft failure is known to be due to coronary artery disease, treatment for acute rejection/graft dysfunction should be initiated with IV methylprednisolone (10–15 mg/kg, maximum 1 g) daily for 3–5 days. Additional therapies may be required, including plasmapheresis. It should be emphasized that treatment of severe acute rejection should not be delayed while awaiting endomyocardial biopsy or biopsy results.

Chronic Rejection or Posttransplantation Coronary Arterial Disease

The terms *chronic rejection* and *posttransplant coronary arterial disease* are generally used synonymously. Coronary disease subsequent to transplantation is an accelerated vasculopathy that is the leading cause of death among late survivors of pediatric heart transplantation. Symptoms of ischemia are often absent, though some children experience episodes of abdominal pain and/or chest pain despite operative denervation of the heart. Syncope and sudden death are also common presentations of graft coronary disease in children. No curative treatment exists for established coronary arterial disease. Diastolic dysfunction tends to develop early. Once overt systolic failure ensues, survival is poor, and consideration should be given to retransplantation.

Infections in patients with coronary arterial disease are caused by pathogens that also cause infection in the non-immunocompromised host.

Common examples include respiratory viruses, *Streptococcus pneumoniae*, and varicella virus. All infections that occur in non-immunocompromised patients can cause greater disease severity in the recipient of a transplanted heart. Of particular note in this respect are infections due to CMV and EBV, which only rarely cause severe disease in the immunocompetent host. Rarely, opportunistic infections are seen due to *Pneumocystis jiroveci* (formerly *Pneumocystis carinii*). Corticosteroids should not be discontinued if they are being used chronically, and stress dosing may be indicated. Broad-spectrum antibiotic coverage is required in any septic transplant recipient until an organism has been identified. When there is clinical and radiographic evidence of pneumonia and deteriorating clinical status, the clinician should maintain a low threshold for performing bronchoalveolar lavage to obtain deep cultures for viruses, fungi, and bacteria. *Pneumocystis jiroveci* should be ruled out when hypoxia occurs and characteristic chest x-ray changes are seen. Respiratory viral pathogens (e.g., respiratory syncytial virus, influenza, parainfluenza, adenovirus) should be sought when evidence of severe respiratory infection is seen in a heart transplant recipient. Primary CMV infection is less problematic in heart transplant patients than in lung transplant recipients. In heart recipients, gastroenteritis, hepatitis, and bone marrow suppression are relatively common findings. Diagnosis is facilitated by evaluation of peripheral blood by PCR or antigenemia (pp65) testing. EBV infection in the immunocompromised host can be asymptomatic or cause a nonspecific viral syndrome, mononucleosis, fulminant "viral sepsis," or posttransplant lymphoproliferative disorder

(PTLD). Therapeutic strategies include reduction or temporary cessation of immunosuppression, antiviral agents, monoclonal antibodies against B-cell antigens (e.g., rituximab), chemotherapy and, rarely, cellular (adoptive) immunotherapy. With the latter, patients are given infusions of autologous cytotoxic T lymphocytes (cultured ex vivo) directed against EBV-specific antigens.

Nonimmune Complications

In addition to the consequences of over- or under-immunosuppression, transplant recipients experience systemic hypertension, hyperlipidemia, glucose intolerance, decreased bone mineral density, bone marrow suppression, and progressive renal dysfunction due to calcineurin inhibitor renal toxicity.

CHAPTER 47 ■ CARDIAC CONDUCTION, DYSRHYTHMIAS, AND PACING

BRADLEY S. MARINO • JONATHAN R. KALTMAN • RONN E. TANEL

THE CARDIAC CONDUCTION SYSTEM

The sinus node is the normal site of impulse formation in the heart. Propagation of the impulse then travels through the atrial myocardium to the atrioventricular (AV) node. Refractoriness of AV node cells is both voltage and time dependent. These characteristics result in slowing of conduction between the atrium and ventricle and potential filtering of rapid or closely coupled beats. From the AV node arises the bundle of His, which penetrates the interventricular septum and divides into right and left bundle branches (fascicles), and the left bundle further divides into an anterior and posterior fascicle. The fascicles propagate the depolarizing wave to the penetrating Purkinje fibers, which carry the electrical depolarization to the ventricular myocardium.

DYSRHYTHMIA MECHANISMS AND CLINICAL CATEGORIZATION

Tachyarrhythmias

Abnormally fast rhythms involve three electrophysiologic mechanisms: (a) *reentry*, (b) *increased automaticity*, and (c) *triggered automaticity* (**Fig. 47.1**). *Reentry* describes the phenomenon of an electrical wave front "reentering" cardiac tissue through which it has already traveled. An electrical impulse will enter the circuit and begin to pass down the two pathways. If that impulse arrives in one limb of the pathway at such

a time that the pathway with the longer refractory period has not recovered from the previous impulse, block will occur in that pathway. If the second pathway has recovered (shorter refractory period), the impulse will propagate down that second pathway. Propagation down that pathway may be slow enough to allow for the recovery of the first pathway, thus allowing the electrical impulse to travel in a retrograde fashion up the first pathway, thereby returning it to the original entry site into the circuit and establish a reentry circuit (a.k.a., *circus movement*). Reentrant arrhythmias typically have a regular rate with an abrupt onset and termination. In addition, this type of dysrhythmia can be provoked by an electrical stimulus, such as a premature atrial or ventricular contraction or by pacing maneuvers and can be terminated by a variety of means, including pacing and direct-current cardioversion.

Automaticity refers to the ability of a cell or group of cells to spontaneously depolarize. When cells outside of the sinus node or AV node develop increased automaticity, they have the potential to suppress the sinus node if their rate of depolarization is greater than that of the sinus node. If these cells fire pathologically in a repetitive fashion, they result in a tachycardia. Automatic tachycardias typically have an irregular rate and a warm-up and cool-down phase, and they are sensitive to the adrenergic state. Unlike reentrant tachyarrhythmias, pacing and direct-current cardioversion do not convert these arrhythmias.

Triggered automaticity results from small oscillations of a cell's membrane potential during or after repolarization. Tachycardias derived from triggered activity share characteristics of both reentrant and

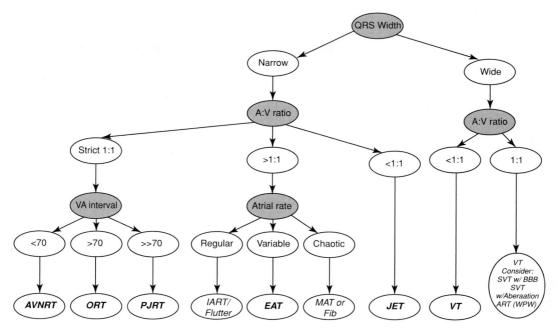

FIGURE 47.1. Diagnostic approach for determining tachycardia mechanism. ART, antidromic recipro-cating tachycardia; AV, atrioventricular; AVNRT, atrioventricular nodal reentrant tachycardia; BBB, bundle branch block; EAT, ectopic atrial tachycardia; IART, intra-atrial reentrant tachycardia; JET, junctional ec-topic tachycardia; MAT, multi-focal atrial tachycardia; ORT, orthodromic reciprocating tachycardia; PJRT, permanent junctional reciprocating tachycardia; SVT, supraventricular tachycardia; VA, ventriculo-atrial; VT, ventricular tachycardia; WPW, Wolff-Parkinson-White. From Walsh EP. Clinical approach to diag-nosis and acute management of tachycardias in children. In: Walsh EP, Saul JP, Triedman JK, eds. *Cardiac Arrhythmias in Children and Young Adults with Congenital Heart Disease.* Philadelphia: Lippincott Williams & Wilkins, 2001, with permission.

automatic arrhythmias. For example, they may be in-duced or terminated with pacing maneuvers, have warm-up and cool-down phases, and are cate-cholamine sensitive.

Postoperative reentrant pathways around surgical scars have been termed *intra-atrial reentrant tachy-cardia* (IART) or *incisional tachycardia*. Reentry may also involve pathways within or leading to the AV node, resulting in AV nodal reentrant tachycardia (AVNRT). The most common reentrant tachycar-dias in the pediatric population are those that in-volve an *accessory pathway*, which is an anomalous electrical connection between atrial and ventricular myocardium across the AV groove. These AV re-ciprocating tachycardias (AVRT) use the accessory pathway (usually the pathway with the longer re-fractory period) and the AV node (usually the path-way with slower conduction) as the two limbs of the reentrant circuit. Wolff-Parkinson-White (WPW) syndrome involves an accessory pathway that can support both antegrade and retrograde conduction (**Fig. 47.2**).

Automatic tachycardias may originate in any of the cardiac segments. Multifocal atrial tachycardia

(MAT), or chaotic atrial rhythm, is derived from mul-tiple atrial foci firing during the same time interval. Increased automaticity near the AV node gives rise to junctional ectopic tachycardia (JET). Finally, some rare types of VT may arise from isolated foci within the Purkinje fibers of the ventricle.

Diagnostic Approach to Tachyarrhythmias

A 12-lead electrocardiogram (ECG) with a long multi-lead rhythm strip, telemetry recording, or Holter monitor is necessary to determine the dys-rhythmia mechanism. Narrow-complex tachycar-dias imply conduction through the normal AV node and His-Purkinje system and are therefore supraventricular in origin. A wide-complex tachy-cardia should be assumed to be ventricular in origin but may also be due to a supraventricular tachycar-dia (SVT) with bundle-branch block, rate-dependent aberrancy, or antidromic reciprocating tachycardia (e.g., WPW).

The relationship of atrial to ventricular complexes is important to the determination of the tachycardia mechanism. If the ratio of P waves to QRS complexes

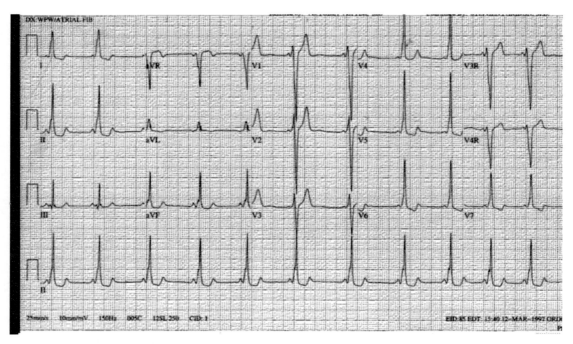

FIGURE 47.2. ECG from a child with Wolff-Parkinson-White syndrome. Note the short PR interval and delta wave.

is 1, then AVNRT or AVRT is likely. Sinus tachycardia may be differentiated from AVNRT or AVRT by a P wave frontal plane axis of 0 to +90 degrees in a normal situs solitus heart. An A : V ratio >1 is diagnostic of a primary atrial tachycardia, although 1 : 1 AV conduction can also occur with a primary atrial tachycardia. If the atrial rate is regular, atrial flutter (or IART) is likely (**Fig. 47.3**). An irregular atrial rate that has a single P-wave morphology different from the sinus P-wave morphology and the axis of which is outside of the 0 to +90-degree range suggests ectopic atrial tachycardia. An irregular atrial rate with 3 or more P wave morphologies suggests MAT. JET may have 1 : 1 VA conduction or VA dissociation with

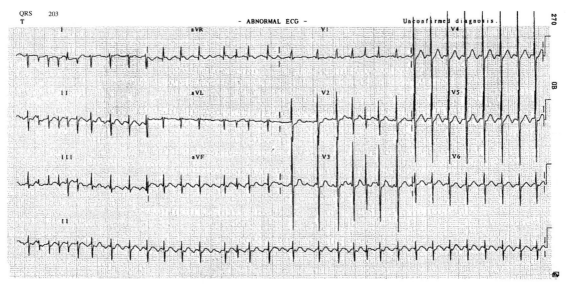

FIGURE 47.3. ECG showing atrial flutter with 2 : 1 conduction in a newborn. Note the typical flutter waves and "saw-tooth pattern" in leads II, III, and aVF.

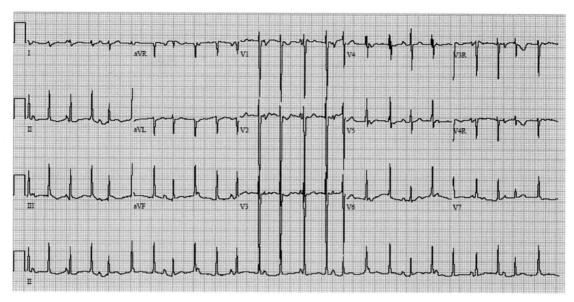

FIGURE 47.4. ECG showing congenital junctional ectopic tachycardia in a newborn. Note the narrow QRS complex with AV dissociation and a ventricular rate that is faster than the atrial rate.

occasional sinus capture and a ventricular rate greater than the atrial rate (**Fig. 47.4**).

Wide-complex tachycardias should be assumed to be ventricular, until proven otherwise. A wide-complex tachycardia with AV dissociation (i.e., no relationship between P waves and QRS complexes) and a ventricular rate greater than the atrial rate is diagnostic of VT. A wide-complex tachycardia with an A : V ratio of 1 can be VT with retrograde conduction or SVT with aberrancy, SVT with bundle-branch block, or antidromic SVT.

Bradyarrhythmias

Bradyarrhythmias result from abnormalities in impulse propagation or sinus node dysfunction (SND). Important features to determine whether a bradyarrhythmia is due to SND or conduction block. include the relationship of P waves to QRS complexes and the PR interval. If the ratio of P waves to QRS complexes is 1 : 1, the PR interval is normal, and the rhythm is atrially derived, then SND is present with sinus bradycardia or ectopic atrial bradycardia. If the PR interval is prolonged, then first degree AV block is present. If the PR interval is prolonging beat to beat, culminating with a dropped QRS complex, then Mobitz type I (Wenckebach) second-degree AV block is present. Intermittent dropped QRS complexes without PR interval prolongation on prior beats indicates Mobitz type II second-degree AV block. Complete

heart block, or third-degree AV block, is present when AV dissociation occurs and the ratio of atrial to ventricular complexes is >1 : 1.

Specific Diagnosis

The most common type of reentrant SVT in children is AVRT, which requires participation of both the atrium and ventricle in the reentrant circuit. AVRT utilizes accessory pathways and includes WPW syndrome, orthodromic tachycardia from concealed bypass tracts, and AVNRT. If SVT goes undetected, the patient may develop congestive heart failure, manifested as tachypnea, diaphoresis, pallor, and lethargy. Older children may complain of symptoms such as palpitations, chest pain, abdominal pain, or dizziness. Syncope may occur if the tachycardia rate is sufficiently fast to impair diastolic filling, resulting in hypotension and cerebral hypoperfusion. Wolff-Parkinson-White (WPW) syndrome is characterized by a short PR interval and delta wave, which represents ventricular pre-excitation prior to normal activation of the AV node and His-Purkinje system. SVT may be either orthodromic reciprocating tachycardia (down the AV node and up the accessory pathway) or antidromic reciprocating tachycardia (down the accessory pathway and up the AV node). Patients with WPW are at an increased risk of atrial fibrillation and sudden death.

The goal of acute therapy for atrioventricular reciprocating tachycardia is to terminate the reentrant circuit and restore sinus rhythm. A patient who presents in shock should be treated with the ABCs of resuscitation (airway, breathing, and circulation). If vascular access cannot readily be obtained and/or the patient is in extremis, then direct-current cardioversion is indicated. Synchronized cardioversion should be performed with an energy dose of 0.5–1 J/kg. The output can be doubled to a maximum of 6 J/kg until the treatment is effective.

In the acute but stable patient with AVRT, first-line therapy is adenosine. Adenosine rapidly interrupts the reentrant circuit at the AV node. Due to the short half-life, adenosine should be administered through a large-bore intravascular catheter placed as close to the heart as possible. Digoxin is effective and especially useful in the patient with decreased myocardial function, but it may take several hours to achieve blood levels to provide pharmacologic cardioversion. Other IV pharmacologic therapies used in the acute setting include β blockers (e.g., esmolol), procainamide, and amiodarone. These medications should be used with caution, as they all have negative inotropic effects. Other therapeutic modalities include transesophageal pacing and vagal maneuvers. Vagal maneuvers for adolescents and older children include the Valsalva maneuver and the headstand. In infants, a bag of ice to the center of the face frequently terminates the SVT by eliciting the diving reflex. While IV calcium-channel blockers are an important therapy for SVT in adults, they are contraindicated in young children, especially in those children <1 year of age or who are receiving β blockers. Hemodynamic collapse and sudden death have been reported in infants treated with verapamil.

Digoxin and calcium-channel blocker are contraindicated in patients with WPW because they may enhance antegrade conduction down the accessory pathway and allow for a more rapid ventricular response during atrial flutter or fibrillation. For SVT refractory to first-line therapy of adenosine or cardioversion, amiodarone, or other agents such as flecainide, procainamide, sotalol, and verapamil can also be employed. An increasingly popular therapeutic modality for recurrent SVT is catheter ablation, using either radiofrequency energy or cryoenergy.

Atrial flutter of infancy is rare. It may present in utero or during the newborn period. As congenital heart defects may coexist with the dysrhythmia, echocardiography is recommended to exclude most commonly atrial septal defect, aneurysm of atrial septum, or Ebstein anomaly. The reentrant circuit of atrial flutter of infancy is generally confined to the right atrium. Characteristic saw-toothed flutter waves are usually present in leads II, III, and aVF. Atrial rates may reach over 400 bpm. AV block with 2 : 1 conduction results in a ventricular response rate of $\geq$200 bpm (**Fig. 47.3**). Atrial flutter in the newborn

is converted to sinus rhythm with medications, transesophageal pacing, or cardioversion. Medications include IV digoxin, procainamide, amiodarone, and sotalol. Procainamide should be used in conjunction with digoxin, as procainamide may slow the flutter rate, resulting in more rapid AV conduction. Digoxin is used to increase the degree of AV block in this setting.

Atrial flutter in patients who have undergone surgery for congenital heart disease is referred to as IART or *incisional atrial tachycardia* to highlight its differences from typical atrial flutter. The surgical procedures that predispose patients to IART generally involve surgery in the atria, including atrial septal defect repair, atrial baffling procedures (Senning or Mustard operation) for D-transposition of the great arteries, and the Fontan operation for the univentricular heart. Atrial rates in IART vary considerably from 150 to 450 bpm, with variable conduction to the ventricle. Symptomatology is related to the ventricular response rate and myocardial function. A fast ventricular response may result in palpitations, syncope, or sudden death. A slower ventricular response rate may result in gradual fatigue or exercise intolerance, especially in the Fontan patient, as AV synchrony may be crucial for adequate cardiac output. If the ventricular response rate is slow enough, patients may be asymptomatic.

Prior to any attempts at converting IART to sinus rhythm, the presence of an atrial thrombus must be ruled out, which usually requires transesophageal echocardiography, especially in older children and adolescents, as transthoracic windows may be inadequate to visualize an intra-atrial thrombus. Acute therapy includes antiarrhythmic medications, transesophageal pacing, and cardioversion. Medications that have been successful in this setting include procainamide, propafenone, amiodarone, and sotalol. An agent to slow AV nodal conduction, such as digoxin, should be used in conjunction with class IA antiarrhythmics, such as procainamide.

Ectopic atrial tachycardia (EAT), or *automatic atrial tachycardia*, arises from a single focus of increased automaticity located within the atria. The firing rate of the ectopic focus is faster than that of the sinus node and overrides the normal sinus node activity. Heart rates can range from 130 to 210 bpm in children and adolescents, but can reach 300 bpm in infants. AV block may occur during the tachycardia but will not interrupt the atrial tachycardia. EAT is associated with conditions that result in atrial dilation, such as AV valve regurgitation and postoperative atrial surgery. In addition, the arrhythmia has been associated with chronic cardiomyopathy and myocarditis. While some cases of EAT spontaneously resolve, most patients require chronic therapy.

Multifocal atrial tachycardia (MAT), or chaotic atrial rhythm, is rare and arises from multiple foci of increased automaticity located within the atria. The tachycardia is defined by the presence of three or more P-wave morphologies. MAT may be confused with atrial fibrillation because of the irregular rhythm and the variable P wave morphologies.

Treatment of an automatic SVT involves decreasing the ventricular response rate by slowing AV conduction and decreasing the automaticity of the abnormal focus or foci. Digoxin and calcium-channel blockers can slow conduction through the AV node, but they also have negative inotropic properties. Calcium-channel blockers should not be used in children <1 year of age. β blockers, which oppose adrenergic stimulation of the focus, may help suppress the tachycardia. Agents such as procainamide, flecainide and propafenone act by decreasing automaticity and prolonging refractoriness. Agents such as amiodarone and sotalol can slow conduction throughout the myocardium, including the abnormal focus. Radiofrequency ablation of the ectopic focus has become an effective means of curing EAT and is the treatment of choice for medically refractory dysrhythmia.

Junctional ectopic tachycardia (JET) occurs as a result of enhanced automaticity in the region of the AV node. JET is characterized by a narrow-complex tachycardia with AV dissociation and a ventricular rate faster than the atrial rate (**Fig. 47.4**). JET also occurs in the immediate postoperative period following surgery for congenital heart disease. Postoperative JET is usually transient, usually lasting up to 72 hrs. Despite its self-limited nature, postoperative JET can cause significant hemodynamic instability. The combination of depressed postoperative myocardial function, tachycardia rates as high as 250 bpm, and loss of AV synchrony may significantly impair cardiac output. Postoperative JET is most commonly seen following repairs that include a ventricular septal defect closure.

For the congenital form of JET, digoxin may slow the tachycardia rate and support cardiac function. Often, a second-line agent is required, with amiodarone being the most successful. Antiarrhythmic therapy may result in enough SND that a pacemaker may be necessary. Ablation therapy is reserved for the most resistant cases of JET because of the high risk for the development of AV block. Postoperative JET can be treated pharmacologically with amiodarone. Digoxin and procainamide may be used rarely as second-line therapies. Other nonpharmacologic measures include controlling fever, hypothermia with core temperatures reduced to 35°C, and sedation. AV sequential pacing to restore AV synchrony and paired ventricular pacing to decrease the effec-

tive heart rate have been used to augment cardiac output. Any wide-complex rhythm should first be considered ventricular in origin. It is inappropriate to use the rate of the tachycardia to determine whether the rhythm is supraventricular or ventricular in origin. Finally, in that many pediatric cardiac surgical procedures result in a prolonged electrocardiographic wave (QRS) duration, usually with a right bundle-branch-block pattern, it is more difficult to determine the mechanism of a wide-complex tachycardia after congenital heart disease surgery. During assessment of a wide-complex tachycardia, two important principles should be considered. The QRS complex should have a prolonged duration in ventricular tachycardia (VT), but this may be subtle in very young children, as normal measurements of the QRS duration vary with age (**Fig. 47.5**). In addition, VT typically has dissociation of the P waves and QRS complexes, with the QRS complexes occurring at a faster rate. However, children may have retrograde AV node conduction during VT, resulting in P waves (inverted) with a 1:1 relationship. If it is not possible to determine the P wave-to-QRS relationship by the surface ECG, recording the atrial activity with a transesophageal electrode catheter or temporary pacing lead placed at the time of cardiac surgery may be helpful.

The patient with a ventricular arrhythmia may be asymptomatic or may present with a cardiomyopathy or cardiac arrest. VT in pediatric patients may be associated with a prior surgical repair, myocarditis, cardiomyopathy of any cause, or primary electrical disease. Some wide-complex rhythms may occur as a result of marked metabolic or pharmacologic effects on the normal conduction system. Although it is appropriate to manage a wide-complex rhythm as a ventricular arrhythmia, other noncardiac etiologies (i.e., hypoxia) should not be overlooked. The mechanisms by which ventricular arrhythmias occur are the same as those that result in supraventricular arrhythmias: reentry, automaticity, and triggered automaticity. The patient should always be evaluated first clinically for signs of adequate perfusion and hemodynamic stability.

Single, premature, ventricular complexes are not uncommon in children and are usually benign in the patient with a structurally normal heart, including patients who have ventricular ectopy in a pattern of bigeminy or trigeminy. Although these patterns may result in a relatively high frequency of ectopic beats, they need not be treated differently in the patient without underlying heart disease. On the other hand, the tenuous patient may be compromised by single, premature, ventricular complexes if ventricular filling is impaired. When a wide-complex tachycardia is irregular, occurs with a gradual onset and termination,

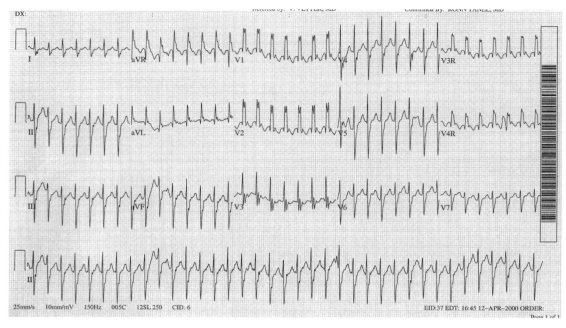

FIGURE 47.5. ECG from an infant with ventricular tachycardia.

and does not respond to cardioversion, an automatic mechanism should be suspected.

Patients with an automatic VT may be treated with either medical therapy to suppress the focus or curative catheter-ablation therapy. The goal of medical therapy is to suppress the active focus or control the rate of the tachycardia. β blockers and verapamil may be very effective and have the benefit of being associated with a lower side-effect profile. Patients with tetralogy of Fallot, aortic stenosis, pulmonary stenosis, and ventricular septal defect have a higher frequency of premature ventricular complexes and higher grade ventricular ectopy than the general population.

Arrhythmogenic right ventricular cardiomyopathy is another less common cause of VT in apparently healthy young people that is thought to be an under-recognized cause of sudden death. The associated VT typically has the morphology of a left bundle-branch block, as the arrhythmia generally arises form the right ventricular outflow tract. The cardiomyopathy involves aneurysmal dilatation and dyskinesis of the right ventricular outflow tract. Cardiac MRI has become the primary method of identifying the anatomic abnormalities.

Patients with hypertrophic cardiomyopathy comprise another group with myocardial disease that is prone to ventricular arrhythmias. Left ventricular outflow tract obstruction may result in ventricular

arrhythmias due to coronary artery insufficiency and myocardial ischemia.

Although cardiac tumors are rare, they are a source of ventricular arrhythmias with an automatic mechanism. Rhabdomyomas are the most common cardiac tumor in pediatric patients and are usually found in those with tuberous sclerosis.

Long-QT syndrome is associated with syncope, cardiac arrest, neurosensory hearing loss, Timothy syndrome, Andersen syndrome, and sudden death. These symptoms are due to the polymorphic VT, torsades de pointes, that occurs as a result of a prolonged refractory period and increased "R-on-T" vulnerability. The electrical abnormality can occur as an inherited congenital problem or due to an acquired metabolic disturbance or medication exposure. As the presenting symptom can be that of a convulsion, all patients with a presumed seizure disorder should have a screening ECG. Other ECG findings include bradycardia, AV block, abnormal T-wave morphology, prominent U waves, and T-wave alternans. Effective therapies include pacing for bradycardia, isoproterenol infusion to avoid pause-dependent episodes of ventricular arrhythmia, lidocaine, magnesium, and β blockers. Long-term therapy is usually addressed with β blockers, mexiletine, pacemaker implantation, and consideration of implantable defibrillators. It is equally important to avoid cardiac stimulants and medications that are known to prolong

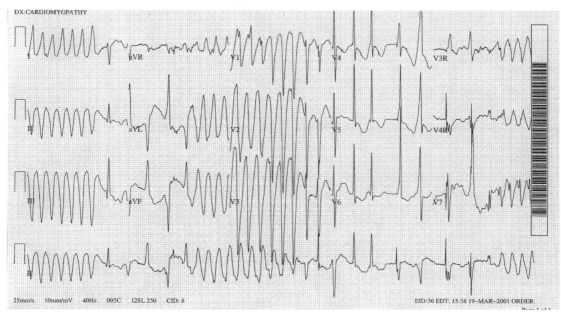

FIGURE 47.6. ECG showing torsades de pointes in a patient with long-QT syndrome.

the QT interval, such as some antiarrhythmic drugs, psychotropic medications, erythromycin, and many antifungal agents. It is important to screen family members, as the presenting symptom of long-QT syndrome may be a life-threatening arrhythmia.

Polymorphic VT should be differentiated from monomorphic VT and is generally more poorly tolerated. Torsades de pointes (**Fig. 47.6**) is recognized by its characteristic pattern of positive and negative oscillations of the QRS complex around the isoelectric baseline, or "twisting of the points." Torsades de pointes should initially be treated with the withdrawal of any aggravating medications and correction of any metabolic abnormalities. Medical therapy should include magnesium supplementation, β-blockers, and lidocaine. Although seemingly counterintuitive, isoproterenol may be beneficial by directly shortening myocardial repolarization times and increasing the heart rate in order to avoid pause-dependent arrhythmias. Patients who experience sustained polymorphic VT with significant hemodynamic compromise despite maximal medical therapy may be candidates for circulatory support with extracorporeal membrane oxygenation.

Ventricular arrhythmias may arise in any condition that can be associated with myocardial inflammation, ischemia, infarction, and myocarditis, such as dilated cardiomyopathy; coronary artery hypoperfusion, such as in Kawasaki disease; anomalous coronary artery; pulmonary hypertension; neuromuscular diseases; generalized myopathies; sepsis; and severe and long-standing hypertension. Patients with

neuromuscular diseases such as Duchenne muscular dystrophy seem to have more ectopy, as their skeletal muscle strength and myocardial contractility decrease. Patients with Becker muscular dystrophy do not appear to exhibit a similar correlation. Ventricular arrhythmias may occur in patients with myotonic dystrophy. Rett syndrome is a neurologic disorder that is associated with sudden death. The diagnosis is usually made in school-aged and adolescent girls who often have abnormalities of repolarization, including a prolonged QT interval, that seem to correlate with the severity of neurologic disease.

Wide-complex rhythms and ventricular arrhythmias are caused by an assortment of systemic causes (**Table 47.1**). Hyperkalemia results in prolongation of the PR interval, QRS widening, and lengthening of the QT interval, with a terminal ECG that resembles a sinusoidal waveform (**Fig. 47.7**). The ECG changes seen with hyperkalemia respond promptly to immediate treatment with calcium, sodium bicarbonate, or glucose/insulin.

Medical management of acute ventricular arrhythmias is usually the first therapeutic option. Synchronized direct-current cardioversion may be used to treat a perfusing ventricular arrhythmia or a wide-complex arrhythmia with an organized electrical pattern. If the rhythm is pulseless or disorganized to the point that distinct QRS complexes cannot be recognized by the defibrillator, asynchronous defibrillation must be delivered immediately.

Bradycardia due to SND may result in sinus bradycardia, junctional bradycardia, ectopic atrial

SYSTEMIC CAUSES OF VENTRICULAR ARRHYTHMIA

Metabolic	Hyperkalemia
	Hypokalemia
	Hypomagnesemia
	Hypocalcemia
	Hypoxia
	Acidosis
Ischemia	Kawasaki disease
Infectious	Systemic viral infections causing myocarditis
	Systemic bacterial infections causing endocarditis
Toxic	Cocaine/catecholamine infusions/ stimulants
	Antiarrhythmic medications
	Digitalis toxicity
	Psychotropic medications
Traumatic	Commotio cordis
	Mechanical irritation/central catheters

bradycardia, and sinus pauses. Bradycardia may also be due to abnormalities of AV conduction, including first-, second-, or third-degree (complete) heart block. Second-degree heart block is further divided into Mobitz type I (Wenckebach) **(Fig. 47.8)**, Mobitz type II, and fixed-ratio AV block. Sinus brady-

cardia may result from increased vagal tone, hypoxia, ischemia, central nervous system disorders with increased intracranial pressure, hypothyroidism, hypothermia, drug intoxication (digoxin, β blockers, calcium-channel blockers), and prior atrial surgery. It is defined by heart rates <100 bpm in the neonate and <60 bpm in the older child.

The clinical manifestations of SND consist of pronounced sinus bradycardia, exercise-induced chronotropic incompetence, and sinus pauses (>2.5–3 secs while awake, dependent on age). When episodes of bradycardia are associated with SVT or atrial flutter or fibrillation, the situation is frequently referred to as "tachy-brady" syndrome. SND has intrinsic causes, including cardiomyopathy, myocarditis, trauma, ischemia, and infarction. A common cause of symptomatic SND in pediatric patients is prior surgery for congenital heart disease, especially the atrial-switch operation, Fontan procedure, and repair of atrial septal defect. Extrinsic SND usually results from autonomic influences such as neurally mediated syncope and carotid sinus hypersensitivity or cardioactive drugs. Symptomatic SND treatment is placement of an atrial pacemaker.

Abnormalities of the AV conduction system can be described by the location of the block within the specialized conduction tissue (His bundle, AV node) or the pattern observed on the surface ECG. First-degree heart block results from slowing of conduction at the level of the AV node and occasionally in the atrium or the His Purkinje system. It may be due to increased vagal tone, digoxin or

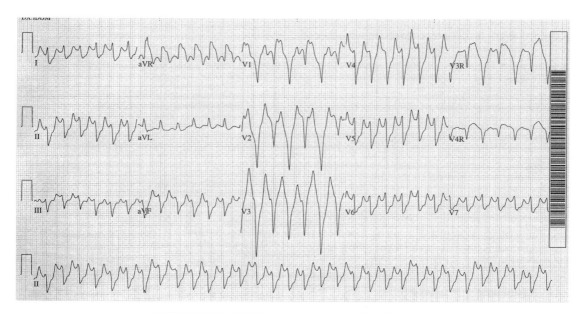

FIGURE 47.7. ECG findings observed with hyperkalemia.

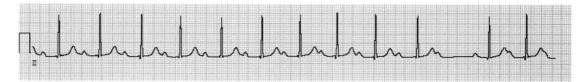

FIGURE 47.8. ECG showing second degree AV block, Mobitz type I, in a child. Note the progressive prolongation of the PR interval before the blocked P wave.

β-blocker administration, viral myocarditis, Lyme disease, hypothermia, electrolyte abnormalities, congenital heart disease, rheumatic fever, or cardiomyopathy. First-degree AV block is characterized by PR-interval prolongation. The rhythm is regular, originates in the sinus node, and has a normal QRS-complex morphology. First-degree AV block as an isolated event does not require investigation or treatment, but it may be the manifestation of an underlying disease state or conduction disturbance.

Second-degree heart block is the failure of an atrial impulse to traverse the AV node and infranodal conduction system and elicit a ventricular response. Mobitz type I, second-degree heart block, or Wenckebach, is defined by a progressive prolongation of the PR interval followed by a P wave that is not associated with a QRS complex (**Fig. 47.8**). Mobitz type II, second-degree heart block is defined by intermittent loss of AV conduction without prior lengthening of the PR interval. This condition is always abnormal and may progress to complete heart block. High-grade second-degree heart block (frequent nonconducted P waves) can be associated with hemodynamic compromise and is treated with pacemaker implantation. Fixed-ratio AV block is a dysrhythmia in which sequential P waves have no subsequent QRS complex, and the repetitive nature results in a pattern of 2:1, 3:1, 4:1, etc., AV block. A normal PR interval with conducted beats is present. A slightly prolonged QRS complex may be seen.

Third-degree heart block is the complete inability of an atrial impulse to be propagated to the ventricles. The ECG demonstrates AV dissociation. The atrial rate is faster than the ventricular rate, and the atrial rhythm and rate are normal for age. If an escape rhythm arises from the AV node (junctional rhythm), the QRS complex is narrow; however, if an escape rhythm arises from the distal His bundle or Purkinje fibers, the QRS complex is wide (idioventricular rhythm). Complete heart block may be congenital or acquired. Congenital complete heart block can be associated with L-transposition of the great arteries (congenitally corrected transposition of the great arteries), heterotaxy syndrome (left atrial iso-

merism), AV canal defect, or maternal systemic lupus erythematosus. Complete heart block due to maternal collagen vascular abnormality results from antibodies crossing the placenta. The fetus and newborn with congenital complete heart block may develop hydrops fetalis. The most common cause of transient and permanent acquired complete heart block is surgery near the AV node. Other causes of acquired complete heart block include cardiomyopathy and Lyme disease.

Treatment of Abnormalities of Atrioventricular Conduction

No intervention is necessary for sinus bradycardia if the cardiac output is maintained. Treatment for hemodynamically significant bradycardia is shown in **Table 47.2**. No treatment is necessary for first-degree or Mobitz type I second-degree heart block. Mobitz type II second-degree heart block, fixed-ratio AV block, and third-degree heart block are always pathologic and abnormal. If the child with complete heart block is hemodynamically unstable, transcutaneous or transvenous pacing can be performed acutely, and permanent transvenous or

TABLE 47.2

TREATMENT FOR HEMODYNAMICALLY SIGNIFICANT BRADYCARDIA

Trendelenburg position (supine with the head lower than the level of the pelvis and feet)
Volume expansion
Pharmacologic interventions
    Anticholinergic agents
        Atropine 0.02–0.04 mg/kg (maximum 1–2 mg)
    β-adrenergic agonists and activators of adenylate cyclase
        Isoproterenol infusion 0.01–2.0 mcg/kg/min
        Epinephrine IV bolus 0.01–0.5 mg/kg, infusion 0.1–0.5 mcg/kg/min
    Glucagon
Digoxin-specific antibody Fab fragments for digoxin toxicity
Temporary transcutaneous or transvenous pacing

epicardial pacemaker placement can be performed later. Third-degree heart block is managed with either ventricular demand pacing or AV sequential pacing. Severe bradycardia may be emergently treated with isoproterenol and temporary pacing.

Placement of temporary atrial and ventricular pacing wires is standard practice with most cardiothoracic surgical procedures that involve cardiopulmonary bypass. Temporary pacing wires are used for pacing patients with SND or AV block, recording atrial electrograms for diagnostic purposes, and overdrive pacing for termination of reentrant arrhythmias. Temporary pacemakers can be configured for either single- or dual-chamber pacing. Standard nomenclature is used to describe pacemaker function and programming. The first three letters of the program refer to the chamber paced, the chamber sensed, and the response to the sensed event, in that order (**Table 47.3**). The fourth and fifth letters refer to advanced programming options that are related to permanent implantable pacemakers. For instance, a VVI pacemaker paces the ventricle, senses the ventricle, and inhibits pacing when an intrinsic sensed ventricular event occurs, thus preventing an R-on-T phenomenon.

Mechanical contraction of the ventricles is most efficient when depolarization occurs down the normal conduction pathway of the His-Purkinje system with AV synchrony. The augmented preload as a result of atrial contraction at the end of ventricular diastole enhances cardiac output. For example, in patients with sinus bradycardia and intact AV conduction, atrial pacing is far more efficient than ventricular pacing alone due to important ventricular contractility mechanics and ventricular-ventricular interactions. Similarly, in patients with AV block, dual-chamber pacing is superior to ventricular pacing alone due to the contribution of AV synchrony to the cardiac output.

Because temporary pacing wires deteriorate over a relatively short period of time, capture thresholds (the minimum amount of amperage required to depolarize the respective chamber of the heart) and sensitivity should be checked on a daily basis, and the pacemaker output should be set to 2–3 times threshold value. Guidelines for pacemaker implantation are published by the American College of Cardiology, American Heart Association, and Heart Rhythm Society and are periodically updated, reflecting the current consensus opinion.

Antiarrhythmic Drugs

For children admitted to the PICU for arrhythmia and the initiation of antiarrhythmic drugs, 5 half-lives of the medication are required to achieve steady-state pharmacologic levels unless a loading dose is administered. During this time, families may be educated about the signs and symptoms of arrhythmia and how to appropriately dose the medication(s). The Vaughn Williams classification of antiarrhythmic drugs is based on pharmacologic effects on the types and phases of the cardiac-cell action potential. The drugs are categorized into four major

---

TABLE 47.3

PACEMAKER CODES FROM THE NORTH AMERICAN SOCIETY OF PACING AND ELECTROPHYSIOLOGY AND THE BRITISH PACING AND ELECTROPHYSIOLOGY GROUP

Position 1	Position 2	Position 3
Chamber paced	Chamber sensed	Response to sensed event
O = none	O = none O	O = none
A = atrium	A = atrium	I = inhibited
V = ventricle	V = ventricle	T = triggered
D = dual (A + V)	D = dual (A + V)	D = dual (T + I)

The first two positions of this code are Chamber Paced and Chamber Sensed. The third position is described as follows:

  D—(dual): In DDD pacemakers, atrial pacing is in the inhibited mode (the pacing device will emit an atrial pulse if the atrium does not contract). In DDD and VDD pacemakers, once an atrial event has occurred (whether paced or native), the device will ensure that an atrial event follows.

  I—(inhibited): The device will pulse to the appropriate chamber, unless it detects intrinsic electrical activity. In the DDI program, AV synchrony is provided only when the atrial chamber is paced. On the other hand, if intrinsic atrial activity is present, no AV synchrony is provided by the pacemaker.

  T—(triggered): Triggered mode is only used when the device is being tested. The pacing device will emit a pulse only in response to a sensed event.

Adapted from Miller RD. *Miller's Anesthesia*, 6th ed. Philadelphia: Elsevier, Inc, 2005.

TABLE 47.4

VAUGHN WILLIAMS CLASSIFICATION OF ANTIARRHYTHMIC DRUGS

Class	Effect	Drugs
I	Sodium-channel blockade	
Subclass IA		Procainamide, disopyramide, quinidine
Subclass IB		Lidocaine, mexiletine, phenytoin
Subclass IC		Flecainide, propafenone, encainide
II	β-adrenergic receptor blockade	Propranolol, esmolol, atenolol, nadolol, carvedilol
III	Potassium-channel blockade	Amiodarone, sotalol, bretylium
IV	Slow, inward, calcium-channel blockade	Verapamil, diltiazem, nifedipine
Other		Digoxin, adenosine

groups, though many current medications have multiple (class) actions (**Table 47.4**).

The class IA agents all carry a risk of proarrhythmia, with the aggravation of existing arrhythmias or the development of new atrial and ventricular arrhythmias, including torsades de pointes. Lidocaine has historically been used for the treatment of complex ventricular ectopy, VT, and ventricular fibrillation. It may also be useful for the emergent treatment of arrhythmias that occur in association with prolonged QT syndrome (torsades de pointes). Lidocaine has no significant effect on the autonomic nervous system, and proarrhythmia is a rare adverse effect. The class IC agents have a relatively high potential for proarrhythmia. Proarrhythmia may lead to cardiac arrest and death, predominantly among patients with underlying heart disease.

Class II agents are used to treat all arrhythmias of abnormal automaticity, especially those that are catecholamine-driven. In addition, they may be used to treat reentry tachycardias by preventing the premature beats that act as initiating events or by affecting AV nodal conduction when that structure is part of the arrhythmia circuit.

The class III agents prolong the action-potential duration. Amiodarone has been incorporated in advanced cardiac life support treatment algorithms after defibrillation and epinephrine for unstable VT or ventricular fibrillation. It is also the principal antiarrhythmic agent for junctional ectopic tachycardia. Sotalol is used in situations similar to those for amiodarone, but it has the advantage of a faster onset of action and a shorter duration of activity.

Class IV antiarrhythmic, specifically verapamil, is used most frequently in pediatric practice for the treatment of arrhythmias. Patients with WPW syndrome should not receive chronic verapamil therapy,

as accessory pathway conduction may be enhanced while AV nodal conduction may be slowed, particularly during atrial tachycardias. Diltiazem is frequently used for control of the ventricular rate during an atrial tachycardia by blocking conduction at the AV node. The calcium-channel blockers are widely used for long-term therapy of pulmonary hypertension, and nifedipine is preferred in those patients, as it has little effect on the sinus node, AV node, and cardiac contractility. Due to its potential for peripheral vasodilation, nifedipine is used for the acute management of hypertension.

Digoxin is a cardiac glycoside that is useful for the treatment of both arrhythmias and congestive heart failure. It is also used to achieve control of ventricular rate during an atrial tachycardia. Digoxin may be used for atrial tachycardia, atrial fibrillation, premature atrial complexes, and blocked premature atrial complexes. Digoxin should not be used in patients with WPW syndrome due to its ability to block the AV node, shorten the accessory-pathway effective refractory period, and potentially enhance antegrade conduction across the accessory connection during an atrial tachycardia. Toxic concentrations can result in increased automaticity and triggered arrhythmias.

Digoxin toxicity can result in almost any type of arrhythmia, but the development of arrhythmias is generally a late indicator of toxicity. For toxicity, the medication should be discontinued. Serum electrolyte abnormalities should be corrected, while atrial and ventricular arrhythmias can be treated with phenytoin or lidocaine. Atropine or a temporary pacemaker can be used to treat bradycardia or AV block. Digoxin-immune, antigen-binding Fab fragments are specific antibodies that may be used to bind digoxin and may be especially helpful in cases of potentially life-threatening toxicity.

Adenosine is useful for terminating SVT caused by a reentry mechanism. It will terminate the reentrant circuit by abruptly blocking the AV node, but the atrial tachycardia will persist with block at the AV node, resulting in a ventricular response to the atrial arrhythmia of <1:1. The effects of adenosine are brief, as the drug is rapidly metabolized with a half-life of <10 secs. Caffeine and the methylxanthines cause competitive and reversible antagonism via the specific adenosine receptor, requiring higher doses of adenosine for clinical effect. Patients with orthotopic heart transplant have a denervation-induced supersensitivity to adenosine.

CHAPTER 48 ■ PREOPERATIVE CARE OF THE PEDIATRIC CARDIAC SURGICAL PATIENT

DAVID L. WESSEL • ALAIN FRAISSE

Optimal preoperative care involves (a) initial stabilization, airway management, and establishment of vascular access; (b) a complete and thorough noninvasive delineation of the anatomic defect(s); (c) resuscitation with evaluation and treatment of secondary organ dysfunction, particularly the brain, kidneys, and liver; (d) cardiac catheterization if necessary—typically for physiologic assessment, interventional procedures such as balloon atrial septostomy or valvotomy, or anatomic definition not visible by echocardiography (e.g., coronary artery distribution in pulmonary atresia with intact ventricular septum or delineation of aorticopulmonary collaterals in tetralogy of Fallot with pulmonary atresia); and (e) surgical management when cardiac, pulmonary, renal, and central nervous systems are optimized. The observed benefits of neonatal reparative operations in patients with two ventricles are numerous (**Table 48.1**). Whereas the neonate may be more labile than the older child, many examples also exist of the enhanced neonatal resilience to metabolic or ischemic injury. At most centers, the approach to neonates with congenital heart disease (CHD) has been toward complete surgical correction rather than palliation in order to avoid the pathophysio-

logic consequences and limits on neonatal growth. This concept has been extended to include the premature newborns. Despite improvements in ventilation, widespread use of surfactant, and prenatal administration of glucocorticoids, infants who are <30 weeks of gestation carry a significant risk of developing bronchopulmonary dysplasia. The coexistence of CHD and bronchopulmonary dysplasia may worsen the clinical course as a result of elevated pulmonary vascular resistance (PVR). Hence, palliative medical or surgical interventions are often preferred management options in premature infants with CHD. However, current experience with increased mortality after palliative surgery supports the notion that early biventricular repair can be achieved with low mortality.

PREOPERATIVE MANAGEMENT AND CARE

A complete history and physical examination are required, directed to the extent of cardiopulmonary impairment, airway abnormalities, and associated extracardiac congenital anomalies. Upper and lower airway problems in patients with Down syndrome, calcium and immunologic deficiencies in patients with aortic arch abnormalities, and renal abnormalities in patients with esophageal atresia and CHD are a few of the associated congenital abnormalities with which the intraoperative team should be familiar. Intercurrent pulmonary infection is a common and significant finding in chronically overcirculated lungs. The presence, degree, and duration of hypoxemia are important details that, in the absence of iron

TABLE 48.1
ADVANTAGES OF NEONATAL REPAIR

Early elimination of cyanosis
Early elimination of congestive heart failure
Optimal circulation for growth and development
Reduced anatomic distortion from palliative procedures
Reduced hospital admissions while awaiting repair
Reduced parental anxiety while awaiting repair

TABLE 48.2

TEN INTENSIVE CARE STRATEGIES TO DIAGNOSE AND SUPPORT LOW CARDIAC OUTPUT STATES

1. Know the cardiac anatomy in detail and its physiologic consequences.
2. Understand the specialized considerations of the newborn and implications of reparative rather than palliative surgery.
3. Diversify personnel to include expertise in neonatal and adult congenital heart disease.
4. Monitor, measure, and image the heart to rule out residual disease as a cause of postoperative hemodynamic instability or low cardiac output.
5. Maintain aortic perfusion and improve the contractile state.
6. Optimize preload (including atrial shunting).
7. Reduce afterload.
8. Control heart rate, rhythm, and synchrony.
9. Optimize heart-lung interactions.
10. Provide mechanical support when needed.

deficiency, are reflected in a raised hematocrit. The nadir of physiologic anemia during infancy may contribute to left-to-right shunting by decreasing the relative PVR. Ten key features required to identify and treat low cardiac output states in the perioperative period are described in **Table 48.2**.

Chest radiography shows heart size, pulmonary vascular congestion, airway compression, and areas of consolidation or atelectasis. The electrocardiogram may reveal rhythm disturbances and demonstrate ventricular strain patterns (ST- and T-wave changes) characteristic of pathologic pressure or volume burdens on the ventricles. Electrolyte abnormalities caused by congestive heart failure and forced diuresis must also be evaluated preoperatively. Severe hypochloremic metabolic alkalosis may occur in some patients. It may be important to discontinue digoxin preoperatively and to avoid hyperventilation and administration of calcium to these patients during induction of anesthesia and preparation for the operating room. The alkalotic, hypokalemic, hypercalcemic, hypotensive, dilated, digoxin-bound myocardium fibrillates with ease.

Accurate echocardiographic anatomic diagnosis is now routine in children without the need for cardiac catheterization. Skilled echocardiographers accurately interpret the alignment of cardiac chambers and great vessels but cannot always visualize an atrial septal defect or ventricular septal defect, although color flow-mapping techniques have vastly improved diagnostic capabilities. An atrial septal defect can be indirectly inferred from right ventricular volume overload and interventricular septal shift.

Distal pulmonary artery architecture and conduits between a ventricle and a great artery are poorly imaged by echocardiography, and pressure gradients in these areas are not always measurable with Doppler techniques. Evaluation of atrioventricular valve regurgitation may be subjective and nonquantitative. Accuracy of echocardiographic diagnosis is limited by an inadequate window for imaging in the obese patient, the older child, and some postoperative patients. Techniques for three-dimensional echocardiography are available that may improve diagnostic capabilities, such as defining the mechanism of valve regurgitation. Doppler measurements add greatly to noninvasive diagnostic capabilities. Measurements of pressure gradients across semilunar valves and other obstructions are frequently accurate but may not always correlate with peak systolic ejection gradients measured at catheterization. As good as echocardiographic diagnosis of anatomic defects and Doppler measurements of pressure gradients and valve function have become, the standard for assessment of physiology when other clinical information is ambiguous or contradictory remains cardiac catheterization. Evaluation of left and right ventricular function in children with CHD is an essential component of the preoperative assessment.

Cardiac Catheterization

When echocardiographic analysis with Doppler measurements and color flow mapping is complete and unambiguous, preoperative assessment may no longer require cardiac catheterization. Catheterization is not typically performed before infant or neonatal operations for ventricular septal defects, complete atrioventricular canal defects, tetralogy of Fallot, interrupted aortic arch, hypoplastic left heart syndrome, or coarctation of the aorta. However, in older patients with complex anatomy (e.g., a single ventricle), physiologic data from catheterization may be essential. This technique allows description of the direction, magnitude, and approximate location of intracardiac shunts. Intracardiac and intravascular pressures are measured to determine the presence of obstructions and whether shunt orifices are restrictive or nonrestrictive. Pressure gradients across sites of obstruction must be considered in light of simultaneous blood flow; a small pressure gradient measured at a time of low cardiac output is misleading.

Normally, oxygen saturation does not significantly change from vena cava to pulmonary artery. In the child with CHD, the superior vena cava gives the best indication of true SvO_2; an increase ("step-up") in saturation of $\geq 5\%$ downstream from the superior vena cava suggests the presence of a left-to-right shunt, which would occur at the level of the right atrium with an atrial septal defect, in the right ventricle with a ventricular septal defect, and in the pulmonary artery with a patent ductus arteriosus. The oxygen consumption of the patient is usually measured by direct calorimetry, as are the saturation values, but subsequent flow and resistance calculations can be in error.

The patient whose aortic blood is fully saturated can be safely assumed to have no significant right-to-left shunting. However, when a right-to-left shunt is present, aortic blood is hypoxemic. Blood samples should also be obtained from the pulmonary veins, left atrium, and left ventricle for oxygen saturation determination and ascertainment of the source of desaturated blood. Pulmonary venous desaturation implies a pulmonary source of venous admixture (e.g., pneumonia, atelectasis, or other pulmonary disease). Intrapulmonary shunting may substantially alter the perioperative plan and the postoperative ventilatory requirements of the patient.

In the presence of a left-to-right shunt and elevated PVR, pressure and saturation measurements are often repeated, with the patient breathing 100% oxygen and/or inhaled nitric oxide to assess both the reactivity of the pulmonary vascular bed and any contribution of ventilation-perfusion abnormalities to hypoxemia. If breathing 100% oxygen increases pulmonary blood flow and dramatically increases Q_p/Q_s (with a fall in PVR), potentially reversible processes such as hypoxic pulmonary vasoconstriction are probably contributing to the elevated PVR. The patient with a high, unresponsive PVR and a small left-to-right shunt despite a large shunt orifice may have extensive pulmonary vascular damage from irreversible obstructive pulmonary vascular disease. If so, surgical repair is usually contraindicated.

Magnetic Resonance Imaging and Angiography

Following the development of electrocardiogram-gated MRI, MRI and MR angiography have emerged as important diagnostic modalities in the evaluation of the cardiovascular system. While ferromagnetic implants near the region of interest might produce artifact, sternal wires and vascular clips produce relatively minor disturbances and therefore MRI can be performed in patients who have undergone previous cardiac surgery. Contraindications include patients with pacemakers, recently implanted endovascular or intracardiac implants, and aneurysm clips on vessels that will be exposed directly to the magnetic field. When MRI is contraindicated or when breath holds cannot be achieved easily in young, nonsedated children, CT scanning with three-dimensional imaging is an interesting alternative in the morphologic assessment of congenital cardiac anomalies.

Assessment of Patient Status and Predominant Pathophysiology

Frequently, congenital heart defects are complex and can be difficult to categorize or conceptualize. Rather than trying to determine the management for each individual anatomic defect, a physiologic approach can be taken. The following questions should be asked:

1. How does the systemic venous return reach the systemic arterial circulation to maintain cardiac output? What intracardiac mixing, shunting, or outflow obstruction exists?
2. Is the circulation in series or parallel? Are the defects amenable to a two-ventricle or single-ventricle repair?
3. Is pulmonary blood flow increased or decreased?
4. Is there a volume load or pressure load on the ventricles?

Severe Hypoxemia

Many of the cyanotic forms of CHD present in the ICU with severe hypoxemia (PaO_2 <50 mm Hg) during the first few days of life but without respiratory distress. Infusion of prostaglandin E_1 (PGE_1) in patients with decreased pulmonary blood flow maintains or reestablishes pulmonary flow through the ductus arteriosus, which may also improve mixing of venous and arterial blood at the atrial level in patients with transposition of the great arteries. Consequently, neonates rarely require surgery while they are severely hypoxemic. During preoperative preparation with PGE_1, neurologic examination and blood chemistry analysis of renal, hepatic, and hematologic function are necessary to assess the effects of severe hypoxemia during or after birth on end-organ dysfunction.

Cyanotic patients who present for surgery after infancy require adequate preoperative and postoperative hydration to prevent the thrombotic problems caused by their high hematocrits. The perioperative team should prepare for significant coagulopathy in the cyanotic patient. Premedication must be given cautiously to avoid causing hypoventilation in these patients.

The common side effects of PGE_1 infusion—apnea, hypotension, fever, excitation of the central nervous system—are easily managed in the neonate when normal therapeutic doses of the drug (0.02–0.05 mcg/kg/min) are used. However, as PGE_1 is a potent vasodilator, intravascular volume frequently requires augmentation. Patients with intermittent apnea resulting from administration of PGE_1 may require mechanical ventilation preoperatively.

PGE_1 usually improves the arterial oxygenation of hypoxemic neonates who have poor pulmonary perfusion due to obstructed pulmonary flow (critical pulmonic stenosis or pulmonary atresia). By providing pulmonary blood flow from the aorta via the ductus arteriosus, an infusion of PGE_1 improves oxygenation and stabilizes the condition of neonates with these lesions. The improved oxygenation reverses the lactic acidosis that may have developed during episodes of severe hypoxia. PGE_1 administration for 24 hrs usually markedly improves the condition of a severely hypoxemic neonate with restricted pulmonary blood flow.

Neonates with transposition of the great arteries must have adequate mixing of oxygenated and deoxygenated blood at the atrial level to achieve appropriate oxygen delivery. To accomplish this, balloon atrial septostomy creates or enlarges an interatrial septal defect, using echocardiographic guidance in most patients. It may also be of considerable value in creating an atrial septal defect in any neonate with left atrial obstruction such as hypoplastic left-heart syndrome with intact atrial septum. For such patients, fenestration of the atrial septum with an intra-atrial stent is sometimes necessary to maintain patency.

Excessive Pulmonary Blood Flow

Excessive pulmonary blood flow is frequently the primary problem of patients with CHD. Children with left-to-right shunts may have chronic low-grade pulmonary infection and congestion that cannot be eliminated despite optimal preoperative preparation. If so, surgery should not be postponed further. Aside from the respiratory impairment caused by increased pulmonary blood flow, the left heart must dilate to accept pulmonary venous return that is several times normal.

In children with severely failing hearts, the body weight is below the third percentile for age, and the child is tachypneic, tachycardic, and dusky in room air. The child may have intercostal and substernal retractions and skin that is cool to the touch. Capillary refill may be prolonged. Expiratory wheezes are usually audible. Medical management with digoxin, vasodilators, and diuretics may improve the patient's condition, but the diuretics may induce a profound hypochloremic alkalosis and potassium depletion, which may persist after surgery.

Obstruction of Left Heart Outflow

These lesions include interruption of the aortic arch, coarctation of the aorta, aortic stenosis, and mitral stenosis or atresia as part of the hypoplastic left heart syndrome. These neonates present with inadequate systemic perfusion and profound metabolic acidosis. The initial pH may be <7.0 despite a low $PaCO_2$. Systemic blood flow is largely or completely dependent on blood flow into the aorta from the ductus arteriosus. Ductal closure in the neonate with these problems causes dramatic worsening of the patient's condition. The patient becomes critically ill or even moribund and requires PGE_1 infusion for survival. PGE_1 allows blood flow into the aorta from the pulmonary artery because it maintains the patency of the ductus arteriosus, thus creating a systemic circulation in the neonate that depends on right ventricular contractile function and ductal patency. Acidosis, metabolic derangements, and renal failure arise if systemic perfusion is inadequate. In addition to PGE_1 infusion, other supportive measures include ventilatory and inotropic support, as well as correction of metabolic acidosis, hypoglycemia, hypocalcemia and other electrolyte abnormalities.

Ventricular Dysfunction

Although patients with large shunts may have complete mixing of systemic and venous blood and only mild-to-moderate hypoxemia as a result of their excessive pulmonary blood flow, the price paid for near-normal arterial oxygen saturation is chronic ventricular dilation and dysfunction as well as pulmonary vascular obstructive disease. Consequently, narrowing the shunt or a staged approach to single-ventricle repair may be indicated before any other elective surgery can be undertaken. Older patients with CHD and poor ventricular function due to chronic ventricular volume overload (aortic or mitral valve regurgitation or long-standing pulmonary-to-systemic arterial shunts) present a different problem, which may be amenable to afterload reduction to some extent. However, in all of these circumstances when the heart is dilated and volume overloaded, a propensity for ventricular fibrillation during sedation, anesthesia, and/or intubation of the airway is seen.

Assessment should include an estimation of the patient's functional limitation as an indicator of myocardial performance and reserve, quantification of the degree of hypoxia and the amount of pulmonary blood flow, and evaluation of PVR. For patients with increased Q_p/Q_s, systemic blood flow should be optimized prior to and during induction of anesthesia but without further augmenting pulmonary blood flow. However, during maintenance and emergence from anesthesia, retraction of the lung, positional changes, and abdominal distension may increase the hypoxemia and compromise the function of a dilated, poorly contractile ventricle. If this sequence occurs during surgery, the management must be altered to improve pulmonary blood flow. Systolic function of the ventricle may be impaired by intrinsic myopathic abnormalities related to drug toxicity, inborn enzyme deficiencies, or acquired inflammatory or infectious disease. Patients with such dilated cardiomyopathies require optimization of ventricular performance, with emphasis on inotropic support and afterload reduction.

PREOPERATIVE MANAGEMENT OF PATIENTS WITH A SINGLE VENTRICLE

Single-Ventricle Anatomy and Physiology

For a variety of anatomic lesions, the systemic and pulmonary circulations are in parallel, with a single ventricle effectively supplying both systemic and pulmonary blood flow. The relative proportion of the ventricular output to either pulmonary or systemic vascular bed is determined by the relative resistance to flow in the two circuits. The pulmonary artery and aortic oxygen saturations are equal, with mixing of the systemic and pulmonary venous return within a "common" atrium. Assuming adequate mixing with normal cardiac output and normal pulmonary venous oxygen saturation, an SaO_2 of 80%–85% with an SvO_2 of 60%–65% indicates a Q_p/Q_s of ~1 and hence a balance between systemic and pulmonary flows. Although "balanced," the single ventricle is still required to receive and eject twice the normal amount of blood: one part to the pulmonary circulation and one part to the systemic circulation. A Q_p/Q_s of >1 implies an intolerable volume burden on the heart. While each of the defects associated with single-ventricle physiology involves specific management issues, they all share common management considerations in balancing flow and augmenting systemic perfusion.

Preoperative Management

Changes in PVR have a significant impact on systemic perfusion and circulatory stability, especially preoperatively, when the ductus arteriosus is widely patent. In preparation for surgery, it is important that systemic and pulmonary blood flow be as well balanced as possible to prevent excessive volume overload and ventricular dysfunction that reduces systemic and end-organ perfusion. For example, a newborn with hypoplastic left-heart syndrome who has an arterial oxygen saturation of >90%, tachypnea, oliguria, cool extremities, hepatomegaly, and metabolic acidosis has severely limited systemic blood flow. Even though ventricular output is increased, the blood flow that is inefficiently partitioned back to the lungs is unavailable to the other vital organs. Immediate interventions are necessary to prevent imminent circulatory collapse and end-organ injury. In this "overcirculated" state, PVR is falling as it should in the normal postnatal state, and the ductus arteriosus is maintained widely patent with prostaglandin infusion to permit unrestricted blood flow from the single right ventricle across the ductus to the systemic bed. Blood flow manipulation of mechanical ventilation and inotrope support may temporarily stabilize the patient, but surgery should not be delayed. Often, the newborn's spontaneous, unassisted ventilatory pattern provides a more stable cardiorespiratory condition than the injudicious use of positive-pressure ventilation and excessive use of vasoactive agents.

Similarly, in a patient with pulmonary atresia and an intact ventricular septum, for example, pulmonary blood flow depends on left ventricular contractile function and ductal patency. As PVR falls, pulmonary blood flow will be excessive and will eventually steal from the systemic circulation. Initial resuscitation involves maintaining patency of the ductus arteriosus with a PGE_1 infusion at a rate of 0.02–0.05 mcg/kg/min. Intubation and mechanical ventilation are not necessary in all patients. Patients are usually tachypneic, but provided the work of breathing is not excessive and systemic perfusion is maintained without a metabolic acidosis, spontaneous ventilation is often preferable to achieve an adequate systemic perfusion and balance of Q_p and Q_s. A mild metabolic acidosis and low bicarbonate level may be present, but this may not specifically indicate poor perfusion and lactic acidosis.

Patients require intubation and mechanical ventilation due to apnea secondary to PGE_1 or the presence of a low cardiac output state or for manipulation of gas exchange to assist balancing pulmonary and systemic flows. An SaO_2 of >90% indicates pulmonary overcirculation (i.e., Q_p/Q_s >1.0). PVR can be increased with controlled mechanical hypoventilation to induce a respiratory acidosis, often necessitating sedation and neuromuscular blockade, and with a low FIO_2 to induce alveolar hypoxia. Ventilation in room air may suffice, but occasionally a hypoxic gas mixture is necessary and is achieved by adding nitrogen to the inspired gas mixture, thereby reducing the FIO_2 to 0.17–0.19. While these maneuvers are often successful in increasing PVR and reducing pulmonary blood flow, it is important to remember that these patients have limited oxygen reserve and may desaturate suddenly and precipitously. Controlled hypoventilation in effect reduces the functional residual capacity and, therefore, oxygen reserve, which is further reduced by the use of a hypoxic inspired gas mixture. An alternate strategy is to add carbon dioxide to the inspiratory limb of the breathing circuit, which will also increase PVR; however, because a hypoxic gas mixture is not used, systemic oxygen delivery is maintained. In practice, manipulating inspired gas concentrations is rarely needed in the current era. Patients who have continued pulmonary overcirculation with high SaO_2 and reduced systemic perfusion despite the above maneuvers require early surgical intervention to control pulmonary blood flow.

Decreased pulmonary blood flow in preoperative patients with a parallel circulation is reflected by hypoxemia with an SaO_2 of <75%. Preoperatively this may be due to restricted flow across a small ductus arteriosus, increased PVR secondary to parenchymal lung disease, or increased pulmonary venous pressure secondary to obstructed pulmonary venous drainage or a restrictive atrial septal defect. Sedation, paralysis, and manipulation of mechanical ventilation to maintain an alkalosis may be effective if PVR is elevated. Nitric oxide may also be used in this situation as a specific pulmonary vasodilator. Systemic oxygen delivery is maintained by improving cardiac output with inotropes and maintaining the hematocrit at >40%. Among some newborns with hypoplastic left-heart syndrome, pulmonary blood flow may be insufficient because the mitral valve hypoplasia in combination with the occasional finding of a restrictive or nearly intact atrial septum severely restricts pulmonary venous return to the heart. The newborn is intensely cyanotic and has a pulmonary venous congestion pattern on chest x-ray. Urgent interventional cardiac catheterization with balloon septostomy or dilation (or stent placement) of a restrictive atrial septal defect may be necessary.

Systemic perfusion is maintained with the use of volume and vasoactive agents. Inotropic support is often necessary because of ventricular dysfunction secondary to shock states associated with a closing ductus arteriosus at the time of presentation. Systemic afterload reduction with agents such as phosphodiesterase inhibitors (e.g., milrinone) may improve systemic perfusion and reduce atrioventricular valve regurgitation in volume-loaded hearts. However, milrinone may also decrease PVR and thus not fully address the imbalance of pulmonary and systemic flows. Oliguria and a rising serum creatinine level may reflect renal insufficiency from a low cardiac output. Necrotizing enterocolitis is a risk secondary to splanchnic hypoperfusion, and the authors prefer not to enterally feed newborns with a wide pulse width and low diastolic pressure (usually <30 mm Hg) prior to surgery, especially in the context of obstructive left heart lesions. It is important to evaluate end-organ perfusion and function, and optimize the patient's condition prior to surgery.

The "Risk Adjustment in Congenital Heart Surgery" classification, which has been shown to predict hospital mortality, classifies 79 open- and closed-heart operations into 6 risk categories. Another international method, called the *Aristotle Score*, is based on the potential for mortality, the potential for morbidity, and the anticipated technical difficulty.

CHAPTER 49A ■ POSTOPERATIVE CARE OF THE PEDIATRIC CARDIAC SURGICAL PATIENT: GENERAL CONSIDERATIONS

DAVID L. WESSEL • ALAIN FRAISSE

ASSESSMENT

Assessment of a child following cardiac surgery begins with review of the preoperative and operative findings, including details of the operative repair and cardiopulmonary bypass (CPB), particularly total CPB or myocardial ischemia (aortic cross-clamp) times, concerns about myocardial protection, recovery of myocardial contractility, typical postoperative systemic arterial and central venous pressures, findings from intraoperative transesophageal echocardiogram, and vasoactive medication requirements. This information will guide subsequent examination, which should focus on the quality of the repair or palliation plus a clinical assessment of cardiac output. In addition to a complete cardiovascular examination, a routine set of laboratory tests should be obtained, including a chest x-ray, 12- or 15-lead electrocardiogram, blood gas analysis, serum electrolytes, lactate, cardiac troponin T, and glucose, an ionized calcium level, complete blood count, and coagulation profile.

Monitoring

All patients should have continuous monitoring of their heart rate and rhythm by electrocardiogram, systemic arterial blood pressure (invasive or noninvasive), oxygen saturation by pulse oximetry, and respiratory rate. Breath-to-breath end-tidal CO_2 monitoring is often routinely used in mechanically ventilated patients to monitor for possible disconnection, misplacement, or obstruction of the endotracheal tube. It is also a useful indicator for acute changes in pulmonary blood flow. Monitoring central venous pressure following cardiac surgery is essential for many patients, except those who undergo the least complex procedures.

Intracardiac or transthoracic left atrial (LA) catheters are often used to monitor patients after complex reparative procedures. LA catheters are especially helpful in the management of patients with ventricular dysfunction, coronary artery perfusion abnormalities, and mitral valve disease. The mean LA pressure is typically 1–2 mm Hg greater than mean right atrial (RA) pressure, which generally varies between 2 and 6 mm Hg in non-postoperative pediatric patients who undergo cardiac catheterization.

TABLE 49A.1

COMMON CAUSES OF ELEVATED LEFT ATRIAL PRESSURE AFTER CARDIOPULMONARY BYPASS

1. Decreased ventricular systolic or diastolic function
   Myocardial ischemia
   Dilated cardiomyopathy
   Systemic ventricular hypertrophy
2. Left atrioventricular valve disease
3. Large left-to-right intracardiac shunt
4. Chamber hypoplasia
5. Intravascular or ventricular volume overload
6. Cardiac tamponade
7. Dysrhythmia
   Tachyarrhythmia, junctional rhythm
   Complete heart block

In postoperative patients, mean LA and RA pressures are both often >6–8 mm Hg. However, they should generally be <15 mm Hg. The compliance of the RA is greater than that of the LA, except in the newborn; therefore, pressure elevations in the RA of older patients with two ventricles are typically less pronounced. Possible causes of abnormally elevated LA pressure are listed in **Table 49A.1**. The causes of abnormally high or low RA, LA, and pulmonary artery (PA) oxygen saturations, which can be measured at the bedside in the ICU, are listed in **Table 49A.2**. Determination of the PA oxygen saturation can be useful in patients with systemic-to-PA collaterals because flow from these vessels into the pulmonary arteries can increase the oxygen saturation.

TABLE 49A.2

CAUSES OF ABNORMAL RIGHT ATRIAL, LEFT ATRIAL, OR PULMONARY ARTERY OXYGEN SATURATION

Location	Elevated O_2 saturation	Reduced O_2 saturation
RA	Atrial level left-to-right shunt Anomalous pulmonary venous return Left ventricular-to-right atrial shunt ↑ dissolved O_2 content ↓ O_2 extraction Catheter tip position (e.g., near renal veins)	↑ Vo_2 (e.g., low CO, fever) ↓ Sao_2 saturation with a normal AV O_2 difference Anemia Catheter tip position (e.g., near CS)
LA	Does not occur	Atrial level right-to-left shunt ↓ Pvo_2 (e.g., parenchymal lung disease)
PA	Significant left-to-right shunt Small left-to-right shunt with incomplete mixing of blood Catheter tip position (e.g., PA "wedge")	↑ O_2 extraction (e.g., low CO, fever) ↓ Sao_2 saturation with a normal AV O_2 difference Anemia

RA, right atrium; Vo_2, oxygenation consumption; CO, cardiac output; Sao_2, arterial oxygen saturation; AV, arteriovenous; CS, coronary sinus; LA, left atrium; Pvo_2, pulmonary vein oxygen tension; PA, pulmonary artery

Low Cardiac Output Syndrome

Myocardial dysfunction following CPB can be caused by the inflammatory response associated with CPB, the effects of myocardial ischemia from aortic cross-clamping, hypothermia, reperfusion injury, inadequate myocardial protection, or ventriculotomy (when performed). Mixed venous oxygen saturation, whole blood pH, and lactate are laboratory measures commonly used to evaluate the adequacy of tissue perfusion and, hence, cardiac output.

Volume Adjustments

After CPB, the factors that influence cardiac output, such as preload, afterload, myocardial contractility, heart rate, and rhythm, must be assessed and manipulated. Volume therapy (increased preload) is commonly necessary, followed by appropriate use of inotropic and afterload-reducing agents. Atrial pressure and the ventricular response to changes in atrial pressure must be evaluated. While 5% albumin solution remains a popular choice because it remains within the vascular compartment longer than does crystalloid, its use may be limited by cost, availability, and risk of transfusion-related events and other morbidities. Alternatives that have recently gained popularity include crystalloid solutions such as 0.9% sodium chloride, balanced electrolyte solutions such as Ringer lactate, and starch-polymer artificial colloids. Selected children with low cardiac output may benefit from strategies that allow right-to-left shunting at the atrial level in the face of postoperative RV dysfunction.

Right Ventriculotomy and Restrictive Physiology

RV "restrictive" physiology in infants and children who have undergone congenital cardiac surgery has been described by echocardiography as persistent antegrade diastolic blood flow into the pulmonary circulation following reconstruction of the RV outflow and occurs in the setting of decreased RV compliance as a result of diastolic dysfunction with an inability to relax and fill during diastole. The RV is usually not dilated in this circumstance, and pulmonary regurgitation is limited because of the higher diastolic pressure in the RV. If RV end-diastolic pressure is sufficiently elevated, the septal position shifts to the left, which decreases LV compliance and function (ventricular interdependence). As a result of the low cardiac output syndrome (LCOS), patients often have cool extremities, are oliguric, and may have a metabolic acidosis. As a result of the elevated RA pressure, hepatic congestion, ascites, increased chest tube losses, and pleural effusions may be evident. These patients may be tachycardic and hypotensive with a narrow pulse pressure. Preload must be maintained, despite elevation of the RA pressure. Significant inotrope support is often required (typically dopamine, 5–10 mcg/kg/min, and/or low-dose epinephrine, <0.05 mcg/kg/min), and a phosphodiesterase inhibitor such as or milrinone is beneficial because of its lusitropic properties. Sedation and even paralysis for a period of 24–48 hrs may assist by minimizing cardiorespiratory work.

Mechanical ventilation may have a significant impact on RV afterload (**Table 49A.3**). Both

TABLE 49A.3

CARDIORESPIRATORY INTERACTIONS OF A POSITIVE-PRESSURE MECHANICAL BREATH

	Afterload	Preload
Pulmonary ventricle	**Elevated** Effect: ↑ RVEDp ↑ RVp ↓ Antegrade PBF ↑ PR and/or TR	**Reduced** Effect: ↓ RVEDV ↓ RAp
Systemic ventricle	**Reduced** Effect: ↓ LVEDp ↓ LAp ↓ Pulmonary edema ↑ Increase cardiac output	**Reduced** Effect: ↓ LVEDV ↓ LAp

RVEDp, right ventricle end-diastolic pressure; RVEDV, right ventricle end-diastolic volume; RVp, right ventricle pressure; RAp, right atrial pressure; PBF, pulmonary blood flow; PR, pulmonary regurgitation; TR, tricuspid regurgitation; LVEDp, left ventricle end diastolic pressure; LVEDV, left ventricle end diastolic volume; LAp, left atrial pressure underinflation and overinflation of the lungs raise pulmonary vascular resistance (PVR) and RV afterload, thereby increasing the amount of pulmonary regurgitation. In addition, an increase in PVR because of hypothermia, acidosis, and either hypoinflation or hyperinflation of the lung will also increase afterload on the RV and pulmonary regurgitation.

Pharmacologic Support

Preload adjustments often do not suffice to provide adequate cardiac output. Use of pharmacologic agents to support cardiac output is common. Common vasoactive drugs used for cardiac patients in the ICU, along with their actions, are listed in **Table 49A.4** and **Table 49A.5**. The less compliant neonatal myocardium, like the ischemic adult heart, may raise its end-diastolic pressure during higher-dose infusions of catecholamines, further impairing ventricular compliance and further reducing ventricular filling. Prophylactic use of high-dose milrinone significantly reduces the development of LCOS T3 supplementation cannot be recommended.

When systemic blood pressure is elevated and cardiac output appears low or normal, a primary vasodilator (**Table 49A.4**) is indicated to normalize blood pressure and to decrease systemic vascular resistance and therefore afterload on the LV. This situation is most often true for the newborn myocardium, which is especially sensitive to changes in afterload and tolerates elevated systemic resistances poorly. The use of nitroprusside may be associated with generation of the toxic metabolites cyanide and thiocyanate, which are produced in a dose-related manner. Nesiritide (synthetic B-type natriuretic peptide) is well tolerated and associated with improvement in diuresis and fluid balance. Fenoldopam is a new dopaminergic agent useful in the treatment of systemic hypertension and may have salutary effects on renal blood flow. It causes systemic vasodilatation, increased renal output, and increased tubular sodium secretion. It has no known chronotropic or inotropic effects on the heart but reduces afterload and may augment urine output in critical ill newborns after cardiac surgery. Levosimendan is a calcium sensitizer that increases cardiac output by increasing stroke volume, decreases cardiac filling pressures, reduces afterload on the ventricles, and has anti-inflammatory properties.

Other Strategies

Newer strategies to support low cardiac output associated with cardiac surgery in children include the use of atrio-*bi*ventricular pacing for patients with complete heart block or prolonged interventricu-

lar conduction delays and asynchronous contraction. Appreciation of the hemodynamic effects of positive- and negative-pressure ventilation may facilitate optimization of cardiac output by adjustments to ventilation. Avoidance of hyperthermia and even induced hypothermia may provide end-organ protection during periods of low cardiac output. In children with LCOS who are resistant to catecholamine administration, a relative adrenal insufficiency has been proposed as a causative factor.

Diastolic Dysfunction

Occasionally, there is an alteration of ventricular relaxation, which is an active energy-dependent process that reduces ventricular compliance. This event is particularly problematic in a patient with a hypertrophied ventricle who is undergoing surgical repair. A gradual increase in intravascular volume to augment ventricular capacity, in addition to the use of low doses of inotropic agents, has proven to provide modest benefit in patients with diastolic dysfunction. Tachycardia must be avoided to optimize diastolic filling time and to decrease myocardial oxygen demands. Milrinone or enoximone is useful under these circumstances, as these agents are noncatecholamine inodilators, with vasodilating and lusitropic (improved diastolic state) properties, in contrast to other inotropic agents.

Managing Acute Pulmonary Hypertension in the ICU

Vasodilators historically reported as useful in pulmonary hypertension (e.g., tolazoline, phenoxybenzamine, nitroprusside, and isoproterenol) had little biologic basis for selectivity or enhanced activity in the pulmonary vascular bed. However, if myocardial function is depressed and the afterload-reducing effect on the LV is beneficial to myocardial function and cardiac output, these drugs may have some value. In addition to drug-specific side effects, they all have the limitation of potentially causing profound systemic hypotension, critically lowering right (and left) coronary perfusion pressure and simultaneously increasing intrapulmonary shunt. Prostacyclin appears to have somewhat more selectivity for the pulmonary circulation, but high doses can precipitate profound systemic hypotension in unstable postoperative patients with refractory pulmonary hypertension. Nitric oxide (NO) is a selective pulmonary vasodilator that can be breathed as a gas and distributed across the alveoli to the pulmonary vascular smooth muscle. iNO can also be used diagnostically in neonates with RV hypertension after cardiac surgery to discern those with reversible vasoconstriction. The

SUMMARY OF SELECTED VASOACTIVE AGENTS: NONCATECHOLAMINES

Agent	Doses (IV)	Noncatecholamines		
		Peripheral vascular effect	Cardiac effect	Conduction system effect
Digoxin (total digitalizing dose)	Premature, 20 mcg/kg Neonate (0–1 mo), 30 mcg/kg Infant (<2 yr), 40 mcg/kg Child (2–5 yr), 30 mcg/kg Child (>5 yr), 20 mcg/kg	Increases peripheral vascular resistance 1–2+; acts directly on vascular smooth muscle.	Inotropic effect 3–4+; acts directly on myocardium.	Slows sinus node slightly; decreases A-V conduction more.
Calcium chloride	10–20 mg/kg/dose (slowly)	Variable; age-dependent. Vasoconstrictor	Inotropic effect 3+; depends on ionized Ca^{2+}.	Slows sinus node; decreases AV conduction.
Calcium gluconate	50–100 mg/kg/dose (slowly)			
Nitroprusside	0.5–5 mcg/kg/min	Donates nitric oxide group to relax smooth muscle and dilate pulmonary and systemic vessels.	Indirectly increases cardiac output by decreasing afterload.	Reflex tachycardia
Nitroglycerin	0.5–10 mcg/kg/min	Primarily venodilator. As a nitric oxide donor, may cause pulmonary vasodilation and enhance coronary vasoreactivity after aortic cross-clamping	Decreases preload; may decrease afterload. Reduces myocardial work related to change in wall stress.	Minimal
Milrinone	50–75 mcg/kg loading dose 0.25–1.0 mc/kg/min maintenance	Systemic and pulmonary vasodilator	Diastolic relaxation (lusitropy); measurable inotropic effect	Minimal tachycardia
Vasopressin	.003–.002 U/kg/min	Potent vasoconstrictor	No direct effect	None known

TABLE 49A.5

SUMMARY OF SELECTED VASOACTIVE AGENTS: CATECHOLAMINES

		Catecholamines				
Agent	Dose range	α	β_1	β_2	Dopa	Comment
Phenylephrine	0.1–0.5 mcg/kg/min	4+	0	0	0	Increases systemic resistance; no inotropy; may cause renal ischemia; useful for treatment of tetralogy of Fallot spells.
Isoproterenol	0.05–0.5 mcg/kg/min	0	4+	4+	0	Strong inotropic and chronotropic agent; peripheral vasodilator; reduces preload; pulmonary vasodilator. Limited by tachycardia and oxygen consumption.
Norepinephrine	0.1–0.5 mcg/kg/min	4+	2+	0	0	Increases systemic resistance; moderately inotropic; may cause renal ischemia.
Epinephrine	0.03–0.1 mcg/kg/min 0.2–0.5 mcg/kg/min	2+ 4+	2–3+ 4+	1–2+ 0	0 0	Beta$_2$ effect with lower doses; best for blood pressure in anaphylaxis and drug toxicity.
Dopamine	2–4 mcg/kg/min 4–8 mcg/kg/min >10 mcg/kg/min	0 0 2–4+	0 1–2+ 1–2+	0 2+ 0	2+ 2+ 0	Splanchnic and renal vasodilator; may be used with isoproterenol; increasing doses produce increasing alpha effect.
Dobutamine	2–10 mcg/kg/min	1+	3–4+	2+	0	Less chronotropy and fewer dysrhythmias at lower doses; effects vary with dose, similar to dopamine; chronotropic advantage compared with dopamine may not be apparent in neonates.

withdrawal response to iNO can be attenuated by pretreatment with the type V phosphodiesterase inhibitor sildenafil (Viagra). The clinical management of postoperative pulmonary hypertension is now well understood (**Table 49A.6**).

Cardiac Tamponade

Cardiac tamponade may occur following cardiac surgery due to compression of the heart within the thorax following blood or serous fluid collection

TABLE 49A.6

CRITICAL CARE STRATEGIES FOR POSTOPERATIVE TREATMENT OF PULMONARY HYPERTENSION

Encourage	Avoid
1. Anatomic investigation	1. Residual anatomic disease
2. Opportunities for right-to-left shunt as "pop off"	2. Intact atrial septum in right-heart failure
3. Sedation/anesthesia	3. Agitation/pain
4. Moderate hyperventilation	4. Respiratory acidosis
5. Moderate alkalosis	5. Metabolic acidosis
6. Adequate inspired oxygen	6. Alveolar hypoxia
7. Normal lung volumes	7. Atelectasis or overdistension
8. Optimal hematocrit	8. Excessive hematocrit
9. Inotropic support	9. Low output and coronary perfusion
10. Vasodilators	10. Vasoconstrictors/increased afterload

or because of swelling of intrathoracic tissues in response to a perioperative systemic inflammatory response. The signs of tamponade include tachycardia, hypotension, narrow pulse pressure, pulsus paradoxus, and high filling pressures on both the left and right sides of the heart. Postoperative tamponade from bleeding immediately after operation is best handled by facilitation of chest tube drainage or re-opening the sternotomy. Some children develop pericardial effusions at other phases of their illness, or postpericardiotomy syndrome. Fluid in the pericardial space may accumulate under considerable pressure, and filling of the heart is impaired. If this problem is left unattended, the transmural pressure in the atria diminishes as the intra-atrial pressures rise, and diastolic collapse of the atria can be observed echocardiographically.

MECHANICAL SUPPORT OF THE CIRCULATION

Despite the expanding options for pharmacologic support, the circulation cannot be adequately supported in some patients in either preoperative or postoperative situations. Mechanical assist devices have an important role in providing short-term circulatory support to enable myocardial recovery and the potential for longer-term support while the patient awaits cardiac transplantation. A variety of assist devices is available for adult-sized patients; however, extracorporeal membrane oxygenation (ECMO) is the predominant mode of support for children. General indications for ECMO support of the circulation are summarized in **Table 49A.7**.

Special Problems for the Cardiac Patient

Diaphragmatic paresis (reduced motion) or paralysis (with paradoxical movement) may precipitate and promote respiratory failure. Topical cooling with ice during deep hypothermia may cause transient phrenic palsy. Increased work of breathing on low ventilator settings, increased Pco_2, and a chest x-ray that reveals an elevated hemidiaphragm are suggestive of diaphragmatic dysfunction. Ultrasonography or fluoroscopy is useful for identifying diaphragmatic motion or paradoxical excursion. Postextubation stridor due to subglottic edema is treated with inhaled alpha agonists. A summary of factors that should be considered in the patient who fails to wean from mechanical ventilation is presented in **Table 49A.8**.

TABLE 49A.7
TYPICAL INDICATIONS FOR EXTRACORPOREAL MEMBRANE OXYGENATION

I. Inadequate oxygen delivery
  A. Low cardiac output
    1. Chronic (cardiomyopathy)
    2. Acute (myocarditis)
    3. Failure of weaning from CPB
    4. Need for preoperative stabilization
    5. Progressive postoperative failure
    6. Refractory pulmonary hypertension
    7. Refractory dysrhythmias
    8. Cardiac arrest
  B. Profound cyanosis
    1. Intracardiac shunting and cardiovascular collapse
    2. Acute shunt thrombosis
    3. Acute respiratory failure exaggerated by underlying heart disease
    4. CHD complicated by other newborn indications for ECMO, such as meconium aspiration syndrome, PPHN, pneumonia, sepsis, respiratory distress syndrome
II. Support for intervention during cardiac catheterization

CPB, cardiopulmonary bypass; CHD, congenital heart disease; PPHN, persistent pulmonary hypertension of the neonate

Weaning from Mechanical Ventilation

Early tracheal extubation of children following congenital heart surgery is not a new concept but has received renewed attention with the evolution of "fast-track" management for cardiac surgical patients. Early extubation generally refers to tracheal extubation within a few hours (i.e., 4–8 hrs) after surgery, though in practice it means the avoidance of routine, overnight mechanical ventilation. Factors to consider when planning early extubation are listed in **Table 49A.9**.

POSTOPERATIVE ISSUES

Though the incidence of seizures in the ICU has dramatically declined in recent years, we treat seizures aggressively when they do occur, using benzodiazepines, phenobarbital, or phenytoin. Intraventricular hemorrhage, which may occur as a consequence of perinatal events or circulatory collapse in the first few days of life, is commonly associated with prematurity.

TABLE 49A.8

FACTORS THAT CONTRIBUTE TO THE INABILITY TO WEAN FROM MECHANICAL VENTILATION AFTER CONGENITAL HEART SURGERY

Residual cardiac defects
   Volume and/or pressure overload
   Myocardial dysfunction
   Low cardiac output state

Restrictive pulmonary defects
   Pulmonary edema
   Pleural effusion
   Atelectasis
   Chest wall edema
   Phrenic nerve injury
   Ascites/Hepatomegaly

Airway
   Subglottic edema and/or stenosis
   Retained secretions
   Vocal cord injury
   Extrinsic bronchial compression
   Tracheobronchomalacia

Metabolic
   Inadequate nutrition
   Sepsis
   Stress response

Risk factors for postoperative renal failure include preoperative renal dysfunction, prolonged bypass time, low cardiac output, and cardiac arrest. Postoperative sepsis and nephrotoxic drugs may cause further damage to the kidneys. Oliguria in the first 24 hrs after complex surgery and CPB is common in neonates and infants until cardiac output recovers and neurohumoral mechanisms abate. While diuretics are commonly prescribed in the immediate postoperative period, the neurohumoral influence on urine output is powerful. Diuresis will usually occur as time elapses after CPB (~24 hrs) and as cardiac output is enhanced through intravascular volume and pharmacologic adjustments. Peritoneal dialysis, hemodialysis, and continuous venovenous hemofiltration provide alternate renal support in patients with severe oliguria and renal failure. The indications for peritoneal catheter placement in the ICU include the need for renal support and the need to reduce intraabdominal pressure from ascites that may be compromising mechanical ventilation. Peritoneal drainage may be significant in the immediate postoperative period as third-space fluid losses continue. Replacement with albumin and/or fresh frozen plasma may be necessary to treat hypovolemia and hypoproteinemia.

Critically ill children often have decreased caloric intake and increased energy demand after surgery; the neonate in particular has limited metabolic and fat

TABLE 49A.9

CONSIDERATIONS FOR PLANNED EARLY EXTUBATION AFTER CONGENITAL HEART SURGERY

Patient factors	Risk factors associated with anatomy and planned surgery
	Limited cardiorespiratory reserve of the neonate and infant
	Pathophysiology of specific congenital heart defects
	Timing of surgery and preoperative management
Anesthetic factors	Premedication
	Hemodynamic stability and reserve
	Drug distribution and maintenance of anesthesia on bypass
	Postoperative analgesia
Surgical factors	Extent and complexity of surgery
	Residual defects
	Risks for bleeding and protection of suture lines
Conduct of bypass	Degree of hypothermia
	Level of hemodilution
	Myocardial protection
	Extent of the inflammatory response and reperfusion injury
Postoperative management	Myocardial function
	Cardiorespiratory interactions
	Neurologic recovery
	Analgesia management

reserves. Total parenteral nutrition can provide adequate nutrition in the early hypercatabolic phases of the early postoperative period. Upper gastrointestinal bleeding and ulcer formation may occur following the stress of cardiac surgery in children and adults. Hepatic failure may occur after cardiac surgery (particularly after the Fontan operation) and is typically characterized by elevated liver enzymes and coagulopathy. Risk factors for necrotizing enterocolitis include (a) left-sided obstructive lesions, (b) umbilical or femoral arterial catheterization/angiography, (c) hypoxemia, and (d) lesions with wide pulse pressures (e.g., systemic-to-pulmonary shunts, patent ductus arteriosus, especially in transposition of the great arteries, and severe aortic regurgitation, all of which may produce retrograde flow in the mesenteric vessels during diastole). Treatment includes continuous nasogastric suction, parenteral nutrition, and broad-spectrum antibiotics. Bowel exploration or resection may be necessary in severe cases.

Low-grade (<38.5°C) fever during the immediate postoperative period is common and may be present for up to 3–4 days, even without a demonstrable infectious etiology. Fever <38.5°C in the immediate postoperative period is usually the result of a systemic inflammatory reaction to surgery rather than active infection, but its course should be closely observed. Despite the increased use of broad-coverage, third-generation cephalosporins, these agents do not seem to be more effective in decreasing postoperative infections. Meticulous catheter insertion and daily care routines along with early removal of indwelling catheters in the postoperative patient may potentially reduce the incidence of sepsis. Mediastinitis occurs in up to 2% of patients who undergo cardiac surgery; risk factors may include delayed sternal closure, early re-exploration for bleeding, or reoperation. Mediastinitis is characterized by persistent fever, purulent drainage from the sternotomy wound, instability of the sternum, and leukocytosis. Staphylococcus is the most common offending organism. Treatment usually involves debridement and irrigation with parenteral antibiotic therapy.

POSTOPERATIVE MANAGEMENT OF PATIENTS WITH A SINGLE VENTRICLE AFTER NEONATAL PALLIATIVE SURGERY

The First Stage of Palliation

Management of patients following the first stage of single-ventricle reconstruction (Stage I Norwood operation) is complex; intensive monitoring is essential, as the clinical status may change abruptly with rapid deterioration (**Table 49A.10**). The type, diameter, length, and position of the shunt will also affect the balance of pulmonary and systemic flows. Generally, a 3.5-mm Blalock-Taussig shunt from the distal innominate artery will provide adequate pulmonary blood flow without excessive steal from the systemic circulation for most full-term neonates. Echocardiography is useful as is cardiac catheterization, which is sometimes necessary. A modification to the Norwood procedure has been introduced that involves placement of a conduit from the RV to the PA confluence (also called a ventriculopulmonary shunt or Sano modification).

Bidirectional Cavopulmonary Anastomosis

The bidirectional cavopulmonary anastomosis is the follow-up surgical procedure in infants after neonatal palliation of single-ventricle anatomy. In this procedure, also known as a *bidirectional Glenn shunt* (BDG), the superior vena cava is transected and connected end-to-side to the right PA, but the pulmonary arteries are left in continuity. Therefore, flow from the superior vena cava is bidirectional into both left and right PAs. This is the only source of pulmonary blood flow, and inferior vena cava blood returns to the common atrium. Performed at between 3 and 6 mos of age, the BDG has proven to be an important early staging procedure for patients with single-ventricle physiology because the volume and pressure load are relieved from the systemic ventricle, yet effective pulmonary blood flow is maintained. $Q_p:Q_s$ is always <1, and the volume load to the single RV is relieved, compared to the volume load with a systemic-to-pulmonary artery shunt. Systemic hypertension is common following a BDG. Treatment with vasodilators may be necessary during the immediate postoperative period and during the weaning process. Following the BDG anastomosis, arterial oxygen saturation should be in the 80%–85% range. Persistent hypoxemia is often secondary to an LCOS and low Svo_2. Treatment is directed at improving contractility, reducing afterload, and ensuring that the patient has a normal rhythm and hematocrit.

Fontan Procedure

Factors that contribute to a successful cavopulmonary connection are shown in **Table 49A.11**. A systemic venous pressure of 10–15 mm Hg and a LA pressure of 5–10 mm Hg (i.e., a transpulmonary gradient of 5–10 mm Hg) are ideal. Early resumption of spontaneous ventilation is recommended to offset the detrimental effects of positive-pressure

TABLE 49A.10

MANAGEMENT CONSIDERATIONS FOR PATIENTS FOLLOWING A NORWOOD PROCEDURE

Scenario	Etiology	Management
SaO_2 ~80% SvO_2 ~60% Normotension	**Balanced flow** $Q_p = Q_s$	No intervention

SaO_2 > 90%
Hypotension
	Overcirculated
	$Q_p > Q_s$
	Low PVR
	Large BT shunt
	Residual arch obstruction
		Raise PVR:
		    Controlled hypoventilation
		    Low FIO_2 (0.17–0.19)
		    Add CO_2 (3%–5%)
		Increase systemic perfusion:
		    Afterload reduction, vasodilation,
		        inotropic support
		    Surgical shunt revision

SaO_2 <75%
Hypertension
	Undercirculated
	$Q_p < Q_s$
	High PVR
	Small, kinked, thrombosed BT shunt
		Lower PVR:
		    Controlled hyperventilation
		    Alkalosis
		    Sedation/paralysis
		Increase cardiac output:
		    Inotrope support
		Hematocrit >40%
		Surgical intervention

SaO_2 <75% Hypotension Low SvO_2	**Low cardiac output** Ventricular failure Myocardial ischemia Residual arch obstruction AV valve regurgitation	Minimize stress response Inotropic support Surgical revision Consider mechanical support Consider transplantation

SaO_2, arterial oxygen saturation; SvO_2, mixed venous oxygen saturation; Q_p, pulmonary blood flow; Q_s, systemic blood flow; PVR, pulmonary vascular resistance; FIO_2, inspired oxygen concentration; BT, Blalock-Taussig

TABLE 49A.11

MANAGEMENT CONSIDERATIONS FOLLOWING A MODIFIED FONTAN PROCEDURE

	Aim	Management
Baffle (right side) Pressure 10–15 mm Hg	Unobstructed venous return	→ or ↑ Preload Low intrathoracic pressure

Pulmonary circulation	PVR <2 Wood units/m_2
	Mean PAp <15 mm Hg
	Unobstructed pulmonary vessels
		Avoid increases in PVR, such as from acidosis,
		    hypo- and hyperinflation of the lung,
		    hypothermia, and excess sympathetic
		    stimulation.
		Early resumption of spontaneous respiration.

Left atrium
Pressure, 5–10 mm Hg
	Sinus rhythm
	Competent AV valve
	Ventricle:
	    Normal diastolic function
	    Normal systolic function
	    No outflow obstruction
		Maintain sinus rhythm.
		→ or ↑ rate to increase CO
		→ or ↓ afterload
		→ or ↑ contractility
		PDE inhibitors useful because of vasodilation
		    and inotropic and lusitropic properties.

PAp, pulmonary artery pressure; PVR, pulmonary vascular resistance; CO, cardiac output; AV, atrioventricular; PDE, phosphodiesterase ventilation. A delivered tidal volume of 10–12 mL/kg with the lowest possible mean airway pressure is appropriate. While it is preferable to wean from positive-pressure ventilation in the early postoperative period, hemodynamic responses must be closely monitored. A normal pH and a $PaCO_2$ of 40 mm Hg should be the goal, and depending on the amount of right-to-left shunt across the fenestration, the arterial oxygen saturation is usually in the 80%–90% range. Alternative methods of mechanical ventilation have also been employed for these patients. High-frequency ventilation has been used successfully, although the hemodynamic consequences of the raised mean intrathoracic pressure must be continually evaluated. Negative-pressure ventilation can be beneficial by augmenting pulmonary blood flow. Nonspecific pulmonary vasodilators, such as sodium nitroprusside, glycerol trinitrate, PGE_1, and prostacyclin, have been used to dilate the pulmonary vasculature in an effort to improve pulmonary blood flow

after a Fontan procedure; however, results vary. PVR may fall, and pulmonary blood flow may increase.

The incidence of recurrent pleural effusions and ascites has decreased since the introduction of the fenestrated baffle technique. (The baffle is the conduit that connects the inferior vena cava to the Glenn shunt, resulting in the "completion" Fontan. Fenestration creates a hole in the medial wall of the baffle to allow flow of some systemic venous blood directly into the atrium and ventricle rather than into the pulmonary circuit, which results in lower systemic venous pressures.)

Atrial flutter and/or fibrillation, heart block and, less commonly, ventricular dysrhythmia, may have a significant impact on immediate recovery, as well as long-term outcome. Sudden loss of sinus rhythm initially causes an increase in LA and systemic ventricular end-diastolic pressure and a fall in cardiac output. The superior vena cava or PA pressure must be increased, usually with volume replacement, to

TABLE 49A.12

ETIOLOGY AND TREATMENT STRATEGIES FOR PATIENTS WITH LOW CARDIAC OUTPUT IMMEDIATELY FOLLOWING THE FONTAN PROCEDURE

Low cardiac output	Etiology	Treatment
Increased TPG Baffle >20 mm Hg LAp <10 mm Hg ↑ TPG >>10 mm Hg	Inadequate pulmonary blood flow and preload to left atrium: Increased PVR	Volume replacement Reduce PVR Correct acidosis

Clinical state:
High SaO_2/Low SvO_2
Hypotension/tachycardia
Core temperature high
Poor peripheral perfusion
SVC syndrome with pleural
  effusions and increased chest
  tube drainage
Ascites/hepatomegaly
Metabolic acidosis
	Pulmonary artery stenosis
	Pulmonary vein stenosis
	Premature fenestration closure
		Inotropic support
		Systemic vasodilation
		Catheter or surgical intervention

Normal TPG Baffle >20 mm Hg LAp >15 mm Hg TPG normal 5–10 mm Hg	Ventricular failure: Systolic dysfunction Diastolic dysfunction	Maintain preload Inotrope support Systemic vasodilation

Clinical state:
Low SaO_2/Low SvO_2
Hypotension/tachycardia
Poor peripheral perfusion
Metabolic acidosis
	AVV regurgitation and/or stenosis
	Loss of sinus rhythm
	↑ Afterload stress
		Establish sinus rhythm or AV synchrony
		Correct acidosis
		Mechanical support
		Surgical intervention, including
		  takedown to BDG and
		  transplantation

LAp, left atrial pressure; TPG, transpulmonary gradient; PVR, pulmonary vascular resistance; SaO_2, systemic arterial oxygen saturation; SvO_2, SVC oxygen saturation; SVC, superior vena cava; AVV, atrioventricular valve; BDG, bidirectional Glenn anastomosis maintain the transpulmonary gradient. Prompt treatment with antiarrhythmic drugs, pacing, or cardioversion is necessary.

Premature closure of the fenestration may occur in the immediate postoperative period, leading to an LCOS with progressive metabolic acidosis and large chest-drain losses from high right-sided venous pressures (**Table 49A.12**). Patients may respond to volume replacement, inotrope support, and vasodilation; however, if hypotension and acidosis persist, cardiac catheterization and removal of thrombus or dilation of the fenestration should occur urgently.

CHAPTER 49B ■ POSTOPERATIVE CARE OF THE PEDIATRIC CARDIAC SURGICAL PATIENT: LESION-SPECIFIC MANAGEMENT

STEVEN M. SCHWARTZ • JOHNNY MILLAR

RESIDUAL LEFT-TO-RIGHT SHUNT

Residual left-to-right shunts can occur after operations that involve repair of septal defects, when preoperative shunts are left unrepaired, or when unrecognized or untreated systemic-to-pulmonary artery shunts (aortopulmonary collaterals) exist. Because of the resultant increase in pulmonary blood flow, residual left-to-right shunts may lead to pulmonary edema, pulmonary hypertension, volume overload of the systemic ventricle and, in certain circumstances, limitations of systemic cardiac output. Common signs or symptoms include a pulmonary outflow or VSD murmur, high systemic atrial pressure, hepatomegaly, and a large heart with increased pulmonary vascularity on chest x-ray.

Atrial level shunts are rarely a problem, unless they are associated with factors that cause LA hypertension, which increases left-to-right shunt flow and pulmonary artery pressure. Congestive heart failure and pulmonary overcirculation secondary to an atrial left-to-right shunt should therefore lead the clinician to carefully evaluate the patient for mitral stenosis or insufficiency, inadequate systemic ventricular size, poor systemic ventricular function, or systemic ventricular outflow tract obstruction with elevated end-diastolic pressure.

Ventricular and vascular shunts are more often problematic, as they are always associated with systemic ventricular volume overload and, often, with pulmonary hypertension. In general, shunts of $Q_p:Q_s$ <1.5:1–2:1 without pulmonary hypertension are well tolerated, but larger shunts result in the clinical syndrome of congestive heart failure. Patients with large preoperative left-to-right shunts generally tolerate residual shunts better than those who were cyanotic before surgery. For example, a patient with a residual VSD following repair of tetralogy of Fallot has gone from a situation in which the LV was essentially volume "underloaded" preoperatively (owing to the contribution of the RV to preoperative cardiac output) to one in which the LV is now volume overloaded.

Residual Systemic Ventricular Outflow Tract Obstruction

Residual systemic ventricular outflow tract obstruction should be looked for after all surgery to relieve outflow obstruction (such as repair of subaortic stenosis, aortic stenosis, or coarctation). Additionally, systemic ventricular outflow obstruction can occur after repair of AV canal defects or after other operations that remove large volume loads from the systemic ventricle when the underlying anatomy includes subvalvar hypertrophy, for example, when a patient with double-inlet LV is converted from a shunted circulation to a Glenn or Fontan. The volume unloading of the ventricle may cause the systemic outflow tract through the bulboventricular foramen to become narrowed. Signs and symptoms of systemic outflow obstruction include an ejection murmur and elevated systemic atrial pressure.

Tricuspid or Mitral Valve Dysfunction

Residual AV valve dysfunction, either insufficiency or stenosis, can occur after any attempted valve repair or when closure of a septal defect unmasks valvar stenosis on one side of the heart. AV valve insufficiency is associated with high atrial pressures on the affected side of the heart. If atrial pressure is being directly monitored, very prominent *v* waves on the tracing will often be observed, and a regurgitant murmur will be heard. Because of the associated ventricular volume overload, signs or symptoms of ventricular failure may be present. AV valve stenosis is also associated with high atrial pressure but with prominent ("cannon") *a* waves. Peripheral (right-sided) or pulmonary (left-sided) edema is common with stenotic lesions and pulmonary hypertension occurs with mitral stenosis. Medical management of AV valve insufficiency is focused on afterload reduction, with inotropic support when needed. Systemic vasodilators promote antegrade cardiac output in the face of mitral (or even aortic) insufficiency, whereas diuretics may be useful in either stenotic or regurgitant lesions.

Right- or Left-ventricular Diastolic Dysfunction

Ventricular diastolic dysfunction should be an expected complication of any operation in which significant ventricular hypertrophy occurs, which most commonly happens after relief of obstructive lesions or in the presence of preexisting diastolic dysfunction. Operations that require a right ventriculotomy in an already hypertrophied RV represent a particularly high risk for postoperative diastolic dysfunction. A ventriculotomy can impair either systolic or diastolic function. Diastolic dysfunction is marked by elevated atrial pressure and has many of the same features as seen in AV valve disease. The presence of a residual atrial shunt in this setting compounds the adverse effects of *left*-sided disease by promoting pulmonary overcirculation. Conversely, an atrial defect can help to maintain cardiac output when the *right* ventricle is noncompliant, although associated cyanosis will occur.

In general, the first-line treatment for diastolic dysfunction is to use fluid to maintain adequate preload, although inotropic agents (such as milrinone) that reduce afterload can also improve diastolic function. Fluid administration can be limited by impairment of oxygenation and lung function with progressive pulmonary edema or by complications of peripheral edema and third-spacing of fluid. Right-sided lesions in particular often respond very well to initial fluid boluses, but the hydrostatic forces in combination with diminished lymphatic drainage due to high venous pressure lead to ascites and to pleural effusions or large amounts of chest tube drainage. If a peritoneal drainage catheter is

not present, progressively higher airway pressure may be necessary to compensate for increased abdominal pressure on the diaphragm and/or loss of effective lung volume. The high airway pressure is transmitted to the pulmonary vasculature because the pulmonary parenchyma is relatively healthy; this, in turn, increases pulmonary vascular resistance (PVR), thereby increasing afterload on the already poorly functioning RV. Raised intra-abdominal pressure and low cardiac output also result in decreased renal perfusion and, eventually, renal failure, further complicating fluid management. A downward spiral thus develops in which cardiac output cannot be readily restored and pulmonary gas exchange as well as fluid and electrolyte management cannot be adequately maintained. Effective treatment can include drainage of effusions or ascites followed by further fluid resuscitation. In severe cases, mechanical support with an RV assist device or ECMO may be necessary. In general, RV diastolic function often improves over several days as the ventricle heals from surgery and becomes more compliant, assuming that the initial operation effectively restored near-normal RV systolic pressure. LV diastolic dysfunction may similarly resolve but is more likely to be associated with prolonged heart failure and/or the need for transplantation.

Pulmonary Hypertension

CPB can provoke pulmonary hypertension in those patients with significant underlying risk. Neonates, patients with pulmonary venous obstruction or mitral valve disease, and those with elevated preoperative pulmonary resistance are at particularly high risk, especially when associated with pain, agitation, suctioning, or hypoventilation. Chronic pulmonary hypertension that is not acutely worsened as a result of CPB can be well tolerated in the postoperative period, whereas acute pulmonary hypertensive crises can precipitate life-threatening symptoms. The presence of a patent foramen ovale, atrial septal defect, ventricular septal defect (VSD), or systemic-to-pulmonary artery shunt causes the main clinical consequence of acute elevations in PVR to be cyanosis because of an increase in right-to-left shunting. Pulmonary hypertension without shunting can cause acute RV failure and low cardiac output without significant changes in saturation. A sudden fall in either blood pressure or saturation in a patient with known pulmonary vascular disease or with significant risk of postoperative pulmonary hypertension should prompt immediate consideration of this diagnosis and institution of treatment when appropriate. The presence of a pulmonary artery pressure-monitoring catheter can help to establish the diagnosis of pulmonary hypertension.

Most commonly, the systemic pressure falls while the pulmonary artery pressure remains unchanged. The increased ratio of pulmonary to systemic arterial pressure is diagnostic of an increase in PVR.

In addition to hypotension or cyanosis, a pulmonary hypertensive crisis in the absence of a right-to-left shunt is usually associated with an acute increase in right atrial pressure because the increase in RV afterload raises diastolic pressure. This pressure increase can also result in shift of the ventricular septum into the LV and a subsequent increase in LA pressure despite the decreased filling of the left side of the heart. Clinical manifestations can include tachycardia, a sudden decrease in lung compliance, and/or onset of bronchospasm. As pulmonary hypertension is exacerbated by hypoxia and hypercarbia, these manifestations can be especially troublesome.

The most effective treatment strategy for those at significant risk of postoperative pulmonary hypertension is prevention. Maintenance of adequate analgesia and sedation, particularly during noxious stimuli such as suctioning, is important. Induction of respiratory alkalosis can be helpful in an acute pulmonary hypertensive crisis, but maintaining a pH above 7.5 for prolonged periods may have adverse consequences for cerebral perfusion. Therefore, a more practical approach is to avoid common problems that lead to hypoxia and respiratory acidosis, such as pneumothorax, right main-stem bronchus intubation, or mucous plugging, and to maintain a pH between 7.4 and 7.5. When prophylactic therapy fails, more aggressive treatment with inhaled NO, sildenafil, bosentan, or even mechanical support may be helpful. Sildenafil and bosentan can be used to transition from inhaled NO to chronic oral therapy for patients with chronic pulmonary vascular disease, as exogenous NO can lead to inhibition of endogenous production. Numerous other IV vasodilators, including calcium-channel blockers, nitrovasodilators, and prostaglandins, have been used but are often limited by the occurrence of systemic hypotension because of lack of pulmonary selectivity. Prostacyclin has shown promise as an agent that may reverse pulmonary vascular changes previously thought to be permanent.

Single-ventricle Lesions: Stage I Palliation

Arterial saturation is essentially an average of the pulmonary and systemic venous saturations weighted by the $Q_p:Q_s$, so that anything that decreases mixed venous saturation, pulmonary venous saturation, or $Q_p:Q_s$ can result in increased cyanosis. Problems in the postoperative period that can lead to diminished oxygen delivery include low systemic cardiac output and/or excessive cyanosis. Poor systemic perfusion or an increased gradient between arterial and mixed venous oxygen saturation suggests a primary problem with total cardiac output or high $Q_p:Q_s$. Cyanosis with preserved hemodynamics suggests either low $Q_p:Q_s$ or a primary pulmonary problem. Increases in systemic vascular resistance can increase blood pressure, $Q_p:Q_s$, and arterial saturation at the expense of systemic perfusion. It has become common practice to use afterload reduction with phenoxybenzamine, milrinone, or nitroprusside to maximize perfusion. Blood pressure can be kept in an acceptable range by improving total cardiac output with β agonists such as low-dose epinephrine or even norepinephrine.

Single-ventricle Lesions: Stage II (Bidirectional Glenn) and Stage III (Fontan) Palliation

The physiology of the bidirectional cavopulmonary anastomosis (Glenn) is that pulmonary blood flow is largely dependent on the resistance of two highly but differentially regulated vascular beds—the cerebral and pulmonary circulations. Both cerebral and pulmonary vasculatures have opposite responses to changes in carbon dioxide, acid-base status, and oxygen, which can make treatment of elevated pulmonary resistance or low arterial saturation particularly challenging. Hyperventilation and alkalosis are effective pulmonary vasodilators; hyperventilation and alkalosis cause cerebral vasoconstriction. As pulmonary blood flow is dependent on venous return via the superior vena cava (largely made up of cerebral blood flow), maneuvers that limit cerebral blood flow may decrease pulmonary flow and exacerbate hypoxemia. Hyperventilation following bidirectional cavopulmonary anastomosis does, in fact, impair cerebral blood flow and decrease arterial saturation. Other frequently used techniques for decreasing pulmonary resistance (such as deep sedation/anesthesia) may also reduce cerebral blood flow and therefore fail to increase pulmonary blood flow, even if they successfully reduce resistance. Inhaled NO may work well in combination with mild hypoventilation for high pulmonary resistance and cyanosis. When the degree of cyanosis is not prohibitive, expectant management with good hemodynamic support and maintenance of hemoglobin will often suffice because saturation tends to slowly improve in the first few days following surgery and again at the time of extubation as long as there are no intervening airway or pulmonary issues occur. Persistent cyanosis should prompt a search for lesions such as decompressing venovenous collaterals that divert superior vena cava blood away from the pulmonary circulation.

Systemic hypertension is a common phenomenon following the Glenn operation, perhaps a response to increased cerebral venous pressure or improved output from a ventricle that has had some of its volume load removed. Acute treatment with vasodilators is often necessary, and blood pressure tends to fall to normal levels over the first few postoperative days. A proportion of patients require more long-term treatment with angiotensin-converting-enzyme inhibitors.

Fontan physiology is a hybrid of bidirectional Glenn and normal cardiovascular physiology. Like the bidirectional Glenn, pulmonary blood flow is dependent on systemic venous pressure, and all pulmonary flow is effective. If the Fontan baffle is fenestrated, a right-to-left shunt may still exist, causing some mild systemic arterial desaturation, but the systemic and pulmonary circulations are largely separated, as with a normal heart. Important issues for the intensive care physician arise when pulmonary artery pressure is elevated, which can occur because the pulmonary resistance is high, in the presence of mechanical pulmonary artery obstruction, or when myocardial dysfunction raises pulmonary venous atrial pressure. Numerous studies demonstrate that elevated pulmonary artery pressure (>10–15 mm Hg) is associated with poor outcome in Fontan patients, largely because it is very difficult to maintain central venous pressure in this range without large third-space losses of fluid. As these fluid losses progress, patients often develop pleural effusions, ascites, and peripheral edema. It then becomes necessary to increase ventilator pressures to maintain adequate functional residual capacity and tidal volume in the face of a full abdomen, heavy chest wall, and smaller effective pleural cavities. Increased airway pressure, particularly in the absence of parenchymal lung disease, effectively raises pulmonary resistance and thus necessitates even higher venous pressures to maintain cardiac output. Furthermore, as central venous and intra-abdominal pressures rise, renal perfusion pressure decreases, especially in the face of low cardiac output and borderline hypotension, as is often the case in this scenario. In general, Fontan fenestration can lower the risk of some of these complications by providing a source of systemic blood flow that is not dependent on passing through the pulmonary circulation. Fenestration can also decrease pulmonary artery pressure enough to reduce third-space losses of fluid.

It is common for postoperative Fontan patients to need large amounts of volume in the first day after surgery. Persistently low central venous and LA pressures strongly suggest the need for volume. Pulmonary artery obstruction should be considered as the cause of low output when LA pressure is low and central venous pressure is high. If central venous pressure is not monitored, large third-space fluid losses with a low or normal LA pressure should raise the suspicion of pulmonary artery obstruction. Even in the presence of a fenestrated Fontan, the capability of the fenestration to preserve cardiac output in the face of anatomic or physiologic obstruction to pulmonary blood flow is significantly limited compared to the situation after the bidirectional cavopulmonary anastomosis. Therefore, limited pulmonary flow can result in low cardiac output and, when a fenestration is present, significant cyanosis. Cyanosis can also result from intrapulmonary arteriovenous malformations (such as occur after the Glenn operation or ventilation-perfusion mismatch related to low cardiac output).

If high pulmonary resistance is responsible for the elevation of central venous pressure, institution of the standard therapies of supplemental oxygen, hyperventilation, and alkalosis are indicated. However, as with the bidirectional Glenn patient, the use of high positive pressures to achieve these ends may be counterproductive. Negative-pressure ventilation can augment stroke volume and cardiac output, and high-frequency jet ventilation may lower $PaCO_2$ at low mean airway pressures. Intravenous vasodilators such as prostacyclin or PGE should be used with caution because of the risk of systemic vasodilation with limited cardiac output. iNO has been reported to be effective in lowering the transpulmonary pressure gradient.

Low cardiac output with high LA and central venous pressures indicates myocardial dysfunction in the patient with Fontan physiology. Myocardial dysfunction can occur from ischemia-reperfusion injury if aortic cross-clamping and cardioplegia are used to create the Fontan baffle. It may also be related to poor preoperative myocardial function. The only effective long-term therapy for low cardiac output with ventricular dysfunction following a Fontan operation is to improve cardiac output and reduce LA pressure. The use of inotropic agents that do not increase ventricular afterload, such as phosphodiesterase inhibitors, dobutamine and low dose epinephrine (≤ 0.05 mcg/kg/min) may be helpful. If systemic blood pressure will tolerate it, aggressive afterload reduction with vasodilating agents may also lower LA pressure significantly. If there is good reason to believe the insult to ventricular function is reversible, mechanical circulatory support can also be effective therapy. Because persistent aortopulmonary collateral vessels can be associated with hemodynamics similar to those of ventricular dysfunction, aggressive assessment and embolization of these vessels may be useful in this situation.

CHAPTER 49C ◼ POSTOPERATIVE CARE OF THE PEDIATRIC CARDIAC SURGICAL PATIENT: EFFECTS OF CARDIOPULMONARY BYPASS

S. ADIL HUSAIN • MARK S. BLEIWEIS

THE EXTRACORPOREAL CIRCUIT

Blood drains from the patient via the right atrium or from both cavae into a cardiotomy reservoir (**Fig. 49C.1**). This drainage is dependent on gravity or can be assisted by a vacuum. Once in the reservoir, blood is pumped through a membrane oxygenator that incorporates a heat exchanger. Subsequently, this oxygenated blood is returned to the patient's systemic bloodstream, usually via a cannula in the aorta, arch vessel, axillary artery, or femoral artery. A filter is usually employed within this arterial line to prevent any embolization of air or other debris into the systemic circulation. In many instances, a hemofilter is used within the circuit for ultrafiltration of the patient's blood volume (**Fig. 49C.1**).

Modern trends in CPB are to miniaturize its components to minimize the amount of prime. This goal is particularly important in neonates and small infants. High prime volumes will lower the infant's hematocrit. A minimal hematocrit of ~25% is usually acceptable for any CPB situation and thus often demands the use of donor blood within the prime. The use of donor blood has potential risks, such as complement activation, transfusion reaction, viral transmission, and electrolyte abnormalities. Hemodilution reduces clotting factors and colloid osmotic pressure and, in turn, promotes the release of stress hormones and inflammatory mediators. As a result of all of these physiologic sequelae, priming volumes should be kept to a minimum, and transfusions avoided.

Although whole blood improves colloid oncotic pressure, as well as levels of circulating clotting factors, it also contains a much higher glucose content. The resulting hyperglycemia has been delineated as a risk factor for neurologic injury. Colloid solutions, such as fresh-frozen plasma and albumin, are commonly used. Priming solutions also contain electrolytes, glucose, calcium, lactate, and buffers (tris hydroxymethyl aminomethane or sodium bicarbonate, THAM). Buffer is added to help maintain appropriate pH. Agents such as mannitol and steroids may also be added to help with osmotic diuresis and as prophylaxis against systemic inflammatory responses.

Bubble oxygenators were the first employed for CPB and functioned by allowing fresh microbubbles to mix with circulating blood, all within an oxygenation column. This direct interface created a traumatic environment for RBCs, which led to increased hemolysis, platelet microaggregation, and an increased release of inflammatory mediators. Membrane oxygenators minimized this interface issue via the use of microporous hollow fibers.

A pumping mechanism is used during CPB to propel the blood through the circuit and back to the infant, and two forms are used—roller pumps and centrifugal pumps. Roller pumps are most widely used in the infant population and consist of two rollers oriented 180 degrees from one another. Blood is displaced in a forward manner, in a continuous nonpulsatile fashion. The centrifugal pump system functions by entrapping blood against spinning curved blades that create a vortex. This mechanism is advantageous as another method to minimize priming volume and to minimize general red cell trauma. The vortex functions in removing any air that could be a source of embolization once the blood returns to the arterial circulation. These pumps are also capable of producing pulsatile flow, which may improve the overall flow through both infant and circuit.

The tubes are constructed with polyvinylchloride and must be large enough to support appropriate flow rates but small enough to minimize pump prime and exposure surface area of the circulating blood. In neonates, 3/16-inch tubing is used for the arterial limbs of the circuit, and 1/4-inch tubing is used for the venous limbs. Heparin-bonded tubing has been utilized by some centers to improve the interface with circulating blood and to reduce the extent of anticoagulation required to safely maintain an infant on CPB. In addition, many have felt that its use impacts the degree of inflammatory response following CPB.

In comparison with adults, infant anatomic abnormalities may involve interrupted aortic arch anatomy, presence of intracardiac shunts, and aortopulmonary collateral circulation. Infants have lower circulating blood volumes that, coupled with their increased oxygen consumption rates, require much higher flow rates, often 200 mL/kg/min.

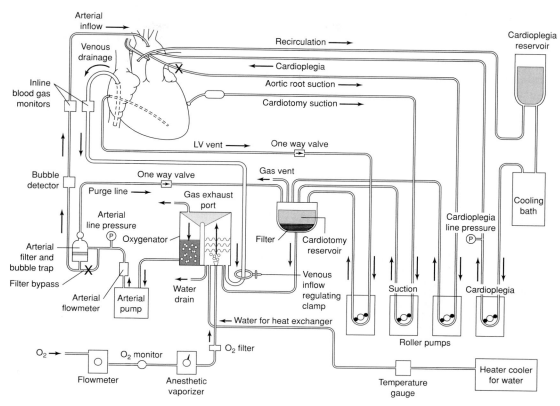

FIGURE 49C.1. Extracorporeal cardiopulmonary bypass circuit.

INITIATION OF CARDIOPULMONARY BYPASS

Heparin must be utilized during CPB, and a bolus dose of 300–400 units/kg is administered. Heparin and its effects upon anticoagulation are monitored intraoperatively by measuring the patient's activated clotting time (ACT). An ACT of >350–400 secs is generally accepted. Heparin resistance may occur in patients with low levels of antithrombin III, and administration of fresh frozen plasma may be employed to counteract this clotting deficiency. Following heparinization and cannulation, CPB is instituted, and blood begins to drain from the patient's heart. Venous drainage is dependent upon the height difference between patient and circuit, the diameter of the venous cannula and line tubing, and whether vacuum assistance is used. Arterial cannula pressure is continuously monitored and may be elevated in cases of a malpositioned or kinked arterial cannula. Once CPB has been instituted without concerns at the cannula level or elsewhere in the circuit, the heat exchanger within the oxygenator can be cooled, and the patient core body temperature can be lowered. Some degree

of hypothermia is implemented in most congenital cardiac surgical procedures that require CPB.

Cardiac Arrest—Myocardial Protection/Ischemia

Cardioplegia is an extremely cold (4°C–8°C) and highly potassium-enriched solution that allows for myocardial cells to be "protected" during periods of ischemia. Because of the high potassium concentration, the decompressed heart is arrested in diastole and, thus, has low myocardial oxygen and metabolic demands. The concept of complete circulatory arrest—actually stopping pump flow—defines the extreme of low-flow rates during CPB.

The effect of hypothermia upon metabolic rate is described using the nomenclature of Q10, which is defined by the difference in metabolic rate (oxygen consumption) at 2 temperatures, 10 degrees apart. It has been reported that infants have a higher Q10 than do adults and thus have a greater metabolic suppression and impact upon oxygen consumption. The technique of deep hypothermic circulatory arrest (DHCA) is beneficial for highly complex intracardiac or aortic arch repairs, especially in the neonatal population. Arrest times of 30 mins at temperatures of 18°C–20°C have been described with overall minimal clinically evident neurologic injury. The risk of neurologic injury rises with increasing arrest times, especially with arrest periods of >45–60 mins.

Low-flow continuous bypass with deep hypothermia is another operative strategy that is based on the premise that some cerebral blood flow is better than no flow. Low-flow bypass in neonates and infants at ~30–50 mL/kg/min can be used in certain surgical scenarios to allow for improved surgical visualization while maintaining cerebral blood flow. Despite its cerebral protective effects, hypothermia can significantly negatively impact other organ systems and strongly influence the postoperative course and management. The major benefit of pulsatile flow seems to be linked to a reduction in circulating vasoconstrictors following CPB. Improved regional perfusion to end organs seems to occur. However, the overall use of pulsatile pumps is limited.

MANAGING ACID-BASE/RESPIRATORY PHYSIOLOGY: α-STAT AND pH-stat

α-stat strategy maintains a pH of 7.40 measured without correction for temperature (37°C), whereas pH-stat recognizes that temperature; more specifically, hypothermia has a significant impact upon pH. With hypothermia, blood pH becomes more alkalotic, and carbon dioxide is added to the circuit (and thus to the patient) to maintain a temperature-corrected pH of 7.40. However, this addition of carbon dioxide increases the intracellular pH and leads to a loss of electrochemical neutrality. More specifically, hydrogen and hydroxyl ions are impacted due to this change in intracellular pH. Cellular enzyme function is thus impacted when using pH-stat.

MANAGEMENT OF ANTICOAGULATION

ACT is the standard variable measured in the operating room to gauge levels of anticoagulation once systemic heparin has been administered. The pediatric population requires an ACT of at least 350–450 secs to maintain appropriate anticoagulation while on CPB. Hemodilution from the priming volume of the circuit and initiation of CPB impact the quantity of factors. Second, ongoing activation of the extrinsic clotting system can result in a consumptive process. Both a quantitative and qualitative platelet dysfunction occurs as these cells are consumed in large numbers and activation occurs, with contact with the surface of the circuit and membrane oxygenator. Hypothermia following separation from bypass may also play a role in platelet dysfunction and the clotting impairment.

Protamine sulfate is a heparin antagonist that is administered (1–1.5 mg/100 units of circulating heparin) in the operating room to reverse the anticoagulation required for CPB. Protamine often results in a transient systemic vasodilatation, which can occasionally produce hypotension and hemodynamic instability. Although rare, more severe protamine reactions can result in severe pulmonary hypertension and may require urgent return to CPB until the process reverses. Vigilant correction of coagulation parameters, platelet dysfunction and counts, and core temperature is critical in the aggressive treatment of postoperative bleeding.

MODIFIED ULTRAFILTRATION

The systemic inflammatory response from CPB and cardiac surgery leads to a marked increase in total body water. This, in turn, can lead to marked tissue edema and increased risk of end-organ dysfunction. Modified ultrafiltration is a technique to remove excess free water, cytokines, and other small molecules, with an additional benefit of hemoconcentrating the patient's blood. In this technique, blood is routed from the aortic cannula and passed through a hemofilter and a heat exchanger. Hemoconcentrated blood is then returned to the venous reservoir, thereby decreasing the need for transfusion of RBCs.

CHAPTER 50 ■ NEUROHORMONAL CONTROL IN THE IMMUNE SYSTEM

KATHRYN A. FELMET

Acute stress causes activation of the sympathetic nervous system (SNS), which leads to epinephrine release; activation of the hypothalamic-pituitary-adrenal (HPA) axis, which leads to cortisol release; and activation of endogenous opioids. Proinflammatory peptides such as vasopressin and prolactin are also released as a part of the stress response. To do so, the central nervous system (CNS) monitors immune function with high acuity, being sensitive to low levels of inflammatory cytokines and to very early mediators of inflammation. Immune-derived cytokines that circulate in the bloodstream and afferent sensory pathways that are carried via peripheral nerves influence CNS signal output and are capable of activating the central stress response (**Fig. 50.1**). Adrenal replacement therapy has gained wide acceptance for its effects on response to circulating catecholamines. Corticosteroids are known to have immunosuppressive affects; however, it is unclear whether the small doses used for adrenal replacement will increase patients' susceptibility to nosocomial infection. Recovery from severe sepsis requires a balance between control of inflammation and activation of the specific or adaptive immune response.

The hypercatabolic state seen in critically ill patients has been attributed in part to growth hormone dysfunction. Trauma, sepsis, and surgery are thought to induce a state of growth-hormone resistance. The hyperglycemic, catabolic state induced by growth-hormone depletion and resistance is compounded by the normal stress response, the effects of immune-derived cytokines, and inadequate calorie delivery in the ICU. Unfortunately, use of exogenous growth hormone in critically ill patients is associated with increased mortality. At physiologic levels, growth hormone is immunostimulatory, but it has immunosuppressive effects at supraphysiologic levels in vitro. Vasopressin has been proposed as a replacement or adjunct to epinephrine in the resuscitation of cardiac arrest and catecholamine-unresponsive shock. Adults with septic shock have low levels of circulating vasopressin, and some evidence suggests that restoring high normal levels of vasopressin may be beneficial in

vasodilatory shock. Children appear to have normal-to-high vasopressin levels.

PATHWAYS OF COMMUNICATION

Signals can travel between the brain and immune system on peripheral nerves or in the form of circulating chemical signals such as hormones or cytokines. Direct neural control of immune function can be extremely rapid, discrete in location, and brief in duration. Humoral control occurs when molecules diffuse to and from the site of action; thus, these signals are slower in onset and termination.

The importance of neural pathways in neuroendocrine-immune (NEI) communication is highlighted by the fact that the vagus nerve senses and regulates inflammation with simple and rapid feedback loops. Vagal efferent fibers, distributed throughout the reticuloendothelial system, modulate the immune response to endotoxin through cholinergic signaling. Endotoxin (lipopolysaccharide) induces macrophages to release cytokines that promote local inflammation and potentiate activation of the specific immune response. Acetylcholine decreases expression of endotoxin-inducible proinflammatory cytokines (IL-1β, IL-6, and IL-18) but does not alter release of the anti-inflammatory cytokine IL-10 (**Table 50.1**). Acetylcholine-dependent downregulation of inflammation is reproduced by stimulation of the vagus nerve.

Bone marrow, thymus, spleen, lymph nodes, and gut-associated lymphoid tissue receive adrenergic, dopaminergic, and peptidergic input. These fibers play a role in controlling blood flow to these organs and thus may regulate lymphocyte traffic.

The main targets of noradrenergic innervation are T cells, macrophages, and mast cells. T cells and other immune cells have β-adrenergic receptors as well as specific receptors for dopamine and a variety of neuropeptides (acetylcholine, substance P, neuropeptide Y, somatostatin, and prolactin). In general, catecholamines are believed to favor Th-2

Efferent Signals

Afferent Signals

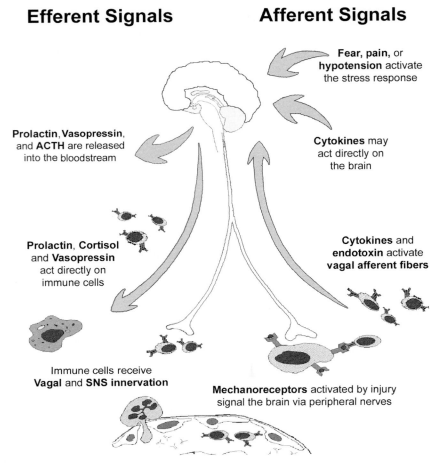

FIGURE 50.1. Bidirectional NEI communication. Stimulation of the acute stress response generates immunosuppressive signals (activation of the hypothalamic-pituitary-adrenal axis, the sympathetic nervous system, and endogenous opioids) and immune-supportive signals (release of proinflammatory peptides such as vasopressin and prolactin). A threat to the homeostatic milieu, in the form of trauma or infection, activates the immune system. Activated immune cells produce cytokines (e.g., TNF-α, IL-1, IL-6), which signal the CNS by stimulating peripheral fibers of the vagus nerve or by circulating directly to the brain. Vagal nerve activity delivers anti-inflammatory signals in response to immune activation. ACTH, adrenocorticotropic hormone; NEI, neuroendocrine immune; SNS, sympathetic nervous system.

cytokines and inhibit cellular immunity by suppressing Th-1 cytokine production. It is interesting to note that in the NEI system, the sympathetic and parasympathetic nervous systems may act synergistically rather than in opposition.

Exogenous opioids and endogenous endorphins have immunosuppressive effects. Opioids induce immune suppression at analgesic doses by binding to classic, naloxone-sensitive opioid receptors in the brain. In addition, immune cells have both classic and nonclassic opioid receptors, but it is unclear to what extent morphine interacts directly with these cells to cause immune suppression in vivo. Acutely, centrally acting morphine activates the SNS, and most of the observed immunosuppressive effects of

morphine may occur via this pathway. Morphine also activates the HPA axis, which may lead to cortisol-mediated immune suppression, particularly during chronic administration. Opioids specific for the χ- or ∂-receptors may induce less immune suppression; therefore, methadone and fentanyl may be slightly less immunosuppressive than morphine. Studies of receptor affinity predict that buprenorphine, hydromorphone, oxycodone, oxymorphone, and tramadol would be the least immunosuppressive. Opioids given locally, as in epidural analgesia, avoid the immunosuppressive complications of systemic administration. Somatostatin analogs (Octreotide) are used in the treatment of gastrointestinal hemorrhage. In addition to decreasing splanchnic blood flow,

TABLE 50.1

PROINFLAMMATORY AND ANTI-INFLAMMATORY CYTOKINES

Produced by		Actions on immune cells	Relevance in critical illness
Proinflammatory cytokines			
TNF-α	APCs, NK cells, T-cells	Local inflammation, endothelial activation	An early mediator of inflammation and shock
IL-1β	APCs, epithelial cells	T-cell activation, macrophage activation	Causes fever and acute-phase protein production
IL-12	B cells, macrophages	Activates NK cells, induces CD4 T-cell differentiation into Th-1-like cells	Suppresses Th-2
IFNγ	Th-1 cells, NK cells	Potent macrophage activation, suppresses Th-2 responses	Low levels associated with increased risk of infection
GM-CSF	Macrophages, T cells	Stimulates growth and differentiation of granulocytes and monocytes	Increases HLA-DR expression, may be clinically useful as an immune stimulant
Anti-inflammatory cytokines			
IL-4	Th-2 cells, mast cells	B-cell activation, suppresses Th-1 cells, IGE switch	Suppresses Th-1 response
IL-10	Th-2 cells, APCs	Potent suppressor of macrophage functions	Suppresses Th-1 response
Other important cytokines			
IL-2	T cells	T-cell proliferation, supports Th-1 cells	Most important proliferative factor for T-cells
IL-6	T cells, macrophages, endothelial calls	T- and B-cell growth and differentiation	Causes fever, and acute-phase protein production levels are related to severity of systemic inflammation
IL-8	Monocytes, endothelial cells	Chemotactic for neutrophils	Levels are related to severity of systemic inflammation
GCSF	Fibroblasts and monocytes	Stimulates neutrophil growth and differentiation	Exogenous GCSF safely increases neutrophil counts but does not alter mortality

APCs, antigen-presenting cells; NK, natural killer; GM-CSF, granulocyte-macrophage colony-stimulating factor; HLA-DR, human leukocyte antigen-DR; GCSF, granulocyte colony-stimulating factor

somatostatin inhibits the release of insulin and decreases secretion and absorption in the gastrointestinal tract. Somatostatin receptors are expressed on peripheral T and B lymphocytes, on activated monocytes, and in hematopoietic precursors. In the bone marrow, somatostatin inhibits proliferation, particularly in response to granulocyte colony-stimulating factor. Somatostatin strongly inhibits interferon gamma production by T cells, thereby decreasing macrophage activation and antigen presentation. Somatostatin also decreases prolactin release by the pituitary, and some of its immunosuppressive effects may occur via this mechanism.

Substance P, a neuropeptide present in afferent nerves in the dorsal horn of the spinal column, was originally discovered to be a mediator of pain sensation. Substance P is powerfully proinflammatory via tumor necrosis factor-α (TNF-α) and IL-12 and plays a role in chronic inflammation. Substance P, gene-related peptide, neuropeptide Y, calcitonin, vasoactive intestinal peptide, pro-opiomelanocortin-related peptides, and β-endorphins are among a growing group of neuropeptides that have been shown to have immunoregulatory function.

Humoral Efferent Pathways

Activation of the HPA axis begins with release of corticotrophin-releasing hormone (CRH) from hypothalamus in response to cortical signals generated by fear, pain, or hypotension or in response to immune-derived signal molecules, especially IL-1β, TNF-α, and IL-6. CRH leads to adrenocorticotropic hormone (ACTH) release by the pituitary, which, in turn, causes cortisol release by the adrenal gland. Cortisol inhibits growth and generally increases catabolism while it enhances protein synthesis in the liver, where acute-phase reactants are generated. Cortisol potentiates the vasoconstrictive action of catecholamines and regulates the distribution of total body water. In the immune system, corticosteroids reduce circulating numbers of lymphocytes, monocytes, and eosinophils by stimulating apoptosis. Corticosteroids stabilize lysosomal membranes, decrease capillary permeability, impair demargination of WBCs and phagocytosis, and decrease release of IL-1, preventing fever. Steroids also support a Th-2 (humoral immunity) over a Th-1 (cellular immunity) phenotype.

Prolactin and vasopressin are the immunostimulatory hormones associated with the CNS response to stress. Release of these hormones occurs simultaneously with HPA-axis activation and SNS activation and thus represents an important counterbalance to the immunosuppressive effects of the stress response. Prolactin, though best known for its role in promoting milk secretion, directly opposes many of the actions of corticosteroids. Prolactin release is stimulated by suckling, IL-1β, IL-2, IL-6, oxytocin, serotonin, and thyrotropin-releasing hormone. In the normal state, prolactin secretion is tonically inhibited by hypothalamic dopamine. The immunosuppressive drug cyclosporine exerts its effect through the prolactin receptor on lymphocytes. Vasopressin is released in response to hypotension and increased serum osmolarity. Peripheral vasopressin favors Th-1 responses. Vasopressin can also potentiate the release of prolactin. Acting centrally, vasopressin causes release of CRH, but it also has effects on the immune system independent of its effect in stimulating the HPA axis.

Afferent Signals: Alerting the Central Nervous System to a Microbial Threat

The immunoregulatory actions of pituitary hormones, vagal nerve activity, and SNS activation occurs in response to information about the current state of immune function that is generated by classic sensory organs and the immune system and synthesized by the brain. The brain is alerted to a microbial threat via both humoral and neural pathways. Cytokines, particularly TNF–α and IL-1β, can act directly, reaching the brain via the bloodstream, or indirectly by stimulating peripheral afferent nerves.

Immune Activation of Afferent Peripheral Nerves

Afferent nerves provide a surveillance system to allow the CNS to monitor immune function. The neural pathway of immune-to-brain communication centers on the vagus nerve. TNF-α and IL-1 released from dendritic cells and macrophages have been shown to stimulate vagal afferents, even at concentrations too low to reach the brain via the bloodstream. Afferent pathways also collect information about infection and injury independent of immune cells. Vagal afferents can be directly stimulated by endotoxin, a bacterial product that leads to TNF-α release. Receptors sensitive to mechanical, thermal, and osmolar changes may also activate vagal sensory fibers, suggesting that the brain can anticipate injury and the resulting inflammation. Inflammation sensed by the vagus nerve increases inflammation-suppressing signals traveling back down the vagus and activates humoral responses via the HPA axis. Humoral pathways of immune-to-brain communications revolve around circulating cytokines.

Peripheral Responses: The Effects of Neuroimmunomodulation

The brain receives information about potential and ongoing immune responses and sends out signals that modulate these responses. The most obvious result of CNS integration of signals from the immune system is a combination of physiologic changes and behaviors associated with recovery, collectively known as *the sickness response*. In response to illness signaled mainly by TNF-α and IL-1, the CNS initiates physiologic changes, including fever, increased WBC count, production of acute phase proteins in the liver, and increased slow-wave sleep, as well as behavioral changes, including decreased feeding and drinking and reductions in activity and social interaction. Alterations in pain sensation are also a part of the sickness response. In the acute phase, the stress response rapidly induces analgesia, presumably by a neural route. Later, inflammatory cytokines induce hyperalgesia, signaling the individual to care for a wound.

Inflammation and Phagocytosis

The *nonspecific immune response*, comprised mainly of inflammation and phagocytosis, is even more evolutionarily conserved than the sickness response. Nonspecific immunity is initiated rapidly by microbial invasion or trauma and serves to limit tissue damage and infection to the wound or site of entry. Inflammation and phagocytic cells comprise the first line of defense and recognition. The inflammatory response leads to vasodilation, increased capillary permeability, and an influx of phagocytes, including blood monocytes, neutrophils, and tissue macrophages. Local coagulation limits hematogenous spread of infection. Phagocytic cells recruited by inflammation produce proinflammatory cytokines.

Corticosteroids, vagal nerve stimulation, SNS activation, and circulating catecholamines are antiinflammatory. Inflammation is potentiated by prolactin and vasopressin. Opioids and corticosteroids suppress phagocytosis. Recovery from sepsis depends on a balance between pro- and anti-inflammatory signals. Inflammation recruits phagocytic cells, some of which are responsible for the initiation of the specific immune response. Antigen-presenting cells such as macrophages and dendritic cells engulf foreign matter and bacteria, break them down into large molecules, and present these molecules as antigens to T lymphocytes. Antigen presentation is the crucial step in initiating adaptive immunity.

Humoral versus Cellular Immunity

An antigen-specific immune response begins when a T lymphocyte recognizes its specific antigen on the surface of an antigen-presenting cell. The T cell begins to activate and proliferate. T-cell proliferation is suppressed by catecholamines and supported by prolactin. Most viral infections stimulate replication of cytotoxic T cells. Helper T cells (Th cells) make cytokines that support other cells. The two lines of

helper cells, Th-1 and Th-2, are mutually inhibitory and direct different types of immune responses. Th-1 cells are stimulated by pathogens that accumulate inside the vesicles of macrophages and dendritic cells. A Th-1 or cell-mediated immune response promotes the microbicidal properties of the macrophage and supports the production of immunoglobulin G (IgG), an opsonizing antibody that facilitates uptake of these pathogens. A Th-1 proinflammatory phenotype is associated with autoimmune disease.

Extracellular spaces are protected by the Th-2 or humoral immune response. In response to extracellular pathogens, Th-2 cells initiate the humoral immune response by activating naïve antigen-specific B cells to produce IgM antibodies. The cytokine profile associated with Th-2 humoral immune response is anti-inflammatory, with IL-4 and IL-10 predominating. The catecholamine and cortisol excess seen in the stress response favors Th-2 responses. Septic patients tend to have increased numbers of Th-2 cells relative to the normal Th-1/Th-2 balance and relative to nonseptic, critically ill controls.

Apoptosis and Lymphocyte Proliferation

A few days into an episode of sepsis, the catecholamine and cortisol excess of the acute phase suppresses the initial hyperinflammatory state, replacing

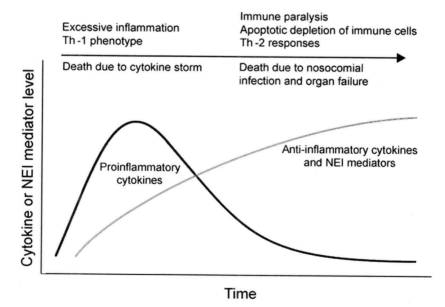

FIGURE 50.2. The acute and prolonged phases of critical illness and sepsis. Early death in sepsis can occur due to overwhelming inflammation with cytokine storm, which causes shock and tissue injury. Therapies directed at decreasing inflammation may be considered during this phase. Resuscitation medications used during this phase, including catecholamines and corticosteroids, are anti-inflammatory. During the prolonged phase of critical illness, patients developed immune paralysis with depletion of lymphoid elements due to apoptosis and decreased antigen-presenting capacity. During this stage, patients are at high risk for secondary infection. Therapies that enhance immune function by activating antigen-presenting cells or by blocking lymphocyte apoptosis may be considered in the future.

it with a state of relative immune suppression. Ideally, immune cells are protected by a balance of the proapoptotic forces of adrenal steroids and the antiapoptotic effects of serum prolactin. Once the acute phase of critical illness has passed, the normal pattern of pituitary hormone release and the normal adrenal response to ACTH are disrupted. As a result, cortisol levels often remain elevated. The balance between pro-apoptotic and anti-apoptotic forces may be further upset in the ICU when patients are treated with prolactin-suppressing dopamine and steroids.

IMMUNE COMPETENCE AND FAILURE IN THE PICU

The acute phase of critical illness is characterized by supranormal release of neuroendocrine mediators from the hypothalamus and pituitary. This secretory activity ensures that short-term goals of blood pressure support and mobilization of fuel substrates are met at the expense of neglecting homeostatic mechanisms, immune function, and cell growth and repair. When a patient's own fight-or-flight response is insufficient to maintain perfusion, shock ensues. During this phase, the anti-inflammatory effect of steroids and catecholamines may be beneficial in many patients. Critically ill patients need a balance between immunosuppressive and immune-supportive signals, between a short-term improvement in blood pressure and long-term cell growth and repair (**Fig. 50.2**, **Fig. 50.3**). In the ICU, an appropriate hormone level cannot be judged with reference to norms established in healthy people.

Catecholamines exert an immunosuppressive effect. Circulating catecholamines have been shown to modulate lymphocyte traffic and circulation in vivo. Within 30 mins of exogenous administration of

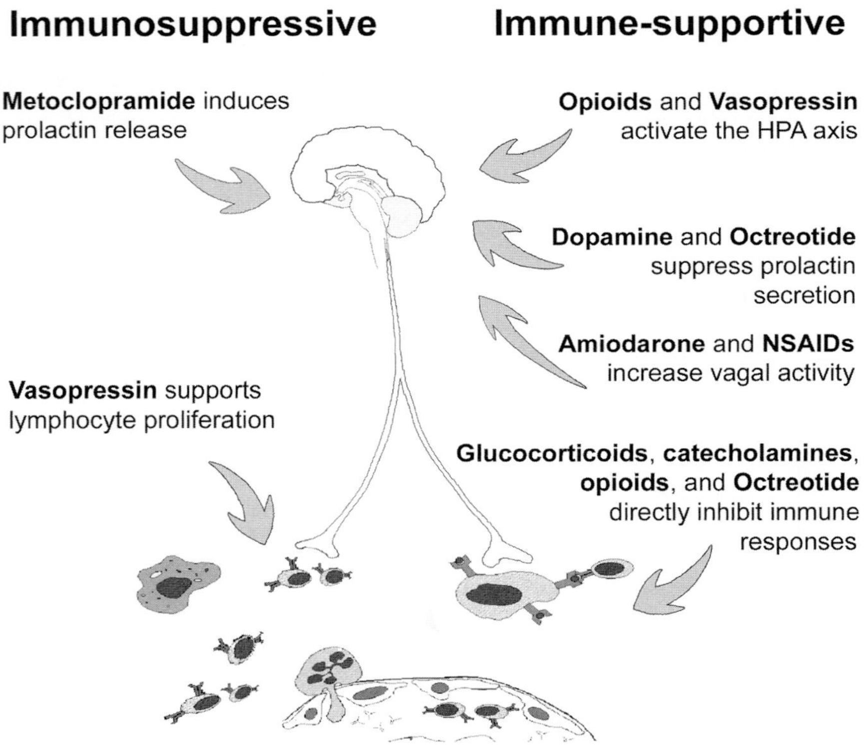

Immunosuppressive

Metoclopramide induces prolactin release

Vasopressin supports lymphocyte proliferation

Immune-supportive

Opioids and **Vasopressin** activate the HPA axis

Dopamine and **Octreotide** suppress prolactin secretion

Amiodarone and **NSAIDs** increase vagal activity

Glucocorticoids, catecholamines, opioids, and **Octreotide** directly inhibit immune responses

FIGURE 50.3. Drugs used in the ICU influence immune function. These commonly used ICU drugs can alter neuroendocrine secretory activity and can bind to immune cells directly. Circulating catecholamines and corticosteroids promote Th-2 type immune responses and are broadly anti-inflammatory and immunosuppressive. Opioids and vasopressin activate the HPA axis, leading to cortisol release. Dopamine and octreotide block the release of the immune-supportive hormone prolactin. Opioids and Octreotide also have direct effects on immune cells, decreasing lymphocyte proliferation and function of antigen-presenting cells. Amiodarone and nonsteroidal anti-inflammatory drugs (NSAIDs) may increase vagal activity, thus increasing anti-inflammatory signals. The only immune-supportive therapies commonly used in the ICU are vasopressin, which supports lymphocyte function, and metoclopramide, which induces prolactin release. HPA, hypothalamic-pituitary-adrenal.

catecholamines, lymphocytes, and NK cells are mobilized, followed by an increase in circulating granulocytes and relative lymphopenia at 3–4 hrs. Prolonged infusion of β agonists may have the opposite effect, reducing numbers and activity of NK cells. In vitro, catecholamines inhibit Th-1 and favor Th-2 responses. Dopamine at doses as low as 1 μg/kg/min has a powerful inhibitory effect on release of the proinflammatory mediator, prolactin and has been shown to decrease lymphocyte proliferation. Dopamine inhibits pulsatile release of growth hormone and thus contributes to the catabolic state observed in critical illness.

Nonsteroidal anti-inflammatory drugs and the antiarrhythmic amiodarone are known to increase vagal activity. Patients with vagal nerve stimulators and patients with transplanted organs have disruptions in their cholinergic anti-inflammatory pathways. Vagus nerve stimulation has been proposed as a mechanism to treat inflammation in inflammatory bowel disease.

Without the effect of the vagus nerve to inhibit TNF-α production in response to endotoxin, transplant patients may have intermittent elevations in inflammatory cytokines. Elevations in TNF-α, also known as *cachexin*, may impact the ability of these patients to gain weight. When the absolute lymphocyte count is persistently <1000, indicators of T- and B-cell function may be measured. T-cell subsets will help identify patients with low CD4 counts who may benefit from early prophylaxis against fungus or *Pneumocystis carinii* pneumonia. Patients with impaired B-cell function, as evidenced by low immunoglobulin levels, may benefit from IV immunoglobulin.

CHAPTER 51 ■ THE IMMUNE SYSTEM

MEREDITH L. ALLEN • NIGEL J. KLEIN • MARK J. PETERS

The *innate* arm of the immune system is present at birth. The recognition systems employed are targeted against highly conserved structures common to large groups of microorganisms, which are achieved through interactions between host-derived pattern recognition receptors and pathogen-associated molecular patterns on microbes. The *adaptive* immune system develops after birth and provides highly specific recognition of both host and foreign antigens, allowing for effective handling of a multitude of microorganisms and the generation of targeted immunologic memory (**Table 51.1**). In addition to severe combined immunodeficiency syndrome, **Table 51.2** outlines congenital immunodeficiency states. A number of defects in the immune system highlight the *balance* between risk of infection and severity of the host response. Four immune networks have been chosen to illustrate this point: complement system, mannose-binding lectin (MBL), endotoxin recognitions, and cytokines (**Fig. 51.1**).

COMPLEMENT SYSTEM

Working in concert with the adaptive immune system, activation of the 3 complement pathways leads to the construction of membrane attack complexes that cause direct lysis and death of the

TABLE 51.1

CHARACTERISTICS OF THE INNATE VERSUS ADAPTIVE IMMUNE SYSTEM

Innate immune system	Adaptive immune system
Older phylogenetically—present in all multicellular organisms	Evolved later—present only in vertebrates
Present from birth	Learned response
Does not require previous exposure	Slower but more definitive
No memory	Memory specific to antigen
Cellular components—phagocytic system (monocytes, macrophages, dendritic cells) and natural killer cells	Cellular components—T and B lymphocytes
Soluble components—cytokines, complement, and acute-phase proteins	Soluble components—immunoglobulins

TABLE 51.2

CONGENITAL IMMUNODEFICIENCY SYNDROMES

Disorder	Chromosome	Gene	Function/defect	Diagnostic test
X-linked chronic granulomatous disease	Xp21	gp91phox	Component of phagocyte NADPH	Nitroblue tetrazolium test gp91phox by oxidase–phagocytic respiratory burst immunoblotting; mutation analysis
X-linked agammaglobulinemia	Xq22	Bruton's tyrosine kinase (Btk)	Intracellular signalling pathways essential for pre-B-cell maturation	Btk by immunoblotting or FACS analysis and mutation analysis
X-linked hyper-IgM syndrome (CD40 ligand deficiency)	Xq26 (CD154)	CD40 ligand	Isotype switching, T-cell function	CD154 expression on activated T cells by FACS analysis mutation analysis
Wiskott-Aldrich syndrome	Xp11	WASP	Cytoskeletal architecture formation, immune-cell motility and trafficking	WASP expression by immunoblotting; mutation analysis
X-linked lymphoproliferative syndrome	Xq25	SAP	Regulation of T-cell responses to EBV and other viral infections	Mutation analysis SAP expression—under development
Properdin deficiency	Xp21	Properdin	Terminal complement component	Properdin levels
Leukocyte-adhesion deficiency type 1	21q22	CD11/CD18	Defective leucocyte adhesion and migration	CD11/CD18 expression by FACS analysis; mutation analysis
Chronic granulomatous disease (recessive)	7q11 1q25 16p24	p47phox p67phox p22phox	Defective respiratory burst and phagocytic intracellular killing	p47phox, p67phox, p22phox, expression by immunoblotting; mutation analysis
Chédiak-Higashi syndrome	1q42	LYST	Abnormalities in microtubule-mediated lysosomal protein trafficking	Giant inclusions in granulocytes; mutation analysis
MHC class II deficiency	16p13 19p12	CIITA (MHC2TA) RFXANK	Defective transcriptional regulation of MHC II molecule expression	HLA-DR expression; mutation analysis
RFX5			13q13	RFX4P
Autoimmune lymphoproliferative syndrome	10q24	APT1 (Fas)	Defective apoptosis of lymphocytes	Fas expression; apoptosis assays; mutation analysis
Ataxia telangiectasia	11q22	ATM	Cell-cycle control and DNA damage responses	DNA radiation sensitivity; mutation analysis
Inherited mycobacterial susceptibility	6q23 5q31 19p13	Interferon g-receptor IL-12 p40 IL-12 receptor b1	Defective IFN-g production and signalling function	Interferon-g receptor expression; IL-12 expression; IL-12 receptor expression; mutation analysis

EBV, Epstein–Barr virus; WASP, Wiskott-Aldrich syndrome protein; MHC, major histocompatibility complex

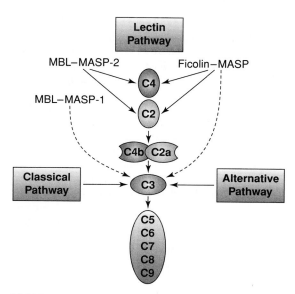

FIGURE 51.1. The complement and lectin pathways. The lectin pathway of complement is activated by MBL and ficolins. On binding to appropriate targets, MBL–MASP-2 complexes cleave C4 and C2 to form C3 convertase (C4bC2a). MBL–MASP-1 complexes may activate C3 directly. Ficolins also work in combination with the MASPs. The classic and alternative pathways also generate C3 convertase enzymes, which cleave C3. The lytic pathway (C5–C9) is common to all 3 routes of C3 cleavage. MBL, mannose-binding lectin; MASP, MBL-associated serine proteases; MASP-1, MBL-associated serine protease-1; MASP-2, MBL-associated serine protease-2. Adapted from Dommett RM, Klein N, Turner MW. Mannose-binding lectin in innate immunity: Past, present and future. *Tissue Antigens* 2006;68(3):193–209.

microorganisms. During activation, opsonic and chemotactic factors are also generated that facilitate the removal of live and dead organisms from the circulation and from tissues. Patients with terminal complement component deficiencies are particularly susceptible to *Neisserial* sp., including *N. meningitidis*; however, paradoxically, these episodes of infection are generally less severe.

Mannose-binding Lectin

MBL is a liver-derived plasma protein that recognizes repeating sugar arrays on the surface of many bacteria, fungi, viruses, and parasites. MBL binds to microbes, such as *Staphylococcus aureus* and *N. meningitides*, and activates complement in an antibody- and C1–complex-independent fashion. In contrast to most complement defects, MBL deficiency is common in the population. Children with reduced levels of MBL are at an increased risk for many minor infections of childhood and for more frequent and

severe infections in the presence of coexisting immunodeficiencies such as caused by chemotherapy for the treatment of cancer. Children who are admitted to intensive care following infection, trauma, or surgery have a greatly increased risk of developing the systemic inflammatory response syndrome (SIRS) in the first 48 hrs of PICU admission if they have MBL deficiency. MBL deficiency may be beneficial in some circumstances. In both animals and humans, MBL deficiency has been shown to reduce the insult following ischemia-reperfusion injury.

Endotoxin Recognition

Perhaps the ultimate "danger-signal" on an invading pathogen is endotoxin or lipopolysaccharide (LPS). Nonspecific protection against LPS can be provided by antibodies directed against the core of endotoxin (EndoCAb). Recognition of LPS is complex and involves multiple receptors and mediators. Functional mutations and polymorphisms of proteins involved in LPS recognition and signaling, including TLR4, CD14, MyD88, IRAK4, and NFκB, have been identified.

Cytokines

IL-10 is an anti-inflammatory cytokine, the levels of which are critical in the modulation of the proinflammatory/anti-inflammatory balance. Functional polymorphisms exist in a number of other genes, the products of which are thought to be important in sepsis, including cytokines, such as tumor necrosis factor (TNF), IL-1, and IL-6, and proteins involved in hemostasis and thrombosis, such as plasminogen activator inhibitor 1 and angiotensin converting enzyme, which has multiple functions, including inflammatory modulation.

THE BALANCE BETWEEN PROINFLAMMATION AND ANTI-INFLAMMATION

Systemic Inflammatory Response Syndrome

SIRS can be induced by any major insult that does not result in immediate death. It is typically defined in terms of alterations in simple clinical or laboratory parameters that arise from this insult. In brief, SIRS is defined by 2 or more of the following: (a) hyperthermia or hypothermia, (b) tachycardia or bradycardia,

(c) tachypnea, or (d) a pathologic alteration in white cell count. When SIRS is the result of suspected or proven infection, it is termed *sepsis*; however, noninfectious causes, such as burns, trauma, surgery, and pancreatitis, can also cause this clinical picture. Mild-to-moderate SIRS is most likely beneficial, for example, both a raised temperature and production of the cytokine TNF facilitate killing of microorganisms. However, a similar response may cause harm, either by being too severe or by spilling over into body compartments where they are not required. Examples include excessive body temperatures raising tissue oxygen demand beyond the available supply and causing rhabdomyolysis, while pathways that involve TNF or IL-6 may contribute to unwelcome myocardial depression.

Excessive Proinflammation?

Overwhelming sepsis such as that seen during the acute presentation of meningococcal septicemia is a powerful reminder to the clinician of the effects of acute immune activation in part; sepsis-induced multiorgan failure results from an excessive unchecked proinflammatory response typified by mediators such as TNF and IL-1. Additional contributions include the proinflammatory T-helper-1 (T_H-1) pattern of immunity associated with cytotoxic T-cell and macrophage activation and suppression of humoral responses. In 1996, Roger Bone suggested that the proinflammatory response does not occur in isolation and that a compensatory anti-inflammatory response syndrome (CARS) is always initiated at the same time. This "arm" of the immune response is typified by such mediators as IL-10 and shares many characteristics with the T-helper-2 (T_H-2) response, involving the suppression of macrophage activation and promotion of antibody production. This important insight raised the concept that wide variability might exist between patients in the nature of the immune response: predominant "proinflammatory" SIRS/T_H-1 in some, and predominant anti-inflammatory response CARS/T_H-2 in others. These responses may lead to multiorgan failure and death via different routes In most cases, the patient's compensatory anti-inflammatory response is proportional to the proinflammatory response and homeostasis is rapidly restored.

Excessive Anti-inflammation: "Acquired Immunoparalysis"

An excessive compensatory anti-inflammatory response, or CARS, to the primary insult leaves patients

in a state of *acquired immunoparalysis*, in which they are unable to produce an adequate immune response to a new threat, such as a nosocomial infection. In part, this inadequacy is attributable to apoptosis of dendritic cells and lymphocytes in response to the CARS/T_H-2 mediators. Several laboratory tests are being used to classify and monitor the immune status of critically ill patients. Most studies use 2 assays to define *acquired immunoparalysis*. One measures the capacity of host monocytes to produce TNF in response to stimulation with endotoxin, while the other measures surface expression of the major histocompatibility complex class II molecule on circulating monocytes (usually the human leukocyte antigen HLA-DR) by flow cytometry. Reduced monocyte surface expression of HLA-DR occurs in critically ill patients over the first few days of ICU admission following surgery, trauma, or sepsis.

Resolution Versus Persistence of the Inflammatory Response

The balance between processes that act to resolve acute inflammation and those that cause it to persist exists. SIRS/T_H-1 responses tend to prolong inflammation and CARS/T_H-2 responses tend to resolve it. A key element in resolving the immune response is effective clearance of microorganisms. This requires the presence of activated polymorphonuclear cells (PMNs, or neutrophils) and other phagocytic cells in the appropriate tissue at the appropriate time, with intact cellular processes for killing and disposing of the bacteria. These cells are powerful agents for resolution of the inflammatory response because bacteria that have been recognized, ingested, and killed by PMNs no longer present an inflammatory stimulus.

Defects in the Removal of Microorganisms

Leukocytes

Chemotherapy-induced neutropenia clearly demonstrates the importance of PMNs. The mechanisms by which activated leukocytes are recruited into inflamed tissues are illustrated in **Fig. 51.2**. This multistep process is modulated by adhesion molecules present on whole cells such as neutrophils, platelets, and endothelial cells. Leukocytes can form complexes with themselves or with other cell types, including platelets and cell fragments, or "microparticles." These complexes then present a wider array

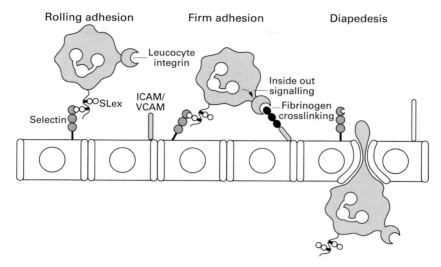

FIGURE 51.2. Mechanism of leukocyte-endothelial interaction. Rolling adhesion mediated by sialyl Lewis x and other glycosylated structures and selectins. Firm adhesion and diapedesis is mediated by integrins and molecules of the immunoglobulin superfamily (chemokines). ICAM, intercellular cell adhesion molecule; VCAM, vascular cell adhesion molecule.

of adhesion molecules than either cell alone. In sepsis, these circulating platelet-neutrophil complexes are reduced, probably due to selective binding to the endothelium and/or migration into the tissues. The potential for these primed platelet-neutrophil complexes to cause tissue injury and initiate thrombus formation is considerable and may explain why the combination of low platelets and neutrophils is a good predictor of poor outcome in meningococcal sepsis.

Chronic granulomatous disease is a rare condition in which patients' leukocytes lack the capacity to generate bacterial killing. These patients are deficient in the enzyme nicotinamide adenine dinucleotide phosphate oxidase, which is required for production of the toxic conditions that effect bacterial killing, and suffer stubborn infections similar to those seen in patients with leukocyte adhesion deficiency or neutropenia. Granuloma formation probably represents a failure to adequately remove microbial products. These lesions paradoxically may necessitate the use of steroids to reduce the ensuing inappropriate inflammatory response.

Effective Removal of Prokaryote and Eukaryote Material for Resolution of Infection and the Inflammatory Response

All of the steps discussed above are required for the effective killing of invading microorganisms and the inflammatory response that they generate. However, for the inflammatory response to resolve, an effective removal of cellular (both host and microbial) debris must also occur without further release of proinflammatory elements, such as endotoxin.

Importantly, "spent" PMNs undergo apoptosis (programmed cell death) after they have performed these useful functions—and, therefore, die "silently" without leaving inflammatory cellular debris. Typically, these apoptotic PMNs are, in turn, phagocytosed by tissue macrophages.

Hemophagocytic Lymphohistiocytosis

Hemophagocytic lymphohistiocytosis (HLH) describes a mix of congenital and acquired conditions in which high fever, lymphadenopathy, hepatosplenomegaly, pancytopenia, liver dysfunction, and CNS dysfunction are often prominent (**Table 51.3**). Typically, these findings are in the context of an acute infection. Abnormally large and activated cells of myeloid origin (hemophagocytes) are typically found on examination of bone marrow.

HLH represents a sustained, systemic inflammatory response following a variety of primary insults (viral, bacterial, or fungal) similar to the way in which SIRS represents a nonspecific final pathway after infection, trauma, burns, and pancreatitis.

Several cellular mechanisms of congenital predispositions to HLH have been identified. Mutations in the genes for perforin are especially important, occurring in 20–40% of HLH cases. Perforin is a protein found in granules of cytotoxic effector cells including natural killer cells and activated lymphocytes. Perforin polymerizes in the membranes of target cells to allow entry of the variety of cytotoxic enzymes that cause target-cell death via apoptosis. Apoptosis allows efficient packaging of toxic

TABLE 51.3

CRITERIA FOR THE DIAGNOSIS OF HEMOPHAGOCYTIC LYMPHOHISTIOCYTOSIS

The diagnosis of HLH is established by fulfilling either or both of the following criteria:

1. A molecular diagnosis consistent with HLH (e.g., PRF mutations, SAP mutations, etc.)

AND/OR

2. Having ≥5 of the following:
   a. Fever
   b. Splenomegaly
   c. Cytopenia (affecting 2 cell lineages, hemoglobin <9 g/dL (or 10 g/dL for infants <4 wks of age), platelets <100,000/mcL, neutrophils <1000 mcL
   d. Hypertriglyceremia (>272 mg/dL) and/or hypofibrinogenemia (<150 mg/dL)
   e. Hemophagocytosis in the bone marrow, spleen, or lymph nodes without evidence of malignancy
   f. Low or absent NK cell cytotoxicity
   g. Hyperferritinemia (>500 ng/mL)
   h. Elevated soluble CD25 (IL-2Ra chain >2400 U/mL)

HLH, hemophagocytic lymphohistiocytosis

material (e.g., infected cells) for phagocytosis while causing the minimum amount of inflammatory stimulus. Lack of perforin prevents access of these enzymes, and the inflammatory stimulus of the infected target cell persists.

Therapies That Can Modulate the Balance between Effective Microbial Killing and the Resultant Inflammatory Response

A proportion of patients who are admitted to the PICU will subsequently be found to have a major defect in their immune system. The vast majority of patients, however, who are either admitted with an infection or who develop an infectious complication while in the PICU will not have been noted to be at an increased risk of either infection or an excessive inflammatory response prior to admission. Limited data indicate that in *Staphylococcal* and *Streptococcal* toxic shock syndromes, the use of IV immunoglobulin and clindamycin could be beneficial. Both agents act to neutralize the effect of exotoxins—IV immunoglobulin by binding to the exotoxins and clindamycin by inhibiting the production of exotoxins.

Possible Therapies for Acute Severe Proinflammation

Glucocorticoids

Glucocorticoids bind to cytoplasmic glucocorticoid receptors, and, via NFκB, act at a transcription level to modulate proinflammatory and anti-inflammatory cytokine levels. Glucocorticoids inhibit production of the proinflammatory cytokines TNF-α, IL-1α, IL-1β, IFN-γ, IL-6, IL-8, IL-12, and granulocyte-macrophage colony-stimulating factor (GM-CSF). In addition, glucocorticoids increase transcription of IL-1ra and IL-10, inhibit neutrophil activation, and suppress the synthesis of phospholipase A2, cyclooxygenase, and inducible nitric oxide synthase.

Large doses of synthetic glucocorticoids (methylprednisolone or dexamethasone) have been investigated in unselected severe sepsis in adults. While some favorable cardiovascular changes were observed, an overall trend toward decreased survival, with high rates of nosocomial infection, was also observed. This effect may be secondary to a steroid-induced state of temporary hyperglycemia. Evidence suggests that uncontrolled hyperglycemia in critically ill patients is associated with a higher mortality, largely through sepsis-driven multiorgan dysfunction. The practice of high-dose steroids in sepsis has largely ceased.

The option of high-dose steroids is being reconsidered in pediatric catecholamine-resistant septic shock, in which the risk of early cardiovascular collapse is greater than that of secondary infection. Observational studies suggest that relative adrenal insufficiency may be common and intensive cardiovascular support alone may be insufficient without replacing adequate doses of hydrocortisone.

At physiologic levels, cortisol supports the vascular adrenergic receptor function and inhibits cytokine-induced nitric oxide synthase, thus potentiating vasoconstriction and myocardial contractility. The use of glucocorticoids has been reconsidered with evidence that adrenal failure or *relative adrenal insufficiency* is common in critically ill adults and children. Physiologic doses of corticosteroids over 5–7 days improve systemic hemodynamics, shorten the duration of shock, and improve survival rates. A similar protocol has also been shown to be beneficial in low cardiac output states. It is not clear whether these doses of steroids have significant anti-inflammatory effects.

Activated Protein C

Recombinant human activated protein C (rhAPC) possesses anticoagulant, profibrinolytic, and anti-inflammatory properties. It is still the only agent to have a positive outcome in a phase III sepsis trial. The Recombinant Human Activated Protein C Worldwide Evaluation in Severe Sepsis demonstrated that treatment with rhAPC was associated with a reduction in the risk of death. It is interesting to speculate that rhAPC may have been more successful than other agents because of its lack of specificity or multiple sites of activity. At present, rhAPC is approved for use only in adult patients with severe sepsis who have a high risk of mortality, as determined by an Acute Physiology and Chronic Health Evaluation II score of ≥25. However, a similar study in children with sepsis-induced cardiovascular and respiratory failure did not show any benefit of rhAPC above placebo for either mortality or time to resolve sepsis-induced organ failures.

Aggressive De-intensification of Patients

Acquired immunoparalysis will present a problem only if the patient's immune system is challenged beyond the residual capacity to respond. Simple best practice of critical care may reduce this risk dramatically and should not be forgotten during the quest for more innovative solutions. Priority should be given to removal of invasive monitoring lines, endotracheal tubes, and urinary catheters at the earliest possible time in the PICU stay to reduce the risk of transient bacteremias in these vulnerable patients.

Stimulating Factors

GM-CSF and granulocyte colony-stimulating factor are naturally occurring cytokines that stimulate the number and antimicrobial function of both neutrophils and monocytes. They have a clear clinical use in the treatment of neutropenia, where their use has been shown to reduce the number of documented infections but not infection-related mortality. Interest has extended from their use in accelerating myeloid cell recovery to take advantage of their immune-enhancing properties. Administration of GM-CSF appears to have minimal side effects, to restore monocyte HLA-DR expression and function, and to assist in reducing sepsis episodes but, to date, it has not been shown to affect mortality.

A possible role of immunonutrients (arginine, glutamine, eicosapentaenoic acid, omega-3 fatty acids) as immunomodulating agents has gained attention. Glutamine is an abundant free amino acid in humans, critical for the integrity and function of metabolically active tissues. Under normal conditions, glutamine is a nonessential amino acid. However, in critical illness, glutamine levels in the body decrease, and its endogenous supply cannot match the increased demand. Glutamine has immunomodulatory properties. Parenteral supplementation with glutamine in adults has been associated with preservation of monocyte HLA-DR expression, decreases in infectious complications, and shortened hospital stay. A mortality benefit has been suggested with enteral feeding with eicosapentaenoic acid, γ-linolenic acid, and antioxidants in adult septic shock cases.

Removal of Inhibitory Plasma Mediators

While IL-10 appears to be playing an important role in acquired immunoparalysis, it is not the only soluble factor that appears to be acting. Attempts to eliminate a wide range of different inhibitory factors (as well as possible proinflammatory mediators) have resulted in case reports of hemofiltration, apheresis, and plasmapheresis in critically ill patients. The ability of any of these therapies to change the level of circulating mediators depends on the method used. Conventional plasma exchange does not consistently affect plasma levels of IL-6, IL-6R, TNF-α, TNF-αR, or C-reactive protein. At present, this therapy remains experimental. By comparison, continuous hemofiltration has been shown to minimally reduce inflammatory mediators (complement activation, plasma thromboxane, and proinflammatory cytokines at high-volume filtration). Retrospective, single-centered studies suggest that the use of continuous renal hemofiltration in critically ill children improves outcome. The mechanism by which this may be acting is uncertain, and while it may be through an immunomodulating effect, it may also be acting to removal of free water, improve fluid balance, and correct acid-base status.

Possible Therapies for Failure of Resolution or Persistence of the Inflammatory Response

Treatments for HLH are well established and consist of high-dose steroid, etoposide, and cyclosporine.

No consensus exists as to the use of these drugs for hemophagocytosis that occurs as part of systemic inflammation in the ICU. It has been proposed that these drugs should be considered in acute inflammatory conditions that are persisting, especially following severe viral infections, such as severe acute respiratory syndrome or H5N1.

A number of agents for inhibiting apoptosis (caspase inhibitors, CD95 inhibitors, and protease inhibitors) are promising.

CHAPTER 52 ■ THE POLYMORPHONUCLEAR LEUKOCYTE IN CRITICAL ILLNESS

M. MICHELE MARISCALCO

Surface proteins may have multiple names, often provided by the group that initially identifies them. However, these proteins may also be formally identified as "human cell differentiation molecules" (HCDM) and given a unique CD (cluster of differentiation) number (www.hla.org).

NEUTROPHIL PHYSIOLOGY

Approximately 100 billion neutrophils leave the bone marrow each day in a healthy adult. The normal ratio of neutrophils to erythroid cells ranges from 2:1 to 3:1. The nucleus contracts from the large, ovoid shape of the promyelocyte to the "band" and, finally, to the 3–5-lobed nucleus of the mature neutrophil. After release in the bloodstream, neutrophils circulate for up to 12 hrs.

The elimination of foreign microorganisms through phagocytosis, generation of reactive oxygen metabolites, and release of microbicidal substances is dependent on the mobilization of neutrophilic granules and secretory vesicles. The mature neutrophil contains 4 granule populations (**Fig. 52.1, Table 52.1**). Exocytosis of granules occurs in reverse order, with secretory granules the easiest to mobilize and the primary granule the least easy, requiring strong phagocytic stimuli.

More than 40 different growth factors, cytokines, and chemokines regulate polymorphonuclear leukocyte proliferation and differentiation and cell fate. The most clinically useful is granulocyte colony-stimulating factor (GCSF). GCSF specifically promotes neutrophil proliferation and maturation and enhances neutrophil microbicidal activity when administered in vivo. GCSF interacts with relatively late hematopoietic progenitors that have already committed to the neutrophil lineage and serves to support their growth and final maturation into functional neutrophils. Granulocyte-macrophage colony-stimulating factor (GM-CSF) acts on progenitors that are committed to produce either neutrophils or monocytes but can also act on granulocyte precursors directly. As with GCSF, it can enhance neutrophil reactivity when given in vivo.

Neutrophils continuously egress from the sinusoids of the bone marrow. Within the circulation, about half of the neutrophils are in the flowing stream; the other half are inaccessible to phlebotomy; the *marginating pool*. In response to stress, exercise, or IV epinephrine, the neutrophils in the marginating pool are released into the circulating pool. The marginating pool of neutrophils is in the postcapillary venules in major organs and in the capillaries of the lungs. Neutrophilia occurs after the administration of glucocorticoids due to mobilization from the marginated pool, increased bone marrow release, and lengthened half-life in circulation. The administration of GCSF shortens the transit time of neutrophils through the marrow, particularly in the post-mitotic pool. In response to inflammatory stimuli or infection, neutrophil production and release significantly increase. IL-6, one of the major regulators of the acute-phase response, induces demargination of intravascular neutrophils and shortens the neutrophil transit in the marrow. However, those neutrophils that are released preferentially sequester in the lung microvessels, are less deformable, and have increased F-actin. "Mature" neutrophils released from the bone marrow have altered function after infection, compared to cells produced during the "noninfected" state. They demonstrate decreased chemotaxis, decreased phagocytosis, and an impaired ability to upregulate CD10, a neutral endopeptidase that is present on only mature granulocytes.

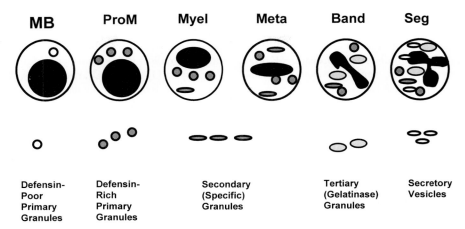

FIGURE 52.1. Neutrophil maturation. Note that granules develop during neutrophil maturation. No further cell division occurs beyond the myelocyte stage. MB, myeloblast; ProM, promyelocyte; Myel, myelocyte; Meta, Metamyelocyte; Seg, segmented (mature) neutrophil.

TABLE 52.1

NEUTROPHIL GRANULE CONTENTS

Protein	Primary (azurophil)	Secondary (specific)	Tertiary (gelatinase)	Secretory vesicle
Membrane Proteins				
Cytochrome b_{558}			+	+
CD11b/CD18 (CR3)		+	+	+
fMLF-R		+	+	+
Alkaline phosphatase				+
CD10				+
CD14				+
CD16 (FcγRIIIb)				+
CD35 (CR1)				+
C1qR				+
Enzymes				
Myeloperoxidase	+			
Proteinase-3	+			
Leukolysin		+	+	+
Collagenase		+		
Gelatinase		+	+	
Anti-microbial peptides				
Lysozyme	+	+	+	
Defensins	+			
BPI	+			
Cathepsins	+			
Lactoferrin		+		
Others				
Haptoglobin		+		
α_1-antitrypsin	+			
$\beta_2$microglobulin		+	+	

CD, cluster of differentiation; CR3, complement receptor 3; fMLF-R, formylmethionine-leucine-phenylalanine receptor; BPI, bacterial permeability increasing factor

Neutrophil Localization in Infection

The endothelium of the nearby postcapillary venule, under the immunologic pressure of pro-inflammatory cytokines, transforms from a nonadhesive surface to one that is proadhesive through the expression of specific ligands on the endothelial surface (**Table 52.2, Fig. 52.2**). The leukocyte integrins are heterodimers composed of α and β subunits. The β subunit may be shared by multiple members of a subfamily, while the α subunit confers specificity. The leukocyte integrins are generally functionally in an "inactive state." Through a process known as "inside-out signaling," the integrins change their conformation and become "active," and ligand recognition can now occur (**Table 52.3**).

Opsonophagocytosis and Microbial Killing

The ingestion and disposal of microbes is a major aspect of neutrophil function. To facilitate recognition of microbes by neutrophils, these targets are covered with serum opsonins, which include proteolytic fragments derived from complement cascade and specific immunoglobulins. Receptors that recognize opsonized bacteria are present on the neutrophil surface (**Table 52.4**).

Ligation of FCγ and/or complement receptors initiates a cascade of biochemical events that results in the exocytosis of granules, the respiratory burst, and phagocytosis. As neutrophil receptors are activated, the plasma membrane "ruffles" and assumes a bipolar configuration, with the formation of a "head," or pseudopod, and "tail," or uropod. The pseudopod surrounds the microbe and fuses at the distal end to form a phagolysosome. The particle is internalized and generally completely surrounded by plasma membrane. Granules join this newly formed vacuole and discharge their contents within seconds. Release of myeloperoxidase from the primary granule is important for oxygen-dependent killing. Release of other granule contents, such as bactericidal/permeability increasing protein, lactoferrin, and defensins, is critical for oxygen-independent killing.

The respiratory burst refers to the coordinated consumption of oxygen and production of metabolites that occurs when neutrophils are confronted with appropriate stimuli, actions that are the basis of all oxygen-dependent killing by neutrophils and other phagocytes. The NADPH oxidase system is a transmembrane electron system in which NADPH, the primary electron donor on the cytoplasmic side of the membrane, reduces oxygen in the extracellular fluid or within the phagolysosome to form superoxide (O_2^-) (**Fig. 52.3**). In turn, 2 molecules of O_2^- can

spontaneously (or enzymatically through superoxide dismutase) form hydrogen peroxide (H_2O_2). While both H_2O_2 and O_2^- can directly kill bacteria, it is the hydroxyl radical (OH$\bullet$) and hypohalous acids produced from O_2^- and H_2O_2, respectively, that are the most injurious to microbes and to healthy tissue/cells, if directly exposed.

Neutrophils have unique pathways that can afford control of gene product at the translational level in response to signals from the environment. Rapid protein synthesis without requirement for new transcription is one of several biologic advantages of "signal-dependent" translation of mRNA that are stored or silent in the basal state. Neutrophils also produce vascular endothelial growth factor. While this growth factor is important in vascular proliferation, it also has a role in the development of sepsis and in the progression of coronary artery lesions in acute Kawasaki disease.

Clearance of Neutrophils

The half-life of neutrophils is <12 hrs in the circulation. Circulating neutrophils undergo apoptosis (programmed cell death) and are removed by the reticuloendothelial system of the spleen and bone marrow. In patients with sepsis, circulating neutrophils have profoundly delayed apoptosis. Neutrophils that migrate to an inflammatory source have a prolonged half-life and increased function. However, these neutrophils do undergo apoptosis and are cleared from the tissue by inflammatory monocytes that have transformed to macrophages. Two apoptotic signal pathways have been characterized: the death receptor and the mitochondrial pathways. Both pathways ultimately result in the activation of caspase 3 and subsequent DNA fragmentation, chromatin condensation, and formation of the apoptotic body. Neutrophils can undergo apoptosis through either mechanism. One signal, phosphatidylserine (PS), is formed during the early stages of apoptosis, as PS is relocated from the inner to the outer surface of the plasma membrane. PS is recognized by a specific PS receptor on the macrophage. Proteinases released by bacteria provide novel mechanisms for an "eat me" signal from the apoptotic neutrophil.

DEFECTS IN NEUTROPHIL NUMBER AND/OR FUNCTION

Congenital Neutropenias

Congenital neutropenias are characterized by low neutrophil count (<200 neutrophils/mcL). *Severe congenital neutropenia* (Kostmann syndrome) appears

TABLE 52.2

ADHESION MOLECULES FOR NEUTROPHIL LOCALIZATION TO INFLAMMATORY SITES

Name	CD classification	Cell expression	Constitutive/ inducible	Ligand
Integrin family				
β_1 Integrins				
$\alpha_2\beta_1$ (VLA-2)	CD49b/CD29	Neutrophil	C/I?	Coll I, Coll IV, LN
$\alpha_4\beta_1$ (VLA-4)	CD49d/CD29	Neutrophil	C/I?	FN, VCAM, JAM2
$\alpha_5\beta_1$ (VLA-5)	CD49e/CD29	Neutrophil	C/I?	FN, Tsp
$\alpha_6\beta_1$ (VLA-5)	CD49f/CD29	Neutrophil	C/I?	N
$\alpha_9\beta_1$		Neutrophil	C/I?	VCAM-1, osteopontin
β_2 Integrins				
$\alpha_L\beta_2$ (LFA-1)	CD11a/CD18	Neutrophil	C	ICAM-1, ICAM-2, ICAM-3, JAM-1
$\alpha_M\beta_2$ (Mac-1, CR3)	CD11b/CD18	Neutrophil	C/I	ICAM-1, C3b, C3bi, Fg, FN, Factor X
$\alpha_x\beta_2$ (p150,95)	CD11c/CD18	Neutrophil	C/I	C3bi, GPIb-IX-V
β_3 Integrins				
$\alpha_V\beta_3$ (Vitronectin Receptor)	CD51/CD61	Neutrophil	C	vWf, VN, FN, Fg, PECAM-1, Tsp, LN, Osp, Coll I, Coll IV
Immunoglobulin gene superfamily				
ICAM-1	CD54	T & B cell; Endo; Epi; hepatocytes, pneumocytes, fibroblasts	C/I	FA-1, Mac-1
VCAM-1	CD102	Endo	I	$\alpha_4\beta_1$, $\alpha_9\beta_1$
JAM-1		Endo, Epi	C	FA-1, JAM-1
Selectins and selectin ligands				
L-selectin	CD62-L	Neutrophil	C	Unknown endo ligand, PSGL-1,
P-selectin	CD62-P	Platelet, Endo	C/I	PSGL-1, E-selectin, GPIb-IX-V
E-selectin	CD62-E	Endo	I	PSGL-1
P-selectin-glycoprotein Ligand 1 (PSGL-1)	CD162	Neutrophil	C	P-selectin, E-selectin, L-selectin

Note that this table focuses primarily on adhesion molecules specifically for neutrophil localization to inflammatory sites.
Inducible adhesion molecules: While ICAM-1 is constitutively expressed on many cell types, its expression can also be induced by the cytokines TNF, IL-1 and IFN-γ after only a brief period (3–4 hrs). E-selectin and P-selectin can be induced on endothelial cells by TNF and IL-1 after 3-4 hrs of stimulation. VCAM-1 is present on endothelial cells only after cytokine stimulation. Its appearance is delayed compared to the other adhesion molecules. Both endothelial cells (Weibel-Palade bodies) and platelets (α granule) contain an intracellular pool of P-selectin, which can be mobilized to the surface after cell activation. Similarly, Mac-1 and p150,95 are constitutively present on neutrophils, but pools are also present in secretory vesicles which can be easily mobilized.
VLA, very late antigen; Coll I, collagen type I; Coll IV, collagen type IV; LN, laminin; FN, fibronectin; VCAM, vascular cell adhesion molecule; JAM, junctional adhesion molecule; Tsp, thrombospondin; LFA, leukocyte functional antigen: ICAM, intercellular adhesion molecule; Fg, fibrinogen; GPIb-IX-V, glycoprotein complex present on platelet surface; vWF, von Willebrand factor; Vn, vitronectin; PECAM-1, platelet-endothelial cell adhesion molecute-1; Osp, osteopontin; Endo, endothelial cell; Epi, epithelial cells

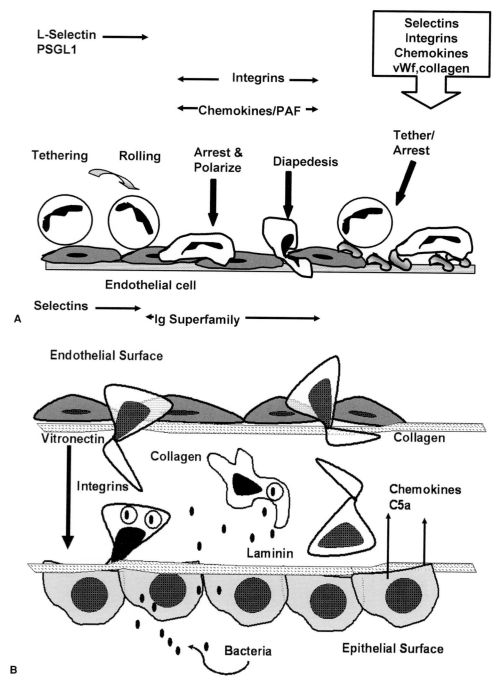

FIGURE 52.2. Neutrophil localization. **A:** In an inflammatory focus, the endothelium, which is normally nonadhesive, becomes proadhesive as a result of activation by cytokines, such as IL-1β and TNF. Neutrophils are tethered from the free-flowing stream and roll on the endothelial lining of the blood vessel, an interaction mediated by all 3 members of the selectin family. The neutrophils slow, arrest, and change shape (polarize). Integrins and their ligands, the immunoglobulin gene superfamily, mediate the transition from rolling to arrest. This transition is also dependent on the production of activating agents by the endothelial surface, such as platelet-activating factor and IL-8. The neutrophils then crawl over the surface of the endothelium until they migrate through the endothelial monolayer. A neutrophil may be tethered by adherent platelets or another adherent leukocyte. Platelets themselves release chemokines which activate

TABLE 52.3

CHEMOTACTIC FACTORS FOR NEUTROPHIL LOCALIZATION

Activating agent	Neutrophil ligand	Source
PAF	PAF receptor	Monocytes, endothelial cells
LTB$_4$	LTB$_4$receptor	Monocytes, neutrophils
C5a	C5a receptor	Anaphylatoxin from complement activation
fMLF	fMLF receptor	Bacteria
C-X-C and CC chemokines		
IL-8 (CXCL8)	CXCR1, CXCR2	Endothelial cells, monocytes, neutrophils, T cells, epithelial cells
GRO-α, MGSA-α (CXCL1)	CXCR2>CXCR1	Epithelial cells
NAP-2 (CXCL7)	CXCR2	Epithelial cells
ENA-78 (CXCL5)	CXCR2	Epithelial cells
MIP-1α (CCL3)	CCR5, CCR1	T cells, monocytes
MIP-1β (CCL4)	CCR5	T cells, monocytes
RANTES (CCL5)	CCR1, CCR3, CCR5	T cells

Chemokines regulate cell trafficking of all types of leukocytes. Chemokines interact with a subset of 7-transmembrane spanning, G-protein-coupled receptors on the neutrophil surface. Chemokines for neutrophils are subdivided into major subfamilies based on the arrangement of the 2 amino-terminal cysteine residues CXC and CC. The CXC family has an amino acid between the 2 cysteine residues; the CC family does not.
PAF, platelet activating factor; LTB$_4$, leukotriene B$_4$; fMLF, formylmethionyl-leucyl-phenylalanine; CXCL, CXC chemokine ligand; CXCR, CXC chemokine receptor; GRO, growth regulating protein; MGSA, melanocyte growth stimulating activity; NAP, neutrophil activating peptides; ENA, epithelial derived neutrophil attractant; MIP, macrophage inflammatory peptide; CCL, CC chemokine ligand; CCR, CC chemokine receptor; RANTES, regulated on activation, normal T-cell expressed and secreted

after birth, with 90% of all children symptomatic within 6 mos. In children with *cyclic neutropenia/cyclic hematopoiesis*, a cyclic fluctuation occurs in all hemapoietic lines, though that of the neutrophil line is most marked. In both of these diseases, the use of GCSF has dramatically improved the outcome.

Defects of Oxidative Metabolism

The most widely recognized and most prevalent defect of neutrophil function is chronic granuloma-tous disease (CGD), a heterogeneous disease that is characterized by recurrent life-threatening infections with bacteria, fungi, and the formation of abnormal granulomata. The defect is in the NADPH oxidase, the enzyme system responsible for the oxidative burst (**Fig. 52.3**). The most common genotype of the CGD are the X-linked mutations of gp91^{phox}. Males are affected, and females are carriers. The most frequent sites of infection are lung, lymph nodes, and liver as well as osteomyelitis, perianal abscess, and gingivitis.

←

FIGURE 52.2. (*Continued*) neutrophils. Platelets may bind directly to von Willebrand factor (vWf) on the endothelial surface or on the basement membrane; alternatively, they may bind to collagen or fibronectin on the exposed basement membrane. **B:** Neutrophil localization in response to bacterial challenge. Bacteria present on the epithelial surface activate the epithelium to produce neutrophil chemokines NAP-2 (CXCL7) and ENA 78 (CXCL5); complement is activated, and the chemotactic factor C5a is produced. The epithelial surface also produces TNF-α and/or IL-1β, promoting the transition of the adjacent endothelial surface from an anti-adhesive to a proadhesive surface. Neutrophils emigrate out of the blood vessel across the endothelial cell lining and crawl through the basement membrane and along the connective tissue. This is mediated by members of the β_1-integrin family and CD11b/CD18 (Mac-1, $\alpha_M\beta_2$). These integrins interact with their specific epitopes in the basement membrane structural proteins (e.g., laminin and vitronectin) and collagen. Neutrophils can continue to emigrate across the epithelial surface. Upon encountering bacteria, neutrophils surround them with plasma membrane, forming a phagolysosome. In the phagolysosome, both oxygen-dependent and oxygen-independent mechanisms are operative resulting in bacterial killing.

TABLE 52.4

TABLE 52.4

RECEPTORS FOR PHAGOCYTOSIS ON NEUTROPHILS

Receptor	CD classification	Ligand
FcγRI	CD64	Fc portion of IgG (high-affinity receptor)
FcγRIIA	CD32	Fc portion of IgG (low-affinity receptor)
FcγRIIIB	CD16	Fc portion of IgG (low-affinity receptor)
FcαRI		Fc of IgA
CR1	CD35	C3b>C4b>C3bi
CR3 (Mac-1)	CD11b/CD18	C3bi
C1qR		C1q

Complement fragments of C3: C3b, C3bi; complement fragment of C4: C4b; C1q is the q subunit of the complement complex 1.
CD, cluster of differentiation

The functional defect is the inability of the NADPH complex to generate superoxide (O_2^-) and the downstream reactive oxygen species (ROS), H_2O_2 and OH, resulting in defective microbial killing and recurrent infections with catalase-positive bacteria. Organisms that produce their own H_2O_2 but do not degrade it (those that are catalase-negative) supply the substrate for the formation of hypohalous acid by the myeloperoxidase released into the phagolysosome by the neutrophil. The overwhelming majority of infections result from *Aspergillus*, *Staphylococcus aureus*, *Burkholderia cepacia*, *Nocardia*, and *Serratia marcescens*.

The cornerstone of treatment of CGD is trimethoprim/sulfamethoxazole prophylaxis. A large, multicentered trial of interferon-γ (IFN-γ)

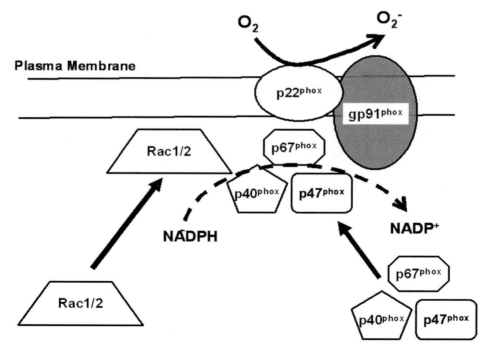

FIGURE 52.3. NADPH oxidase components and activation. On activation of the neutrophil, the 3 cytosolic components of the NADPH oxidase (p67^{phox}, p47^{phox}, and p40^{phox}) plus either Rac1 or Rac2 are translocated to the membrane of the phagocytic vacuole. The p47^{phox} binds to the membrane component of the NADPH oxidase, cytochrome b_{558} (gp91^{phox} plus p22^{phox}). The NADPH oxidase transfers an electron from NADPH to O_2 to form superoxide (O_2^-). The unstable superoxide is converted to hydrogen peroxide, either spontaneously or by superoxide dismutase.

demonstrated 70% fewer infections, compared to placebo. In severe infections, granulocyte infusions have been used; while they are potentially life saving, they may also complicate the ICU course. A potential transfusion hazard may exist in X-linked CGD patients.

Defects of Leukocyte Adhesion and Trafficking

Leukocyte adhesion deficiency-1 (LAD-1) is an autosomal recessive disorder with mutations in the common chain of the β_2 integrin CD18, which results in a deficiency in number or function of adhesion molecules Mac-1 (CD11b/CD18), LFA-1 (CD11a/CD18), and p150,95 (CD11c/CD18) on the cell surface. Neutrophils cannot adhere and transmigrate to the inflammatory focus. In addition, as Mac-1 is also the complement receptor 3, severely reduced complement-mediated phagocytosis occurs (**Table 52.2**, **Table 52.4**). With this severe type, children usually present within the first months of life with omphalitis and delayed cord separation. They have severe infections, impaired pus formation, and impaired wound healing. They have neutrophilia at baseline, but with infections, the neutrophil count may rise > 100,000/mcL. In LAD-2 or congenital disorder of glycosylation IIc (CDGIIc), defects occur in glycosylation. Selectins must be appropriately glycosylated for full function (**Fig. 52.2A**, **Table 52.2**).

Other Associated Defects in Neutrophil Function

Newborn infants, whether born at term or very premature, have peripheral blood counts similar to older children and adults. However, they differ dramatically from adults in their response to sepsis. The profound, sustained neutrophilia with sepsis seen in adults is not found in neonates and premature infants. Instead, neonates and premature infants frequently become neutropenic during infection due to low neutrophil cell mass and an apparent inability to increase the proliferation of the early progenitor pool. Defects in phagocyte function are present in children with protein calorie malnutrition.

NEUTROPHILS AND CRITICAL ILLNESS

In human sepsis, neutrophil chemotaxis to the bacterial product fMLF and leukotriene B$_4$ (an arachidonic acid-derived chemotactic factor) is diminished. In patients with sepsis and multiple organ failure, chemo-

tactic response to the chemokine IL-8 is also reduced. The loss of motility corresponds to reduction in the surface expression of the receptor for IL-8, CXCR2, but not CXCR1. Neutrophil Mac-1 (CD11b/CD18) was upregulated in the patients with sepsis and correlated with increased levels of IL-8, compared to normal volunteers. Neutrophils from patients with sepsis have increased spontaneous oxidative burst activity. In traumatized patients, chemotaxis is delayed, spontaneous oxidative burst activity is increased, oxidative activity is diminished with further stimulation, and opsonophagocytosis is decreased. The effects of "critical illness" on the neutrophil may not be due as much to the "illness" per se but rather the release of factors that themselves result in a pool of neutrophils with increased inflammatory characteristics. Neutrophils produced and circulating under such conditions contribute to organ injury.

Transfusion-related Acute Lung Injury

The neutrophil is the effector cell in transfusion-related acute lung injury (TRALI). For TRALI to develop, "two hits" must occur. The first results in activation of the endothelium, and a normal anti-adhesive surface becomes pro-adhesive for neutrophils. Neutrophils become activated and sequestered in the lung. This first hit can occur from sepsis, trauma, and massive blood transfusion. The second hit is the infusion of specific antibodies directed against antigens on the neutrophil surface and/or biologic modifiers in the stored blood component, which activate the adherent or trapped neutrophils in the lung, causing neutrophil-endothelial injury, capillary leak, and acute lung injury (ALI). Differentiating TRALI from transfusion-associated circulatory overload (hydrostatic pulmonary edema) may be difficult and may require more invasive studies, such as measurement of the left atrial pressure. Blood component and donor management strategies have been suggested to prevent TRALI, including the avoidance of blood products from individuals with known leukocyte antibodies, leukoreduction of blood components, shortening the storage time of cellular components to reduce accumulation of cytokines and other biologic response modifiers, and washing cellular components prior to transfusion.

Neutropenia and the ICU

In a Cochrane Review, the use of colony-stimulating factors in patients with febrile neutropenia due to cancer chemotherapy reduced the amount of time spent in the hospital and time for neutrophil recovery, but no clear survival benefit was seen.

Recommendations regarding the use of GCSF in neutropenic critically ill patients must be individualized. In those neutropenic children with proven or suspected fungal infections in whom mortality is high, GCSF appears prudent. If neutropenic patients have sepsis (bacteremia and organ failure) along with neutropenia, again GCSF would be indicated. However, those who have pneumonia or another pulmonary process and neutropenia may be at risk of developing worsening respiratory status with the use of GCSF, and withholding GCSF or continuous infusion should be considered.

Even though a number of studies have been conducted in both neonates and adults, none contain conclusive evidence that either GCSF or GM-CSF improves outcome in the non-neutropenic patient. GCSF or GM-CSF in the non-neutropenic ICU patient should only be used in the context of therapeutic trials. Granulocyte transfusions all but disappeared in the 1980s and 1990s. Little therapeutic benefit was observed, and reports surfaced regarding adverse pulmonary responses with granulocyte transfusions. In neonates, in one trial of granulocyte transfusion compared to IV immunoglobulin, a reduction in mortality was associated with granulocyte transfusion.

Critical Care Therapies and Neutrophil Function

Mechanical stretch of the alveolar epithelium can lead to production of pro-inflammatory cytokines, in particular chemokines for neutrophils. In ALI, the use of conventional ventilation strategy (compared to a protective ventilation strategy) for as little as 36 hrs resulted in increased production of plasma IL-6 and bronchoalveolar fluid, which activated donor neutrophils. In premature infants, the use of mechanical ventilation resulted in activation of circulating neutrophils and monocytes, as measured by increased CD11b/CD18 compared to infants treated with nasal continuous positive airway pressure (CPAP). Mild hypothermia (32°C–34°C) is advocated in adult patients after cardiac arrest and possibly for traumatic brain injury. However, several lines of evidence suggest that hypothermia increases mortality in patients with sepsis and trauma and that hypothermia favors wound infections.

In cardiopulmonary bypass and extracorporeal membrane oxygenation (ECMO), interaction of the blood elements with the oxygenator membrane and the mechanical stress of the circuit on the cells result in an acute inflammatory process that is dependent on complement activation, production of platelet-activating factor and other arachidonic intermediates, and activation of the kallikrein system. Neutrophils are activated with increased oxidative burst, and myeloperoxidase, elastase, and lactoferrin are found in the plasma. Leukocyte filtration systems for cardiopulmonary bypass or leukocyte depletion of blood used in ECMO circuits are useful to prevent injury induced by activated leukocytes.

Barbiturates, midazolam, and propofol all have profound effects on neutrophils. All inhibit respiratory burst, and barbiturates inhibit chemotaxis, opsonophagocytosis, and intracellular killing. While anesthesia-relevant concentrations may have minimal effects, the considerably higher concentrations used in the ICU place patients potentially at risk for increased infections.

Pentoxifylline and Cyclic AMP Modulators

Pentoxifylline, a xanthine derivative, is a phosphodiesterase inhibitor used in adult patients for treatment of claudication. With the discovery that it also decreases tumor necrosis factor (TNF) gene transcription in sepsis, pentoxifylline has attracted fresh attention as an anti-inflammatory agent. It has numerous functions, including preventing the development of necrotizing enterocolitis in neonates by preserving small vessel function, preventing endothelial dysfunction in sepsis, enhancing prostacyclin release, and attenuating the release of thromboxane. Pentoxifylline increases erythrocyte and leukocyte deformability, presumably by increasing cyclic AMP levels. Methylxanthines suppress neutrophil chemotaxis, superoxide anion production, phagocytosis, and degranulation. In a metaanalysis of 2 single-centered, randomized, placebo-controlled trials of pentoxifylline in neonatal sepsis as an adjunct to antibiotics, all-cause mortality was reduced with the use of pentoxifylline, and no adverse events were found. Though the data are still limited, pentoxifylline should be considered in neonates with sepsis as an adjunct to antibiotic therapy.

The elevation of intracellular cyclic AMP results in decreased neutrophil adhesion, demonstrated with type IV phosphodiesterase inhibitors (rolipram) and the β_2 agonist isoproterenol but not with type III phosphodiesterase inhibitors (milrinone). Neutrophils, monocytes, eosinophils, and mast cells have β_2-adrenergic receptors. Activation of neutrophil β_2-adrenergic receptors results in decreased IL-8–induced chemotaxis. Catecholamines, including epinephrine, norepinephrine, dobutamine, and dopamine, depress neutrophil phagocytic ability and production of ROS. Thus, many of the agents used commonly in the ICU can have direct suppressive effects on neutrophil function at the pharmacologic doses achieved.

Corticosteroids

The main anti-inflammatory effects of corticosteroids result from changes in the function of macrophages, monocytes, and granulocytes, including the decreased production of anti-inflammatory cytokines, inhibition of arachidonic acid metabolism, and decreased granulocyte adherence and migration. Lymphocyte number and function are also markedly affected by corticosteroids.

Modulating Neutrophil Function

Anti-integrin Therapy

With the critical role of neutrophils in pathophysiologic diseases, such as shock, acute respiratory distress syndrome, and ischemia-reperfusion injury, a number of therapies to block neutrophil adhesive function have been proposed and produced. Numerous animal studies have demonstrated that anti-adhesive strategies are, in fact, successful. At least in theory, such strategies should also be beneficial in critically ill humans. Initial enthusiasm with this paradigm has given way to a number of negative human studies and a cautious reappraisal of the concept. Studies in traumatic shock, stroke, burns, myocardial infarction, and transplant have demonstrated no benefit of β_2-integrin, LFA-1, or ICAM-1 blockade in humans. Use of anti-α_4 or anti-$\alpha_4\beta_7$ therapy in inflammatory bowel disease, asthma, multiple sclerosis, and anti-$\alpha_L\beta_2$ in psoriasis has been more successful. These latter therapies do not target neutrophils per se, but other leukocytes—primarily lymphocytes.

Platelet Activating Factor Inhibition

Platelet activating factor (PAF) is a potent phospholipid synthesized by a large number of cells. Its functions are mediated through receptors that are located on a surface of a variety of cells, including the neutrophil. PAF is implicated in necrotizing enterocolitis in infants, asthma, systemic lupus erythematosus, rheumatoid arthritis, and Crohn disease. Neither the use of PAF acetylhydrolase (which increases the breakdown of PAF) nor the use of a PAF receptor antagonist has been demonstrated to decrease mortality in severely septic patients, though a substantial reduction in organ dysfunction has been achieved.

Neutrophil Elastase Inhibition

When neutrophils have reduced deformability, such as occurs in sepsis, severe trauma, and ALI, they potentially are trapped in capillaries. These neutrophils may then secrete neutrophil elastase, reactive oxygen products, and other soluble mediators of tissue injury. A selective inhibitor of neutrophil elastase, sivelestat, attenuates leukocyte adhesion in pulmonary capillaries and attenuates the decreased neutrophil deformability in animal models of sepsis. In humans with ALI, sivelestat infusion for 5 days also attenuated diminished neutrophil deformability. In a phase III multicentered, randomized, controlled trial of sivelestat in adult patients with ALI, no difference between sivelestat and placebo was seen in mortality or ventilator-free days at 28 days. An increase in mortality in the sivelestat group at 180 days was seen.

Activated Protein C

Despite multiple clinical trials of immunomodulatory therapies in severe sepsis through the years, only one has significantly affected outcome in adult patients. Surprisingly, that drug is the activated form of the naturally occurring anticoagulant protein C [drotrecogin alpha (activated), Xigris]. Activated protein C (APC) decreased death by 20% in the Recombinant Human Activated Protein C Worldwide Evaluation in Severe Sepsis (PROWESS) trial, which included 1690 patients. If administered on day 1 of multiorgan failure, the drug had a greater effect on survival than if administered on day 2. In patients with sepsis and single-organ failure, APC did not improve outcome, and an increased risk of bleeding was associated with APC. A trial of APC in children with severe sepsis was halted early, as no benefit was detected with its use, though serious bleeding events were not greater with its use.

That the PROWESS trial demonstrated a benefit in adult patients with severe sepsis but other anticoagulant therapy trials have had no effect suggests that the role of APC may reside less in its role as an antithrombotic and more in its role as an anti-inflammatory. In human models of endotoxemia, at best an incomplete model of sepsis, APC had minimal effect on hemodynamics, inflammation, thrombin generation, and fibrinolysis. However, it inhibited leukocyte accumulation in the airspaces of subjects who received intrabronchial administration of endotoxin. Neutrophils express the endothelial protein C receptor (EPCR) on their plasma membrane. Treatment of neutrophils in vitro with APC inhibited neutrophil chemotaxis but had no effect on respiratory burst, bacterial phagocytosis or apoptosis. Incubation of neutrophils and platelets in plasma from patients with sepsis resulted in increased adhesion to endothelial monolayers and self-aggregation, compared to incubation in plasma obtained from normal subjects. The addition of APC abrogated this increase in adhesion and aggregation, and the effect could be reversed by low-dose heparin.

CHAPTER 53 ■ THE IMMUNE SYSTEM AND VIRAL ILLNESS IN THE CRITICALLY ILL

LESLEY DOUGHTY

Viral infections, such as HIV, deplete lymphocyte subsets, thereby creating vulnerability to opportunistic pathogens. The immune defects progressively worsen until death. As such, HIV represents the most extreme example of immunomodulation induced by viral infection. The effect of this viral infection on immune function is well understood; however, the effect of common viral infections, such as influenza A and B, respiratory syncytial virus (RSV), parainfluenza, adenovirus, enterovirus, and cytomegalovirus (CMV), on host immunity is less well appreciated. Disruption of mucosal/epithelial protective barriers important for tissue homeostasis and infection prevention can provide a portal of entry for bacteria. This aspect of viral infection has long been appreciated and thought to be the critical event in creating a permissive state for secondary bacterial infection. In addition to increasing the risk of bacterial infection, viruses have been implicated in exacerbations of, and morbidity from, diseases such as asthma and a variety of autoimmune diseases.

Viral replication can directly injure mucosal and epithelial protective barriers by causing cell lysis upon replication and release (**Table 53.1**). The immune response to microbial pathogens consists of several phases. The earliest and least specific is the innate immune response, followed by a pathogen-specific adaptive immune response that leads to immunologic memory. These phases of immune response include activation of diverse cellular and humoral mediators, many of which are common to many types of infections. The immune response to viral infection involves mechanisms similar to immune responses to bacterial infections, as well as unique mechanisms. Recognition of viruses by the innate immune system begins by the host recognition of viral pathogen-associated molecular patterns (PAMPs) through their interaction with pattern recognition receptors such as the Toll-like receptors (TLRs), thereby initiating the immune response. Viral PAMPs include virion proteins, hemaglutinin, double-stranded RNA produced during replication of many viruses, F protein from RSV, single-stranded RNA, and viral DNA. TLRs 2, 3, 4, 7, 8, and 9 have been implicated in responses to viral PAMPs. In fact, the initial cellular reactions to viral PAMPs are very similar to those initiated by bacterial PAMPs (**Fig. 53.1**). The innate response is critical for containment of viral particles and initiation of the adaptive, or antigen-specific, immune response that is necessary for viral eradication and immunologic memory. Binding to TLRs initiates intracellular signal transduction, which leads to production of inflammatory cytokines, including interferons alpha and beta (IFN-α/β), IFN gamma (IFN-γp, TNF-α, IL-12p70, IL-10), and many chemokines that facilitate trafficking of cells to sites of viral invasion.

IFNs activate natural killer (NK) cells and macrophages, induce maturation of dendritic cells, and upregulate proteins that are important in antigen presentation to T cells that are critical for antigen-specific immunity. Macrophages and dendritic cells can bind to synthesized intracellular viral peptides via the major histocompatibility complex (MHC) I and extracellular viral peptides via MHC II. Once activated by viruses, these cells mature as they migrate to draining lymph nodes, where they present viral antigens to CD4 T cells via MHC I and II. Antigen-activated CD4 and dendritic cells are critical for stimulation of CD8 cytotoxic T cells and B cells. Dendritic cells can present viral antigens to CD8 T cells via MHC I molecules inducing an antigen specific proliferation of CD8 T cells. Cytotoxic CD8 T cells can eliminate virus (a) by further induction of another essential antiviral cytokine, IFN-γs (b) by lysis of virus-infected cells via the release of perforin (a membrane pore-forming protein important for cytotoxicity), and (c) by induction of apoptosis through Fas ligand with Fas (CD95) on the virus-infected cells. A result of this immune cascade is eradication of the virus, production of antibodies specific for multiple viral peptides, and creation of memory T cells and B cells important in protection against subsequent infection with the same virus.

Viral infection can compromise antibacterial function, thereby creating a permissive state for bacterial superinfection (**Table 53.2**). Antibacterial functions altered during and/or following viral infection include diminished neutrophil and macrophage recruitment and activation and reduced phagocytic function, with reduced bacterial killing and containment; augmented neutrophil apoptosis; dendritic cell dysfunction with poor antigen presentation; suppressed CD4 T cell proliferation; altered cytokine production with excess IL-10 and IL-4 (Th2) and decreased IFN-γ (Th1) (in RSV); reduced

TABLE 53.1

MECHANISMS OF BACTERIAL ADHERENCE TO HOST CELLS DURING VIRAL INFECTION

Respiratory epithelial disruption	Loss of mucociliary function
	Basement membrane exposure
Bacterial features	Fimbriae
	Capsule
Expression of viral glycoproteins	Neuraminidase (influenza/parainfluenza)
	Hemagglutinin (influenza/parainfluenza)
	Glycoproteins F and G (RSV)
Upregulation of host cell receptors	CD14, CD15, and CD18
	PAFR
	Complement protein C3
	Fimbriae-associated receptors
	IgA translocating receptor
	Pentameric IgM
Proteins from injured ECM	Fibrinogen
Other	Coupling bacteria to epithelium by RSV
	Altered bacterial adhesins

RSV, respiratory syncytial virus; PAFR, platelet activating factor receptor; ECM, extracellular matrix
Adapted from Hament JM, Kimpen JL, Fleer A, et al. Respiratory viral infection predisposing for bacterial disease: A concise review. *FEMS Immunol Med Microbiol* 1999;26:189–95.

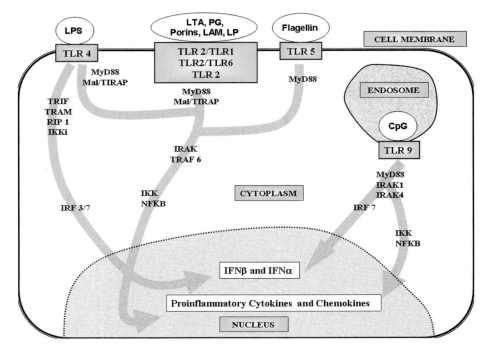

FIGURE 53.1. Early signaling initiated by bacterial pathogen-associated molecular patterns (PAMPs). Pattern recognition receptors (PRRs) recognize many components of bacteria, providing early signaling to initiate inflammatory responses to invading pathogens. The signaling pathways are shared by many Toll-like receptors (TLRs); however, the specificity of each differs, providing the ability to respond to a diverse range of pathogens. Considerable overlap between signaling pathways exists, leading to common endpoints, such as nuclear factor κB (NFκB) activation, which leads to induction of inflammatory cytokines and chemokines. Induction of IFN-α, IFN-β, and other interferon-inducible genes occurs by binding of TLR-2, -4, and -9 ligands.

TABLE 53.2

IMMUNOMODULATORY EFFECTS OF VIRAL INFECTIONS

Cell type	Decreased	Increased
Macrophages	MHC expression Activation and recruitment Phagocytosis Bacterial killing Antigen presentation	Inflammatory cytokines
Neutrophils	Bacterial killing	TLR-2 expression Apoptosis
Dendritic cells	Altered IFN-α/β production Altered IFN-γ signaling MHC expression Antigen presentation	Apoptosis
NK cells	Activation	
T cells	CD4 proliferation CD8 cytotoxicity Th-2 cytokines Regulatory T-cell activation DTH response	Th-1 cytokines Apoptosis
Other	Bone marrow suppression Complement activation	

MHC, major histocompatibility complex; TLR, Toll-like receptor; DTH, delayed-type hypersensitivity

cell-mediated immunity and CD8 T cell cytotoxicity; and activation of suppressive regulatory T cells (CD4+CD25+) (**Table 53.2**). Viruses that are implicated in inducing a state of immunosuppression include measles, CMV, herpes viruses, and HIV. Measles infection suppresses many aspects of the immune response, leading to profound vulnerability of the host to secondary infections. This immune modulation can persist many weeks (up to 6 months in some cases) after resolution of the acute measles infection and presence of the virus. As with other viral infection, triggers for these effects include expression of measles viral proteins, including hemagglutinin, fusion proteins H and F, measles virus nucleoprotein, and the nonstructural proteins C and V.

In most immunocompetent people, CMV causes asymptomatic or very mild illness, and, in some, it causes a mononucleosis-like syndrome. In immunosuppressed individuals, it can cause severe/fatal disease involving liver, lung, gastrointestinal tract, and CNS. In addition to its direct pathology, CMV is a virus capable of modulating the immune response, permitting its persistence in a latent state. In recipients of orthotopic liver transplant, CMV disease (primary or reactivated) frequently precedes bacteremia and/or invasive fungal disease. The use of anti-CMV treatments (ganciclovir or anti-CMV

IgG) after transplantation reduces the incidence of invasive fungal disease.

The association between viral infection and bacterial infection has been repeatedly described for the following sequences: respiratory viruses such as influenza, RSV, and parainfluenza with a secondary bacterial pneumonia; varicella with toxic shock syndrome or necrotizing fasciitis; measles with bacterial pneumonia; and influenza with meningococcemia or toxic shock. Other viruses, including rotavirus and enterovirus, have also been associated with bacterial co-infection. Antecedent and/or concurrent influenza infection has been strongly associated with secondary bacterial pneumonia, which has historically carried with it severe morbidity and high mortality. In addition, a possible role is emerging for antecedent viral infections, including influenza in severe community-acquired, methicillin-resistant *Staphylococcal aureus* pneumonia. The incidence of severe group A β hemolytic streptococcal (GAβHS) disease also occurs coincident with influenza epidemics.

The first significant change induced by viral infection is often disruption of protective epithelial barriers as a result of diversion of cell machinery to intracellular viral formation and replication, often with direct lysis of infected cells. When protective epithelial barriers are disrupted, protective mucous and mucociliary dysfunction can occur, as can exaggerated bacterial adherence to exposed basement membrane elements, permitting penetration into deeper tissues (**Table 53.1**). Bacterial adherence is facilitated in areas where epithelium has been denuded. Mechanisms of bacterial adherence to infected/disrupted epithelium can be nonspecific, as exemplified by bacteria binding to fibrinogen and fibronectin-binding protein of the exposed extracellular matrix, seen with GAβHS in influenza A infection. Examples of bacterial adherence during viral infection include enhanced fimbriae-mediated and capsule-mediated binding of nontypeable *H. influenzae*, GAβHS, and *N. meningitidis* to alveolar epithelial cells infected with RSV or influenza A. Native host cell-surface protein/receptor expression (including platelet-activating factor receptor, CD14, CD15, and CD18) can be upregulated during many viral infections. The best characterized glycoproteins are hemagglutinin and neuraminidase (NA), which are expressed on the host cell surface during influenza and parainfluenza infections. Hemagglutinin binds to sialic acid residues of host glycoproteins on the

host cell surface. NA is critical for replication of influenza and parainfluenza because it cleaves sialic acid residues from host glycoproteins during viral budding from infected cells, facilitating release of newly synthesized virus. These sialic acid residues on host proteins provide protection against bacterial adherence and, once cleaved by NA, bacteria can adhere and invade. Other viral glycoproteins implicated in susceptibility to bacterial superinfection include glycoproteins F and G, which are inserted into the host cell membrane during RSV infection.

Respiratory viral infections can precipitate acute asthma exacerbations in children. Athmatics are more susceptible to rhinoviral infections, and viral replication in bronchial epithelial cells obtained from asthmatics is increased. Induction of apoptosis of virus-infected host cells is a critical event in the innate antiviral response because early apoptosis of virus-infected host cells prevents establishment and spread of virus and promotes phagocytosis of infected cells. Upregulation of mediators, and activation of cells (e.g., IgE and eosinophil) that are associated with asthma exacerbations is summarized in **Figure 53.2**.

A. Normal Host

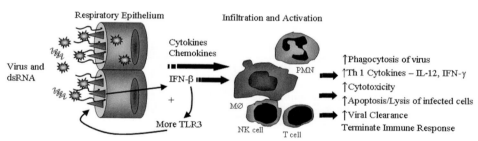

B. Asthmatic Host

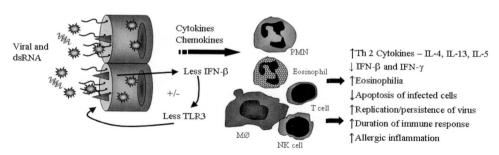

FIGURE 53.2. The antiviral immune response in asthma. Viruses infect respiratory epithelium and dsRNA (released during replication of most viruses) signals through TLR-3, which is constitutively expressed on epithelial cells. Both lead to production of a multitude of cytokines and chemokines, including IFN-β by epithelial cells. IFN-β upregulates TLR-3, leading to further induction of IFN-β. IFN-β also induces IFN-α both of which are pleiotropic cytokines that activate a multitude of inflammatory cells, kinases, and regulatory proteins critical for viral containment. **A:** Under normal circumstances, activation and infiltration of inflammatory cells lead to a proinflammatory response, including Th1 cytokines, which are also important for viral clearance. Effective killing/apoptosis of infected cells occurs, promoting viral clearance and resolution of inflammation. **B:** Respiratory epithelial cells from asthmatics produce less IFN-β and TLR-3. Inflammatory cell stimulation is different with infiltration of eosinophils, a Th-2 response with less IFN-γ, longer survival of infected cells, and delayed viral clearance.

TABLE 53.3

IMMUNE DYSFUNCTION IN CRITICAL ILLNESS STATES, INCLUDING TRAUMA/POST-SURGICAL, BURN INJURY, SEPTIC SHOCK, BRAIN INJURY, MALNUTRITION, AND MULTIPLE TRANSFUSIONS

Affected immune cell	Immune defect
Macrophage/dendritic cells	Increased anti-inflammatory cytokines
	Decreased proinflammatory cytokines
	Decreased HLA-DR
	Decreased antigen presentation
	Decreased phagocytosis
	Decreased NO and ROI
	Decreased PBMC response to LPS
Neutrophils	Decreased adhesion molecules
	Decreased NO, PAF, ROI
	Decreased chemotaxis
	Decreased phagocytosis
	Decreased degranulation
	Decreased lysosomal activity
NK cells and lymphocytes	Th1 to Th2 shift
	Poor response to mitogens
	Increased apoptosis
	Decreased cytotoxicity
	Decreased Ig production
	Anergy

HLA-DR, human leukocyte antigen-DR; NO, nitric oxide; ROI, reactive oxygen intermediates; PBMC, peripheral blood mononuclear cells; LPS, lipopolysaccharide; PAF, platelet activating factor; Ig, immunoglobulin
Adapted from Doughty L. Modulation of the immune response in critical illness/injury. In: Doughty L, Linden P, eds. *Immunology and Infectious Disease.* Norwell, MA: Kluwer Academic Publishers, 2003:115–54.

Viral infection has been thought to be among the triggers for exacerbation of autoimmune disease, as well as a potential etiology. A frequently hypothesized mechanism is referred to as *molecular mimicry*, in which the immune response to viral infection cross-reacts with self-antigens, resulting in activation of T and B cells, which causes formation of self-reactive auto-antibodies that are capable of mediating tissue injury. Alternatively, viruses such as CMV, during primary or reactivated disease, can activate antigen-presenting cells and/or virus-specific T cells, inducing cytokines and chemokines that can activate preexisting autoreactive T cells in susceptible individuals. This phenomenon is called *bystander activation. Epitope spreading* is a mechanism that involves exposure of damaged self-proteins during viral infection, resulting in anti–self-immune responses to proteins that, prior to damage, are not considered foreign.

Generally, the therapy for autoimmune exacerbations includes pulse steroids and adjustment of other anti-inflammatory regimens. Viral infections, either primary or reactivated, are known to be significant pathogens in the context of immunosuppressed states (bone marrow and solid organ transplants).

Reactivation of latent viral infections, such as CMV, EBV, HSV, HHV 6, and HHV-7, can occur during stressed states, particularly in the presence of inflammatory cytokine production. The immune defects associated with critically ill patients are listed in **Table 53.3**. Data indicate that reactivation of human herpes virus of many types (CMV, EBV, HSV, HHV) can occur with fairly high prevalence in critically ill patients who have been traditionally considered "immunocompetent," as well as in the immunosuppressed populations.

CHAPTER 54 ■ IMMUNE MODULATION AND IMMUNOTHERAPY IN CRITICAL ILLNESS

MARK W. HALL

The immune response and its proper regulation by the host is critical for the mounting of a successful defense against invading pathogens and for facilitating healing and repair of injured tissues. Much of the morbidity seen in the ICU, however, is a direct consequence of abnormal regulation of this immune response. The classic example of this maladaptive scenario is the case of septic shock, whereby an overly robust proinflammatory response causes far more tissue damage than the original infection that initiated it. At the same time, it is important to appreciate that pathology also occurs when the pendulum swings in the other direction. It is intuitive that children with underactive immune systems as the result of chemotherapy or treatment with immunosuppressive medications are at high risk for the development of infectious complications. Perhaps less intuitive is the notion that an overactive endogenous compensatory anti-inflammatory immune response can follow a proinflammatory insult and can result in significant morbidity and mortality *without* the influence of exogenous immunosuppressants.

The cytokines tumor necrosis factor (TNF)-α, IL-1β, and interferon (IFN)-γ are pro-inflammatory cytokines released by innate immune cells (TNF-α, IL-1β) and lymphocytes (IFN-γ) in response to an inflammatory stimulus. The signaling pathways associated with the production of proinflammatory cytokines in immune cells include the mitogen-activated protein kinase and NFκB pathways. The cytokine that has been most reliably associated with adverse outcomes in the setting of proinflammatory disease is IL-6, likely because IL-6 is released in response to more potent proinflammatory cytokines and, therefore, serves as a *marker* for inflammation. IL-6, while an inducer of the acute phase response, has significant anti-inflammatory properties of its own. More potent anti-inflammatory cytokines, produced by both innate and adaptive immune cells, include IL-10 and transforming growth factor (TGF)-β. Innate immune cells include neutrophils, monocytes, macrophages, and dendritic cells, while adaptive immune cells include T and B lymphocytes.

The classic signs and symptoms of severe septic disease, including fever, altered vascular tone, and increased capillary permeability, are largely the result of the effects of pro-inflammatory cytokines rather than the offending pathogen itself.

Multiple studies have investigated attacking the inflammatory pathways. It should be noted that significant overlap exists between the inflammatory and hemostatic pathways. Activated protein C (APC) is an endogenous protein with anti-thrombotic, profibrinolytic, and anti-inflammatory properties. Recombinant human (rh) APC (rhAPC) has recently been studied in adults and children who had severe sepsis, with mixed results. In the subset of adults with the most severe illness (APACHE II scores ≥ 25 or ≥ 2 organ failure *and* an absence of risk factors for severe bleeding, including recent surgery), rhAPC was shown to significantly reduce mortality, compared to placebo. The pediatric phase III trial that followed, with resolution of organ failure as the primary outcome variable, was stopped at its planned interim analysis for lack of efficacy. No widely accepted indication currently exists for the use of rhAPC in pediatric septic disease.

It was once thought that methylprednisolone or dexamethasone would, by virtue of their anti-inflammatory properties, have beneficial effects in the setting of the proinflammatory storm of sepsis. Two meta-analyses published in the mid-1990s concluded that the use of these drugs was associated with an *increased* risk of mortality from sepsis in adults. Two more recent meta-analyses demonstrated a survival *benefit* associated with the use of a 5–7-day course of low-dose hydrocortisone (200–300 mg/day) in adults with severe sepsis or septic shock. The benefits of hydrocortisone are likely due to the fact that it has far less glucocorticoid (immunosuppressive) activity and far more mineralocorticoid (hemodynamic supporting) activity than either methylprednisolone or dexamethasone (**Table 54.1**).

Another approach to the restoration of immunologic homeostasis is the bulk removal of inflammatory mediators through hemofiltration, membrane adsorption, plasmapheresis, or plasma exchange. An advantage of most of these techniques is that no single mediator is targeted; rather, large concentrations of cytokines can be removed at once. Disadvantages include the need for dedicated large-bore IV access, exposure to blood products (plasma exchange), and the likely need for relatively long-term therapy. In fact, most prospective studies of extracorporeal therapies in sepsis have been small, involved short-term treatment (1–2 days) and have been largely

TABLE 54.1

RELATIVE POTENCIES OF CORTICOSTEROIDS

Drug	Anti-inflammatory (immunosuppressive)	Mineralocorticoid
Dexamethasone	30	0
Methylprednisolone	5	1
Hydrocortisone	1	5

unsuccessful in demonstrating improved outcomes. Of these therapies, plasmapheresis and plasma exchange have shown the most promise in prospective trials, perhaps because plasma exchange involves the replacement of patient plasma with donor plasma, thereby both removing unwanted mediators and replacing potentially deficient ones.

Reduction of inflammation and inhibition of the fibroproliferative phase of acute respiratory distress syndrome (ARDS) seem to be reasonable therapeutic goals in the management of this syndrome. While the use of glucocorticoids in patients without infection who have unresolving ARDS is still defensible (particularly in the second week of illness), the practice is currently being viewed with considerable equipoise. To date, no studies have been performed to address this question in the pediatric population.

Exposure of leukocytes and complement to the tubing and membranes associated with extracorporeal procedures, including cardiopulmonary bypass (CPB), is known to induce a potent proinflammatory response. The administration of glucocorticoids to the patient and/or bypass pump has been shown to reduce neutrophil activation and proinflammatory cytokine release. The serine protease inhibitor aprotinin is frequently used to mitigate postoperative bleeding after CPB. Aprotinin has also been shown to reduce proinflammatory cytokine production after bypass, with a potentially synergistic effect with glucocorticoids, although its use is being scrutinized. Attempts to effect bulk removal of proinflammatory cytokines through modified ultrafiltration during CPB have yielded variable results.

Major inflammatory insults typically result in a compensatory anti-inflammatory response syndrome characterized by reduction in cell-surface marker expression on innate immune cells and increased production of anti-inflammatory cytokines, including IL-10 (**Fig. 54.1**). *Immunoparalysis*, has been quantified in 2 major ways. First, surface expression of the class II major histocompatibility complex molecule HLA-DR, important in antigen presentation, has been shown to be reduced in circulating monocytes from patients with compensatory anti-inflammatory response syndrome. Severe reduction in HLA-DR expression, such that <30% of circulating monocytes are strongly HLA-DR+ by flow cytometry, is characteristic of immunoparalysis. A more functional measure of innate immune capability is the ex vivo LPS-induced TNF-α production assay. In this test, an aliquot of whole blood is incubated with a standard concentration of LPS and TNF-α production

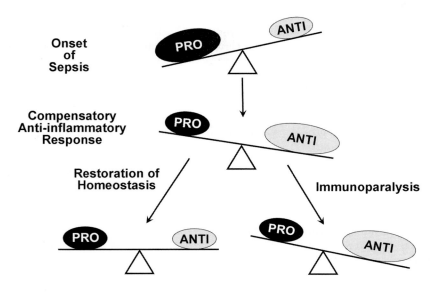

FIGURE 54.1. Schematic of the development of immunoparalysis following a proinflammatory insult.

TABLE 54.2

COMMONLY USED NON–ANTIBODY-BASED IMMUNOSUPPRESSIVE AGENTS

Class	Drug	Target	Nonimmune toxicities
Glucocorticoids	Methylprednisolone Dexamethasone Prednisone	Inhibition of proinflammatory and cell-proliferation gene transcription in lymphocytes and other immune cells	Hypertension, hyperglycemia, impaired wound healing, neuromuscular weakness, growth impairment
Calcineurin inhibitors	Tacrolimus (FK506) Cyclosporine A (CsA)	Inhibition of T cell signaling pathways	Nephrotoxicity, CNS toxicity (including seizures), tremor, hypertension, hyperglycemia (FK506), hirsutism (CsA)
TOR protein kinase inhibitor	Sirolimus	Inhibition of T and B cell proliferation	Hyperlipidemia, hypertension, thrombocytopenia, rash
Antimetabolite	Azathioprine Mycophenolate mofetil	Purine synthesis inhibition	Bone marrow suppression, diarrhea, cholestasis

is measured in the supernatant. When immunoparalysis exists, there is a skewing toward a Th-2-like immune phenotype with high levels of circulating IL-10. Immunoparalysis has also been reported in the context of post-transplantation immunosuppressive regimens. The laboratory measures of immunoparalysis described above represent evidence that some patients' compensatory anti-inflammatory response, while initially an adaptive attempt to restore immunologic homeostasis, can progress to a maladaptive state, which can be thought of as a type of secondary immunodeficiency. It appears that the duration of immunoparalysis is crucial. Transient immunoparalysis for only 1 or 2 days is well tolerated. If severe, innate immune dysfunction persists for as little as 3–5 days, however, numerous prospective reports have shown an association with the development of secondary infection and death in adult and pediatric critical illness. In 2005, improved monocyte function and enhanced clearance of infection were demonstrated in a prospective, randomized, controlled trial of GM-CSF in 40 non-neutropenic septic adults. Across-the-board administration of immunostimulating agents to critically ill patients is unlikely to yield improvements in outcomes. It is quite likely that the most benefit from IFNγ or GM-CSF therapy, for example, would be seen in the subpopulation of patients with immunoparalysis. To give these agents to a child with a robust innate immune response could conceivably be harmful. Unfortunately, no overt marker of immunoparalysis can be detected on the basis of physical exam or blood counts. It is, therefore, critically important that standardized assays of innate immune function be employed to survey for immunoparalysis and target patients who may benefit from inclu-

sion in prospective trials of immunostimulatory agents.

Impairment of immune function in the ICU is frequently the result of overt iatrogenic or endogenous inhibition of the immune response. Immunosuppressive medications continue to be the mainstay of treatment for children with cancer, transplantation, autoimmunity, and other chronic inflammatory diseases (**Table 54.2**). Accordingly, these patients are known to be at high risk for morbidity and mortality due to infection complications. Similarly, children with primary (congenital) and secondarily acquired (e.g., HIV) immunodeficiencies pose a management challenge for the ICU practitioner. An overarching principle in the care of children with overt immunodeficiency is to remove the offending immunosuppressive agent whenever possible and/or to administer the appropriate immunologic supplementation to the deficient child. Obvious examples of this principle include the withholding of chemotherapy from a child with sepsis and the administration of IV immunoglobulin (IVIG) to a hypogammaglobulinemic child.

THE NEUTROPENIC PATIENT

Severe, prolonged neutropenia most commonly results from the administration of myelosuppressive chemotherapy in the context of cancer treatment but can also be seen with infection-induced marrow failure and as an unintended side effect of numerous drugs, including antibiotics. Absolute neutrophil count of <500 cells/mm^3 is associated with increased incidence of sepsis and death in patients with malignancy. Prophylaxis against Pneumocystis pneumonia and candidal infections with trimethoprim/sulfamethoxazole and fluconazole, respectively, should be considered in this population when patients are critically ill. Use of the drug granulocyte colony-stimulating factor (GCSF) has become the standard of care in the treatment of cancer patients with fever and neutropenia. Administration of GCSF results in increased myelopoiesis and neutrophil maturation. The National Comprehensive Cancer Network now advocates the use of a colony-stimulating factor in patients with a 20% risk of developing this condition. Another therapeutic option for the treatment of severely neutropenic children with life-threatening infection is the administration of donor leukocytes via granulocyte transfusion. Donor leukocytes can induce a potent proinflammatory response following infusion. A 2005 Cochrane Database meta-analysis concluded that evidence to support or contraindicate the use of granulocyte transfusion therapy is inconclusive, but subgroup analysis suggested that patients who received $>1 \times 10^{10}$ cells per dose fared better than those receiving lower doses.

THE LYMPHOPENIC PATIENT

Lymphopenia frequently accompanies critical illness and has been associated with increased risk of death in the settings of adult sepsis and pediatric multiorgan dysfunction syndrome. It is especially important to note that the definition of lymphopenia varies by age, with infants and toddlers requiring more robust lymphocyte numbers to remain immunocompetent (**Table 54.3**). Causes of lymphopenia in the PICU include drug-related marrow failure (including chemotherapy), infection-induced bone marrow suppression, HIV infection, and lymphocyte loss via chylothorax drainage. One potential consequence of lymphocyte depletion is a lack of antibody production by B cells. Assessment of quantitative immunoglobulin levels can identify patients with hypogammaglobulinemia who may benefit from replacement with IVIG. While the role of IVIG in the empiric management of critical illness in the *absence* of low IgG levels is somewhat controversial. It is noteworthy that many therapies commonly used in the practice of critical care medicine may themselves promote or exacerbate lymphopenia. Glucocorticoids, for example, are potent inducers of lymphocyte apoptosis. Dopamine use is associated with the development of lymphopenia, presumably through its inhibitory effect on the neuroendocrine axes, most notably prolactin, which is known to be a necessary growth factor for lymphocytes. Other vasoactive agents should be considered instead of dopamine.

THE TRANSPLANT PATIENT

Patients who have undergone transplantation are placed in the double bind of taking medicines that place them at high risk for the development of infection, without which they are likely to reject their allograft. Multidrug regimens, including calcineurin inhibitors, corticosteroids and other immunosuppressives (e.g., mycophenolate or azathioprine), are frequently employed to shut down the adaptive immune response against the transplanted organ, often with significant systemic toxicities. The suppressive effects of these regimens are not limited to the adaptive immune response and inhibit the innate response as well, with reductions in monocyte function associated directly or indirectly with calcineurin inhibition. Lastly, most transplantation regimens rely on plasma drug levels and end-organ toxicity to drive dose titration rather than on direct measures of immune function. Several strategies can be employed to promote improved outcomes in the transplant patient with critical illness. First, antimicrobial prophylaxis is crucial for the prevention of secondary infection. Perhaps the most comprehensive set of recommendations in this regard comes from the Centers for Disease Control Guidelines for Preventing Opportunistic Infection in Hematopoietic Stem Cell Transplant Recipients (**Table 54.4**). Second, the use of antibody-based immunosuppressive regimens, including anti–IL-2 receptor antibodies, has been shown to be an effective anti-rejection strategy without the systemic toxicity profiles of drugs, such as cyclosporine and tacrolimus. Lastly, the ICU practitioner can rapidly taper the exogenous immunosuppression to allow for a more robust immune response in the setting of suspected or proven infection. A major impediment to the optimal titration of immunosuppressive therapy in transplant patients is the reliance on drug levels as the primary indicator of immunosuppression. While plasma tacrolimus levels of <10 ng/mL and cyclosporine A levels of <200 ng/mL can be generally thought of as mildly-to-moderately

TABLE 54.3

CENTERS FOR DISEASE CONTROL DEFINITIONS OF SEVERE REDUCTIONS IN CD4+ COUNT IN CHILDREN

Age	CD4+ count (cells/mm^3)
<1 year	<750
1–5 years	<500
6–12 years	<200

Adapted from MMWR *Recomm Rep* 1995;44(RR-4):1–11.

TABLE 54.4

ROUTINE PREVENTIVE REGIMENS FOR PEDIATRIC HEMATOPOIETIC STEM CELL TRANSPLANT RECIPIENTS

Infection	Indication	First-line drug
Bacterial infections	Severe hypogammaglobulinemia (serum IgG level <400 mg/dL) at <100 days after transplant	IVIG 400 mg/kg/mo (or as needed to keep IgG level >400 mg/dL)
Candida species	Allogeneic recipients or high-risk autologous recipients from transplant to engraftment or until 7 days after ANC >1000 cells/mm^3	Fluconazole 3–6 mg/kg/day PO or IV (6 mo–13 yrs); or 400 mg PO or IV daily (>13 yrs). Max dose 600 mg/day
Cytomegalovirus	All patients from engraftment through day 100	Ganciclovir 5 mg/kg/dose IV every 12 hrs for 5–7 days, followed by 5 mg/kg/dose IV daily for 5 days/week
Pneumocystis jirovecii pneumonia	Allogeneic recipients or high-risk autologous recipients until 6 months post-transplant (longer if immunosuppression continued or GVHD)	Trimethoprim/sulfamethoxazole (TMP/SMX; 150 mg TMP/ 750 mg SMX) PO twice daily 3 times weekly. [Alternative regimens available; see MMWR *Recomm. Rep* 2000;49(RR10):1–128.]
Herpes simplex virus	Seropositive patients from the beginning of conditioning therapy until engraftment	Acyclovir 250 mg/m^2/dose IV every 8 hrs or 125 mg/m^2/dose IV every 6 hrs
Varicella zoster virus	Post-exposure prophylaxis in actively immunosuppressed patients	Varicella-zoster immunoglobulin 125 units/10 kg body weight IM (max dose 625 units)
Methicillin-resistant *Staphylococcus aureus*	Known MRSA carriers	Mupirocin calcium ointment 2% to nares twice daily for 5 days or to wounds daily for 2 weeks

Recommendations include vaccination against influenza, respiratory syncytial virus, *Streptococcus pneumoniae*, and *Haemophilus influenzae* type b.
IgG, immunoglobulin G; IVIG, IV immunoglobulin; ANC, absolute neutrophil count; GVHD, graft-versus-host disease; IM, intramuscularly; MRSA, methicillin-resistant *Staphylococcus aureus*
Adapted from MMWR *Recomm. Rep* 2000;49(RR10):1–128.

immunosuppressive, functional assays of the immune response, such as ex vivo LPS-induced TNF-α production capacity, have the potential to serve as more relevant targets for titration of these potent drugs.

IV IMMUNOGLOBULIN

A meta-analysis of IVIG use for the treatment of suspected or proven infection in critically ill neonates showed no effect on mortality with empiric use. It did show, however, that mortality risk was lowered when IVIG was used in the setting of proven infection. A 2004 meta-analysis of high-quality adult studies failed to show a reduction mortality risk when IVIG was empirically used in the treatment of sepsis. However, in a 2005, prospective, randomized, controlled trial in children <2 years of age with sep-

sis, 3 days of polyclonal IVIG treatment resulted in improved survival to discharge and in shorter durations of PICU stay. Interestingly, it appears that IVIG may be of particular benefit in the setting of severe invasive group A strep infection. A subset of IVIG trials has employed a product that is enriched in the IgM fraction of immunoglobulin. Evidence suggests that IgM-enriched IVIG may be beneficial in postoperative sepsis in adult patients, though a multicentered, randomized, controlled trial failed to show benefit in the setting of chemotherapy-induced neutropenic sepsis.

IMMUNONUTRITION

Another approach that has been taken to effect immunomodulation in the ICU is through

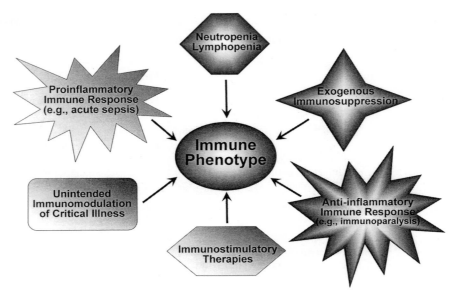

FIGURE 54.2. The patient's overall immune phenotype is determined by the net effects of pro-inflammatory and anti-inflammatory forces acting to influence the inflammatory balance. Many of these forces are occult, necessitating immune monitoring.

immunonutrition. With this strategy, patients are provided with nutritional supplementation that, in the course of metabolism, has an effect on the immune response. The 2 substrates that have been the focus of the most investigation are the n-3 polyunsaturated fatty acids (PUFA) and the amino acid arginine. The n-3 PUFAs, including docosahexaenoic, eicosapentaenoic, and α-linoleic acid, are thought to promote an anti-inflammatory immune state through at least 2 mechanisms. Arginine is thought to promote a more vigorous immune response through augmentation of intracellular killing and lymphocyte function. A 2001 meta-analysis of 22 studies in critically ill adults concluded that arginine supplementation resulted in *higher* mortality in treated patients, though its use was associated with a lower overall infection rate. More recent studies have explored the use of combined formulas, including both n-3 PUFAs, arginine, and other supplements, in critically ill adults and children.

THE IMPACT OF CRITICAL ILLNESS ON INFLAMMATION

In addition to overt immunosuppression with drugs (e.g., tacrolimus) and endogenous phenomena (e.g., immunoparalysis), other drugs routinely used in the ICU have profound immunologic effects. Catecholamines, for example, can enhance (α receptors) or inhibit (β receptors) the immune response. Bacteriocidal antibiotics can transiently exacerbate the inflammatory response due to release of bacterial components at the time of cell death. Conversely, β-lactams can lead to immunodeficiency through bone marrow suppression, while macrolides are known to impair proinflammatory cytokine production. Opioids are inducers of lymphocyte and macrophage apoptosis and can induce the anti-inflammatory cytokine TGF-β. Insulin is thought to have significant anti-inflammatory properties both through reduction of hyperglycemia-induced proinflammatory cytokine production and through direct inhibition of the NFκB pathway. Even furosemide is thought to be immunologically active, resulting in attenuation of the inflammatory response in mononuclear cells.

Hepatic failure, with its associated impairment of cytokine clearance, is frequently associated with a proinflammatory state. Uremic plasma from patients with renal failure has been shown to induce apoptosis in innate and adaptive immune cells. Hyperglycemia, the control of which is now the target of prospective clinical trials in the PICU, has been clearly shown to be a potent activator of the NFκB pathway in innate immune cells. Conversely, the endogenous stress-induced cortisol response, though less immunosuppressive than some exogenous glucocorticoids, inhibits proinflammatory cytokine production in leukocytes (**Fig. 54.2**).

Perhaps the most important method of immunomodulation is that achieved through immunization. Prevention of disease, rather than its treatment, should continue to be the highest goal of the medical community. We should therefore continue to advocate for routine immunization against organisms such as *Haemophilus influenzae*, *Streptococcus pneumoniae*, and *Neisseria meningitis*. Similarly, high-risk children should receive prophylaxis against respiratory syncytial virus and influenza.

CHAPTER 55 ■ IMMUNOLOGY OF CANCER AND PRIMARY IMMUNE DEFICIENCY SYNDROMES

BRANDT P. GROH • JENNIFER A. McARTHUR • SACHIN S. JOGAL • ROBERT F. TAMBURRO

The clinical features common to the majority of congenital immune deficiencies are presented in **Tables 55.1** and **55.2**. Defects predominantly affecting antibody production and function include isolated immunoglobulin (Ig) M deficiency, isolated IgA deficiency, and IgG subclass deficiencies. Antibody defects predispose patients to sinopulmonary infections with encapsulated organisms, such as Streptococcus pneumoniae (S. pneumoniae) and *Haemophilus influenzae*. The patient who presents with a severe pneumonia that has been poorly responsive to antibiotic therapy deserves quantitative assessment of immunoglobulin levels.

X-LINKED AGAMMAGLOBULINEMIA

Infection symptoms peak at ~7 months of age, and the majority present between 3 and 5 years of age. A presentation with recurrent and refractory sinopulmonary infections is the rule, usually involving extracellular pyogenic bacteria, such as pneumococci, streptococci, meningococci, *H. influenzae*, and *Pseudomonas aeruginosa*. Infections with fungal pathogens and even *Pneumocystis jiroveci* (formerly *Pneumocystis carinii*) are occasionally reported. In addition, children with X-linked agammaglobulinemia (XLA) have a unique susceptibility to enteroviral infections. Recognition of hypoplastic lymphoid tissue in the setting of invasive infection should heighten suspicion of a disorder such as XLA. Mature B cells, which comprise the bulk of tonsillar and lymphoid follicular tissue, are virtually absent from the circulation. Plasma cells and immunoglobulins are consequently also lacking, such that immunoglobulin levels are <10% of normal and antigen specific responses cannot be demonstrated. An early clue to immunoglobulin deficiency is the finding of a low total protein level in the presence of a normal albumin level on routine blood analysis, as gammaglobulin comprises the largest fraction of the total protein measurement. The absence of mature B cells in the peripheral blood, demonstrated by flow cytometry analysis of B-cell surface markers (CD19 and/or CD20) in the presence of normal T-cell numbers, is virtually diagnostic of XLA in a male. The finding of protein antigen unresponsiveness by specific titers to diphtheria and tetanus toxoid after vaccination in conjunction with normal T-cell function (demonstrated by delayed-type hypersensitivity testing or lymphocyte proliferation assays), lends additional diagnostic certainty such that genotyping is not necessary in the majority of cases.

Therapy has evolved from intramuscular gammaglobulin replacement to IV replacement to the relatively new option of subcutaneous replacement. In the intensive care setting, gammaglobulin replacement therapy can be helpful in the control and clearance of severe infections, and IV administration at physiologic replacement doses of 400–500 mg/kg is most appropriate. Concurrent IgA deficiency mandates the use of IgA-depleted IV immunoglobulin (IVIG) to minimize the risk of anaphylaxis. Children with a known diagnosis of IgG deficiency may benefit from supplementary gammaglobulin at the time of infection. In spite of consistent IgG replacement therapy, a significant proportion of XLA patients' progress to bronchiectasis, and chronic antibiotic therapy is recommended for this subset of patients.

TABLE 55.1

CLINICAL FEATURES COMMON IN IMMUNODEFICIENCY

Usually present
Recurrent upper respiratory infections
Severe bacterial infections
Persistent infections with incomplete or no response to therapy

Often present
Failure to thrive or growth retardation
Paucity of lymph nodes and tonsils
Infections with unusual organisms
Skin lesions (e.g., rash, telangiectasias, abscesses, warts)
Recalcitrant thrush
Clubbing
Diarrhea and malabsorption
Persistent sinusitis, mastoiditis
Recurrent bronchitis, pneumonia
Autoimmune disorders
Hematologic abnormalities (aplastic anemia, hemolytic anemia, neutropenia, thrombocytopenia)

Occasionally present
Weight loss, fevers
Chronic conjunctivitis
Periodontitis
Lymphadenopathy
Hepatosplenomegaly
Severe viral disease
Adverse reaction to vaccines
Bronchiectasis
Urinary tract infections
Delayed umbilical cord separation (>30 days)
Chronic stomatitis
Granulomas
Lymphoid malignancies

From Stiehm ER, Ochs HD, Winkelstein JA. *Immunologic Disorders in Infants and Children*, 5th ed. Philadelphia: Elsevier Saunders, 2004, with permission.

COMMON VARIABLE IMMUNODEFICIENCY

Common variable immunodeficiency (CVID) describes an XLA-like condition with later onset, generally during the second or third decades of life, although earlier presentations may occur throughout the pediatric age range. Total IgG levels in CVID are <2 standard deviations below the mean for age but generally not as low as those found in XLA. Also in contrast to XLA, IgM and IgA levels may be normal. Patients present in a fashion similar to XLA, with recurrent sinopulmonary disease related to encapsulated organisms. Sarcoidosis-like pulmonary granulomas and lymphoid hyperplasia may complicate the interpretation of pulmonary infections. Malabsorp-

tive symptoms should prompt a work-up to exclude *Giardia lamblia* infection and autoimmune enteritis, similar to celiac enteropathy and/or inflammatory bowel disease. Impaired vaccine responses, in particular to diphtheria and tetanus toxoid antigens, are most helpful in defining this disorder. Treatment involves antibody replacement, again with care to use IgA-depleted products in IgA-deficient patients. Patients with granulomatous disease have been treated with corticosteroids and, more recently, with etanercept after careful consideration of malignant and infectious etiologies.

TRANSIENT HYPOGAMMAGLOBULINEMIA OF INFANCY

A number of premature and, occasionally, term infants develop an exaggerated hypogammaglobulinemia at the natural nadir of maternal immunoglobulin between 6 and 9 months of age. While immunoglobulin values in these infants overlap with those of immune-deficient infants, normal antigen responses can eventually be demonstrated, and most of these infants mature to have normal immunologic function. Normalization of IgG levels can be expected at between 2 and 4 years of age. Upper respiratory infections are common in these infants, and only rarely can IVIG use be justified to treat more invasive infections. The occurrence of invasive infections and the need for IVIG therapy should prompt reconsideration of a mild XLA phenotype, early onset CVID, or a combined immunodeficiency.

Hyper-IgM Syndrome

These males generally present in infancy with upper and lower respiratory tract infections. Diarrhea is another common presenting symptom, often associated with *cryptosporidium* infection. Cytopenias, lymphoid hyperplasia, inflammatory bowel disease, and seronegative arthritis are not infrequent manifestations of autoimmune disease in hyper-IgM patients, reflecting T-cell dysfunction. For that reason, many authors classify the hyper-IgM syndrome as a combined immune deficiency. Significant early mortality from chronic liver disease and malignancy has justified trials of stem cell transplantation for these patients.

22q11.2 Deletion Syndrome

Infants with DiGeorge syndrome (DGS) and velocardiofacial syndrome have a characteristic 22q11.2

deletion and frequently manifest T-cell deficiency due to lack of normal thymic development.

Severe Combined Immunodeficiency Disease

Severe combined immunodeficiency disease (SCID) is the prototype of combined immunodeficiencies. Infants usually present in the first month of life with refractory oral candidiasis and persistent viral infections. *P. jiroveci* is a frequent cause of morbidity and mortality in this group of infants. Absolute lymphopenia below 2000 cells/mm^3 is a common laboratory finding, even on cord blood specimens. Flow cytometry will generally indicate very low absolute CD3 or T-cell numbers. Maternal T-cell engraftment, however, may dramatically affect the fetal T-cell population; thus, clinical suspicion of SCID can justify lymphocyte proliferation assays regardless of lymphocyte counts. B cells and NK cells may be present or absent, depending on the specific defect. The intensive care of an infant suspected of or known to have SCID should include strict isolation and the use of only irradiated, cytomegalovirus-negative, and leukocyte-depleted blood products. The infant with SCID may benefit from aggressive antiviral therapies in addition to antibiotics and IVIG. An immunologist or hematologist should be involved early in the care of these infants to facilitate arrangements for HSCT, which remains the most successful therapy for SCID. CID at the less severe end of the spectrum involves variable degrees of T- and B-cell dysfunction.

Wiskott-Aldrich Syndrome

Wiskott-Aldrich syndrome (WAS) is an X-linked disorder that often presents with the classic triad of eczema, thrombocytopenia, and immunodeficiency. Boys present with bleeding within the first year of life, often in the nursery, with bloody diarrhea or prolonged oozing from a circumcision. Platelets in WAS patients are abnormally small and defective, as compared to the relatively large and functionally normal platelets seen in immune thrombocytopenic purpura. Infections often involve encapsulated organisms related to the inability to produce antibodies in response to polysaccharide antigens. IgM levels are typically low, as reflected by low isohemagglutinin (blood group) antibodies. Autoimmune phenomena are common manifestations of T-cell dysfunction in WAS. While IVIG therapy and splenectomy may help to maintain platelet counts and minimize infections, an HLA-matched HSCT from a sibling or from a cord blood bank offers the best chance of long-term survival.

Ataxia Telangiectasia

Patients with ataxia telangiectasia present with delayed ambulation and speech, followed by deterioration of gross and fine motor skills. Cerebellar ataxia and oculocutaneous telangiectasias become evident at ~7 years of age. Frequent pulmonary infections may be related to subtle antibody defects or swallowing dysfunction and aspiration. Deficiencies in both humoral and cellular immunity have been reported.

X-linked Lymphoproliferative Disease

The often life-threatening presentation of X-linked lymphoproliferative disease (XLP), or Duncan disease, represents an abnormal immune response to Epstein-Barr virus (EBV) infection. Classically, patients present with massive lymphadenopathy, hepatic necrosis, and bone marrow failure, much like posttransplant lymphoproliferative disease. The diagnosis of XLP is facilitated by positive EBV serology and, more specifically, blood or tissue polymerase chain reaction assays. Bone marrow examination will often indicate hemophagocytosis. Etoposide and rituximab have proven useful in the therapy of acute lymphoproliferation in patients diagnosed prior to EBV exposure.

Immune Deficiency, Polyendocrinopathy, X-linked Syndrome

The defining clinical characteristics of immune deficiency, polyendocrinopathy, X-linked syndrome are enteropathy, eczematoid rash, and early endocrinopathy, most often, diabetes mellitus. Patients will present prior to diagnosis with a serious infection, usually *Staphylococcus*, *Candida*, or cytomegalovirus. Autoimmune cytopenias and splenomegaly are also frequently noted at presentation. Therapy with sirolimus may be more effective than other forms of immunosuppression for the autoimmune manifestations of this disorder.

Disorders Associated with Primary Neutropenia

Severe congenital neutropenia, also known as Kostmann syndrome, and cyclic neutropenia commonly respond to treatment with granulocyte colony-stimulating factor (GCSF). Patients with severe congenital neutropenia have profound neutropenia (an absolute neutrophil count [ANC] of <500

TABLE 55.2

SUMMARY OF PRIMARY IMMUNE DEFICIENCY DISORDERS

Category	Name	Type of deficiency	Gene	Primary organisms	Usual sites	Treatment	Associated findings
Humoral	1. X-linked agamma-globulinemia	Absent or low levels of all immunoglobulins	BTK	Encapsulated bacteria Enteroviruses	Sinopulmonary GI	IVIG, Antibiotics as needed ? gene therapy	Respiratory failure Bronchiectasis Sepsis, Diarrhea
	2. Common variable immunodeficiency	Low levels of IgG ± low IgA, IgM	ICOS, TACI	Encapsulated bacteria	Sinopulmonary GI	IVIG, Antibiotics as needed	T-cell dysfunction Autoimmunity
	3. Transient hypogam-maglobulinemia	Low levels of immunoglobulins until age 4 years	Unknown	Encapsulated bacteria	Sinopulmonary	None	None
	4. Hyper IgM	Low levels of IgG and IgA Neutropenia	CD154, CD40 AICDA, UNG NEMO	Encapsulated bacteria, PCP Cryptosporidium	Sinopulmonary Lymph nodes GI, Liver	IVIG, Antibiotics as needed TMP-SMX	PCP, autoimmunity Chronic liver disease, Cancer
Cellular	22q11.2 Deletion syndrome (DGS/velocardiofacial syndrome)	Thymic hypoplasia Absence of mature T-cells	T-box 1 (?)	Candida Viruses PCP	MM Skin Lung	Antifungals as needed, TMP-SMX, ? thymic transplant	Congenital heart disease, Hypopara-thyroidism Hypocalcemia
Combined disorders	1. Severe combined immunodeficiency	Dysplastic thymus, low or absent levels of immunoglobulins Lymphopenia	IL2R gamma JAK3, RAG1/2 ZAP-70, PNP ADA, IL-7	Encapsulated bacteria Candida Viruses PCP	Sinopulmonary MM Skin Liver, GI Blood	IVIG, TMP-SMX Antibiotics, Antivirals, Antifungals HSCT ? gene therapy	Fatal without HSCT, enzyme replacement or gene therapy
	2. Wiskott-Aldrich syndrome	Low levels of IgA and IgM, B- and T-cell dysfunction	WASP	Encapsulated bacteria, PCP Candida, Viruses	Sinopulmonary MM Skin	IVIG Antibiotics as needed HSCT	Eczema, Bleeding, Thrombocytopenia HSM, Malignancy Autoimmunity
	3. Ataxia telangiectasia	Low levels of IgA and IgG$_2$ Cutaneous anergy	ATM	Encapsulated bacteria	Sinopulmonary	IVIG Antibiotics as needed	Muscle weakness, Ataxia, Malignancy Telangiectasias
	4. X-linked lympho-proliferative disorder	T- and B-cell dys-function, low immunoglobulins	SH2D1A	EBV	Sinopulmonary Lymph nodes Liver	Rituximab or Etoposide acutely IVIG, HSCT	Lymphadenopathy Hepatic necrosis HLH, Malignancy
	5. Immune deficiency; polyendocrinopathy, X-linked (IPEX)	T-regulatory cell dysfunction	FoxP3	Staph, Gram (-) bacteria, PCP Candida, CMV	Sinopulmonary MM, Skin GI	Steroids, Sirolimus Antibiotics as needed, ? HSCT	Growth failure IDDM, eczema rash Autoimmunity
	6. Immuno-osseous dysplasias	Variable T- and B-cell defects	Unknown	Viral, primarily varicella	Skin Lung	IVIG, Antibiotics as needed, ? HSCT	Autoimmunity
Neutropenia	1. Severe congenital neutropenia	Neutrophil maturation defect	ELA2?	Pyogenic bacteria	Skin, MM Lymph node Blood	GCSF	Agranulocytosis, MDS/AML
	2. Cyclic neutropenia	Neutrophil maturation defect	ELA2?	Pyogenic bacteria	Skin, MM Lymph node	GCSF	Periodic fevers Aphthous ulcers

	Defect	Gene/molecule	Organisms	Sites	Treatment	Features
3. Primary autoimmune neutropenia	Antibody directed against neutrophil	Unknown	Pyogenic bacteria	Sinopulmonary Skin	Antibiotics, TMP-SMX, GCSF	URI, May resolve by age 3
4. Schwachman-Diamond syndrome	Neutropenia, T-, B-, and NK-cell abnormalities	SBDS	Pyogenic bacteria	Sinopulmonary	GCSF Antibiotics as needed	Pancreatic insuffi-Ciency Leukemia Skeletal anomalies Pancytopenia, MDS
Neutrophil dysfunction						
1. LAD-1/LAD-2	Abnormal neutrophil migration	CD18/ Sialyl-Lewis X	Staph species, Gram (-) bacteria, Fungi	Skin, Lymph node, MM Liver, Bone	Antimicrobials HSCT Oral fucose-LAD2	Gingivitis, impaired wound healing, UC separation delayed
2. Hyper-IgE syndrome	Impaired chemotaxis T-, B- cell dysfunction	Unknown	Staph species Strep species	Skin, Lung (abcesses with pneumatoceles)	Staph prophylaxis, Antibiotics as needed, ? IVIG	Skeletal/connective tissue abnormalities Eczema, ↑ eosinophil
3. Chronic granulomatous disease	Oxidative burst and bactericidal activity impaired	gp91phox p-22phox p47-phox p67-phox	Staph species Catalase (+) bacteria Fungi	Sinopulmonary Lung Liver, GI Skin, MM	Antifungal prophylaxis, TMP-SMX, IFN-γ HSCT	Intestinal and bladder obstruction Osteomyelitis, Liver abscesses
4. Chediak-Higashi syndrome	Abnormal degranulation	YST	Pyogenic bacteria	Sinopulmonary Skin	Ascorbic acid, Folate, Antibiotics as needed	Bleeding, albinism, HLH, peripheral neuropathy
Complement						
1. Hereditary angioedema	Low C2, C4 and C1-INH	C1-INH	None	GI, Upper respiratory tract	Steroids, C1-INH replacement, FFP	Abdominal crises Airway obstruction
2. C1, C2, C3, C4	Low component levels	C1, C2, C3, C4	Encapsulated organisms	Skin Blood	Antibiotics as needed	Lupus-like syndrome
3. C5-9	Absent membrane attack complex	C5-9	Meningococci	Blood Meninges	Vaccination, Early antibiotic therapy	Recurrent meningitis
4. Properdin deficiency	Unstable C3 and C5 convertases	PFC	Meningococci	Blood Meninges	Vaccination, Early antibiotic therapy	Recurrent meningitis
5. Mannan binding lectin deficiency	Impaired MASP-activation	MBL	Various bacteria	Sinopulmonary Meninges Blood	Antibiotics as needed	Autoimmunity ↑ SIRS/severity ? Kawasaki disease
Toll-like receptors						
EDA-ID IRAK-4 deficiency	Impaired TLR signaling	NEMO IRAK-4	Gram (+) bacteria	Sinopulmonary Blood	Antibiotics as needed	Recurrent sepsis

BTK, Bruton's tyrosine kinase; GI, gastrointestinal; Ig, immunoglobulin; IVIG, IV immunoglobulin; ICOS, inducible T-cell costimulator gene; TACI, transmembrane activator and calcium-modulating and cyclophilin ligand interactor; AICDA, activation-induced cytidine deaminase; UNG, uracil DNA glycosylase; NEMO, nuclear factor κB essential modulator; PCP, *Pneumocystis jiroveci* pneumonia; MM, mucous membrane; TMP-SMX, trimethoprim-sulfamethoxazole; PNP, polynucleotide phosphorylase; ADA, adenosine deaminase; HSCT, hematopoietic stem cell transplant; WASP, Wiscott-Aldrich syndrome protein; HSM, hepatosplenomegaly; EBV, Epstein-Barr virus; CMV, cytomegalovirus; HLH, hemophagocytic lymphohistiocytosis; IDDM, insulin dependent diabetes mellitus; GCSF, granulocyte colony-stimulating factor; MDS/AML, myelodysplastic syndrome/acute myelocytic leukemia; SBDS, Shwachman Bodian Diamond syndrome; URI, upper respiratory infections; UC, umbilical cord; C1-INH, C1 esterase inhibitor; MBL, binding lectin; SIRS, systemic inflammatory response syndrome; TLR, Toll-like receptor; IRAK, IL-1-receptor-associated kinase.

neutrophils/m^3), and they experience recurrent bacterial infections beginning in the first year of life. Infections are commonly caused by *S. aureus* and *P. aeruginosa*. Cyclic neutropenia is a rare autosomal-dominant (AD) disorder. Patients with cyclic neutropenia experience recurrent episodes of severe neutropenia that last 3–6 days and occur in cycles of every 14–36 days. Although these patients may be asymptomatic, during neutropenic cycles they may develop aphthous ulcers, gingivitis, stomatitis, and cellulitis, and they are at increased risk of mortality from serious infection.

Autoimmune neutropenia may be either primary or secondary. Secondary autoimmune neutropenias are associated with inflammatory diseases, such as rheumatoid arthritis (i.e., Felty syndrome) and systemic lupus erythematosus. Often, these patients will have additional hematologic abnormalities, such as thrombocytopenia and/or hemolytic anemia. Successful treatment and control of the underlying disease is the most effective therapy for the neutropenia.

Primary autoimmune neutropenia most commonly begins in the newborn period and is frequently diagnosed within the first several months of life. These patients have significant neutropenia at presentation, with an ANC often <500–1000 neutrophils/m^3. However, severe infections, such as pneumonia, sepsis, and meningitis, are relatively uncommon. The treatment for patients with a benign form of autoimmune neutropenia may simply be antibiotics as needed to treat infections or antibiotic prophylaxis with such agents as trimethoprim-sulfamethoxazole. For patients with serious infections, GCSF has been found to be beneficial and is considered first-line therapy.

Shwachman-Diamond syndrome is a rare autosomal disorder associated with neutropenia, exocrine pancreatic insufficiency, skeletal abnormalities, recurrent infections, and occasionally, pancytopenia and is caused by a mutation in the gene encoding the Shwachman-Bodian-Diamond syndrome protein. The neutropenia associated with this disorder may be persistent or cyclic. Moreover, in addition to neutropenia, these patients may also have abnormalities of T-cell, B-cell, and NK-cell lymphocytes. GCSF therapy is useful in this condition to reduce the risk of serious infection. These children are at increased risk of myelodysplasia and leukemia independent of the use of GCSF.

Disorders of Neutrophil Function

In addition to disorders associated with an absolute decrease in the number of neutrophils, several conditions have been identified in which neutrophil function is compromised. For example, in leukocyte adhesion disorders, neutrophils are unable to bind appropriately to the endothelial surface, complete diapedesis, and migrate to the site of infection. Leukocyte adhesion deficiency type 1 is caused by genetic mutations encoding CD18, the γ-subunit of the neutrophil adhesion molecule LFA-1. The neutrophils of patients with this disorder are unable to adhere appropriately to the endothelial surface and, therefore, are unable to migrate toward the site of infection. Patients often present with recurrent, severe infections and may have a history of delayed umbilical cord separation.

Hyper-IgE syndrome (HIES or Job syndrome) is an immunodeficiency characterized by recurrent staphylococcal infections, eczema, recurrent respiratory infections with persistent pneumatoceles, elevated IgE levels, eosinophilia, abnormal cytokine and chemokine expression, and T-cell dysfunction. Neutrophil chemotaxis may be impaired in some patients. Patients have been described as having coarse facial features, joint hyperextensibility, osteopenia and prolonged retention of primary teeth, but the features may be quite variable. The only treatment known to be of clear benefit is antibiotic prophylaxis against staphylococcal infections though IVIG may be of benefit in individual patients.

Chronic granulomatous disease (CGD) is caused by a mutation in any of the 4 structural genes of the NADPH oxidase apparatus. The majority of cases are inherited in an X-linked recessive manner, while the others are autosomal recessive (AR). The disease is characterized by recurrent infections of the skin, lungs, and liver, as well as by excessive granuloma formation that can obstruct the gastrointestinal or genitourinary tract. Most infections are caused by *S. aureus*, *Burkholderia cepacia*, *Aspergillus* species, *Nocardia* species, and *Serratia marcescens*. *S. aureus* liver abscesses are highly suspicious for the diagnosis of CGD. Patients with CGD are most susceptible to catalase-positive micro-organisms. The diagnosis of CGD can be made by laboratory tests that analyze superoxide formation, such as the nitroblue tetrazolium test, or by flow cytometry with dihydrorhodamine dye. Patients with CGD are commonly treated with the prophylactic antimicrobials trimethoprim-sulfamethoxazole and itraconazole to prevent bacterial and fungal infections, respectively. Severe glucose-6-phosphate dehydrogenase deficiency and myeloperoxidase deficiency, both of which present with a milder phenotype of CGD.

Immunodeficiencies may also result from defective formation of neutrophil granules. Chediak-Higashi syndrome, an AR disorder, is the best characterized of these disorders. Neutrophils from these patients have impaired chemotaxis, and they are characterized by large perinuclear granules. In addition, elastase and cathepsin G may be absent from their neutrophil granules. Patients with Chediak-Higashi disease have abnormalities in both the hematologic and neurologic systems. Clinical features include recurrent bacterial infections, peripheral nerve disorders, mental retardation, autonomic dysfunction, partial albinism, silver-colored hair, and platelet dysfunction.

COMPLEMENT DEFICIENCY

The complement system is a key component of innate immunity, acting to protect the host from microorganisms. Complement may be activated via 3 distinct pathways, all of which require activation of the complement protein C3 (**Fig. 55.1**). Strict control of the complement system is essential to prevent complement-mediated destruction of host tissues. C1 esterase inhibitor (C1-INH) is a glycoprotein that recognizes and inactivates activated C1r and C1s. Because it is consumed during the process of inactivation, high levels of C1 inhibitor must be produced, requiring the activation of 2 gene sites. In fact, deficiency of C1-INH results in hereditary angioedema. Hereditary angioedema is a rare AD disorder which presents with recurrent episodes of subcutaneous or submucosal angioedema that

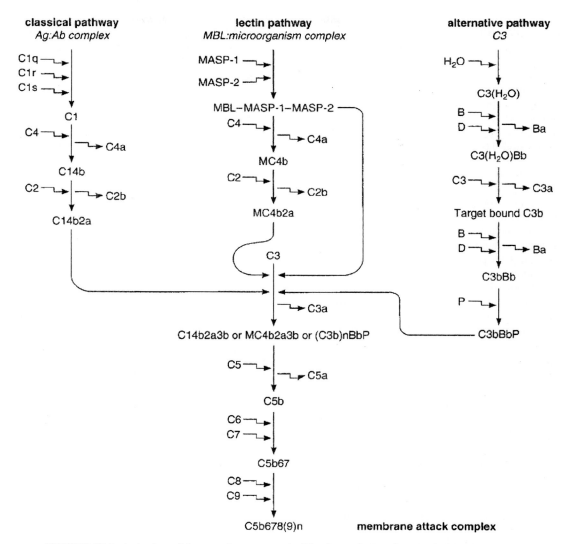

FIGURE 55.1. Activation of the complement cascade. The figure depicts the complement components involved in activation of the three pathways of the complement cascade. From Cunnion KM, Wagner E, Frank MM. Complement & Kinin. In: Parslow TG, Stites DP, Terr AI, et al., eds. *Medical Immunology*. New York: McGraw-Hill, 2001:175–88, with permission.

primarily affects the upper respiratory or gastrointestinal tracts. Clinical manifestations of this edema include limb swelling, painful abdominal crises, and life-threatening airway obstruction. The edema generally persists for 1–5 days. Analysis of C1-INH levels, both antigenic and functional, are most commonly used to establish the diagnosis. Analysis of C1q levels can help to differentiate between hereditary and acquired angioedema. The scenario in which the critical care provider is most likely to encounter hereditary angioedema is in the setting of acute laryngeal edema causing upper airway obstruction or with intestinal obstruction. Treatment options include antifibrinolytic agents, C1-INH-concentrate infusions, and fresh-frozen plasma, if C1-INH is not available.

An increased susceptibility to invasive infection is a prominent feature of many patients with inherited complement deficiencies. Although complement protects against a variety of pathogens, patients with complement deficiency are most susceptible to bacterial infections. Moreover, the specific type of infection tends to be associated with the component of the complement cascade that is deficient. *Neisseria meningitides* is the most common pathogen among patients with X-linked properdin deficiency. Vaccination with the tetravalent meningococcal vaccine may be particularly important for properdin-deficient patients. In addition to an increased susceptibility to infections, complement-deficient patients are at increased risk for rheumatologic disorders, most notably, systemic lupus erythematosus.

MBL is a soluble pathogen-recognizing molecule that is capable of binding to microbes and activating complement via MASPs. Low levels of MBL have been reported in children deficient in opsonizing activity and with increased susceptibility to infection. Among critically ill patients, MBL deficiency appears to increase susceptibility to sepsis and septic shock.

TOLL-LIKE RECEPTORS

Impaired toll-like receptor (TLR) signaling has been reported to be associated with immunodeficiency. TLRs are surface and intracellular pattern recognition receptors critical to the identification of invading microbes by recognizing the PAMPs of the microorganisms. The TLR–PAMP interaction triggers a complex signaling cascade that ultimately results in the activation of NFκB and activated protein-1. X-linked anhidrotic ectodermal dysplasia with immunodeficiency is caused by mutations in the NEMO gene. These patients may present with ab-

sent or conical teeth, dry skin due to absence or decreased number of eccrine sweat glands, and hypohidrosis with sparse scalp and eyebrow hair due to abnormal development of ectoderm-derived structures. In addition, these children experience an increased susceptibility to a wide variety of severe infections.

HEMOPHAGOCYTIC LYMPHOHISTIOCYTOSIS AND MACROPHAGE ACTIVATION SYNDROME

Hemophagocytic lymphohistiocytosis (HLH) and macrophage activation syndrome (MAS) comprise a spectrum of disorders related to defective NK cells or cytotoxic T cells. Both disorders have similar clinical features. MAS is typically seen in patients with autoimmune disease and often resolves with aggressive treatment of the underlying autoimmune disorder. HLH requires much more aggressive therapy, often including HSCT. Familial forms of HLH may also be associated with an immunodeficiency, most notably Chediak-Higashi syndrome, Griscelli syndrome type 2, and XLP. Although acquired HLH is usually associated with infections, it may also occur with malignancy, inborn errors of metabolism, and after HSCT. Patients with HLH typically present with high and prolonged fevers associated with hepatosplenomegaly. Neurologic symptoms, a rash, and lymphadenopathy may also occur. An infectious source may or may not be found. The infections typically associated with HLH are viruses, especially EBV, but bacteria and protozoa have also been described as triggering agents. Corticosteroids are used to help decrease cytokine and chemokine production. Cyclosporine A is used for its ability to inhibit activation of T lymphocytes. Etoposide is used for its toxicity to monocytes and histiocytes.

MAS has the same clinical presentation as HLH, but MAS is more responsive to immunosuppressive therapies. MAS presents in patients with systemic onset juvenile idiopathic arthritis (SOJIA), as well as in the context of several other connective tissue and autoinflammatory diseases. Management of MAS involves withdrawal of potentially hepatotoxic medications, including nonsteroidal anti-inflammatory medications, administration of high-dose pulse corticosteroids (methylprednisolone 30 mg/kg, maximum 1 g/day), and additional treatment with cyclosporine A for rapidly progressive and refractory cases. A decrease in platelet count combined with a coagulopathy similar to disseminated intravascular coagulopathy and hepatic dysfunction form a very sensitive and specific triad of the diagnosis of MAS. Clinical criteria, which are less specific, include CNS dysfunction, evidence of hemorrhage, and hepatomegaly. The demonstration of hemophagocytosis is not required for diagnosis, but hemophagocytosis in a bone marrow aspirate from a patient with SOJIA is virtually diagnostic of MAS.

IMMUNODEFICIENCY AND CANCER PREDISPOSITION

Several inherited immunodeficiency disorders have an increased risk of cancer, including WAS, ataxia telangiectasia, SCID, Kostmann syndrome, and XLP. In addition, patients with acquired immunodeficiencies, such as those with the acquired immunodeficiency syndrome and those receiving immunosuppressive therapy following organ transplantation, also have an increased susceptibility to cancer. This association of immunodeficiency with a predisposition to cancer suggests that an intact immune system provides a surveillance mechanism to eliminate transformed cancer cells from the body.

IMMUNE DYSFUNCTION ASSOCIATED WITH HEMATOPOIETIC STEM CELL TRANSPLANT

Immunosuppression is common with most antineoplastic therapy; however, it would appear to be most severe in the setting of allogeneic HSCT, owing primarily to the fact that the process requires the near-complete replacement of the host lymphohematopoietic system. For replacement to successfully occur, intense immunosuppression of the host is required—a host who is likely immunocompromised as a result of underlying disease and previous therapy. Thus, HSCT patients will be profoundly immunocompromised until effective immune reconstitution occurs. Immune reconstitution, however, is a complex and prolonged process. In fact, although neutrophil engraftment may occur early in the posttransplant period, complete immune reconstitution requires months to years. B-cell recovery tends to occur before T-cell reconstitution. Graft-versus-host disease (GVHD) is particularly detrimental to immune reconstitution. The process is directly toxic to the thymic microenvironment. GVHD may also impair negative selection of T cells that react to host antigens.

CHAPTER 56 ■ PRINCIPLES OF ANTIMICROBIAL THERAPY

PHILIP TOLTZIS • JEFFREY L. BLUMER

Three categories of infected patients are typically found in the PICU (**Table 56.1**). Therapeutics is the discipline within pharmacology dealing with the use of drugs in the prevention or treatment of disease. From a pharmacologic perspective, three key determinants of effective therapy exist: pharmacokinetics, pharmacodynamics, and pharmaceutics (**Fig. 56.1**). A number of procedures are available for testing the in vitro susceptibility of various microorganisms to anti-infective drugs. These procedures have

been well established for bacteria, less so for fungi, and poorly developed for other infectious agents. Susceptibility to the antibacterial effects of antibiotics is usually assessed by determining the minimal concentration, of drug required to inhibit bacterial growth, termed the *minimum inhibitory concentration*, or MIC. MIC values provide some indication of the potency of the antibiotic against the infecting bacterial pathogen. Although anti-infective adverse events remain rare, some of the more unusual side effects of

TABLE 56.1

MICROORGANISMS COMMONLY IMPLICATED IN INFECTIONS IN THE PICU

Type of Infection	Microorganisms
Community-acquired	<u>Bacteria:</u> *Streptococcus pneumoniae, Neisseria meningitidis., Staphylococcus aureus, Streptococcus pyogenes, Bordetella pertussis,* group B streptococcus[a], *Listeria*[a], enteric Gram-negative bacilli[a,b], atypical respiratory tract bacteria <u>Viruses:</u> Herpes simplex[a], enterovirus[a], respiratory viruses
Nosocomial	<u>Bacteria:</u> Coagulase-negative staphylococcus, *S. aureus, Enterobacteriaceae, Pseudomonas, Acinetobacter, Nocardia, Clostridium difficile* <u>Fungi:</u> *Candida* <u>Viruses:</u> Respiratory and enteric viruses
Immunocompromised host	<u>Bacteria:</u> Coagulase-negative staphylococcus, *S. aureus,* viridans streptococcus, *Corynebacteria, Enterobacteriaceae, Pseudomonas, Acinetobacter* <u>Fungi:</u> *Candida, Aspergillus,* non-*Aspergillus* molds, *Cryptococcus,* endemic fungi, *Pneumocystis jiroveci* <u>Viruses:</u> Herpesvirus family, adenovirus, respiratory viruses <u>Parasites:</u> Toxoplasma, enteric parasites

[a] Seen in infants <2 months of age.
[b] Primarily associated with urosepsis.

these drugs can assume enormous clinical importance in critically ill infants and children (**Table 56.2**). Four pharmacodynamic issues must be considered: (a) the expected variability in response when the same dose of drug (normalized to body weight) is administered to all patients; (b) the pharmacodynamic variables that are linked to microbiologic effect; (c) the amount of free fraction of drug that reaches the site of infection; and (d) the overarching effect of resistance.

When the pharmacokinetics of antibiotics is studied in healthy infants and children, given a fixed weight-adjusted dose, the results are always characterized by large inter-individual variations in key pharmacokinetic parameter estimates, such as apparent volume of distribution, area under the plasma concentration-versus-time curve (AUC), and clearance. These inter-individual variations, in turn, result in wide ranges in elimination half-life ($t_{1/2}$) and maximum and minimum plasma concentrations (C_{max} and C_{min}). Thus, at a given dose of antibiotic, it is likely that a population of children exists for whom either the peak concentration is too low or the time

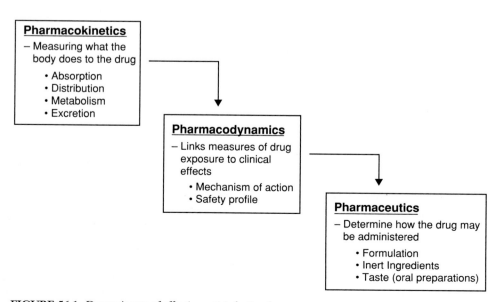

FIGURE 56.1. Determinants of effective anti-infective therapy.

TABLE 56.2

EXAMPLES OF CLINICALLY IMPORTANT UNUSUAL SIDE EFFECTS ASSOCIATED WITH ANTI-INFECTIVE AGENTS

Drug	Adverse event
Aminoglycosides	Apnea; respiratory depression
Thiomethyltetrazole-containing cephalosporins	Hypoprothrombinemia
Carboxypenicillins and acylureidopenicillins	Inhibition of platelet aggregation
Metronidazole	Peripheral neuropathy
Amphotericin	Hyponatremia
Amphotericin	Anemia
Ceftriaxone	Biliary sludge/colic
Carboxy- and acylureidopenicillins	Exacerbation of CHF
Vancomycin	Hypotension 2° histamine release
Ganciclovir, acyclovir	Crystalluria
Sulfonamides, voriconazole	Stevens-Johnson syndrome
Chloramphenicol	Cardiogenic shock
Azoles	Liver failure
Acyclovir	Neutropenia

that the effective concentration remains above the MIC for the suspected or documented pathogen is too short. In each case, in the absence of actually monitoring drug concentrations, a built-in failure rate appears to be associated with the use of "standard" dosing regimens.

The antibiotics in use currently sort themselves into either "time-dependent" or "concentration-dependent" killers. The activity of the first group is determined by the time that the antibiotic concentration at the site of the infection exceeds the MIC for the infecting bacteria (denoted $T > MIC$). For the second group, the functional activity is driven by the relationship between the concentration achieved at the site of the infection relative and the MIC (**Table 56.3**). For both time-dependent and concentration-dependent antibiotics, it is the free form of the drug that is active.

THE PENICILLINS

The β-lactams are bactericidal and have an excellent record for safety. As a result, they are often the first choice for empiric therapy of both hospital- and community-acquired infections. β-lactam antimicrobial agents include the penicillins, cephalosporins, carbapenems, and monobactams. All have a β-lactam ring, with variable rings and side chains. When

bacteria develop resistance to β-lactam antibiotics, it is most often due to their ability to elaborate a β-lactamase enzyme. Some of the enzyme activities involved in this cell wall synthesis are found in a group of proteins called *penicillin-binding proteins* (PBP). As each new penicillin was introduced, bacterial strains rapidly acquired β-lactamases with the ability to hydrolyze them; this was especially a problem among Gram-negative bacteria. A group of β-lactam compounds, many of which were devoid of antibacterial activity, were synthesized as β-lactamase inhibitors (e.g., clavulanic acid). It was found that these could be combined with β-lactam antibiotics, resulting in a combination that was therapeutically active against β-lactamase-producing organisms.

Protein binding varies markedly from a low of ~17% for ampicillin to >90% for nafcillin. Few of these drugs undergo any significant metabolism, though some, including ampicillin, nafcillin, ticarcillin, mezlocillin, and piperacillin, display significant hepatic elimination. However, most excretion is via the kidney. Virtually all of the parenteral penicillins penetrate into the cerebrospinal fluid in concentrations that are adequate to treat meningitis when a meningeal inflammation is present. As with all β-lactam antibiotics, the drug concentrations must remain above the MIC for the infecting organism in order for the drug to be effective. Therefore, parenteral penicillins must be administered on a very

TABLE 56.3

MODE OF ANTIBACTERIAL ACTION: THE PHARMACOKINETIC-PHARMACODYNAMIC INTERFACE

Drug class	Mode of bacterial killing	Pharmacodynamic determinant
β-Lactams Monobactam Carbapenems Linezolid Macrolides Clindamycin	Time-dependent	T > MIC
Aminoglycosides Fluoroquinolones Metronidazole	Concentration-dependent	C_{max}/MIC
Fluoroquinolones Glycopeptides Azithromycin	Concentration- and time-dependences	AUC/MIC

MIC, minimum inhibitory concentration; AUC, area under the plasma concentration-versus-time curve

frequent basis, usually every 4 hrs or by prolonged infusions (e.g., 2–3 hrs) for serious infections.

The major toxic effects associated with the penicillins are allergic reactions. It is often possible to substitute other β-lactam agents for a penicillin with minimal risk of cross-reactivity. Other adverse events include alterations in platelet function by carbenicillin and ticarcillin; interstitial nephritis, noted especially with the penicillinase-resistant antistaphylococcal penicillins; hypokalemia and platelet functional impairment seen with the antipseudomonal and extended spectrum penicillins; and bone marrow suppression, particularly neutropenia, observed with prolonged use of virtually all of the penicillins. The only drug–drug interactions of note is that with probenecid, which competes with the penicillins for renal tubular secretion. This interaction is employed clinically to prolong the elimination half-life of penicillin or ampicillin.

THE CEPHALOSPORINS

Unlike the natural penicillins, the first-generation cephalosporins are active against both Gram-positive and Gram-negative bacteria as well as being acid stable and resistant to β-lactamase hydrolysis by the early β-lactamases. The activity of these agents against Gram-negative rods is somewhat variable. They are most commonly used for surgical prophylaxis and skin and orthopedic infections. Members of this generation include cephalothin and cephalexin.

The second-generation cephalosporins, such as cefuroxime and cefprozil, were synthesized to broaden coverage against respiratory pathogens and to provide some additional Gram-negative activity. For infections of the respiratory tract they possess therapeutic activity against *S. pneumoniae*, *Streptococcus pyogenes*, *Haemophilus influenzae*, and *Moraxella catarrhalis*. The cephamycin group of antibiotics, cefoxitin and cefotetan, are generally less potent than the second-generation cephalosporins against respiratory pathogens but have clinically significant anaerobic activity. The third-generation cephalosporins, including ceftriaxone, cefotaxime, and ceftazidime, have become among the most widely used drugs for the empiric treatment of infants and children with moderate-to-severe infections. They have greatly improved activity against Gram-negative organisms. Unfortunately, with the increased Gram-negative spectrum and potency, these agents have less Gram-positive potency than the first-generation cephalosporins. Ceftazidime is the only member of the group with activity against *Pseudomonas* and has only marginal activity against Gram-positive pathogens. Cefepime is a fourth-generation cephalosporin with Gram-positive potency and Gram-negative spectrum including *P. aeruginosa*. Cephalosporins currently available do not have reliable activity against enterococci, MRSA, coagulase-negative staphylococci, and *Listeria monocytogenes*.

The cephalosporins demonstrate varying degrees of protein binding, ranging from ~10% for cefazolin to >90% for ceftriaxone. By administering ceftriaxone as a single daily dose, an initial bolus of free drug distributes rapidly to tissues due to the saturation of the protein-binding sites, followed by a continual release of active drug from bound reservoirs over 24 hrs. Of the four generations of cephalosporins, only the drugs in the third and fourth generations penetrate into the cerebrospinal fluid reliably so that they can be used to treat bacterial meningitis. Several of the third generation have sufficient biliary excretion to make them useful in the treatment of hepatobiliary infections. Because the elimination of the cephalosporins is mainly renal, renal function necessitates dosing modifications. In addition, because of its high degree of protein binding and related concerns about bilirubin displacement, ceftriaxone is not recommended for the treatment of infants in the first month of life. The cephalosporins are the safest class of antibiotics and perhaps the safest class of drugs available in medicine today. Gastrointestinal side effects are most common. Allergic reactions also occur but are not as frequent as those seen with the penicillins. The cross-reactivity of cephalosporins in patients with documented penicillin allergy is somewhat higher than in the general population. Other adverse reactions that have been associated with cephalosporins include positive Coombs reactions, bone marrow suppression, thrombocytosis, acute tubular necrosis, and mild transaminase elevations; these are all rare. Ceftriaxone has been associated with the formation of biliary sludge in the gallbladder, may lead to cholecystitis. Cefoperazone and cefotetan have been implicated in bleeding due to hypoprothrombinemia.

The cephalosporins are the drugs of choice for the empiric treatment of infants and children with moderate to severe infections. In the newborn period, ampicillin plus cefotaxime has become a standard regimen for the treatment of infants with suspected sepsis and/or meningitis. Ceftriaxone has become the standard therapeutic intervention for such children admitted to the hospital beyond the first month of life. Ceftazidime and cefepime have become standard agents for empiric therapy in critically ill children, those with fever and neutropenia, and those with nosocomially acquired infections in the ICU.

THE MONOBACTAMS: AZTREONAM

The spectrum of antibacterial activity of aztreonam is limited to aerobic Gram-negative bacteria resembling the aminoglycoside antibiotics in its activity without the renal toxicity. It is administered by intramuscular or IV administration and is well distributed into most body fluids and tissues, including achieving effective antibacterial concentrations in the cerebrospinal fluid of patients with bacterial meningitis.

Approximately 30%–50% of the drug is bound to plasma protein. Aztreonam is eliminated from the body by both hepatic and renal mechanisms. The drug does not precipitate allergic reactions in patients allergic to penicillin.

CARBAPENEMS

Imipenem, the prototype carbapenem, binds to all of the PBPs. These drugs possess a broad spectrum of antibacterial activity against aerobic and anaerobic Gram-positive and Gram-negative pathogens. As such, they arguably are among the broadest antibacterial agents currently available. The carbapenems are highly resistant to degradation by both plasmid and chromosomally mediated β-lactamases, although bacteria expressing carbapenemases have emerged. *Pseudomonas spp.*, in particular, may acquire resistance to the carbapenems. Like other β-lactam antibiotics, these drugs are well distributed in most body fluids and tissues, including the central nervous system (CNS) in patients with meningitis. Approximately 20% of imipenem and meropenem are bound to plasma proteins, while ertapenem is highly and saturably protein bound. Imipenem and meropenem are excreted by the kidney. For clinical use, imipenem is administered along with a competitive inhibitor of dehydropeptidase I, cilastatin. Meropenem and ertapenem are resistant to degradation by the dehydropeptidase enzyme. The adverse effect profile of carbapenems is similar to other β-lactam antibiotics. Additionally, seizures have been reported in some patients with reduced renal function who are receiving high-dose therapy with imipenem.

The carbapenems are safe and effective in pediatric patients with community-acquired respiratory tract infections, skin and soft tissue infections, uncomplicated urinary tract infections, and intra-abdominal infections, as well as in the treatment of serious infections in hospitalized patients. As such, they offer a therapeutic alternative for the treatment of Gram-negative bacterial sepsis in the immunocompromised patient, the treatment of nosocomial infections in critically ill children, and in the treatment of patients who have failed therapy with other broad-spectrum antibiotics or antibiotic combinations.

THE AMINOGLYCOSIDE ANTIBIOTICS

The aminoglycosides include amikacin, gentamicin, kanamycin, neomycin, netilmicin, streptomycin, and tobramycin. The most stable aminoglycoside against the effects of inactivating enzymes is amikacin, followed by tobramycin and gentamicin. The amino-glycosides are not metabolized by the body and are excreted completely unchanged by the kidney. The aminoglycosides do not cross the blood–brain barrier well. The relationship between serum aminoglyco-side concentration and clinical outcome is question-able. The most commonly recognized adverse effects associated with aminoglycoside administration are ototoxicity and nephrotoxicity. Allergic reactions, in-cluding rash, fever, and eosinophilia, are uncommon. Aminoglycoside-associated neuromuscular blockade causing weakness of skeletal muscles is a very uncom-mon adverse reaction but may precipitate respiratory depression.

The aminoglycoside agents are used predomi-nately to treat serious infections by aerobic Gram-negative bacilli, including those caused by more resistant organisms, such as *Pseudomonas spp.* Amino-glycosides also are indicated in the treatment of se-rious enterococcal infections. While not suscepti-ble to the aminoglycosides alone, many enterococci are killed synergistically when an aminoglycoside is added to penicillin or ampicillin. The levels of amino-glycoside necessary to produce synergy may not be as high as those required when the drugs are used alone to treat Gram-negative infections. Synergy between an aminoglycoside and a β-lactam or glycopeptide drug can also be exploited in the treatment of serious infections due to other Gram-positive organisms, in-cluding viridans streptococci, group B streptococci, *S. aureus*, and coagulase-negative staphylococci.

GLYCOPEPTIDES AND OTHER ANTIBIOTICS FOR GRAM-POSITIVE BACTERIA

Vancomycin has no utility in the treatment of Gram-negative bacterial infections. The poor oral bioavail-ability is exploited with the drug's oral use in the treatment of *Clostridium difficile* antibiotic-associated colitis; 55% of vancomycin is bound to plasma pro-tein. Vancomycin distributes to most body fluids and tissues, although because of its large molecular size, penetration into some infected spaces, particularly devitalized wounds, may be marginal. Vancomycin is not metabolized and is excreted unchanged from the body by the kidney. A large number of adverse effects have been associated with vancomycin admin-istration, but most have been attributed to impuri-ties in earlier pharmaceutical formulations. Newer, more pure formulations are safer. The "red-man syn-drome," characterized by flushing, pruritus, tachy-cardia, and an erythematous rash, is associated with the rapid IV administration of vancomycin. The

syndrome is due to vancomycin-induced histamine release. Pretreatment with antihistamine and slowing the vancomycin infusion rate reduce the frequency and severity of this reaction. Ototoxicity and nephro-toxicity have long been attributed to vancomycin therapy, but the true incidences of these adverse ef-fects are very low. Drug interactions with vancomycin include the possible additive ototoxic and nephro-toxic effects with other drugs known to cause these toxicities.

Vancomycin therapy is indicated for the treat-ment of infections caused by MRSA and coagulase-negative staphylococci. The drug may also be used as an alternative to β-lactam therapy in the treat-ment of streptococcal and staphylococcal infections in children who are allergic to penicillin. Dalba-vancin possesses more potent in vitro activity against many Gram-positive organisms compared with van-comycin and has a very prolonged terminal half-life that allows once-per-week IV dosing. Daptomycin has in vitro activity against virtually all clinical iso-lates of *S. aureus*, coagulase-negative staphylococci, and enterococci. Linezolid possesses activity against most isolates of Gram-positive bacteria and is avail-able in both a parenteral and oral preparations.

MACROLIDE/AZALIDE ANTIBIOTICS

Erythromycin, clarithromycin, and azithromycin are active against many community-acquired respira-tory pathogens, most notably pneumococcus, *My-coplasma*, *Legionella*, and *Chlamydia*. They are the drugs of choice for eradication of *B. pertussis*. Once in the bloodstream, these agents are widely dis-tributed throughout the body. Their high intracellu-lar concentrations enhance their effectiveness against intracellular pathogens such as *Chlamydia* and *Le-gionella*. The most common adverse effect associ-ated with erythromycin use is gastrointestinal dis-comfort. More serious adverse effects associated with erythromycin administration include hepatic toxi-city, ototoxicity, and cardiac toxicity. Prolongation of the QT interval and ventricular tachyarrhyth-mias are most common manifestation. None of these more serious side effects have been noted with clar-ithromycin or azithromycin. Drugs that are reported to result in clinically important drug interactions with macrolides include carbamazepine, corticosteroids, cyclosporine, warfarin, and theophylline.

QUINOLONES

The fluoroquinolone agents that are currently mar-keted are not labeled for use in patients <18 years of age. Their unique properties may offer important and perhaps life-saving therapy for selected pediatric patients. The second-generation quinolones ciprofloxacin and levofloxacin are effective against many Gram-negative pathogens, including *P. aeruginosa*, and indeed were the first oral antibiotics available for Pseudomonas infections. However, they have marginal activity against *S. pneumoniae*, limiting their use in pneumonia. Newer-generation quinolones have largely maintained their activity against Gram-negative bacteria but have improved their activity against pneumococcus. They also have activity against the atypical respiratory pathogens *Mycoplasma pneumoniae* and *Chlamydia pneumoniae*, rendering them excellent choices for both community- and hospital-acquired respiratory tract infection. Oral bioavailability approaches 100%, offering the clinician an enteral option for the treatment of serious Gram-negative bacterial infections in the patient who lacks IV access. These drugs are primarily metabolized by the liver and do not require substantial dose adjustments in patients with mild-to-moderate renal functional impairment. In contrast, dosage adjustments may be necessary for most quinolone drugs in patients with liver disease. Nausea, abdominal distress, headache, and dizziness appear to be the most common adverse events in adults. Less common adverse effects have included skin rash, photosensitivity reactions, and CNS manifestations, including depression, hallucinations, and seizures. Some quinolones have been associated with prolongation of the QT interval. The most important quinolone-associated adverse effect pertinent to pediatric patients is the possibility of drug-induced arthropathy. Concomitant enteral administration of quinolones with divalent and trivalent cation-containing antacids, sucralfate, and iron substantially reduces the oral absorption of quinolone antibiotics.

ANTIFUNGAL AGENTS

Polyenes

The polyenes in current use include nystatin and colloidal and lipid-associated amphotericin B. Amphotericin B has activity against *Candida*, *Aspergillus*, non-*Aspergillus* molds, *Cryptococcus*, and the endemic fungal pathogens such as *Histoplasma*, *Blastomyces*, *Coccidioides*, and *Sporothrix*. Rare organisms resistant to amphotericin include *Candida lusitaniae* and the molds *Aspergillus terreus* and *Pseudallescheria boydii*. The organs with the highest concentrations of amphotericin are liver, kidney, and lung, with little drug detectable in bronchial secretions and

brain. Nevertheless, amphotericin B has been used successfully for selected fungal infections of the CNS, particularly those due to *Cryptococcus* and *Coccidiomycosis*, although advanced cases frequently require intraventricular instillation of drug. The infusion-related toxicities of amphotericin B include fever, chills, rigors, nausea and vomiting, arthralgias, and myalgias. These toxicities are uncomfortable but usually not dangerous, although occasionally they may be associated with hypotension and dysrhythmias. Small studies have supported the administration of antipyretics and meperidine prior to amphotericin B infusion, and hydrocortisone with the amphotericin itself, to reduce infusion-related symptoms. Dose-related toxicities correlate with cumulative end-organ exposure to drug and include nephrotoxicity, resulting in potassium, magnesium, and bicarbonate wasting, and anemia. Observational studies suggest that the incidence of nephrotoxicity can be lessened by sodium loading prior to infusion.

Lipid-associated formulations of Amphotericin B deoxycholate have been introduced to enable higher dosing with fewer side effects. The three available lipid formulations are liposomal amphotericin B (LAmB), amphotericin B colloidal dispersion (ABCD), and amphotericin B lipid complex (ABLC). Typically, the lipid formulations are infused at a dose several-fold higher than that employed with conventional amphotericin B deoxycholate (3–5 mg/kg/dose versus 0.5–1 mg/kg/dose of the conventional drug).

The Azoles: Miconazole, Ketoconazole, Fluconazole, Itraconazole and Voriconazole

Drug-drug interactions with other agents metabolized by certain CYP450 isoforms are prominent and common to all of the azoles. They are especially prominent with voriconazole. Several of the interactions are clinically important in the patient who is likely to require antifungal therapy, including those receiving benzodiazepines, long-acting barbiturates, phenytoin, tacrolimus, sirolimus, cyclosporine, warfarin, rifampin, omeprazole, calcium-channel blockers, and hydrochlorothiazide. Other untoward side effects of the azoles are mild and are composed primarily of constitutional symptoms such as nausea, abdominal pain, and headache. Mild elevations of hepatic transaminases are common, but significant elevations occur infrequently and, unlike with ketoconazole, fulminant hepatitis with the newer azoles is rare. Voriconazole is associated with distinct side effects not noted with other azoles such as: visual disturbances, rash and, rarely, Stevens-Johnson syndrome or toxic epidermal necrolysis. Fluconazole is cleared by the kidneys, and dose adjustment in renal failure is necessary. Itraconazole and posaconazole are highly protein bound; consequently, neither is dialyzed or enters the CNS efficiently. Mechanisms of azole resistance include (a) overexpression of multidrug efflux pumps with subsequent extrusion of the drug from the intracellular environment of the fungus and (b) alterations of the target enzyme lanosterol 14α-demethylase or other enzymes in the synthetic pathway for ergosterol. Fluconazole-resistant isolates of *Candida* usually remain susceptible to voriconazole and posaconazole.

Fluconazole remains the major alternative to amphotericin in the treatment of serious infections due to *Candida spp.* It has a wide distribution with excellent penetration into virtually all body compartments, including the CNS. *C. krusei* is intrinsically resistant to fluconazole, as are some isolates of *C. glabrata*. Acquired fluconazole resistance in *C. albicans* and other non-albicans species, such as *C. tropicalis* and *C. parapsilosis*, remains uncommon. Fluconazole has no clinically relevant activity against *Aspergillus* or other molds. In contrast to fluconazole, itraconazole possesses in vitro activity against most *Aspergillus spp.* and the endemic fungi. Voriconazole has in vitro activity against virtually all *Candida spp.*, including those resistant to fluconazole; against *Aspergillus spp.*, including the polyene-resistant species *A. terreus*; and most of the endemic fungi. It also is active against some but not all of the non-*Aspergillus* molds. Notably, voriconazole is not active against zygomycetes. Currently, the drug is used most prominently in the treatment of invasive aspergillosis. Posaconazole possesses the broadest activity of all of the azoles, including virtually all *Candida spp.*, cryptococcus, nearly all *Aspergillus spp.*, and non-*Aspergillus* molds, including many *Fusarium spp.* and *P. boydii.* It is also active against zygomycetes, including *Rhizopus* and *Mucor.*

Echinocandins

Caspofungin, micofungin, and anidulafungin exhibit a spectrum limited to *Candida* and *Aspergillus spp.* including *C. krusei* and *C. glabrata* and *C. lusitaniae.* They have also been tested as empiric antifungal therapy in febrile neutropenia. These three echinocandins are not absorbed orally and all are available only as IV preparations. They are highly protein bound and have poor penetration into the CNS. Caspofungin and micofungin are both metabolized in the liver and excreted in an inactive form in

the bile and urine. Dosage adjustment is suggested for moderate-to-severe hepatic insufficiency. Only a very small proportion of active drug is excreted in the kidneys, and dosing need not be altered for renal failure. Anidulafungin is slowly degraded in human plasma, and the degradation products are then excreted in the bile. Preliminary studies indicate that this drug may be safely dosed in both renal and hepatic insufficiency without adjustment. The echinocandins are poor substrates for the cytochrome CYP450 enzymes, with relatively few drug–drug interactions. The most frequent adverse effect is pain and phlebitis at the injection site.

Combination Antifungal Therapy

The difficulty inherent in curing a patient of invasive fungal disease suggests that combinations of agents may be superior to single-agent therapy. Some theoretical concerns have given pause to this strategy. In particular, the use of azoles decreases the synthesis of ergosterol, the molecular target of the polyenes, suggesting that the combination may be antagonistic. Clinical experience suggests that such antagonism is uncommon and that combination of one class with another usually leads to synergistic or additive effects.

ANTIVIRAL AGENTS

Viruses are obligate intracellular organisms, and antiviral drugs work intracellularly. Therefore, traditional pharmacokinetic studies that measure the pattern of drug in the intravascular compartment may not reflect the more relevant intracellular kinetics. Moreover, in contrast to antibacterial drugs, in vitro susceptibility tests are not standardized for antiviral agents, and in many instances, they correlate poorly with clinical efficacy. The response of the host to an antiviral agent is more strongly associated with the integrity of the host immune system than with the intrinsic properties of the drug.

Acyclovir

Acyclovir has in vitro and clinical activity against herpes simplex virus type 1 (HSV-1), HSV type 2 (HSV-2), and varicella-zoster virus (VZV). The principal toxicity is renal impairment that is potentiated by rapid infusion. Slow administration while maintaining adequate hydration is usually adequate to avoid nephrotoxicity. Occasionally, patients experience disorders of the CNS such as agitation, confusion, or hallucinations. Acyclovir has demonstrated utility in the treatment of HSV encephalitis and neonatal herpes. It is also the treatment of choice for HSV infections in immunocompromised patients. The drug also has been effective in the treatment of VZV infection in the immune-suppressed patient, a condition marked by widespread disease that involves the lungs and abdominal viscera. Acyclovir is effective in suppressing reactivation of latent HSV when given prophylactically to selected hosts, including HSV-seropositive bone marrow transplant patients.

Ganciclovir

Ganciclovir has activity against HSV-1, HSV-2, VZV, CMV, and human herpes virus 6 (HHV-6). Neutropenia is the most frequently encountered adverse effect of ganciclovir. Ganciclovir is the established agent of choice in the treatment of CMV infections. Like all herpes viruses, CMV converts to a state of latency after the initial infection and may reactivate throughout the life of the host. In some patients, particularly those with CMV pneumonitis, ganciclovir therapy is augmented with IV immune globulin with high titers of antibody against CMV. Recent emphasis has been placed on using ganciclovir as prophylaxis against multiorgan infection in transplant recipients. Ganciclovir is the first-line therapy for disseminated HHV-6 disease. Resistance to ganciclovir has been reported in both HSV and CMV. Resistant isolates are generally susceptible to foscarnet and cidofovir.

Cidofovir

Cidofovir possesses in vitro antiviral activity against: HSV-1 and HSV-2, CMV, VZV, EBV, HHV-6, HHV-7, HHV-8, adenovirus, the human papilloma, polyoma viruses, the poxviruses, including monkeypox, smallpox, and vaccinia. Nephrotoxicity may be reduced by the administration of probenecid before and at 3 hrs and 8 hrs after cidofovir infusion and by generous IV hydration. The use of cidofovir is indicated in immunocompromised patients, particularly those who have received bone marrow transplant.

Foscarnet

Foscarnet has activity against: HSV-1, HSV-2, VZV, CMV, HHV-6, and hepatitis B virus. Foscarnet has poor oral bioavailability and must be administered intravenously. The drug has a large volume of distribution and adequate CNS penetration. Dosing adjustment is required for patients with diminished renal function. The principal toxicity of foscarnet is renal impairment. The nephrotoxicity can be reduced by hydration prior to and during infusion. A second commonly reported side effect of foscarnet is derangement of calcium, phosphate, potassium, and magnesium. The most frequently reported side effects are depression of ionized calcium and hyperphosphatemia. Penile and vulvar ulcerations have been reported during foscarnet therapy, possibly due to exposure of these surfaces to high concentrations of active drug in the urine.

CHAPTER 57 ■ BACTERIAL SEPSIS AND MECHANISMS OF MICROBIAL PATHOGENESIS

NEAL J. THOMAS • ROBERT F. TAMBURRO • MARK W. HALL • SURENDER RAJASEKARAN • JOHN S. VENGLARCIK

An International Consensus Conference on Pediatric Sepsis and Organ Dysfunction defined pediatric-specific definitions for systemic inflammatory response syndrome SIRS, sepsis, severe sepsis, and septic shock (**Table 57.1**). Certain conditions predispose to sepsis with certain bacteria (**Table 57.2**). Gram-positive (GP) bacteria depend on the production of powerful exotoxins (e.g., tetanus, botulism, diphtheria); with Gram-negative (GN) bacteria,

it is principally the cell wall component LPS of the outer envelope that is implicated in pathogenesis of sepsis. Most of the toxicity of endotoxin resides in the innermost core region, which consists of lipid A. The production of soluble extracellular toxins is one of the hallmarks of disease caused by some GP bacteria. The list is extensive, but examples include the toxins of clostridial species (gas gangrene, antibiotic-associated colitis), diphtheria (*Corynebacterium*

TABLE 57.1

DEFINITIONS OF SYSTEMIC INFLAMMATORY RESPONSE SYNDROME, INFECTION, SEPSIS, SEVERE SEPSIS, AND SEPTIC SHOCK

SIRS
The presence of at least 2 of the following 4 criteria, one of which must be abnormal temperature or leukocyte count:

- Core temperature of >38.5°C or <36°C
- Tachycardia, defined as a mean heart rate >2 SD above normal for age in the absence of external stimulus, chronic drugs, or painful stimuli;
  OR otherwise unexplained persistent elevation over a 0.5–4-hr period
  OR for children <1 yr old: bradycardia, defined as a mean heart rate <10th percentile for age in the absence of external vagal stimulus,
  β-blocker drugs or congenital heart disease; or otherwise unexplained persistent depression over a 0.5-hr period
- Mean respiratory rate >2 SD above normal for age or mechanical ventilation for an acute process not related to underlying neuromuscular disease or the receipt of general anesthesia
- Leukocyte count elevated or depressed for age (not secondary to chemotherapy-induced leukopenia) or >10% immature neutrophils

Infection
A suspected or proven (by positive culture, tissue stain, or polymerase chain reaction test) infection caused by any pathogen OR a clinical syndrome associated with a high probability of infection. Evidence of infection includes positive findings on clinical exam, imaging, or laboratory tests (e.g., WBCs in a normally sterile body fluid, perforated viscus, chest x-ray consistent with pneumonia, petechial or purpuric rash, or purpura fulminans).

Sepsis
SIRS in the presence of, or as a result of, suspected or proven infection

Severe Sepsis
Sepsis plus one of the following: cardiovascular organ dysfunction OR acute respiratory distress syndrome OR 2 or more other organ dysfunctions

Septic Shock
Sepsis and cardiovascular organ dysfunction

From Goldstein B, Giroir B, Randolph A. International Consensus Conference on Pediatric Sepsis. International pediatric sepsis consensus conference: definitions for sepsis and organ dysfunction in pediatrics. *Pediatr Crit Care Med.* 2005;6:2–8, with permission.

diphtheriae), food poisoning (*Bacillus cereus, S. aureus*), and anthrax (*Bacillus anthracis*). A superantigen (SAg), toxin-1 is found in toxic shock syndrome. Concentrations of <0.1 pg/mL of a bacterial SAg are sufficient to stimulate the T lymphocytes in an uncontrolled manner, resulting in fever, shock, and death.

The invasiveness of *Fusobacterium necrophorum* in the context of Lemierre syndrome, also called postanginal sepsis, can be explained by the production of the proteolytic enzymes endotoxin, leukocidin, and hemagglutinin. Disruption of the mucosal barrier of the oropharynx leads to hypoxia and tissue destruction, which creates the oxygen-free environment required to maintain the low oxidation-reduction potential necessary for bacterial proliferation. Furthermore, the family to which Fusobacterium belongs has been associated with thromboembolic phenomena that are a consequence of the lipid A moiety of their LPS. The pathogenesis of postanginal sepsis then can best be understood

in terms of Virchow's triad, specifically that damage to the endothelium of the internal jugular vein, alteration of normal blood, and blood hypercoagulability lead to vascular thrombosis. The anatomy of the lateral pharyngeal space allows invasion of the internal jugular vein either by direct extension or by lymphatic or hematogenous spread from the peritonsillar vessels.

HOST DEFENSE

Most innate immune cells (monocytes, macrophages, dendritic cells, natural killer cells, neutrophils) constitutively express receptors that are capable of sensing molecules that are frequently expressed by pathogenic organisms. These bacterial pathogen-associated molecular patterns (PAMPs) include ligands such as LPS, LTA, and peptidoglycan. Activation of an innate immune cell does not require previous exposure to a PAMP, or priming. Each exposure

TABLE 57.2

CLINICAL CONDITIONS THAT PREDISPOSE THE HOST TO SPECIFIC BACTERIA

Condition	Bacteria
Asplenia Polysplenia	*Streptococcus pneumoniae* *Salmonella*
Sickle cell disease	*Streptococcus pneumoniae* *Salmonella*
Nephrotic syndrome	*Streptococcus pneumoniae*
HIV/AIDS	*Streptococcus pneumonia* *Haemophilus influenzae* type b *Staphylococcus aureus* *Pseudomonas aeruginosa*
Complement deficiencies C5, C6, C7, C8, C9	*Neisseria meningitidis* *Neisseria gonorrhoeae*
Iron overload	*Yersinia enterocolitica* *Listeria monocytogenes* *Vibrio vulnificus*
Neutropenia	*Streptococcus viridans*

HIV, human immunodeficiency virus; AIDS, acquired immune deficiency syndrome

has the potential to result in a robust response, thus standing in contrast to the adaptive immune system, which responds to repeat exposures to the same antigen with increasing speed and vigor. PAMP recognition and subsequent activation of the inflammatory response occur via several groups of intracellular and extracellular receptors, the best characterized being the Toll-like receptors (TLRs). Binding of a ligand to the TLR complex (the TLR itself plus co-stimulatory molecules found at or near the cell membrane) results in the initiation of a cascade of intracellular protein phosphorylation, ultimately resulting in the translocation of transcription factor nuclear factor-κB (NFκB) to the nucleus, where transcription of proinflammatory gene elements is initiated. Another family of molecules structurally similar to the TLRs are leucine-rich repeat regions (LRRs) thought to be important in PAMP binding but located in the intracellular compartment. Variously termed NLRs (NACHT-LRRs) and CATERPILLARs, this family contains the NOD subfamily of intracellular receptors that are known to bind to diaminopimelic acid found in GN bacteria (NOD1) and muramyl dipeptide seen in GP species (NOD2).

The adaptive immune system is composed of T and B lymphocytes. First, each lymphocyte is programmed through gene rearrangement to respond to a distinct antigenic stimulus, in contrast to monocytes, for example, which are all capable of sensing LPS through their TLR4 receptor complexes. Second, the activation of lymphocytes typically requires assistance in the form of antigen presentation by innate immune cells. Third, the adaptive immune response is frequently characterized by the development of memory cells that are capable of generating a more rapid and robust antibody response upon repeat exposure to a given antigen. The relevance of the adaptive immune response to critical illness is highlighted by an association between apoptosis in lymphoid organs and sepsis mortality. Prolonged lymphopenia and apoptosis-associated depletion of lymphoid organs has also been demonstrated to be strongly associated with death from nosocomial sepsis in the setting of pediatric multiple organ dysfunction syndrome (MODS). T cells can be generally thought of as belonging to one of two classes, CD4+ helper T cells (Th) and CD8+ cytotoxic T cells. In the presence of proinflammatory mediators, naïve T cells typically develop into Th-1 cells, which promote the proinflammatory response through the production of cytokines such as interferon (IFN)-γ, IL-2, and granulocyte-macrophage colony-stimulating factor. In the presence of antiinflammatory mediators, T-cell differentiation is skewed toward the Th-2 phenotype. Th-2 cells elaborate cytokines, including IL-4, IL-10, and IL-13, which inhibit the innate immune response and promote the production of antibodies by B cells.

Inflammatory Imbalance and the Sepsis Syndrome

In large part, it is the action of the immune system, not the bacteria themselves, that is responsible for morbidity and mortality from bacterial sepsis. When confined to a local region, the effects of proinflammatory cytokines such as vasodilation and increased capillary permeability are beneficial in that they allow for recruitment and activation of effector immune cells to eliminate infection. When the immune response is overly robust, these mediators spill over into the systemic circulation, resulting in the classic signs and symptoms of bacterial sepsis. A host of polymorphisms have been identified that code for inflammatory molecules and protein products essential for host defense, including polymorphisms for TNF-α, TNF-β, Fc-γ receptors, mannose-binding lectin, TLRs, IL-1, IL-1RA, IL-6, IL-10, plasminogen activator inhibitor 1 (PAI-1), and heat shock proteins.

Any device that breaches the skin barrier and remains in place creates the potential for

TABLE 57.3

ENVIRONMENTAL CONDITIONS THAT PREDISPOSE THE HOST TO SPECIFIC BACTERIA

Organism	Environmental source
Listeria monocytogenes	Food, especially dairy and pork products
E. faecium	Commercial chicken and meat products
Clostridium perfringens	Soil
Salmonella	Poultry, pork, beef, egg, and dairy products
Yersinia	Pork, chitterlings (pork intestines), and dairy products
Vibrio vulnificus	Seawater and undercooked seafood (clams, oysters, and mussels)

contamination of the device and subsequent bacteremia. Most endemic transmission follows the route of nose to hand to device from either the patient or the healthcare worker. The widespread but often necessary use of indwelling central venous catheters in the ICU lends itself to a large number of nosocomial bloodstream infections. GP bacteria, largely *Staphylococcus*, are usually present on the patient's skin before placement of the device. In contrast, healthcare workers introduce GN organisms present on their hands during manipulation of IV devices. Virtually all closed-system urinary catheters are colonized by 7 days after placement, and open systems are colonized much sooner. Some bacteria associated with sepsis are linked to exposure to specific environmental sources (**Table 57.3**). Identifying a source can be difficult but is important in preventing other cases.

Bacterial Pathogenesis

In critically ill patients, increased intestinal permeability leads to translocation of the bacteria of the intestinal lumen, as well as their toxins, into the bloodstream. Moreover, the injury to the mucosa caused by ischemia may be exacerbated by reperfusion, with increased formation of reactive oxygen species, which may result in further intestinal injury and increased intestinal permeability. Intestinal lymphatics are the major route by which intestine-derived proinflammatory or toxic factors reach the systemic circulation. Bacterial translocation, once believed to be the simple movement of bacteria and toxins across the lining of the intestines into the systemic circulation secondary to increased intestinal permeability, is now known to be a much more complex process. Splanchnic hypoperfusion and intestinal injury can result in the gut becoming a cytokine-generating organ. These nonbacterial, inflammatory mediators then access distant organ systems via mesenteric lymphatics, rather than the portal circulation.

Selective decontamination, aimed at minimizing the risk of nosocomial infection, involves the use of oral nonabsorbable and systemic antibiotics to eliminate potentially pathogenic, aerobic bacteria from the oropharynx, stomach, and intestines, while at the same time, causing minimal effect on indigenous anaerobic flora. In this way, potentially pathogenic bacteria that may be colonizing the gastrointestinal tract are eradicated, while the indigenous flora remain, which provides further protection against secondary colonization. Although its efficacy remains controversial, meta-analyses have demonstrated a decrease in nosocomial respiratory infections after selective decontamination. Data suggest that the combination of oral and systemic antibiotics is more effective.

Physiology and Pathophysiology of Sepsis

In GN infections, it is the monocyte-macrophage that first responds to endotoxin. Endotoxin first binds to LPS-binding protein, an acute-phase protein produced by the liver. The endotoxin-LPS-binding protein complex acts as the ligand for CD14 (a cell-surface receptor on mononuclear cells), and signal transduction results in monocyte/macrophage activation, leading to cytokine release. It has become clear that GP processing is more complex. Several human proteins have the ability to bind endotoxin, which is "shuttled" between them and CD14. It appears that the CD14 mechanism is not limited to endotoxin-LPS-binding protein but that it is a pattern-recognition molecule that can also respond to components of the GP bacterial cell wall, such as peptidoglycan and LTA.

The activation of monocytes by GP components leads to the production of the proinflammatory cytokines, particularly TNF-α and IL-1, and then to other mediator cascades, including the complement and coagulation pathways, inflammatory prostanoids, and production of reactive oxygen intermediates. Both GP and GN microbial components bind to pattern recognition receptors such as the TLRs. LPS in combination with LPS binding protein interacts with CD14 and the trimolecular complex binds with TLR4. The result of this binding is usually the activation of several intracellular pathways that lead to the activation of transcription proteins (e.g., NF$\kappa\beta$ and activator protein-1) that are implicated in the expression of widespread effector molecules such as cytokines. Proinflammatory molecules such as interleukins and TNF-α seek to eradicate invading microorganisms by stimulating inflammation, accomplished by orchestrating cellular and humoral responses that lead to increasing vascular permeability, increasing adherence to endothelium, and exerting chemotactic effects, all of which encourage migration of leukocytes to the primary site of infection. In addition, cytokines stimulate the proliferation of B-cell and T-cell lymphocytes.

Favorable trends in survival have been observed in a variety of clinical trials of sepsis with anti-inflammatory agents. Anti-inflammatory agents for sepsis generally appeared to benefit patients with GN organisms as the cause of sepsis.

Pathophysiology of Septic Shock

The macrophages are among the first cells to come in contact with the pathogen. The excessive, unregulated, prolonged stimulation of the macrophage in conjunction with other active cells, such as the leukocyte and the endothelium, leads to the release of proinflammatory mediators such as TNF-α and IL-1 (**Fig. 57.1**). When activated systemically or in the presence of endothelial damage, neutrophils become mediators of microvascular injury. Distinct phases occur during this process, which include rolling, firm adhesion, activation, aggregation, and migration through cell junction into tissue.

Endothelial dysfunction is a sentinel event in the pathogenesis of septic shock. The dysfunction is a result of injury that occurs due to production of oxygen free radicals, arachidonic acid metabolites, complement activation, platelet aggregation, and monocyte

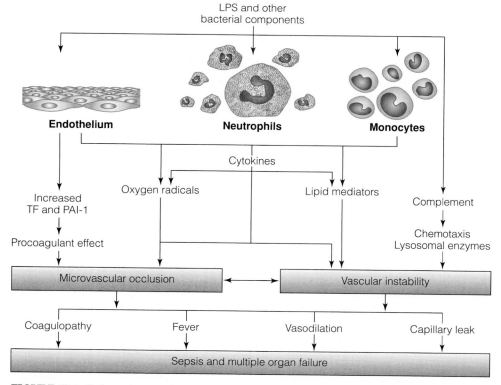

FIGURE 57.1. Pathogenic networks in shock. Lipopolysaccharide (LPS) and other microbial components simultaneously activate multiple parallel cascades that contribute to the pathophysiology of acute respiratory distress syndrome and shock. The combination of poor myocardial contractility, impaired peripheral vascular tone, and microvascular occlusion leads to tissue hypoperfusion and inadequate oxygenation and, thus, organ failure.

production of cytokines. In addition, the endothelium is capable of generating its own inflammatory mediators in a process known as "activation of the endothelium," which involves a change from anticoagulant to procoagulant and the production of vasoactive substances such as nitric oxide along with adhesion molecules. These changes result in increased microvascular permeability, edema, and eventually systemic hypotension from fluid losses. The production of nitric oxide, kinins, and vasoactive peptides leads to peripheral vasodilation, which causes decreased vascular resistance or "warm shock."

Myocardial dysfunction, once considered a preterminal event, is common in sepsis. Human septic myocardium is characterized by reversible biventricular dilation, increased end-diastolic volume, decreased ejection fraction, and diminishing response to volume resuscitation and catecholamine resistance. Humoral factors, including TNF-α and IL-1β, in synergy with nitric oxide, are largely responsible for this phenomenon. The concept of altered oxygen supply dependency and a strategy of driving the circulation with fluids and high-dose inotropes to achieve "supranormal" levels of oxygen delivery and consumption resulted in adverse outcomes when applied to critically ill patients with organ failure.

Septic shock includes signs of bioenergetic derangements, with increases in mixed venous oxygen saturation (Svo$_2$) and lactate. Because increasing severity of sepsis may be associated with a progressive fall in tissue oxygen consumption with a rise in tissue oxygen tension, the bioenergetic derangement is likely one of reduced cellular use of oxygen rather than tissue hypoxia. The Svo$_2$ reflects the balance between local oxygen supply and demand. The elevated values found in sepsis imply abnormally reduced cellular utilization of oxygen, thereby accounting for the elevation in Svo$_2$. It is now also appreciated that sepsis-induced lactic acidosis may arise from increased activity of muscle Na,K-ATPase pumps, rather than from anaerobic metabolism secondary to inadequate tissue perfusion. Skeletal muscle has been shown to be a leading source of lactate production through exaggerated aerobic glycolysis rather than through tissue hypoxia.

The mitochondria control the amount of oxygen consumed by the cells via the process of oxidative phosphorylation. Mitochondrial activity is controlled by numerous extrinsic factors, including levels of ATP, local partial pressure of oxygen, and reactive oxygen species. Numerous hormonal influences (e.g., thyroid hormones, leptin, catecholamines, and corticosteroids) also mediate their actions partly through influencing mitochondrial respiration. Nitric oxide and its metabolite peroxynitrite are potent inhibitors of the electron transport chain, with variable duration effects depending on the levels produced. Sepsis is the classic condition in which large amounts of nitric oxide are generated systemically. There is an inhibitory effect of nitric oxide on mitochondria in septic patients. Apart from respiratory complex inhibition, physical damage to mitochondria occurs that varies across organs and depends on sepsis severity.

Decreased TNF-α activity is thought to lead to immunoparalysis and blockade by drugs such as etanercept and infliximab, now being utilized in children with collagen vascular diseases and after transplantation, can create features of immunoparalysis and decreased TNF-α activity, which may account for an increased susceptibility to infections in these patients.

CLINICAL PRESENTATION AND DIFFERENTIAL DIAGNOSIS

The classic triad of clinical signs of sepsis is change in temperature (either hyperthermia or hypothermia), tachypnea and tachycardia, and change in mental status. It is important to recognize the lack of hypotension in this triad. Children can have severe sepsis and septic shock without hypotension. The addition of basic laboratory parameters can help to confirm the diagnosis but are unnecessary at the initial stages of resuscitation.

Septic shock, most commonly a combination of distributive, hypovolemic, and cardiogenic shock, by definition, requires manifestations of decreased organ perfusion. Whereas a change in mental status is the most obvious symptom to note on a brief physical examination, other symptoms include decreased urine output, delayed capillary refill, or an increased base deficit, most likely representing an increased serum lactate.

The hemodynamic alterations that can occur with bacterial sepsis are varied. As the ages of children cared for in the PICU range from newborns to young adults, children must be categorized to determine parameters that signify abnormal. Recent definitions published by the International Consensus Conference on Pediatric Sepsis stratified children into age groups listed in **Table 57.4**, based on defining categories of children that are clinically and physiologically meaningful.

While certain children, especially those in whom sepsis is recognized early in the course of infection, can present with the classic adult picture of "warm," vasodilated shock signified by an increase in cardiac output and a decrease in systemic vascular resistance, most children will present with "cold" shock, with an increase in systemic vascular resistance and a

TABLE 57.4

AGE-SPECIFIC VITAL SIGNS AND LABORATORY VARIABLES

Age group	Heart rate, beats/min		Respiratory rate, breaths/min	Leukocyte count, leukocytes $\times 10^3$/mm	Systolic blood pressure (mm Hg)
	Tachycardia	Bradycardia			
0 days–1 wk	>180	<100	>50	>34	<65
1 wk–1 mo	>180	<100	>40	>19.5 or <5	<75
1 mo–1 yr	>180	<90	>34	>17.5 or <5	<100
2–5 yrs	>140	NA	>22	>15.5 or <6	<94
6–12 yrs	>130	NA	>18	>13.5 or <4.5	<105
13 to <18 yrs	>110	NA	>14	>11 or <4.5	<117

Lower values for heart rate, leukocyte count, and systolic blood pressure are for the 5th percentile, and upper values for heart rate, respiration rate, or leukocyte count for the 95th percentile.
From Goldstein B, Giroir B, Randolph A; International Consensus Conference on Pediatric Sepsis. International pediatric sepsis consensus conference: definitions for sepsis and organ dysfunction in pediatrics. *Pediatr Crit Care Med.* 2005;6:2–8, with permission.

decrease in cardiac output, requiring inotropic support as opposed to a vasopressor.

A leukocytosis occurs due to demargination of polymorphonuclear cells (PMNs) and increased production and release of immature PMNs from the bone marrow. Neutropenia develops when the PMNs are consumed peripherally as they attach to endothelial cells and become ensnared in peripheral capillaries. Platelet count is likely to decrease early due to increased peripheral consumption and increase later as a result of reactive thrombocytosis. Acute-phase proteins, including C-reactive protein, amyloid, α_1-acid glycoprotein, haptoglobin, fibrinogen, ceruloplasmin, and α_1-antitrypsin, are produced in response to IL-1 and IL-6 stimulation. The levels of albumin, prealbumin, transferrin, and retinol-binding protein fall. As these factors are produced in proportion to the cytokine stimulation, they will mirror the intensity of the process. Due to uptake of iron and zinc by liver cells and inflammatory cells, serum levels fall, while copper levels increase in response to higher concentrations of ceruloplasmin. The low iron will manifest as a mild anemia that can be seen in individuals with considerable inflammation. Sepsis places considerable stress on the host. Accelerated use of energy sources leads to an increase in free fatty acids, hyperglycemia, and the catabolism of amino acids. Coagulation abnormalities are common. Fibrinogen, factor V, and factor VIII levels are decreased. Prothrombin time is prolonged in 50%–75% of patients with disseminated intravascular coagulation, the partial thromboplastin time is prolonged in 50%–60% of cases, fibrin degradation products are present in most patients with disseminated intravascular coagulation, and D-dimer is elevated in 90% of patients and is more specific than fibrin degradation products. The peripheral smear will demonstrate microangiopathic changes.

Differential Diagnosis

In the first 3 months of life, *E. coli* and *S. agalactiae* are the most common causes of sepsis, with the risk of *E. coli* declining each month. *L. monocytogenes* has a much lower incidence than the other two. Other agents to be considered include enterococcus, coliforms, and nontypable *H. influenzae*. Rarely, Hib and *S. pneumoniae* can also be seen in this age group. In the context of the PICU, *S. aureus* and *Pseudomonas* should be considered. Candidemia is common in premature infants but unusual in otherwise healthy infants. Viruses can also present in a fashion indistinguishable from a bacterial process in young infants, especially herpes simplex. Varicella, influenza, adenovirus, and respiratory syncytial virus can cause serious, life-threatening infections. In certain circumstances, a TORCH complex (toxoplasma, rubella, cytomegalovirus, and herpes simplex virus) agent should be considered. Rarely, SIRS can be seen with the intravascular infusion of lipids alone. In older otherwise healthy children and adolescents, *S. pneumoniae* and *N. meningitidis* are the most commonly seen bacterial causes of sepsis, with Hib now quite rare. *Salmonella* species should be considered in the presence of significant diarrhea, and *S. aureus* or Group A streptococcus should be considered in the presence of cellulitis, a skeletal infection, or indwelling catheter. *P. aeruginosa* should be suspected with erythema gangrenosum, and a variety of GN bacilli can be isolated in the patient with impaired immunity. In patients with a history of a tick bite, Rocky Mountain spotted fever and *Ehrlichia* should be suspected. Certain foods are linked with pathogens (**Table 57.3**). Other unusual pathogens such as *Sphingomonas paucimobilis* are being seen more frequently. A child with acquired immune deficiency syndrome and disseminated

Mycobacterium avium complex may develop sepsis syndrome. Abdominal catastrophes should raise the possibility of an anaerobic infection. Leptospirosis, brucellosis, and tularemia are rare and linked to specific exposures. Fungal infections have become much more common as a cause for sepsis and are associated with a high mortality rate. In the immunocompromised patient, a variety of viral entities can present as a life-threatening infection: primary herpes simplex, disseminated varicella, and adenovirus. Rabies virus must be considered, especially if the patient had contact with a bat or raccoon. Bioterrorism has resurrected the threat of smallpox. Severe Kawasaki disease, Steven Johnson syndrome, drug reactions, juvenile rheumatoid arthritis, pancreatitis, and systemic lupus erythematosus can all masquerade as sepsis. Other causes of SIRS include trauma, burns, and autoimmune disorders. Past problems and procedures, recent medications, travel, and potential exposures can all aid in the diagnosis. Children with neutropenia often manifest symptoms consistent with SIRS without being infected.

Diagnosis

The most important aspect of the evaluation of the patient with suspected sepsis is the procurement of adequate bacterial cultures from all possible, relevant sources—blood; cerebrospinal fluid (meningitis and encephalitis); urine (urosepsis); stool (enteric fever); respiratory secretions and pleural fluid (pneumonia and empyema); skin lesions (cellulitis and abscesses); vaginal (toxic shock syndrome), synovial (arthritis and osteomyelitis), and peritoneal (ruptured viscus) fluid—preferably before the administration of antimicrobial agents. One blood culture set is rarely advisable or sufficient, 2 blood culture sets are usually adequate when bacteremia is due to a pathogen not likely to be a contaminant, 3 blood culture sets are usually adequate when a continuous bacteremia is suspected, and 4 blood culture sets are reasonable when the anticipated pathogen is likely to be a common contaminant such as coagulase-negative staphylococci. More important is the appropriate dilution of blood to broth; the ideal is 1:5 dilution to decrease the effect of sodium polyanetholesulfonate, which inhibits phagocytosis and serum bactericidal activity but can also decrease the growth of some pathogens. The recommended amount of blood per culture for different age groups is as follows: 1–2 mL in neonates, 2–3 mL in infants, 3–5 mL in children, and 10–20 mL in adolescents. Viral cultures can yield significant information if obtained with the appropriate method and materials. Sites suitable for sampling include conjunctiva, nasopharynx, urethra, vagina, and vesicles

or ulcers on skin and mucous membranes. Blood and cerebrospinal fluid can be sent for viral culture, but results are usually disappointing and better detection methods are available. The one exception would be a blood culture for human immunodeficiency virus in a newborn.

DNA amplification by polymerase chain reaction is revolutionizing the diagnosis of infectious diseases. It is particularly useful in detecting herpes simplex infection of the central nervous system in newborns by examining cerebrospinal fluid for viral DNA. Similarly, a polymerase chain reaction test is available for enterovirus in the cerebrospinal fluid. This technology is helpful in diagnosing bacterial infections that take a long time to grow in culture, such as *Mycobacterium tuberculosis* and *Borrelia burgdorferi*, and in diagnosing rickettsial infections in which treatment is needed acutely but antibodies may take weeks to develop in the serum.

CLINICAL MANAGEMENT AND TREATMENT

Fluid resuscitation with >40 mL/kg (average 60 mL/kg) in the first hour of treatment conferred a dramatic survival advantage to children with septic shock, compared to those who received less fluid in the same time frame. While it should be made clear that administration of antibiotics should *in no way* take precedence over proper management of the airway, breathing, and circulation, recent evidence strongly suggests that the early use of appropriate empiric antimicrobial agents can significantly reduce morbidity and mortality from severe sepsis. While this may seem intuitive, debate continues regarding the use of empiric broad-spectrum antibiotics versus the concomitant desire to reduce patient exposure to broad-spectrum agents for fear of promoting antibiotic resistance. It is now generally recommended that a de-escalating approach to the use of empiric antimicrobial agents be adopted, with broad-spectrum agents being transitioned to the narrowest possible spectrum drugs once culture and sensitivity data are known. Empiric antibiotic therapy must be tailored to provide coverage for community-acquired or nosocomial pathogens (for children who have been hospitalized for >48 hrs or who are at high risk for developing nosocomial infection), taking into account regional, hospital, and unit-specific resistance patterns.

The American College of Critical Care Medicine (ACCM) published clinical practice parameters for hemodynamic support of pediatric and neonatal patients in septic shock in 2002. The ACCM clinical practice parameters define shock by clinical parameters (hypothermia *or* hyperthermia, altered mental status, and abnormal peripheral vasodilation *or* vasoconstriction), hemodynamic variables (inadequate organ perfusion pressure), and SvO_2. Within the first 5 mins of the diagnosis of shock, the child's airway and breathing should be maintained and IV access established. Continuous pulse oximetry, cardiorespiratory monitoring, urine output measurement, and frequent vital-sign assessment are necessary. Isotonic fluid boluses (normal saline or colloid) should be administered IV in 20 mL/kg aliquots up to and over 60 mL/kg in the next *15 mins*, while the patient is monitored for hypoglycemia and hypocalcemia if the shock state is not reversed. If shock persists despite the administration of 60 mL/kg of IV fluid, the authors recommend establishing arterial and central venous access and initiating therapy with a dopamine infusion. If the shock state is not reversed with a dopamine dose of 10 mcg/kg/min, it is recommended to transition to an epinephrine infusion in the setting of vasoconstrictive (cold) shock or norepinephrine for vasodilatory (warm) shock. The former is characterized by poor peripheral pulses, prolonged capillary refill, and diminished peripheral pulses compared to central pulses. Patients with warm shock demonstrate bounding peripheral pulses, erythematous skin, and instantaneous capillary refill. Children with septic shock, in contrast to adults, frequently present in cold shock with low cardiac output and high systemic vascular resistance, and children who present in warm shock often transition to cold shock over the first 48 hrs of illness. Thus, titration of inotropic or vasopressor support should be based upon frequent reassessment of the child's hemodynamic state.

Should either type of shock state be persistent despite adequate intravascular volume status and an appropriate inotrope or vasopressor regimen, the authors recommend consideration of the use of hydrocortisone for empiric treatment of adrenal insufficiency. Factors that favor the use of hydrocortisone include prior corticosteroid use, purpura fulminans, HIV infection, and chronic pituitary or adrenal abnormalities. A random cortisol level of <18 mcg/dL with shock is consistent with adrenal insufficiency. The guidelines indicate that this point in the algorithm should be reached *within 60 mins* of the diagnosis of shock if it is not reversed with fluid and catecholamine therapy.

Should shock continue to be present in the second hour of resuscitation, the ACCM guidelines recommend therapies based upon the patient's clinical, hemodynamic, and oxygen use phenotype. Patients with normal blood pressure who demonstrate cold shock and an SvO_2 of <70% should be treated with

after-load reduction with careful attention to preservation of preload. Children who demonstrate low blood pressure, cold shock, and an SvO_2 of <70% should be treated with titration of epinephrine and ongoing optimization of volume status. Lastly, children who are hypotensive but are persistently vasodilated should undergo additional volume loading, with consideration given to the use of vasopressin as an adjunct vasoconstrictor. Should these maneuvers fail to reverse shock, the authors recommend placement of a pulmonary artery catheter (PAC) to direct ongoing therapy to maintain normal perfusion pressure and maintain the cardiac index between 3.3 and 6 L/min/m^2. For children with refractory shock, a final recommendation is given to consider the use of extracorporeal membrane oxygenation as a rescue therapy for life-threatening septic shock.

Other Therapies for Acute Management of Sepsis

Activated protein C (APC) is an endogenous molecule with antithrombotic, profibrinolytic, and anti-inflammatory properties. The use of recombinant human (rh) APC has reduced mortality in a specific subset of adults with severe sepsis. However, a pediatric phase III follow-up study aimed at promoting resolution of organ dysfunction was stopped at its planned interim analysis due to lack of efficacy. Currently no widely accepted pediatric indication exists for rhAPC in the treatment of pediatric bacterial sepsis. Extracorporeal therapies such as hemofiltration, plasmapheresis, and plasma exchange represent another approach to the acute restoration of inflammatory homeostasis in sepsis. IVIG use for the treatment of neonatal infection shows no effect on mortality with empiric use but does show a reduction in mortality risk when used in the context of proven infection. IVIG use in adult sepsis does not reduce mortality. Three days of polyclonal IVIG therapy results in improved survival to discharge and shorter length of ICU stay. Both retrospective and prospective evidence suggests that IgM-enriched IVIG may be beneficial in adult postoperative patients with severe sepsis.

Multiorgan Dysfunction

Although the progression of sepsis to MODS is poorly understood, it is highly likely that poor perfusion, hypoxia, hyperglycemia, and acidosis all contribute to the process. The risk of mortality increases with each additional organ system failure. Serious abnormalities of liver function, coagulation, and CNS function tend to occur hours to days after the onset of sepsis.

Ventilation Strategies

Timely intubation and mechanical ventilation based on clinical parameters rather than laboratory indices are crucial, as intubation and mechanical ventilation reduce respiratory-muscle oxygen demand and decrease the risk of aspiration and cerebral anoxia from a catastrophic event. Based on data from adult patients, lung-protective ventilation should be used. Multiple trials have now shown the benefit of a high positive end-expiratory pressure and low-tidal-volume approach. The goal of mechanical ventilation is to maintain a reasonable level of oxygenation while keeping the fraction of oxygen in inspired gas (FiO_2) below 0.6, allowing for some hypercapnia with the buffered pH >7.25. Nonconventional modes of ventilation, such as airway-pressure-release ventilation and high-frequency ventilation, may be required to support oxygenation and minimize lung toxicity.

Cardiac Monitoring

The ACCM task force recommends the use of PACs in dopamine-resistant patients based on studies that demonstrated safety and some benefit, including one study which demonstrated that a large number of subjects were receiving incorrect cardiovascular therapy after fluid resuscitation. Given the concerns regarding PACs and the improvements in echocardiography, it is possible that echocardiography will assume an expanding role in the management of septic shock.

Transfusion

Transfusion of packed RBCs must be implemented judiciously and with caution, as evidence suggests that a liberal transfusion practice in adults is associated with a higher mortality. In stable, critically ill children, a restrictive transfusion threshold of hemoglobin 7 g/dL does not increase adverse outcomes compared to a more liberal threshold of hemoglobin 9 g/dL. The results of these and other trials may influence the opinions of the ACCM task force, which currently recommends transfusion if the hemoglobin is <10 mg/dL. Importantly, patients with cardiovascular disease, low cardiac output, severe arterial hypoxemia, low mixed-venous saturation, and/or persistent lactic acidosis may need higher hemoglobins.

Nutrition

A hypermetabolic state such as sepsis, in concert with bed rest and inactivity, may result in malnutrition. Enteral nutrition has been advocated as a means of reducing villous atrophy with increased intestinal permeability, with consequent reduction in the incidence of gut translocation and septic complications. Early enteral feeding of critically ill children on vasoactive drugs and mechanical ventilation is feasible and well tolerated. Patients with sepsis who require pressors and narcotics often have a degree of gastroparesis and thus may benefit from transpyloric feeding, which may be associated with a shorter time interval to full-strength feeds and a decreased incidence of nosocomial pneumonia. The European Society of Parenteral and Enteral Nutrition recommends that if critically ill patients are not expected to be feeding within 3 days, enteral nutrition should be commenced. Enteral feedings have many theoretical advantages, including gastric pH buffering, avoidance of the use of parenteral-nutrition catheters, preservation of gut mucosa, avoidance of the introduction of bacteria and toxins from the gastrointestinal tract into the circulation, a more physiologic pattern of enteric hormone secretion, the ability to administer a complete, nutritional mixture that includes fiber, and lower costs. While generally thought to be beneficial in critically ill patients, enteral immunonutrition with L-arginine, omega-3 fatty acids, zinc, and selenium is harmful in severe sepsis.

Glycemic Control

Maintaining a tight control on serum glucose has been shown to be beneficial in a number of adult studies. The etiology of the hyperglycemia is unclear, as hyperglycemia in pediatric septic shock has been shown to be due to hypoinsulinemia rather than insulin resistance. Children are generally more prone to hypoglycemia when treated with insulin; therefore, insulin therapy should be used cautiously. The impact of tight glucose control in critically ill children is presently undergoing study.

IDENTIFYING THE SOURCE OF INFECTION AND SOURCE CONTROL OF INFECTION

Sources of infection, such as surgical wounds and indwelling foreign bodies (central venous catheters, ventriculoperitoneal shunts, urinary catheters, etc.) should be carefully scrutinized. Blood cultures should be obtained for all patients with sepsis. If the patient has a central line, both peripheral and catheter cultures should be sent to the lab. The length of time to bacterial growth and the colony count often determine if the catheter is the infectious source. A colony count that is 5–10 times greater from the catheter compared to the peripheral blood is indicative of an infected device. A quantitative culture that yields at least 100 CFu/mcL is diagnostic of a central venous catheter infection. If bacteremia persists with appropriate antibiotics, the catheter should be removed. In cases of immunocompromised states, intra-abdominal infections, or oral/neck infections, anaerobic cultures should also be considered. Other sites should be evaluated such as pleural fluid or empyema; a diagnostic thoracentesis may be performed for fluid culture. Exudate from sites of soft-tissue infection should be cultured. If the patient has an abscess, aspiration may be indicated for diagnostic purposes.

Source control of infection encompasses all of the adjunctive physical measures that can control a focus of infection and modify factors that promote microbial growth or impair host antimicrobial defenses.

Antimicrobial Control of Infection

A third-generation cephalosporin will usually provide sufficient empiric coverage as first-line therapy. A β-lactam antibiotic with an aminoglycoside is also as efficacious. If an anaerobic infection is suspected, the addition of metronidazole or clindamycin is appropriate. For children with indwelling catheters, prosthetic materials or potential infections with methicillin-resistant *S. aureus*, vancomycin should be added. Vancomycin is also indicated in the treatment of bacterial meningitis or sepsis in areas with high levels of penicillin-resistant pneumococcus and in neutropenic patients with fever in whom coagulase-negative *staphylococci* and *Streptococcus viridans* are predominant pathogens. If a CNS infection is suspected, appropriate dosing is indicated to allow CNS penetration.

Hyperbaric Oxygen

Hyperbaric oxygen is the administration of 100% oxygen at 2–3 times the atmospheric pressure at sea level in a chamber, which can result in arterial oxygen tension in excess of 2000 mm Hg and oxygen tension in tissue of almost 400 mm Hg. Hyperbaric oxygen has been used as an adjunct to wound care and infection control in myonecrosis, necrotizing fasciitis, and refractory osteomyelitis. For treatment of

wounds that do not respond to debridement or antibiotics, most protocols average 90 mins with 20–30 treatments.

Prevention of Sepsis

Nosocomial infections contribute significantly to hospital-associated morbidity, mortality, and costs. The rate of catheter-related bloodstream infections has been reported at 7.3 per 1000 catheter days. The Society of Critical Care Medicine, in collaboration with multiple other organizations, published guidelines which emphasized the following areas: (a) educating and training healthcare providers who insert and maintain catheters; (b) using maximal sterile barrier precautions during central venous catheter insertion; (c) using a 2% chlorhexidine preparation for skin antisepsis; (d) avoiding routine replacement of central venous catheters as a strategy to prevent infection; (e) using antiseptic/antibiotic-impregnated, short-term central venous catheters if the rate of infection is high despite adherence to other strategies; and (f) removing the catheter as soon as possible.

High-risk Patient Populations

There is an increased rate of central catheter infections, ventilator-related pneumonia, and urinary catheter-related urinary tract infections in children with burns. Burn patients are predisposed to sepsis for a number of reasons: (a) a global decrease in cellular immune function is associated with burns; (b) neutropenia is common, neutrophil function is depressed, and T-cell transcription is altered; (c) these patients are at risk for increased gut permeability; and (d) bacteremia may occur with wound manipulations.

Injury-related infections are primarily wound, intra-abdominal, and CNS infections, while nosocomial infections include respiratory, bloodstream, and urinary tract infections. The nosocomial infections are most common among mechanically ventilated trauma victims, head-injured patients, and those who require prolonged immobilization or hospitalization. The propensity for nosocomial infection fits well with the currently accepted paradigm of the immune response to traumatic injury in which traumatic injury and the initial resuscitation are followed by SIRS, which may lead to early MODS.

HIV-infected children are also at increased risk of viral, bacterial, and fungal sepsis, and the case fatality rate for nonopportunistic infections may be greater for them than in non–HIV-infected children. Prior to the advent of highly active antiretroviral therapy (HAART), primary bacterial infection rates and nosocomial infection rates were very high. The use of HAART in many parts of the world has resulted in an ever-growing cohort of clinically stable HIV-infected children, with low viral loads and normal CD4 T-lymphocyte counts.

Children born without a spleen or who have impaired splenic function secondary to disease or splenectomy are at significantly increased risk of life-threatening bacterial sepsis. In addition to appropriate immunization, antimicrobial prophylaxis is recommended for all children <5 years of age and for at least 2 years after splenectomy. Children with sickle cell disease are at high risk of serious bacterial infection, in large part, from functional asplenia.

Neutropenic bacteremia appears to occur more frequently among leukemia patients. Patients with solid tumors may also receive myeloablative therapy; however, usually less so. Hematologic parameters, particularly neutropenia (absolute neutrophil count <500), have long been used to identify oncology patients at risk for sepsis, with a well-established relationship between decreased leukocytes and an increased risk of infection. It has been shown that temperature >39.0°C in neutropenic cancer patients increases the likelihood that the patient is bacteremic.

Prophylaxis

Prophylaxis is the use of antimicrobial drugs in the absence of suspected or documented infection to decrease the incidence of infection in high-risk populations. The use of prophylactic antibiotics has been categorized into 3 major indications. First, antibiotic prophylaxis may be indicated for children because of exposure to specific pathogens, such as *N. meningitides*. Close contacts of all people with invasive meningococcal disease are at high risk and should receive prophylaxis, ideally within 24 hrs of diagnosis of the primary case. For most children, rifampin is the drug of choice. Rifampin chemoprophylaxis may also be indicated for close contacts of invasive Hib disease. The second major indication for antimicrobial prophylaxis is to prevent infections of vulnerable body sites; the periprocedure use of antibiotics to prevent bacterial endocarditis in children with specific cardiac lesions is a well-established example of this form of prophylaxis. The final form of prophylactic antibiotic use is to prevent infections in high-risk patient populations. For example, the use of antibiotic prophylaxis is recommended for all asplenic children <5 years of age, regardless of immunization status. Children with sickle cell disease and children with HIV also should be treated with prophylactic antibiotics.

CHAPTER 58 ■ CRITICAL VIRAL INFECTIONS

RAKESH LODHA • SUNIT C SINGHI • JAMES D. CAMPBELL

DENGUE HEMORRHAGIC FEVER AND DENGUE SHOCK SYNDROME

Dengue fever (DF) is an acute febrile illness characterized by biphasic fever, myalgia, arthralgia, and rash. Dengue hemorrhagic fever (DHF) is characterized by abnormalities in hemostasis and marked leakage of plasma from the capillaries; the latter may lead to dengue shock syndrome (DSS). DF and DHF are caused by infection due to any of the 4 serotypes of dengue viruses, which are arboviruses that belong to the family Flaviviridae. Dengue viruses are transmitted to humans through the bites of infective female *Aedes vexans* mosquitoes. After virus incubation of 8–10 days, an infected mosquito is capable,

during probing and blood feeding, of transmitting the virus to susceptible individuals for the rest of its life. Infected female mosquitoes may also transmit the virus to their offspring. Diseases that may mimic DHF/DSS are reviewed in **Tables 58.1, 58.2, 58.3 and 58.4**. Children with DHF/DSS show increasing hematocrit, decreased platelet counts, and increased white cell counts with relative lymphocytosis; however, they may have leukopenia. The peripheral smear may show transformed/atypical lymphocytes.

The treatment of DF is symptomatic and consists of fever management, fluid replacement, and close monitoring for clues to progression to DHF/DSS. No specific antiviral drugs have been shown to be efficacious. Fever may be treated with paracetamol or acetaminophen. Salicylates and other nonsteroidal anti-inflammatory drugs should be avoided, as these

TABLE 58.1

GRADING OF DENGUE HEMORRHAGIC FEVER

Grade	Clinical features	Bleeding manifestations	Hemodynamic status
Grade I	Fever accompanied by nonspecific constitutional symptoms	A positive tourniquet test and or easy bruising	Tachycardia ± normal BP, pulse pressure
Grade II	Fever accompanied by nonspecific constitutional symptoms	Spontaneous bleeding, usually in the form of skin or other hemorrhages	Tachycardia ± normal BP, pulse pressure
Grade III (DSS)	Same as Grades I/II, may present with cold peripheries	Spontaneous bleeding may be present	Circulatory failure manifested by a rapid, weak pulse, narrowing of pulse pressure, or hypotension, with cold clammy skin and restlessness
Grade IV (DSS)	Same as Grades I/II; may present with cold peripheries. May have features suggestive of organ hypoperfusion	Spontaneous bleeding may be present	Profound shock with undetectable blood pressure or peripheral pulse

DSS, dengue shock syndrome; BP, blood pressure

may predispose a child to mucosal bleeds and salicylates have been associated with Reye syndrome. In an epidemic setting, all patients with DF require regular monitoring by a primary care physician for early detection of DHF. The primary care physician/healthcare worker should monitor the patient for clinical features of DHF/DSS along with hematocrit and platelet counts, if possible. Any patient who develops cold extremities, restlessness, acute abdominal pain, decreased urine output, bleeding, or hemoconcentration should be admitted to a hospital. Children with a rising hematocrit and thrombocytopenia without clinical symptoms should also be admitted. Children should be encouraged to improve their oral fluid intake, when possible. Electrolyte/carbohydrate solutions, such as WHO oral rehydration salt solutions, are preferred over plain water or other fluids. The management discussed here is based on guidelines issued by the WHO. Early recognition of these conditions is crucial for decreasing case fatality rates. In the hospital, children without hypotension (DHF grades I and II) should be given Ringer lactate infusion at the rate of 7 mL/kg over 1 hr. After 1 hr, if the hematocrit decreases and vital parameters improve, fluid infusion rate may be decreased to 5 mL/kg over the next hour and to 3 mL/kg/hr for 24–48 hrs. When the patient is stable, as indicated by normal blood pressure, satisfactory oral intake, and urine output, the child can be discharged. If at 1 hr, the hematocrit is rising and vital parameters do not show

TABLE 58.2

DIAGNOSTIC TESTS FOR DENGUE HEMORRHAGIC FEVER

Period	Tests
Within first 5 days of onset of fever	Viral isolation from blood (inoculated either in suckling mice or in various tissue cultures of mammalian or mosquito origin)
After defervescence/in convalescent phase	Serologic tests: IgM: MAC ELISA, strip test IgG: hemagglutination inhibition test, strip test

IgM, immunoglobulin M; MAC-ELISA, IgM antibody-capture enzyme-linked immunosorbent assay; IgG, immunoglobulin G.

TABLE 58.3

VARIOUS VIRAL HEMORRHAGIC FEVERS

Disease	Virus	Vector	Geographic areas
Crimean-Congo hemorrhagic fever	Congo virus	Ixodid ticks (*Hyalomma*)	Bulgaria, western Crimea, Rostov-on-Don and Astrakhan regions, Pakistan, Afghanistan, Arabian Peninsula, South Africa, Oman, southern Russia
Kyasanur Forest disease	Kyasanur forest disease virus	Ticks	Mysore State, India
Omsk hemorrhagic fever	Omsk virus	Ticks	South central Russia, northern Romania
Rift Valley fever	Rift valley fever virus	Mosquitoes	North, Central, East, and South Africa, Saudi Arabia, Yemen
Argentine hemorrhagic Fever	Junin virus	Rodent	Argentina
Bolivian hemorrhagic fever	Machupo virus	Rodent	Amazonian Bolivia
Lassa fever	Lassa virus	Rodent (*Mastomys*)	Nigeria, Sierra Leone, Liberia
Marburg disease	Marburg virus	Unknown	Congo Republic, Germany, Yugoslavia Zimbabwe, Kenya, South Africa
Ebola hemorrhagic fever	Ebola virus	Unknown	Northern Zaire, southern Sudan, Uganda, Central and West Africa
Hemorrhagic fever with renal syndrome	Hanta virus	Rodents (*Apodemus agrarius, Clethrionomys glareolus, Apodemus flavicollis*)	Japan, Korea, Far Eastern Siberia, north and central China, European and Asian Russia, Scandinavia, Czechoslovakia, Romania, Bulgaria, Yugoslavia, Greece
Yellow fever	Yellow fever virus	Mosquitoes (*Aedes* and *Haemogogus*)	Tropical areas of Africa and the Americas

improvement, fluid infusion rate is increased to 10 mL/kg over the next hour. In case of no improvement, the fluid infusion rate is further increased to 15 mL/kg over the third hour. If no improvement is observed in vital parameters and hematocrit at the end of 3 hrs, administration of plasma infusion (10 mL/kg) or colloids should be initiated (**Fig. 58.1**). Once the hematocrit and vital parameters are stable, the infusion rate is gradually reduced and discontinued over 24–48 hrs.

VIRAL HEMORRHAGIC FEVERS

Viral hemorrhagic fevers (VHF) are summarized in **Table 58.3**. The clinical features of different types of viral hemorrhagic fevers are summarized in **Table 58.4**. In all VHF, the virus can be recovered during the early febrile stage. The viruses are readily identified by electron microscopy, with a filamentous structure that differentiates them from all other known agents. The viruses of hemorrhagic fever with renal syndrome (HFRS) can be recovered from acute-phase serum or urine by inoculation into tissue culture. A variety of antibody tests using viral subunits are becoming available. Serologic diagnosis depends on demonstrating seroconversion (i.e., a 4-fold or greater increase in immunoglobulin G antibody titer in acute and convalescent serum samples taken 3–4 weeks apart). Handling blood and other biologic specimens is hazardous and must be performed by specially trained personnel. For those hemorrhagic fever viruses that can be transmitted from person to person (Ebola, Marburg, Lassa, and Crimean-Congo hemorrhagic fever viruses), avoiding close physical contact with infected people and their body fluids

TABLE 58.4

CLINICAL FEATURES OF VIRAL HEMORRHAGIC FEVERS

Disease	Incubation period	Clinical features	Case fatality
Crimean-Congo hemorrhagic fever	3–12 days	Fever, severe headache, myalgia, abdominal pain, anorexia, nausea, and vomiting; erythematous facial or truncal flush and injected conjunctivae; hemorrhagic enanthem on the soft palate and a fine petechial rash on the chest and abdomen. Large areas of purpura and bleeding from gums, nose, intestine, lungs, or uterus may be seen. Hepatomegaly in absence of icterus. In severe illnesses, CNS symptoms and signs may be seen	2%–50%
Kyasanur Forest disease	3–8 days	Severe myalgia, prostration, and bronchiolar involvement; often presents without hemorrhage but occasionally with severe gastrointestinal bleeding, bronchopneumonia, acute renal failure, and focal liver damage, meningoencephalitis	3%–10%
Omsk hemorrhagic fever	3–8 days	Moderate epistaxis, hematemesis, and a hemorrhagic enanthem but no profuse hemorrhage, bronchopneumonia	1%–10%
Rift Valley fever	3–6 days	Fever, headache, prostration, myalgia, anorexia, nausea, vomiting, conjunctivitis, and lymphadenopathy, purpura, epistaxis, hematemesis, and melena	~ 1%
Argentine, Venezuelan, and Bolivian hemorrhagic fever and Lassa fever	~ 7–14 days	Fever, headache, diffuse myalgia, anorexia, sore throat, dysphagia, cough, oropharyngeal ulcers, nausea, vomiting, diarrhea, pains in chest, abdomen, pleuritic chest pain; tourniquet test may be positive. Hypovolemic shock may be accompanied by pleural effusion and renal failure; respiratory distress (airway obstruction, pleural effusion, or congestive heart failure); neurologic symptoms, seizures	10%–40%
Marburg disease and Ebola hemorrhagic fever	4–7 days	Headache, malaise, drowsiness, lumbar myalgia, vomiting, nausea, and diarrhea. Maculopapular eruption, often hemorrhagic, dark red enanthem on the hard palate, conjunctivitis, and scrotal or labial edema. Gastrointestinal hemorrhage in severe illness. Hypotension and coma in severe cases. Disseminated intravascular coagulation and thrombocytopenia are seen in most patients	Marburg disease: 25% Ebola hemorrhagic fever: 50%–90%
Hemorrhagic fever with renal syndrome (Hanta, Puumala)	9–35 days	Fever, petechiae, mild hemorrhagic phenomena, mild proteinuria. Thrombocytopenia, petechiae, proteinuria. Hypotension may follow defervescence. Hemoconcentration, ecchymoses, oliguria. Confusion, extreme restlessness. Fatal cases may manifest retroperitoneal edema and marked hemorrhagic necrosis of the renal medulla	5%–10%
Yellow fever	3–6 days	Abrupt onset. Fever, headache, severe myalgias, diarrhea, vomiting, severe prostration, conjunctival suffusion, photophobia, cervical and axillary adenopathy, and more rarely, splenomegaly or hepatosplenomegaly. Papulovesicular lesions involving the soft palate and pulmonary manifestations are frequent during the first stage of the illness. The second stage of the illness is associated with neurologic involvement. Hemorrhagic manifestations are similar to those observed with other viral hemorrhagic fevers	<10%

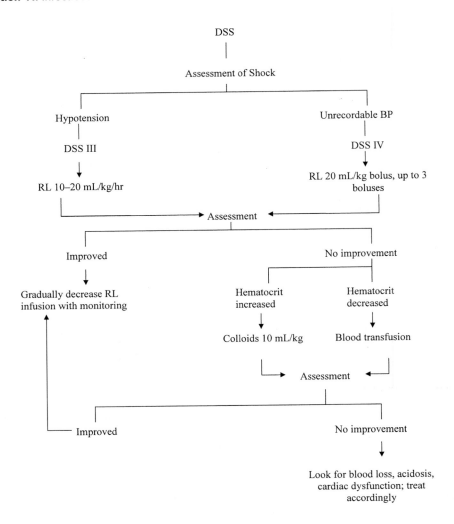

DSS, Dengue shock syndrome; BP, blood pressure, RL, Ringer's lactate;

FIGURE 58.1. Treatment of dengue shock syndrome.

is the most effective way of controlling the spread of disease. Infection control techniques include barrier nursing, isolating infected individuals, and wearing protective clothing. Other infection control recommendations include proper use, disinfection, and disposal of instruments and equipment (needles, thermometers, etc.) used in treating or caring for patients with VHF.

VHF isolation precautions include the following:

1. Isolation of the patient (universal, contact, droplet)
2. Wearing of protective clothing in the isolation area, in the cleaning and laundry areas, and in the laboratory; protective gear should include a scrub suit, gown, apron, 2 pairs of gloves, mask, head cover, eyewear, and rubber boots
3. Cleaning and disinfecting spills, waste, and reusable equipment safely
4. Cleaning and disinfecting soiled linens and laundry safely
5. Using safe disposal methods for nonreusable supplies and infectious waste
6. Providing information about the risk of VHF transmission to health facility staff; reinforcing use of VHF isolation precautions with all health facility staff

Ribavirin administered IV is effective in reducing mortality in Lassa fever and HFRS. The principle involved in management of all of these diseases, especially HFRS, is the reversal of dehydration, hemoconcentration, renal failure, and protein, electrolyte, or blood losses. The management of hemorrhage should be individualized. Transfusions of fresh blood and platelets are frequently given. Good results have been reported in a few patients after the administration of clotting factor concentrates.

HIV INFECTION IN THE CRITICALLY ILL CHILD

HIV infection has become an important contributor to childhood morbidity and mortality, especially in many developing countries. The pandemic has undone many of the significant gains in child health. Increasing numbers of infants and children with HIV infection/AIDS are being admitted to PICUs, particularly in certain geographic areas, and a significant proportion of these patients may be first diagnosed during their PICU stay. Most patients are admitted because of respiratory infections and respiratory failure, septic shock, and CNS disorders. As the number of children receiving antiretroviral therapy increases, severe complications of therapy may also become indications for PICU admission. Specific infection control, nutritional, and medicolegal strategies will facilitate safe, effective delivery of care to HIV-infected infants and children in the PICU. Perinatal treatment of HIV-infected mothers with antiretroviral drugs has dramatically decreased these rates. Heat treatment of factor VIII concentrate and HIV antibody screening of donors has virtually eliminated HIV transmission to children with hemophilia. Blood donor screening has dramatically reduced, but not eliminated, the risk of transfusion-associated HIV infection. Although HIV can be isolated rarely from saliva, it is in very low titers (<1 infectious particle/mL) and has not been implicated as a transmission vehicle.

Before highly active antiretroviral therapy (HAART) was available, 3 distinct patterns of disease were described in children. HIV-infected children have changes in the immune system that are similar to those in HIV-infected adults. CD4 cell depletion may be less dramatic because infants normally have a relative lymphocytosis. Therefore, for example, a value of 1500 CD4 cells/mm^3 in children <1 year of age is indicative of severe CD4 depletion and is comparable to <200 CD4 cells/mm^3 in adults. B-cell activation occurs in most children early in the infection, as evidenced by hypergammaglobulinemia associated with high levels of anti-HIV-1 antibody.

The clinical manifestations of HIV infection vary widely among infants, children, and adolescents. The HIV classification system is used to categorize the stage of pediatric disease via 2 parameters: clinical status (**Table 58.5**) and degree of immunologic impairment (**Table 58.6**).

The most common HIV-related diseases that lead to PICU admission are respiratory infections and respiratory failure, septic shock, and disorders of the CNS. Pneumocystis pneumonia is common in HIV-infected children with severe immunodeficiency, and if untreated, is universally fatal. *Pneumocystis jiroveci* (previously *P. carinii*) pneumonia (PCP) is one of the commonest AIDS-defining illnesses in children in the US and Europe. Even if a child develops PCP while on prophylaxis, therapy may be started with trimethoprim/sulfamethoxazole. Despite hypergammaglobulinemia, HIV-infected children are at risk for severe and recurrent bacterial infections. The common pathogens for community-acquired pneumonia are *Streptococcus pneumoniae*, *Haemophilus influenzae*, and *Staphylococcus aureus*. However, in children with severe immunosuppression and in hospital-acquired infections, Gram-negative organisms, such as *Pseudomonas aeruginosa*, gain importance. Sick children with pneumonia should be treated with parenteral antibiotics. Choices of appropriate antibiotics are often made based on local patterns of etiologies and susceptibilities. In many settings, an appropriate choice would be a combination of a broad-spectrum cephalosporin and an aminoglycoside. In areas where a large proportion of *Staphylococcus aureus* isolates are resistant to antistaphylococcal antibiotics (MRSA or methicillin-resistant *Staphylococcus aureus*), the empiric inclusion of vancomycin, clindamycin, linezolid, or other drugs to which community-acquired MRSA is usually susceptible should be considered. As *P. jiroveci* pneumonia cannot be excluded at the outset in most HIV-infected children with severe respiratory infections, cotrimoxazole should be added unless another diagnosis has been definitively made.

Coexistent tuberculosis (TB) and HIV infections accelerate the progression of both diseases. HIV-infected children are more likely to have extrapulmonary and disseminated TB; the course is also likely to be more rapid. All HIV-infected children with active TB should receive longer duration of antitubercular therapy; a 9–12-month therapy is preferred.

Pulmonary disease with *Mycobacterium Avium-intracellulare* is uncommon in children with HIV infection, despite immunosuppression. The common symptoms and signs include persistent fever, failure to thrive, night sweats, lymphadenopathy, organomegaly, and refractory anemia. The pulmonary lesions are usually limited to lymphadenopathy and localized parenchymal lesions. The diagnosis

TABLE 58.5

CLINICAL CATEGORIES OF HUMAN IMMUNODEFICIENCY VIRUS INFECTION

Clinical category N
Children who have no signs or symptoms considered to be the result of HIV infection or who have only one of the conditions listed in Category A

Clinical category A
Children with 2 or more of the conditions listed below but none of the conditions listed in Categories B and C.

Lymphadenopathy ($\geq$0.5 cm at >2 sites; bilateral = 1 site
Hepatomegaly
Splenomegaly
Dermatitis
Parotitis
Recurrent or persistent upper respiratory infection, sinusitis, or otitis media

Clinical category B
Children who have symptomatic conditions other than those listed for Category A or C that are attributed to HIV infection. Examples of conditions in clinical Category B include but are not limited to:

Anemia (<8 g/dL), neutropenia (<1000/mm^3), or thrombocytopenia (<100,000/mm^3) persisting for at least 30 days
Bacterial meningitis, pneumonia, or sepsis (single episode)
Candidiasis, oropharyngeal (thrush), persisting for >2 months in children >6 months of age
Cardiomyopathy
Cytomegalovirus infection, with onset before 1 month of age
Diarrhea, recurrent or chronic
Hepatitis
HSV stomatitis, recurrent (>2 episodes within 1 year)
HSV bronchitis, pneumonitis, or esophagitis, with onset before 1 month of age
Herpes zoster (shingles) involving at least 2 distinct episodes or >1 dermatome
Leiomyosarcoma
Lymphoid interstitial pneumonia
Nephropathy
Nocardiosis
Persistent fever (lasting >1 month)
Toxoplasmosis, onset before 1 month of age
Varicella, disseminated

Clinical category C
Serious bacterial infections, multiple or recurrent (i.e., any combination of at least 2 culture-confirmed infections within a 2-year period), of the following types: septicemia, pneumonia, meningitis, bone or joint infection, or abscess of an internal organ or body cavity (excluding otitis media, superficial skin or mucosal abscesses, and indwelling catheter-related infections)
Candidiasis, esophageal or pulmonary (bronchi, trachea, lungs)
Coccidioidomycosis, disseminated (at site other than, or in addition to, lungs or cervical or hilar lymph nodes)
Cryptococcosis, extrapulmonary
Cryptosporidiosis or isosporiasis with diarrhea persisting >1 month
Cytomegalovirus disease, with onset of symptoms at age >1 month (at a site other than liver, spleen, or lymph nodes)
Encephalopathy (at least one of the following progressive findings present for at least 2 months in the absence of a concurrent illness other than HIV infection that could explain the findings):
failure to attain or loss of developmental milestones, or loss of intellectual ability, verified by standard developmental scale or neuropsychologic tests; impaired brain growth or acquired microcephaly demonstrated by head circumference measurements or brain atrophy demonstrated by CT or MRI (serial imaging is required for children <2 years of age); acquired symmetric motor deficit manifested by 2 or more of the following: paresis, pathologic reflexes, ataxia, or gait disturbance
HSV infection causing a mucocutaneous ulcer that persists for >1 month; or bronchitis, pneumonitis, or esophagitis for any duration affecting a child >1 month of age
Histoplasmosis, disseminated (at a site other than, or in addition to, lungs or cervical or hilar lymph nodes)
Kaposi sarcoma
Lymphoma, primary, in brain
Lymphoma, small, noncleaved cell (Burkitt syndrome), or immunoblastic or large cell lymphoma of B-cell or unknown immunologic phenotype
Mycobacterium TB, disseminated or extrapulmonary
Mycobacterium, other species or unidentified species, disseminated (at a site other than, or in addition to, lungs, skin, or cervical or hilar lymph nodes)
Mycobacterium avium complex or Mycobacterium kansasii, disseminated (at site other than, or in addition to, lungs, skin, or cervical or hilar lymph nodes)
Pneumocystis jiroveci pneumonia
Progressive multifocal leukoencephalopathy
Salmonella (nontyphoid) septicemia, recurrent
Toxoplasmosis of the brain with onset at >1 mo of age
Wasting syndrome in the absence of a concurrent illness other than HIV infection that could explain the following findings:
(a) Persistent weight loss >10% of baseline, *OR*
(b) Downward crossing of at least 2 of the following percentile lines on the weight-for-age chart (e.g., 95th, 75th, 50th, 25th, 5th) in a child at least 1 year of age, *OR*
<Fifth percentile on weight-for-height chart on 2 consecutive measurements at least 30 days apart, *PLUS*
  (i) Chronic diarrhea (i.e., at least 2 loose stools per day for >30 days), *OR*
  (ii) Documented fever (for at least 30 days, intermittent or constant)

HIV, human immunodeficiency virus; HSV, herpes simplex virus; TB, tuberculosis
From Centers for Disease Control and Prevention. 1994 Revised classification system for human immunodeficiency virus infection in children less than 13 years of age. *MMWR* 1994;43:6–8.

TABLE 58.6

IMMUNOLOGIC CATEGORIES BASED ON AGE-SPECIFIC CD-4 T LYMPHOCYTE COUNTS IN CHILDREN WITH HIV INFECTION

Immunologic categories	Age of child					
	<12 mos		1–5 yrs		6–12 yrs	
	Cells/mm^3	%	Cells/mm^3	%	Cells/mm^3	%
1 No evidence of suppression	≥1500	≥25	≥1000	≥25	≥500	≥25
2 Moderate suppression	750–1499	15–24	500–999	15–24	200–499	15–24
3 Severe suppression	<750	<15	<500	<15	<200	<15

From Centers for Disease Control and Prevention. 1994 Revised classification system for human immunodeficiency virus infection in children less than 13 years of age. *MMWR* 1994;43:6–8.

of disseminated disease primarily depends on isolation of the organism from blood. Current therapy for disseminated *Mycobacterium Avium-intracellulare* infection involves use of a combination of clarithromycin or azithromycin with ethambutol.

Infections caused by respiratory syncytial virus, influenza, and parainfluenza viruses result in symptomatic disease more often in HIV-infected children, in comparison to noninfected children. Infections with other viruses, such as adenovirus and measles virus, are more likely to lead to serious sequelae than are the previously mentioned viruses. As respiratory syncytial viral infection most often occurs in children in the first 2 yrs of life, during which many may not be severely immunocompromised, the severity of illness may not be different from the non–HIV-infected children. In children with AIDS, disseminated cytomegalovirus is a known opportunistic infection, but pneumonia caused by this virus is rare.

Pulmonary fungal infections usually present as a part of disseminated disease in immunocompromised children. Primary pulmonary fungal infections are uncommon. Pulmonary candidiasis should be suspected in any HIV-infected child with lower respiratory tract infection that does not respond to the common therapeutic modalities. A positive blood culture supports the diagnosis of invasive candidiasis.

Lymphoid interstitial pneumonitis (LIP) has been recognized as a distinctive marker for pediatric HIV infection and is included as a Class B condition LIP is characterized by nodule formation and diffuse infiltration of the alveolar septae by lymphocytes, plasmacytoid lymphocytes, plasma cells, and immunoblasts. LIP is usually diagnosed in children with perinatally acquired HIV infection when they are >1 year of age, unlike with PCP. Most children with LIP are asymptomatic. Reticulonodular pattern, with or without hilar lymphadenopathy, that persists on chest x-ray for 2 mos or greater and that is unresponsive to

antimicrobial therapy is considered presumptive evidence of LIP. Care should be taken to exclude other possible etiologies. A definitive diagnosis of LIP can be made only by histopathology. Early disease is managed conservatively. The effect of antiretrovirals on LIP is probably limited. Steroids are indicated if children with LIP have symptoms and signs of chronic pulmonary disease, clubbing and/or hypoxemia. Treatment usually includes an initial 4–12-week course of prednisolone (2 mg/kg/d), followed by a tapering dose, using oxygen saturation and clinical status as a guide to improvement. This treatment is then followed by chronic low-dose prednisolone.

A variety of microbes can cause gastrointestinal disease, including bacteria (*Salmonella*, *Campylobacter*, *Mycobacterium avium intracellulare* complex), protozoa (*Giardia*, *Cryptosporidium*, *Isospora*, microsporidia), viruses (cytomegalovirus, herpes simplex virus, rotavirus), and fungi (*Candida*). The protozoal infections are most severe and can be protracted in children with severe immunosuppression. Children with cryptosporidium infestation can have severe diarrhea that leads to hypovolemic shock, which may merit admission to the PICU. AIDS enteropathy, a syndrome of malabsorption with partial villous atrophy not associated with a specific pathogen, is probably the result of direct HIV infection of the gut. Chronic liver inflammation is relatively common in HIV-infected children. In some, hepatitis caused by cytomegalovirus, hepatitis B or C viruses, or *Mycobacterium avium* complex (MAC) may lead to liver failure and portal hypertension. It is important to recognize that several of the antiretroviral drugs (e.g., didanosine) and protease inhibitors may also cause reversible elevation of transaminases.

Neurologic disease presents as progressive encephalopathy with loss or plateau of developmental milestones, cognitive deterioration, impaired

TABLE 58.7

INDICATIONS FOR INITIATION OF HIGHLY ACTIVE ANTIRETROVIRAL THERAPY IN HIV-INFECTED CHILDREN

Clinical category		CD4 percentage		Plasma viral load	Recommendation
AIDS (clinical category C)[a]	OR	15% (immune category 3)[b]		Any value	Initiate HAART
Mild-to-moderate symptoms (clinical category A or B)[a]	OR	15%–25% (immune category 2)[b]	OR	>100,000 copies/mL	Consider initiating HAART
Asymptomatic (clinical category N)[a]	AND	>25% (immune category 1)[b]	AND	<100,000 copies/mL	Usually HAART is deferred, and the child is monitored.

HAART, highly active antiretroviral therapy
[a] See Table 58.5.
[b] See Table 58.6.
From Working Group on Antiretroviral Therapy and Medical Management of HIV-Infected Children. *Guidelines for the Use of Antiretroviral Agents in Pediatric HIV Infection*. National Institutes of Health (NIH). US. Nov 3, 2005.

brain growth that results in acquired microcephaly, and symmetric motor dysfunction. CNS infections (meningitis due to bacterial pathogens, fungi, such as *Cryptococcus*, and a number of viruses) may be responsible for clinical presentations that are indications for PICU admission. CNS toxoplasmosis is exceedingly rare in young infants but may occur in HIV-infected adolescents; the overwhelming majority of these cases have serum IgG antitoxoplasma antibodies as a marker of infection.

Cardiac abnormalities in HIV-infected children are common, persistent, and often progressive; however, most are subclinical. Electrocardiography and echocardiography are helpful in assessing cardiac function before the onset of clinical symptoms.

Nephropathy is an unusual presenting symptom of HIV infection, more commonly occurring in older symptomatic children. Nephrotic syndrome is the most common manifestation of pediatric renal disease, with edema, hypoalbuminemia, proteinuria, and azotemia with normal blood pressure. Polyuria, oliguria, and hematuria have also been observed in some patients.

All infants born to HIV-infected mothers test antibody-positive at birth because of passive transfer of maternal HIV antibody across the placenta. Specific viral diagnostic assays, such as HIV DNA or RNA PCR, HIV culture, or HIV p24 antigen immune dissociated p24 (ICD-p24), are essential for diagnosis of young infants born to HIV-infected mothers. By 6 months of age, the HIV culture and/or PCR identifies all infected infants, who are not having any continued exposure due to breast feeding. HIV DNA PCR is the preferred virologic assay in developed countries. Plasma HIV RNA assays may be more sensitive than DNA PCR for early diagnosis, but data are limited. HIV culture has similar sensitivity to HIV DNA PCR; however, it is more technically complex and expensive, and results are often not available for 2–4 weeks, compared to 2–3 days with PCR. The p24 antigen assay is less sensitive than the other virologic tests.

The indications for initiation of HAART are detailed in **Table 58.7**. Availability of antiretroviral therapy has transformed HIV infection from a uniformly fatal condition to a chronic infection, with which children can lead a near-normal life. The currently available therapy does not eradicate the virus and cure the child; it rather suppresses the virus replication for extended periods of time. The 3 main groups of drugs are nucleoside reverse transcriptase inhibitors (NRTI), nonnucleoside reverse transcriptase inhibitors (NNRTI), and protease inhibitors (PI). HAART is a combination of 2 NRTIs with a PI or an NNRTI (**Table 58.8**). Some complications of antiretroviral therapy, such as lactic acidosis, severe pancreatitis, and Stevens Johnson syndrome, may require care in the PICU.

The staff in the PICU should always adhere to universal precautions, regardless of the presence or absence of known or suspected HIV infection in their patients. In case of exposure, the staff should follow the standard guidelines for postexposure prophylaxis (PEP). The majority of HIV exposures will warrant a 2-drug regimen, using 2 NRTIs [zidovudine and lamivudine or emtricitabine (FTC)] or 1 nucleotide reverse transcriptase inhibitor and 1 NRTI (tenofovir and lamivudine or emtricitabine). The U.S. Public Health Service now recommends that expanded PEP regimens be PI-based. The PI preferred for use in expanded PEP regimens is lopinavir/ritonavir (LPV/RTV). Other PIs acceptable for use in

ANTIRETROVIRAL DRUGS COMMONLY USED IN CHILDREN

Drug	Dose	Side effects
Nucleoside reverse transcriptase inhibitors		
Abacavir	3 mos–13 yrs: 8 mg/kg/dose q 12 hrs >13 yrs: 300 mg/dose q 12 hrs (max: 300 mg/dose)	Hypersensitivity
Didanosine	0–3 mos: 50 mg/m^2/dose q 12 hrs 3 mos–13 yrs: 90–150 mg/m^2 q 12 hrs (max: 200 mg/dose) >13 yrs: <60 kg: 125-mg tablet q 12 hrs >13 yrs: >60 kg: 200-mg tablet q 12 hrs (higher dose for powder preparations)	Peripheral neuropathy, pancreatitis, abdominal pain, diarrhea
Lamivudine (3TC)	1 mo–13 yrs: 4 mg/kg q 12 hrs >13 yrs: <50 kg: 4 mg/kg/dose q 12 hrs >13 yrs: >50 kg: 150 mg/kg/dose q 12 hrs	Pancreatitis, neuropathy, neutropenia
Stavudine (d4T)	1 mo–13 yrs: 1 mg/kg q12 hrs >13 yrs: 30–60 kg: 30 mg/dose q 12 hrs >13 yrs: >60 kg: 40 mg/dose q 12 hrs	Headache, gastrointestinal upset, neuropathy
Zalcitabine	<13 yrs: 0.01 mg/kg/dose q 8 hrs >13 yrs: 0.75 mg q 8hrs	Rash, peripheral neuropathy, pancreatitis
Zidovudine	Neonates: 2 mg/kg q 6 hrs 3 mos–13 yrs: 90–180 mg/m^2 q 6–8 hrs >13 yrs: 200 mg q 8 hrs or 300 mg q 12 hrs	Anemia, myopathy
Nonnucleoside reverse transcriptase inhibitors		
Nevirapine (NVP)	2 mos–13 yrs: 120 mg/m^2(max 200 mg) q 24 hrs for 14 d, followed by 120–200 mg/m^2 q 12 hrs OR <8 yrs: 7 mg/kg q 12 hrs >8 yrs: 4 mg/kg q 12 hrs >13 yrs: 200 mg q 24 hrs for 14 d; then increase to 200 mg q 12 hrs if no rash or other side effects	Skin rash, Steven Johnson syndrome
Efavirenz	>3 yrs: 10–<15 kg: 200 mg q 24 hrs 15–<20 kg: 250 mg q 24 hrs 20–<25 kg: 300 mg q 24 hrs 25–<32.5 kg: 350 mg q 24 hrs 32.5–<40 kg: 400 mg q 24 hrs >40 kg: 600 mg q 24 hrs	Skin rash, central nervous system symptoms, increased transaminase levels
Protease inhibitors		
Amprenavir	4–16 yrs & <50 kg: 22.5 mg/kg q 12 hrs (oral solution) OR 20 mg/kg q 12 hrs (capsules) >13 yrs & >50 kg: 1200 mg q 12 hrs (capsules)	
Indinavir	500 mg/m^2 q 8 hrs >13 yrs: 800 mg q 8 hrs	Hyperbilirubinemia, nephrolithiasis
Lopinavir/ ritonavir	6 mos–12 yrs: 7–<15 kg: 12 mg/kg lopinavir OR 3 mg/kg ritonavir q 12 hrs with food; 15–40 kg: 10 mg/kg lopinavir OR 2.5 mg/kg ritonavir q 12 hrs with food >12 yrs: 400 mg lopinavir OR 100 mg ritonavir q 12 hrs with food	Diarrhea, fatigue, headache, nausea, and increased cholesterol and triglycerides
Nelfinavir	<13 yrs: 50–55 mg/ kg q 12 hrs >13 yrs: 1250 mg q 12 hrs (max 2000 mg)	Diarrhea, abdominal pain
Ritonavir	<13 yrs: 350–400 mg/m^2 q 12 hrs (starting dose: 250 mg/m^2) >13 yrs: 600 mg q 12 hrs (starting with 300 mg)	Bad taste, vomiting, nausea, diarrhea, rarely, hepatitis
Saquinavir	50 mg/kg q 8 hrs >13 yrs: soft gel capsules, 1200 mg q 8 hrs	Diarrhea, headache, skin rash

Data from Working Group on Antiretroviral Therapy and Medical Management of HIV-Infected Children. *Guidelines for the Use of Antiretroviral Agents in Pediatric HIV Infection.* Bethesda, Maryland: National Institutes of Health, Nov. 3, 2005.

expanded PEP regimens include atazanavir, fosamprenavir, ritonavir-boosted indinavir, ritonavir-boosted saquinavir, and nelfinavir. Although side effects are common with NNRTIs, efavirenz may be considered for expanded PEP regimens, especially when resistance to PIs in the source person's virus is known or suspected. Caution is advised when efavirenz is used in women of childbearing age because of the risk of teratogenicity. PEP should be initiated as soon as possible, preferably within hours rather than days of exposure. If a question exists concerning which antiretroviral drugs to use or whether to use a basic or expanded regimen, the basic regimen should be started immediately rather than delay PEP administration. PEP should be administered for 4 weeks, if tolerated.

MEASLES

The virus can easily be inactivated by heat, ultraviolet light, lipid solvents, and extremes of pH. All measles strains are antigenically homogeneous. The measles virus is spread from an infected individual to a new host by the respiratory route via aerosolized droplets of respiratory secretions. Close person-to-person contact can facilitate transfer of nasal secretions of a patient to the nose of the host. Of the various organ systems involved, the most prominent are the lungs and the brain. The first sign of infection is usually high fever, which begins ~8–12 days after exposure and lasts 1–7 days. During this initial stage, the child may develop coryza (runny nose), cough, red and watery eyes, and an enanthem—small white Koplik spots usually found on the buccal mucosa near the molars. Children are usually very irritable. After several days of fever, a rash develops, usually beginning on the face (often in the hairline) and upper neck. The rash is initially erythematous and maculopapular; typical of measles rash is the coexistence of discrete and confluent red maculopapules. Microvesicles may be seen on the top of the erythematous base. Over a period of ~3 days, the rash proceeds downward, eventually reaching the hands and feet. The rash lasts for 5–6 days and then fades. The rash occurs, on average, at day 14 after exposure to the virus, with a range of 7–18 days. Pharyngitis, cervical lymphadenopathy, diarrhea, vomiting, laryngitis, and croup may also occur during the illness.

Atypical measles, a clearly defined clinical syndrome that occurred in previously vaccinated individuals (specifically those who received a killed measles vaccine that is no longer available) after exposure to natural measles, is no longer seen. This illness was characterized by high fever, petechial rash, and pneumonitis and was caused by immune complex deposition. It had a different progression of the rash (cephalad from the extremities).

Primary viral involvement of the lungs is characterized by hyperinflation and fluffy perihilar infiltrates. Infants with measles-associated lower-respiratory tract infections may present with features suggestive of bronchiolitis. Although measles virus itself can lead to severe pulmonary disease, secondary bacterial pneumonias are caused by *H. influenzae*, *S. pneumoniae*, and *S. aureus*.

Measles virus can result in 3 different forms of CNS infections. Acute progressive brain disease, also referred to as inclusion body encephalitis, reflects a direct attack by the virus under conditions of yielding cell-mediated immunity. The postinfectious acute disease is interpreted to reflect an autoimmune reaction. Symptoms of encephalitis usually develop in the second week of illness. Some children may have rapid deterioration, and marked increase in intracranial pressure and herniation may occur. SSPE is a rare CNS disease with progressive degenerative loss of intelligence, behavioral difficulties, and seizures.

The differential diagnosis of measles includes all illnesses in which erythematous maculopapular rash occurs, such as rubella, erythema infectiosum, roseola infantum, enteroviral infections, infectious mononucleosis, *Mycoplasma pneumoniae* infections, and drug reactions. The typical course and pattern of rash usually allow the diagnosis to be made clinically.

Children who require hospitalization must be managed for the complications and treated with a dose of 200,000 IU of vitamin A. The WHO and UNICEF recommend vitamin A for all children with measles in regions where vitamin A deficiency is common. The dose should be repeated after 24 hrs.

NONPOLIO ENTEROVIRAL INFECTIONS

Enteroviruses include polioviruses, coxsackieviruses, and echoviruses. Newer enteroviruses are classified by numbering. Although >60 different serotypes have been identified, 11 account for the majority of disease

Enteroviral infections vary from mild to fatal illnesses. The spectrum of mild illnesses includes nonspecific febrile illness, common cold, pharyngitis, herpangina, stomatitis, and parotitis. Croup may be caused by coxsackie and echovirus infections; however, this illness is milder when compared to croup caused by influenza and parainfluenza viruses. The respiratory tract infection may result in bronchitis, bronchiolitis or pneumonia; these are caused by coxsackie and echovirus infections. Various serotypes of coxsackie and echoviruses have been implicated in causation of pericarditis and myocarditis. Neurologic illness is a frequent manifestation of infection with enteroviruses; the most common illness is aseptic meningitis. Encephalitis, paralytic disease due to infection of anterior horn cell infection, Guillain-Barré syndrome, transverse myelitis, and cerebellar ataxia may occur. The genitourinary manifestations include nephritis, orchitis, and epididymitis. Arthritis and myositis may be caused by coxsackie virus infections. Skin rashes are common with enterovirus infections and may be maculopapular, morbilliform, petechial, or small vesicles. A common distribution is on the palms, soles, and oral mucosa, leading to the so-called hand-foot-mouth syndrome.

The clinical presentation may be mistaken for bacterial infections or other viruses that cause similar illnesses. The diagnosis of enterovirus infection can be confirmed by virus isolation and detection. The samples may be collected from the nasopharynx, throat, stool, rectal swab, blood, urine, and cerebrospinal fluid (CSF).

The mainstay of care is supportive treatment. IV immunoglobulin has been used in neonates with severe disseminated infection and is used for children with persistent CNS infection due to immune deficiencies that cause hypogammaglobulinemia. Children with enteroviral infections require universal and contact precautions when admitted to healthcare facilities.

SEVERE VARICELLA INFECTIONS

Varicella (chickenpox) can result in severe manifestations, such as pneumonia, hepatitis, encephalitis, and disseminated intravascular coagulation, particularly in certain groups: neonates, pregnant women, adolescents, adults, and the immunocompromised. Varicella-zoster virus (VZV) establishes life-long latency in the dorsal root ganglia after the primary infection. Reactivation of virus leads to zoster (shingles), which is usually characterized by a pruritic vesicular rash in a dermatomal pattern in immunocompetent patients. Zoster may manifest as a more severe illness in immunocompromised patients and can involve multiple dermatomes and viscera.

Transmission of varicella occurs by either airborne droplets or contact with secretions or infected vesicular fluid. The incubation period is between 10 and 21 days. Chickenpox is characterized by a rash, low-grade fever, and malaise. Patients may have prodromal constitutional symptoms 1–2 days before the onset of rash. The rash, which evolves from maculopapules to pruritic vesicles to crusts, often initially appears on the trunk or face and spreads over days to involve the entire body. Groups, or crops, of skin lesions, which number on average 250–500 in the unvaccinated child, progress from macules to vesicles to crusts. Simultaneously having lesions in various stages of evolution is a clinical hallmark of chickenpox.

Secondary bacterial complications can occur in skin, soft tissues, and other sites and is often caused by group A *Streptococcus* (GAS) and *Staphylococcus aureus*. Varicella is a particularly important risk factor for severe invasive GAS infections in previously healthy children. A GAS infection should be considered in any child with varicella who also has localized skin findings of erythema, warmth, swelling, or induration and in any child with varicella who becomes febrile after having been afebrile, who has a temperature of >39°C beyond day 3 of illness, or who has any fever beyond day 4 of illness. When present, GAS infections are usually painful, and initially, the amount of pain is frequently out of proportion to the clinical findings.

VZV pneumonia often occurs in immunocompromised adults and in those with chronic lung disease. Varicella pneumonia usually presents 1–6 days after the onset of the rash and is associated with tachypnea, chest tightness, cough, dyspnea, fever, and occasionally, with pleuritic chest pain and hemoptysis. Chest symptoms may start before the appearance of the skin rash. Physical findings are often minimal, and chest x-rays typically reveal nodular or interstitial pneumonitis. Findings of VZV pneumonia on chest x-ray consist of multiple 5–10-mm, ill-defined nodules that may be confluent and fleeting. The small, round nodules usually resolve within a week after the disappearance of the skin lesions but may persist for months. Usually resolving in 3–5 days in milder disease, the small nodules may persist for several weeks in widespread disease. The lesions calcify and can persist as numerous, well-defined, randomly scattered, 2–3-mm dense calcifications. High-resolution CT of the chest in patients with varicella pneumonitis usually shows 1–10-mm, well-defined and ill-defined nodules that are diffuse throughout both lungs. Nodules with a surrounding halo of ground-glass opacity, patchy ground-glass opacity, and coalescence of nodules are also seen.

Encephalitis is another serious complication of varicella infection.

SEVERE HERPES SIMPLEX VIRUS INFECTIONS

Herpes simplex virus (HSV) infection is one of the most common human viral infections and frequently involves the skin, mucous membranes, and the genitalia. Immunocompetent patients with HSV infection usually have asymptomatic or mild disease, while immunocompromised patients have a higher risk of disseminated disease, with involvement of multiple organ systems. Herpes simplex encephalitis (HSE) is a life-threatening manifestation of HSV infection of the CNS. HSV pneumonia, particularly in immunocompromised patients, carries a high mortality. The diagnosis of this and other infections caused by the herpes virus family are made difficult by the phenomenon of latency. Extensive cutaneous and visceral dissemination of HSV is seen in certain children with immune deficiencies, such as severely malnourished children, transplant recipients, patients with malignancies or other conditions that require immunosuppression, patients on high-dose steroid therapy, AIDS patients, burn patients or patients with other immunodeficiencies, particularly those affecting T lymphocytes. Disseminated disease in these patients may manifest as a sepsis-like syndrome with fever or hypothermia, leukopenia, hepatitis, disseminated intravascular coagulation, and shock and often results in death.

Neonatal herpes may manifest in 1 of 3 ways. The least severe form is disease limited to skin, eyes, and mucous membranes (SEM disease), which presents usually between days 5 and 19 of life. Disseminated HSV is rapidly progressive and has a high mortality rate. It also usually has onset before the third week of life. Neonatal HSV disease may also be localized to the CNS. Clinicians may fail to make an early diagnosis because children often have no associated cutaneous findings. Cutaneous HSV infections can be diagnosed rapidly by microscopic examination of stained scrapings from the vesicles for giant cells and intranuclear inclusions (Tzanck smear). HSV PCR has been found to be as sensitive as viral culture for diagnosis of cutaneous HSV infection and has the advantage of allowing rapid diagnosis. PCR of the CSF is the method of choice for diagnosis of HSE, but CSF PCR results can be negative in the first 72 hrs following illness onset. Neonatal herpes may occur in the absence of skin lesions; therefore, if the infection is suspected, swabs of the mouth, nasopharynx, conjunctiva, rectum, skin lesions, mucosal lesions, and urine should be promptly taken and submitted for virus culture. Evidence of disseminated or CNS infection should be sought using liver function tests, complete blood cell count, CSF analysis, and chest x-ray, if respiratory abnormalities are present. Microscopic examination, culture and PCR assay of bronchoalveolar lavage fluid may help in the diagnosis of HSV pneumonia.

Serious HSV infections require treatment with IV acyclovir. The recommended dose for HSE is 10 mg/kg every 8 hrs for 21 days. It is also recommended that all patients with HSE undergo a CSF PCR for HSV at the end of 14 days to document elimination of replicating virus. Neonatal and disseminated forms of HSV also require treatment with IV acyclovir. The dose recommended for neonatal HSV encephalitis and neonatal disseminated infection is 20 mg/kg every 8 hrs for 21 days, while SEM disease requires treatment for 14 days. The drug of choice for acyclovir-resistant HSV strains is IV foscarnet.

CHAPTER 59 ■ CENTRAL NERVOUS SYSTEM INFECTIONS

PRATIBHA D. SINGHI • SUNIT C. SINGHI • CHARLES R.J.C. NEWTON • JAKUB SIMON

The main features of CNS infections are fever, headache, and altered sensorium. Focal neurologic signs may also be seen. However, these symptoms and signs are nonspecific and can be seen in noninfectious CNS syndromes as well. Acute meningitis syndrome presents as acute onset over a few hours to a few days of fever, headache, vomiting, photophobia, neck stiffness, and altered sensorium. In subacute or chronic meningitis, the onset is usually gradual, often without any evident predisposing condition. Fever is often present but tends to be lower than in acute meningitis. Progression is slower over a few weeks.

Acute encephalitis may be diffuse or focal. In diffuse encephalitis, alteration of sensorium is predominant and occurs earlier in the course of disease than in acute meningitis. Seizures are seen more frequently than with meningitis and often during the initial phase of disease.

Many systemic infections involve the CNS, and CNS symptoms may be the presenting feature in

TABLE 59.1

CEREBROSPINAL FLUID CHARACTERISTICS IN MENINGITIS

Characteristics	Viral	Bacterial	Tubercular
WBC/mm^3	N (<5) or raised to 10–100	Raised 100 to >1000	Raised 100–1000
Predominant cell type	Lymphocytes	Neutrophils	Lymphocytes
Glucose CSF: serum	N (<0.6) or decreased to <0.4	Decreased to <0.4 or much lower	Decreased to <0.4 or lower
Protein mg/dL	N (<50) or up to 100	Raised 100 to >500	Raised 100–500

WBC, white blood cell; N, normal; CSF, cerebrospinal fluid

some cases. For example, shigellosis, typhoid fever, malaria, rickettsial diseases, and infective endocarditis may involve the CNS. It is therefore important to consider systemic infection as a possible underlying cause in children with encephalopathy.

Acute disseminated encephalomyelitis (ADEM), transverse myelitis, optic neuritis, and multiple sclerosis are disorders of demyelination of the CNS (collectively referred to as *idiopathic inflammatory diseases of the CNS*) that may present global or focal neurologic deficits days to weeks after recovery from an infectious illness, suggesting an autoimmune phenomenon triggered by infection or vaccine.

PRINCIPLES OF CLINICAL MANAGEMENT

The usual cerebrospinal fluid (CSF) characteristics of meningitis are listed in **Table 59.1**. Neuroimaging, electroencephalogram (EEG), and other studies may add to the diagnosis. Drainage of abscesses and obtaining CNS tissue for histopathology are occasionally required.

As with any other serious illness, management starts with the primary survey to ensure immediate attention to the basic airway, breathing, and circulation (ABCs) of life support before looking for an etiologic diagnosis. A secondary survey, with particular attention to the neurologic examination, meningeal signs, and assessment of the severity of coma, if present, is then undertaken. The physical examination in a child with meningitis is mainly geared toward excluding focal neurologic pathology, determining whether the child has clinically significant elevation of intracranial pressure (ICP), finding any source of infection elsewhere in the body (e.g., sinusitis, otitis, pneumonia), and identifying any other etiologic clues, such as rashes or skin lesions.

Children with a Glasgow Coma Scale score of <8, pharyngeal hypotonia, poor gag reflex, and loss of

swallowing reflex require intubation and supplemental oxygen. Appropriate techniques should be used to minimize potential increases in ICP associated with endotracheal intubation. Clinical signs and laboratory data that warrant admission of a child with meningitis to the PICU are listed in **Table 59.2**. Antimicrobial therapy must be administered promptly and, owing to limited penetration into the CSF, at high doses. With increasing severity of illness and raised ICP, the cerebral blood flow (CBF) decreases, especially in the subcortical white matter. ICP must be maintained within a narrow range in children with meningitis. Although ICP monitoring is not routinely recommended, it may be considered in those

TABLE 59.2

CHECKLIST OF CLINICAL SIGNS AND METABOLIC DATA THAT WARRANT ADMISSION OF A CHILD WITH MENINGITIS TO THE PICU

Clinical signs	Metabolic data
Glasgow Coma scale <8	Significant metabolic acidosis
Airway instability	Hypoxemia
Poor/irregular respiratory effort	Hypercapnia
Respiratory distress	Hyponatremia
Hyperventilation	Anemia
Poor perfusion/hypotension	Neutropenia
Oliguria/anuria	Other: Falciparum parasitemia >5%
Hypertension/bradycardia	
Abnormal posturing	
Impaired pupillary response	
Deranged liver/renal functions	
Abnormal doll's eye movements	
Abnormal motor response	
Focal neurodeficits	
Cranial nerve palsy	
Seizures	
Purpura/bleeding diathesis	

children with CNS infection who have clinical signs of moderate-to-severe increase in ICP. Seizures are controlled with IV benzodiazepines, generally diazepam or lorazepam.

Fever, diminished intake, and vomiting may lead to significant dehydration and hypovolemia. Capillary leak secondary to sepsis can further add to hypovolemia. Diabetes insipidus may rapidly lead to hypovolemia and hypernatremia due to urinary free-water loss. The syndrome of inappropriate secretion of antidiuretic hormone may lead to free-water retention, hypo-osmolality, and hyponatremia. Empiric fluid restriction in children with CNS infection is not justified. Fluid therapy should be aimed at maintaining normovolemia and normal blood pressure, thereby maintaining adequate cerebral perfusion. Hyponatremia should be identified early and corrected slowly over 36–48 hrs with normal saline or, occasionally, with 3% saline.

BACTERIAL MENINGITIS

Most organisms that cause bacterial meningitis are transmitted by the respiratory route. They colonize the nasopharyngeal mucosa. To survive in the blood-stream, the pathogens must overcome the host defense systems of circulating antibodies, complement-mediated bacterial killing, and neutrophil phagocytosis. The blood–brain barrier normally protects against meningeal invasion. Cerebral edema in bacterial meningitis may be vasogenic, cytotoxic, or interstitial. Severe brain edema can cause herniation of brain tissue and compression of the brainstem due to increased ICP. The ICP may also increase because of excessive intracerebral hypertension, including the development of obstructive hydrocephalus, cerebritis, cerebral infarction and cerebral venous thrombosis, status epilepticus, and syndrome of inappropriate secretion of antidiuretic hormone.

The presentation in neonates and infants is generally nonspecific with fever, poor feeding, vomiting, lethargy, irritability, high-pitched cry, and seizures. Fever may be absent in very small infants and in severely malnourished babies. The anterior fontanel is full and often bulging, and separation of sutures may be seen. The typical presentation in older children is with acute onset of fever, headache, vomiting, anorexia, photophobia, and altered sensorium. A history of preceding upper respiratory or gastrointestinal infection is often present. On examination, signs of meningeal irritation (stiffness and pain on flexion of the neck), a positive Kernig sign, and positive Brudzinski sign are seen. Older children may adopt a tripod posture with arms held back and straight on sitting surface. Seizures may be the presenting

feature. Raised ICP is common in bacterial meningitis. It often manifests with progressive impairment of sensorium with deepening coma, headache, vomiting, and Cushing triad (abnormalities in ventilation, hypertension, bradycardia). Focal signs may be due to subdural collection, cortical infarction, or cerebritis. Patients with meningococcemia may present with a maculopapular rash, which rapidly progresses into a petechial rash. Rashes can occasionally be seen in *H. influenzae* or pneumococcal meningitis. A child with meningitis should also be examined for other sites of infections, such as pneumonia, otitis media, endocarditis, sinusitis, pyoderma or joint infections.

Meningitis in neonates and very young infants may present as nonspecific septicemia, without any symptoms and signs of CNS involvement. Lumbar puncture (LP) should be done in all such cases to exclude meningitis. In older infants, febrile seizures are the most important differential diagnosis. Cerebral malaria is an important differential diagnosis in developing countries, particularly in endemic regions. In children with raised ICP and focal signs, cerebral abscess, focal encephalitis, such as herpes, intracranial bleeds, and other space-occupying lesions must be excluded. Urgent neuroimaging is warranted in such cases. Early recognition of bacterial meningitis is important for optimal outcome. The World Health Organization (WHO) Integrated Management of Childhood Illness referral criteria for meningitis include lethargy, unconsciousness, inability to feed, stiff neck, and seizures. Definitive diagnosis of meningitis is made by analysis and culture of the CSF. LP should be undertaken in all cases of suspected meningitis unless one of the following contraindications is present: raised ICP (unequal pupils, blood pressure/heart rate changes, abnormal respiratory pattern, deep coma/deteriorating consciousness), focal neurologic symptoms or signs (obtain a CT to exclude space-occupying lesion), shock/cardiorespiratory instability, thrombocytopenia (platelet count <40,000/mm^3/coagulation disorder), or local infection at LP site. Antibiotics should, however, be administered in all cases of suspected meningitis even if the LP is delayed. A proper history and clinical examination are sufficient in most cases to decide the safety of performing an LP, though CT scans are sometimes necessary to rule out pathologies such as mass lesions. It must be remembered that a normal CT does not rule out raised ICP. The characteristic CSF findings in bacterial meningitis are increased opening pressure, polymorphonuclear pleocytosis, decreased glucose, and increased protein concentration. A cloudy CSF under pressure can be considered diagnostic of bacterial meningitis. Normal CSF in children has 0–5 mononuclear cells/mm^3 (lymphocyte and monocytes);

polymorphonuclear cells are very rarely seen. Presence of a single polymorphonuclear cell in the clinical setting of meningitis should be considered significant. In neonates, the upper limit of normal extends to a white blood cell (WBC) count of 20–30 WBC/mm^3, although the mean count is generally 5–10 WBC/mm^3. The CSF glucose is <40 mg/dL and a ratio of serum to blood glucose of <0.4 is suggestive of bacterial meningitis in children >2 months of age; in term neonates, a ratio of <0.6 is considered abnormal. The LP may occasionally be traumatic; a grossly traumatic CSF can be used for culture alone. With less traumatic LPs, prediction of meningitis can often be made. A predicted CSF white cell count is calculated using the formula:

$$\text{CSF WBC (predicted)} = \text{CSF red blood cell (RBC)} \times (\text{blood WBC/blood RBC})$$

The Gram stain is a quick, inexpensive, accurate method for organism identification. The positivity of the Gram stain depends on the number of organisms in the CSF. Acridine orange stain is a fluorochrome that stains the nucleic acid of some bacteria so that they appear bright red orange when seen under a fluorescent microscope. It stains the intracellular bacteria better than the Gram stain and may be positive even when the Gram stain is negative. It has been suggested that in the absence of other tests, empiric diagnosis of bacterial meningitis can be made if the CSF shows cells >300/mm^3 with polymorphs >60% and sugar <50% of the blood level, or an absolute value of <30 mg/dL. Although tubercular meningitis may occasionally have an acute presentation, generally the symptoms are more prolonged; evidence of tuberculosis (TB) elsewhere in the body, such as lungs, abdomen, and fundus for choroid tubercles, should be investigated. It is not always possible in children to differentiate between viral and bacterial meningitis based on clinical symptoms or even after blood or CSF analysis using routine investigations. Rapid diagnostic tests—ELISA—PCR assays, and latex agglutination are useful in providing early diagnosis. Serum and CSF CRP levels can help in discriminating between bacterial and viral meningitis. Several complications may occur with meningitis (**Table 59.3**).

The diagnosis of meningitis is made by clinical presentation and CSF analysis. In the early stages of meningitis, CT may show meningeal enhancement and widening of basal cisterns. A CT scan at presentation is necessary to exclude other pathologies in a child with focal neurologic signs. Later in the illness, CT scan is performed to look for complications if a child does not show clinical improvement, has sudden unexplained deterioration, new-onset seizures or focal neurologic signs, signs of raised ICP, persistent

TABLE 59.3

COMPLICATIONS OF BACTERIAL MENINGITIS

Raised ICP
Seizures
Subdural empyema
Infarcts
Cerebritis
Hydrocephalus
Cranial nerve involvement
Brain abscess
Sensorineural deafness
Disseminated intravascular coagulation

fever, or enlarging head. Routine ultrasound of the head in infants with open fontanel detects most complications early.

If bacterial meningitis is suspected, treatment should be instituted without delay. CSF, blood, and pertinent cultures should ideally be taken before starting antibiotics, but if specimens are difficult to obtain, therapy should be started and specimens obtained later. The Infectious Disease Society of America guidelines for empirical and specific antimicrobial therapy and the recommended dosages of the antimicrobials are shown in **Table 59.4**, **Table 59.5**, and **Table 59.6**.

The American Academy of Pediatrics recommends the use of dexamethasone in *H. influenzae* meningitis: a dose of 0.4 mg/kg, 12 hourly for 2 days. In developing countries, most children receive antibiotics before a diagnosis of meningitis is made, and corticosteroid administration before or with the first dose of antibiotics is rarely possible. As dexamethasone may mask the presentation of underlying infections (e.g., brain abscess, tubercular meningitis, or meningitis due to resistant bacteria), delaying their diagnosis and treatment, routine administration of steroids cannot be recommended in developing countries. The use of human IV immunoglobulin is particularly important for children who have immunoglobulin deficiencies and for neonates who have a limited immunologic response, such as those with group B streptococcus meningitis. Isolation of children with meningitis caused by *H. influenzae* or *N. meningitidis* until they have received effective antimicrobial therapy for 24 hrs is recommended to prevent spread of infection. For *H. influenzae* meningitis, rifampin prophylaxis (20 mg/kg once daily for 4 days) is recommended for all household contacts if at least one unvaccinated contact is <4 years old; rifampin prophylaxis for the index case is not needed if ceftriaxone was used but is needed if ampicillin and/or chloramphenicol were used, as they do not eradicate *H. influenzae*. In treating meningococcal

TABLE 59.4

RECOMMENDATION FOR EMPIRICAL ANTIMICROBIAL THERAPY FOR PURULENT MENINGITIS BASED ON PATIENT AGE AND SPECIFIC PREDISPOSING CONDITION

Predisposing factor	Common bacterial pathogens	Antimicrobial therapy
Age		
<1 mo	*Streptococcus agalactiae, Escherichia coli, Listeria monocytogenes, Klebsiella species.*	Ampicillin plus cefotaxime or ampicillin plus an aminoglycoside
1–23 mos	*S. pneumoniae, N. meningitidis, S. agalactiae, H. influenzae, E. coli*	Vancomycin plus a third-generation cephalosporin[a,b]
2–50 yrs	*N. meningitidis, S. pneumoniae*	Vancomycin plus a third-generation cephalosporin[a,b]
>50 yrs	*S. pneumoniae, N. meningitides, L. monocytogenes.* Aerobic Gram-negative bacilli	Vancomycin plus ampicillin plus a third-generation cephalosporin[a,b]
Head trauma		
Basilar skull fracture	*S. pneumoniae, H. influenzae,* group A β–hemolytic streptococci	Vancomycin plus a third-generation cephalosporin[a]
Penetrating trauma	*S. aureus,* coagulase-negative staphylococci (especially *S. epidermidis*), aerobic Gram-negative bacilli (including *P. aeruginosa*)	Vancomycin plus cefepime, vancomycin plus ceftazidime, or vancomycin plus meropenem
Postneurosurgery	Aerobic Gram-negative bacilli (including *P. aeruginosa*), *S. aureus,* coagulase-negative staphylococci (especially *S. epidermidis*)	Vancomycin plus cefepime, vancomycin plus ceftazidime, or vancomycin plus meropenem
CSF shunt	Coagulase-negative staphylococci (especially *dermidis*), *S. aureus,* aerobic Gram-negative bacilli (including *P. aeruginosa*), *Propionibacterium acnes*	Vancomycin plus cefepime[c], vancomycin plus ceftazidime[c], or vancomycin plus meropenem[c]

[a] Ceftriaxone or cefotaxime.
[b] Some experts would add rifampin if dexamethasone is also given.
[c] In infants and children, vancomycin alone is reasonable unless Gram stains reveal the presence of Gram-negative bacilli.
From Tunkel AR, Hartman BJ, Kaplan SL, et al. Practice guidelines for the management of bacterial meningitis. *Clin Infect Dis* 2004;39:1267–84 with permission.

disease, rifampin prophylaxis (10 mg/kg, 12 hourly for 2 days) is recommended for household and daycare contacts to prevent secondary cases and to reduce nasopharyngeal carriage. A single intramuscular dose of ceftriaxone (125 mg for children <12 yrs and 250 mg for older children and adults) has been found to be better than oral rifampin for eliminating meningococcal group A nasopharyngeal carriage. A single oral dose of 500 mg of ciprofloxacin or 500 mg of azithromycin may be used for adults.

ASEPTIC AND TUBERCULAR MENINGITIS

Aseptic meningitis is a clinical syndrome of meningeal inflammation in which common bacterial agents cannot be identified in the CSF. In general,

aseptic meningitis is characterized by a benign clinical course and a lack of long-term sequelae; however, some cases may be associated with significant morbidity. Enteroviruses are the most common etiologic agents for aseptic meningitis (**Table 59.7**).

Tubercular meningitis (TBM) is the most serious complication of TB, especially in children. It is fatal without effective treatment and is associated with significant morbidity even with treatment. CNS TB may take a number of forms, including TBM, tuberculomas, tubercular abscesses, and, rarely, myeloradiculopathy. Multidrug resistance is increasingly common. The brainstem and various cranial nerves, particularly III, VI and VII, are surrounded by the exudates. The exudate accumulates mostly at the base of the brain and interferes with the normal flow of CSF, leading to hydrocephalus. Vasculitis, infarction, and hydrocephalus result in severe brain damage. The clinical presentation of TBM is generally

TABLE 59.5

RECOMMENDATION FOR SPECIFIC ANTIMICROBIAL THERAPY IN BACTERIAL MENINGITIS BASED ON ISOLATED PATHOGEN AND SUSCEPTIBILITY TESTING

Microorganism, susceptibility	Standard therapy	Alternative therapies
Streptococcus pneumoniae Penicillin MIC <0.1 mcg/mL	Penicillin G or ampicillin	Third-generation cephalosporin[a], chloramphenicol
0.1–1.0 mcg/mL[b]	Third-generation cephalosporin[a]	Cefepime (B-II), meropenem (B-II)
≥ 2.0mcg/mL	Vancomycin plus a third–generation cephalosporin[a,c]	Fluoroquinolone[d] (B-II)
Cefotaxime or Ceftriaxone MIC ≥1.0 mcg/mL	Vancomycin plus a third–generation cephalosporin[a,c]	Fluoroquinolone[d] (B-II)
Neisseria meningitis Penicillin MIC <0.1 mcg/mL	Penicillin G or ampicillin	Third-generation cephalosporin[a] Chloramphenicol
0.1–1.0 mcg/mL	Third-generation cephalosporin[a]	Chloramphenicol, fluoroquinolone, meropenem
Listeria monocytogenes	Ampicillin or penicillin G[e]	Trimethoprim-sulfamethoxazole, meropenem (B-III)
Streptococcus agalactiae	Ampicillin or penicillin G[e]	Third-generation cephalosporin[a] (B-III)
Escherichia coli and other *Enterobacteriaceae*[g]	Third-generation cephalosporin (A-II)	Aztreonam, fluoroquinolone, meropenem, trimethoprim-sulfamethoxazole, ampicillin
Pseudomonas aeruginosa[g]	Cefepime[e] or ceftazidime[e] (A-II)	Aztreonam[e] ciprofloxacin[e] meropenem[e]
Haemophilus influenzae β-Lactamase negative	Ampicillin	Third-generation cephalosporin[a], cefepime, chloramphenicol, fluoroquinolone
β-Lactamase positive	Third-generation Cephalosporin (A-I)	Cefepime (A-I), chloramphenicol, fluoroquinolone
Staphylococcus aureus Methicillin susceptible	Nafcillin or oxacillin	Vancomycin, meropenem (B-III)
Methicillin resistant	Vancomycin[f]	Trimethoprim-sulfamethoxazole, linezolid (B-III)
Staphylococcus epidermidis	Vancomycin[f]	Linezolid (B-III)
Enterococcus species Ampicillin susceptible	Ampicillin plus gentamicin	
Ampicillin resistant	Vancomycin plus gentamicin	
Ampicillin and vancomycin resistant	Linezolid (B-III)	

All recommendations are A-III, unless otherwise indicated.
[a] Ceftriaxone or cefotaxime.
[b] Ceftriaxone, cefotaxime-susceptible isolates.
[c] Consider addition of rifampin if the MIC of ceftriaxone is >2 mcg/mL.
[d] Gatifloxacin or moxifloxacin.
[e] Addition of an aminoglycoside should be considered.
[f] Consider addition of rifampin.
[g] Choice of a specific antimicrobial agent must be guided by in vitro susceptibility test results. MIC, minimal inhibitory concentration.
From Tunkel AR, Hartman BJ, Kaplan SL, et al. Practice guidelines for the management of bacterial meningitis. *Clin Infect Dis* 2004;39:1267–84, with permission.

TABLE 59.6

RECOMMENDED DOSAGES OF ANTIMICROBIAL THERAPY IN PATIENTS WITH BACTERIAL MENINGITIS (A-III)

	Total daily dose (dosing interval in hours)			
	Neonates, age in days			
Antimicrobial agent	0–7[a]	8–28[a]	Infants and children	Adults
Amikacin[b]	15–20 mg/kg (12)	30 mg/kg (8)	20–30 mg/kg (8)	15 mg/kg (8)
Ampicillin	150 mg/kg (8)	200 mg/kg (6–8)	300 mg/kg (6)	12 g (4)
Aztreonam				6–8 g (6–8)
Cefepime			150 mg/kg (8)	6 g (8)
Cefotaxime	100–150 mg/kg (8–12)	150–200 mg/kg (6–8)	225–300 mg/kg (6–8)	8–12 g (4–6)
Ceftazidime	100–150 mg/kg (8–12)	150 mg/kg (8)	150 mg/kg (8)	6 g (8)
Ceftriaxone			80–100 mg/kg (12–24)	4 g (12–24)
Chloramphenicol	25 mg/kg (24)	50 mg/kg (12–24)	75–100 mg/kg (6)	4–6 g (6)[c]
Ciprofloxacin				800–1200 mg (8–12)
Gatifloxacin				400 mg (24)[c]
Gentamicin[b]	5 mg/kg (12)	7.5 mg/kg (8)	7.5 mg/kg (8)	5 mg/kg (8)
Meropenem			120 mg/kg (8)	6g (8)
Moxifloxacin				400 mg (24)[d]
Nafcillin	75 mg/kg (8–12)	100–150 mg/kg (6–8)	200 mg/kg (6)	9–12 g (4)
Oxacillin	75 mg/kg (8–12)	150–200mg/kg (6–8)	200 mg/kg (6)	9–12 g (4)
Penicillin G	0.15 mU/kg (8–12)	0.2 mU/kg (6–8)	0.3 mU/kg (4–6)	24 mU (4)
Rifampin		10–20 mg/kg (12)	10–20 mg/kg (12–24)[e]	600 mg (24)
Tobramycin[b]	5 mg/kg (12)	7.5 mg/kg (8)	7.5 mg/kg (8)	5 mg/kg (8)
TMP-SMZ[f]			10–20 mg/kg (6–12)	10–20 mg/kg (6–12)
Vancomycin[g]	20–30 mg/kg (8–12)	30–45 mg/kg (6–8)	60 mg/kg (6)	30–45 mg/kg (8–12)

[a] Smaller doses and longer intervals of administration may be advisable for very low-birth weight neonates (<2000 g).
[b] Peak and trough serum concentrations must be monitored.
[c] Higher dose recommended for patients with pneumococcal meningitis.
[d] No data on optimal dosage required in patients with bacterial meningitis.
[e] Maximum daily dose of 600 mg.
[f] Dosage based on trimethoprim component.
[g] Maintain serum, though concentrations of 15–20 mcg/mL.
TMP-SMZ, trimethoprim-sulfamethoxazole
From Tunkel AR, Hartman BJ, Kaplan SL, et al. Practice guidelines for the management of bacterial meningitis. *Clin Infect Dis* 2004;39:1267–84, with permission.

insidious, with low grade fever, poor feeding, irritability, headache, and vomiting, followed by neck rigidity and altered sensorium. Occasionally it may be rapid, particularly in infants and young children who may experience symptoms for only a few days before the onset of acute hydrocephalus, seizures, and cerebral edema. More commonly, the signs and symptoms progress slowly over several weeks and can be divided into 3 stages (**Table 59.8**). Differentiation of TBM from partially treated bacterial meningitis is a common problem in developing countries. The CSF is generally clear or straw colored in TBM, with a cell count of 10–500 cells/mm³, predominantly lymphocytes, although in a few cases polymorphonuclear leukocytes may be present. A "cobweb" formation in the CSF on prolonged standing is highly suggestive of TBM. The CSF glucose is typically <40 mg/dL, and the protein is elevated (generally up 150–200 mg/dL but may increase to 1000–2000 mg/dL). Low CSF chloride is no longer considered diagnostic of TBM. Identification or isolation of mycobacterium on smear or culture is the gold standard for diagnosis of TBM. Radiometric culture gives early results. CSF PCR, adenosine deaminase levels, enzyme-linked immunosorbent assay (ELISA), and other antigen or antibody detection tests have been reported to be useful with varying degrees of sensitivity and specificity. Positive results support, but negative results do not exclude, the diagnosis of TBM.

Neuroimaging is extremely valuable in the diagnosis of tubercular meningitis, particularly because isolation of acid fast bacilli is not possible in

TABLE 59.7

COMMON INFECTIOUS CAUSES OF ASEPTIC MENINGOENCEPHALITIS

Organism	Disease			Diagnosis		
	Infectious					
	Parenchyma	Meninges	Postinfectious	Culture	PCR	Serology
Virus						
Adenoviruses	+	+		Y		Y
Arboviruses	++	+				Y
Enteroviruses	+++	++++	+	Y	Y	
Herpes viruses	+++	+	+	Y	Y	Y
Human immunodeficiency viruses	+	+		Y	Y	Y
Influenza A and B viruses	++	+		Y	Y	
Japanese encephalitis virus	++	+	+		Y	
Lymphocytic choriomeningitis virus	+	+			Y	
Measles	+	+	+	Y		Y
Mumps	++	+	+	Y		Y
Rubella	+	+	+	Y		Y
Rabies	+	+		Y		
Bacteria						
Bartonella henselae	+	+		Y	Y	Y
Bordetella pertussis	+	+		Y	Y	Y
Borrelia burgdorferi (Lyme disease)	++	+		Y	Y	
Brucella spp.	+	+		Y		Y
Chlamydia spp.	+	+	Y	Y	Y	
Ehrlichia spp.	+	+			Y	Y
Leptospira spp.	++	+		Y	Y	Y
Mycobacteria spp.	++	+	Y	Y		
Mycoplasma spp.	++	+	+	Y	Y	Y
Rickettsia spp.	++	+			Y	
Treponema pallidum	++	+		Y	Y	
Fungi						
Aspergillus fumigatus	+	+		Y	Y	Y
Blastomyces dermatitidis	+	+		Y		Y
Candida spp.	+	++		Y		
Cryptococcus neoformans	+	+		Y		Y
Coccidioides immitis	+	+		Y		Y
Histoplasma capsulatum	+	+		Y		Y
Others						
Toxoplasma gondii	+	+			Y	Y
Entamoeba histolytica	+	+			Y	Y
Acanthamoeba	+	+		Y		Y
Trichinella	+	+			Y	
Naegleria	+	+		Y		

Y, yes; + , relative frequency of involvement

many cases. The CT scan characteristically shows thick basilar enhancement, parenchymal enhancement, hydrocephalus, cerebral edema, early focal ischemia, or infarcts and, sometimes, silent tuberculomas. MRI scan shows similar findings and may detect additional posterior fossa lesions, which may not be detected by CT. Brain involvement has been shown in MRIs of patients with miliary TB without symptoms or signs of CNS involvement. CT or MRI of the brain may, however, be normal during early stages of disease. CT signs of TBM were found to be less prominent in HIV-infected versus noninfected children. Corroborative evidence of TB elsewhere in the body, especially pulmonary involvement on chest

CLINICAL STAGING OF PATIENTS WITH TUBERCULOUS MENINGITIS

Stage I (early) (days to weeks)	Nonspecific symptoms and signs (fever, headache, irritability, malaise)
	Lethargy or alteration in behavior
	No neurologic deficits
	No clouding of consciousness
Stage II (intermediate) (weeks to months)	Meningeal irritation
	Minor neurologic deficits (cranial nerve deficits)
Stage III (late) (months to years)	Abnormal movements
	Convulsions
	Stupor or coma
	Severe neurologic deficits (hemiplegia, paraplegia, decerebration)

x-ray and choroid tubercles on funduscopy, gastric aspirates for acid-fast bacilli, and family screening for identification of contact, may aid in the diagnosis.

Initial treatment regimens for TBM use either 3 or 4 drugs. All regimens include isoniazid and rifampicin. Pyridoxine is recommended for infants, children, and adolescents who are being treated with isoniazid and who have nutritional deficiencies or symptomatic HIV. The WHO recommends a 4-month continuation phase for TBM in its Guide-lines for National Programmes. The regimens recommended by the WHO, the American Thoracic Society, and the Indian Academy of Pediatrics for CNS TB are listed in **Table 59.9**. Corticosteroids are used with antitubercular therapy, as they reduce the neurologic sequelae of all stages of TBM, especially when they are administered early in the course of disease. Dexamethasone is administered IV for the first few days, followed by 1–2 mg/kg/day oral prednisolone, generally given for an initial 6 weeks and

TABLE 59.9

RECOMMENDED TREATMENT REGIMENS FOR CENTRAL NERVOUS SYSTEM TUBERCULOSIS

Therapy	WHO	American thoracic society	Indian academy of pediatrics
Initial	HRZS	HRZE daily for 2 mo	HRZE or (HRZS) daily for 2 mos
Continuation Phase	Daily for 2 mos HR for 4 months	*OR* daily for 2 wks followed by twice weekly[a] for 6 wks HR daily *OR* twice weekly for 10 mos	HRE daily for 10 mos

Doses for antitubercular drugs for children[b]		
	Daily dose mg/kg/24 hrs	**Twice weekly dose mg/kg/dose**
Isoniazid (max)	10–15 (300 mg)	20–30 (900 mg)
Rifampin (max)	10–20 (600 mg)	10–20 (600 mg)
Pyrazinamide (max)	15–30 (2.0 g)	50–70 (2 g)
Ethambutol (max)	15–25 (1.0 g)	50 (2.5 g)
Streptomycin (max)	20–40 (1.0 g)	25–30 (1.5 g)

[a] All intermittent therapies to be monitored by directly observed therapy (DOT) for the duration of therapy.
[b] WHO recommends somewhat lower doses; it does not recommend twice weekly doses.
H, isoniazid; R, rifampicin; Z, pyrazinamide; S, streptomycin; E, ethambutol

tapered off over 2–3 weeks. Shunt surgery is often necessary in children with TBM who develop hydrocephalus. Paradoxic response, including development of tuberculomas in children is known even after up to 1 year on standard treatment for TBM. The clinical signs and symptoms may sometimes be severe; corticosteroids are helpful in such cases. Rarely, drug resistance may develop during treatment and is suspected when a patient with TBM shows worsening or cord involvement. Additional antitubercular drugs and steroids are used.

ENCEPHALITIS AND MYELITIS

The term *encephalitis* denotes inflammation of brain parenchyma. Encephalitis caused by direct infection of the CNS is called *primary encephalitis*. Clinically, symptoms and signs of cortical or brainstem involvement, such as seizures and altered sensorium, are seen. Acute inflammatory demyelination that occurs in temporal association with a systemic viral infection or immunization but without direct viral invasion in the CNS is called *postinfectious encephalitis*. As the spinal cord may also be involved, it is referred to as ADEM. Clinically, symptoms and signs of white matter involvement in addition to gray matter involvement are often seen. Pathologically, demyelination and perivascular aggregation of immune cells in the CNS are noted but not evidence of virus or viral antigen, suggesting an autoimmune etiology. The term *encephalopathy* refers to signs of diffuse cerebral dysfunction and can involve dysfunction that does not have an inflammatory component. The most common causes of neonatal encephalitis is HSV, enterovirus or adenovirus. Intrauterine infections, such as cytomegalovirus, rubella, and toxoplasma, may involve the brain but generally do not present as acute encephalitis. In childhood, the most common causes of epidemic encephalitis are arthropod-borne viruses (arboviruses) and enteroviruses. The common etiologies of acute encephalitis are listed in **Table 59.7**. Arbovirus encephalitis in North America generally occurs in the late summer and fall. Enteroviruses are endemic in the developed and developing world, with higher transmission rates in summer and fall. Most enteroviral infection is asymptomatic, and meningitis is more common than encephalitis.

Most viruses that cause encephalitis simultaneously involve the meninges, causing "meningoencephalitis," while some viruses (e.g., rabies) do not have significant meningeal involvement (**Table 59.10**). In neonates, encephalitis generally presents with nonspecific symptoms and signs of systemic sepsis, including fever, poor feeding, irritability, lethargy, seizures, or apnea. History of maternal

TABLE 59.10

DIFFERENTIAL DIAGNOSIS OF ACUTE ENCEPHALITIS/MENINGOENCEPHALITIS ACUTE DISSEMINATED ENCEPHALOMYELITIS

Infectious
   Bacterial meningitis
   Tuberculous meningitis
   Cerebral malaria
   Cryptococcal meningoencephalitis
   Brain abscess
Metabolic
   Hepatic coma
   Reye syndrome
   Uremia
   Hypoglycemia
   Hyposmolar or hypersomolar states
   Organic acidemias
   Amino acidopathies
   Urea cycle defects
   Fat oxidation defects
   Mitochondrial disorders
   Acute intermittent porphyria
Toxic
   Shigellosis
   Salmonella
   Drugs
   Lead encephalopathy
   Carbon monoxide poisoning
   Pertussis
Vasculitic
   Systemic lupus erythematosus
   Polyarteritis nodosa
Other
   Benign raised intracranial pressure
   Trauma
   Nonconvulsive status epilepticus
   Neoplasms
   Cerebrovascular accidents

fever in the peripartum may be present in some cases of enterovirus or adenovirus infections. The usual presentation of encephalitis in older children is with acute-onset fever, headache, seizures, behavioral changes, and rapid alteration in sensorium, progressing to coma. A prodromal illness with myalgias, fever, anorexia, and lethargy, reflecting the systemic viremia, may be seen in some cases. Alteration in sensorium, the hallmark of encephalitis, generally occurs early and progresses rapidly, as compared to meningitis. Seizures are common and may be generalized or focal. The neurologic symptoms may vary from subtle to severe, and depending on the degree of meningeal involvement, symptoms and signs of meningitis, including photophobia, vomiting, and stiff neck, may be present. Associated spinal cord involvement (myelitis) may cause flaccid paraplegia with abnormalities of the deep tendon reflexes. A history of recent travel, exposure to persons with infections, and insects or animal bites should be obtained. A history of focal seizures, personality changes, and aphasia suggests herpes encephalitis. Fever with severe pharyngitis and fatigue may indicate Epstein-Barr virus EBV encephalitis. Fever, parotitis, and dysphagia suggest mumps encephalitis. Fever, conjunctivitis, and the characteristic rash of measles indicate measles encephalitis. History of a dog bite or bat exposure with characteristic behavioral changes and predominant bulbar involvement suggests rabies. The furious type of rabies with agitation, characteristic hydrophobia, or hypersalivation is much more common than the "paralytic" or "dumb" type with flaccid ascending paralysis. Exposure to kittens suggests *Bartonella henselae* (cat-scratch) encephalitis. Encephalitis in summer with a suggestive rash is seen with Rocky Mountain spotted fever (petechial), entero viruses, arboviruses (maculopapular), and Lyme disease (erythema migrans). Epidemics of Japanese Encephalitis (JE) generally occur after the rainy season during mosquito breeding periods; signs and symptoms of basal ganglia involvement are further diagnostic clues. Fever and the presence of focal signs help in distinguishing encephalitis from encephalopathies secondary to metabolic problems and toxins. Children with Reye syndrome present with afebrile encephalopathy following a prodrome of nausea and vomiting. They have mild hepatomegaly, hypoglycemia, some elevation of liver transaminases with mild hyperbilirubinemia (serum bilirubin <5 mg/dL), and elevated blood ammonia levels. A biphasic illness, with antecedent viral illness, rash, or immunization followed by sudden onset meningoencephalitis with multifocal motor deficits indicates ADEM.

Given the more significant outcome of encephalitis, compared to aseptic meningitis, aggressive determination of etiology is often sought. The CSF can be obtained by LP once the child is hemodynamically stable, the ICP is not significantly elevated, and focal lesions have been excluded. In general, CSF findings in encephalitis are nonspecific and CSF abnormalities seldom correlate with clinical or histologic severity of encephalitis. CSF cell count and protein are generally slightly elevated or may be normal, and the glucose concentration is often normal. Very rarely, subarachnoid hemorrhage from occult trauma or a vascular malformation may be considered. A very low CSF glucose is unusual in viral encephalitis, and other causes, including bacterial and tubercular meningitis, must be considered. PCR has replaced viral culture for identification of HSV and enteroviruses from the CSF and is available for cytomegalovirus, EBV, varicella zoster virus, human herpes virus (HHV)-6, HIV, influenza, adenovirus, *Mycoplasma*, *Mycobacteria*,

Rickettsia, and others. Serology may be helpful. EEG may be complementary to neuroimaging in the diagnosis of encephalitis and may help in distinguishing generalized from focal encephalitis. In generalized encephalitis, the EEG typically shows diffuse slowing with high voltage slow waves; occasionally, spikes and spike wave activity may be seen. In focal encephalitis, focal EEG abnormalities, including focal slow waves or spikes, may be seen. The EEG is particularly helpful in HSV encephalitis, wherein characteristic periodic lateralizing discharges (PLEDS) may be seen. Characteristic cytoplasmic inclusions in monocytes, known as *morulae*, are seen in ehrlichiosis. Finding of malarial parasites in the smear helps to confirm a diagnosis of cerebral malaria. Chest x-ray may help in the diagnosis of TB, mycoplasma, or legionella. A full-thickness skin biopsy from the nape of the neck, where numerous hair follicles are located, can help diagnose rabies. MRI is the diagnostic modality of choice in differentiating acute infectious encephalitis from ADEM. In ADEM, the MRI shows multiple patchy areas of involvement of the white matter and, at times, the deep gray matter of the brain; the spinal cord may also be involved in some cases. Demyelination is best seen in T_2-weighted and FLAIR images. The CT scan may help to exclude a bleed or a space-occupying lesion in a suspected case.

CNS infections, particularly meningoencephalites, are the most common cause of refractory status epilepticus in the PICU. Specific antimicrobial therapy should be initiated as soon as an etiologic agent is reasonably suspected or identified. Bacterial, fungal, and parasitic etiologies of encephalitis require specific antimicrobial therapy. Antiviral therapy is important for treatment of HSV encephalitis and must be administered promptly in all suspected cases. Cytomegalovirus encephalitis requires ganciclovir or foscarnet. Amantadine and rimantadine are effective against influenza A, whereas oseltamivir and zanamivir are effective against both influenza A and B. Highly active antiretroviral therapy is available for HIV infection. No specific antiviral therapy is available for enteroviral and arboviral encephalitis. Passive immunity in the form of IV immune globulin may be helpful in immunocompromised individuals who cannot mount an effective immune response.

HERPES ENCEPHALITIS

HSV is the most common cause of fatal sporadic encephalitis in childhood. Intrauterine infection may manifest in the neonate with skin vesicles or scarring and involvement of the eyes (e.g., chorioretinitis or optic atrophy) and brain (e.g., microcephaly or encephalomalacia). Clinical presentation of disseminated disease is similar to bacterial sepsis.

Symptoms start approximately a week after birth and include poor feeding, lethargy, irritability, and seizures and may sometimes progress to shock with multiorgan failure.

HSE in children generally presents acutely with fever, headache, vomiting, and focal seizures, followed within a few days by alteration in sensorium. Neck stiffness may occur in some cases. At times, preceding nonspecific influenza like symptoms of malaise, lethargy, or mild irritability may be present. Behavioral and personality changes and difficulty with speech may be noted in some children. Focal neurologic abnormalities develop in most cases, generally reflecting involvement of the temporal or frontal lobes. Raised ICP with papilledema, transtentorial herniation, and hemodynamic instability follows. Focal signs and personality changes may provide etiologic clues. HSE has no other specific clinical markers. Presence of herpetic skin lesions has no correlation with concurrent encephalitis. The course of HSE is generally rapid and may be fatal unless specific therapy is started early.

It may not be possible to differentiate HSE from other causes of encephalitis on the basis of clinical features alone. A number of conditions may mimic HSE, including other viral encephalitis, such as EEE, JE, western equine encephalitis, St. Louis encephalitis, EBV, and other viral infections. The differential diagnosis should also include bacterial and fungal infections (e.g., early brain abscess) and other infections, including tubercular, rickettsial, toxoplasma, and collagen vascular diseases. In the absence of skin lesions, making a clinical diagnosis of herpes is problematic, particularly in neonates. Swab cultures from conjunctiva, nasopharynx, and rectum may detect early infection. The MRI is not as helpful in neonates as in older children because of diffuse involvement and high brain-water content of the neonatal brain. PLEDS on EEG, if seen, add to the diagnosis but are not specific for herpes. Identification of HSV in the CSF by PCR has become the gold standard for diagnosis of HSE. MRI is often the first diagnostic investigation, as LP may be contraindicated in children with raised ICP and focal signs. Involvement of inferofrontal and mediotemporal lobes with gyral swelling and cerebral edema is characteristic. The MRI is much more sensitive than CT and detects changes earlier than CT in cases of HSE. If an MRI facility is not immediately available, a CT scan may be obtained. Low-density areas in a unilateral medial temporal lobe and insular cortex are seen. Small areas of hemorrhage may also be seen in these regions. The CT may appear normal in very early phases of the disease, and abnormalities may be visible only after 4–5 days of illness.

In children, acyclovir, 30 mg/kg/day divided q8 hrs for 14–21 days, is the treatment of choice, whereas for neonatal HSE, 60 mg/kg/day divided q8 hrs for 21 days is recommended.

JAPANESE ENCEPHALITIS

JE is an arthropod-borne encephalitis and is the most common form of epidemic and sporadic encephalitis in the tropical region of Asia. The epidemics generally occur after the rainy season in rural areas with rice fields. JE is a zoonotic disease maintained by a pig-mosquito-pig and bird-mosquito-bird cycle. JE affects mainly children and young adults. The incubation period is 5–15 days, and most infections are either asymptomatic or mildly symptomatic. JE infection that progresses to encephalitis often starts acutely with fever, headache, tiredness, nausea, vomiting, and diarrhea and progresses within a few days to confusion, irritability, and coma. The onset may be abrupt, with high fever, chills, and seizures, with rapid progression to altered sensorium and neurodeficits. The presence of extrapyramidal symptoms and signs in a child with encephalitis strongly suggests the diagnosis of JE. If CSF can be obtained safely, lymphocytic pleocytosis with moderate elevation of protein and a normal glucose may be seen. The CSF may be acellular or show polymorphonuclear predominance in early stages. The virus can be isolated from the CSF. Viral antigens can be detected in the CSF by indirect immunofluorescence assay. Viral antibodies can be detected by rapid serologic assays, such as IgM-capture ELISA (MAC-ELISA) and IgG-ELISA. Monoclonal antibodies (mabs) have also been used for diagnosis, and real-time PCR for JE is available but not yet routinely used. Diffuse slowing is commonly seen on EEG. Theta and delta coma, burst suppression, and occasionally epileptiform activity are suggestive. CT scans show hypodense areas in the thalamus, basal ganglia, midbrain, and brainstem MRI scans show abnormal signals that are hypointense on T_1-weighted and hyperintense on T_2-weighted images that involve the thalami and basal ganglia bilaterally are characteristic. Vaccination against JE is the most effective way of preventing epidemics. Mosquito control measures that employ larvicidal and adulticidal techniques have been used for this and other mosquito-borne diseases. Water management systems with alternate drying and wetting in rice fields and the use of "neem" products as fertilizers suppress the breeding of culcine vectors.

ACUTE DISSEMINATED ENCEPHALOMYELITIS

ADEM is an inflammatory demyelinating disorder of the CNS that usually follows infections or, less frequently, immunization. The common preceding infections are respiratory and gastrointestinal viral illnesses; however, ADEM has been reported following many viral and bacterial infections and immunization. Most cases have an acute meningoencephalitic presentation with fever, headache, and irritability, progressing rapidly to altered sensorium and, often, an abrupt multifocal neurodeficit. Ataxia is predominant in some cases, and extrapyramidal symptoms, such as choreoathetosis or dystonia, may occur in others. In the affected limbs, the muscle tone is generally increased with increased stretch reflexes, upgoing plantar reflexes and, at times, clonus. A clinical definition of ADEM has recently been put forth by the Brighton collaboration of the Centers for Disease Control and Prevention (http://www.brightoncollaboration.org/internet/en/index.html). One of 3 levels of diagnostic certainty may be established with the presence of encephalopathy or focal/multifocal. CNS findings on MRI imaging that are consistent with ADEM. CSF may show pleocytosis or may be normal and is not helpful in making a diagnosis of ADEM. RBCs may be seen in cases of hemorrhagic encephalitis. Elevated CSF HSV or Lyme titers do not exclude the possibility of associated ADEM. The MRI scan is the diagnostic modality of choice. The lesions are best visualized on T_2-weighted or proton density sequences. Multiple large confluent centrifugal white matter lesions seen generally at the junction of deep cortical gray and subcortical white matter are characteristic. The mainstay of treatment is IV methylprednisolone given in a dose 20–30 mg/kg/day for 3–5 days. Improvement may be observed in some cases within hours but usually occurs over several days. Generally a taper of oral steroids for 3–6 weeks is used. Concern over treatment with steroids in light of HSE in the differential is occasionally raised. Plasmapheresis and IV immune globulin 2 g/kg/day for 2–3 days have also been used, especially in cases in which meningoencephalitis cannot be excluded and it is feared that corticosteroids might worsen the course of infection.

BRAIN AND SPINAL CORD ABSCESS

Abscess in the brain and spinal cord can occur as a primary event or, occasionally, as a complication of bacterial meningitis. The common pathogens include anaerobic bacteria, Gram-negative organisms, streptococci, and staphylococci. The inflammation and edema progress over a few days to weeks, leading to central necrosis with formation of a surrounding capsule of inflammatory granulation tissue. The first stage, "early cerebritis" is followed by "late cerebritis," in which central liquefaction necrosis is surrounded by an area of neovascularization and fibroblastic infiltration, forming an ill-defined beginning of a capsule. The necrotic center shrinks, and the fibroblastic capsule becomes well formed. The fourth phase is late capsule formation, in which a dense fibrous capsule is surrounded by reactive astrocytes and glial cells, marked edema, and neovascularization. Abscesses secondary to ear infection are located generally in the unilateral temporal lobe or cerebellum, and those following sinusitis are located in the frontal lobe. In children with cyanotic heart disease, abscesses are generally seen in the distribution of the middle carotid artery. The classic triad of fever, headache, and vomiting seen in adults is seen in only half of childhood cases. An LP is often contraindicated in a child with brain abscess because of the risk of cerebral herniation. Confirmation of the etiologic organism is achieved by aspiration of the abscess and analysis and culture of the aspirated contents. Other sources of organism identification, such as blood culture or aspiration from sinuses or mastoids, should also be considered. A CT scan or MRI with contrast is warranted in all suspected cases. Contrast-enhanced CT scan shows a characteristic ring-enhancing lesion with central hypodensity and surrounding edema in a mature abscess. In early cases of cerebritis, the ring enhancement may be incomplete. The MRI is more sensitive than CT in diagnosis of cerebritis. In countries where TB is endemic, a pyogenic abscess must be differentiated from a tubercular abscess. Tubercular abscesses are generally seen at the base of the brain, especially in the cerebellum. MR spectroscopy may sometimes be necessary to differentiate an abscess from a neoplasm.

Antibiotic therapy with surgical drainage or excision of the abscess is required in most cases. In children, aspiration under CT guidance is used more frequently because of the low mortality and morbidity associated with the procedure. Empiric antibiotic therapy before organism identification typically consists of a broad-spectrum combination of agents to cover anaerobic, Gram-negative, and staphylococcal species. Cefotaxime or any other third- or fourth-generation cephalosporin with metronidazole is generally used. If *S. aureus* is suspected or identified, vancomycin should be added.

SUBDURAL EMPYEMA

Subdural empyema is a suppurative collection in the subdural space. It is an important focal intracranial infection that is often a complication of acute bacterial meningitis. The diagnosis of a subdural empyema is made by neuroimaging. A contrast-enhanced, crescent-shaped, hypodense lesion, at times with loculations, is characteristic. Purulent collections are hyperintense to the CSF in both T_1- and T_2-weighted images. Analysis of the subdural fluid obtained by subdural tap or surgical drainage reveals a purulent fluid with marked leukocytosis. Organism identification can be performed by Gram stain and culture. An LP is often contraindicated.

Removal of the purulent collection and IV administration of appropriate antibiotic therapy in high doses for 3–6 weeks in warranted. Antibiotics are chosen according to the suspected source of infection. Surgical removal of adjacent source of infection, such as chronic otitis media or osteomyelitis, is also necessary.

EPIDURAL ABSCESS

A cranial epidural abscess is a collection of suppurative material between the dura and the cranium. Spinal epidural abscesses also occur. Children with a cranial epidural abscess present with fever, headache, vomiting, neck rigidity, focal seizures, and focal neurodeficits, including hemiparesis. Children with spinal epidural abscess present with fever, back pain, and symptoms and signs of spinal cord compression. Localized tender swelling may be found at the site of the pain. Progression may lead to bladder and bowel involvement. A sensory level may be seen in late cases. MRI is more sensitive than CT and shows an enhancing lenticular collection between the dura and the cranium or the cord. If spinal epidural abscess is suspected, the entire spine should be scanned, as multiple abscesses may be present. Plain radiographs of the spine and contrast myelography have no role in diagnosis.

Treatment involves surgical drainage, appropriate antibiotics, and supportive management. As *S. aureus* is a common pathogen, the initial antibiotic therapy consists of a combination of antibiotics to cover staphylococci and Gram-negative organisms. Once the abscess is drained and the organism identified, the appropriate antibiotic therapy is administered IV for 4–6 weeks.

CSF SHUNT INFECTION

CSF shunts are placed by neurosurgeons to relieve pressure from CSF accumulation and brain parenchymal displacement when hydrocephalus is present. CSF shunts may direct CSF from the ventricles to the peritoneum (ventriculoperitoneal), atrium (ventriculoatrial), or to the outside world (externalized). Ventriculoperitoneal shunts are the most common. More than two-thirds of all shunt infections are caused by staphylococcal species. Shunts may become infected by several mechanisms: colonization at the time of surgery; breakdown of the surgical wound or of the skin that overlies the shunt, which allows direct access of microbes to the shunt; retrograde infection from the distal end through transluminal passage of bacteria; and hematogenous seeding and infection of CSF shunts, which occurs infrequently.

Most children present with fever, headache, vomiting, lethargy, irritability, and change in mental status. Occasionally, seizures, cranial nerve palsies, visual deficits, and neck rigidity may be seen. The classic symptoms of infection, such as fever and pain, may be absent in some cases.

The prerequisites for a diagnostic label of shunt infection are no meningitis/ventriculitis and a sterile CSF culture at the time of shunt placement, shunt in place for at least 24 hrs, and a positive CSF culture obtained from the shunt/LP. The gold standard for diagnosis of shunt infection is the isolation of organism from culture of the shunt or of the fluid in contact with it. Certain patients, even in the absence of infection, may have an elevated CSF white count, generally eosinophilic, probably due to a hypersensitive reaction to the presence of shunt tubing. A positive CSF Gram stain and culture are diagnostic and extremely important in deciding the course of treatment. Ultrasonography in neonates and young infants may show ventriculitis or a "CSFoma," which strongly suggest infection. A CT scan or MRI is useful if early postoperative scans are available for comparison. An increase in ventricular size because of associated shunt malfunction is often seen. Various management regimens have been used, but a combination of antibiotics, shunt removal, and external drainage is perhaps most effective. Use of prophylactic antibiotics before and after surgery helps in reducing subsequent shunt infection.

FUNGAL INFECTIONS OF THE CENTRAL NERVOUS SYSTEM

Most patients with a fungal infection of the CNS have some predisposing deficiency in immune response, very often caused by neutropenia, lymphoreticular malignancy, lymphoma, malnutrition, use of immunosuppressive drugs, potent broad-spectrum antibiotic therapy, or AIDS due to HIV. The large number of fungi that can infect the CNS are shown in **Table 59.11** and **Table 59.12**. Clinical manifestations may be due to meningitis, meningoencephalitis,

TABLE 59.11

FUNGAL INFECTIONS THAT MAY BE SUSPECTED IN PRESENCE OF VARIOUS PREDISPOSING FACTORS

Predisposing factor	Fungus most likely to cause infection
Prematurity	*Candida albicans*
Primary immunodeficiency (e.g., CGD, SCID)	*Candida, Cryptococcus, Aspergillus*
Corticosteroids	*Cryptococcus, Candida*
Cytotoxic agents	*Aspergillus, Candida*
Secondary immunodeficiency (e.g., AIDS)	*Cryptococcus, Histoplasma*
Iron chelator therapy	*Zygomycetes*
Intravenous drug abuse	*Candida*, Zygomycetes
Ketoacidosis, renal acidosis	Zygomycetes (Mucor)
Trauma, foreign body	*Candida*

CGD, chronic granulomatous disease; SCID, severe combined immunodeficiency; AIDS, acquired immunodeficiency syndrome

or focal lesions due to infarction or abscess. Fungal meningitis predominantly involves the base of the brain. These infections have some characteristic clinical features, such as new-onset seizures and insidious onset may help.

FUNGAL MENINGITIS

The common causes are *C. neoformans, C. immitis, Candida,* and *Aspergillus.* Clinical manifestations of fungal meningitis are less stereotyped than the manifestations of bacterial meningitis. Rhinocerebral syndrome is a major presentation of zygomycosis (Rhizopus and Mucor), often in patients with poorly controlled diabetes. It presents with orbital pain, nasal discharge, and facial edema. Proptosis and visual loss may occur. Involvement of carotids may cause hemiparesis. Subsequently, trigeminal nerve and adjacent brain may be involved—classically found in mucormycosis, in which blackish necrotic areas are seen in the palate and nasal turbinates. Aspergillosis or mucormycosis may produce sudden onset of neurodeficit due to vasculitis. In the presence of a predisposing condition, such as HIV infection, children who present with fever with or without CNS signs should have an LP for CSF analysis and culture. CSF examination usually reveals high proteins, low glucose, and mononuclear leukocytosis ranging between 20 and 500 cells/mm³. Direct microscopic examination of CSF mixed with India ink on a slide is helpful in identification of encapsulated cryptococci. Latex agglutination test using CSF is highly specific for cryptococcal meningitis. The test is diagnostic and may be positive early in the infection, even when culture is negative. Complement fixating antibody is

useful to diagnose some fungal infections. CT and MRI scans show the basal involvement, associated abscess, and areas of infarction.

Amphotericin B remains the most used and successful drug for fungal infections of CNS (**Table 59.13**). Lipid formulation of Amphotericin B, such as liposomal amphotericin B (AmBisome) 4 mg/kg/day or more, may be a better alternative to conventional amphotericin B, especially in the setting of renal dysfunction. Penetration into the CSF and early favorable clinical experience make voriconazole the drug of choice in CNS aspergillosis and scedosporiosis. Caspofungin is fungicidal against *Candida* spp. and active against *Aspergillus.* Activity against *Fusarium, Rhizopus,* and *Trichosporon* is limited. In cryptococcal meningitis, amphotericin B plus flucytosine has proven successful.

PARASITIC INFECTIONS

Some of the parasites that can involve the CNS and their clinical manifestations are listed in **Table 59.14**. In any case of suspected parasitic infection, the most important etiologic clue is obtained by a detailed history, particularly related to travel to, or immigration from, endemic areas. Some parasitic infections, such as falciparum malaria, manifest clinically within a few days, whereas others, such as neurocysticercosis, may manifest several months or even years after infection. It is important to inquire about both recent travel and past travel to endemic areas. History of suggestive mode of acquisition, such as blood transfusion for malarial parasite, bathing in a pond for *Naegleria,* exposure to tsetse fly for African trypanosomiasis, or Reduviid bug for American

TABLE 59.12

GEOGRAPHIC DISTRIBUTION, PREDISPOSING HOST CHARACTERISTICS, PRIMARY PATHOGENIC MECHANISM, AND PREDOMINANT CLINICAL SYNDROME OF VARIOUS FUNGAL CENTRAL NERVOUS SYSTEM INFECTIONS

Fungus	Distribution	Primary pathogenesis	Predisposing host characteristic	Usual clinical syndrome
1. *Cryptococcus neoformans* variety *neoformans*, variety *gatti*, variety *grubii*	Worldwide Common in Australia, Southeast Asia, Central Africa, California.	Pulmonary infection from inhalation of small yeast (basidiospore) Dissemination involves CNS in 30%–50%; often meningitis	Impaired cell-mediated immunity	Meningitis Meningoencephalitis Cryptococcoma
2. *Coccidioides* (*C. immitis*)	South and Central America, Southern US Occasional	Pulmonary infection from inhalation of arthroconidia. Dissemination in 0.2%; Up to 30% have meningitis; Also involves thoracic and lumber spine	Impaired cell-mediated immunity	Meningitis
3. *Histoplasma* (*H. capsulatum*)	Parts of US Rare	Inhalation of spores, dissemination rare; of these, 10%–25% have CNS infection, more in patients with AIDS	Impaired cell-mediated immunity	Meningitis
4. *Blastomycosis* (*B. dermatitidis*)	Parts of US Rare	Inhalation of spores from soil leads to primary granulomatous lesion of lung, skin: Dissemination in up to 1/3 of patients.	No prominent risk factor or immune defect	Meningitis
5. *Candida* (*C. albicans, C. tropicalis* & others)	Normal flora of body Common	Pulmonary or GI primary, Hematogenous dissemination, CNS involvement in 50% with dissemination; most often leads to meningitis in infants. Direct inoculation via trauma, VP shunt placement, indwelling catheter	Patients with impaired cell-mediated immunity, neutropenia, prematurity, broad-spectrum antibiotics, corticosteroid therapy, hyperalimentation, malignancy, indwelling catheters, diabetes, abdominal surgery, thermal injury	Meningitis commonly, Abscess
6. *Aspergillus* (*A. fumigatus, A flavus, A terreus*)	Ubiquitous Occasional	Hematogenous spread in immunocompromised host from pulmonary primary. Direct extension from paranasal sinus or following head trauma. Surgery	Immunocompromised host (graft-versus-host disease, neutropenia)	Infarct, abscess
7. *Zygomycosis* (Mucor)	Ubiquitous Infection only in immunocompromised occasional	Direct extension to CNS from nasal or paranasal sinuses through tissue plains leading to rhinocerebral disease. Hematogenous, rarely. Angioinvasive, causes cerebrovascular occlusion and infarction.	Diabetes, diabetic ketoacidosis, Immunosuppressive therapy, IV drug users, malignancy, deferoxamine chelation therapy, renal acidosis.	Infarct, Abscess

CNS, central nervous system; AIDS, acquired immune deficiency syndrome; VP, ventriculoperitoneal

TABLE 59.13

ANTIFUNGAL THERAPY RECOMMENDED IN COMMON FUNGAL CNS INFECTION

Fungus	Antifungal agent	Dose	Route	Duration
Cryptococcus neoformans	Amphotericin B; + 5-FC, then Fluconazole	0.7–1 mg/kg/day q 24 hrs 100–150 mg/kg/d q6 hrs 10 mg/kg/loading, then 5–6 mg/kg/d qd	IV PO PO PO	2 wks 2 wks 8–10 wks HIV patients: indefinite Non-HIV patients: 6 mos–1 yr
Candida albicans and other	Amphotericin B ± 5-FC then Fluconazole	0.7–1 mg/kg/day q24 hrs 100–150 mg/kg/d q6 hrs 10 mg/kg loading, then 5–6 mg/kg/d qd	IV PO PO/IV	2 wks 4–6 wks
Aspergillus fumigatus	Amphotericin B ± 5-FC OR Voriconazole	1–1.5 mg/kg/day q24 hrs 100–150 mg/kg/day q6 hrs 6 mg/kg, 2 doses 12 hrs apart, then 4 mg/kg q12 hr[a]	IV PO IV/PO	initial 6 mos to 1 yr
Coccidioides immitis	Amphotericin B, then fluconazole	0.7–1 mg/kg/d 10 mg/d loading then 5–6 mg/kg/d	IV PO	4 wks lifelong

[a] By IV infusion, 5 mg/mL strength, maximum rate 3 mg/kg/hr. 5-FC levels should be monitored 2–4 hrs after oral dose after 3–4 days, with target peak 40–60 mcg/mL.

TABLE 59.14

COMMON PARASITIC CNS INFECTIONS

Parasite	Clinical manifestations
Protozoa	
■ *Plasmodium falciparum*	Cerebral malaria
■ Amoeba	Meningitis/meningoencephalitis
Entamoeba histolytica	Meningitis/meningoencephalitis
Acanthamoeba	Meningoencephalitis
Naegleria	
■ *Trypanosoma brucei (rhodesiense or gambiense) cruzi*	
■ *Toxoplasma gondii*	
Helminths (worms)	
Cestodes (flatworms)	
	Seizures/meningoencephalitis
■ *Taenia solium* (Neurocysticercosis)	Mass lesion with raised ICP
■ *Echinococcus* (hydatid cyst) (multilocularis/granulosus)	Solitary/multiple
	Seizures
Nematodes (roundworms)	
	Meningoencephalitis
■ *Trichinella*	Meningoencephalitis
■ *Strongyloides*	Seizures
■ *Ascaris*	

trypanosomiasis, is also important. Underlying immune status of the child, such as HIV-positive status, corticosteroid therapy, and asplenia, may indicate possible specific opportunistic parasitic diseases, such as toxoplasmosis. *Entamoeba histolytica* is transmitted by the fecal-oral route. Trypanosoma are transmitted by vectors, including the tsetse fly in Africa and Reduviid bug in Central and South America. *T. brucei* is the etiologic agent of African trypanosomiasis (also known as African sleeping sickness), and *T. cruzi* is the etiologic agent of American trypanosomiasis (Chagas disease). *Toxoplasma gondii* is acquired most commonly by ingestion of oocysts present in cat feces or through ingestion of tissue cysts of contaminated meat that is undercooked. Echinococcosis is caused by a larval form of the tapeworm *Taenia echinococcus*. Cystic echinococcosis is caused by *Echinococcus granulosus*, found worldwide in association with sheep herding. Nematodes, such as *Trichinella* and *Ascaris*, are found in soil in tropical areas with poor sanitation. *Strongyloides* is also endemic in tropical climates with poor sanitation, but infection occurs by penetration through exposed skin.

The clinical presentation of parasitic CNS disease varies considerably based on the causative agent. Symptoms of acute meningitis or meningoencephalitis are most typical, with fever, headache, vomiting, photophobia, neck stiffness, and altered sensorium. New onset seizures are another common clinical presentation, as in neurocysticercosis (NCC). Cystic echinococcal infection may present insidiously over years with a slowly enlarging cyst, causing headache and progressing toward neurologic deficit and herniation. The CSF may be diagnostic in certain cases, such as finding of free-floating amoebae in the case of *Naegleria* or Giemsa stain for trypanosomiasis. A positive serology in serum or CSF may suggest NCC; rise in specific IgM titer for toxoplasmosis is highly suggestive. PCR studies are also available for some parasites. Various investigations may be of use in diagnosis, such as blood film for malaria or presence of eosinophilia for helminths. Neuroimaging may reveal characteristic findings, such as a scolex seen within the cyst in NCC. The presence of a round, thin-walled cyst filled with fluid isointense to CSF suggests hydatid due to *Echinococcus*, whereas small, ring-enhancing lesions (particularly in deep gray matter) in a child with HIV suggest toxoplasmosis.

NEUROCYSTICERCOSIS

NCC is the most common parasitic infection of the CNS and an important cause of epilepsy in the tropics. The clinical presentations are variable and depend on the stage and location of cysts. Most cases present with seizures, and approximately one-third of cases have symptoms and signs of raised ICP. NCC is caused by infestation of the CNS with encysted larvae of *Taenia solium*. Humans acquire intestinal infection (taeniasis, tapeworm) from pigs by ingestion of undercooked pork infected with *T. solium* cysticerci. Cysticercosis in humans is acquired through the feco-oral route by ingestion of contaminated raw vegetables or food prepared by carriers of tapeworms. The clinical presentation of NCC is variable and depends on the stage and location of the cysts; it is classified into parenchymal and extraparenchymal types.

The common clinical manifestations of parenchymal neurocysticercosis include (a) seizures, (b) raised ICP with headache and vomiting, (c) focal neurodeficits, and (d) encephalitis: Extraparenchymal involvement is rare in children and includes (a) obstructive hydrocephalus or chronic meningitis, (b) subarachnoid involvement, (c) spinal involvement, and (d) ophthalmic involvement. The "gold standard" for diagnosis of NCC is pathologic confirmation through biopsy or autopsy. Practically, the diagnosis rests mainly on neuroimaging. The characteristic CT picture consists of small, low-density, ring or disc-enhancing lesions, with perilesional edema. The scolex appears as a bright, high-density, eccentric nodule in these cysts and is pathognomonic of NCC. In subarachnoid NCC, the CT findings include hydrocephalus, tentorial enhancement, and occasionally, infarcts. MRI is more sensitive than CT for visualization of extraparenchymal cysts and identification of scolex. On T1-weighted images, live cysts are seen as round lesions, either isointense or slightly hyperintense to the CSF, with a scolex that is hyperintense or isointense to white matter. On T2-weighted images, the cysts are isointense to CSF and the perilesional edema appears bright.

A child with an encephalitic presentation requires intensive care management similar to any other encephalitis. IV steroids are used to reduce the cerebral edema and anticonvulsants to control the seizures. Cysticidal therapy is not used in the acute phase, as it may provoke a further inflammatory response and worsen the edema. It may be considered later in select cases once the edema subsides and the child is stable. Praziquantel and albendazole are the 2 drugs that have been found effective against *T. solium* cysticerci. Surgery for cyst removal has been used in ophthalmic NCC. Shunt placement is necessary in cases with hydrocephalus; use of steroids and albendazole reduces shunt failure.

CEREBRAL MALARIA

Cerebral malaria (CM) is a clinical syndrome characterized by CNS dysfunction associated with

TABLE 59.15

PARENTERAL ANTIMALARIAL TREATMENT OF CEREBRAL MALARIA

Drug	Route	Loading dose	Maintenance dose
Quinidine gluconate	IV	15 mg base/kg (24 mg/kg salt) in normal saline over 4 hrs OR 6.25 mg base/kg (10 mg salt/kg) over 2 hrs	7.5 mg base/kg (12 mg salt/kg) infused over 4 hrs, q 8–12 hrs with ECG monitoring OR 0.0125 mg base/kg/min (0.02 mg salt/kg/min) as a continuous infusion for 24 hrs
Quinine dihydrochloride	IV	20 mg salt/kg over 2–4 hrs	10 mg salt/kg over 2–4 hrs every 8–12 hrs until able to take orally
Quinine dihydrochloride	IM	20 mg salt/kg (dilute IV formulation to 60 mg/mL) given in 2 injection sites (anterior thigh)	10 mg salt/kg q 8–12 hrs until able to take orally
Artemether	IM	3.2 mg/kg	1.6 mg/kg/day for a minimum of 5 days
Artesunate	IV/IM	2.4 mg/kg	1.2 mg/kg after 24 hrs, then 1.2 mg/kg/day for 7 days

IV, intravenous; IM, intramuscular
Parenteral therapy should be given for at least 72 hrs before changing to oral medication. Total therapy should be at least 7 days, and a parenteral antimalarial should be used in conjunction with another antimalarial of a different class.

Plasmodium falciparum infection. The parasites are transmitted by anopheline mosquitoes. CM should be suspected in any child who has visited or even transiently landed at an airport in an endemic area and develops CNS symptoms, such as headache and mental status changes. Children with malaria usually have a history of fever, headache, irritability, restlessness, or drowsiness. Vomiting and, to a lesser extent, diarrhea are common and may contribute to dehydration or electrolyte depletion. Falciparum malaria is associated with a distinctive retinopathy, which includes retinal hemorrhages, retinal whitening, color changes in the vessels, and less frequently papilledema. These features are associated with sequestration in the brain and help to differentiate CM from other causes of encephalopathy. The liver is often enlarged and may be slightly tender. Splenic enlargement, which may not be present on admission, usually occurs a few days into the illness. Spontaneous bleeding from the gastrointestinal tract occurs in nonimmune individuals. Hypoglycemia is a common complication of severe falciparum malaria, particularly CM. Metabolic acidosis, a prominent feature of CM in both nonimmune adults and African children, is mainly caused by lactic acid. The WHO has adopted the following strict criteria for the diagnosis of CM: (a) a patient is unable to localize a painful stimulus (such as pressure on the sternum) at least 1 hr after last seizure; (b) asexual parasites are present in the peripheral blood; and (c) other causes of

encephalopathy (e.g., meningitis, encephalitis, or hypoglycemia) are excluded. Blood smears must be examined every 6 hrs for 48 hrs to exclude this infection. Rapid diagnostic tests may be helpful, particularly in the absence of positive blood smear. Hypoglycemia and a lactic acidosis are the major metabolic complications. Hypoxemia is associated with pulmonary edema and infections. Renal impairment is common. Hyponatremia is mainly caused by salt depletion. Hypoalbuminemia is also common and may result in low plasma calcium concentrations. Hypophosphatemia is a feature of severe malaria and may be exacerbated by glucose therapy.

Any child with features of severe falciparum malaria should be treated with parenteral antimalarial therapy (**Table 59.15**). At present, the drugs of choice for treatment of severe falciparum malaria are the cinchona alkaloids (quinine and its diastereomer quinidine) and the artemisinin compounds. Since quinine for IV administration is unavailable in the US, quinidine is used. Side effects are common, particularly cinchonism (tinnitus, hearing loss, nausea, restlessness, blurred vision). Serious cardiovascular side effects, such as hypotension and cardiac arrhythmias, may occur if the drugs are administered undiluted and too rapidly. The Q-T interval should be monitored during the infusion. Artemisinin compounds (artesunate, artemether, arteether) are fast-acting and act against all blood stages, reducing the time to parasite clearance and fever resolution in comparison to the cinchinoid alkaloids. A second antimalarial drug should be combined with the parenteral antimalarial to prevent the emergence of resistance to the former. They can be used in parasites that are relatively resistant to the cinchinoids, to shorten the course of therapy, or for the treatment of nonsevere falciparum malaria. Atovaquone-proguanil (Malarone^{TM}) is useful in this context. Antibiotics (clindamycin) are effective against the blood stages but should not be used as primary antimalarial drugs. The spread of chloroquine-resistant strains of *P. falciparum* has severely limited the use of chloroquine, and it should not be used in the treatment of severe falciparum malaria. Likewise, the spread of resistance to the sulfonamides (sulfadoxine, sulfalene, cotrimoxazole) has limited their usefulness. Exchange transfusions may be helpful in the management of CM in patients who have a parasitemia in excess of 10% or who are deteriorating in spite of conventional treatment. Vitamin K and cryoprecipitate should be administered if a patient has a bleeding diathesis. Seizures must be treated promptly with benzodiazepines and a prophylactic anticonvulsant, such as phenytoin or Phenobarbital. A CT or MRI scan should be completed to exclude brain swelling before an LP is performed. If brain swelling is detected, ICP monitoring should be considered. Steroids appear to be deleterious, increasing the incidence of bleeding without any beneficial effect on outcome. Secondary bacterial infections should always be suspected, and broad-spectrum antimicrobial treatment should be started as soon as a complicating infection is suspected. Severe falciparum malaria is a multisystem disease, and advice from hematologists, infectious disease specialists, and nephrologists may be needed. A reference center, such as the Center for Disease Control in Atlanta, should be contacted for current information (http://www.cdc.gov/Malaria/diagnosis_treatment/tx_clinicians.htm) about antimalarial therapy.

Currently, no vaccine is available for malaria. Prophylaxis for travelers involves taking an oral antimalarial such as mefloquine or atovaquone-proguanil.

CHAPTER 60 ■ NOSOCOMIAL INFECTIONS IN THE PEDIATRIC INTENSIVE CARE UNIT

JOHN P. STRAUMANIS

A *nosocomial infection* is any infection that a patient acquires within the hospital setting that is not present at admission. *Community-acquired infections* are those present at the time of admission. *Surgical site infections* (SSIs) are associated with the surgical procedure. *Colonization* is the growth or presence of potentially infectious organisms in a cavity, on a surface, in tissue, in body fluids, or with a medical device, without causing a host reaction, a clinically adverse event, or disease. Nosocomial infection rates may be noted as a percentage of patients, number of infections per 100 patients, or number of infections per 1000 device days. The National Nosocomial Infection Surveillance (NNIS) System of the Centers for Disease Control and Prevention (CDC) reports SSIs in terms of number of infections per 100 procedures. For children, the top three nosocomial infections are bloodstream infections, pneumonia, and urinary tract infections (UTIs). The location of the hospital also plays a role, with an increased risk of nosocomial infection being noted in developing nations (**Table 60.1**). Younger children, particularly neonates, have the highest risk of infection. Patients who are immunosuppressed from chemotherapy, human immunodeficiency virus infection, or steroid use, patients who are receiving parenteral nutrition with high glucose concentrations and lipid, increased length of stay, prior antimicrobial therapy, and device utilization ratios, understaffing, and RBC transfusions are all independent risk factors for acquiring nosocomial infections.

ISOLATION PRECAUTIONS

Standard precautions should be used at all times and are designed to prevent the practitioner from coming in contact with potentially infectious bodily fluids. The most important standard precaution is hand hygiene. Soap and water hand washing is considered the gold standard. Use of waterless antiseptic agents is appropriate. Hand hygiene must be practiced both

TABLE 60.1

COMPARISON OF DEVICE USE AND RATES OF DEVICE-ASSOCIATED INFECTION IN THE ICUS OF THE U.S. NATIONAL NOSOCOMIAL INFECTION SURVEILLANCE SYSTEM AND THE INTERNATIONAL NOSOCOMIAL INFECTION CONTROL CONSORTIUM

Variable	US NNIS ICUs 1992–2004	INICC ICUs 2002–2005
Rate of device use[a]		
Mechanical ventilators	0.43 (0.23–0.62)	0.38 (0.19–0.64)
CVCs	0.57 (0.36–0.74)	0.54 (0.22–0.97)
Urinary catheters	0.78 (0.65–0.90)	0.73 (0.48–0.94)
Rate per 1000 device[a]		
Ventilator-associated pneumonia	5.4 (1.2–7.2)	24.1 (10.0–52.7)
CVC-associated bloodstream infection	4.0 (1.7–7.6)	12.5 (7.8–18.5)
Catheter-associated UTI	3.9 (1.3–7.5)	8.9 (1.7–12.8)
Proportion of device-associated infections with resistance, %[b]		
MRSA	59	84
Ceftriaxone-resistant *Enterobacteriaceae*	19	55
Ciprofloxacin-resistant *Pseudomonas aeruginosa*	29	59
Vancomycin-resistant enterococci	29	5

[a] Overall (pooled) and 10th to 90th percentile range for US NNIS teaching hospitals; overall (pooled) and range of individual countries for the INICC hospitals.
[b] Overall (pooled) data from NNIS, 1992–2004 (300 hospitals) and from INICC, 2002–2005.
Data from National Nosocomial Infections Surveillance (NNIS) System Report, data summary from January 1992 through June 2004, issued October 2004. *Am J Infect Control* 2004;32:470–85; and from Rosenthal VD, Maki DG, Salomao R, et al. Device-associated nosocomial infections in 55 intensive care units of 8 developing countries. *Ann Intern Med* 2006;145(8):582–91, with permission.
NNIS, National Nosocomial Infection Surveillance System; INICC, International Nosocomial Infection Control Consortium; CVC, central venous catheter; UTI, urinary tract infection; MRSA, methicillin-resistant *Staphylococcus aureus*

before and after patient contact, even if gloves are worn. Barriers such as gloves, masks, eye protection, and nonsterile gowns should be worn when contact with bodily fluids or secretions is likely.

Transmission-based precautions are aimed at protection against transmission of infectious organisms from patients with documented or suspected infection, as well as from those colonized with specific organisms. These additional precautions are over and above the standard precautions and are based on route of transmission: contact, droplet, or airborne transmission (**Table 60.2**). *Contact precautions* are used for a wide variety of organisms that spread by direct contact with the patient or indirect contact via fomites such as toys, stethoscopes, and unwashed hands. Contact isolation should include single-patient rooms or cohorting, gowns, and gloves in addition to standard precautions. *Droplet precautions* are used for organisms that spread short distances (<3 feet away) from the patient via coughing or sneezing. Droplet isolation includes single-patient rooms or cohorting of patients with the same organism. Healthcare providers should wear masks with eye shields in addition to following standard precautions. *Airborne precautions* include additional safeguards to be taken for organisms

such as tuberculosis, measles, and varicella that are transmitted by air currents. Patients should be in private rooms with negative air flow. For measles and varicella isolation, susceptible healthcare providers should avoid contact if possible. For other organisms that require airborne precautions, a fitted respirator should be worn by all who enter in the patient's room (**Table 60.3**). The air-supplying respirators provide the greatest protection but are expensive and require high amounts of maintenance to ensure proper functioning. Air-purifying respirators filter air through a cartridge that must be selected based on the type of hazard (bacterial or chemical) to which the wearer will be exposed. The N95 respirators are the most commonly used in healthcare settings. "95" identifies the mask as having the ability to filter at least 95% of particles, with a median diameter of 0.3 microns or greater. Oil-resistant masks and oil-proof masks are designated "R" and "P," respectively. The personal protective equipment that should be worn is determined by the organism being isolated. To ensure the maximal effect of the protective equipment, it must be donned and removed in the proper order. The CDC has recommendations for healthcare facilities available at: www.cdc.gov/ncidod/dhqp/pdf/guidelines/Enviro_guide_03.pdf.

TABLE 60.2

TRANSMISSION-BASED ISOLATION RECOMMENDATIONS FOR SPECIFIC INFECTIOUS ORGANISMS AND ILLNESSES

Contact precautions	Droplet precautions	Airborne precautions
Clostridium difficile	Adenoviruses	*Mycobacterium tuberculosis*
Conjunctivitis, viral and hemorrhagic	Diphtheria	Rubeola (measles) virus
Diphtheria (cutaneous)	*Haemophilus influenzae* type b (invasive)	Varicella-Zoster virus
Enteroviruses	Hemorrhagic Fever viruses	During aerosol-generating procedures such as intubation, nebulized therapy, and bronchoscopy
Escherichia coli O157:H7 and other Shiga toxin-producing *E. coli*	Influenza	Severe acute respiratory syndrome
Hepatitis A virus	Mumps	Viral hemorrhagic fevers
Herpes simplex virus (neonatal, mucocutaneous, or cutaneous)	*Mycoplasma pneumoniae*	Consider for influenza
Herpes zoster (localized with no evidence of dissemination)	*Neisseria meningitidis* (invasive)	
Impetigo	Parvovirus B19 during the phase of illness before onset of rash in immunocompetent patients	
Major (noncontained) abscess, cellulitis, or decubitus ulcer	Pertussis	
Multidrug-resistant organisms as determined by local infection control	Plague (pneumonic)	
Parainfluenza virus	Respiratory syncytial virus (beneficial during large outbreaks)	
Pediculosis (lice)	Rubella	
Respiratory Syncytial Virus	Severe acute respiratory syndrome	
Rotavirus	Streptococcal pharyngitis, pneumonia, or scarlet fever	
Scabies		
Shigella		
Staphylococcus aureus (cutaneous or draining wounds)		
Viral hemorrhagic fevers (Ebola, Lassa, or Marburg)		

Some organisms may include more than one type of isolation. This list is not all-inclusive.
Data from American Academy of Pediatrics. Infection Control for Hospitalized Children. In: Pickering LK, Baker CJ, Long SS, et al, eds. *Red Book: 2006 Report of the Committee on Infectious Diseases*, 27th ed. Elk Grove Village: American Academy of Pediatrics, 2006:153–64.

SURVEILLANCE CULTURES

In communities that have high levels of resistant organisms, it may be worth screening for these infections at admission such as methicillin-resistant *Staphylococcus aureus* (MRSA). The admission screening is most commonly performed by culturing the anterior nares, but other sites such as wounds or skin lesions, catheter sites, tracheostomies, and the umbilicus in neonates can be used. Following admission screening, surveillance screening is performed to identify new, hospital-acquired infections. Once a patient is identified as being colonized with MRSA, he or she should be isolated, informed of his or her colonization status, and considered for treatment to clear the colonization. This approach has been used for MRSA colonization and infections but could be used for a variety of organisms if the frequency in the community or hospital warrants it. Cohorting of patients with the same organism and the staff caring for them may be beneficial.

CATHETER-RELATED BLOODSTREAM INFECTIONS

Tunneled central venous catheters have a lower risk of infection compared to percutaneously inserted lines.

TABLE 60.3

CLINICAL SYNDROMES OR CONDITIONS THAT WARRANT PRECAUTIONS IN ADDITION TO STANDARD PRECAUTIONS TO PREVENT TRANSMISSION OF EPIDEMIOLOGICALLY IMPORTANT PATHOGENS PENDING CONFIRMATION OF DIAGNOSIS[a]

Clinical syndrome or condition[b]	Potential pathogen[c]	Empiric precaution[d]
Diarrhea		
Acute diarrhea with a likely infectious cause	Enteric pathogens[e]	Contact
Diarrhea in patient with history of recent antimicrobial use	*Clostridium difficile*	Contact
Meningitis	*Neisseria meningitidis*	Droplet
Rash or exanthems, generalized, cause unknown		
Petechial or ecchymotic with fever	*N. meningitidis*	Droplet
Vesicular	Varicella virus	Airborne and contact
Maculopapular with coryza and fever	Measles virus	Airborne
Respiratory tract infections		
Pulmonary cavitary disease	*Mycobacterium tuberculosis*	Airborne
Paroxysmal or severe persistent cough during periods of pertussis activity in the community	Bordetella pertussis	Droplet
Viral infections, particularly bronchiolitis and croup, in infants and young children	Respiratory syncytial virus or parainfluenza virus	Contact and droplet
Risk of multidrug-resistant microorganisms[f]		
History of infection or colonization with multidrug-resistant organisms	Resistant bacteria	Contact
Skin, wound, or urinary tract infection in a patient with a recent hospital or nursing home stay in a facility in which multidrug-resistant organisms are prevalent	Resistant bacteria	Contact
Skin or wound infection		
Abscess or draining wound that cannot be covered	*Staphylococcus aureus*, group A streptococcus	Contact

[a] Infection control professionals are encouraged to modify or adapt this table according to local conditions. To ensure that appropriate empiric precautions are implemented, hospitals must have systems in place to evaluate patients routinely according to these criteria as part of their preadmission and admission care.
[b] Patients with the syndromes or conditions listed may have atypical signs or symptoms (e.g., pertussis in neonates, absence of paroxysmal or sever cough in adults). The clinician's index of suspicion should be guided by the prevalence of specific conditions in the community and clinical judgment.
[c] The organisms listed in this column are not intended to represent the complete or even most likely diagnoses but, rather, possible causative agents that require additional precautions beyond Standard Precautions until they can be excluded.
[d] Duration of isolation varies by agent (see Garner JS. Hospital Infection Control Practices Advisory Committee. Guidelines for isolation precautions in hospitals. *Infect Control Hosp Epidemiol* 1996;17:53–80).
[e] These pathogens include shiga toxin-producing *Escherichia coli* including *E. Coli* O157:H7, *Shigella* organisms, *Salmonella* organisms. *Campylobacter* organisms, hepatitis A virus, enteric viruses including rotavirus, and *Cryptosporidium* organisms.
[f] Resistant bacteria judged by the infection control program on the basis of current state, regional, or national recommendations to be of special clinical or epidemiologic significance.
From American Academy of Pediatrics. Infection Control for Hospitalized Children. In: Pickering LK, Baker CJ, Long SS, et al, eds. *Red Book: 2006 Report of the Committee on Infectious Diseases*. 27th ed. Elk Grove Village: American Academy of Pediatrics, 2006, with permission.

Tunneled lines, with or without cuffs, are generally used for long-term access. Guidelines from the CDC have set criteria for diagnosing bloodstream infections that involve intravascular catheters. A *catheter-related bloodstream infection* is either a bacteremia or fungemia documented with at least one peripherally obtained blood culture that is obtained from a vein and not a catheter. Clinical evidence of an infection, including a host response, must be present that cannot be attributed to any source other than the catheter. The growth of an organism in the bloodstream must be documented by (a) positive semi-quantitative or quantitative cultures of a catheter segment with an organism identical in species and antibiogram as isolated from a peripheral blood culture, (b) simultaneously drawn peripheral and line quantitative blood cultures with >5:1 ratio in catheter blood versus peripheral blood colony counts, or (c) a differential in timing of culture positivity of >2 hrs between the catheter and peripheral blood culture, where the catheter culture is positive first. A *catheter-associated bloodstream infection* has less rigorous criteria and requires the presence of a central line being in place during the 48 hrs prior to the drawing of the positive culture and compelling evidence that the infection is related to the line. The most common route of infection for percutaneous lines in the ICU is migration of skin organisms down the external surface of the catheter to the bloodstream; this can be greatly influenced by catheter care and the patient's own bacterial flora. Other sources of line-associated infection can be grouped into the following categories: (a) hematogenous spread from distant sites with increased risk

due to biofilm and clot formation on the catheter surface, which is influenced by type of catheter material and the presence of antiseptic or antibiotic coatings; (b) infection via contaminated infusate; (c) colonization of the catheter hub; (d) transducer or IV tubing contamination; or (e) contamination of the catheter prior to insertion. Two blood cultures should be obtained when a catheter-related infection is suspected, and at least one, if not both, should be drawn percutaneously. Once the decision has been made to remove the line, the catheter tip should be sent for quantitative or semiquantitative cultures; qualitative broth cultures are not recommended (**Fig. 60.1**). Exchanging the catheter over a guidewire minimizes the risks associated with the placement of the line at a new site; however, it does not lower the risk of infection. It may not be necessary to remove the catheter in patients

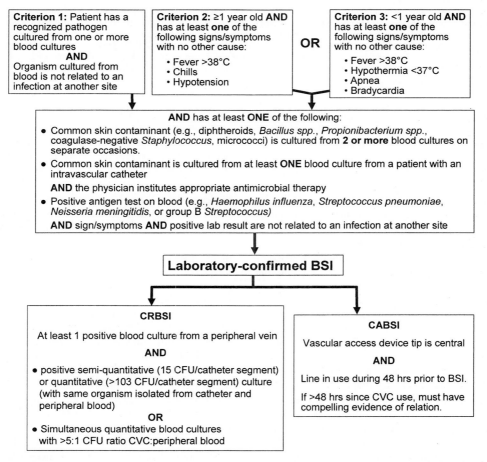

FIGURE 60.1. Bloodstream infection (BSI) diagnostic flow diagram. A catheter-related BSI (CRBSI) can also be confirmed with at least 1 positive blood culture from a peripheral vein and a differential time to positivity at least 2 hrs earlier for a central-line culture. CABSI, Catheter-associated BSI; CFU, colony-forming units; CVC, central venous catheter. From Stockwell JA. Nosocomial infections in the pediatric intensive care unit: Affecting the impact on safety and outcome. *Pediatr Crit Care Med.* 2007;8(2 Suppl): S21–S37, with permission.

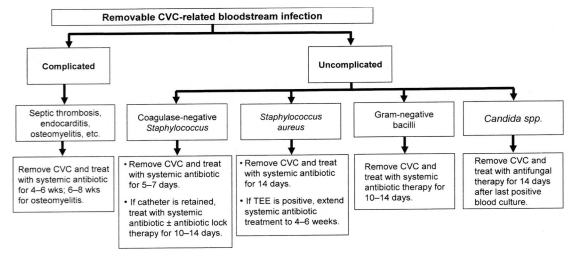

FIGURE 60.2. Approach to the management of patients with nontunneled central venous catheter–related bloodstream infection. Duration of treatment will depend on whether the infection is complicated or uncomplicated. The catheter should be removed, and systemic antimicrobial therapy should be initiated, except in some cases of uncomplicated catheter-related infection due to coagulase-negative staphylococci. For infections due to Staphylococcus aureus, transesophageal echocardiography (TEE) may reveal the presence of endocarditis and help to determine the duration of treatment. From Mermel LA, Farr BM, Sherertz RJ, et al. Guidelines for the management of intravascular catheter-related infections. Clin Infect Dis 2001;32(9):1249–72, with permission.

without evidence of persistent bloodstream infection or if there is a culture-positive, coagulase-negative staphylococcal infection in the absence of local or metastatic infectious complications. For both conditions, appropriate antibiotic therapy is indicated (**Fig. 60.2**). Some authors have reported successful treatment of central line infections without removal of the device. Such management should include close observation of the clinical condition, with prompt removal if clinical deterioration occurs. Regardless of the culture results, if the child does not respond or worsens within the first 3 days of antibiotic therapy, the line should be removed.

Thorough hand washing prior to insertion is basic clinical practice. Skin preparation should be performed with a 2% aqueous chlorhexidine gluconate solution. Where a 2% solution of chlorhexidine is not available, povidone-iodine or 70% alcohol should be used. Chlorhexidine preparations should not be used on infants <2 months of age due to possible absorption through the immature skin. After adequate skin preparation, full-barrier precautions, which include a large sterile or full-body drape, long-sleeved sterile gown, cap, mask, and sterile gloves, should be taken. Chlorhexidine-impregnated sponge dressing at the site of catheter insertion decreases bloodstream infections. A higher number of lumens increases infection risk. Teflon and polyurethane catheters are associated with fewer line-related infections. Additional antimicrobial resistance can be imparted by

coating or impregnating central venous catheters with antiseptics or antibiotics. The antimicrobial activity decreases over time. An infection rate >3.3 per 1000 catheter days may favor the added cost of these catheters in adults where the average NNIS bloodstream-infection rate ranges from 2.9–5.9 infections per 1000 catheter days. Catheters impregnated internally and externally with the antibiotics minocycline and rifampin have shown even lower infection rates. Replacement at a new site carries all of the risks associated with insertion and does not lower the cumulative risk of infection. Routine replacement of arterial lines is not recommended. The routine replacement of central venous catheters is not recommended due in part to the limited number of vascular sites in children. Routine replacement of tubing and infusion sets has been proven to decrease the risk of catheter infection. Tubing for peripheral and central lines should be changed no more frequently than every 72 hrs for routine fluids. Infusion sets used for blood, blood products, and lipid infusions should be changed within 24 hrs of starting the infusion. For arterial lines, the tubing and the transducer should be changed at 96-hr intervals. Common sense would dictate changing stopcocks with tubing changes and when soiled or potentially contaminated.

In adult studies, the subclavian site has significantly lower infection risk than does the internal jugular site. However, this risk must be balanced by the increased risk of complications as well as operator experience and expertise. A higher colonization rate at the femoral site with an increased risk of catheter infection has been reported in the adult population but has not been found in studies of pediatric patients, in which femoral sites were associated with fewer mechanical complications and had an equivalent infection rate when compared to catheters at other sites. The type of line inserted must be determined by the patient's needs and the infectious risks associated with the line (**Table 60.4**).

The risk factors identified for nosocomial infections associated with extracorporeal membrane oxygenation (ECMO) are prolonged ECMO support, support for cardiac disease, undergoing a major surgical procedure immediately prior to or while on ECMO, and having an open chest while on ECMO. The nosocomial infections associated with ECMO include wound infections of the neck and chest, bloodstream infections, UTIs, and respiratory infections.

TABLE 60.4

DESCRIPTION OF VASCULAR ACCESS DEVICES AND RISK OF INFECTION

Catheter type	Entry site	Length	Comments
Peripheral venous catheters (short)	Usually inserted in veins of forearm or hand	<3 in	Phlebitis with prolonged use; rarely associated with bloodstream infection
Peripheral arterial catheters	Usually inserted in radial artery; can be placed in femoral, axillary, brachial, posterior tibial arteries	<3 in	Low infection risk; rarely associated with bloodstream infection
Midline catheters	Inserted via the antecubital fossa into the proximal basilic or cephalic veins; does not enter central veins	3–8 in	Anaphylactoid reactions have been reported with catheters made of elastomeric hydrogel; lower rates of phlebitis than short peripheral catheters
Nontunneled CVCs	Percutaneously inserted into central veins (subclavian, internal jugular, or femoral)	≥8 cm, depending on patient size	Account for most CRBSIs
Pulmonary artery catheters	Inserted through a Teflon introducer in a central vein (subclavian, internal jugular, or femoral)	≥30 cm, depending on patient size	Usually heparin bonded; similar rates of bloodstream infection as CVC; subclavian site preferred to reduce infection risk
PICCs	Inserted into basilic, cephalic, or brachial veins and enter the superior vena cava	≥20 cm, depending on patient size	Lower rate of infection than nontunneled CVCs
Tunneled CVCs	Implanted into subclavian, internal jugular, or femoral veins	≥8 cm, depending on patient size	Cuff inhibits migration of organisms into catheter tract, lower rate of infection than nontunneled CVC
Totally implantable	Tunneled beneath skin and have devices that are subcutaneous-port accessed with a needle; implanted in subclavian or internal jugular vein	≥8 cm, depending on patient size	Lowest risk for CRBSI; improved patient self-image; no need for local catheter site care; surgery required for catheter removal
Umbilical catheters	Inserted into either umbilical vein or umbilical artery	≤6 cm, depending on patient size	Risk for CRBSI similar to catheters placed in umbilical vein versus artery

CVC, central venous catheter; CRBSI, catheter-related bloodstream infection; PICC, peripherally inserted central catheters
From O'Grady NP, Alexander M, Dellinger EP, et al. Guidelines for the prevention of intravascular catheter-related infections. The Hospital Infection Control Practices Advisory Committee, Center for Disease Control and Prevention, *US. Pediatrics* 2002;110(5):e51, with permission.

NOSOCOMIAL RESPIRATORY INFECTIONS

The definition of ventilator-associated pneumonia (VAP) is the development of a new pneumonia at least 48 hrs after initiation of mechanical ventilation. Independent risk factors for the development of VAP in children are immunodeficiency, immunosuppression, neuromuscular blockade, neuromuscular weakness, burns, steroid administration, total parenteral nutrition, antibiotic use, longer ICU lengths of stay, use of indwelling catheters, use of H_2-receptor-blocker therapy, reintubation, transport out of the ICU while intubated, the presence of a nasoenteric tube, in-line nebulizers and manipulation of ventilator circuits. The pediatric NNIS VAP rate (January 1992 through June 2004) is 2.9 episodes per 1000 ventilator days. Although length of time with an endotracheal tube in place increases the risk of nosocomial pneumonia, the greatest risk is during the first 2 weeks of intubation. The bacterial organisms identified most often are Gram-negative bacilli, followed by Gram-positive organisms. Viruses, predominantly RSV, are the most common cause of nosocomial respiratory infections. Fungal infections are exceedingly rare but may occur in children who are immunosuppressed, especially if they frequently receive broad-spectrum antibiotics. The diagnosis of VAP in children can be made on clinical grounds without the use of bronchoscopy (**Table 60.5**). Endotracheal tube cultures are inaccurate due to colonization of the endotracheal tube and upper airway. For adults and older children, bronchoalveolar

TABLE 60.5

CLINICAL CRITERIA FOR DIAGNOSING VENTILATOR-ASSOCIATED PNEUMONIA BY AGE

	All patients	1–12 Yrs of age	<12 mos of age
Chest x-ray	At least 2 serial chest x-rays with new or progressive and persistent infiltrate or consolidate or cavitation that develops later than 48 hrs postinitiation of mechanical ventilation		
Additional criteria	At least one of the shaded criteria *and* at least two of the nonshaded criteria	At least 3 of the criteria below	Worsening gas exchange *and* at least 3 of the criteria below
Temperature	>38°C without other recognized cause	>38.4°C or <37°C without other recognized cause	Temperature instability without other recognized cause
WBC count	<4000/mm³ OR >12,000/mm³	<4000/mm³ OR >15,000/mm³	<4000/mm³ OR >15,000/mm³ and band forms >10%
Altered mental status	If >70 years of age without other recognized cause	N/A	N/A
Sputum/secretions	New onset purulent sputum **OR** change in the character of sputum **OR** increased respiratory symptoms		
Respiratory symptoms	New onset or worsening of cough, dyspnea, or tachypnea		Apnea, tachypnea, increased work of breathing, or grunting
Auscultation findings	Rales or bronchial breath sounds		Wheezing, rales, or ronchi
Cough	N/A as separate criteria	N/A as separate criteria	+
Worsening oxygenation or ventilation	Present	Present	Required criteria
Heart rate	N/A	N/A	<100 beats/min OR >170 beats/min

CXR, chest x-ray; WBC, white blood cell count; N/A, not applicable
Modified from Wright ML, Romano MJ. Ventilator-associated pneumonia in children. *Semin Pediatr Infect Dis* 2006;17(2):58–64.

TABLE 60.6

COMMONLY UTILIZED PEDIATRIC VENTILATOR-ASSOCIATED PNEUMONIA BUNDLE ITEMS

Items to prevent iatrogenic spread of infection
Adherence to good hand hygiene practices
Use of universal precautions
Use of appropriate isolation techniques based on infectious organism (proven or suspected)

Items to prevent aspiration of gastric contents
Elevate the head of the bed between 30 and 45 degrees
Monitor/drain gastric contents

Items to improve oral hygiene
Oral rinsing/cleaning with chlorhexidine (0.12%)
Use of toothbrush and oral swabs in daily oral care

Items to decrease endotracheal tube risk factors
Use of in-line suction equipment where appropriate and available
Suction of the hypopharynx prior to endotracheal suctioning and repositioning

Items to avoid contamination of respiratory equipment
Dedicated oropharyngeal suction equipment
Prevention of accumulation of respiratory circuit condensates
Prevention of contamination of ventilation equipment

Items to decrease the duration of mechanical ventilation
Daily readiness for extubation trials
Neuromuscular blockade holidays

Adapted from Curley MA, Schwalenstocker E, Deshpande JK, et al. Tailoring the Institute for Health Care Improvement 100,000 Lives Campaign to pediatric settings: The example of ventilator-associated pneumonia. *Pediatr Clin North Am* 2006; 53(6):1231–51.

lavage and protected-specimen brush collection has been used with success.

Adult studies provide increasing evidence that subglottic drainage of secretions significantly diminishes the risk of VAP (**Table 60.6**). These specialized endotracheal tubes are both expensive and not yet available for the majority of the pediatric population because of size limitations. The findings of these studies have led to the practice of suctioning the hypopharynx to clear secretions in pediatric patients. The use of constant, high-dose sedation should be avoided, and appropriate sedation scales should be used. If neuromuscular blockade is being used, it is reasonable to intermittently hold the paralyzing agents if clinically appropriate. Another potential, albeit unproven, element of a pediatric VAP bundle should be the daily assessment as to whether or not the patient can be extubated (**Fig. 60.3**). Pa-

tients managed with noninvasive ventilation have a shorter ICU length of stay and a decreased mortality rate. When appropriate, noninvasive ventilation should be considered as a potential method by which to decrease VAP risk. Sinusitis is a risk factor for the development of pneumonia. Patients in intensive care are uniquely at risk for developing a nosocomial sinus infection because of supine positioning, decreased sinus drainage due to positive-pressure ventilation, and nasal placement of therapeutic devices that obstruct sinus drainage.

The risk factors of contracting an RSV nosocomial infection are young age, especially neonates; underlying chronic illness such as cardiac or pulmonary disease; a long hospitalization; overcrowding or staff shortages; and hospitalization during the RSV endemic season. An additional source of nosocomial RSV infection is healthcare workers. The most common modes of transmission of RSV from one person to another are via either large-droplet aerosols or adherence to fomites. As large droplets can only travel short distances (<1 meter), they require close person-to-person contact. Fomites pose the greatest risk of transmission in a hospital setting. RSV can survive and remain infectious on nonporous surfaces for 6–12 hrs.

Personal protective equipment appeared to be quite effective in preventing acquisition of severe acute respiratory syndrome (SARS). It was found that consistent wearing of either a simple surgical mask or an N95 respirator was more effective than inconsistent use, with a 13% versus 56% infection rate respectively. Additional infection control measures used to prevent large-droplet transmission of infectious agents during the SARS outbreak included "physical space interventions" such as separation of patients, methods to decrease infectious aerosols during at risk therapies, and environmental decontamination and containment. Intubation, continuous positive-airway pressure, and nebulization therapy increase the transmission of SARS.

NOSOCOMIAL URINARY TRACT INFECTIONS

The NNIS nosocomial urinary tract rate is 4.0 infections per 1000 catheter days. The nosocomial UTI risks are: increased duration of catheterization, female gender, absence of systemic antibiotics, and disconnection of the catheter-collecting tube junction. Strategies to prevent or decrease nosocomial UTIs include minimizing exposure to urinary catheters by using them only when truly indicated, using a sterile insertion technique, maintaining uninterrupted use of a closed collection system, and removing the device as soon as possible—ideally in <3 days.

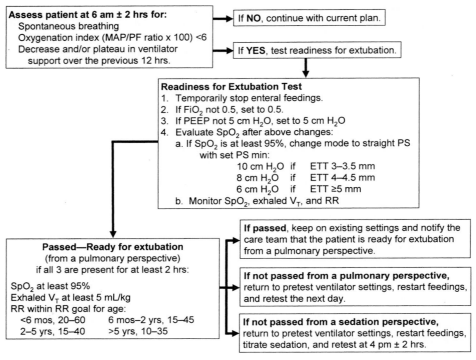

FIGURE 60.3. Daily test for patient readiness for extubation. In this model, prescreening for suitability for extubation is assessed over a 2-hr period. If prescreening criteria are met, feeds are held, and the patient is brought to low ventilator settings for a trial on pressure support ventilation. If the patient does well based on preset criteria, extubation is considered. MAP, mean arterial pressure; PF ratio, PaO_2/FiO_2 ratio; PEEP, positive end-expiratory pressure; ETT, endotracheal tube; PS, pressure support; V_T, tidal volume; RR, respiratory rate. From Curley MAQ, Arnold JH, Thompson JE, et al. Clinical trial design: Effect of prone positioning on clinical outcomes in infants and children with acute respiratory distress syndrome. J Crit Care 2006;21:23–32; with permission.

NOSOCOMIAL GASTROINTESTINAL INFECTIONS

Nosocomial diarrhea is defined as loose stools that occur >48 hrs after admission, a stool frequency of at least two per 12 hrs, and no identified noninfectious cause of the loose stools. Outside the PICU, viral etiologies as a group predominate and are usually similar organisms as those seen in the community, such as rotavirus, adenovirus, and Norwalk virus. The most common organism isolated in the PICU is *Clostridium difficile*. The organisms responsible for nosocomial diarrhea are typically spread by the fecal-oral route. Good hand hygiene and contact precautions are paramount to this effort. The viruses that cause diarrheal illnesses can survive on fomites and other surfaces for several hours, and the spores of *C. difficile* can survive for more than a day on inanimate surfaces.

The etiology of necrotizing enterocolitis is multifactorial; however, nosocomial, epidemic outbreaks do occur in NICUs. Affected centers used infection control measures that focused on preventing orofecal transmission to limit the epidemic, including strict use of hand washing, the use of gloves, isolation of the infected newborns, cohorting of cases, and the closing of some units. Identified organisms in outbreaks have been *E. coli*, *K. pneumoniae*, *Enterobacter cloacae*, *Clostridium butyricum*, *C. difficile*, *S. epidermidis*, *Coronavirus*, *Rotavirus*, and echovirus.

SURGICAL SITE INFECTIONS

Nosocomial infections of the CNS usually involve a surgical site or the presence of a foreign body. The risk of a SSI from a ventricular shunt with zero risk categories is 4.42 per 100 operations. Other CNS operations have a combined SSI rate of 1.53 per 100 operations. Several risk factors for infection include repairs of syndromic craniosynostosis, an oblique facial cleft, more complicated preoperative diagnosis, an increased duration of surgery, closure of the overlying skin under tension, the presence of more than 4 surgeons during the operative procedure, associated medical conditions, and previous surgical procedures, including tracheotomy and ventriculoperitoneal shunt. The infection rates in epidural catheters for pain management range from 0% to 0.7%. Possible sources of epidural catheter infection include skin contamination, introduction of bacteria by the needle or catheter, hematogenous spread, or contamination of the infusate. Risk of infection can be reduced with attention to aseptic technique during placement, adequate skin preparation, and disinfection prior to placement, and maintenance of appropriate dressings is an important safety measure to prevent infection of the catheter and the epidural space. The duration of catheter use increases the risk of infection. The incidences of dressing contamination, cellulitis, and bacterial colonization are more common in caudally placed catheters than in lumbar catheters.

Adult rates of SSIs following cardiovascular surgery are between 1.5 and 2.3 infections per 100 operations. More than half of the infections in children are caused by *S. aureus*, followed in frequency by coagulase-negative staphylococci, enterococci, and *Enterobacter spp.* Debridement when appropriate and IV antibiotics are the therapies administered. Risk factors for SSI have been identified and can be divided into preoperative, intraoperative, and postoperative categories. Preoperative risks include younger age at time of surgery, a higher American Society of Anesthesiologists score, a longer preoperative inpatient length of stay, a prior sternotomy, and an elevated leukocyte band count. Intraoperative factors are the duration of the surgery, cardiopulmonary bypass, and circulatory arrest. Postoperative factors include failed primary closure of the chest, low cardiac output, infection at another site, and the duration of use of mechanical ventilation, central venous line, and urinary catheter.

Mediastinitis, defined by purulent discharge in the mediastinal space necessitating surgical debridement, positive cultures from the mediastinal space, or sternal instability in the presence of positive blood cultures has an incidence ranging from 0.04% to 3.9%. Mediastinitis occurs at a mean of 11 days following sternotomy, with Gram-positive infections occurring later than Gram-negative infections—13 versus 6.5 days, respectively. Delayed sternal closure was found to be an independent risk factor.

VECTOR-BORNE INFECTIONS

Nosocomial transmission of traditionally vector-borne infections such as malaria and dengue fever is possible in the hospital setting. Malaria has been reported to be transmitted via blood transfusions, organ transplantation, needle stick injuries, improper use and cleaning of medical devices such as glucometers and catheters, misuse of multidose vials, and open wounds. Dengue fever has been transmitted by needle stick injuries and bone marrow transplantation. Nosocomial transmission of vector-borne infections should be considered if the patient has not traveled to endemic areas of the world.

CHAPTER 61 ■ INTERNATIONAL AND EMERGING INFECTIONS

TROY E. DOMINGUEZ • CHITRA RAVISHANKAR • MIRIAM K. LAUFER

INTERNATIONAL INFECTIONS

When a child who has been abroad is evaluated for an illness, many infections cannot be distinguished on clinical grounds alone (**Table 61.1**).

Malaria

Malaria is transmitted by a bite from the female anopheline mosquito. The areas of the world affected are illustrated in **Figure 61.1**. Four species of Plasmodium cause malaria infections in humans, of which P. falciparum is most common. The Anopheles mosquito injects sporozoites into the human during the process of taking a blood meal. The sporozoites immediately travel to the liver. In the hepatic stage, which lasts 1–2 weeks, the parasites undergo asexual reproduction and become schizonts; no symptoms are associated with this exoerythrocytic life-cycle stage. When the schizonts in the liver rupture, merozoites emerge into the bloodstream and

TABLE 61.1

CAUSES OF SYSTEMIC FEBRILE ILLNESS AMONG RETURNED TRAVELERS

Diagnosis	Caribbean	Central America	South America	Sub-Saharan Africa	South or Central Asia	Southeast Asia
Malaria	+	++	++	+++	++	++
Dengue	++	++	++	−/+	++	++
Mononucleosis	+	+	+	+	+	+
Rickettsia				+*	+/−	+
Typhoid fever	+	+	+	−/+	++	+

Adapted from Freedman DO, Weld LH, Kozarsky PE, et al. Spectrum of disease and relation to place of exposure among ill returned travelers. *N Engl J Med* 2006;354:119–30.

begin the erythrocytic stage of infection that is associated with clinical disease. Merozoites infect erythrocytes and mature into trophozoites; these become schizonts. Rupture of infected red blood cells (RBCs) that contain the schizont forms produces more merozoites capable of invading more RBCs. Sequestration in the brain microcirculation is associated with the most dreaded complication of infection—cerebral malaria.

The initial presentation of uncomplicated malaria is a nonlocalizing febrile illness with fever, chills, headache, and diaphoresis. Other common symptoms include nausea, vomiting, diarrhea, malaise, myalgias, dizziness, diarrhea, and dry cough. The World Health Organization (WHO) has suggested clinical features to help identify patients at high risk of death (**Table 61.2**). Patients with any impairment of consciousness should be treated as if they have

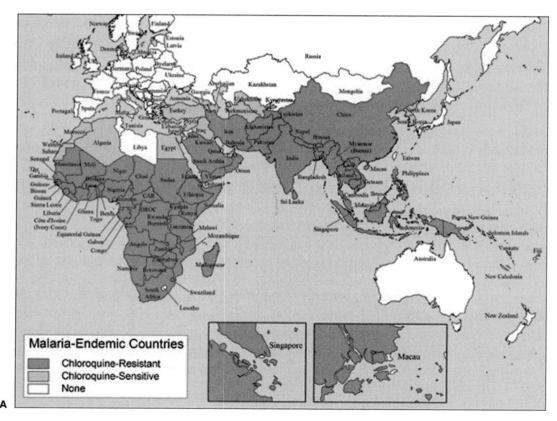

A

FIGURE 61.1. Distribution of malaria (all species). From the US Centers for Disease Control and Prevention, http://wwwn.cdc.gov/travel/yellowBookCh4-Malaria.aspx.

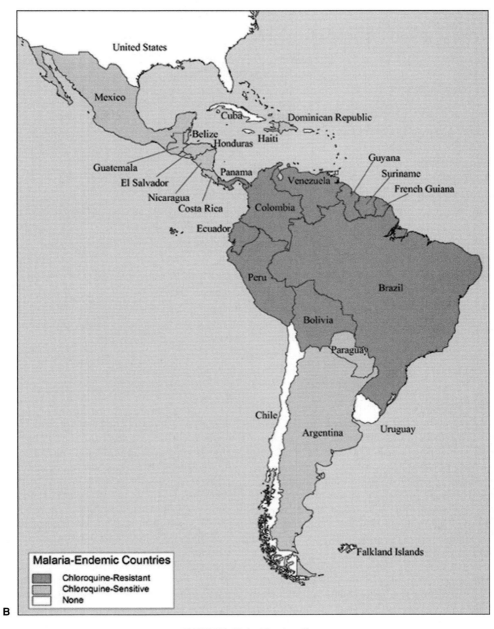

FIGURE 61.1. (*Continued*)

cerebral malaria. Severe malarial anemia is an important, life-threatening form of severe disease in young children from endemic areas. Hypoglycemia, acidosis, and pulmonary edema also complicate severe disease and are associated with a poor outcome. The severe manifestations that are more common in adults are: jaundice and hepatic dysfunction, acute respiratory distress syndrome (ARDS), and renal dysfunction. Other severe complications include

hypotension with shock, splenic rupture in children with hypersplenism and disseminated intravascular coagulation. Hypersplenism is is known as *hyperreactive malarial splenomegaly* or *tropical splenomegaly syndrome*. Blackwater fever (hemoglobinuria, hemolysis, renal failure) and algid malaria (cardiovascular collapse, shock, hypothermia) are rarely seen in children.

Laboratory findings in patients with severe malaria include: thrombocytopenia, hyperbilirubinemia,

TABLE 61.2

DEFINITION OF POOR PROGNOSTIC SIGNS IN SEVERE MALARIA

Prostration	Inability to sit in a child who was previously able to sit. In infants, can be defined as unable to feed.
Impaired consciousness	Coma that lasts at least 30 mins after a seizure, with no other cause identified (e.g., meningitis, hypoglycemia). Impairment may be less severe.
Respiratory distress (acidotic breathing)	In the absence of abnormalities on auscultation or radiography, normal oxygen saturation
Multiple convulsions	>2 in 24 hrs
Circulatory collapse	Hypotension with cold, clammy skin
Pulmonary edema	Not due to volume overload
Abnormal bleeding	Spontaneous mucosal bleeding or laboratory evidence of disseminated intravascular coagulopathy
Jaundice	Detected clinically or >3 g/dL (50 mcmol/L)
Hemoglobinuria	Macroscopic
Severe anemia	Normocytic anemia with hemoglobin <5 g/dL or hematocrit <15%
Hypoglycemia	<40 g/dL or 2.2 mmol/L
Acidosis	Arterial or capillary pH <7.3 or bicarbonate <15 mmol/L
Renal impairment	Urine output <0.5 mL/kg/hr, failure to respond to rehydration, creatinine >3.0 mg/dL
Hyperlactatemia	>5 mmol/L
Hyperparasitemia	>4%–5% in nonimmune children and adults

anemia, and elevated hepatic transaminases. The white blood cell (WBC) count can be normal or low with a left shift. Other nonspecific markers of inflammation such as C-reactive protein and erythrocyte sedimentation rate are usually elevated. Coagulation abnormalities may be present due to disseminated intravascular coagulation. The diagnosis of malaria is established by examining three sets of thick and thin blood smears stained with a 3% Giemsa stain 12–24 hours apart.

For uncomplicated malaria, the decision for specific antimicrobial therapies depends upon the infecting species and the geographic source of the infection. The appropriate therapies for uncomplicated disease are listed in **Table 61.3**. Patients with any signs of severe disease should initially be treated with parenteral therapy. Quinine is the mainstay of therapy in endemic areas, although it is not available in the US. Quinidine is the recommended drug in the US. If no quinidine can be located in an emergency situation, providers can contact Eli Lilly Company (800-821-0538).

Malaria smears should be repeated every 8 hrs when patients have signs or symptoms of severe disease. Quinine and quinidine are slow-acting medications, and it is common for parasites to increase in the blood for the first 24 hrs after initiation of

therapy. Outside the US, artemisinin-derivatives are being used to treat severe disease. They are more rapid-acting than quinine and quinidine and have significantly less adverse effects. The combination of artemether–lumefantrine is sold in Europe as Riamet. If hypoglycemia is present, it should be corrected with dextrose infusions. In patients with impaired consciousness or any other suspicion of cerebral malaria, volume resuscitation should proceed cautiously, as cerebral edema is common. Albumin has been shown to be more beneficial than saline among comatose children with severe malaria. Potassium levels may fall. Packed RBC transfusions are indicated for patients with symptomatic anemia. The CDC recommends considering exchange transfusion if the parasite density is >10% or in the presence of cerebral malaria, non-volume overload pulmonary edema, or renal insufficiency.

Typhoid

Typhoid fever is an enteric fever syndrome caused by *Salmonella enterica* serotype. These organisms are carried only by humans, and transmission usually occurs via contaminated food or water. *S. typhi* is a Gram-negative rod in the family *Enterobacteriaceae*.

TABLE 61.3

TREATMENT OF UNCOMPLICATED AND SEVERE MALARIA

Diagnosis	Therapy
Uncomplicated malaria with *P. falciparum* or unknown species: chloroquine sensitive (*only* Central America west of the Panama Canal, Haiti, Dominican Republic)	**Chloroquine phosphate** 10 mg base/kg initial dose, followed by 5 mg base/kg at 6, 24, and 48 hrs Total dose 25 mg base/kg Maximum adult dose: 1,500 mg base
Uncomplicated malaria with *P. falciparum* or unknown species: chloroquine resistant (all regions except for those mentioned above)	**Quinine sulfate** 8.3 mg base/kg po tid for 3–7 days Maximum adult dose: 542 mg base/dose PLUS one of the following for 7 days **Doxycycline** 2.2 mg/kg po bid Maximum adult dose: 100 mg/dose **Tetracycline** 25 mg/kg/day divided qid Maximum adult dose 250 mg/dose **Clindamycin** 20 mg/kg/day divided tid **Atovaquone-proguanil** Adult tabs: 250 mg atovaquone/100 mg proguanil Pediatric tablets: 62.5 mg atovaquone/25 mg proguanil Doses given once per day for 3 days: 5–8 kg: 2 pediatric tabs 9–10 kg: 3 pediatric tabs 11–20 kg: 1 adult tab 21–30 kg: 2 adult tab 31–40 kg: 3 adult tabs >40 kg: 4 adult tabs **Mefloquine** 15 mg salt/kg po initial dose, followed by 10 mg salt/kg po 6–12 hrs after initial dose. Total dose: 25 mg salt/kg Maximum adult dose: 1,250 mg salt
Complicated/severe malaria	**Quinidine gluconate** *Continuous infusion*: 6.25 mg base/kg IV over 1–2 hrs, followed by 0.0125 mg base/kg/min continuous infusion for at least 24 hrs *Every 8-hr dosing*: 15 mg base/kg over 4 hrs, followed by 7.5 mg base/kg every 8 hrs Switch to oral therapy when parasite density is <1%. Complete 3–7 days of quinidine therapy *PLUS* **doxycycline, tetracycline, or clindamycin** as above. If patient cannot tolerate oral medication, doxycycline or clindamycin may be administered intravenously.

The typical presentation of typhoid fever is fever, chills vomiting, anorexia, myalgia, and nonfocal abdominal pain. The fever rises slowly, and as it reaches its peak, it is sustained, unlike the paroxysms of fever typical of malaria. Physical examination often reveals hepatosplenomegaly and abdominal pain. Rose spots are the typical rash of typhoid fever. They are 2–4 mm wide blanching erythematous papules usually found on the trunk. Relative bradycardia in the face of high fever is typical. An "apathetic affect" is common, and intermittent episodes of confusion can occur in the absence of direct infection of the CNS.

Altered mental status is a manifestation of typhoid encephalopathy, one of the severe complications of typhoid fever. Seizures may occur in young children. The WBC count is often slightly low, although young children may have leukocytosis. Mild increases in liver function tests are common. In severe disease, coagulopathy may be present, with thrombocytopenia and signs of disseminated intravascular coagulopathy.

The differential diagnosis depends on the precise travel and exposure history of the patient. Malaria is frequently the leading alternative diagnosis because typhoid and malaria coexist in many regions, and they are among the leading causes of fever without localizing signs in returned travelers. The pattern of fever may distinguish the two diseases: In typhoid, the fever rises gradually and is sustained, while malaria is associated with sudden onset paroxysms of fever. However, treatment for both infections may be indicated as evaluation is underway. Other diseases to consider include bacterial sepsis of other etiologies, leptospirosis, rickettsial disease, dengue, hepatitis, Epstein-Barr virus, typhus, brucellosis, and tularemia.

The diagnosis of typhoid fever is made when large-volume blood cultures are collected during the first week of illness. Bone marrow culture is more sensitive than standard blood culture. Recommended therapies for typhoid fever are listed in **Table 61.4**. Severe disease requires parenteral therapy for a minimum of 10 days. There is a benefit of dexamethasone for treatment of severe typhoid with delirium, obtundation, or shock (3 mg/kg infusion over 1 hr, followed by 1 mg/kg every 6 hrs for 8 doses). If dexamethasone is administered, providers should be aware that further intestinal complications may be masked. Severe intestinal bleeding or perforation requires hemodynamic stabilization and surgery. In cases of perforation, the intestine should be explored for additional sites of perforation. Excretion of *S. typhi* can persist beyond the clinical illness.

Chagas Disease

Trypanosoma cruzi is the etiologic agent causing Chagas disease. The reduviid bug (kissing bug) is responsible for transmitting the disease to human via feces contamination after a bite or through feces contamination of conjunctiva or mucosa. Housing conditions are important for disease transmission, as the reduviid bugs usually live in the cracks within the walls of mud and straw houses found in rural and poor urban areas. Transfusion-associated *T. cruzi* is another important mode of disease transmission in countries (e.g., Brazil) with a high prevalence of disease.

The initial symptoms of infection with *T. cruzi* are nonspecific and often unrecognized. Beginning 6–10 days after exposure and lasting up to 2 mos, patients may develop general malaise. Other associated physical findings may include hepatosplenomegaly, lymphadenopathy, rash, and edema. The reduviid bug has a predilection for biting on exposed areas during sleep so that the bite occurs in the periorbital or perioral areas and can produce a characteristic swelling of the eyelid and face. Abnormalities in the heart can develop during the acute illness, and abnormalities on electrocardiogram and chest radiography are common although generally do not produce symptomatic disease. After acute infection, most patients enter a prolonged asymptomatic period, known as the *indeterminate phase* and remain in this phase for the rest of their lives. Chagas cardiomyopathy is consistent with a diffuse process. Patients present with chest pain, dizziness, and peripheral edema. Chest x-rays show cardiomegaly in all chambers of the heart. The typical electrocardiographic finding is a right bundle-branch block. Megaviscera syndrome, due to neuronal loss in the gastrointestinal tract, leads to megaesophagus and megacolon. The presenting symptom of megaesophagus is dysphagia, although this occurs late in the disease. The finding on upper gastrointestinal contrast studies is diagnostic. Megacolon is associated

TABLE 61.4

TREATMENT OF TYPHOID FEVER

	Drug	Dose	Duration
Empiric	Ceftriaxone	60 mg/kg/day	7–14
Fully susceptible	Ciprofloxacin or ofloxacin	15 mg/kg/day	5–7 days
	Amoxicillin (second line)	75–100 mg/kg/day	14 days
	Trimethoprim-sulfamethoxazole (second line)	8/40 mg/kg/day	14 days
Multidrug resistant	Ceftriaxone	60 mg/kg/day	10–14 days
	Azithromycin	8–10 mg/kg/day	7 days
	Ciprofloxacin or ofloxacin (nalidixic acid *susceptible* infection)	15 mg/kg/day	5–7 days
	Ciprofloxacin or ofloxacin (nalidixic acid *resistant* infection)	20 mg/kg/day	10–14 days

with constipation and the palpation of a fecaloma on examination. Barium enema can be used to confirm the diagnosis.

Reactivation of *T. cruzi* infection can occur in immunocompromised patients, including those with human immunodeficiency virus (HIV) infection or those receiving immunosuppressive therapy and in children who are infected before 2 years of age. The CNS is the most common site of reactivation. Trypanosome invasion of the brain forms chagoma masses, causing patients to present with headache, fever, cognitive changes, focal neurologic impairment, and seizures. The second most commonly affected site during reactivation is the heart. Cardiac reactivation manifests as acute myocarditis or cardiomyopathy. During the acute phase, parasitemia can be detected in the bloodstream on stained smears or microscopic examination of anticoagulated blood or buffy coat. Organisms may also be visualized in infected organs, including lymph nodes, bone marrow, and pericardial fluid. During the indeterminate, chronic phase, the diagnosis can be made by serology. Polymerase chain reaction (PCR) is very sensitive.

Treatment of Chagas disease is most beneficial during the acute phase of the infection. For those with end-organ damage due to chronic infection, treatment has not been demonstrated to improve outcomes. The two effective treatment regimens are nifurtimox (8–10 mg/kg/day, divided 3 times per day) for 90–120 days or benznidazole (5–10 mg/kg/day in 2 divided doses) for 30–90 days. Patients who weigh <40 kg require higher doses—up to 12 mg/kg/day of nifurtimox and 7.5 mg/kg/day of benznidazole. Common side effects include hypersensitivity, bone marrow suppression, and peripheral neuropathy and may require suspension of treatment with benznidazole. Weight loss, gastrointestinal distress, and psychiatric disturbance may result from treatment with nifurtimox. Availability of these drugs varies by country. Only nifurtimox, produced by Bayer in Germany, is available in the US through the Drug Service of the CDC.

Human African Trypanosomiasis

Trypanosoma brucei is the organism responsible for human African trypanosomiasis (HAT) of which there are two types: West and East African sleeping sickness. The transmission to humans occurs after a bite from the tsetse fly that results in wound contamination by infected saliva. Other mechanisms of disease transmission in both areas include blood transfusions, contaminated needles, or congenital transmission. *Trypanosoma* are parasitic protozoa that are single-celled flagellates transmitted by biting insect vectors.

The presentation of HAT can be divided into an early, or hemolymphatic, stage and a late, or encephalitic, stage. The difference between the two stages is the presence of CNS involvement. Lumbar puncture demonstrates an increased number of monocytes and an elevated protein level. A white blood cell count >5 cells/mcL is considered positive for CNS disease. Occasionally foamy plasma cells, the pathognomonic Mott morula cells, are found in the cerebrospinal fluid (CSF). Brain imaging may show basal ganglia involvement such as seen in Parkinson disease, ventriculomegaly, and asymmetric white-matter abnormalities. Electroencephalography in encephalopathic patients may be abnormal, but findings are not pathognomonic. The differential diagnosis includes malaria, tuberculosis, HIV, leishmaniasis, toxoplasmosis, typhoid, and viral encephalitis. Definitive diagnosis is made by visualizing trypomastigotes in the blood or tissue. Aspiration of enlarged lymph nodes has a high yield. Thick and thin blood smears are prepared with Geimsa stains, similar to malaria smear preparation.

Treatment regimens vary based on the infecting organism and stage of illness. *T. b. gambiense* can usually be distinguished from *T. brucei rhodesiense* based on the patient's travel or exposure history. Any patient with evidence of trypanosomiasis and a CSF WBC count >5 cells/mm^3 is considered to have late disease, regardless of clinical neurologic status. First-line treatment of the hemolymphatic stage is parenteral pentamidine for *T. brucei gambiense* and IV suramin for *T. brucei rhodesiense*. As use of suramin carries a risk of anaphylactic shock, a test dose must be given first. Eflornithine is only useful for late *T. brucei gambiense* disease; however, convulsions may occur and bone marrow toxicity is common. For CNS disease, IV melarsoprol is effective for both varieties of HAT.

Leptospirosis

Leptospirosis is a bacterial disease caused by the spirochete *Leptospira interrogans*. Infections can range from being asymptomatic to causing an influenza-like illness to causing hemorrhage, renal failure, and death. Leptospires are carried by a variety of wild and domestic animals, including rodents, dogs, and livestock. Transmission frequently occurs due to contact with infected water or moist soil. The most common scenario is flooding of urban areas or fields, leading to the spread of infected excreta and exposure of the human population.

Most infections caused by Leptospira result in an asymptomatic or mild infection. The clinical is biphasic consisting of an acute (septicemic) phase that usually lasts 1 week, followed by an immune phase. During the acute phase, the most common symptom is fever, often with chills, and other common symptoms include headache, conjunctival suffusion, myalgia, nausea, and vomiting. Myalgias can be severe. Mild changes in mental status may occur without meningitis. A pretibial papular rash may develop. Jaundice occurs in less than half the identified cases of leptospirosis during the acute phase. The severe icteric form of the disease, Weil disease, may develop as a progression from the initial febrile episode or as a distinct separate phase from the first. It is characterized by jaundice, renal failure, and hemorrhage. Serum bilirubin levels are elevated out of proportion to transaminase levels. Renal failure usually occurs during the second week of the illness. Pulmonary symptoms occur irregularly and may take the form of dyspnea or cough or may be severe with hemorrhage and ARDS. Thrombocytopenia is common but is not usually associated with disseminated intravascular coagulopathy. The most common diagnostic method is serology using the microscopic agglutination test. Diagnosis of leptospirosis can be made through direct visualization of the organism. PCR can detect Leptospira from clinical samples and may be a rapid, reliable strategy where the assay is available.

Antimicrobials with demonstrated in vivo efficacy against leptospirosis are penicillin, doxycycline, ceftriaxone, and cefotaxime. Doxycycline has typically been reserved for mild or moderate disease. However, in areas endemic for both leptospirosis and rickettsiosis, cephalosporin or doxycycline therapy may be preferable to penicillin therapy because of their activity against co-infecting rickettsia. The Jarisch-Herxheimer reaction (release of endotoxin from large-scale death of bacteria that can follow administration of an antimicrobial in certain diseases) can occur with the initiation of β-lactam therapy.

Hantavirus

Human disease begins with inhalation of infected particles that reach the bronchioles or alveoli. Viremia develops with damage to the characteristic endothelial surfaces. Hemorrhagic fever with renal syndrome (HFRS) is characterized by fever, renal failure, and hemorrhage. The disease has been described to have 5 phases: (1) febrile, (2) hypotensive shock and hemorrhage, (3) oliguric, (4) diuretic, and (5) convalescence. The differential diagnosis is broad and depends on the exposure history of the patient. For patients who have traveled to Asia, rickettsial disease, dengue virus, and leptospirosis are possible infectious causes. The mild noninfectious etiologies, including renal disease and renal vein thrombosis,

might not be easy to differentiate from mild common viral illnesses. Severe HFRS may be confused with hemolytic uremic syndrome, but the former lacks a microangiopathic, hemolytic anemia.

The incubation period for hantavirus pulmonary syndrome (HPS) due to the Sin Nombre virus is usually 1–2 weeks but may be much shorter or longer after exposure to infected excreta. HPS consists of 3 phases: a prodromal phase that lasts 3–6 days, a cardiorespiratory phase that lasts 7–10 days, and a convalescent phase. The most consistent laboratory evaluation abnormality is thrombocytopenia. The differential diagnosis includes community-acquired bacterial and viral pneumonias, septic shock with ARDS, initially acute gastroenteritis, leptospirosis, septicemic plague, Colorado tick fever, tularemia, relapsing fever, Rocky Mountain fever ("spotless"), Legionnaire disease, ehrlichiosis, Q fever, coccidioidomycosis, and histoplasmosis. Cardiac shock with high peripheral vascular resistance points toward a viral hemorrhagic fever rather than septic shock. A history of peridomestic and/or recreational contact with rodent-infested structures is present in most cases. The diagnosis of any Hantavirus infection is based on IgM which is almost always present at the time of clinical symptoms, and IgG levels rise early and peak during the first week of illness. Ribavirin is of questionable value in the treatment of HPS but may be of some value in HFRS.

Poliomyelitis

The peak incidence of poliovirus infections occurs in the summer and fall in temperate climates, with infections occurring year-round in tropical climates. Four types of infection with poliovirus occur: inapparent infection, abortive infection, nonparalytic infection, and paralytic poliomyelitis. Risk factors for paralytic disease with poliovirus infection include older age, pregnancy, recent diphtheria/pertussis/tetanus vaccination, physical exercise at the time of infection, trauma at the time of infection, and tonsillectomy. Infection is spread primarily via the fecal-oral route. Nonparalytic cases of poliomyelitis have evidence of CNS injury without paralysis, including meningismus, muscle spasms, and CSF that suggests aseptic meningitis. Paralytic poliomyelitis is life-threatening in the event that respiratory insufficiency develops. Paralytic symptoms may not begin for several days after the prodrome. Signs such as toxicity, irritability, higher fever, anxiousness, and the presence of diminished superficial reflexes may herald the onset of paralysis. Weakness may progress over a period of 3–5 days to flaccid paralysis with loss of deep-tendon reflexes. Patients with paralytic poliomyelitis are classified into 3 clinical groups: (1) those children with pure spinal poliomyelitis without cranial nerve involvement but with muscular weakness and/or paralysis, (2) individuals with pure bulbar poliomyelitis that have weakness or paralysis of cranial nerves IX, X, and/or XII primarily, and (3) Bulbospinal disease which demonstrate a combination of features. The diagnosis of poliomyelitis is confirmed by poliovirus recovery from the stool and/or oropharynx. The differential diagnosis includes Guillain-Barré syndrome, other enterovirus infections, acute disseminating encephalomyelitis, rabies, botulism, West Nile virus, Ebstein-Barr virus, and other causes of aseptic meningitis or encephalitis. The presence of flaccid paralysis and lack of significant sensory changes is helpful in ruling out other diseases.

Treatment of children with paralytic poliomyelitis is primarily supportive with a focus on monitoring and management of associated respiratory failure. In patients with bulbar or bulbospinal poliomyelitis, maintenance of airway patency with suctioning and positioning is of importance to ensure adequate ventilation and prevent aspiration of secretions and pneumonia. Patients with spinal poliomyelitis who have significant weakness or paralysis of the muscles of respiration may require mechanical ventilation. Given the prolonged time to recovery or residual paralysis that occurs in some patients, tracheostomy may be necessary. Analgesia may be necessary in those patients with significant myalgia or headaches. Constipation can also be problematic and require the use of laxatives. Physical and occupational therapists and physiatrists should be involved to assist with proper positioning, splinting, and therapies to facilitate recovery and prevent contractures.

EMERGING INFECTIONS

West Nile Virus

The strongest risk factor for the development of West Nile neuroinvasive disease (WNND) and death is advanced age (age >70 yrs). With the increasing prevalence of the WNV, other modes of viral transmission have been identified, including blood transfusion, breast feeding, organ transplantation, and transplacental infection. WNV is sustained through an enzootic cycle between birds and mosquitoes. Infection to humans occurs when they are bitten by infected mosquitoes. In West Nile fever, an abrupt onset of fever occurs, with symptoms that may include headache, myalgia, nausea, vomiting, abdominal pain, or diarrhea. Additionally, sore throat, cough, and maculopapular rash have been

described. Most cases have resolution of symptoms within 1 week, but milder symptoms of malaise and fatigue may persist for several weeks. In patients with WNND, other causes of aseptic meningitis should be considered, including infections with enterovirus and other viruses in the Flavivirus family. The presentation with acute muscle weakness may suggest a diagnosis of Guillain-Barré syndrome. Other treatable infections, including herpesvirus infection or bacterial meningoencephalitic, should be considered as well. The presence of WNV nucleic acid can be detected using reverse-transcriptase PCR and provides strong evidence of infection.

Avian Influenza

The reservoir for Avian influenza is birds. Influenza A viruses are defined by two major surface glycoproteins: hemagglutinin and neuraminidase (NA). Antigenic drift, changes within the same viral subtype, is responsible for the annual occurrence of influenza epidemic, whereas antigenic shift, with the circulation of a new subtype, has led to pandemics. The presenting signs and symptoms may vary, depending on the specific type of avian influenza viral infection. Gastrointestinal symptoms, including diarrhea (with or without blood), vomiting, and abdominal pain, are common and may precede the respiratory illness, although the degree of gastrointestinal involvement may vary. Almost all patients have signs and symptoms of pneumonia, including dyspnea, increased respiratory rate, and crackles on auscultation. As the disease progresses, patients develop ARDS and multiorgan failure, including cardiac dysfunction. Low WBC count, especially lymphopenia, leukopenia, and thrombocytopenia, is a common laboratory finding.

As the signs and symptoms of avian influenza viral infection are nonspecific, the most important trigger for consideration of the diagnosis is the potential for exposure, including travel to an area where infection is endemic and contact with poultry, ill birds, or other another individual with avian influenza. The WHO tracks cases of human and bird infections and their geographic distribution (http://www.who.int/csr/disease/avian_influenza/en/). Throat swabs have higher yield than nasal swabs. The commonly available kits to identify influenza A may detect the presence of H5/N1 in a minority of cases. The H5N1 viruses are sensitive to the NA inhibitors oseltamivir and zanamivir. The standard dose is given for 5 days: 30 mg twice per day for children ≤15 kg, 45 mg twice a day for those >15–23 kg, 60 mg twice a day for those >23–40 kg, and 75 mg twice a day for those >40 kg. Common adverse effects are nausea and vomiting. Oseltamivir prophylaxis is recommended for 7–10 days after the last exposure in cases of high-to-moderate risk exposures. Oseltamivir is preferred over zanamivir because it is easier to administer. Zanamivir is administered by oral inhalation of a dry powder, making drug delivery difficult in intubated patients and potentially less effective if distributed unevenly in the respiratory system, as can occur in patients with significant lung disease who may not achieve high enough levels in the blood to treat systemic disease. Zanamivir may be preferable for prophylaxis or for less severely ill patients. The appropriate infection control measures (standard, contact, airborne, and eye) should be instituted.

Severe Acute Respiratory Syndrome

At this writing, no cases of severe acute respiratory syndrome (SARS) have been reported to the CDC or the WHO since 2004. The disease appears to be transmitted through droplet or fomite contact of the mucous membranes of the respiratory system. Quarantine measures have been effective, as no instances of transmission have been reported prior to the onset of symptoms. In some outbreaks, some individuals appear to be "super-spreaders," where a few cases result in a disproportionate number of transmissions. The etiology of SARS has now been established to be a novel coronavirus (SARS-CoV).

The disease course in SARS is triphasic: (a) Patients initially present with myalgia, fever, malaise, and chills/rigors after an incubation period of ~4–7 days; (b) development of persistent fever with cough, oxygen desaturation, chest pain, tachypnea, and dyspnea as they develop bronchopneumonia; and (c) progression to ARDS. A key component of treatment is the use of infection control procedures to control spread of disease through droplets, aerosolization, and fomites.

CHAPTER 62 ■ TOXIN-RELATED DISEASES

SUNIT C. SINGHI • M. JAYASHREE • JOHN P. STRAUMANIS • KAREN L. KOTLOFF

The toxin produced at the site of infection and/or colonization spreads systemically and causes typical disease. Important toxin-producing bacteria and the life-threatening systemic diseases caused by them are listed in **Table 62.1**.

TETANUS

Tetanus is a potentially fatal disease characterized by hypertonia, muscle spasms, and autonomic instability caused by action of tetanospasmin (commonly called *tetanus toxin*), a potent neurotoxin elaborated by the organism *Clostridium tetani* (*C. tetani*). Disease is initiated when *C. tetani* spores enter a breach in the skin or mucosa and typically occurs after acute injury to soft tissue, particularly with deep penetrating or puncture wounds or lacerations, in which anaerobic bacterial growth is facilitated. After entering the body, tetanospasmin enters the nervous system at the neuromuscular junction of the lower motor neurons. The incubation period, i.e., the time interval between spore inoculation and symptom onset, may vary from 2 days to months (average 2 weeks). Tetanus

typically evolves as one of four clinical forms: generalized, localized, neonatal, or cephalic.

Generalized Tetanus

The most common form of tetanus is generalized tetanus, which manifests with classic trismus or

TABLE 62.1

COMMON TOXIN-PRODUCING BACTERIA AND THE LIFE-THREATENING SYSTEMIC DISEASES THEY CAUSE

Corynebacterium diphtheria	Diphtheria
Clostridium tetani	Tetanus
Clostridium botulinum	Botulism
Clostridium perfringens	Gas gangrene, food poisoning
Clostridium difficile	Antibiotic-associated colitis
Staphylococcus aureus	Toxic shock syndrome
Streptococcus pyogenes (group A streptococcus)	Toxic shock syndrome

"lockjaw," as tetanus is commonly called, followed by *risus sardonicus* (a facial grimace that results from hypertonia of the orbicularis oris), generalized muscle rigidity, hyperreflexia, dysphagia, opisthotonos, and spasms. The body assumes an opisthotonic position that resembles decorticate posturing (without loss of consciousness) with flexion of the arms and extension of the legs. The muscle spasms are caused by a sudden burst of tonic contraction of muscles and are very painful. Pharyngeal spasms lead to severe dysphagia. If prolonged, spasms may lead to rhabdomyolysis and its complications: laryngeal obstruction, acute respiratory failure, and cardiac arrest. Spasms are more prominent in the first 2 weeks, and their severity may increase during this period. Rigidity may last beyond the occurrence of spasms and autonomic disturbances, which usually occur some days after the spasms and reach a peak during the second week of the disease. Sympathetic overactivity, associated with elevated plasma norepinephrine and epinephrine concentrations, causes fluctuating heart rate, peripheral pallor, labile hypertension, and fever with profound sweating. Parasympathetic involvement may manifest as excessive salivation and increased bronchial secretions as well as bradycardia and sudden cardiac arrest in severe tetanus. Recovery usually begins after 3 weeks and takes ~4 weeks.

Localized Tetanus

Occasionally, muscle rigidity, often in association with muscle weakness, may remain localized at the site of spore inoculation. Symptoms may be mild and self-limited, persistent (partially immune hosts), or progress to generalized tetanus.

Neonatal Tetanus

Neonatal tetanus is a generalized form of tetanus that develops through contamination of the umbilical stump in infants born to inadequately immunized mothers. The contamination may be caused by use of unsterile instruments to cut the cord or by unhygienic cord care practices (e.g., applying soil or cow dung dressing to the stump) that are prevalent in certain populations. The first signs are poor sucking and excessive crying, followed by variable degrees of trismus, risus sardonicus, and repeated generalized muscle spasms. Apnea may result from spasm of respiratory muscles. The baby cannot be nursed and, unless appropriate treatment is available, is at high risk for death. If the baby survives, spasms subside by the late second or early third week, and swallowing returns by the end of 4 weeks.

Cephalic Tetanus

Cephalic tetanus is an uncommon localized form of disease that is often associated with otitis media and head injuries and affects the cranial nerves. Facial paresis is usually present. A coexisting aerobic infection, often caused by *S. aureus* may be present.

Diagnosis and Differential Diagnosis

The diagnosis of tetanus is made on clinical grounds alone. On insertion of a spatula (or tongue blade) that touches the posterior pharyngeal wall, if the patient gags and expels the spatula, the test is negative for tetanus; if the patient bites the spatula because of reflex masseter spasms, the test is positive for tetanus. Trismus caused by peritonsillar and odontogenic abscesses and abdominal rigidity caused by local trauma or peritonitis can be excluded by history and examination. Dystonic reactions to dopamine blockade usually cause torticollis and oculogyric crises. However, spasms are not seen. Benztropine or diphenhydramine can be administered to rule out such a reaction. Meningitis, meningoencephalitis, and tuberculous meningitis, which cause generalized hypertonia, neck rigidity, and tonic seizures, may sometimes mimic tetanus but can be differentiated by the presence of impaired mental status. Hypocalcemic tetany involves limb muscles more than the trunk and is associated with positive Chvostek and Trousseau signs. Poisoning with strychnine, a direct antagonist of glycine receptors, closely resembles generalized tetanus. Trismus is absent and abdominal muscles are less rigid in strychnine poisoning. Stiffman syndrome has an insidious onset; hypertonia involves face and jaw muscles minimally and improves during sleep.

Hypoxemia that leads to respiratory failure is a major cause of death. Patients who are treated in the ICU are particularly prone to respiratory complications related to the use of mechanical ventilation, nosocomial infection, urinary tract infection related to indwelling catheters and wound sepsis, and gastrointestinal hemorrhage. If the serum creatine kinase level is high or myoglobin is detected in the urine, hydration with normal saline and urinary alkalinization with sodium bicarbonate should be considered. A proposed protocol for management of severe grades of tetanus appears in **Table 62.2** and **Table 62.3**. The role of pyridoxine is controversial, and corticosteroids are not advised.

Supportive treatment in a patient with tetanus should include maintenance of airway and ventilation, proper gastrointestinal function, skin integrity, and prevention of complications of respiratory dysfunction, such as atelectasis. Endotracheal intubation

TABLE 62.2

SUGGESTED PROTOCOL FOR TETANUS MANAGEMENT (STEPS IN MANAGEMENT)

A. Stabilization in Emergency Room
1. Assess airway and ventilation, prepare for endotracheal intubation using rapid-sequence intubation technique, if generalized rigidity or spasm.
2. Obtain samples for electrolytes, blood urea, creatinine, creatinine kinase, and urinary myoglobin. If clinically indicated, perform neuroimaging and a lumbar puncture to rule out other diagnosis.
3. Determine and record the portal of entry, incubation period, period of onset, immunization history, and severity grade.
4. Administer diazepam IV, starting with 0.2 mg/kg to control spasms and decrease rigidity. If this compromises the airway or ventilation, intubate using rapid-sequence induction technique.
5. Transfer the patient to a dark isolated room in the ICU.

B. Early management in PICU: First week
1. Administer human tetanus immune globulin (HTIG; 500 units), IM; and tetanus toxoid (0.5 mL) IM, at different sites.
2. Consider intrathecal administration of HTIG (1000 IU).
3. Start crystallin penicillin (100,000 IU/kg/day, q 6 hrs, IV) for 10–14 days or metronidazole (50 mg/kg, IV q 8 hrs) for 7–10 days.
4. Initiate airway management: endotracheal intubation. Perform a tracheostomy if spasms produce any degree of airway compromise or difficulty in managing secretions.
5. Débride the wound under local anesthesia.
6. Establish a nasogastric tube for feeding.
7. Start continuous monitoring of heart rate, blood pressure, and cardiac rhythm.
8. Continue benzodiazepine infusion (in incremental doses as needed) to control spasms and achieve sedation. If adequate control of spasm is not achieved, initiate neuromuscular junction blockade with vecuronium 0.1 mg/kg/hr. Continue benzodiazepine for sedation.
9. Administer magnesium IV to achieve a serum magnesium concentration of 4–8 mEq/L (2–4 mmol/L).

C. Continuing management in PICU: Next 2–3 weeks
1. Control sympathetic hyperactivity with IV propranolol or labetalol. Administer fluids, dopamine, or norepinephrine as and when needed to maintain hemodynamic stability. Avoid diuretics and blood.
2. With sustained bradycardia, atropine is useful; a pacemaker may be needed.
3. Use water or air mattress, if possible, to prevent skin breakdown.
4. Maintain benzodiazepines until neuromuscular junction blockade is no longer necessary. Taper the dose over 14–21 days.
5. Maintain serum magnesium, if used, until spasms are no longer present.

D. Convalescent stage
1. Active physical therapy. Supportive psychotherapy.
2. Administer another dose of the appropriate tetanus toxoid.

should be performed in all patients who have generalized rigidity on arrival, even in absence of frequent spasms, as the disease is likely to progress in severity for 10–14 days after onset. Strict asepsis, meticulous mouth care, chest physiotherapy, and regular endotracheal tube care are essential to prevent atelectasis, lobar collapse, and pneumonia.

Energy demand is high in patients with tetanus because of muscular spasms, excessive sweating, and associated sepsis. Therefore, adequate caloric intake should be ensured as early as possible. Enteral feeding, with head elevated to 30–45 degrees, is preferred. Gastrointestinal hypomotility or paralytic ileus may develop as a result of immobility and treatment with morphine. If patients cannot tolerate enteral feedings, parenteral nutrition becomes necessary. The complications of immobility caused by heavy sedation and paralysis must be minimized. Special water or air mattresses to allow turning the patient with minimal stimulation and to prevent the development of pressure ulcers are preferred. Passive range-of-motion exercises must be instituted early to maintain muscle strength, prevent deformities, and stimulate circulation.

Psychosocial care is important for paralyzed patients. It is essential to keep them comfortable and anticipate their needs. Patients who are anxious or in pain have reflex increases in heart rate and blood pressure. Patients' family members should be allowed to participate in the patients' care.

Prevention

Tetanus is preventable with proper use of tetanus toxoid and human tetanus immunoglobulin (HTIG).

TABLE 62.3

PHARMACOLOGIC TREATMENT OF TETANUS

Drug	Dose	Major side effects	Contraindication	Duration
ANTIBIOTICS				
Penicillin G	100,000–200,000 IU/kg IV in 4 divided doses	Local pain, inflammation at IM injection site, hypersensitivity, may potentiate effects of tetanus toxin due to its GABA agonist effect.	Documented hypersensitivity	7–10 days
Metronidazole	30–40 mg/kg/day IV q 6 hrs; max, 4 g/day	Neurotoxicity in the form of dizziness, vertigo; rarely, convulsions.	Documented hypersensitivity	7–10 days
CONTROL OF SPASMS				
Benzodiazepines				
Diazepam	0.2 mg/kg initial dose through IV infusion, stepped up rapidly in increments until spasms are controlled; usually, 1 mg/kg/hr. Change to enteral route in 4–6 divided doses through nasogastric tube; max. 2 mg/kg/hr	Respiratory depression, hypotension secondary to vasodilation and myocardial depression. Glycols and benzyl alcohol used as preservatives in IV preparation are toxic when very high doses of diazepam are used.	Shock, respiratory depression	Full doses for 2–3 weeks; then, gradually tapered off over 2 weeks
Midazolam	0.1–0.3 mg/kg/hr as IV infusion	Respiratory depression, hypotension	Shock	
Lorazepam	0.15 mg/kg loading dose, followed by 1–2 mcg/kg/min.	Respiratory depression, hypotension, toxic glycols or benzyl alcohol used as preservatives.	Hypotension, shock	
Neuromuscular Blocking Agents				
Pancuronium	Initial dose 0.08–0.1 mg/kg; then as IV infusion 0.1 mg/kg/hr or 0.5–1.7 mcg/kg/min	Tachycardia, hypertension, and increased cardiac output due to intrinsic sympathomimetic activity. Delayed recovery from paralysis and need for prolonged ventilation.	Known hypersensitivity and lack of access to mechanical ventilation	Shortest possible
Vecuronium	Initial dose 0.08–0.1 mg/kg; then as IV infusion 0.1 mg/kg/hr or 0.5–1.7 mcg/kg/min	Minimal cardiovascular side effects. The drug is considered "cardiovascularly clean." Complications related to prolonged use are similar to pancuronium.	Used cautiously in presence of hepatic or renal disease.	Shortest possible

(Continued)

TABLE 62.3

PHARMACOLOGIC TREATMENT OF TETANUS (CONTINUED)

Drug	Dose	Major side effects	Contraindication	Duration
Atracurium	Initial dose 0.5 mg/kg, followed by infusion of 4–12 µg/kg/min	Increases bronchial secretions, itching and wheezing due to histamine release.	Safe in hepatic and renal disease unlike vecuronium and baclofen.	Shortest possible
Intrathecal baclofen	No definite guidelines. Average bolus dose for patients <55 years is 1000 mcg. Infusion through an epidural catheter placed in the L3–L4 space for prolonged therapy.	Drowsiness, sedation coma, respiratory depression, hypersensitivity. Side effects increase with repeated boluses. Reversible on stopping therapy.	Known hypersensitivity. Used with caution in presence of respiratory depression and altered sensorium.	7–14 days
CONTROL OF AUTONOMIC INSTABILITY				
Propranolol	0.5–1 mg/kg/day in 3–4 divided doses. Increased gradually every 3–5 days to 1–5 mg/kg/day, max. 8 mg/kg/day	Bradycardia, hypotension, congestive heart failure, pulmonary edema, hypoglycemia, hyperglycemia, bronchospasm, agranulocytosis.	Known hypersensitivity, asthma/chronic obstructive pulmonary disease, cardiogenic shock, bradycardia, pulmonary edema	6–8 weeks
Labetalol	IV 0.2–0.5 mg/kg/dose, titrated to effect, max 20 mg/dose. Oral 4 mg/kg/day in 2 divided doses, max 20 mg/kg/day	Bradycardia, hypotension, congestive heart failure, bronchospasm, rash, dizziness, reversible myopathy (very rarely)	Known hypersensitivity, asthma, cardiogenic shock, bradycardia, pulmonary edema	6–8weeks
Morphine	0.01–0.1 mcg/kg/min as IV infusion or 0.1 mg/kg IV every 4–6 hrs	Respiratory depression hence caution in patients with respiratory compromise. Bronchoconstriction, vomiting, and hypotension.	Used with caution in advanced liver and renal disease and in known asthmatic.	7–10 days
Magnesium Sulfate	25–50 mg/kg/dose IV as an hourly infusion, max dose ~2 g/dose, repeated every 6 hrs, depending on the clinical response and serum magnesium	Hypocalcemia, weakness, sedation, paralysis, hypotension, and bradyarrhythmias. Serum magnesium levels must be monitored closely, as clinical signs may be missed in a sedated and paralyzed patient.	Compromised renal function	Maintain serum magnesium at ~4–8 mEq/L
Clonidine	Initial 5–10 mcg/kg/min in divided doses every 8–12 hrs. Increase to 5–25 mcg/kg/min every 6 hrs gradually	Hypotension, bradycardia, headache, dizziness, fatigue, respiratory depression, Reynaud phenomenon.		

Active immunization of all survivors of tetanus with tetanus toxoid is imperative to prevent reinfection and further illness. The total amount of toxin produced during disease is inadequate to mount an immune response; therefore, patients with newly diagnosed tetanus must be actively immunized.

Recommendations for primary immunization depend on the age of the patient. A total of 5 doses of combined diphtheria tetanus-pertussis vaccine at ages 2, 4, 6, 15–18 months, and 5 years are recommended during primary childhood immunization. The vaccine may be given simultaneously with hepatitis-B and *Haemophilus influenzae* type b (Hib) vaccines. A booster dose of tetanus toxoid is recommended every 10 years. Postinjury prophylaxis is not required in people who have received a tetanus toxoid booster dose within the previous 5 years. Children who have received partial immunization need only the remaining doses from the schedule, rather than to restart from the first dose. "Tetanus prone" wounds are contaminated with dirt, saliva, feces or are puncture wounds (including unsterile injections, missile injuries, burns, frostbite, avulsions, and crush injuries). If an individual who sustains a tetanus-prone wound has an uncertain history of vaccination or received the last dose of tetanus toxoid 5 years or more before injury, he or she should receive 1 dose of HTIG and 3 doses of tetanus toxoid—2 doses 2 months apart, followed by a third one after 6 months. HTIG should also be given to immunodeficient patients with a tetanus-prone wound. If doubt exists, a wound should be considered to be tetanus-prone. In children, the dose of HTIG should be 500 units to achieve adequate antibody concentration (0.1 IU/mL). Tetanus toxoid and HTIG should be administered at different sites in different syringes to avoid interaction between the two.

DIPHTHERIA

Diphtheria is an acute localized infection of skin or respiratory mucous membranes caused by toxin-producing strains of *Corynebacterium diphtheriae*. It is characterized by a pseudomembrane in the throat and a systemic illness that results from absorption of toxin. Onset of symptoms may be insidious or abrupt after an incubation period of 2–5 days. Both sore throat and fever are almost universal. Cough and stridor may be presenting features in unimmunized children with an acute fulminant course. Pseudomembrane, fever, "bull neck," upper-respiratory tract infection and obstruction are common symptoms. The characteristic thick adherent fibrinous pseudomembrane on the respiratory epithelium looks dull and grayish and bleeds easily on touch. It may be found on the palate, pharynx, tonsils, epiglottis, and larynx or may extend to the tracheobronchial tree. Other forms of diphtheria may be seen less commonly. Cutaneous diphtheria infection typically presents as a chronic nonhealing ulcer with a gray membrane.

Upper airway obstruction is seen in "severe disease" owing to soft tissue edema and necrosis, dislodgement of pharyngeal membrane, and bleeding into the airway. The airway should be secured early, as rapid progression of the membrane may preclude a later opportunity. Myocarditis may be identified by the presence of troponin T. Myocarditis is seen at the end of the second week of illness but may be seen as early as 5 days after the onset of upper respiratory disease in unimmunized patients. Diphtheria toxin has a high affinity for the conduction system of the heart, and prolonged PR interval is frequent. Bradyarrhythmias in the form of bundle-branch blocks progress to complete heart blocks are more common than tachyarrhythmias.

Diphtheritic polyneuropathy usually occurs after a latent period of 3–16 weeks after the onset of acute diphtheria, but this sequence can vary from 4 days to 3–5 weeks. The neuropathy involves the motor cranial nerves (III, IV, VI, VII, IX, and XII) and the peripheral nerves and is predominantly motor in character. In severe cases, respiratory and abdominal muscles may be involved. Weakness usually begins proximally and spreads distally. Typically, palatal paralysis (nasal twang, dysphonia, and regurgitation of fluids) occurs in the second week; ocular palsies (loss of accommodation, squint, and diplopia) in the third week, and generalized motor weakness after 3–6 weeks of illness. Autonomic disturbances, such as tachycardia, hypotension, or hypertension and hyperhidrosis may be seen.

The diagnosis of diphtheria and indication for initiating antitoxin therapy should be based on clinical grounds. The definition recommended by the WHO for a probable clinical case is "an illness characterized by laryngitis or pharyngitis or tonsillitis, *and* an adherent membrane of the tonsils, pharynx and/or nose." Other conditions that can give rise to a membranous tonsillopharyngitis include acute streptococcal pharyngitis, candidiasis, Vincent angina, infectious mononucleosis, and agranulocytosis (mucositis). At the beginning of the illness, diphtheria can look like any type of tonsillitis, with only a small spot of membrane on the tonsil. Pharyngeal co-infection with group A streptococci (GAS) is common in diphtheria. Presumptive rapid diagnosis is usually obtained with methylene blue and Gram stain of pharyngeal smear. *C. diphtheriae* is seen as club-shaped, Gram-positive, pleomorphic bacillus with terminal swellings, arranged in a Chinese letter pattern.

Diphtheroids that are normal commensals in the throat may give rise to a false-positive test. Isolation of *C. diphtheriae* from a clinical specimen or fourfold or greater rise in serum antibody is necessary for confirmation of diagnosis. Successful isolation of *C. diphtheriae* depends on proper collection of swabs and transport to the laboratory. The laboratory must be alerted to the suspicion of diphtheria. Because most microbiology labs in the US lack the expertise and materials to reliably identify diphtheria, US practitioners should contact their local health department or the Centers for Disease Control and Prevention for guidance on correct handling of specimens. Polymerase chain reaction detection of sequences from the toxin A subunit and enzyme immunoassay for toxin have also been developed. A chest x-ray and echocardiography should be obtained to assess the cardiac size and contractility, respectively. Platelet counts are obtained to detect thrombocytopenia, serum electrolytes, and blood urea nitrogen are obtained to assess renal injury.

Principles of Clinical Management

Attention must first be given to the airway, breathing, and circulation (ABCs). Once these are stabilized, antitoxin therapy must be initiated immediately after taking appropriate specimens for culture. Airway problems must be anticipated in children who present with extensive disease and bull-neck. Use of accessory muscles of respiration is an indication for immediate airway management. Airway should be secured early, as rapid progression of membrane may preclude a later opportunity.

Patients with respiratory-tract diphtheria should be placed in strict isolation, which should be maintained until therapy has been completed and 2 cultures obtained at least 24 hrs apart after completion of antibiotic therapy are both negative. In situations in which initial cultures are negative due to prior antibiotic therapy, patients should be isolated until completion of antibiotic therapy.

Diphtheria antitoxin acts by neutralizing the unbound toxin and prevents its binding to the cell membrane surface receptor cells. The dose of the antitoxin varies from 20,000–120,000 units, depending on the site of primary infection, the extent of pseudomembrane, and the delay between onset and seeking of medical advice. The usual recommended dose is 20,000–40,000 units for faucial diphtheria of <48-hr duration, 40,000–80,000 units for faucial diphtheria of >48-hr duration or laryngeal infection, and 60,000–120,000 units for severe toxic state with bull-neck. Therapy is usually given IV over 30–60 mins. Extensive late or complicated disease should always

be treated with doses at the higher end of the range. As antitoxin is a horse serum preparation, it may provoke severe hypersensitivity reactions. A test dose of 50–100 units is recommended 30 mins prior to giving the therapeutic dose. If any untoward reactions are observed, desensitization must be accomplished before the full dose is given.

In tox$^+$ infections, antimicrobial therapy eradicates organism, limits toxin production, and prevents locally invasive disease. However, antibiotics are adjuncts and not a substitute for antitoxin. Although *C. diphtheriae* is susceptible to a variety of antibiotics in vitro, only penicillin and erythromycin are recommended. Acceptable regimens include IV or IM aqueous crystalline penicillin G (100,000–150,000 units/kg/day in 4 divided doses), IM procaine penicillin G (300,000 units for patients who weigh <10 kg and 600,000 for patients who weigh >10 kg every 12 hrs; OR 25,000–50,000 units/kg/day in 2 divided doses), or erythromycin 50 mg/kg/day (maximum, 2 g/day, orally or parenterally) in 4 divided doses. Therapy is given for 10–14 days. Erythromycin is the most effective drug for elimination of the carrier state. Antibiotic treatment usually renders patients noninfectious within 24 hrs. Untreated patients are infectious for 2–3 wks. Of the treatment options available for diphtheritic myocarditis, neither carnitine nor pacing has been conclusively proven to be of any benefit. The incidence of myocarditis and mortality are reduced after DL-carnitine therapy (100 mg/kg/day in 2 divided doses orally for 4 days). The severe systolic dysfunction that accompanies bundle branch blocks and complete heart blocks remains refractory to pharmacologic stimulation and inotropes.

Clinical diphtheria does not confer natural immunity. Patients who recover from diphtheria should begin or complete active immunization with diphtheria toxoid during convalescence. Persons who have had close contact with diphtheria should have cultures obtained from nose, throat, and skin lesions and receive daily checks for development of signs of diphtheria for 7 days. Contacts, regardless of immunization status, and carriers should receive oral erythromycin (40–50 mg/kg/day; maximum, 2 g/day) for 7–10 days or IM benzathine penicillin (one dose of 0.6 mega units for patients <5 years of age and 1.2 mega units for those >5 years). The immunization status of the carriers and contacts should be assessed, and booster doses or primary series should be administered as needed. A total of 5 doses of combined diphtheria-tetanus-pertussis vaccine at ages 2, 4, 6, 15–18 months, and 5 years are recommended during primary immunization. Carriers should be placed in strict isolation (for respiratory tract colonization) or contact isolation (for cutaneous colonization) until at least two cultures taken 24 hrs apart at least

2 weeks after cessation of therapy are negative for *C. diphtheriae*. If cultures remain positive, a course of erythromycin should be repeated.

HUMAN BOTULISM

Human botulism is caused by the neurotoxin produced by *Clostridium botulinum* and, rarely, by *C. baratii* and *C. butyricum*. The organism and its spores are found in all types of soil; in aquatic sediment from streams, lakes, and coastal waters; in the digestive system of fish and mammals; and in the viscera of shellfish and crabs. Purified botulinum toxin type A is commercially available and is used for cosmetic indications, hyperhidrosis, cervical dystonia, and strabismus. Five specific forms of the disease are seen in humans. Inhalation botulism does not occur naturally but could potentially result from a biological warfare application. All of the toxin types block the release of acetylcholine from nerve endings. The toxin does not cross the blood-brain barrier but does affect the neuromuscular junction, parasympathetic nerve endings, autonomic ganglia, and acetylcholine sympathetic nerve endings.

INFANT BOTULISM

Infant botulism is due to ingestion of *C. botulinum* spores. Infant botulism is rarely if ever seen after the age of 1 year. Where the source has been identified, it has typically been isolated in soil, honey, or household dust. Most cases of infant botulism have an insidious onset. The most common symptom is constipation, which may be identified only in hindsight after presentation with more severe symptoms. No evidence of infection, such as fever, leukocytosis, or positive cultures in the absence of a complicating infection, is observed. The classic presentation is that of cranial nerve palsies associated with symmetric descending weakness in the face of a normal sensorium. Fatigue is noted on repetitive muscle contraction and can be elicited by repeated examination of the pupillary light reflex, with slowing of the pupil's constriction over 2–3 mins. Deep tendon reflexes diminish as the paralysis worsens. Autonomic effects are responsible for the constipation and may occasionally cause hypertension. Affected infants have a floppy appearance, poor head control, expressionless faces, and ptosis. A subset of infant botulism cases has a more rapid course of progression that has been implicated as one potential cause of SIDS.

Diagnosis leading to treatment must be made on clinical grounds to avoid delays in potential disease-shortening therapies. Electromyography (EMG) may be helpful in confirming the diagnosis. In most but not all patients, the stool samples will have an assay positive for toxin or a culture positive for *C. botulinum*. With the appearance of lethargy due to hypotonia, sepsis is a common admitting diagnosis. Infectious causes, such as sepsis, pneumonia, meningitis, and encephalitis, can be ruled out quickly due to the lack of fever, leukocytosis, or signs of inflammation. CSF studies will be normal to aid in ruling out meningitis, encephalitis, Guillain-Barré syndrome, and poliomyelitis. The weakness in polio is usually asymmetric, which further differentiates it from infant botulism. Myasthenia gravis should not be considered without a history of maternal disease. Encephalopathy as seen in heavy-metal poisoning or metabolic diseases is not associated with a normal electroencephalogram, as would be expected in botulism. Normal electrolytes, acid-base status, ammonia, and liver transaminases eliminate electrolyte abnormalities, hepatic dysfunction, and metabolic disease from the differential diagnosis. Thyroid function testing will be normal, ruling out hypothyroidism. Spinal muscular atrophy has a very similar presentation but can be differentiated by the EMG findings, the presence of tongue fasciculations and, definitively, by positive genetic testing.

Once the diagnosis of infant botulism is clinically made, specific therapy should be given as soon as possible, without delaying for confirmatory testing. Human botulism immune globulin as a single dose of 50 mg/mL is reserved for the treatment of infant botulism. Equine botulinum toxin used in adult forms of botulism should not be given to infants, as it is ineffective and confers a sensitization and anaphylaxis risk. In the US, information on how to obtain botulism immune globulin can be obtained from the California Department of Health Services' Infant Botulism Treatment and Prevention Program at www.infantbotulism.org or by calling 510-231-7600. The overall goal of supportive treatment is to prevent nosocomial infections, skin breakdown, malnutrition, and airway complications until recovery of the neuromuscular junction is complete. Antibiotics are not indicated unless a complicating infection is involved. If antibiotics are used, aminoglycosides in particular should be avoided due to the risk of worsening the degree of weakness by effects on the neuromuscular junction. Monitoring of vital capacity, negative inspiratory force, the child's ability to adequately protect the airway, and arterial blood gases will help to determine the need for mechanical ventilation. Once intubation is required, the risks and benefits of tracheotomy must be carefully weighed. Most children can be managed without tracheotomy. Nutrition should be given enterally via nasojejunal or nasogastric feeding tubes, as indicated.

Food-Borne Botulism

Unlike infant botulism, food-borne botulism is caused by the ingestion of food contaminated with preformed botulinum toxin. The conditions for germination and growth of *C. botulinum* in food are fairly strict. Large outbreaks are usually associated with restaurants whereas small outbreaks or single cases are usually related to home-prepared foods, such as home-canned vegetables, fruits, and fish products.

The initial symptoms of food-borne botulism are abdominal pain, nausea, vomiting, and diarrhea. Constipation is not seen until after the onset of neurologic symptoms, which occur 1–5 days after consumption of the toxin but usually within 18–36 hrs. The first symptoms to occur are dry mouth due to autonomic nervous system involvement, diplopia from cranial nerve paralysis, and dilated pupils. These bulbar palsies progress to involve the facial muscles and then the muscles of the oropharynx, with symptoms of ptosis, facial droop, depressed gag reflex, dysphagia, dysarthria, and dysphonia. Cranial nerve involvement is complete once the neck muscles become involved. The paralysis continues to descend in a proximal-to-distal pattern, with diaphragmatic involvement typically prior to that of the lower extremities.

The diagnosis of botulism is based on the recognition of the clinical syndrome. An isolated case, as would be seen with the index case or if affected individuals presented to different hospitals, has a limited differential diagnosis. Common diagnoses entertained in botulism cases are Guillain-Barré syndrome, cerebrovascular accident, myasthenia gravis, tick paralysis, and other intoxications, such as carbon monoxide, organophosphates, and mushrooms. The evaluation of these illnesses with CSF studies, cranial imaging, and Tensilon test will be negative in cases of botulism. An EMG may be helpful in making the diagnosis of botulism. Confirmatory testing is warranted but should not delay treatment with antitoxin.

Antitoxin is the most important treatment modality. As the binding of the toxin at the neuromuscular junction is irreversible, the goal is to treat the patient with the equine-derived antitoxin before respiratory symptoms become severe enough to require prolonged ventilation. The dose of the trivalent antitoxin for both adults and children is one vial diluted 1:10 in normal saline and given IV over 30–60 mins. Prior to administration, skin testing with horse serum is recommended. If skin testing is not performed, pretreatment with antihistamines and steroids is recommended. The respiratory status should be closely monitored for deterioration, even after administration of the antitoxin. Vital capacity must be monitored and mechanical ventilation may be necessary. The paralysis associated with botulism can be lengthy; therefore, tracheotomy may be considered for severely affected individuals. Regardless, careful attention must be paid to preventing complications, such as nosocomial infections, skin breakdown, and neuromuscular injury from disuse, which are associated with prolong intensive care admissions.

Wound Botulism

Wound botulism is an extremely rare disease, but it has been reported in children. The classic at-risk wound is a crush injury, puncture wound, or gross trauma to an extremity. Toxin is released from bacteria in the wound into the bloodstream, producing neurologic symptoms as described for food-borne botulism. Inflammation, fever, and leukocytosis are often absent in wound botulism, making the diagnosis potentially more difficult. The diagnosis should be considered in a patient who presents with classic symptoms and an at-risk wound. Even wounds that do not appear to be infected should be explored with swabs, and wound exudates and tissue samples should be sent for anaerobic cultures and serum toxin levels. Prompt treatment with antitoxin as described for food-borne botulism is indicated, even before laboratory results are available.

Adult (Intestinal) Botulism

Intestinal botulism has a pathophysiology similar to infant botulism and a similar presentation. It is very rare and only occurs in patients with severe alteration of their intestinal bacterial flora, which favors the germination and growth of ingested spores. As a result, the onset of symptoms is more insidious than that seen in infant botulism. The diagnosis should be considered in immunosuppressed patients with the classic neuromuscular findings. Treatment is with botulinum antitoxin, as described in the food-borne botulism section. Confirmatory testing should include stool and serum for toxin, obtained prior to antitoxin administration, as well as stool cultures.

Toxic Shock Syndrome

Staphylococcal Toxic Shock Syndrome

Staphylococcal toxic shock syndrome (TSS) has two forms: menstrual and nonmenstrual. More than 99% of menstrual TSS cases are associated with tampon use. Nonmenstrual TSS has been described in nonmenstruating women, in children, and in men and is associated with *S. aureus* colonization of nasal packing or focal infection, such as wound infection, soft tissue infections, lymphadenitis, sinusitis, tracheitis, empyema, abscesses, infection after burn, abortion,

TABLE 62.4

CENTERS FOR DISEASE CONTROL AND PREVENTION CLINICAL CASE DEFINITION OF STAPHYLOCOCCAL TOXIC SHOCK SYNDROME

An illness with the following clinical manifestations:
- Fever: temperature $\geq$38.9°C (102°F)
- Rash: diffuse macular erythroderma
- Desquamation: 1–2 weeks after onset of illness, particularly palms and soles
- Hypotension: systolic blood pressure $\leq$90 mm Hg for adults or less than fifth percentile by age for children <16 years of age; orthostatic drop in diastolic blood pressure $\geq$15 mm Hg from lying to sitting, orthostatic syncope, or orthostatic dizziness
- Multisystem involvement: 3 or more of the following:
    Gastrointestinal: vomiting or diarrhea at onset of illness
    Muscular: severe myalgia or creatine phosphokinase level at least twice the upper limit of normal for laboratory
    Mucous membrane: vaginal, oropharyngeal, or conjunctival hyperemia
    Renal: blood urea nitrogen or creatinine at least twice the upper limit of normal for laboratory or urinary sediment with pyuria ($\geq$5 leukocytes per high-power field) in the absence of urinary tract infection
    Hepatic: total bilirubin, serum glutamic-oxaloacetic transaminase (SGOT), or serum glutamic-pyruvic transaminase (SGPT) at least twice the upper limit of normal for laboratory
    Hematologic: platelets <100,000/mm^3
    Central nervous system: disorientation or alterations in consciousness without focal neurologic signs when fever and hypotension are absent
- Negative results on the following tests, if obtained:
    1. Blood, throat, or cerebrospinal fluid cultures (blood culture may be positive for *S. aureus*)
    2. Rise in titer to Rocky Mountain spotted fever, leptospirosis, or measles

Case classification
Probable: A case with five of the six clinical findings described above
Confirmed: A case with all six of the clinical findings described above, including desquamation, unless the patient dies before desquamation occurs

Adapted from Centers for Disease Control and Prevention. Case definition for public health surveillance *MMWR* 1990;39:38–9.

---

animal and insect bites, osteomyelitis, etc. Menstrual TSS occurs during or within 2 days of onset or termination of menses. Nonmenstrual TSS is encountered in association with focal staphylococcal infections. The onset is abrupt. The Centers for Disease Control and Prevention has established a set of diagnostic criteria based on clinical and laboratory findings (**Table 62.4**). The differential diagnosis of TSS is broad (**Table 62.5**).

To ensure adequate perfusion of vital organs, volume replacement with appropriate crystalloids and colloids is a must. Vasoactive therapy may be required to normalize blood pressure and to improve perfusion once volume repletion is accomplished. Hypoproteinemia may worsen peripheral edema, but colloids should be used with extreme caution in a setting of leaky capillaries. Children are more likely to require respiratory support. Infected wounds and necrotizing skin lesions should be débrided immediately. All packings and foreign objects, including retained tampons, should be removed. Abscesses should be drained and irrigated.

Parenteral administration of a β-lactamase-resistant, antistaphylococcal antibiotic is recommended after appropriate cultures have been taken. Cloxacillin, oxacillin, or nafcillin in combination

TABLE 62.5

DIFFERENTIAL DIAGNOSIS IN TOXIC SHOCK SYNDROME

Infectious	Noninfectious
Acute viral syndrome	Kawasaki disease
Acute gastroenteritis	Acute rheumatic fever
Acute pyelonephritis	Systemic lupus
Legionnaire disease	erythematosus
Leptospirosis	Thrombophlebitis
Lyme disease	Tumor
Meningococcemia/	Hematoma
meningococcal meningitis	Hemolytic uremic
Typhus	syndrome
Streptococcal scarlet fever	
Rocky Mountain spotted fever	
Septic shock	

Adapted from Herzer CM. Toxic shock syndrome: Broadening the differential diagnosis. *J Am Board Fam Pract* 2001; 14:131–6.

with aminoglycosides are the first-line agents. Clindamycin or vancomycin can be used in patients who are allergic to penicillin. Addition of clindamycin in severe cases will halt toxin production. Antibiotics do not shorten the duration of acute illness. Eradication of toxigenic strains of *S. aureus* may require prolonged antibiotics. IV immunoglobulin (IVIG), 1 g/kg for 2 days, is suggested for severe cases. Corticosteroids are not effective. Several reports of recurrent menstrual and nonmenstrual TSS can be found in the literature. Failure to eradicate colonization with *S. aureus* predisposes the patient to recurrent nonmenstrual TSS.

Streptococcal TSS

Streptococcal TSS (STSS) is a severe, potentially fatal form of infection caused by invasive GAS. It is characterized by early shock and multiorgan failure. Whereas staphylococcal TSS is often associated with colonization, GAS TSS most often accompanies invasive GAS infection. In children, STSS commonly occurs after varicella or during the use of nonsteroidal anti-inflammatories; in others, the focus could be pharyngitis. Onset is abrupt with fever, vomiting, diarrhea, and early shock, just as with staphylococcal TSS. In STSS associated with necrotizing fasciitis, pain is the most common initial symptom; it is severe and out of proportion to physical findings and usually involves an extremity or the abdomen. Influenza-like syndrome, consisting of fever, nausea, vomiting, and diarrhea, may occur. Hypotension may be a presenting sign or develop shortly after presentation. Hypothermia may occur in patients with shock. Confusion is present in >50% of the patients. Erythematous rash as seen in staphylococcal TSS is seen in only 10% cases of STSS. Soft-tissue infection, such as localized swelling and erythema, which often progress to necrotizing fascitis and myosi-tis, require surgical débridement, fasciotomy, or amputation.

Renal involvement is indicated by the presence of hemoglobinuria and by serum creatinine values that are usually >2.5 times normal; creatine kinase level is useful in detecting deeper soft-tissue infections. Mild leukocytosis may be seen as in any other infection, but more striking is the left shift. Hypocalcaemia, hypoalbuminemia, and elevated liver transaminases are commonly found at the time of admission. Bacteremia is common in STSS.

The goals of management are removal of the source of toxin (appropriate antibiotic therapy and surgical debridement of necrotic tissues), neutralization of toxin (IVIG therapy), and aggressive supportive therapy for shock (fluids and vasopressors) and multiorgan failure. GAS remains sensitive to penicillin. It has been suggested that failure of penicillin is because of the Eagle effect. Penicillin and other β-lactams are more efficacious against rapidly growing bacteria. An antibiotic combination of high-dose penicillin and clindamycin should be given when concomitant invasive GAS infection is suspected. Depending on the clinical presentation, particularly if it includes necrotizing fasciitis, empirical simultaneous coverage for Gram negatives, anaerobes, and possibly *S. aureus* might be considered until a specific organism is identified. IVIG is usually given in a dose of 1 g/kg for 2 days at the slightest suspicion of STSS. Volume deficits are massive due to external and interstitial loss, combined with peripheral vasodilatation and peripheral pooling. Vasopressors are required after adequate volume replenishment as in any septic shock. Most patients with STSS require tracheal intubation and mechanical ventilation for septic shock and for complicating acute respiratory distress syndrome. The role of hyperbaric oxygen in STSS remains uncertain.

CHAPTER 63 ■ OPPORTUNISTIC INFECTIONS

SUSHIL K. KABRA • MATTHEW B. LAURENS

Opportunistic infections are infections that usually do not cause disease in a person with a healthy immune system but can affect people with a poorly functioning or suppressed immune system because of immunodeficiency or immunosuppression (**Table 63.1**).

CYTOMEGALOVIRUS INFECTION

Cytomegalovirus (CMV) is in the herpes virus group and may be a co-pathogen with other opportunistic organisms, including *Pneumocystis jiroveci* (*P. jiroveci*) and *Aspergillus* (*A.*) species, especially in AIDS

TABLE 63.1

CONDITIONS PREDISPOSING AN INDIVIDUAL TO OPPORTUNISTIC INFECTIONS

Major defects in immune system	Clinical conditions	Infections/clinical manifestations
B-cell defects (humoral deficiencies)	Agammaglobulinemia, hypogammaglobulinemia, selective IgA deficiency, IgG subclass deficiencies, common variable immune deficiency, hyper-IgM syndrome	Infections with *Staphlococcus aureus*; encapsulated organisms, such as *Streptococcus pneumoniae*, *Haemophilus influenzae*; and Gram-negative organisms, such as pseudomonas species Arthritis due to echoviruses, coxsackieviruses, adenoviruses, and *Ureaplasma urealyticum* Infections due to *Pneumocystis carinii* pneumonitis, and *Cryptosporidium*
T-cell defects (cell-mediated immunity)	Thymic dysplasia (DiGeorge syndrome), defective T-cell receptor, defective cytokine production, T-cell activation defects, CD8 lymphocytopenia	Disseminated viral infections due to herpes simplex, varicella-zoster, and CMV Progressive pneumonia caused by parainfluenza, respiratory syncytial virus, cytomegalovirus, varicella, and *Pneumocystis carinii* Superficial and systemic fungal infections; and parasitic infections. Severe mucocutaneous candidiasis; Disseminated BCG disease after BCG vaccination
Combined B-cell and T-cell defects	Severe combined immunodeficiency, Omenn syndrome, Wiskott-Aldrich syndrome, ataxia telangiectasia, hyper-IgE syndrome	Infections caused by bacteria, fungi, or viruses Chronic diarrhea, mucocutaneous or systemic candidiasis, *P. carinii* pneumonitis, and CMV early in life Infections with *S. pneumoniae* or *H. influenzae* type b, *P. carinii* Late onset recurrent sinopulmonary infections from bacteria and respiratory viruses Recurrent episodes of *S. aureus* abscesses of the skin, lungs, and musculoskeletal system
Abnormalities in phagocytic system	Inadequate numbers (congenital or acquired), chronic granulomatous disease, leukocyte adhesion deficiency, Chédiak–Higashi syndrome	Recurrent pyogenic and fungal infections due to *Pseudomonas*, *Serratia marcescens*, and *S. aureus*, and fungi such as *Aspergillus* and *Candida present as* cellulitis, perirectal abscesses, or stomatitis Pulmonary infection, suppurative adenitis, subcutaneous abscess liver abscess, osteomyelitis and sepsis due to fungi or bacteria (*Staphylococcus*) Gastric outlet obstruction, urinary tract obstruction, and enteritis or colitis History of delayed cord separation and recurrent infections of the skin, oral mucosa, and genital tract, predisposed to development of ecthyma gangrenosum and pyoderma gangrenosum
Disorders of the complement system	Disorders involving any one of the complement components, asplenia, splenic dysfunction due to hemoglobinopathies, splenectomy	Infections due to *Salmonella* spp and encapsulated bacteria including *Streptococcus pneumoniae* and *Haemophilus influenzae*. These agents can cause sepsis, pneumonia, meningitis, and osteomyelitis
Infections that occur with acquired immunodeficiencies	HIV and other virus infections, cancer chemotherapy, immunosupressive therapy after organ transplant, diabetes mellitus, sickle cell disease, severe malnutrition	Similar to cell-mediated immune deficiency Neutropenic patients: infections due to Gram-positive cocci and Gram-negative organisms, such as *P. aeruginosa*, *E. coli*, and *Klebsiella* Fungal infections due to *Candida* and *Aspergillus* in prolonged neutropenia

CMV, cytomegalovirus; BCG, Bacille Calmette-Guérin

TABLE 63.2

CLINICAL MANIFESTATIONS OF CYTOMEGALOVIRUS INFECTION

Organ involved	Susceptible hosts	Clinical features
Mononucleosis syndrome	Immunocompetent and Immunosuppressed persons	Fever, severe malaise, headache, myalgia, abdominal pain with diarrhea
	Reactivation infection in Immunosuppressed	Less common features: interstitial pneumonitis, myocarditis and pericarditis, arthralgias and arthritis, maculopapular rashes, adrenal insufficiency, splenic infarction, ulcerative colitis and proctitis, Guillain-Barré syndrome, and meningoencephalitis
Respiratory system	Congenital immunodeficiency, AIDS, organ or marrow transplantation, or malignancy.	Fever, dry; nonproductive cough, dyspnea, retractions, wheezing, and hypoxia, which require ventilatory support
		Co-infection with other pathogens, especially Gram-negative enteric bacteria and fungal pathogens in transplant recipients and *Pneumocystis carinii* in patients with AIDS
Eyes	Severe immunosuppression, especially in BMT recipients and patients with AIDS	Rapidly progressive retinitis with white perivascular infiltrates, hemorrhage, with a necrosis.
		Peripheral retinitis
		Conjunctivitis, corneal epithelial keratitis and disk neovascularization.
Liver and hepatobiliary system	Recipients of bone marrow, liver, heart, and lung transplant and patients with cancer or AIDS	Fever, thrombocytopenia, and lymphopenia or lymphocytosis with mild hepatomegaly.
		Occasionally granulomatous hepatitis
		Jaundice and hyperbilirubinemia usually do not occur
Gastrointestinal system	Patients with AIDS and those with organ transplant	Esophagitis, gastritis, gastroenteritis, pyloric and small bowel obstruction, duodenitis, colitis, proctitis, pancreatitis, hemorrhage, and acalculous cholecystitis
Central nervous system syndrome	Patients with AIDS and those with organ transplant	Meningoencephalitis headache, photophobia, nuchal rigidity memory deficits, and inability to concentrate
		Ascending paralysis caused by myelitis, with or without vasculitis or necrosis
		Polyradiculopathy in patients with AIDS
Other organs systems	Renal and heart transplant patients AIDS patients	Myocarditis: heart failure, cardiomegaly, electrocardiographic abnormalities, and poor left ventricular function on echocardiography
		Endocrinopathy: Addison's disease

patients and patients after bone marrow transplant (BMT). CMV as an opportunistic infection is recognized more commonly and has varying clinical manifestations (**Table 63.2**). CMV is diagnosed by serology, polymerase chain reaction (PCR), antigenemia, and viral culture. Documentation of primary infection (that usually causes disease) by seroconversion or viremia in a previously seronegative patient is important. Either quantitative serologic PCR for CMV

or CMV pp65 antigenemia may be used to monitor viral loads during antiviral therapy. Among recipients of solid organ transplant, 2000–5000 genome copies/mL of plasma is identified as a useful cutoff value to determine significant risk of CMV disease.

In the immunocompetent host, no treatment is indicated. It is suggested only in severe or life-threatening disease. For immunocompromised hosts, IV antiviral ganciclovir (5–7.5 mg/kg/day) is given for

2–3 weeks, followed by maintenance treatment 3–5 times a week by IV or oral route (5 mg/kg/day). For transplant recipients, different regimens of antiviral agents, immunoglobulins, and combinations are used at different centers for treatment of CMV. Preemptive therapy is an alternative in allogeneic BMT recipients, for whom regular lab screening with antigenemia or PCR determines the need for initiation of antiviral therapy. In recipients of renal transplant, prophylactic antiviral therapy is recommended (a) when the donor or recipient is seropositive and antilymphocyte treatment is part of the immunosuppressive regimen and (b) for seronegative recipients of grafts from seropositive donors.

Varicella-Zoster Virus Infection

Varicella-zoster virus (VZV) is a DNA virus that typically causes benign infections of the skin and mucous membranes. It may cause both varicella and zoster in the normal host. However, in certain groups, including neonates, cancer and BMT patients, patients with AIDS and congenital defects of cell-mediated immunity, and organ transplant patients, VZV can lead to visceral dissemination and pneumonia. Varicella pneumonia may be complicated by acute respiratory distress syndrome, rhabdomyolysis, acute hepatitis, and disseminated intravascular coagulation. CNS complications of VZV include cerebellar ataxia, encephalitis, ischemic strokes and CNS vasculitis. Ocular manifestations include: conjunctivitis, keratitis, iridocyclitis, panuveitis, and acute retinal necrosis. Varicella infection in immunocompromised hosts may cause fulminant hepatic failure, myocarditis, arrhythmias, and progression to dilated cardiomyopathy and endocarditis.

Herpes zoster can be diagnosed based on physical findings, vesicle scrapings, serology, or PCR. Scraping of vesicles in the first few days after their appearance is likely to yield identification of the virus. After a vesicle is unroofed, the fluid can be sent for viral culture as well as direct fluorescent antibody. The Tzanck smear of vesicle scrapings will show multinucleated giant cells but is not specific for VZV.

Susceptible persons exposed to varicella should be given immune globulin (either varicella zoster immune globulin or IVIG up to 92 hrs after exposure). The VZIG dose is 1.25 mL (125 IU) for every 10 kg of body weight, with a maximum dose of 6 mL (625 IU) (up to 72 hrs after exposure). Those who are susceptible include:

- Immunocompromised children without history of varicella or varicella immunization
- Susceptible pregnant women

- Newborn infants whose mothers had onset of chickenpox within 5 days before delivery or within 48 hrs after delivery
- Hospitalized premature infants ≥28 weeks gestation whose mothers lack a history of chickenpox or serologic evidence of protection
- Hospitalized premature infants <28 weeks gestation or ≥1000 g birth weight, regardless of maternal history or serologic status

Significant exposures include:

- Residents of the same household
- Face-to-face indoor playmates
- For varicella, hospital exposure in the same multi-bed room or adjacent beds in a large ward, face-to-face contact with an infectious staff member or patient, or visit by a person deemed contagious
- For zoster, intimate contact (touching or hugging) with a contagious person
- For newborns, onset of maternal chickenpox ≤5 days before delivery or within 48 hrs after delivery; immune globulin is not indicated if the mother has zoster

Exposure to varicella merits airborne and contact precautions from 8 until 21 days after the onset of rash in the index case and for 28 days after exposure to the index case in those treated with VZIG or IVIG. For those who have received high-dose immune globulin (400 mg/kg or greater) within 3 weeks prior to exposure, a second dose is not indicated.

Treatment of varicella in immunocompetent children with increased risk for moderate-to-severe varicella should be considered candidates for oral therapy with acyclovir. Famciclovir and valacyclovir are licensed (in the United States) for treatment of varicella in adults but not in pediatric patients. Immunocompromised patients should receive IV acyclovir (1500 mg/m^2/day in 3 divided doses for children and 30 mg/kg/day for adolescents). Oral, high-dose acyclovir (80 mg/kg/day in 4 divided doses) can be considered in patients who are mildly immunosuppressed and at lower risk for developing severe varicella. The use of VZIG or IVIG is indicated for immunocompromised persons who are exposed and have not shown benefit in those who have established disease. Varicella vaccine is a live-attenuated preparation of the varicella virus.

Herpes Virus Type 6

Human herpes virus 6 (HHV-6) is a DNA virus that is the etiologic agent for roseola and is among the most widespread of the human herpesviruses. In immunocompetent children, HHV-6 causes exanthem subitum, febrile episodes without skin rash, and non–Epstein-Barr and non-CMV infectious mononucleosis. HHV-6 infection occurs in recipients of BMT and solid-organ transplants. HHV-6–associated pneumonia involves immunocompromised patients, especially those who have received a BMT or who have been infected by HIV. Testing for HHV-6 includes serology, culture, immunohistochemistry, and nucleic acid assays.

While treatment is not indicated in healthy children, those who are immunocompromised may experience severe disease. Drugs commonly used when indicated are ganciclovir, valganciclovir, acyclovir, valacyclovir, cidofovir, and foscarnet.

Candidiasis

Acute disseminated candidiasis occurs in immunocompromised hosts. Frequent sites of infection in patients with disseminated candidiasis include lungs, kidneys, liver, spleen, and brain. Organisms may disseminate via the hematogenous route to the tissues of one or more organs. The clinical features are nonspecific in infants and children and are similar to those with sepsis caused by other organisms. Presence of ocular lesions of endophthalmitis and maculopapular rash in an immunocompromised state suggest a possibility of candidal sepsis. The skin lesions consist of generalized rashes or discrete, firm, erythematous papules that measure 0.5–1 cm in diameter. A nodular center is often surrounded by an erythematous halo. Candidiasis may involve bones, joints, heart, and CNS. Osteomyelitis of bones may develop in young infants and children. Cardiac involvement may be in the form of endocarditis, myocarditis, or arrhythmia. CNS involvement may occur in disseminated candidiasis and is more common in preterm infants and young children.

Oral candidiasis can be an early sign of illness or disease progression in HIV/AIDS. The sites commonly involved are buccal mucosa and dorsal and lateral surfaces of tongue. Submucosal edema and bleeding occur while plaques are removed. Esophageal candidiasis is one of the important clinical manifestations of candidal infection in immunocompromised hosts. Gastrointestinal candidiasis may occur in children with immunodeficiency disorders and cancer and after surgery. The airway from pharynx to bronchi may be involved. Renal involvement in children causes microabscesses, papillary necrosis, calyceal distortion, and obstruction due to fungal ball or perinephric abscesses.

Diagnosis of *Candida* infections is based on clinical findings and tissue and body fluid culture. Mucocutaneous candidiasis is diagnosed clinically and can be confirmed with Gram stain and culture. Endoscopy is useful for diagnosis of esophageal candidiasis. Tissue samples can be stained and cultured, and the addition of potassium hydroxide to specimens may help to identify yeast and pseudohyphae. For retinal candidal infections, ophthalmologic examination identifies characteristic findings. Candidal infections in solid organs may be seen on CT or ultrasound studies. In contrast-enhanced CT, fungal microabscesses usually appear as multiple round, discrete areas of low attenuation, generally ranging from 2 to 20 mm.

The treatment of candidiasis, published by the Infectious Disease Society of America, includes first-line therapy of amphotericin B and fluconazole, which are approved for use in pediatrics. Caspofungin is indicated for first-line treatment in adults. Other therapies that have been developed for use in candidiasis include micafungin, anidulafungin, posaconazole, and voriconazole. Fluconazole therapy should also be used in clinically stable patients in ICUs where the predominant candidal pathogen is *C. albicans*. For other species of *Candida*, empiric therapy with amphotericin B can be initiated while awaiting culture results. For severe disease, including meningitis, osteomyelitis, and endocarditis, a combination of amphotericin B and flucytosine is an option. The length of antifungal therapy for candidemia is 14 days, starting from the first negative blood culture. Another mainstay in the treatment of invasive candidiasis is the removal of infected vascular lines and hardware. All candidemic patients should have a dilated eye examination by an ophthalmologist to look for signs of invasive ocular disease, as this would require prolonged antifungal therapy. In the adult ICU setting, invasive candidiasis can be prevented by fluconazole prophylaxis.

Pneumocystis Jiroveci

P. jiroveci, earlier known as *Pneumocystis carinii*, is a eukaryotic microorganism. Patients at higher risk for *P. jiroveci* pneumonia include infants with severe malnutrition; children with primary immunodeficiencies, hematologic malignancies, or HIV infection; recipients of solid organ or BMTs; patients who receive high-dose corticosteroids; and patients with inflammatory or collagen-vascular disorders who receive immunosuppressive therapy. Organisms appear to be abundant in AIDS patients and can usually be identified in sputum, bronchoalveolar lavage (BAL) fluid, or even gastric lavage samples. Despite rapid (80–100/mins), shallow respirations, auscultation of the chest frequently shows absence of adventitious sounds. Pneumocystic pneumonia (PCP) is diagnosed through direct identification of organisms from lung tissue or induced sputum specimens.

While identification of organisms from lung biopsy specimens is the gold standard for diagnosis, other methods of identification may be adequate.

The first-line treatment of PCP is with trimethoprim-sulfamethoxazole (TMP-SMZ) given either intravenously or orally, regardless of previous prophylactic regimen. The initial dosage is 15–20 mg/kg/day of the trimethoprim component, divided every 6–8 hrs. With good clinical response, the dosage can be decreased to 10–15 mg/kg/day, divided every 6–8 hrs. Second-line treatments include oral dapsone with oral or IV TMP-SMZ, oral atovaquone, or IV pentamidine isethionate. Treatment duration is 21 days. For extrapulmonary pneumocystosis, IV therapy is preferred for initial treatment. For patients who present with moderate-to-severe disease (PaO$_2$ <70 mm Hg or A-a O$_2$ gradient >35 mm Hg), early corticosteroid administration is also indicated and should be started within the first 72 hrs of therapy. The recommended regimen is oral prednisone, 40 mg twice daily for days 1–5, then 40 mg daily for days 6–10, and 20 mg daily for days 11–20. Treatment failure occurs if no clinical improvement is seen despite 4–8 days of appropriate therapy. It is anticipated that patients will have deterioration after the first 3–5 days of treatment due to the inflammatory response generated. Patients who do not tolerate TMP-SMZ may be treated with pentamidine, 4 mg/kg/day by IV route once daily. Other drugs include trimethoprim/dapsone combination, pyrimethamine/sulfadoxine combination, clindamycin, primaquine, and atovaquone. Prevention of PCP includes appropriate prophylaxis. For HIV-positive patients with CD4 counts of <200/mm^3, daily prophylaxis with TMP-SMZ is indicated. If this therapy cannot be tolerated, second-line therapies should be used, including dapsone, dapsone and pyrimethamine, atovaquone, or aerosolized pentamidine. Prophylaxis should continue until the CD4 count is >200/mm^3 for 3 months.

Invasive Aspergillosis

Aspergillus is a group of ubiquitous fungal organisms found in soil and other settings, including the hospital environment. Susceptible hosts include recipients of lung, bone marrow, and liver transplants; those who have received treatment for malignancy, chronic granulomatous disease, or HIV infection; and those on immunosuppressive chemotherapy. Disseminated aspergillosis, defined as infection of 2 or more noncontiguous organs, is the most severe form of clinical aspergillosis. Invasive pulmonary aspergillosis is manifested most commonly as necrotizing bronchopneumonia or hemorrhagic infarction, although single or multiple abscesses, granulomata, or lobar infiltrates are occasionally present. Cutaneous aspergillosis is a common manifestation of invasive disease in immunocompromised children secondary to hematogenous dissemination or local spread. In disseminated *Aspergillus* infection, fungal endophthalmitis may be an important finding. Patients may have pain, photophobia, and diminished visual acuity. Examination of the retina shows retinal hemorrhage, focal retinitis, and vitreitis. Orbital cellulitis may occur even in immunocompetent patients secondary to invasive sinusitis. Infection spreads locally through destroyed orbital walls and may involve the retro-orbital space. Aspergillosis of the CNS may result from direct spread from the paranasal sinuses or, more commonly, from widespread dissemination in immunosuppressed patients. *Aspergillus* endocarditis may occur during open heart surgery or as part of disseminated disease.

The mainstay for diagnosis of invasive aspergillosis is chest x-ray. Older children and adults are more likely to show the classic cavitation and air crescent formation than young children. Identification from tissue culture renders a definitive diagnosis and is isolated readily from lung, sinus, and skin biopsy specimens. If allergic aspergillosis is suspected clinically, results of *Aspergillus*-specific IgE serology, eosinophilia, and a positive skin test can provide evidence for the diagnosis.

High-dose amphotericin B (1–1.5 mg/kg/day) is the treatment of choice for invasive aspergillosis. The duration of therapy is 4–12 weeks. Lipid formulations of amphotericin B should be considered when the patient is refractory to conventional amphotericin, or when conventional amphotericin causes toxic effects. Itraconazole can also be considered for children whose isolate is susceptible, but safety and toxicity data in children are lacking. Caspofungin and voriconazole are alternative therapies.

Mucormycosis

Mucormycosis is an acute and often fatal infection caused by a fungus of the Mucorales order of the Zygomycetes class. The organisms that cause mucormycosis may involve lungs, brain, sinuses, kidneys, and skin. Pulmonary involvement may present with persistent fever, chest pain, hemoptysis, and weight loss. Cavitation may occur. Diagnosis of zygomycosis is achieved through a high level of suspicion and aggressive pursuit of tissue culture. Invasive testing procedures, including fine-needle aspirates of lesions in deep tissue, transbronchial biopsies of pulmonary lesions, sinus tissue samples, scrapings of mucocutaneous lesions, or samples of deep tissue lesions, yield diagnostic results. Various methods can be used to detect Mucorales, including treatment with potassium hydroxide, Gomori's methenamine-silver staining, hematoxylin and eosin staining, and periodic acid-Schiff staining. Histopathologic specimens show evidence of vascular invasion. CT of the chest may identify infiltrates suggestive of Mucorales that are not seen on chest x-ray.

The mainstays of treatment include treatment of the underlying medical condition, reduction of immunosuppression, antifungal therapy, and surgical debridement. After the patient is diagnosed, predisposing factors such as hyperglycemia and metabolic acidosis should be corrected. Amphotericin B is the drug of choice for the treatment of mucormycosis, although higher doses are necessary due to resistance.

Cryptococcosis

Cryptococcosis is a fungal disease of humans and animals caused by *Cryptococcus neoformans* (*C. neoformans*). Infection is thought to be acquired by inhalation of fungus into lungs, where the infection mostly goes unnoticed, and it has strong predilection for the CNS. The increasing number of cases of HIV-related cryptococcosis over time paralleled the AIDS epidemic. The other conditions that predispose for cryptococcosis include malignancies, organ transplantation, primary immune deficiencies, and corticosteroid therapy. The disease primarily presents as subacute or chronic meningitis, although involvement of other organs (liver, spleen, skin, lymph node, eye, bones, adrenals, and ears) is variably seen. Disseminated cryptococcosis may present with cough or chest pain, weight loss, fever, hemoptysis, hepatosplenomegaly, and cutaneous findings (e.g., ulcers, nodules, vesicles, abscesses, papules and cellulitis).

The diagnosis of cryptococcal pulmonary infection is suggested by characteristic clinical and radiographic findings, sputum culture, serologic assays for IgG and IgM, and serologic testing for cryptococcal polysaccharide antigen by latex agglutination. Even in asymptomatic patients, chest x-ray findings of diffuse infiltrations with hilar adenopathy may be seen. Sputum culture results are more likely to be positive in patients with AIDS than in those without severely depressed T-cell function. The definitive diagnosis of cryptococcus is via biopsy or fine-needle aspiration. Cryptococcal meningitis is suggested by visualization of encapsulated yeast cells in cerebrospinal fluid using India ink stain.

Immunocompetent patients with isolated pulmonary disease usually clear the organism without antifungal agents. However, as a small risk of dissemination is present, these patients should be treated with fluconazole. For immunocompromised patients with isolated pulmonary disease, cerebrospinal fluid and serum should be evaluated for evidence of disseminated disease. Patients with disseminated disease (including meningitis) should be treated with a combination of amphotericin B and flucytosine for at least 2 weeks or until cerebrospinal fluid testing is negative, continuing with amphotericin B for an additional 4 weeks of therapy. Patients who are immunosuppressed should be treated for a longer course of therapy. Children who are HIV-positive should continue on fluconazole after treatment of their primary infection for life-long suppressive therapy.

Histoplasmosis

Histoplasmosis is a systemic disease caused by the dimorphic fungus *Histoplasma capsulatum*. In children, histoplasmosis occurs exclusively as an acute, progressive, life-threatening infection. Most of these infections develop in children with acquired or congenital cellular immune deficiency. Histoplasmosis is an AIDS-defining opportunistic infection. Clinical manifestations of disseminated histoplasmosis include prolonged, unexplained fever, respiratory complaints, abdominal pain, weight loss, and diarrhea. Liver, spleen, and lymph nodes may be enlarged. Skin may show mucocutaneous lesions, maculopapular rash, papules, nodules, pustules, and ulcerative lesions. Children may present with meningitis or encephalitis and focal brain lesions.

The diagnosis of histoplasmosis is made via culture, fungal stain, antigen detection, and serologic tests for antibodies. Blood cultures are more likely to yield organism if the lysis-centrifugation technique is utilized. Rapid results of antigen testing of pulmonary, CSF, urine, and blood are fairly sensitive for disseminated disease, with sensitivity being higher in urine than blood. The only drawback is that cross-reactivity can occur with penicilliosis, paracoccidioidomycosis, blastomycosis, and African histoplasmosis. Fungal silver or Wright stain can be used on peripheral blood or tissue culture to diagnose histoplasmosis.

No treatment is indicated for immunocompetent children with primary pulmonary histoplasmosis, as the disease usually follows a self-limited course. For complicated disease in children, including those who are immunocompromised, the treatment is with Amphotericin B (the standard therapy for serious infections), followed by itraconazole for long-term suppressive therapy. Those with HIV who become infected with *H. capsulatum* should be placed on itraconazole therapy for life. For isolated pericarditis, drainage of pericardial fluid and nonsteroidal anti-inflammatory drugs are the mainstays of therapy—no antifungals are indicated.

Nontuberculous Mycobacteria

Nontuberculous mycobacteria rarely cause disease in otherwise healthy individuals. Lymphadenitis is the most common manifestation of infection due to nontuberculous mycobacteria. The majority of patients present with an enlarged palpable mass and preceding constitutional symptoms. The lymph node involvement may be multiple, with the most common site being the cervical region. Cases of disseminated *M. avium* complex with gastrointestinal tract involvement have been reported in HIV-infected children and hematopoietic stem cell transplant recipients. If atypical mycobacterial disease is suspected, samples should be sent for acid-fast bacillus (AFB) smear and culture, as well as DNA-probe testing. For suspected pulmonary disease, 3 sputum specimens obtained on 3 different days should be sent for AFB smear and culture. PCR testing is becoming the gold standard for detection of atypical mycobacterial infection and should be performed on at least one sputum specimen and any AFB smear-positive specimen.

For lymphadenitis due to *M. avium intracellulare* or other atypical mycobacteria, surgical excision, if complete, is sufficient without antimicrobial therapy. If excision is not possible or incomplete, therapy with clarithromycin or azithromycin should be considered. For pulmonary disease due to *mycobacterium avium intracellulare*, the treatment of choice includes clarithromycin or azithromycin, ethambutol, and rifabutin. Amikacin or streptomycin may be added in case of cavitary pulmonary disease. This therapy should be continued until the patient is culture negative for 12 months. For salvage therapy, rifabutin and amikacin and/or levofloxacin should be used.

Mycobacterium Tuberculosis

HIV and TB form a lethal combination, each speeding the other's progress. HIV weakens the immune system. TB can occur in HIV-infected individuals at any CD4 count, which is in contrast to other opportunistic infections that generally occur when CD4 counts significantly decline. If purified protein derivative testing is utilized, a positive test for those who are immunosuppressed is defined as induration >5 mm in diameter. While a positive purified protein derivative test without evidence of clinical disease (e.g., absence of pulmonary symptoms or chest

x-ray findings) indicates latent TB infection, the additional x-ray findings and pulmonary symptoms are consistent with TB. Evaluation for pulmonary TB should include a chest x-ray or CT scan. In addition, sputum or gastric aspirate samples should be sent for AFB smear and culture for patients with pulmonary symptoms, cervical lymphadenopathy, or abnormalities on chest x-ray. For children and adolescents with suspected TB, the best test is the early-morning gastric aspirate, obtained on awakening via a nasogastric tube on 3 separate days, or induced sputum using hypertonic saline inhalation by nebulizer. If a sample returns positive for AFB, confirmation via culture or PCR is required, as other mycobacteria can give positive results for this test. Evaluation for nonpulmonary TB includes AFB smear and culture of suspected sterile body sites.

Latent TB infection is managed with a single drug regimen, depending on the resistance pattern in particular geographic regions or the index case. For isoniazid-susceptible latent TB, the child is treated with isoniazid once daily for 6–9 months. In cases with isoniazid resistance, rifampin may be given once daily for 6 months. The recommended treatment for TB disease in patients who are HIV-positive includes a 6-month regimen, using isoniazid, rifampin (or rifabutin), pyrazinamide, and ethambutol for the first 2 months, and isoniazid and rifampin for next 4 months. The key therapeutic principles that underlie the treatment of HIV-TB are (a) treatment of TB always takes precedence over the treatment of HIV infection, (b) in patients who are already on highly active antiretroviral therapy (HAART), it must be continued with appropriate modifications in both HAART and antituberculosis treatment, and (c) in patients who are not receiving HAART, the need for, and timing of, initiation of HAART should be decided on an individual basis after assessing the short-term risk of disease progression and death, based on CD4+ count and type of TB. Treatment of TB that is not associated with HIV infection should be based on drug resistance in the index case, in the local geographic area, or in the country of origin for imported cases. The local health department maintains data on local patterns of TB resistance and can advise if a 3- or 4-drug regimen should be used. Local health departments should also be notified of any new case of TB so that investigation and testing of contacts can begin. The WHO has recommended category-based treatment for children in high-endemic areas. Monitoring for treatment success is essential for treatment of TB. For patients with evidence of pulmonary TB, sputum specimens should be obtained monthly until 2 consecutive specimens are negative. Patients should be followed clinically and radiographically for evidence of treatment success. Routine laboratory testing is not indicated to monitor for adverse medication effects unless elevated transaminase levels are noted at baseline.

Though most children with TB are not contagious (except those with cavitary lesions, positive sputum AFB smears, laryngeal involvement, pulmonary infection, or suspected congenital infection), they are often exposed by a visiting family member who is infectious. For this reason, many hospitals attempt to place these children in a negative-pressure room, with caregivers using particulate respirators. The local health department should be immediately informed when a child tests positive for TB. In countries with universal Bacille Calmette-Guérin vaccination programs, immunocompromised children who are in contact with adults whose sputum smear is positive for TB should be treated with isoniazid prophylaxis for 6–9 months.

Toxoplasmosis

Toxoplasmosis is a parasitic infection. *Toxoplasma gondii* (*T. gondii*) infects cats and other animals and secondarily infects humans, causing congenital toxoplasmosis during intrauterine infection.Owing to the increasing number of patients with AIDS and immunosuppressed transplant patients, disseminated *T. gondii* has emerged as a potentially fatal pathogen. Common presentations include fever, encephalitis, pneumonia, myocarditis, and bone marrow suppression.

The diagnosis of infection due to toxoplasma is made through clinical presentation with confirmation either through serologic methods (reserved for immunocompetent hosts) or molecular methods, such as PCR. In infants and other immunocompromised patients (i.e., HIV patients) with a suspected diagnosis of toxoplasma, sera should be sent for PCR testing. Pregnant females who test positive for toxoplasma-specific IgG can be further tested for IgG avidity.

Infants with toxoplasmosis may be treated with sulfadiazine, pyrimethamine, and folinic acid for a minimum of 12 months. Steroids should be considered for infants with elevated CSF protein and chorioretinitis. Intensive monitoring of ophthalmologic, neuroradiologic, and CSF parameters should be part of their follow-up.

Cryptosporidium Infection

Cryptosporidium spp. is a major cause of diarrheal disease in both immunocompetent and immunodeficient individuals. The most severe disease is seen in individuals with defects in the T-cell response. Children with HIV infection, primary immunodeficiencies (most notably severe combined immunodeficiency syndrome), and acute leukemia are at risk for cryptosporidiosis. Immunocompromised patients, including children with severe malnutrition, suffer from severe and prolonged watery diarrhea. Cryptosporidium may cause cholangitis (particularly sclerosing cholangitis), pancreatitis, and respiratory symptoms. Cryptosporidium may also cause respiratory symptoms. In most patients with respiratory symptoms, co-infection with typical or atypical mycobacterium occurs. Immunoflourescence microscopy and enzyme-linked immunoassays are the methods of choice for identifying cryptosporidium in stool.

Infection in immunocompetent persons is self-limiting and does not require treatment. However, in the immunocompromised, treatment is indicated. The current therapy for immunocompromised children with cryptosporidiosis, in addition to electrolyte management and replacement of fluids, is nitazoxanide. The suggested doses of nitazoxanide are 500 mg twice daily for 3 days in adults and adolescents, 200 mg twice daily for 3 days in children aged 4–11 years, and 100-mg doses twice daily for 3 days in children aged 1–3 years.

CHAPTER 64 ■ PRINCIPLES OF NUTRITION AND METABOLISM

MURAYA GATHINJI • Z. LEAH HARRIS

The metabolic response of critically ill individuals, adult and children, is characterized by an increase in resting energy expenditure (REE). Defined as the amount of calories required by the body during a nonactive, 24-hr period, the REE (calories per day) represents 70%–80% of the calories used by the body. The REE is synonymous to the *resting* metabolic rate, which defines the energy released to maintain normal, basal physiologic functioning. A more sophisticated measurement, the *basal* metabolic rate, represents the amount of energy expended while at rest at a neutral temperature and under fasting conditions (12-hr fast). The REE is useful in optimizing nutrition management for the patient. While critically ill individuals have a greater REE than healthy controls and have an increased caloric need over their "resting" state, a formula by which to derive REE is useful to prevent the underfeeding or overfeeding of individuals. A common calculation for predicted energy expenditure uses the Harris-Benedict equations, which take into account gender, age, height, and weight. Other equations include the Food and Agriculture/World Health Organization/United Nations University equation and the Schofield-height/weight (Schofield-HW) equation (**Table 64.1**).

As the large variations in critically ill children can lead to inaccuracy in predictions when using these equations, the most accurate assessment of REE requires that it be measured. Energy expenditure can be measured indirectly with a metabolic cart, using an analysis of expired gases to derive the volume of air that passes through the lungs, the amount of oxygen extracted from it (V_{O_2}) and the amount of carbon dioxide that is expelled into atmosphere (V_{CO_2}) as a by-product of metabolism. An additional formula to represent V_{O_2} and V_{CO_2} is the respiratory quotient (RQ), which measures the inherent composition and utilization of carbohydrates, fats, and proteins as they are converted to energy substrate units that can be used by the body as energy. The RQ represents the ratio of carbon dioxide produced to the amount of oxygen consumed by the individual: $(RQ) = V_{CO_2}/V_{O_2}$.

TABLE 64.1

EQUATIONS FOR CALCULATING RESTING ENERGY EXPENDITURE

Harris-Benedict Equations (calories/day)
Male: $66.5 + [13.8 \times weight (kg)] + [5.0 \times height (cm)] - [6.8 \times age (years)]$
Female: $655.1 + [9.6 \times weight (kg)] + [1.8 \times height (cm)] - [4.7 \times age (years)]$

FAO/WHO/UNU (calories/day)
Male (3–10 yrs): REE = $[22.7 \times weight (kg)] + 495$
Female (3–10 yrs): REE = $[22.5 \times weight (kg)] + 499$
Male (10–18 yrs): REE = $[12.2 \times weight (kg)] + 746$
Female (10–18 yrs): REE = $[17.5 \times weight (kg)] + 651$

Schofield-HW (calories/day)
Male (3–10 yrs): REE = $[19.6 \times weight (kg)] + [1.033 \times height (cm)] + 414.9$
Female (3–10 yrs): REE = $[16.97 \times weight (kg)] + [1.618 \times height (cm)] + 371.2$
Male (10–18 yrs): REE = $[16.25 \times weight (kg)] + [1.372 \times height (cm)] + 515.5$
Female (10–18 yrs): REE = $[8.365 \times weight (kg)] + [4.65 \times height (cm)] + 200$

RESPIRATORY QUOTIENT

The REE ~70% of total energy expenditure is due to the basal physiologic processes; 20% comes from physical activity and another 10% from digestion of macronutrients in the form of food. RQ ranges from 1.0 (representing the value expected for pure carbohydrate oxidation) to ~0.7 (the value expected for pure fat oxidation). The physiologic range of RQ is 0.67–1.3. When RQ is >1.0, it is recommended to decrease the total calorie intake or decrease the carbohydrate-to-fat ratio in these situations. An RQ of <0.81 indicates a greater oxidation of fat, which may indicate a need to increase the total calorie intake or increase the carbohydrate-to-fat ratio.

In critically ill children, underfeeding results in nutrient depletion, protein-energy malnutrition, decreased immunocompetence, and increased morbidity and mortality. Overfeeding may induce thermogenesis, hepatic fat deposition, and increased carbon dioxide production. The severity of illness affects energy metabolism.

KEY NUTRIENTS

Nutrition is used to modulate the immune response, minimize oxidative stress, normalize gut integrity, and maintain glycemic control. As a simple, inexpensive indicator of potential morbidity, albumin remains the recommended lab value to obtain for nutritional assessment. Infants and children rely on the metabolism of macronutrients—carbohydrates, fats, and protein—to meet their energy demands. Energy produced per gram of substrate metabolized is as follows:

- Carbohydrate   4–5 kcal/g
- Protein   4–5 kcal/g
- Fat   9 kcal/g

The percentage of carbohydrate as a percentage of total body weight is relatively constant (0.4%). Differences in fat reserve/composition (infant, 14%; child, 17%; adult, 19%) and protein (infant, 11%; child, 15%; adult, 18%) are substantial. Clearly, children have half of the protein stores and one-third of the fat stores of adults and thus have much less available at times of injury or illness. Current recommendations for energy and protein requirements in healthy individuals are:

- Infants   2.2 g/kg/d protein, 120 kcal/kg/d total calories

- Children   1.0 g/kg/d protein, 70 kcal/kg/d total calories
- Adults   0.8 g/kg/d protein, 35 kcal/kg/d total calories

Glucose

Glucose production in children is critical to meet their energy demands, especially during illness. Glucose is the preferred energy substrate for the brain, red blood cells, and renal medulla. Without adequate carbohydrate replacement, the catabolism of the diaphragm and intercostal muscles causes additional compromise of respiratory function in an already ill child. The estimation for carbohydrate requirement is 200–300 g/day, based on a need of 3–6 mg/kg/min in the critically ill (26).

Fats

Fats are listed in six categories: total fat, saturated fatty acid, monounsaturated fatty acid, polyunsaturated fatty acid, trans-fatty acid, and dietary cholesterol. Critically ill children who do not receive lipids develop essential fatty acid deficiencies within a week (prevented by administration of linoleic acid [4.5% total calories] and linolenic acid [0.5% total calories]). Free fatty acids interfere with leukocyte function, and hyperlipidemia is associated with decreased oxygenation in premature infants who receive IV fat infusions. Neonates have a theoretical risk of IV lipid displacing unconjugated bilirubin and causing kernicterus. Restricting the infusion of lipid to 2–3 g/kg/day protects against bilirubin displacement.

Proteins

Unlike provision of the storage of fat, the body has no storage depots of protein. Newborns have a protein turnover twice as active as adults: 6.7 g/kg/day versus 3.5 g/kg/day. Burns, trauma, and extracorporeal membrane oxygenation cause protein turnover to increase further. A 100% increase in urinary nitrogen excretion is seen with bacterial sepsis in infants, and a 100% increase in protein breakdown is seen if they require extracorporeal membrane oxygenation support. Amino acid supplementation has been shown to be successful in restoring negative protein balance, but limited data exist that detail the optimal amount of protein to deliver. To provide adequate amino acids for wound healing, for protein synthesis, and for preserving skeletal muscle mass, the quantity of amino acid delivered should be:

- Low-birth-weight infants   3–4 g/kg/day
- Term neonates   2–3 g/kg/day
- Children   1.5 g/kg/day

Protein administration >6 g/kg/day is associated with toxicity to the liver and kidneys and should be avoided. Infants should receive 43% of protein as essential amino acids, and children should receive 36%. While infants should receive a minimum of 30% of their calories from fat, children should receive a maximum of 30% of total calories from fat and no more than 10% of their calories from saturated or unsaturated fats.

Micronutrients

Micronutrients are required in small amounts, compared to macronutrients, and are classified as *vitamins*: A (retinol), B_1 (thiamin), B_2 (riboflavin), B_3 (niacin), B_5 (pantothenic acid), B_6 (pyridoxine), B_7 (biotin), B_9 (folate), B_{12} (cobalamin or cyanocobalamin), C, D, E (tocopherol), and K. Other classifications are *trace elements/minerals* (zinc, iron, copper, selenium, fluoride, iodine, chromium, molybdenum, cobalt, and manganese) and *amino acids* (glutamine, arginine, homocysteine). The significance of these micronutrients lies in their unique disease states, discovered as a result of their deficiency. Divided into fat-soluble (vitamins A, D, E, and K) and water-soluble (vitamins B and C), vitamins are organic compounds required by humans in small amounts from the diet.

Vitamin A deficiency is the leading cause of blindness in developing nations. A deficiency of B_1 results in beriberi, which has three forms: (a) dry beriberi, peripheral neuropathy; (b) wet beriberi, neurologic and cardiovascular abnormalities (congestive heart failure); and (c) cerebral beriberi, Wernicke disease. Cataracts and migraine headaches have been ascribed to decreased levels of riboflavin. Niacin deficiency may occur with administration of isoniazid, inadequate absorption of tryptophan (Hartnup disease), or inadequate synthesis of niacin from tryptophan (carcinoid syndrome). The late stage of severe niacin deficiency is known as *pellagra*, the symptoms of which are dermatitis, diarrhea, dementia and, if untreated, death. Infant seizures are associated with pyridoxine deficiency, in which seizures are the final manifestation. Irritability, depression, and confusion can frequently occur with this disorder. The signs and symptoms of biotin deficiency include an erythematous scaly skin eruption distributed around the eyes, nose, mouth, and perineum and alopecia, conjunctivitis, and neurologic abnormalities. "Biotin deficiency facies" is composed of a rash around the eyes, nose, and mouth, along with an unusual distribution of facial fat. In biotin-deficient infants, the neurologic findings are hypotonia, lethargy, and developmental delay. In adults, the neurologic findings are lethargy, depression, hallucinations, and paresthesias of the extremities. Folate deficiency manifests with bone marrow abnormalities: megaloblastic or macrocytic anemia and hypersegmented neutrophils. Cyanocobalamin and methylcobalamin deficiency can cause anemia (usually macrocytic megaloblastic anemia) or demyelination (numbness, tingling, ataxia). Scurvy, seen in severe vitamin C deficiency, is fatal if left untreated.

Vitamin D_3 (cholecalciferol) is synthesized in the skin after it is consumed in the diet or after exposure to ultraviolet light. It is then transported to the liver, where it is hydroxylated to the form 25-hydroxycholeclaciferol (calcidiol). An additional hydroxylation occurs in the kidneys, producing 1,25-dihydroxycholecalciferol (calcitriol), which is the active form of the vitamin. Severe vitamin D deficiency is seen in the PICU as rickets, osteopenia, or osteoporosis—all due to failure of the bone to mineralize. The main cause of vitamin D deficiency is inadequate intake; rarely, it is secondary to inadequate exposure to ultraviolet light. Vitamin E deficiency is seen in children with fat malabsorption syndromes (cystic fibrosis, pancreatic insufficiency, gastrectomy, Crohn disease, and cholestatic liver disease), very-low-birth-weight neonates, and abetalipoproteinemia. Vitamin E deficiency presents with ataxia, peripheral neuropathy, myopathy, and a pigmented retinopathy. Vitamin K-dependent coagulation factors are synthesized in the liver. Newborn infants are the most susceptible to vitamin K deficiency and hence bleeding; they therefore receive vitamin K injections shortly after birth.

Trace Elements and Minerals

The following are considered essential micronutrients: cobalt, copper, chromium, fluorine, iron, iodine, manganese, molybdenum, selenium, and zinc. Nickel, tin, vanadium, silicon, and boron have been classified as important micronutrients. Aluminum, arsenic, barium, bismuth, bromine, cadmium, germanium, gold, lead, lithium, mercury, rubidium, silver, strontium, titanium, and zirconium are all found in plant and animal tissue; however, their importance is still being determined.

Recent interest has been generated utilizing coenzyme Q_{10} (ubiquinone) in the management of pediatric cardiomyopathy. In the role as a substrate to enhance cellular energy production, exogenous coenzyme Q_{10} (idebenone) has been used in adults with promising results with heart failure with or without cardiomyopathy.

IMMUNONUTRITION

Enteral nutrition results in a decrease in infectious complications in critically ill adults and reduced hospital costs. Three areas of the immune defense system represent targets for specific nutritional manipulation: the mucosal barrier, cellular immunity, and the inflammatory response. Glutamine-supplemented enteral or parenteral solutions are associated with increased mucosal thickness, improved integrity of the mucosal barrier, and reduced bacterial translocation across the enterocyte mucosal barrier. Glutamine supplementation has been associated with heat shock protein (hsp70) induction, reduced heat shock-induced cell death, fewer bloodstream infections, lower incidence of pneumonia, restoration of mucosal IgA, enhanced bacterial clearance in peritonitis, and enhanced production of both intestinal and hepatic glutathione stores. Arginine is a unique substrate for the signaling molecule nitric oxide, which is formed by the oxidation of L-arginine by nitric oxide synthase. Three separate nitric oxide isoenzymes have been characterized: inducible nitric oxide, endothelial nitric oxide, and neuronal nitric oxide. Inducible nitric oxide plays a significant role as an immunomodulator. Early studies documented the effect of enteral arginine on increased lymphocyte and monocyte proliferation and enhanced T-helper cell formation. Multiple studies in wound healing have shown a significant improvement in results with patients on arginine supplementation (25–30 g/dose), such as enhanced protein synthesis, improved wound healing, increased nitrogen balance, increased insulin-like growth factor 1 levels, and enhanced immuno-activity. While it may appear that arginine would enhance immune function, clinical studies suggest that NO potentiates the systemic inflammatory response in patients with sepsis and is associated with worse outcomes.

During catabolic stress or protein malnutrition, de novo nucleotide biosynthesis is severely impaired. Rapidly dividing cells are the most sensitive to this loss, and immune cells appear to be exceptionally susceptible. Omega-3 polyunsaturated fatty acids (PUFAs) modulate and downregulate inflammatory eicosanoids and prostaglandin E1 production. PUFAs are also called *essential fatty acids* because they are not synthesized by the human body and must be obtained in our diet. A standard diet supplemented with EPA and γ-linoleic acid may result in shorter lengths of ventilation and improved respiratory mechanics. The branched-chain amino acids include leucine, isoleucine, and valine. Leucine possesses protein-regulatory properties and is responsible for decreased protein degradation.

Immune-enhancing diets are recommended for those who should receive early enteral nutrition such as patients who are moderately or severely malnourished (albumin <3.5 g/dL), undergo elective gastrointestinal surgery, or have suffered blunt and penetrating torso trauma.

In a blinded, prospective, randomized, controlled clinical trial, early feeding with an enteral formula supplemented with glutamine, arginine, omega-3 PUFAs, and antioxidants resulted in a more favorable effect on nitrogen balance, decreased gastric colonization rates, and a decreasing trend in nosocomial infections. No difference was observed in length of stay or mortality. However, a more careful analysis of the data suggests a trend for increased mortality among the immunonutrition-fed group. A clear position on the effectiveness and safety of immuno-enhanced diets for both children and adults has yet to be determined.

BEST PRACTICES IN NUTRITION THERAPY

Even small feed volumes significantly maintain normal gut flora, minimize bacterial overgrowth, decrease the rate of drug-resistant bacteria emergence, and reduce bacterial translocation. Macronutrients and micronutrients are essential ligands for the signaling process critical for cellular responses to illness. Hypermetabolism and skeletal muscle breakdown during critical illness are only a fraction of the documented catabolism that occurs during illness.

Macronutrient values appear to provide the most accurate serum markers of nutrition status. Albumin, prealbumin, transferrin, and retinol-binding proteins represent the four proteins most commonly measured to assess protein malnutrition and extrapolated to reflect total body nutrient needs.

Serum protein half-lives:

Albumin (3.5–5.5 g/dL)	20 days
Transferrin (200–400 mg/dL)	8 days
Prealbumin (16–35 mg/dL)	2 days
Retinol-binding protein (2.6–7.6 mg/dL)	10 hrs

It is clear that early implementation of a nutritional regimen improves clinical outcomes, decreases infection rate, and reduces hospital stay. Secondary hepatobiliary dysfunction is associated with parenteral feeds. Parenteral nutrition does not confer the gastric-stimulated gut peristalsis or neutralization of gastric acid that protects from both ulcer development and bacterial translocation that is accomplished with enteral feeds. Whereas adult ICU feeding protocols start at a rate of 25 mL/hr and target a gastric intraluminal volume of <100 mL to indicate an excessive gastric residual after 4 hours of feeding, pediatric protocols require volume and rate adjustment based on patient size and age.

The reduction in gastric motility associated with critical illness and an increased risk for pulmonary aspiration appears to be another barrier to early feeding. Transpyloric feeding is well tolerated and desired calories are reached more rapidly, and patients require less sedation.

CHAPTER 65 ■ NUTRITIONAL SUPPORT IN THE CRITICALLY ILL CHILD

WERTHER BRUNOW DE CARVALHO • HEITOR PONS LEITE

The systemic inflammatory response includes activation of the sympathetic nervous system and the hypothalamic-pituitary-adrenal axis. These responses are characterized by changes in glucose metabolism and lipids, along with increased protein turnover and breakdown, which result in increased energy expenditure and a negative nitrogen balance and lead to muscle protein loss. Hypermetabolic and hyperdynamic states are characterized by hyperthermia, tachycardia, tachypnea, hyperglycemia, and an increase in oxygen consumption and in cardiac index. The stress response peaks on the third or fourth day after injury, reversing in 7–10 days. Continued hypermetabolism results in a rapid process of malnutrition and immunologic dysfunction, leading to multiorgan dysfunction in some cases. Critically ill, malnourished children are less able to handle substrate, liquid, and solute overload. The most common absorptive disturbances involve carbohydrates (particularly lactose) and fats.

OBJECTIVES OF NUTRITIONAL SUPPORT

The objective of the initial phases of nutritional support is to attenuate losses due to hypercatabolism, allowing the patient to maintain body mass and organic functions without overloading metabolism, the cardiovascular system, or the respiratory muscles. Once metabolic stress has been resolved, energy supply should be increased to achieve anabolism.

Fluid Intake

Daily assessment of weight, urinary osmolality, diuresis volume, and fluids balance provides a good estimation of hydration state. Fever, increased ambient temperature, hypermetabolism, and liquid loss through diarrhea or digestive juices all imply further water loss and call for increased water intake. A significant weight loss from one day to the next tends to reflect abnormal liquid loss, and conversely, marked weight gain may be the result of excessive water intake. Fluid losses through diarrhea or ileostomy drainage should be replaced daily.

Energy Intake

The main components of energy expenditure in children are base metabolism, growth, and activity. Basing the energy intake of a critically ill child on the predicted requirements of a healthy child (90–110 kcal/kg/day) lends to a risk of overfeeding. Overfeeding predisposes to increased respiratory quotient, risk of steatosis and hepatic cholestasis, and increased risk of infection. Hence, for sedated infants in intensive care, the caloric requirement during acute metabolic stress is limited to that needed to reach basal metabolic rate plus a stress factor, which, depending on the clinical situation, is between 1.1 and 1.2. The basal metabolic rate in newborns and infants is ~50–55 kcal/kg/day and falls steadily until adolescence to 25 kcal/kg/day.

TABLE 65.1

DAILY ELECTROLYTE REQUIREMENTS BY PARENTERAL ROUTE

Electrolyte	Neonates	Infants/Children	Adolescents
Sodium	2–5 mEq/kg	2–6 mEq/kg	Individualized
Chloride	1–5 mEq/kg	2–5 mEq/kg	Individualized
Potassium	1–4 mEq/kg	2–3 mEq/kg	Individualized
Calcium	3–4 mEq/kg	1–2.5 mEq/kg	10–20 mEq
Phosphorus	1–2 mmol/kg	0.5–1 mmol/kg	10–40 mmol
Magnesium	0.3–0.5 mEq/kg	0.3–0.5 mEq/kg	10–30 mEq

Adapted from ASPEN. Board of Directors and The Clinical Guidelines Task Force. Guidelines for the use of parenteral and enteral nutrition in adult and pediatric patients. *JPEN* 2002;26(1):97SA–128SA.

Parenteral Nutrition

Previously well-nourished patients without likelihood of receiving effective enteral nutrition in 5–7 days are candidates for parenteral nutrition. It is recommended that commencement of parenteral nutrition not be delayed to beyond 48 hrs in severely malnourished patients or neonates who are not receiving enteral nutrition, provided they are hemodynamically and metabolically stable.

Nutritional need is the main factor that determines access route, with preference given to the peripheral venous route when use will be <2 weeks. Usually, peripheral veins can support solutions with glucose concentrations of up to 12.5%; this limit does not take into account solution osmolarity and is valid only for IV solutions that contain glucose and electrolytes in quantities equivalent to basal needs. In parenteral nutrition solutions, amino acids and electrolytes in addition to glucose contribute to the final osmolarity of the solution. Concentrations of glucose >8% generally have osmolarity of >600 mOsm/L, independent of amino acid concentration. In the case of intermediate concentrations between 6% and 8%, raised osmolarities are found when amino acid concentrations are ≥10%. Notably, even infusions of solutions with osmolarity of ~600 mOsm/L have been associated with thrombophlebitis in peripheral veins. The tolerated osmolarity by normal-flow peripheral veins is 820 mOsm/kg for 8 hrs, 690 mOsm/kg for 12 hrs, and 550 mOsm/kg for 24 hrs. Superficial veins, due to their low flow, are prone to sclerosis or phlebitis during hypertonic solution infusion, as well as leakage of solution and consequent injury to the subcutaneous tissue. High-osmolarity solutions should be administrated through a central vein.

Electrolyte Intake

Electrolyte intake must also replace abnormal losses that occur in situations associated with alterations in water and electrolytic balance, such as sepsis, malnutrition, and refeeding syndrome. Malnutrition leads to losses in intracellular potassium, magnesium, and phosphorus and increases in sodium and water. Monitoring of sodium, phosphorus, potassium, and calcium serum levels is integral to routine care. The demand for phosphorus is greater in children because it is needed for the formation of new tissues, a state that puts a critically ill patient with severe malnutrition at higher risk of developing hypophosphatemia. The recommended amounts of electrolytes by parenteral route are shown in **Table 65.1**.

Glucose

The maximum rate of glucose that can be oxidized by adults and adolescents is 5 mg/kg/min. Excessive intake of calories in the form glucose can give rise to increased metabolic rate, hyperglycemia, and hepatic alterations. Glucose intake that exceeds 18 g/kg/day (equivalent to a 12.5 mg/kg/min infusion rate) in neonates can lead to lowered energy benefit, increased hepatic lipogenesis, and increased CO_2 production. The glucose infusion rate in full-term newborns required to prevent hypoglycemia is between 3 and 4 mg/kg/min. Acute stress and corticotherapy are conditions that call for reduced glucose intake. Hyperglycemia may trigger glycosuria with osmotic diuresis, hampering immunologic function and healing, and may be associated with intracranial hemorrhage and worse neurologic prognosis in patients with cranioencephalic trauma.

Lipids

The main fatty acids are ω-3, ω-6 series polyunsaturated fatty acids (PUFAs), monounsaturated fatty acids belonging to the ω-9 series, and those from medium and short chains. IV lipid emulsions ensure provision of essential fatty acids and allow caloric intake to be increased without the need or inconvenience of greater glucose intake. Conventional emulsions are essentially composed of soybean oil and phospholipids from egg yolk as emulsifying agents and are available in 10% and 20% concentrations. They contain long-chain triglycerides (LCTs) or a mixture of these with medium-chain triglycerides (MCTs) in equal ratio. Emulsions of 20% concentrations are more easily cleared in patients receiving high doses of lipids, an advantage over lower-concentration emulsions. Two other types of emulsions have become available: One is an olive oil- and soy oil-based emulsion.

Children in metabolic stress have increased serum levels of triglycerides, fatty acids, and glycerol due to increased lipolysis. Elevated concentrations of plasma triglycerides (>200 mg/dL) saturate the lipoprotein lipase system. Infusion of lipid emulsions in high doses has been reported to impair function and hemodynamics, with inflammatory changes, edema, and surfactant alterations in adults with acute lung injury.

Particularities in Premature Neonates

In newborn infants who cannot receive sufficient enteral feeding, IV lipid emulsions should be started no later than on the third day of life but may be started on the first day of life. Preterm infants who weigh <1000 g deserve special attention because of their limited tolerance to IV lipids. IV lipid infusion can reduce arterial PO_2 through the following mechanisms: (a) changes in ventilation:perfusion ratio, which alters, and (b) the deposition of fat in the capillary-alveoli membrane. This effect is minimized by slowing the infusion of lipid emulsion over 20–24 hrs. Fatty acids compete with bilirubin for binding sites on albumin. Icteric premature newborns should be started on 0.5 g/kg/day doses, increasing after bilirubin levels fall or on determination of free fatty acid levels. No increase in fatty acid and free bilirubin concentrations have been seen after lipid intake of up to 3 g/kg/day. Liver function tests should be monitored when lipid emulsions are given. If evidence of progressive hepatic dysfunction or cholestasis is seen, a decrease in lipid administration should be considered, especially if there are other concurrent morbidities (e.g., sepsis, thrombocytopenia). Serum triglyceride concentrations should be monitored and a reduction of parenteral lipid dosage considered.

Points Warranting Attention

- Infant diets should supply 30% of energy in lipid form, where 1–2% of energy intake is derived from linoleic acid and 0.5% is derived from α-linolenic acid.

- Parenteral lipid intake should usually be limited to a maximum of 3–4 g/kg/day (0.13–0.17 g/kg/hr) in infants and 2–3 g/kg/day (0.08–0.13 g/kg/hr) in older children.

- In premature neonates, lipid emulsion should be started after 24 hrs of life at a dose of 0.5 g/day up to a maximum of 3 g/kg/day.

- Lipid emulsions should be administered over 24 hrs.

- Infusion of lipid emulsions as 3-in-1 solutions (protein, sugar, lipid in same container) is not recommended, particularly when calcium concentrations exceed 8.5 mEq/L, as the mixture is not complete and the stability of the emulsion may be impaired. Administration in the Y or 3-route tap connection is also not recommended, as the mixture in low-caliber tubes is also incomplete.

- Heparin does not improve utilization of IV lipids and should not be given with lipid infusion on a routine basis, unless indicated for other reasons.

- Lipid emulsions should be protected by validated light-protected tubing during phototherapy to decrease the formation of hydroperoxides.

Amino Acids

Recommended intakes of parenteral protein are 2.5–3 g/kg/day for neonates, 2–2.5 g/kg/day for infants, 1–1.2 g/kg/day for older children, and 0.8–1 g/kg/day for adolescents. The proportion of protein as caloric source should represent 8–15% of total energy intake, attaining 20% or more in hypercatabolic states. To promote anabolism, the nitrogen:nonprotein calorie ratio must lie between 1:150 and 1:250, or between 1:90 and 1:150 in hypercatabolism. One gram of protein provides 4 kcal; 1 g of protein corresponds to 0.16 g of nitrogen or 1 g nitrogen, is contained in 6.25 g of protein. Parameters for monitoring of protein intake are levels of serum urea, ammonia, total protein, arterial blood gas, and nitrogen balance. Administration of excessive quantities of amino acids can lead to acidosis, respiratory discomfort, uremia, hyperammonemia, hepatic dysfunction, increased oxygen consumption, and cholestatic icterus.

Particularities in Premature Neonates

The majority of premature infants tolerate parenteral amino acid intake of 1.5–2.0 g/kg/day in the first day of life, sufficient to avoid protein catabolism. In premature infants who receive parenteral nutrition with solutions standardized for adults, immaturity of metabolic pathways may result in toxic concentrations of plasma amino acids such as phenylalanine and methionine, along with deficiency in others such as cysteine, tyrosine, and taurine. Parenteral amino acid solutions for neonates have been

TABLE 65.2

DAILY TRACE ELEMENT REQUIREMENTS BY PARENTERAL ROUTE

Element	Newborns (mcg/kg) Preterm	Full term	<5 years (mcg/kg)	Older children and adolescents
Zinc	400	300	100	2–5 mg
Copper	20	20	20	200–500 mcg
Selenium	2.0	2.0	2–3	30–40 mcg
Chromium	0.20	0.20	0.14–0.2	5–15 mcg
Manganese	1.0	1.0	2–10	50–150 mcg
Iodide	1.0	1.0	1.0	

Adapted from Greene H.L, Hambidge K, Schanler R, et al. Guidelines for the use of vitamins, trace elements, calcium, magnesium and phosphorus in infants and children receiving total parenteral nutrition: Report of the Subcommittee on Clinical Practice Issues of the American Society for Clinical Nutrition. *Am J Clin Nutr* 1988;48:1324–42.

developed to achieve an amino acid plasma profile akin to that obtained in children with normal growth who are breastfed. No differences in nitrogen retention, growth or the incidence of cholestasis are seen between infants who receive pediatric amino acid solutions and those who receive the standard solution. Pediatric solutions appear to be beneficial during the neonatal period in that they include taurine and contain greater amounts of semi-essential amino acids such as cysteine and tyrosine, along with lower quantities of phenylalanine and methionine. Micronutrient needs are summarized in **Table 65.2** and **Table 65.3**.

Enteral Nutrition

The enteral route is preferable, as it prevents intestinal atrophy and reduces infectious complications when compared with parenteral nutrition. Furthermore, it is less expensive.

Enteral nutrition is indicated in the presence or risk of malnutrition, when the oral intake proves insufficient to prevent weight loss but when gastrointestinal tract use is viable. In this context, conditions that justify the enteral route include prematurity, mechanical pulmonary ventilation, severe malnutrition, hypermetabolic states, and neurologic diseases. Delay of enteral nutrition can be harmful; very early commencement during mesenteric hypoperfusion may cause intestinal necrosis. Parameters that indicate adequate intestinal function are presence of bowel sounds, absent abdominal distension or vomiting, and a small quantity of gastric residue. As measurement of blood perfusion from the digestive tract using gastric tonometry is not routinely performed, signs of adequate intestinal perfusion in the critical patient include stabilized vital signs, no continuous requirement for administration of fluid volume or vasoactive drugs, and a normalized acid-base balance and serum lactate. Enteral use is not advised when high doses of α-adrenergic drugs and neuromuscular blockers are used.

Potential Renal Solute Load

The potential renal solute load (PRSL) is the quantity of endogenous or dietary solutes that must be excreted by urine if none are used in new tissue

TABLE 65.3

DAILY VITAMIN REQUIREMENTS BY PARENTERAL ROUTE

Vitamin	Preterm infants (kg/body weight)	Children and full-term infants (total dose)
A (UI)	1640	2300
E (mg)	2.8	7
K (mcg)	80	200
D (UI)	160	400
C (mg)	25	80
Thiamin (mg)	0.35	1.2
Riboflavin (mg)	0.15	1.4
Pyridoxine (mg)	0.18	1.0
Niacin (mg)	6.8	17
Pantothenic acid (mg)	2.0	5
Biotin (mcg)	6.0	20
Folate (mcg)	56	140
B12 (mcg)	0.3	1.0
Vitamin K (mcg)		200
Carnitine	20	2–10 mcg/kg

Adapted from Greene H.L, Hambidge K, Schanler R, et al. Guidelines for the use of vitamins, trace elements, calcium, magnesium and phosphorus in infants and children receiving total parenteral nutrition: Report of the Subcommittee on Clinical Practice Issues of the American Society for Clinical Nutrition. *Am J Clin Nutr* 1988;48:1324–42.

synthesis or excreted by extrarenal routes. It consists of nonmetabolizable dietary components, especially electrolytes, in excess of needs and nitrogenous compounds that result from protein metabolism. The actual renal solute load (RSL) is PRSL minus the proportion of PRSL excreted by extrarenal routes and nutrients used for new tissue synthesis. Except in the presence of diarrhea, extrarenal losses are nominal and may be ignored. PRSL is an important consideration in maintaining water balance in the following circumstances: (a) during acute illness, when fluid intake is decreased, especially if the illness is accompanied by fever; (b) when a calorie-dense diet is fed; (c) when environmental temperature is elevated; or (d) when renal concentrating ability is decreased, as in chronic renal disease and diabetes insipidus. An understanding of osmolarity is another key factor, as high-osmolarity formulas may cause diarrhea when administered through duodenal or jejunal routes. The American Academy of Pediatrics recommends that osmolarity of infant formulas for oral or intragastric administration be lower than 460 mOsm/kg.

Infants

Maternal milk is indicated as the exclusive food source in infants up to 6 months of age. After 6 months, solid foods are introduced, and maternal milk is continued up to at least the age of 12 months or older. Contraindications of maternal milk are maternal infections caused by passive microorganisms transmittable through maternal milk, a number of innate metabolism errors, or other conditions that cause intolerance to the components of human milk; galactosemia or tyrosinemia; mother's exposure to foods, drugs, or environmental agents that, when excreted by human milk, can harm the infant. Infant formulas are recommended in situations where maternal breastfeeding is precluded. The caloric density of infant formulas is 0.67 kcal/mL, the same as human milk.

Formulas

Cow's milk formulas fulfill the nutrient needs of healthy children when used exclusively up to the age of 4–6 months. Their main carbohydrate source, as in maternal milk, is lactose. Protein levels are generally 1.5 times that of maternal milk, and the ratio of whey protein to casein is 60:40, similar to human milk.

Soy formulas are indicated for children with cow's-milk protein or lactose intolerance. In term infants, soy formulas promote growth and bone mineralization to the same degree as cow's milk-based formulas. They are milk free and have sucrose and hydrolyzed starch carbohydrates. They contain minerals and vitamins in greater quantities than milk-based formulas to compensate for the presence of possible mineral absorption antagonists such as soy phytates.

Protein hydrolysate formulas are processed by enzymatic hydrolysis of different protein sources, such as bovine casein/whey and soy, with the hydrolysate consisting of free amino acids, dipeptides, and tripeptides that do not require additional digestion. These formulas are lactose free, and their carbohydrate source is tapioca starch, corn syrup, or corn starch. Fats are provided by a blend of MCTs and LCTs in varying amounts. They are recommended for children who are intolerant to whole-milk formulas because of decreased intestinal length, absorptive capacity, or pancreatic or hepatobiliary diseases. These formulas might be considered during the systemic inflammatory response, when alterations in permeability and reduction of the absorptive surface of the intestinal epithelium take place.

Amino acid-based formulas are indicated for patients who have protein hypersensitivity unresponsive to hydrolyzed protein formulas. Nutrients, such as glutamine, arginine, ω-3 chain fatty acids, probiotics, nucleic acids, and antioxidants have immunostimulating properties. Immunonutrition may reduce the rate of infectious complications in trauma and perioperative adult patients, however overstimulation of the inflammatory response by an immune-enhancing diet may be harmful for the critically ill.

Nutrition for Premature Newborns

In feeding premature infants, it should be considered that immaturity of the digestive function and increased growth rate together with their limited energy reserves make this group particularly sensitive to overfeeding. Nutrition through enteral tube feeding using expressed breast milk taken from the mother of the premature infant has benefits over artificial formula use. The use of supplements to maternal milk has been recommended in very-low-weight, premature newborns because they offer increased calcium, phosphorus, proteins, and calorie content and allow for greater weight gain. When use of maternal breast milk is not possible, a special formula for preterm newborns may be used. These formulas have added nutrients but lack the digestion facilitators and protective factors present in maternal milk.

Low duodenal lipase and biliary acid activity in premature neonates reduce absorption of fats ingested to 65%–70%. In this respect, maternal milk is particularly advantageous because it contains its own lipase, which aids triglyceride digestion. MCTs are added to formulas for premature infants in an attempt to reverse the tendency of poor fat absorption. To compensate for lower carbohydrate absorption and digestion that results from lactase deficiency, these formulas, besides lactose, also contain additional glucose polymer. Premature infants, due to their needs for higher quantities of protein and owing to their limited metabolizing capacity, run the risk of developing uremia, metabolic acidosis, and neurologic disturbances if protein intake exceeds metabolic capacity. Formulas developed for premature infants yield higher calorie (0.81 kcal/mL), protein, vitamin, and mineral levels, along with lower lactose levels than formulas for term children. Use of these formulas in indicated up to the postnatal age of 9 months.

Children Aged 1 to 10 Years

At an energy density of 1 kcal/mL, formulas for children aged 1–10 years vary in osmolarity from 300 to 650 mOsm/L and are lactose free. Vitamin and trace elements can be met with a total intake of 950–2000 mL. Patients with fluid restriction may require vitamin and trace element supplementation. Isotonic formulas are preferred for pediatric patients because they allow transpyloric tube feeding.

Children Older than 10 Years

Children older than 10 years can be fed adult formulas. These formulas are not suitable for young children because of the elevated renal solute load and inadequate vitamin levels. Children whose calorie and protein needs are elevated due to severe trauma or burn injury may receive high-nitrogen and high-calorie formulations (1.5 kcal/mL).

NUTRITIONAL AND METABOLIC MONITORING

Anthropometric measures are useful to assess nutritional alterations prior to hospital admission and to document long-term therapeutic effects, but they do not accurately reflect the acute nutritional alteration present under conditions of metabolic stress. Weight and height measurements should be set against a reference standard, preferably those by the National Center for Health Statistics of the Centers for Disease Control and Prevention or the World Health Organization, and weight-height charts should be employed as needed. On ascertaining weight, patients should be properly hydrated.

Laboratory Monitoring

Prealbumin has a half-life of 2 days. Ideally, it should be assessed together with C reactive protein to provide a reference parameter for the magnitude of inflammatory response. Triglyceride levels in serum or plasma should be monitored in patients who receive lipid emulsions, particularly in those with significant risk for hyperlipidemia (e.g., sepsis, trauma, liver or renal diseases, use of steroids, extremely low-birthweight infants). In children with slightly elevated hypertriglyceridemia (175–225 mg/dL), steady increases in infusion rates are recommended. At moderately elevated concentrations (225–275 mg/dL), infusion rates should be reassessed without further increase until levels have normalized. At concentrations that exceed 400 mg/dL, it is recommended that infusion be halted for 12–24 hrs and then resumed at 0.02–0.04 g/kg/hr.

Acute stress and corticotherapy are conditions that require careful glucose monitoring. Hyperglycemia may trigger glycosuria with osmotic diuresis, hamper immunologic function and wound healing, and possibly be associated with intracranial hemorrhage and a worsened neurologic prognosis in patients with cranioencephalic trauma. It has been demonstrated that tight control of glucose levels (between 80 and 110 mg/dL) using insulin reduced mortality among adults in the ICU. Peak blood glucose and duration of hyperglycemia are associated with increased mortality.

Measured Energy Expenditure

At present, the only accurate method by which to determine daily energy expenditure in the critical care setting is to measure it with indirect calorimetry, which allows the assessment of energy expenditure for adequate energy supply, monitoring of the volume of oxygen consumption during weaning from mechanical ventilation, and measurement of the respiratory quotient. Only patients who are hemodynamically stable with an inspired F_{IO_2} of <0.6, no air leaks around the endotracheal tube, adequate sedation, no fever, and no anaerobic metabolism can be adequately measured. When it is not possible to perform indirect calorimetry, energy expenditure can be calculated using a predictive formula.

COMPLICATIONS OF ENTERAL AND PARENTERAL NUTRITION

Mechanical complications may occur when administering total parenteral nutrition (TPN) immediately subsequent to catheter insertion and include pneumothorax, hemothorax, hematoma, and tracheal puncture. Other late complications are linked to catheter blockage, catheter migration, or to vein thrombosis.

Septic complications may be exogenous in nature (extraluminal, with cutaneous microorganisms, and intraluminal, with microorganisms introduced within the vein) or endogenous, stemming from germ-contaminated intravascular catheters. Exogenous-type infections are the most frequent. The propensity of infections is linked to glucose overadministration, with hyperglycemia being an initial risk factor for infectious complications.

Hypernatremia (sodium >145 mmol/L) is associated with excessive sodium intake and consequent cellular dehydration. Hyponatremia (sodium <135 mmol/L) occurs with sodium depletion or water intoxication. Hypokalemia may result from insufficient intake or increased losses of potassium (vomiting, diarrhea, digestive fistula, malnutrition). Treatment consists of increased potassium intake. Hyperkalemia is caused by excessive potassium intake coupled with low renal potassium excretion, and treatment consists of reduction in potassium intake and use of ion-exchange resins, diuretics (furosemide), and sodium bicarbonate. Hypophosphatemia is the result of inadequate phosphorus intake or an increase in phosphorus intracellular shift and uptake during the anabolic protein phase. It represents a frequent complication in malnourished patients during the refeeding process. Treatment consists of increasing phosphorus intake. Hypocalcemia occurs due to insufficient intake or excessive losses of calcium, or poor intestinal absorption, or it is concomitant with hypomagnesemia.

Routine measurement of levels of calcium, phosphorus, and alkaline phosphatase is useful for detecting signs of metabolic bone disease. Generally, alkaline phosphatase serum levels are high and phosphorus levels are low in children with osteopenia. Calcium levels are typically maintained at the expense of bone reabsorption, though the presence of acute and chronic acid-base disturbances may influence this calcium level control. Treatment of hypocalcemia consists of increasing calcium intake and correcting associated fluid and electrolyte disturbances: metabolic or respiratory alkalosis, hypomagnesemia, and hyperkalemia, possibly using vitamin D. Hypercalcemia occurs due to excessive calcium or vitamin D intake or immobilization or insufficient intake of phosphates. Hypomagnesemia occurs due to insufficient intake or excessive losses of magnesium (chronic diarrhea, digestive fistula or malnutrition). Hypermagnesemia may occur in the presence of renal insufficiency.

Intolerance to lipid use may occur in children who are preterm, septic, or malnourished, have hepatic or renal insufficiency, or are receiving steroids.

The use of some medicines that contain lipids (e.g., propofol and amphotericin B) may contribute a sufficient quantity of energy in relation to total daily intake and may increase the possibility of hyperlipemia. High levels of triglycerides may also be attributed to carnitine deficiency, as premature newborns younger than 34 weeks have a limited stock of carnitine.

The safety margin for administration of amino acids is wide, having minimal likelihood of causing an impact on blood ammonia levels. However, ammonia levels in children who present with hepatic failure must be carefully monitored and controlled. Preterm newborns have lower levels of albumin, prealbumin, and retinol-binding protein than do full-term newborns. When the patient presents with normal renal function and hydration, monitoring blood urea nitrogen levels is adequate on a 3-g/kg/day intake of amino acids. Blood urea can be used as a marker for amino acid intolerance. It has been suggested that an increase in blood urea nitrogen levels is a direct reflection of increased quantities of amino acids being available and is evidence of efficient nitrogen use and retention.

Patients on TPN at risk of iron deficiency include premature newborns, those with low or no enteral intake, and chiefly, those who present with poor absorption or fluid loss. Iron can be administered using oral, intramuscular, or parenteral routes for prophylaxis or treatment. Iron overload is linked to increased risk of sepsis in malnourished children who have low transferrin levels and is associated with increasing requirements for vitamin E. Zinc deficiency is seen in patients with severe diarrhea, poor absorption, digestive fistula, and insufficient zinc intake present with characteristic cutaneous lesions (enteropathic acrodermatitis). Low selenium can cause cardiomyopathy, whereas excessive intake leads to toxic manifestations, such as alopecia, headache, nausea, and garlic-like breath odor. Manganese is a frequent ingredient in parenteral nutrition solutions and is present in sufficient quantities to meet daily requirements; with long-term administration, it can lead to toxic symptoms from a buildup. Manganese intoxication may provoke parkinsonian-like symptoms, with muscle weakness, stiffness, trembling, ataxia, asthenia, and speech difficulties. Several parenteral component-nutrition solutions contain aluminium; any additional supply of aluminium raises risk of toxicity in children on TPN.

Cholestasis

If prolonged TPN is predicted (>2 weeks), hepatic function tests should be performed, particularly in

GASTROINTESTINAL COMPLICATIONS OF ENTERAL NUTRITION

Complication	Probable cause	Prevention/treatment
Diarrhea	Overly fast infusion	↓ infusion speed.
	High-osmolarity diet	↑ dilution or change of formula.
	Lactose intolerance	Use lactose-free formula.
	Formula with high lipid level	↓ level of fat in the diet.
	Food intolerance	Use hydrolyzed protein formula.
	Medicines (metoclopramide, aminophylline, erythromycin, sorbitol, xylitol, magnesium, phosphorus)	Do not use antidiuretics; consider vancomycin or metronidazole orally.
	Change in intestinal flora due to antibiotic therapy	Avoid medicine administration via tube. Aseptic preparation and administration technique; infusion flask must not remain exposed to ambient temperature for >8 hrs.
	Bacterial and diet contamination	Choose ready diets and closed infusion systems.
Abdominal distension	Use of antiacids and antibiotics, overly fast infusion; hypertonic formula or with high fat level, narcotic use, ileus.	Consider suspending drugs ↓ flow or volume of infusion; consider formula change; review use of drugs causing gastric atonia.
Nausea and Vomiting	Multifactorial	↓ flow; consider change of formula; exclude infectious process.
Intestinal Obstipation	Diet poor in residues; dehydration	Consider fiber-rich diet; maintain adequate hydration.

very low-weight neonates, to obtain measurements that might suggest the likelihood of hepatic disease or cholestasis. Increased bilirubin and transaminase are late indicators of cholestasis. The earliest indicator, albeit nonspecific, is γ-glutamyl transpeptidase, and its specificity increases when it is used in conjunction with alkaline phosphatase. The supply of at least some nutrition enterally is important, especially in children on TPN for long periods, as small quantities of food have trophic effects on the intestine, reduce bacterial translocation, improve gastric motility, and promote biliary flow.

METABOLIC COMPLICATIONS OF ENTERAL NUTRITION

Complication	Probable cause	Prevention/treatment
Hyperglycemia	Metabolic stress	↓ infusion rate; monitor glycosuria and glycemia
Dehydration	High-osmolarity diets, inadequate liquid intake	Monitor electrolytes, urea, hematocrit ↓ protein intake ↑ liquid intake
Hypokalemia	Anabolism and intake shortage; losses through diarrhea, digestive juices, or diuretic use	Frequent monitoring of potassium
Hyperkalemia	Renal insufficiency; metabolic acidosis	↓ potassium intake, treat underlying cause
Hypernatremia	Hypertonic formulas; inadequate liquid intake	Consider formula change; ↑ liquid intake
Hypophosphatemia	Refeeding of the severely malnourished; use of antiacids	Frequent monitoring of phosphate.
Hypercapnia	Hypercaloric diet with high level of carbohydrates in patients with respiratory insufficiency	↑ proportion of lipids as caloric source

Overfeeding Syndrome

Overfeeding is associated with fatty infiltration of the liver, hyperglycemia, hypertriglyceridemia, increased metabolic rate, and electrolyte disturbances. Furthermore, in cases with increased glucose and caloric intake, increases in oxygen uptake, in CO_2 production, and in CO_2 retention may be seen in children with pulmonary or cardiac insufficiency. Hypermetabolic and malnourished patients are more susceptible to these respiratory problems. Another potential complication of overfeeding with glucose is an increase in infectious complications, as hyperglycemia represents a risk factor for infection.

Complications of Enteral Nutrition

The total aspirated gastric volume is considered a simple measure for assessing gastrointestinal motility in critically ill patients. Nevertheless, increased gastric, residual volume may not accurately express low gastric emptying. Postpyloric feeds may address some feeding intolerances. Diarrhea has been attributed to a series of factors such as food osmolarity, formula type, low serum albumin concentration, and medication interactions. Simultaneous use of some medications, particularly antibiotics, is often the cause of diarrhea in enteral nutrition. Reducing suppression of gastric acidity and providing interruption of feeding, thereby allowing pH to fall and help to prevent excessive bacterial growth during enteral nutrition, may help. It has also been suggested that, occasionally, alimentation-containing fibers may improve enteral nutrition-related diarrhea.

The most frequent mechanical, gastrointestinal, and metabolic complications, along with their probable causes and corresponding treatments are summarized in **Table 65.4** and **Table 65.5**, respectively.

Interaction among Medications and Nutrients

A number of medications are incompatible with enteral diets (see **Table 65.4**) and may cause tube blockage when given in parallel. Thus, both the benefit and efficacy of the drug given may be affected. The most common example is phenytoin, which upon continued use causes deficiencies in folate, vitamin B_{12}, and calcium.

CHAPTER 66 ■ THE ACUTE ABDOMEN

EDUARDO SCHNITZLER • TOMAS IÖLSTER • RICARDO D. RUSSO

INTRODUCTION

The *acute abdomen* is a term used to define a syndrome that is characterized by signs and symptoms of intra-abdominal disease. Accurate clinical assessment is essential so as to diagnose the underlying pathology and avoid unnecessary surgical treatment.

CLINICAL PRESENTATION

The clinical history and physical examination, essential for the diagnosis, together with laboratory tests and imaging studies, will determine the probable diagnosis and guide the initial management.

There are four basic processes that are classic for acute abdomen: infection or inflammation, obstruction, perforation, and ischemia. The infection-inflammation or obstruction can usually be resolved with an adequate diagnosis and treatment, with or without surgical intervention. Perforation and ischemia are processes that lead to severe disease where early surgical intervention may be lifesaving. Any of these processes can progress to multiorgan failure.

A volvulus-associated bowel ischemia usually progresses quickly to a life-threatening situation; also an acute appendicitis if unrecognized or treated inappropriately may lead to a critical condition. Other diseases such as pneumonia, gastroenteritis, hepatitis, renal colic, vertebral disk inflammation, pericarditis and some osteoarthritis may present with abdominal symptoms and should be considered among the differential diagnosis of abdominal pain or acute abdomen in children. The presentation and sequence of symptoms such as fever, vomiting, diarrhea, constipation, urinary symptoms or pelvic symptoms in female teenagers are important for the diagnosis. When possible, localization and radiation of the pain should be sought. Taking an accurate history is essential for the diagnosis, and it should include previous medical pathologies, previous surgery, chronic drug therapy, recent trauma, or possibility of accidental ingestion of harmful substances in young children. Inspection may reveal significant findings such as distension, masses, hernias, surgical scars, or other alterations in the skin. The presence of petechiae, purpura, or rash may be suggestive of a systemic disease. Auscultation should precede palpation so as to avoid modification of the peristalsis by the external stimulation. Bowel sounds are typically altered during abdominal pathology;, however, sometimes findings may not be classic, and they may be absent in mild diseases or may be present even during intra-abdominal catastrophes. Abdominal percussion helps to differentiate between gaseous distension (tympanic) and distension due to masses or ascites (dull). Abdominal palpation should be gentle, and the child's attention should be distracted. Palpation should be systematic,

beginning with a superficial examination in the most distant quadrant from the site of maximum pain and then move slowly toward the painful area. Rebound tenderness is an indication of serious intra abdominal pathology. Examination of the inguinal and scrotal regions is essential so as to detect possible hernias or changes in the scrotal bag filling. Digital rectal examination should not be used routinely and is recommended only for situations in which occult blood, local masses, or rectal lesions need to be ruled out. Ecchymoses with discoloration in the periumbilical region (Cullen's sign) or a dirty green discoloration in both flanks (Turner's sign) have been reported in severe conditions such as ruptured extrauterine pregnancy and acute pancreatitis respectively. Other severe lesions such as bowel ischemia or retroperitoneal hemorrhage may have similar findings. The presence of severe abdominal distension or board-like rigidity and the degree of dehydration or the presence of shock will guide the initial resuscitation and will define the need for urgent surgical intervention (**Figure 66.1**).

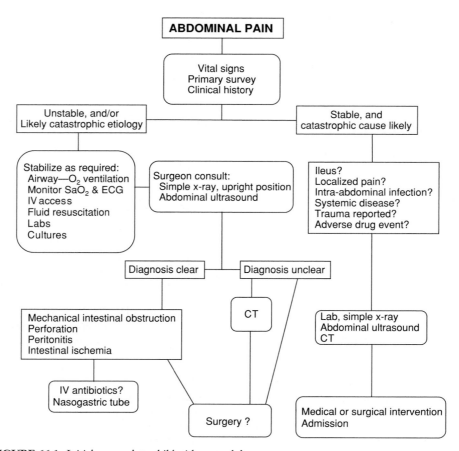

FIGURE 66.1. Initial approach to child with acute abdomen.

PRINCIPLES OF CLINICAL MANAGEMENT

If the child is clinically unstable or there is suspicion of an intra-abdominal catastrophe, initial priorities should include the establishment of an adequate airway, gas exchange, and circulation. Two peripheral venous accesses should be established as fast as possible, with one preferably above the diaphragm, and blood and urine samples should be obtained for full blood count, clotting, biochemistry, blood samples to the blood bank, blood cultures, and urine studies. Fluid boluses should be administered rapidly until appropriate perfusion has been established, and IV antibiotics treatment should be initiated whenever sepsis is suspected. Early surgical review and initial imaging studies such as abdominal x-ray or CT scan or abdominal ultrasound will guide the first therapeutic decisions.

Monitoring of pulse oximetry, heart rate, ECG, and noninvasive blood pressure are essential to guide the therapy. Pelvic examination is indicated for adolescents whose pain is suggestive of gynecologic pathology. The plain abdominal x-ray is useful for the diagnosis. In some diseases such as intussusception, the distribution of air, the presence of an opacity in the upper abdomen obscuring the caudal border of the liver, or on the contrary, the presence of air or opacities suggestive of feces in the cecum may help to confirm or rule out the diagnosis, although specificity and sensitivity are low. Bowel obstruction, renal lithiasis, pneumoperitoneum and pneumatosis intestinalis (**Fig. 66.2**) can be evaluated well by plain x-ray. Although air or barium contrast studies of the colon have been considered the standard diagnostic tests for intussusception, many authors consider the abdominal ultrasound to be the elective initial study when this diagnosis is suspected. Ultrasound is the preferred method to study the biliary duct, delineate abdominal masses, and distinguish appendix inflammation from other intra-abdominal or pelvic pathology. The double-contrast CT scan helps to determine the size, location, and relation of an intra-abdominal mass to other organs, and it is also useful to study the cause of an intestinal obstruction, to evaluate the pancreas and retroperitoneal and pelvic pathology. In adult and pediatric emergency medicine, the practice is to avoid giving analgesia in patients with abdominal pain before the surgeon's evaluation; however, other authors suggest that morphine can reduce the intensity of the abdominal pain without adversely affecting the diagnosis of appendicitis.

If perforation, peritonitis, or ischemic bowel compromise is suspected, immediate surgical intervention is necessary. If bowel obstruction is suspected,

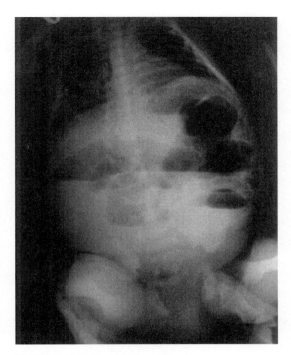

FIGURE 66.2. Paralytic ileus. Enteritis.

the placement of a nasogastric tube is always necessary. The critically ill child receiving mechanical ventilation is usually sedated and may be receiving muscle relaxants. In this situation, physical examination may not reflect the abdominal pathology, and a high degree of suspicion is essential. Clinical worsening, persistence of signs of infection or inflammation, increased nasogastric fluid losses, or persistence of ileus should be considered as possible markers of underlying abdominal pathology. Frequent clinical examination and serial imaging studies will indicate the need of more invasive procedures.

SPECIFIC PATHOLOGIES

Bowel Obstruction

Bowel obstruction is a mechanical blockage to the transit of the intestinal contents. This barrier may be either intrinsic (intraluminal or from the bowel wall) or due to extrinsic compression. The first one may include obstruction secondary to *Ascaris lumbricoides* (still existent in developing countries) or obstruction as a consequence of intussusception, whereas causes of extrinsic compressions may include postsurgical adhesions or incarcerated hernia.

Congenital causes of small-bowel obstruction include annular pancreas, malrotation-volvulus, malrotation-Ladd bands, Meckel diverticulum with volvulus or intussusception, inguinal hernia, and intestinal duplication. Duodenal or ileal atresias are congenital causes diagnosed during the newborn period. The most frequent causes of acquired obstructions are postsurgical adhesions and intussusception. Crohn's disease may also be a cause of small-bowel obstruction. Less frequent causes include duodenal hematoma and superior mesenteric artery syndrome.

Congenital obstructions of the colon include Hirschsprung's disease, pseudo-obstruction, volvulus, and colonic duplication. In the immediate neonatal period, imperforate anus or colonic atresia may be diagnosed. As acquired causes, Crohn's disease and toxic megacolon associated with ulcerative colitis need to be mentioned. In patients with cystic fibrosis, acquired obstructive syndromes in the distal ileon or in the colon may be present.

Clinical presentation may include cramping abdominal pain, nausea, bilious vomits, and absence of intestinal transit when the obstruction is complete. Cramping abdominal pain is changed to continuous pain once intestinal ischemia commences to develop. Typically symptoms are more sudden, intense, and progressive than in ileus wherein symptoms are less intense and have a slower progression. The patient with mechanical obstruction presents with severe pain and systemic signs such as tachycardia, sweating, and occasionally shock. The abdomen is usually distended, and there are increased bowel sounds. Plain abdominal x-ray may reveal air fluid levels in the small bowel, dilated small-bowel or colon loops, intestinal wall edema, or minimal intestinal gas distal to the obstruction. Upright position is necessary to visualize air-fluid levels (see **Fig. 66.2**). Abdominal CT scan is the study of choice to identify less clear causes of obstruction or to evaluate the presence of ischemia. Postponing surgery for more than 24 hrs in a complete obstruction increases the risk of ischemia and intestinal resection.

Intussusception

Intussusception represents the most common cause of acute abdomen in infancy and preschool children. It occurs when one segment of the intestine (proximal) is telescoped into the adjacent segment (distal). Meckel diverticulum, intestinal polyps, hemangioma, mucosal haemorrhage, and lymphoma are causes of lead points.

The classic clinical picture occurs in a previously healthy infant who presents with severe paroxysmal colicky pain accompanied by drawing up of the legs and intense weeping. Initially, the child recovers between episodes; however, if the diagnosis is delayed, progressive lethargy occurs in most cases. Emesis is usually present, and normal stools may be present during the initial phase. Passage of red-currant-jelly stool or presence of blood in rectal examination may happen during the first 12 hrs but may also occur later. A slightly tender sausage-shaped mass may be palpable in the sub-hepatic region of the abdomen. The initial diagnosis depends on clinical examination and may be confirmed by means of abdominal ultrasound. Ultrasound may show a tubular mass in the longitudinal views or a doughnut or target sign in transverse images. Other traditional diagnostic alternatives, especially indicated when ultrasound is not available, include the plain abdominal x-ray and the enema contrast study that combines the diagnostic and therapeutic procedures.

Nonsurgical reduction is contraindicated when symptoms have been present during >48 hours or in the presence of shock, peritoneal irritation, perforation, pneumatosis, or ultrasound findings predictive of failure or suggestive of the presence of a lead point. When nonsurgical reduction fails or is not possible, urgent laparotomy is the rule. Need of surgical reduction, bowel resection, and complications are directly related to the time elapsed since the onset of symptoms.

Peritoneal Adhesions

Postsurgical adhesions may produce folding or strangling of the bowel loops or less frequently may predispose to intestinal volvulus secondary to loop distension and peritoneal shortening. The presence of fever, leucocytosis, or peritoneal signs are suggestive of intestinal ischemia. Usual treatment includes NG tube placement, hydration and presurgical antibiotic therapy. Many patients recover spontaneously without need of surgery.

Others Causes of Intestinal Obstruction

A child with incarcerated hernia presents with a sudden attack of irritability, rejection to feed, and irritability and, when it can't be reduced or there are signs of incarceration or ischemia, urgent surgical consultation is indicated.

The patients with Crohn's disease may present with signs or symptoms of intestinal obstruction produced by the intestinal strictures that may affect the small bowel or the colon. The challenge in these patients is to resolve if the symptoms are linked to the chronic inflammatory disease and can be resolved by intensifying the treatment or if they need surgical intervention. The diagnosis is established with colonoscopy. The CT scan and MRI may help to identify transmural lesions and to exclude strictures.

The tumors usually present as abdominal masses and not as acute episodes of intestinal obstruction. The neuroblastomas originated in the suprarenal gland are the most frequent abdominal tumors in infants, and they usually present as a large abdominal mass, rarely the presence of intratumoral bleeding, or the intestinal compression may cause an acute abdomen. The Wilms tumor, due to its retroperitoneal origin, may grow significantly without compressing other structures. Lymphomas are the third most frequent tumor in children. These are aggressive and diffuse tumors and may present with abdominal pain, vomiting, diarrhea, distension, and occasionally intussusception, peritonitis, or ascitis. Meckel's diverticulum may also be a cause of bowel obstruction by acting as a lead point in intussusception, by formation of adhesions or internal hernias, and it may also produce loop volvulus. Hirschsprung's disease or congenital aganglionic colon is usually diagnosed during the neonatal period owing to the presence of meconial ileus. However, in some cases, this sign may be absent, and presentation may be later with or without signs of acute presentation that may include enterocolitis, bowel obstruction, and sepsis. The enterocolitis is precipitated by bowel dilation, increased intraluminal pressure, compromise of the intestine blood flow, and alterations in the mucosal barrier added to the bacterial proliferation. The diagnosis is established by anorectal manometry and rectal mucosal biopsy. Children with chronic intestinal pseudo-obstruction present symptoms within the first months of life, including abdominal distension, vomiting, chronic constipation, failure to thrive, diarrheic episodes, and abdominal pain.

Intestinal Ischemia

Bowel ischemia frequently arises as a result of the progression of acute pathology which is secondary to anatomic malformations, such as malrotation or progression of a complete mild intestine volvulus. Intestinal mucosal ischemia may occur during or after cardiac surgery in children. Much less frequently, arterial mesenteric thrombosis or venous occlusive thrombosis is reported as causes of intestinal ischemia or gangrene. Colonic ischemia may be secondary to vasculitic processes such as the hemolytic uremic syndrome. Patients with severe bowel ischemia progress from mucosal ischemia to transmural necrosis and bowel perforation. Midgut volvulus with malrotation may cause one of the most severe forms of bowel ischemia **(Fig. 66.3)**. This diagnosis should be suspected in infants and children with severe abdominal

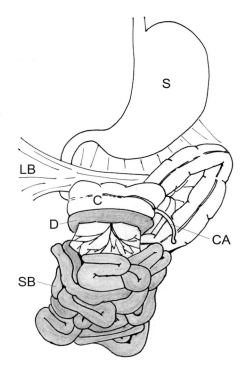

FIGURE 66.3. Volvulus. S, stomach; LB, Ladd bands; C, colon; CA, appendix; D, duodenum; SB, small bowel.

pain and bilious vomiting. The mesenteric vessels are fixed in this structure and are left at risk of a future volvulus. When this happens, intestinal ischemia and necrosis develop rapidly. A child admitted with intestinal ischemia or necrosis is usually in shock, may or may not present abdominal distension depending on the localization of the volvulus, and the abdominal wall may appear to be blue. The classic radiologic findings are the double bubble sign that shows an abdomen with scarce intestinal air with two air bubbles, one in the stomach and one in the duodenum; air fluid levels; abnormal position of the cecum; and absence of distal air. Contrast studies under fluoroscopic control or abdominal CT scan are the elective diagnostic procedures. Treatment is always surgical.

Primary Peritonitis

Primary peritonitis is a peritoneal infection with no apparent intra-abdominal pathology such as perforation, abscesses, or other intra-abdominal sources of infection. In previously healthy children, the history and signs are similar to peritonitis due to suspected appendix perforation, and it is often an intraoperative diagnosis. Primary peritonitis is usually caused by a single organism, the most frequent being *Streptococcus pneumoniae*, group A streptococci, and *Escherichia coli* or other enteric bacteria. The presence of polymicrobial flora or anaerobes is an indicator of perforation and secondary peritonitis.

In children with ascites caused by cirrhosis, portal hypertension or nephrotic syndrome, the diagnosis of primary depends on a high degree of suspicion and should be sought in the presence of fever, increased ascites, or a worsening clinical condition. The most frequent causative agents are enterococcus, streptococcus, staphylococcus, or enteric bacteria such as *E. coli or Klebsiella pneumoniae*.

In children with ascites caused by cirrhosis or nephrotic syndrome, the disease may have an insidious progression, and clinical findings may be similar to those found in children with ascites and without primary peritonitis. Other times, especially in patients with nephrotic syndrome, spontaneous peritonitis may present with severe hypovolemic shock.

Ascitic fluid can reveal a white cell count >250 cells/mcL; >50% polymorphonuclear predominance confirms the diagnosis. Initial empiric antibiotic treatment includes ceftriaxone or cefotaxime in combination with aminoglycosides. In patients with peritoneal dialysis, the diagnosis of primary peritonitis should be suspected in the presence of fever, local signs in the entry site of the cannula, or changes in the characteristics of the dialysate. Confirmed, probable, or possible diagnosis is defined by the presence of >100 white cells/mcL (polymorphonuclear >50%) with or without organisms on Gram stain or culture or symptoms of peritoneal inflammation. The empiric antibiotic treatment depends on the predominant infections in each center. Local treatment adding antibiotic to the dialysate (gentamicin or vancomycin) is possible.

Secondary Peritonitis

Secondary peritonitis is produced by the entrance of bacteria into the peritoneal cavity through a perforation or rupture of the intestinal wall or other viscus as a consequence of obstructive, ischemic, or inflammatory processes. In postpuberal females, bacteria such as *Neisseria gonorrhoeae* and *Chlamydia trachomatis* may invade the pelvic cavity through the fallopian tubes.

The clinical picture includes high fever, diffuse abdominal pain, and vomiting, and the physical findings are the rebound tenderness, wall rigidity, and diminished or absent bowel sounds.

In severe cases, systemic inflammatory response may cause hypovolemia due to third spacing, shock, or acute respiratory distress syndrome. Laboratory tests may show leukocytosis, and the erect abdominal x-ray may show free air in the abdominal cavity, ileus,

and signs of obstruction or obliteration of the psoas shadow.

As secondary peritonitis is caused by rupture of a hollow viscus, the typical microbiologic finding is polymicrobial flora. The most frequent pathogens include enteric gram-negative bacteria (*E. coli*, *Klebsiella*, *Enterobacter*, etc) and anaerobes (*Bacteroides fragilis*, *Clostridium spp*, and others). The site of perforation conditions the inoculum and type of bacteria. The majority of the secondary peritonitis occurrences are a consequence of appendicular inflammation and are conditioned by community pathogens. Therefore, these infections are usually sensitive to antibiotics effective against Gram-negative and anaerobe bacteria. The recovery depends on an adequate and timely surgery and the addition of a broad spectrum antibiotic treatment.

Tertiary Peritonitis

Tertiary peritonitis is defined by the appearance of peritonitis after the failure of more than one surgical procedure undertaken to control an intra-abdominal focus of infection. It is characterized by the presence of nosocomial polymicrobial flora such as coagulase negative staphylococci, candida, enterococcus, pseudomona, or enterobacter. Many times it is not possible to differentiate between a colonization of the peritoneal cavity by these pathogens and an invasive infection. These infections occur as a consequence of alterations in the peritoneal defense mechanisms, and the fluid collections may not be clearly purulent.

Intra-abdominal abscesses may develop in intra-abdominal viscera such as liver, spleen, kidneys, pancreas, or uterine annexes and in the interintestinal, periappendiceal, subhepatic, pelvic, and retroperitoneal spaces. Intra-abdominal abscesses may be community-acquired infections such as those secondary to appendicular infection, or they may be the consequence of complications related to surgical procedures.

The treatment of all patients with intra-abdominal sepsis includes respiratory and hemodynamic stabilization. Initial empiric antibiotic therapy depends on the suspicion of a community acquired or nosocomial infection. Combined regimens of an aminoglycosides (amikacin or gentamicin) and clindamycin or metronidazole or the association of a third- or fourth-generation cephalosporin with an antianaerobe antimicrobial (ceftriaxone + clindamycin or metronidazole) are the most frequently used. Adequate focus control refers to the surgical removal or drainage of the primary cause. Together with the surgeon and with the help of the imaging studies, the source of infection should be identified so as to proceed to its resolution. Antibiotic treatment without drainage of the source may be effective only for small abscesses.

Interloop abscesses and fluid collections may be recurrent or persistent sources of infections wherein antibiotics have poor penetration. The usefulness of closed drains of the peritoneal cavity to prevent abscesses is arguable. The resolution of these collections is achieved by ultrasound or CT-guided needle aspiration or with laparotomy.

Fistulae are abnormal epithelized ducts that connect two hollow viscera or a hollow viscus with the skin. Fistulae may happen in the context of an intestinal operation and in the presence of an inflammatory process. During the development of a fistula and before it finally connects to the skin or to another viscus, the conduct may act as an occult source of infection. The best way to study the tract is by injecting hydrosoluble contrast material through a catheter that is introduced into the external opening and obtaining a radiographic sinogram (fistulogram).

Enteritis

We will not describe necrotizing enterocolitis of the newborn, a severe and frequent complication in neonatal intensive units, in this chapter. However, it should be considered when premature babies or post-surgical newborns are admitted to the PICU.

Intestinal infections may be caused by a wide variety of enteropathogenic organisms including bacteria, viruses, and parasites. There are two basic types of acute infectious diarrhea: (a) inflammatory, caused by bacteria that invade the intestinal wall, and (b) noninflammatory, produced by enterotoxins, villous lesions (virus) or parasitic or bacterial adherences. The inflammatory diarrheas present with fever and gastrointestinal symptoms such as vomiting, bloody diarrhea, severe abdominal pain, and tenesmus. The finding of leukocytes in the feces indicates the presence of an invasive or cytotoxic producing organism such as Salmonella, Shigella, *Campylobacter jejuni*, enteroinvasive *E. coli*, *Clostridium difficile*, or *Yersinia enterocolitica*. In the presence of bloody diarrhea, stools should be sent to the laboratory for culture and testing for some toxins. When hemolytic uremic syndrome is suspected, it may be confirmed by the growth of *E. coli* 0.157 and the finding of verotoxins in the stools. However, the suspicion of *C. difficile* calls for the performance of adequate cultures and a search for the toxins. Enteric infections may present extraintestinal complications such as neurologic manifestations. Shigella infections may associate bloody diarrhea with seizures and fever. In previously healthy hosts, the presence of bloody diarrhea caused by the verotoxin-producing *E. coli* 0157 may develop into a hemolytic uremic syndrome. In this disease, the classic triad consisting of microangiopathic hemolytic anemia, thrombocytopenia, and oligoanuria may be associated with severe complications of the gastrointestinal tract, mainly severe ischemic lesions in the colon.

Neutropenic Enterocolitis

In children with oncologic diseases receiving chemotherapy or during the course of a bone marrow transplant, the onset of abdominal pain and fever have to alert investigators about process such as typhlitis or neutropenic enterocolitis. The presence of an intra-abdominal infectious process in these children, usually localized in the right lower quadrant, implies a therapeutic dilemma wherein surgical treatment may have infectious and hemorrhagic risks due to the cytopenia. Neutropenic enterocolitis or typhlitis is a gastrointestinal complication of chemotherapy that may be life-threatening. It is more frequent during the treatment of lymphomas or leukemias and also with the use of new chemotherapy drugs for the treatment of solid tumors, bone marrow transplantation conditioning, immunosuppressor therapy for transplants, and AIDS. The term *typhlitis* defines an inflammation of the cecum that may extend to the terminal portion of the ileum and the ascending colon. The pain may be localized in the right iliac fossa, or it may be diffuse with peritoneal reaction. Other symptoms that may be present include aqueous or bloody diarrhea, abdominal distension, and vomiting. Symptoms appear between 10 and 14 days after the chemotherapy.

The plain abdominal x-ray may show signs compatible with obstruction, but the diagnosis is confirmed by ultrasound or CT scan. These may show a thickening of the walls of the cecum or other involved areas with mucous edema, fat or mesenteric infiltration, pneumatosis, and free cavity fluid. The treatment includes broad-spectrum antibiotics, nasogastric tube, intestinal rest, parenteral nutrition, and close observation.

Acute Pancreatitis

An inflammation of the pancreas can cause an acute abdomen, and it constitutes a life-threatening disease when it is severe or in the presence of local complications such as necrosis, pseudocysts, and pancreatic abscesses. Trauma, structural anomalies, and multisystemic diseases are the most frequent causes. Mild inflammations may cause abdominal pain and moderate increases of the amylase, and the child usually presents acutely ill with nausea, vomiting, and abdominal pain. The pain is usually epigastric and may irradiate toward the back in adult patients. Abdominal distension and muscular guarding, irritability, hemodynamic compromise, fever, jaundice, ascites, hypocalcemia, and pleural effusion may be present. The diagnosis should be raised in children with acute abdomen and/or SIRS without a clear cause or in the presence of probable etiologic factors. The diagnosis is confirmed by an increased serum amylase and lipase of at least three times their normal value (>300 U/L and 900 U/L, respectively). Pancreatic enzymes may also be elevated in other situations including perforated gastroduodenal ulcers, intestinal perforation or occlusion, peritonitis, acidosis, and renal failure.

Ultrasound and CT scan are the diagnostic studies that are used to confirm the diagnosis, evaluate the etiology and search for complications. The plain abdominal x-ray may reveal indirect signs such as sentinel loop, ileus, blurring of the psoas, transverse colon dilation, or pancreatic calcification, whereas the chest x-ray may show basal infiltrates, diaphragmatic elevation pleural effusion, or pulmonary edema. The CT scan is the most useful study to confirm the diagnosis and to exclude other causes of acute abdomen. The use of contrast allows the identification.

Treatment includes early fluid resuscitation, hemodynamic stabilization, and adequate oxygen administration. Nasogastric tube insertion is necessary so as to relieve the symptoms, especially in patients with gastric atony. There is no clear evidence of the role of prophylactic antibiotic treatment in the prevention of infection of the necrotic areas. Infection of these necrotic areas is the most severe local complication and is associated with high mortality.

Feeding can be started once the symptoms settle and the levels of pancreatic enzymes decrease. The effects of feeding should be controlled by clinical examination and the serum enzyme levels. Parenteral nutrition should be started in severe cases. One of the most frequent complications during the course of the disease is the formation of pseudocysts. They are followed-up with ultrasound and are usually asymptomatic and have a spontaneous resolution. Local infection should be suspected in the presence of fever, leukocytosis, pain, or abdominal guarding. The CT scan is used during the follow-up and to guide invasive draining procedures.

Ileus

Ileus is defined as an intestinal dysmotility in the absence of a mechanical obstruction. Signs and symp-

toms include diminished or absent bowel sounds, failure to pass stools or flatus, abdominal distension, vomiting, or increased volume through the nasogastric tube or an increased gastric residual volume during enteral feeds. The presence of ileus may provoke severe consequences such as ischemia, perforation, or compartment syndrome. Increased air in the small bowel, intestinal distension, or air-fluid levels are signs suggestive of ileus. The abdominal CT can differentiate ileus from mechanical obstruction. The most frequent cause of ileus is intestinal manipulation during abdominal surgery. The ileus may extend from 3 to 5 days after a major intra-abdominal surgery. The presence of ileus predisposes to vomiting and aspiration pneumonia, intestinal ischemia, fluid and electrolyte imbalances, sepsis, and difficulty in reestablishing nutrition. Narcotics inhibit peristalsis. The generation of tolerance to opioids for their analgesic effect does not include the gastrointestinal effect; therefore, higher doses lead to worse constipation. Severe hypokalemia, exogenous catecholamines, general anesthetics, and a diversity of medicines such as benzodiazepines, calcium channel-blocking agents, and anticholinergics may be involved in the development of ileus. Enteral nutrition should not be used in the hemodynamically unstable patient. During resuscitation, the use of vasoactive drugs may further reduce the splanchnic flow. Enteral nutrition should be delayed until perfusion has been reestablished.

Gastric decompression with a nasogastric tube during ileus is an indication for avoiding the risk of vomiting and aspiration pneumonia and to improve the intestinal flow. The use of peridural anesthesia with bupivacaine is one of the known strategies for patients.

Acute Cholecystitis

Acute cholecystitis may be associated with total parenteral nutrition, hemolytic diseases, or cystic fibrosis. The laboratory findings are nonspecific and may include leukocytosis, elevated bilirubin, gamma-glutamyltranspeptidase, and enzymatic mobilization (AST, ALT). Ultrasound is the most useful diagnostic test. The absence of gallstones does not rule out the diagnosis. Initial treatment of acute cholecystitis consists in the administration of antibiotics that are effective against gram negatives, enterococcus, and anaerobes.

Pseudomembranous Colitis

Clostridium difficile is a gram-positive, anaerobic, spore-forming rod that can be responsible for the development of colitis. It usually affects patients who are receiving or have received antibiotics during the previous 3 weeks. The diagnosis is confirmed by means of stool culture and stool assays for toxins. An infrequent but very severe complication is the toxic megacolon. The treatment for *C. difficile* infection includes vancomycin via the oral or nasogastric routes (10 mg/kg/dose) 6 hourly (maximum dose, 500 mg) during 7 days. In the presence of toxic megacolon, the addition of IV metronidazole (8 hourly) is recommended. Broad-spectrum antibiotics should be stopped or avoided if possible to stimulate the recovery of the endogenous flora.

Toxic Megacolon

Toxic megacolon presents as an acute abdomen with abdominal distension, fever, hemodynamic involvement, alterations in the level of consciousness, hypoalbuminemia, electrolyte disbalances, leukocytosis, and thrombocytopenia. It may progress to septic shock and multiple organ failure. The treatment includes circulatory and hydration optimization, ventilatory support when necessary, intravenous antibiotics, hydrocortisone 1.5 mg/kg/dose 6 hourly (up to 100 mg 6 hourly), and digestive decontamination with nonabsorbable antibiotics via the nasogastric tube (polymyxin, tobramycin, and Amphotericin B). Factors that favor intestinal hypomotility, such as hypokalemia or hyperglycemia, should be corrected, and the use of drugs that inhibit the peristaltic activity should be discontinued when possible. Probiotics via enteral feeds may be useful. Indications of surgery include progression to multiorgan failure, tomographic signs of progression, or signs of peritonitis or perforation.

Abdominal Compartment Syndrome

Abdominal compartment syndrome (ACS) is defined as the presence of abdominal distension with an intra-abdominal pressure >15 mm Hg, accompanied by at least three of the following signs: oliguria or anuria, respiratory decompensation, (reduction of the thoracic compliance with increased CO_2 or decreased PaO_2/FIO_2), hypotension or shock, and metabolic acidosis. The hemodynamic and respiratory functions and the urinary output improve within the first hour after decompressive surgery. The measurement of the intra-abdominal pressure is achieved by means of a T-piece with a three-way stopcock placed between urinary catheter and the pressure tubing followed by the injection of 25–50 mL of sterile isotonic sodium chloride solution through the distal stopcock and into the urinary catheter and then opening the stopcock to the transducer.

Diabetic ketoacidosis may present abdominal pain and vomiting associated with polyuria, glucosuria, ke-

tonuria, acidosis, and hyperglycemia. The child may present a tense abdomen with guarding and absent bowel sounds simulating an acute abdomen.

Acute porphyries are hereditary and acquired diseases in which the activity of the enzymes responsible for the heme biosynthesis pathways is partially or completely deficient. One of the clinical types, the acute intermittent porphyria, may present with nausea, vomiting, abdominal pain, diarrhea, constipation, or ileus.

Rheumatologic Diseases

The children and adolescents with rheumatologic diseases sometimes may need intensive care due to digestive hemorrhage or intra-abdominal complications. In systemic lupus erythematosus (SLE) the incidence of gastrointestinal compromise ranges between 20% and 40%. The digestive hemorrhages usually present as a complication of steroid or nonsteroidal anti-inflammatory therapy. Among the abdominal complications, ischemic lesions due to mesenteric vascular compromise may be observed. Other complications include perforations, intussusception, intestinal volvulus, or colonic strictures. Episodes of acute pancreatitis have been described in patients with SLE, juvenile rheumatoid arthritis, and Kawasaki disease. Episodes of primary peritonitis without evidence of infection or perforation have been described in patients with familial Mediterranean fever, SLE, Still disease, and juvenile rheumatoid arthritis.

Henoch-Schönlein purpura affects small vessels, and it is the most frequent cause of non-thrombocytopenic purpura in children. The association of colicky abdominal pain, arthralgia or arthritis, edema in dependent or distensible areas, palpable non-thrombocytopenic purpura, and proteinuria are the basis of the diagnosis. A severe abdominal pain may be sometimes the only symptom, and recognizing the diagnosis can avoid unnecessary surgery. The pain is usually colicky, and it may be accompanied by fecal occult blood or hematemesis. The renal compromise may be demonstrated by the presence of isolated hematuria or proteinuria or by the presence of findings compatible with glomerulonephritis. The treatment with steroids has been associated with a fast improvement of the gastrointestinal or neurologic complications; however, the use of steroids with the initial symptoms has not shown to reduce the risk of renal compromise or the frequency of gastrointestinal complications.

Kawasaki disease may present initially with signs and symptoms of an acute abdomen but not accompanied by sufficient signs for the diagnosis of Kawasaki disease (elevated fever, leukocytosis, and accelerated erythrosedimentation rate).

Sickle cell disease is a hereditary disease that presents chronic hemolytic anemia and recurrent episodes of pain as cardinal manifestations. The episodes of acute pain, previously called sickle cell crisis, are based on the occlusion of the bone marrow vascular bed that leads to bone infarction and release of inflammatory mediators. Severe abdominal pain can be one of the clinical manifestations.

CHAPTER 67 ■ FULMINANT HEPATIC FAILURE AND TRANSPLANTATION

PIERRE TISSIÈRES • DENIS J. DEVICTOR

FULMINANT HEPATIC FAILURE

One accepted definition proposed by the King's College group defines fulminant hepatic failure (FHF) in children as "a multi-systemic disorder in which severe impairment of liver function, with or without encephalopathy, occurs in a patient with no recognized underlying chronic liver disease" (**Table 67.1**). Speed in determining the etiology of the FHF and providing a diagnosis is essential. In the newborn, the clinical spectrum of metabolic FHF is characterized by the association of coagulopathy, hypoglycemia, lactic acidosis, failure to thrive, and irritability, but jaundice is frequently lacking at the time of FHF diagnosis. Association of hypoglycemia, lactic acidosis, neurologic, muscle, and renal tubular abnormalities in an infant should raise the suspicion for mitochondrial diseases. Diagnosis of fulminant Wilson disease is based on the presence of hemolytic anemia, elevated serum and urinary copper levels, low ceruloplasmin (normal in 15% of cases), low alkaline phosphatase in regard to the elevated bilirubin (total bilirubin to alkaline phosphatase <1 mcmol/IU), and the presence of Kayser-Fleischer rings on slit-lamp eye examination. Renal function is frequently impaired. Hepatitis A is the most frequently encountered infective FHF (1.5%–3%) in infants and children and represents a public health challenge in endemic regions. Neonatal herpes simplex infection is well known to produce devastating FHF associated with encephalitis in the first week after birth.

Acetaminophen overdose is the most common cause of toxic FHF. It is more frequently encountered in adults and teenagers (intentional overdose) than in children (inappropriate dosage regimen). Sodium valproate-induced FHF has a significant resemblance to Reye syndrome and mitochondrial cytopathy. Volatile anesthetics (halothane, enflurane, isoflurane, sevoflurane) cause FHF in children. Other drugs, such as carbamazepine, sulfasalazine, antituberculosis drugs, and recreational drugs (ecstasy, cocaine), are involved in drug-induced FHF. Mushroom-induced FHF can occur after ingestion of a wide variety of mushrooms, including *Amanita phalloides* and *Lepiotae* species. Phosphorus and carbon tetrachloride intoxication are other potential causes of FHF.

In the newborn and infant, giant-cell hepatitis may cause FHF. It is associated with an immune hemolytic anemia (positive Coombs test) and can evolve to FHF if immunosuppressive therapy is not initiated. In older children, autoimmune hepatitis can be diagnosed if autoantibodies (antiendoplasmic reticulum, antismooth muscle, or anticytosolic antibodies) are recovered in the plasma. Leukemia and other lymphoproliferative syndromes with massive hepatic infiltration may cause FHF in children. In the newborn, familial lymphohistiocytosis may present as FHF with hypofibrinogenemia, coagulopathy, elevated liver enzymes and, sometimes, jaundice. Associated hyponatremia, hypertriglyceridemia, high ferritin level, pancytopenia, cerebrospinal fluid lymphocytosis, and signs of hemophagocytosis on marrow smear obtained after bone marrow transplantation are highly suggestive. Macrophage activation syndrome is increasingly recognized as a cause of FHF, and an association with a viral trigger should be suspected.

Veno-occlusive disease of the liver (i.e., hepatic vein occlusion after bone marrow transplantation or chemotherapy), Budd-Chiari syndrome (i.e., obstruction of the hepatic venous outflow) or "cardiac liver" (left heart hypoplasia) may initially display an FHF. A reversible hepatic insufficiency occurs

TABLE 67.1

DIAGNOSTIC WORKUP

GENERAL WORKUP

Na, K, Cl, Phos, Mg, Ca, BUN, creatinine, LDH, lactate, ammonia, blood gas; complete blood count; Coombs test, Blood, urine and CSF culture; blood group determination, AST, ALT, alkaline phosphatase, γ-glutaryl transferase, total and conjugated bilirubin, α-fetoprotein. Prothrombin time, partial thrombin time, fibrinogen, factor II, V, VII, IX, X activity, D-dimer.

METABOLIC WORKUP

Tyrosinemia	Urine succinyl acetone, wrist x-ray
Galactosemia	Red cell galactose-1-phosphate uridylyl transferase activity (spot test)
Hemochromatosis	Ferritin level, extrahepatic iron deposition, i.e., salivary gland (biopsy, NMR)
OTC deficiency	Orotic acid
Wilson disease	Serum ceruloplasmin, serum, and urinary copper, Kayser-Fleischer rings
Reye syndrome and fatty-acid oxidation disorders	Urinary and blood organic acid chromatography, carnitine and fatty-acid level
Mitochondrial cytopathy	Mitochondrial DNA, muscle and liver biopsy for quantitative respiratory chain enzyme determination. CSF lactate, creatinine kinase, echocardiography

INFECTIOUS WORKUP

Hepatitis A, B; HHV-1, 2, 6; CMV; EBV; VZV; echovirus; adenovirus; enterovirus; parvovirus B19	Viral serology, keep frozen serum, PCR (blood, CSF), stool culture
Treponema pallidum (syphilis)	VDRL (maternal if newborn)

OTHER

Familial lymphohistiocytosis and macrophage activating syndrome	Blood triglycerides, cholesterol, ferritin, bone marrow analysis
Autoimmune	Coombs test, autoantibodies, biopsy
Intoxication	Acetaminophen level, salicylate level, keep frozen urine and blood
Vascular	Echocardiography

NMR, nuclear magnetic resonance; OTC, ornithine transcarbamylase; HHV, human herpes virus; CMV, cytomegalovirus; EBV, Epstein-Barr virus; VZV, varicella-zoster virus; PCR, polymerase chain reaction; CSF, cerebrospinal fluid; VDRL, venereal disease research laboratory test

frequently after cardiogenic shock, septic shock, multiorgan failure, or any significant hypoperfusion state.

Clinical Manifestations

In the newborn, symptoms are nonspecific, sometimes only related to an altered general condition, failure to thrive, and vomiting, whereas in older children, most have jaundice associated with hepatic encephalopathy. In viral-induced FHF, jaundice is preceded by symptoms such as fever, myalgia, arthralgia, and nausea. Thereafter, jaundice worsens, liver enzymes become increasingly elevated, and prothombin time becomes prolonged before hepatic encephalopathy appears, underscoring hepatic dysfunction secondary to significant viral destruction of the liver. In some cases, in which initial viral-induced cytolytic effect and jaundice are minimal, a delayed improvement (days to weeks) is followed by a recurrence secondary to a viral-induced autoimmune response that is frequently associated with fever, anorexia, abdominal pain, vomiting, and encephalopathy. In some cases, such as after drug/toxin or metabolic-induced FHF, encephalopathy or bleeding can occur before the occurrence of the jaundice. Hepatic encephalopathy is a reversible chemical and neurophysiologic status that occurs when liver function is altered. There is a difference between hepatic encephalopathy that occurs in chronic liver disease and acute hepatic encephalopathy that occurs during FHF, which is often associated with cerebral edema and intracranial hypertension. Hepatic encephalopathy can occur a few hours to days after jaundice appears. In the newborn, hepatic encephalopathy is nonspecific and can be reflected only by behavioral changes, agitation, and a high-pitched cry. These signs may precede the development of brisk reflexes, clonus, and appearance of a coma with hypertonia, agitation, and pupillary abnormalities (sluggish

GRADES OF HEPATIC ENCEPHALOPATHY

I	Changes in behavior, minimal change in level of consciousness, altered sleep (hypersomnia, insomnia, inversed sleep cycle in the newborn)
II	Spaciotemporal disorientation, drowsiness, inappropriate behavior, obvious asterixis
III	Marked confusion, stuporous, respond or not to auditory stimuli, decerebrate posturing to pain, asterixis usually absent
IV	Comatose, unresponsive to pain, decorticate posturing

Adapted from Atterbury CE, Maddrey WC, Conn HO. The West Haven criterion. Neomycin-sorbitol and lactulose in the treatment of acute portal-systemic encephalopathy. A controlled, double-blind clinical trial. *Am J Dig Dis* 1978;23:398–406.

then fixed), followed by a deeper coma with hypotonia and brainstem coning. Hepatic encephalopathy is classified into 4 grades using a modification of the West Haven criteria (**Table 67.2**). Status epilepticus may complicate hepatic encephalopathy. Diagnostic workup is directed toward establishing a diagnosis and characterizing the severity of liver failure (see **Table 67.1**).

Perioperative complications of FHF are listed in **Table 67.3**. Renal failure may be secondary to hypovolemia, acute tubular necrosis, or a functional renal failure, as in hepatorenal syndrome. Hepatorenal syndrome, defined as a progressive renal insufficiency in patients with liver disease, is characterized by a low urine sodium output and elevated urinary-to-plasma ratios for creatinine and osmolarity. In patients with FHF, type 1 hepatorenal syndrome is defined as a rapid and progressive renal impairment characterized by renal cortical vasoconstriction and corticomedullary redistribution of renal blood flow. Recognized risk factors are low mean arterial blood pressure and dilutional hyponatremia. Hepatorenal syndrome may be precipitated after digestive bleeding, septicemia, and dehydration. Nephrotoxic drugs such as aminoglycosides should be avoided. Tubular nephropathy is frequently observed and results in low blood phosphate, magnesium, and potassium. If renal failure occurs, dialysis should not be delayed. Continuous, rather than discontinuous, renal replacement therapy is preferred. Evidence is limited to support the potential utility of *N*-acetylcysteine in improving renal function as part of the management of FHF. Use of terlipressin, for type-I hepatorenal syndrome, even at a low dose, is not recommended due to the risk

PREOPERATIVE AND EARLY POSTOPERATIVE COMPLICATIONS OF FULMINANT HEPATIC FAILURE

Preoperative	Postoperative
Cerebral edema	Cerebral edema
Intracranial hypertension	Intracranial hypertension
Circulatory collapse	Hypovolemia, hemorrhage
Dysrhythmia	Myocardial dysfunction
Hypoxemia, ARDS	Hypoxemia, ALI-VILI, ARDS
Renal failure	Renal failure
Hemostasis disorders	Anemia, thrombocytopenia, leucopenia
Disseminated intravascular coagulopathy	Hemostasis disorders
Metabolic and electrolyte disorders (hypoglycemia, hypokalemia, hyponatremia, hypophosphatemia, hypomagnesemia), lactic acidosis, hyperammonemia, kernicterus	Disseminated intravascular disorders, electrolyte disorders
Bleeding disorders (gastrointestinal, cerebral)	Abdominal compartment syndrome, Acute pancreatitis, bleeding disorders, hemorrhage (abdominal), primary graft nonfunction, graft vascular anastomosis stenosis/thrombosis, acute graft rejection
Bacterial sepsis	Bacterial and fungal sepsis

ARDS, acute respiratory distress syndrome; ALI, acute lung injury; VILI, ventilator-induced lung injury of increased cerebral blood flow, hyperemia, and intracranial hypertension. Hepatorenal syndrome will reverse in most cases after liver transplantation.

Pulmonary edema is related to neurogenic pulmonary edema coupled with fluid overload (syndrome of inappropriate antidiuretic hormone, hyperaldosteronism). In addition, ventilation-perfusion mismatch (loss of vasoconstrictive hypoxia mechanism due to circulating vasodilatory substances) occurs and results in severe refractory hypoxemia. The hemodynamic profile of FHF patients is characterized by cardiac hyperkinesia with elevated cardiac indices and low systemic vascular resistances. Adrenal insufficiency is frequently found in adults with FHF and is associated with hemodynamic instability.

Severity of systemic inflammatory response syndrome may be correlated with progression of hepatic encephalopathy, development of respiratory failure, disseminated intravascular coagulopathy, renal failure, acute pancreatitis, and multiorgan failure. Risk of developing sepsis in the course of FHF is elevated, which may be related to a decreased immune response to pathogens and may be aggravated by invasive procedures inherent in the critically ill condition.

Severe hypoglycemia frequently occurs in FHF patients as a result of impaired glycogen storage, decreased gluconeogenesis, hyperinsulinism (decreased insulin degradation and increased insulin resistance), and increased glucose use (anaerobic metabolism) should be recognized early. Fat and protein stores are used, leading to breakdown of muscle and adipose tissue. Glucagon and growth hormone levels are increased, which further increases catabolism. Energy expenditure in FHF is elevated. Hyponatremia, hypokalemia, hypophosphatemia, and hypomagnesemia can be found in patients with FHF. Kernicterus may precipitate hepatic encephalopathy and appear if plasma direct bilirubin is >26 mg/dL, especially if blood-brain barrier permeability is increased (acidosis, hypoxemia).

Patients should be admitted to the ICU if they show signs of clinical or electric hepatic encephalopathy, if F.V activity decreases below 50%, PT index decreases to <50% (PT index = standard PT/observed PT × 100), and/or if significant lactic acidosis (>2.0 mEq/L), and/or renal failure, and/or intractable hypoglycemia occur.

Some causes of FHF may respond to a specific therapy (**Table 67.4**). In the infant, congenital galactosemia and hereditary fructose intolerance can lead to FHF that is reversible within a week if galactose and fructose are removed from the diet. Acute hepatic manifestations of hereditary tyrosinemia can occur early in life and are usually triggered by infection. Acetaminophen is a dose-related hepatotoxin, with most ingestion that exceeds 150 mg/kg leading to FHF. **Figure 67.1** is an acetaminophen toxicity nomogram.

Treatment of cerebral edema should include (a) lowering endogenous nitrogen intake (by limiting

TABLE 67.4

RECOMMENDED SPECIFIC THERAPIES

Cause	Treatment	Quality of evidence
Hereditary tyrosinemia	Nitisinone (NTBC or 2-(2-nitro-4-trifluoromethylbenzoyl)-1,3-cyclohexanedione) 1 mg/kg/day orally in 2 doses	II-1
Neonatal hemochromatosis	Deferoxamine 30 mg/kg/day IV in 3 doses Selenium 2–3 mcg/kg/day IV N-acetylcysteine 140 mg/kg then 70 mg/kg orally or IV α-tocopherol polyethylene glycol succinate 20 UI/kg/day orally	II-3/III
Herpetic hepatitis	Acyclovir 150 mg/m^2/day IV	I
Acetaminophen poisoning	Activated charcoal 1 g/kg orally	I
	N-acetylcysteine 150 mg/kg IV in 15 min, then maintenance dose 50 mg/kg over 4 hrs, followed by 100 mg/kg administered over 16 hrs	II-1
Mushroom poisoning	Penicillin G 300,000–1 million units/kg/day IV Silymarin 30–40 mg/kg/day IV or orally	II-3

Quality of evidence: I, randomized, controlled trials; II-1, controlled trials without randomization, II-2, cohort or case-controlled analytic study; II-3, multiple time series, dramatic uncontrolled experiments; III, expert opinions

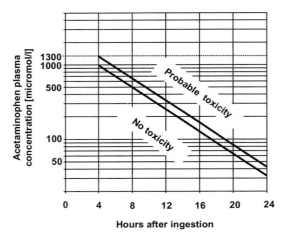

FIGURE 67.1. Acetaminophen intoxication nomogram. The time coordinates refer to time of ingestion. Blood level drawn before 4 hrs may not represent peak value. The graph should be used only in relation to a single, acute ingestion. The lower solid line, 25% below the standard nomogram, is included to allow for possible errors in acetaminophen plasma assays and estimated time from ingestion. Acetaminophen concentration conversion: 1 mg/L = 6.6 mcmol/L. Adapted from Rumack BH. Acetaminophen overdose in young children. Treatment and effects of alcohol and other additional ingestants in 417 cases. *Am J Dis Child* 1984;138:428–33.

bleeding and infection and preventing slowed intestinal transit) or exogenous nitrogen intake (by keeping protein delivery below 0.5 g/kg/day and avoiding unjustified fresh frozen plasma administration) and (b) administration of oral or rectal lactulose (10–15 mL/kg, titrated to result in 2–4 daily soft stools), an osmotic cathartic nonabsorbable disaccharide. Neomycin is not recommended and should not be used, as it may precipitate renal failure. Ornithine aspartate and sodium benzoate have been proposed to decrease serum ammonia, as in Reye syndrome and in urea cycle defects, but hemofiltration remains the main treatment of acute hyperammonemia. In patients with signs (decerebrate posturing, pupillary abnormalities) or measured intracranial hypertension, treatment with mannitol (0.25–0.5 g/kg bolus) is recommended. Hyperventilation to reduce $PaCO_2$ to 30 mm Hg is known to quickly lower ICP. Barbiturate use (thiopental, pentobarbital) may be considered for severe intracranial hypertension. Moderate hypothermia (32°C–34°C; 89.6°F–93.2°F) prevents increases in ICP during liver transplantation for FHF. Corticosteroids and flumazenil are not recommended.

In the absence of bleeding, it is not recommended to correct homeostasis, because doing so will interfere with the evaluation of liver function (F.V activity, PT). An exception would be if an invasive procedure is planned, such as placement of a central venous catheter. In these cases, procedures can be performed under cover of platelet or administration of activated recombinant F.VII if profound thrombopenia ($<10,000/mm^3$) is observed. Activated recombinant F.VII induces hemostasis at the site of injury independent of the presence of F.VIII or F.IX. It is recommended for the treatment of bleeding episodes and for the prevention of bleeding in patients with congenital F.VII deficiency who are undergoing surgery or an invasive procedure. The recommended dosage is 15–30 mcg/kg every 4–6 hrs until hemostasis is achieved. Administration of fresh-frozen plasma is hampered by the risk of volume and protein overload and should be thoughtfully evaluated. Vitamin K is routinely administered intravenously. Patients with FHF are at risk for gastrointestinal bleeding. Histamine-2 receptor blockers should be avoided because of their effect on the CNS. Sucralfate is therefore preferred. No study has evaluated proton-pump inhibitors for gastrointestinal bleeding prophylaxis in FHF patients.

Hypovolemia may be present at admission, but fluid resuscitation should be monitored carefully in regard to volume overload, especially if renal failure occurs. Vasoplegia will generally respond to α-adrenergic agents that should be used as a first-line drug for hypotension once intravascular volume has been restored. As adrenal insufficiency can occur in FHF, hydrocortisone may be beneficial if hemodynamic instability occurs. Although myocardial dysfunction is unusual, echocardiographic examination may help to appreciate pulmonary pressure, preload condition, and contractility. Continuous glucose administration (frequently up to 1 g/kg/hr) is necessary and often requires a central venous line to deliver high-concentration dextrose in a smaller volume. Phosphate, magnesium, and potassium supplementation is common. Enteral nutrition (gastric, duodenal), and stress ulcer prevention should be initiated early. Protein intake should be limited to 0.5 g/kg/day. Finally, branched-chain amino acids are not recommended. Liver support devices have been developed to circumvent the lack of efficient treatment for FHF. The latest generation of liver support techniques can be divided into ex vivo whole-organ perfusion (animal or human), bioartificial liver support using hepatocytes, "detoxification" methods, or a combination of these techniques.

Emergency liver transplantation remains the only treatment of end-stage FHF in children. Transplantation decisions rely on the cause and severity of FHF, the potentiality of spontaneous liver regeneration, and the comorbidities, especially the development of permanent neurologic damage and, ultimately, death. In adults, the most commonly used transplantation criteria are those developed at King's College in London and Beaujon's Hospital in Paris. However, these criteria fail to be adequate in children. In children, etiology is a critical determinant of outcome. Fulminant Wilson disease and undetermined FHF carry the worst prognosis and require emergency liver transplantation, whereas hepatitis A-induced and acetaminophen-induced FHF have significant spontaneous recovery without transplantation. Emergency liver transplantation should be discussed if hepatic encephalopathy is higher than grade II associated with F.V activity <20% or prothrombin index <20% (PT index = standard PT/observed PT × 100). These levels should be adjusted for the age of the patient (in infants, encephalopathy could be unapparent). Other criteria that suggest emergency liver transplantation include a rapid decrease in liver size, seizures, ascites, hepatorenal syndrome, a fibrinogen level <1 g/L, bilirubinemia >23 mg/dL, worsening lactic acidosis, and hyperammonemia >150 mmol/L.

Malignant disease, such as leukemia, lymphoproliferative syndrome, lymphohistiocytosis, and some mitochondrial respiratory chain disorders, as well as the patient's end-stage intracranial hypertension or uncontrolled multiorgan failure, are contraindications to transplantation.

Neurologic awakening from coma is the key element in early postoperative evaluation, as it determines the success of overall management (see **Table 67.3**). Early circulatory resuscitation may be required due to bleeding. It is not unusual to have depressed cardiac outflow associated with inadequate preload. Intra-abdominal pressure monitoring is required, especially in small receiver-to-donor weight ratio, because intra-abdominal hypertension and/or abdominal compartment syndrome will precipitate vascular thrombosis, liver hypoperfusion, graft failure, oliguria, lactic acidosis, and respiratory restrictive syndrome. High ventilatory pressure may alter respiratory function and gas exchange and decrease abdominal wall compliance, increasing intra-abdominal pressure and potentially affecting graft perfusion. Postoperative hemofiltration may effectively control water balance and serve to supplement temporary renal failure. Electrolyte homeostasis is particularly important, as hypophosphatemia may interfere with extubation success.

TRANSPLANTATION

The most common indication for pediatric liver transplantation is biliary atresia and patients with progressive disease despite the Kasai procedure. Infants with dysfunctional portoenterostomies may develop recurrent bacterial cholangitis, ascites, portal hypertension, hypersplenism, gastrointestinal bleeding (varices), and liver failure. Other causes include Alagille syndrome, progressive familial intrahepatic cholestasis (Byler syndrome), α-1 antitrypsin deficiency, Wilson disease, tyrosinemia, type IV glycogen storage disease, Crigler-Najjar syndrome, inborn errors of bile acid synthesis, and urea cycle defects.

Use of calcineurin inhibitors, cyclosporine, sirolimus, tacrolimus, and chimeric humanized monoclonal antibodies (basiliximab and daclizumab) has drastically improved graft survival. Immunosuppressive protocols vary among centers. The degree of immunosuppression will determine the risk of rejection and hematologic, renal, and neurologic complications of overdosage. Daily determination of calcineurin blood level is essential because it will help in dosing immunosuppressive therapy. Multiple commonly used medications interact with calcineurin inhibitor pharmacokinetics, as displayed in **Table 67.5**.

One of the most feared postoperative complications is primary graft nonfunction, which requires

TABLE 67.5

DRUG INTERACTION WITH CALCINEURIN INHIBITORS

Increase blood level		Decrease blood level	
Increased absorption	**Decreased metabolism**	**Decreased absorption**	**Increased metabolism**
Grapefruit juice	Ketoconazole	Phenytoin	Corticosteroids
Octreotide	Fluconazole	Carbamazepine	
Metoclopramide	Itraconazole	Barbiturates	
	Quinolones	Imipenem	
	Ganciclovir		
	Acyclovir		
	Trimethoprim-sulfamethoxazole		

emergency retransplantation. It usually occurs within the first 48 hrs, and diagnosis is based on absence of neurologic awakening, hepatic encephalopathy, hemorrhagic diathesis, increasing liver enzymes, lactic acidosis, and vasoplegic shock. Vascular thrombosis is the main postoperative complication that will cause graft loss. Hepatic artery thrombosis occurs usually within the first 30 days after transplantation and can occur with fulminant allograft failure, biliary obstruction, or sepsis. Successful thrombectomy is possible if hepatic artery thrombosis diagnosis is made before graft necrosis occurs. Biliary complications are particularly frequent after hepatic artery thrombosis because the hepatic artery offers most of the vascularization to the bile duct. Early portal vein thrombosis occurs usually within the first week (median, 2 days) after transplantation and requires emergency thrombectomy in most cases. Children with biliary atresia have an increased risk of portal vein thrombosis (20%), and deficiencies of anticoagulant proteins (proteins C and S and antithrombin III) should be excluded. Refractory ascites may indicate a portal thrombosis or stenosis or stenosis of suprahepatic veins. As a minor vascular gradient may precipitate extensive ascites, investigational technical limits as well as high intravascular volume may mask a small but significant vascular stenosis, and this should be considered when vascular investigations of refractory ascites are performed. Biliary complications (anastomosis stricture, biliary sludge, and recurrent cholangitis) do not significantly affect immediate postoperative care. Rising serum bilirubin and alkaline phosphatase may signify acute rejection, although biliary expression of rejection is usually a late event. Viral infection (cytomegalovirus, Epstein-Barr virus, and adenovirus) should be considered, as it may precipitate liver rejection. Liver biopsy is the key for diagnosis, and histologic findings of acute rejection are a mixed portal inflammatory infiltrate, predominantly mononuclear cells associated with portal and central vein endotheliitis and bile duct damage. The primary treatment is a short course of high-dose methylprednisolone, which is effective in treating rejection in 80% of cases.

Patients, due to their immunosuppressed condition, are at risk of developing nosocomial and opportunistic infection. In addition, the patient's preoperative condition may be a risk factor for sepsis. Children with chronic cholestasis have increased risk for bacterial peritonitis and recurrent cholangitis. Bacterial sepsis occurs in the immediate posttransplant period and is more frequently due to Gram-negative enteric organisms, *Enterococcus spp.* and *Staphylococcus spp.* Fungal sepsis (*Candida spp.*, *Aspergillus spp.*) may occur in the early posttransplant period and hold an elevated mortality if severe infection occurs, making monitoring of colonization index and early treatment mandatory. Frequent postoperative prophylactic regimens include acyclovir, amphotericin B, a β-lactam antibiotic, and trimethoprim-sulfamethoxazole. Although viral and opportunistic infections may occur later after transplantation, Epstein-Barr virus, cytomegalovirus, herpes simplex virus, and adenovirus can cause early infection.

Perioperative trauma may result in digestive perforation in 20% of children with biliary atresia. Acute pancreatitis may occur in <2% of children who undergo liver transplantation but is associated with high mortality (50%). Postoperative cardiopulmonary failure (restrictive or obstructive) cardiomyopathy (oxalosis, chronic cholestasis) and pulmonary hypertension (hepatopulmonary syndrome, pulmonary vein stenosis in Alagille syndrome) may be encountered.

CHAPTER 68 ■ INTESTINAL AND MULTIVISCERAL TRANSPLANTATION

GEOFFREY J. BOND • KATHRYN A. FELMET • RONALD JAFFE • KYLE A. SOLTYS • ROBERT H. SQUIRES, JR. • DOLLY MARTIN • RAKESH SINDHI • KAREEM ABU-ELMAGD • GEORGE V. MAZARIEGOS

Diseases associated with loss of intestinal function can be divided into surgical and nonsurgical etiologies. The indications for transplantation in the case experience at the University of Pittsburgh and Children's Hospital of Pittsburgh are listed in **Table 68.1**.

Parenteral nutrition (PN) is the standard of care for patients with intestinal failure who are unable to maintain a normal nutritional fluid balance and electrolyte state by use of the gastrointestinal tract alone. Intensive care of children with intestinal and

TABLE 68.1

INDICATIONS FOR COMPOSITE AND ISOLATED INTESTINAL TRANSPLANTATION

Pediatric patients	Adult patients
Volvulus	Trauma
Gastroschisis	Superior mesenteric artery
Necrotizing	thrombosis
enterocolitis	Crohn disease
Intestinal atresia	Desmoid tumor
Pseudo-obstruction	Volvulus
Microvillus inclusion	Familial polyposis
disease	Gastrinoma
Intestinal polyposis	Budd-Chiari disease
Hirschsprung disease	Intestinal adhesions
Trauma	Pseudo-obstruction
	Inflammatory bowel disease
	Radiation enteritis

combined intestinal and liver failure can generally be divided into two categories: (a) need for PN and associated vascular access issues and (b) development of liver disease. The success of the intestinal or multivisceral transplantation depends in large measure on the health and nutritional status of the transplant recipient.

PARENTERAL NUTRITION DEPENDENCE

The central lines of patients with short-gut syndrome can become infected by external contamination of the line and by translocation of bacteria across a gut with inadequate barrier function. Because patients have been repeatedly exposed to broad-spectrum antibiotics and because intestinal stasis may contribute to bacterial overgrowth, infections that result from bowel translocation may be multiply resistant. Fungal infections occur more commonly in this patient group compared to the general population. Enteric feedings may help to preserve intestinal mucosa barrier function and decrease infectious complications. The combination of adrenal insufficiency, relative immune deficiency, and the intestinal transplant candidate's requirement for invasive procedures creates a dangerous susceptibility to severe sepsis and septic shock.

Patients with severe liver failure may have a hyperdynamic state at baseline but a blunted contractile response to stress. Both systolic and diastolic ventricular function may be impaired. Clinical experience indicates that children with cirrhotic cardiomyopa-

thy may not tolerate a large-volume fluid challenge. Resuscitation should be appropriately aggressive but with careful attention to signs of intravascular volume overload, as patients may have concomitant hepatopulmonary or hepatorenal syndrome. Palpation of the liver may not be a reliable indicator of intravascular volume overload in patients with cirrhosis; instead, clinicians must often rely on changes in central venous pressure, development of rales on lung exam, and changes on chest x-ray. Echocardiogram can be used in difficult cases to assess cardiac filling and function. In patients with advanced liver disease, albumin may be preferable to crystalloid as a resuscitation fluid to avoid worsening anasarca. High salt loads (e.g., normal saline) should be avoided in established liver disease.

Inotropic or vasopressor agents should be used if clinical signs suggest that the child is intravascularly replete. Low diastolic blood pressures are associated with advanced liver disease. Early septic shock in these children follows a vasodilatory pattern commonly seen in adults and may respond to vasopressor agents. In patients with catecholamine unresponsive septic shock, adrenal function should be evaluated. In some cases it may be appropriate to treat adrenal insufficiency empirically (hydrocortisone bolus and intermittent dosing or continuous infusion) while results of these tests are pending.

When infections cannot be cleared, it may be necessary to remove and replace lines. As children who await intestinal transplant are dependent on central access, meticulous care must be given to prevention of infection and preservation of line sites when possible. Intestinal transplant candidates are at high risk for forming clots around central lines that can become occlusive and persist after line removal. Although failure of clotting is a more obvious sign of liver dysfunction, patients with liver failure are also unable to synthesize anticoagulating factors, such as protein C, protein S, and antithrombin III.

LIVER FAILURE

Coagulopathy, portal hypertension with ascites and hepatomegaly, variceal bleeding, hypoalbuminemia, hyperbilirubinemia, hyperammonemia with hepatic encephalopathy, and hepatorenal and hepatopulmonary syndrome may all be seen. Intestinal transplant candidates with cirrhosis and liver failure have increased abdominal girth due to organomegaly and ascites. In children, particularly infants <1 year of age, the abdominal contents, especially an enlarged liver, may impinge on lung volumes and impede respiration. Although the problem is easily overcome with positive-pressure ventilation, mechanical ventilation should be considered as a last resort, as it brings with it the problems of sedation, respiratory muscle deconditioning, and ventilator-associated pneumonia. Drainage of ascitic fluid may relieve symptoms. Relief is usually temporary, as the circumstances that lead to the fluid collection persist. The indications for peritoneal drainage must be weighed against the risk of infection. Additionally, rapid drainage of large volumes of peritoneal fluid may lead to intravascular hypovolemia and shock.

Combined liver and intestinal transplant patients and multivisceral transplant patients often have some degree of renal dysfunction that renders them sensitive to fluid overload. Repeated infections with fungus and Gram-negative organisms expose these patients to multiple nephrotoxic agents. Additionally, episodes of septic shock can expose the kidney to low flow states, causing acute tubular necrosis. Hepatorenal syndrome is a very late finding in liver failure but can contribute to renal insufficiency. In cases of severe or recurrent bleeding, plasma exchange (plasmapheresis) and judicious use of recombinant factor 7 have been successful in correcting coagulopathy without fluid overload. Plasma exchange may also have a role as a liver support therapy.

THE TRANSPLANT OPERATION

Obtaining vascular access, especially when the liver requires transplantation, can be problematic in these patients who have multiple thrombosed veins. Innovative therapies, including reopening venous channels and intra-arterial perfusion, may be necessary. Access issues are best determined prior to the patient's going to the operating room due to the time constraints involved in minimizing the cold ischemic time of the allograft. Even so, time is often spent at the beginning of the procedure establishing appropriate access. The recipient operation consists of removal of the failed organs after exposure of the vascular anatomy, followed by allograft implantation.

POSTTRANSPLANTATION MANAGEMENT

The immunosuppression regimens include a number of drugs. Currently, thymoglobulin is given as 7.5 mg/kg in divided doses of 5 mg/kg before allograft reperfusion and 2.5 mg/kg after reperfusion in children. Methylprednisolone is given as a bolus (2 mg/kg/IV) as premedication for the lymphocyte depleting agent to limit the cytokine reaction, but this drug is not used routinely postoperatively. Rejection is treated with optimization of tacrolimus levels, supplemental corticosteroids, and monoclonal or polyclonal antibody if necessary. Additional or alternative agents have occasionally been used, including azathioprine, rapamycin, cyclosporin, and mycophenolate mofetil.

Pretransplantation status, postoperative graft status, sepsis, inability to close the abdominal wall, and the presence of diaphragmatic weakness or paralysis must be considered in formulating a plan for weaning the intestine transplant patient from the ventilator. Pain management is a serious complicating factor, as many chronic patients have been on long-term pain medications and obtaining the appropriate level of analgesia may be difficult.

Recipients of intestinal grafts receive prophylactic, broad-spectrum IV antibiotics. Antiviral prophylaxis currently includes a 2-week course of IV ganciclovir (5 mg/kg twice daily IV).

Cytomegalovirus (CMV)-specific hyperimmune globulin (CytoGam) (150 mg/kg IV at 2, 4, 6, and 8 weeks after transplantation and 100 mg/kg/dose IV at 12 and 16 weeks after transplantation) and oral ganciclovir for 90 days is given in CMV-negative recipients of CMV-positive allografts. Oral administration of trimethoprim-sulfamethoxazole (80 mg orally 3 times weekly) is used for the lifetime of the patient as prophylaxis against *Pneumocystis carinii* pneumonia. Bacterial translocation most commonly occurs during episodes of acute rejection, when the mucosal barrier of the allograft has been immunologically damaged, or in enteritis associated with Epstein-Barr virus infection.

The normal intestine is pink and nonedematous and occasionally demonstrates contractions. Changes in the ileal stoma postoperatively should be promptly investigated and vascular, technical, or immunologic causes ruled out. Routine endoscopic surveillance is used to assess graft integrity and for the diagnosis of intestinal rejection. Normal stomal output is 40–60 mL/kg/day. No reliable serum test exists for monitoring function intestinal grafts. While PN is continued in the early postoperative weeks, enteral nutrition is introduced once integrity of the gastrointestinal tract has been demonstrated by contrast study, usually at 1 week after transplantation.

Graft Rejection

Clinically, intestinal allograft rejection may be asymptomatic or present with fever, abdominal pain, distention, nausea, vomiting, and a sudden increase or decrease in stomal output. The stoma may be normal

TABLE 68.2

PEDIATRIC INTESTINAL TRANSPLANTATION: CYTOMEGALOVIRUS DISEASE, POSTTRANSPLANTATION LYMPHOPROLIFERATIVE DISEASE, AND REJECTION BY ERA

Years	Drugs	CMV rate	PTLD rate	Rejection rate
1990–1995	Tacrolimus/Steroids	25%	43%	81%
1995–1997	Cyclophosphamide	60%	20%	79%
1997–1998	Tacrolimus/Steroids	13%	25%	
1998–2001	Daclizumab	4%	22%	79%
2002–2005	Thymoglobulin preconditioning protocol	8%	8%	46%

CMV, cytomegalovirus; PTLD, posttransplantation lymphoproliferative disease

in appearance or lose its normal velvety appearance and become friable or ulcerated. Chronic rejection is observed in ~15% of patients. The presentation may include weight loss, chronic diarrhea, intermittent fever, or gastrointestinal bleeding. Acute rejection occurs in ~50% of patients with the use of a preconditioning protocol (see **Table 68.2**). Lower overall immunosuppression use has subsequently resulted in a concomitant reduction in CMV and Epstein-Barr virus disease.

Mild graft rejection in most cases responds to IV methylprednisolone, with optimization of tacrolimus levels to 15 ng/mL. Antibody therapy with OKT3 is used when rejection has progressed despite a steroid taper or as the initial therapeutic agent in cases of severe mucosal injury and crypt damage.

Biliary Complications

With the modification in donor technique, allowing preservation of the donor duodenum and entire pancreas, and maintenance of the hepaticopancreaticobiliary system, biliary and pancreatic complications from leaks and strictures from anastomoses have been avoided. However, a group of these patients has been identified who have signs and radiologic evidence of obstruction, perhaps from ampulla of Vater dysfunction. This obstruction can occur months to years after transplantation and can be managed via percutaneous transhepatic cholangiography with balloon dilation and/or endoscopic retrograde cholangiopancreaticogram and stenting or incision of the ampulla. In modified multivisceral grafts, continuity of the biliary axis is surgically reestablished, either via a Roux-en-Y enteric loop or duct-to-duct in bigger donors and recipients. Correspondingly, these grafts can develop biliary system-related surgical complications (i.e., leaks and obstructions).

Infection

Fungal infections are more common after heavy treatment for rejection, extensive antibiotic usage, intestinal leaks, and multiple surgical explorations. The current incidence of CMV infection is ~8% (see **Table 68.2**). Clinical presentation is usually with enteritis. Successful clinical management has been accomplished in the majority of episodes, using ganciclovir alone or ganciclovir in combination with CMV-specific hyperimmunoglobulin. A CMV-positive donor graft transplanted into a CMV-negative recipient is a significant risk factor for CMV disease, but monitoring of CMV polymerase chain reaction with preemptive therapy has allowed the successful use of CMV-mismatched organs.

Presentation of posttransplantation lymphoproliferative disease (PTLD) may include asymptomatic findings at routine endoscopy, Epstein-Barr virus enteritis and systemic symptoms, bleeding, lymphadenopathy or tumors. PTLD has decreased in incidence to <10% (see **Table 68.2**) under current immunosuppression. Therapy includes reduction of immunosuppression, antiviral therapy using ganciclovir, acyclovir, and/or hyperimmunoglobulin; rituximab (anti-CD20 monoclonal antibody); and chemotherapy.

Graft-Versus-Host Disease

Skin changes consistent with graft-versus-host disease were diagnosed by histopathologic criteria in ~5% of cases and confirmed by immunohistochemical studies visualizing donor cell infiltration into the lesions on two occasions or by flow cytometry detecting elevated donor cell chimerism in peripheral blood.

CHAPTER 69 ■ CRITICAL ASPECTS OF INTESTINAL DISORDERS

ARISTIDES BALTODANO • MEHRENGISE K. COOPER

SMALL INTESTINE

The net effect of passage through the small intestine is absorption of most of the water and electrolytes (sodium, chloride, potassium) and essentially all dietary organic molecules (including glucose, amino acids, and fatty acids). Through these activities, the small intestine not only provides nutrients to the body but plays a critical role in water and acid-base balance. The absorption of virtually all nutrients into blood entails breaking down large supramolecular aggregates into small molecules that can be transported across the epithelium. The microvillus border of intestinal epithelial cells is referred to as the "brush border." Several types of bacteria produce toxins that strongly, often permanently, activate the adenylate cyclase, leading to elevated levels of cAMP and causing the chloride channels to essentially become stuck in the "open position." The result is massive secretion of water that is manifested as severe diarrhea. Cholera toxin, produced by cholera bacteria, is the best-known example of this phenomenon. The transporter that carries glucose and galactose into the enterocytes is the sodium-dependent hexose transporter, known as SGLUT-1. Glucose is transported out of the enterocyte through a different transporter (GLUT-2) in the basolateral membrane.

LARGE INTESTINE

The mucosa of the large intestine is devoid of villi. It has numerous crypts that extend deeply and open onto a flat luminal surface. Mucus-secreting goblet cells are much more abundant in the colonic epithelium than in the small intestine. The large intestine absorbs water, sodium ions, and chloride ions and secretes bicarbonate ions and mucus. Water is absorbed in response to an osmotic gradient. The colonic epithelium is actually more efficient at absorbing water than the small intestine, and sodium absorption in the colon is enhanced by aldosterone. Secretion of bicarbonate ions into the lumen aids in neutralization of the acids generated by microbial fermentation in the large gut. Goblet cells are abundant in the colonic epithelium, and they secrete mucus in response to tactile stimuli from luminal contents as well as parasympathetic stimuli from pelvic nerves. Fermentation is the enzymatic decomposition and utilization of foodstuffs, particularly carbohydrates, by microbes. The large intestine does not produce its own digestive enzymes but contains huge numbers of bacteria that have the enzymes to digest and utilize many substrates.

The GI tract has a nervous system called the *enteric nervous system*. It lies entirely in the wall of the gut, beginning in the esophagus and extending all the way to the anus. The enteric nervous system is composed mainly of two plexuses: (a) an outer plexus that lies between the longitudinal and circular muscle layers, called the *myenteric plexus* or Auerbach plexus, and (b) an inner plexus, called the *submucosal plexus* or Meissner plexus, which lies in the submucosa. The myenteric plexus mainly controls GI movements, and the submucosal plexus mainly controls GI secretion and local blood flow.

GASTROINTESTINAL PERFUSION

Several vasodilator substances affect GI blood flow, including cholecystokinin, vasoactive intestinal peptide, gastrin, and secretin. Some of the GI glands release kallidin and bradykinin into the gut wall. These kinins are powerful vasodilators that are believed to cause much of the increased mucosal vasodilation that occurs along with secretion. Decreased oxygen concentration in the gut wall can increase intestinal blood flow. The decrease in oxygen can also lead to an increase of adenosine, a vasodilator. Stimulation of the parasympathetic nerves going to the stomach and lower colon increases local blood flow at the same time that it increases glandular secretion. Sympathetic stimulation causes intense vasoconstriction of the arterioles with greatly decreased blood flow. After a few minutes of this vasoconstriction, the flow often returns to almost normal by means of a mechanism called *autoregulatory escape*. The local metabolic vasodilator mechanisms that are elicited by ischemia overcome the sympathetic vasoconstriction and, therefore, redilate the arterioles.

THE GUT AS AN IMMUNE SYSTEM

Saliva contains peroxidase, which inhibits the growth of bacteria, and lysozyme, which lyses bacteria and enhances phagocytosis. The mucous layer provides a barrier that separates bacteria from the villous surface of the small intestine. The bile acids (chenodeoxycholic and cholic acids) possess antibacterial qualities. Cryptdins are low-molecular-weight proteins that are derived from the Paneth cells in the crypts of Lieberkühn. The primary cellular barrier of the gut that restricts luminal antigens from encountering the immune system is the single layer of gut epithelium. Two different classes of pattern recognition receptors are involved. The Toll-like receptors (TLRs) are usually associated with cell membranes and the nucleotide-binding oligomerization domain (Nod) molecules. Signaling through Nod or TLR activates the transcription factor nuclear factor κB, leading to proinflammatory gene expression. Healthy individuals possess an abundant and highly active gut immune system that is tightly regulated to prevent excessive immune responses to foods and gut bacteria.

NEUTROPENIC ENTEROCOLITIS (TYPHLITIS)

Typhlitis is a life-threatening oncologic emergency that occurs in the presence of neutropenia, often in the induction phase of chemotherapy for leukemia. It is an inflammatory process of the GI tract that presents as NEC in the cecum and ascending colon. Abdominal ultrasound typically reveals a right lower-quadrant inflammatory mass, bowel wall edema, and pericecal fluid or soft-tissue inflammation. CT may be the preferred diagnostic modality over ultrasound and plain abdominal films. Barium enema and colonoscopy can be hazardous and may be contraindicated, as they can precipitate perforation. The syndrome is characterized on CT scan by bowel wall thickening, inflammation, and the presence of peritoneal fluid and other areas of edema. As chemotherapy can alter the GI mucosa in cases of gastritis and esophagitis, it can also decrease the integrity of the colon, causing tissue alteration and inflammation and precipitating the invasion of bacteria, which results in septicemia. Necrosis can result in bowel perforation, seen as pneumatosis intestinalis on plain x-rays, especially with an infectious process. Treatment must be broad-spectrum antimicrobial, encompassing coverage for Gram-negatives, -positives, anaerobes, and fungus.

Neutropenic enterocolitis should be suspected in any severely neutropenic patient (absolute neutrophil count <500/mL) who presents with fever and abdominal pain, particularly in the right lower quadrant, with or without rebound tenderness. Symptoms of typhlitis include right-sided abdominal pain; watery, bloody diarrhea; abdominal distention; and fever. Vomiting, anorexia, and possible hematemesis are also hallmark signs, with guarding and positive peritoneal signs found on physical exam. Typhlitis represents an emergency, as it could lead to bowel obstruction or perforation, necessitating an immediate surgical referral. Treatment for the child with typhlitis includes obtaining serial abdominal x-rays, CT, or ultrasounds; ensuring bowel rest; administering broad-spectrum antibiotics; monitoring and managing fluids and electrolytes; and providing nutrition in the form of total parenteral nutrition.

HYPOMOTILITY

Postoperative ileus, defined as the functional inhibition of propulsive bowel activity after surgery, irrespective of pathogenic mechanism, is common, especially after abdominal laparotomy. Like opiates, dopamine has been shown to impair GI motility. This negative effect can be seen at doses as low as 5 mcg/kg/min and worsens with increasing rates of infusion. Other commonly used medications that cause GI hypomotility are phenothiazines, diltiazem, verapamil, and drugs with anticholinergic side effects. If necessary, nasogastric suction and/or rectal tubes and, in intractable cases, colonoscopy can be used to decompress the GI tract. Rectal tubes have been associated with complications, including discomfort, local ulceration, infection, and perforation of rectum. Prokinetic agents, such as erythromycin, have been shown to promote gastric emptying in patients receiving mechanical ventilation and should be considered once mechanical obstruction is excluded. Low-dose erythromycin (1–3 mg/kg) effectively stimulates gastric antral motility. A total daily dose of 20 mg/kg/day divided in 3–4 doses per day, by mouth, is generally used for prokinetic effects. Metoclopramide is another prokinetic agent that is useful in the treatment of gastroduodenal hypomotility.

DIARRHEA

Diarrhea is defined as a change in bowel habit for the individual child that results in substantially more

TABLE 69.1

CAUSES OF DIARRHEA IN ICU PATIENTS

Enteral nutrition
  Hyperosmolar formulas
  High infusion rates
  Dietary lipids
Infection
  Viruses (*Rotavirus, adenovirus, calicivirus, astrovirus*)
  Bacteria (*Salmonella* spp., *shigella* spp., *C. difficile, C. jejuni, E. coli* O157H:, *Yersinia* spp.)
  Parasites (*Aeromonas* spp., *G. lamblia, Cryptosporidium* spp.)
Medications
  Antacids
  H_2-Receptor antagonists
  Antibiotics
Hypoalbuminemia
  Particularly those with chronic severe hypoalbuminemia (<2.6 g/dL)
Prolonged fasting (>5 day)

Adapted from Mutlu GM, Mutlu EA, Factor P. GI complications in patients receiving mechanical ventilation. *Chest* 2001;119:1222–41.

frequent and/or looser stools. The etiology of diarrhea in the ICU is probably multifactorial (**Table 69.1**). Reducing the rate of tube feeds generally improves diarrhea, probably by reducing the carbohydrate load to the gut. Dilution of enteral formulas may not be helpful, especially if the patient is receiving an iso-osmolar tube feeding. Luminal excess of bile acids may be a cause of diarrhea in ICU patients. The administration of bile acid–binding agents improves diarrhea. Liberal use of antibiotics in ICU patients predisposes patients to antibiotic-associated diarrhea. *C. difficile* is associated with significant morbidity and even mortality if fulminant colitis or toxic megacolon (TM) develops. The classic example of secretory diarrhea is that induced by cholera and *Escherichia coli* enterotoxins. Osmotic diarrhea has a reduced volume of stool per day, a lower sodium content, a pH of <5, tests positive for reducing/nonreducing sugars, and usually responds to fasting. Hypoalbuminemia has been implicated as a predisposing factor for diarrhea in critically ill patients, especially those with a serum albumin level <2.6 g/dL and those with chronic malnutrition.

After documenting increased stool frequency and volume, gross stool examination must be conducted to detect blood, leukocytes, mucus, ova, and parasites. Presence of leukocytes suggests presence of invasive or toxin-producing microorganism bacteria in the gut, such as *Shigella, Salmonella, Campylobacter jejuni*, invasive *E. coli, C. difficile, Yersinia enterocolitica,*

Vibrio parahaemolyticus, and possibly *Aeromonas* or *Plesiomonas shigelloides*. Cultures for enteric pathogens and enzyme-linked immunosorbent assay for viral pathogens and *C. difficile* toxin are recommended. Osmotic or secretory causes of diarrhea must be ascertained. Patients should be placed on regimens of enteric precautions and empiric antibiotic therapy while the laboratory tests are pending. If the clinical evolution of the child with diarrhea does not suggest *C. difficile*, other common causes of diarrhea (**Table 69.1**) must be ruled out and treated accordingly. Diarrhea is a common cause of fluid loss, dehydration, and electrolyte disorders.

Following are clinical presentations of dehydration. *Mild dehydration* (3% in older children and 5% in infants): normal or increased pulse rate, decreased urinary output, thirst, and normal physical examination. *Moderate dehydration* (6% in older children and 10% in infants): tachycardia, little or no urine output, irritability/lethargy, sunken eyes and fontanelle, decreased tears, dry mucous membranes, mild tenting of the skin, delayed capillary refill, cool and pale skin. *Severe dehydration* (>9% in older children and >15% in infants): rapid and weak pulse, decreased blood pressure, no urine output, very sunken eyes and fontanelle, no tears, parched mucous membranes, tenting of the skin, very delayed capillary refill, cold and mottled skin. Most patients have isotonic dehydration and, therefore, have normal serum sodium values. The water deficit in liters can be estimated as the percent dehydration multiplied by the patient's weight in kilograms. The sodium and potassium deficits are estimated from the water deficit.

For acute dehydration of <3-day duration, a relatively greater loss of the extracellular fluid (ECF) and electrolyte deficits occurs and can be estimated using:

$$\text{Sodium deficit (mEq)} = \text{water deficit (L)} \times 110 \text{ mEq/L}$$

$$\text{Potassium deficit (mEq)} = \text{water deficit (L)} \times 30 \text{ mEq/L}$$

For more prolonged dehydration, of >3-day duration, relatively more intracellular fluid is lost, and electrolyte deficits can be estimated using:

$$\text{Sodium deficit (mEq)} = \text{water deficit (L)} \times 80 \text{ mEq/L}$$

$$\text{Potassium deficit (mEq)} = \text{water deficit (L)} \times 60 \text{ mEq/L}$$

Initial therapy requires administration of 20–40 mL/kg of 0.9% saline or Ringer lactate in the first hour to expand the ECF volume. Rapid administration of larger quantities (60–100 mL/kg) may be necessary to restore circulation. Once ECF volume is expanded and renal perfusion is restored, treatment can be changed to a slower rate to replace maintenance requirements, remaining deficit fluids, and any ongoing abnormal losses. Acidosis is readily corrected when circulation is restored. Because restoration of volume status usually stops production of metabolic acidosis, correction of pH is rarely needed. If bicarbonate losses are large and need to be corrected, the HCO_3 deficit can be estimated using:

$$HCO_3 \text{ deficit (mEq)} = 0.5 \text{ (L/kg)} \times \text{weight (kg)} \times$$
$$[\text{desired } HCO_3 \text{ (mEq/L)} - \text{current } HCO_3 \text{ (mEq/L)}]$$

When the intravascular volume is reestablished, it is appropriate to plan the fluid therapy for the first 24 hrs.

Isonatremic dehydration (serum sodium concentration 130–150 mEq/L) is the most common form of diarrheal dehydration in children. In isonatremic dehydration, water and sodium are lost in physiologic proportion (isotonic loss), thus maintaining the serum sodium concentration within the normal range. In isotonic dehydration, the entire fluid deficit is corrected over 24 hrs.

If possible, oral rehydrating therapy should be started as soon as tolerated, usually 6–12 hrs after parenteral therapy has begun, and continued for the remaining 24 hrs to replace deficit fluids. If IV fluid therapy is warranted, the total amount of water and electrolyte deficits is determined, and appropriate fluids are selected. IV fluid administration can then proceed, using three solutions. One of the solutions can contain the "deficit replacement" for water and electrolytes, the second can contain "maintenance" water and electrolyte fluid, and the third, a fluid with the appropriate water and electrolyte concentrations to address the "ongoing" losses. A two-solution strategy combines the fluid and electrolyte needs both for half of the "deficit" and one-third of the "maintenance," and again, a second fluid is used for replacing "ongoing" losses. One-half of the deficit replacement fluid can be administered over the first 8 hrs, along with one-third of the maintenance fluid. Using the two-solution method, adjustments may be necessary for the next 16 hrs, with a combination of water and electrolytes to address the other half of the "deficit" and the other two-thirds of the "maintenance" fluids.

The potassium concentration of the maintenance solution must be tailored, depending on the clinical situation. Potassium is not usually included in the IV fluids until the patient voids. Half of the total fluid is given over the first 8 hrs; previous boluses are subtracted from this volume. The remainder is given over the next 16 hrs. It is important to consider ongoing fluid losses of the patient. The child with copious diarrhea must receive an additional replacement solution (the ongoing loss replacement), or the rehydration will not be complete. Ongoing losses from diarrhea can vary in their electrolyte concentration. Sodium losses may range from 10 to 90 mEq/L, and potassium losses may range from 10 to 80 mEq/L.

HYPONATREMIC DEHYDRATION

Hyponatremic dehydration (serum sodium concentration <130 mEq/L) occurs when sodium loss is disproportionately greater than the water loss. Because serum osmolality is low, water shifts from ECF into the intracellular fluid, making the symptoms of ECF volume contraction more severe than in the other forms of dehydration. In addition, some patients develop symptoms, predominantly neurologic, from the hyponatremia. The initial goal in treating hyponatremia is correction of intravascular volume depletion with isotonic fluid (normal saline or Ringer lactate). Hyponatremic dehydration requires replacement of sodium and water losses. The excess sodium deficit can be calculated using the following formula:

$$\text{Excess Na deficit (mEq)} = 0.6 \text{ (L/kg)} \times \text{weight (kg)} \times$$
$$[\text{desired Na (mEq/L)} - \text{present Na concentration (mEq/L)}]$$

This is the amount of sodium that should be added to the sodium deficit calculated from the electrolyte deficits based on the fluid loss. It is not necessary to increase the sodium beyond 135 mEq/L, as "overcorrection" is associated with an increased risk of central pontine myelinolysis. The risk of this condition also increases with overly rapid correction of the serum sodium concentration. The risk in children is not clear, but it is prudent to avoid increasing the sodium by >10–20 mEq/L every 24 hrs.

As with isotonic dehydration, half of the deficit replacement fluid can be administered over the first 8 hrs, along with one-third of the maintenance fluid. Again, potassium delivery is adjusted based on the initial serum potassium and the patient's renal function. Potassium is not given until the patient voids. Patients with neurologic symptoms (e.g., seizures) from hyponatremia must receive an acute infusion of hypertonic (3%) saline to rapidly increase the serum sodium concentration to 120 mEq/L. The above formula for excess sodium deficit can be used with 120 mEq as the desired sodium concentration. The calculated amount of Na in mEq needed to raise the Na level to 120 mEq/L can be given as a bolus of 3% normal saline, with each 2 mL of 3% normal saline containing 1 mEq of Na.

HYPERNATREMIC DEHYDRATION

Hypernatremic dehydration (serum sodium concentration >150 mEq/L) occurs when the lost fluid contains less sodium than water (hypotonic fluid). Because of the ECF hyperosmolality, water is osmotically moved from intracellular fluid into the extracellular space. Hypernatremia can cause serious neurologic damage, including hemorrhage and thrombosis. Children with hypernatremia often appear less ill than children with a similar degree of isotonic dehydration. Urine output may be preserved longer, and less tachycardia may occur. Children with hypernatremic dehydration are often lethargic but irritable. Hypernatremia may cause fever, hypertonicity, and hyperreflexia.

Treatment of hypernatremic dehydration may cause significant morbidity and mortality. Generation of idiogenic osmoles occurs within the brain during the development of hypernatremia. These idiogenic osmoles increase the osmolality within the cells of the brain, providing protection against brain-cell shrinkage caused by movement of water out of cells into the hypertonic ECF. However, these idiogenic osmoles dissipate slowly during correction of hypernatremia. With overly rapid lowering of the extracellular osmolality during correction of hypernatremia, an osmotic gradient may be created that causes water movement from the extracellular space into the cells of the brain, producing cerebral edema. Symptoms of the resultant cerebral edema can range from seizures to brain herniation and death. To minimize the risk of cerebral edema during correction of hypernatremic dehydration, the guideline is that serum sodium concentration should not decrease more than 12–15 mEq/L every 24 hrs. Severe hypernatremic dehydration may need to be corrected over 3–4 days.

The initial management of hypernatremic dehydration requires restoration of the intravascular volume with normal saline. Ringer lactate should not be used because it is more hypotonic than normal saline (Ringer lactate has 100 mL more free water per liter than normal saline) and may cause too rapid a decrease in the serum sodium concentration, especially if multiple fluid boluses are necessary. To avoid cerebral edema when correcting hypernatremic dehydration, the fluid deficit is corrected slowly. The rate of correction depends on the initial sodium concentration. Under these circumstances, the free water deficit (FWD) can be estimated using an estimate of the total body water (TBW in liters = 0.6 L/kg × weight in kg) and the following equation:

$$FWD \text{ in liters} = TBW - TBW \left(desired\ Na\ /\ current\ Na \right)$$

The FWD is subtracted from estimated total fluid deficit (in liters = % dehydration × wt in kg) to produce the solute fluid deficit (SFD).

$$SFD \text{ in liters} = Total\ fluid\ deficit - FWD$$

The SFD is used to calculate the amount of electrolytes that have been lost. All of the SFD (and electrolytes) are replaced in the first 24 hrs, while only one-third of the FWD is replaced in the first 24 hrs, and the other two-thirds are replaced in the second 48 hrs. Unlike patients with isotonic or hyponatremic dehydration, the fluid is not run at a faster rate during the first 8 hrs. The choice and rate of fluid administration are not nearly as important as vigilant monitoring of the serum sodium concentration and adjustment of the therapy based on the result. The rate of decrease of the serum sodium concentration is roughly related to the "free water" delivery, although variation between patients is considerable.

C. DIFFICILE AND PSEUDOMEMBRANOUS COLITIS

Most stools from patients with antibiotic-associated pseudomembranous colitis (PMC) contain the *C. difficile* organism as well as its cytotoxin. Disease as a result of *C. difficile* represents a wide spectrum, ranging from asymptomatic carriage, asymptomatic cases, mild nonspecific diarrhea, antibiotic-associated colitis without pseudomembrane formation, PMC, and fulminant colitis. Endoscopy can detect the typical plaque-like lesions of the pseudomembrane.

Treatment with vancomycin is effective but is associated with a relapse rate of up to 20%. Cholestyramine, an anion-exchange resin that binds *C. difficile* toxins, is an alternative to vancomycin. It is more likely to result in primary treatment failure than vancomycin but is less likely to be followed by relapse. Metronidazole and bacitracin can also be used to treat PMC. Oral metronidazole has efficacy similar to that of oral vancomycin in mild and moderate cases. Loperamide, diphenoxylate hydrochloride with atropine, and opioids should be avoided because they can adversely affect the ability to clear the toxins. Fever, systemic manifestations, and severe diarrhea generally improve within 1–2 days of therapy, but diarrhea may last for 4–5 days.

INTESTINAL ISCHEMIA

Splanchnic hemodynamics may be impaired by mechanical ventilation, particularly when a high level of positive end-expiratory pressure is used, as well as by shock and other hypoperfusion/reperfusion states. Abdominal compartment syndrome (ACS) results from intra-abdominal hypertension (IAH). Its main features include abdominal distention and IAH, refractory oliguria or anuria, decreased cardiac output and hypotension secondary to reduced venous return from the lower part of the body, and markedly reduced thoracic compliance. Life-threatening IAH has been described in neonates born with gastroschisis and omphalocele, when primary closure of the abdominal defect was attempted. ACS can develop at an intra-abdominal pressure (IAP) of >17 mm Hg in children and IAP >25 in adults. Patients are diagnosed as having ACS when they have increasing abdominal distention with IAP >15 mm Hg, accompanied by at least three of the following major criteria: oliguria (urine output <1 mL/kg/hr) or anuria refractory to volume expanders or diuretics, hemodynamic instability or hypotension refractory to volume expanders, reduced chest compliance leading to increasing $PaCO_2$ and decreasing PO_2/FIO_2 ratio and requiring higher FIO_2 and ventilatory pressures; and metabolic acidosis with a base deficit >6 mmol/L. IAP is measured as urinary bladder pressure with the patient supine. Once the diagnosis is made, the patients must undergo emergency abdominal decompression.

TOXIC MEGACOLON

Toxic megacolon (TM) is defined as an acute dilation of the colon due to diffuse inflammation or necrosis of the bowel wall in the absence of mechanical obstruction. The crucial features of this disorder are that the dilation results from inflammatory colitis and that it is accompanied by systemic manifestations or toxicity. TM is most frequently associated with idiopathic inflammatory bowel disease, including ulcerative colitis, Hirschsprung disease (congenital megacolon), infectious colitis (amebiasis, salmonellosis, shigellosis, *Campylobacter* and *Yersinia* bacteria), chronic constipation (intestinal dysmotility), and antibiotic-associated PMC.

Signs of colitis, including diarrhea (often bloody), fever, chills, and abdominal cramping, are the predominant clinical features before the onset of TM. The criteria for the clinical diagnosis of TM in adults is radiographic evidence of colonic dilation plus any three of the following: fever >101.5°F (>38.6°C), heart rate >120 beats/min, white blood cell count >10.5 (>10^9/L), or anemia. Patients should furthermore have one of the following criteria: dehydration, mental changes, electrolyte disturbances, or hypotension. No criteria have been developed for children; however, infants and children with TM seem to be toxic, with fever (>39°C), dehydration,

and marked colon dilation (diameter of >1.5 times the width of the vertebra body of the first lumbar spine on plain abdominal radiographs).

A surgical consultation should be obtained on admission, and the patient should be assessed daily by both medical and surgical teams. Complete blood counts, electrolytes, and serial abdominal plain films are reviewed every 12 hrs initially and then daily as the patient improves. Anemia, dehydration, and electrolyte deficits, particularly hypokalemia, may aggravate colonic dysmotility and should be aggressively treated. The bowel should be completely rested, and a nasogastric tube (or long intestinal tube) should be placed initially to decompress the GI tract. Broad-spectrum antibiotics are recommended to reduce septic complications and in anticipation of peritonitis resulting from perforation.

NECROTIZING ENTEROCOLITIS

The characteristic feature of necrotizing enterocolitis (NEC) is bowel wall necrosis of variable length and depth. NEC mainly affects infants in NICUs, and both sporadic cases and nosocomial outbreaks have been described. Clinical evidence of GI and systemic illness is outlined in **Table 69.2**. The management of infants with NEC is initially medical, consisting of remaining in a nothing-by-mouth status for ~10–14 days, orogastric drainage for decompression, IV fluids, and broad-spectrum antibiotics, as well as blood-product transfusion, if necessary. Absolute indications for operation are pneumoperitoneum, intestinal necrosis, or gangrene obtained on paracentesis. Relative indications include deterioration of clinical condition, oliguria, hypotension, metabolic acidosis, thrombocytopenia, leucopenia, leukocytosis, ventilatory failure, portal venous gas, fixed abdominal masses, persistently dilated bowel loops, or erythema of the abdominal wall.

GASTROINTESTINAL BLEEDING

Anatomically, the ligament of Treitz, located at the end of the duodenum and beginning of the jejunum, provides the division between the origins of the upper- and lower-GI tracts; upper bleeds originate proximal to the ligament, and lower bleeds originate distally. Upper-GI tract bleeding typically presents with hematemesis and melena, though with massive acute bleeding, fresh blood may be passed per rectum. Melanotic stools are black, tarry, and contain partially digested blood, giving rise to an offensive smell. When bleeding occurs from the lower GI tract, fresh blood is passed per rectum or mixed

TABLE 69.2

BELL'S CRITERIA FOR NECROTIZING ENTEROCOLITIS

Stage	Classification	Systemic signs	Intestinal signs	Radiologic signs
I	Suspected	Temperature instability, apnea, bradycardia, lethargy	Increased residuals, mild abdominal distension, emesis, guaiac + stool or bright red rectal bleeding	Normal or intestinal dilation, mild ileus
II	Definite	Mild metabolic acidosis, mild thrombocytopenia	Absent bowel sounds, ± abdominal tenderness, ± abdominal cellulitis, or RLQ mass	Intestinal dilation, ileus, pneumatosis intestinalis, ± portal venous gas
III	Advanced	Hypotension, bradycardia, apnea, respiratory and metabolic acidosis, DIC, neutropenia	Peritonitis, marked abdominal distension, and tenderness	Ascites ± pneumoperitoneum

RLQ, right lower quadrant; DIC, disseminated intravascular coagulation

in with stools, and both melena and hematochezia may be present (maroon-colored stools). Where ischemia has occurred (i.e., intussusception), red, "currant jelly" stool may be seen, which is stool that consists of mucus (products of inflammation) and blood. Black stools that are negative for occult blood must

not be mistaken for melena. The causes of upper- and lower-GI bleeding in children by age category are listed in **Table 69.3**.

Massive upper-GI bleeding may arise due to esophageal or gastric varices, vascular anomalies, and gastric or duodenal ulcer disease. Substantial

TABLE 69.3

CAUSES OF GASTROINTESTINAL BLEEDING IN CHILDREN

Upper GI bleeding

Neonates/Infants	*Child*	*Adolescent*
Swallowed maternal blood	Esophagitis	Esophagitis
Esophagitis	Mallory-Weiss syndrome	Mallory-Weiss syndrome
Gastritis	Gastritis	Gastritis
Ulcer/erosions—gastric/duodenal	Ulcer—gastric/duodenal	Ulcer—gastric/duodenal
Vascular malformation	*Helicobacter pylori* infection	*Helicobacter pylori* infection
Vitamin K deficiency	Arteriovenous malformations	Arteriovenous malformations
	Esophageal or gastric varices	Esophageal or gastric varices
	Adverse drug reactions—NSAIDs	Adverse drug reactions—NSAIDs
	Portal hypertension	Portal hypertension
	Swallowed epistaxis	

Lower GI bleeding

Neonates/Infants	*Child*	*Adolescent*
Swallowed maternal blood	Polyps	Infectious enterocolitis
Anal fissures	Hereditary illness	Inflammatory bowel disease
Upper-GI bleed	Intussusception	Arteriovenous malformation
Milk protein allergy	Infectious enterocolitis	Polyps
Necrotizing enterocolitis	Meckel diverticulum	Hereditary illness
Hirschsprung enterocolitis	Hemolytic uremic syndrome	Hemolytic uremic syndrome
Malrotation and volvulus	Henoch-Schönlein purpura	
Infectious enterocolitis	Inflammatory bowel disease	

NSAID, nonsteroidal anti-inflammatory drugs

TABLE 69.4

MANAGEMENT OF ACUTE GASTROINTESTINAL BLEEDING

Stabilization
Airway breathing circulation
Continuous monitoring of vital signs
Central venous pressure in severe cases or when
    volume status unclear or critical

Diagnosis
Source of bleeding
    Nasal, oral, abdominal, and rectal examinations
    Nasogastric aspiration to differentiate upper from
        lower and to assess for ongoing bleeding
    Emesis or gastric contents and stool tests for blood
Imaging studies
    Plain abdominal film
    Abdominal ultrasound
    Upper endoscopy
    Lower endoscopy
    Contrast CT
    Nuclear medicine studies
    Angiography
Laboratory tests
    Complete blood counts
    Coagulation studies
    Fibrinogen D-dimers
    Serum urea nitrogen/creatinine
    Liver function tests
    C-reactive protein
    Stool for white cells
    Stool for culture

Therapeutic interventions
Stop feeding
Neutralize acid
Institute pharmacotherapy
    Octreotide
    Vasopressin
    Activated Factor VII
Invasive Techniques
    Endoscopic resection, cautery, sclerosis, or band
        ligation
    Arteriography and embolization
    Transjugular intrahepatic portosystemic shunt
    Surgery

---

lower-GI bleeding can occur in inflammatory bowel disease, Henoch-Schönlein purpura, intussusception, Meckel diverticulum, vascular anomalies, intestinal duplications, and infectious colitis. Significant bleeding may also arise from GI infections, as a result of critical illness (stress-induced GI bleeding) and as an adverse reaction to drugs, including corticosteroids (more predominantly seen in neonates), nonsteroidal anti-inflammatory drugs, and the newer COX-2 inhibitors. Options in the management of acute GI bleeding are summarized in **Table 69.4**.

Where possible, endoscopy is the investigation of choice and may have therapeutic options as well. Where NEC is suspected, plain abdominal x-ray will show characteristic features of intramural gas or portal air. For suspected intussusception, ultrasound characteristically shows a target lesion of the telescoping small bowel. Contrast CT scans of the abdomen have been used to localize acute lower-GI bleeding points. (99m)Tc(technium)-labeled red blood cells and (99m)Tc-sulphur colloid allow localization of bleeding points when there is active bleeding as low as 0.1 mL/min in the lower GI tract. Large-bore IV access is essential. Saline solution or water at room temperature may be used, via gastric lavage, to determine whether bleeding continues or has resolved. Enteral feeding regimens should be stopped and parenteral feeding commenced in acute situations. Gastric-acid prophylaxis should begin when feedings are held, and enteral feeding should be recommenced as soon as possible. Transfusion with blood and clotting factors (i.e., activated Factor VII) may be necessary for either acute or prolonged chronic bleeding. The somatostatin analog, octreotide (1–2 mcg/kg/hr), has been used to control variceal bleeding due to portal hypertension. IV vasopressin 0.01 (U/kg/min) has been used for GI bleeding.

Bleeding sources such as polyps may be removed using sigmoidoscopy. Thermal or laser coagulation can be applied to lesions with upper-GI endoscopy. Endoscopic emergency sclerotherapy and variceal band ligation are useful for acute variceal bleeding. A beneficial interventional radiology treatment for uncontrolled variceal bleeding in children is the placement of a transjugular intrahepatic portosystemic shunt. Surgery may be indicated in circumstances in which, despite pharmacologic and nonoperative management, bleeding continues.

One of the reasons for a high rate of stress-ulcer bleeding in critically ill children with severe illness or CNS injury is that gastric pH is lower and more difficult to control. Critically ill children who may benefit from stress-ulcer prophylaxis include those with two of the following: respiratory failure, coagulopathy, and a Pediatric Risk of Mortality score of ≥ 10 (when duration of mechanical ventilation is likely to be ≥ 48 hrs). Bleeding is a common occurrence in children with inflammatory bowel disease but usually is not severe. Where colitis is severe and unresponsive to conservative medical management (typically IV corticosteroids and cyclosporin), tacrolimus has been shown to have benefit in the short term. When bleeding is acute and severe, it may be possible to identify the bleeding points by colonoscopy or angiography; however, emergency surgery is often inevitable.

Chronic liver disease leads to portal hypertension and can be complicated by life-threatening GI bleeding. Esophageal varices are the major cause of bleeding in this group, with variceal bleeding dependent upon the height of portal pressure. Bleeding duodenal ulcers have been found concurrently in children with portal hypertension, especially in those who have had a previous variceal bleed. Therefore, it is important to consider both varices and duodenal ulcers as a source of bleeding in children with liver disease.

Infectious agents may cause GI bleeding to different degrees. Organisms associated with bloody diarrhea include Rotavirus, *Salmonella* spp., *Shigella* spp., *Yersinia*, enterohemorrhagic *E. coli*, and *C. difficile*. An uncommon complication of intestinal tuberculosis is GI bleeding after the formation of ulcers in the small bowel and colon. CMV causes a colitis, which may result in severe GI bleeding. *Helicobacter pylori* infection is usually not associated with severe GI side effects. In adults, it is commonly associated with the development of gastric and duodenal ulcers. Diagnosis is confirmed by *H. pylori*–specific IgG, breath tests for urea production, and endoscopic biopsy. Duodenal ulceration is far less common in children. Young children infected with enterohemorrhagic *E. coli* develop bloody diarrhea and the hemolytic uremic syndrome due to the production of verocytotoxins, in particular after infection with *E. coli* 0157.

These patients require resuscitation from GI bleeding and require renal supportive therapy. Continuous venovenous hemofiltration can be used to provide renal support in critically ill patients.

Gastrointestinal Bleeding in Immunocompromised Patients

GI bleeding is the most common presentation of GI CMV disease; the majority of patients infected with CMV in the GI tract are immunocompromised. Another associated feature is fever. At endoscopy, characteristic abnormalities are seen. Treatment is with ganciclovir as first-line therapy. Immunocompromised patients are more susceptible to infections, including those due to opportunist organisms. CMV is a well-recognized cause of massive lower-GI hemorrhage in patients with HIV infection. Bone marrow transplant recipients and those who have received solid-organ transplants are at greater risk of GI complications, including GI bleeding.

Critically ill children after liver and intestinal transplantation develop stress-related GI bleeding. Omeprazole suspension delivered by nasogastric instillation was effective at acid neutralization and preventing GI bleeding as a complication in children with liver or intestinal transplants.

SECTION VIII ■ RENAL, ENDOCRINE, AND METABOLIC DISORDERS

CHAPTER 70 ■ ADRENAL DYSFUNCTION

ABEER HASSOUN • SHARON E. OBERFIELD

Three main classes of hormones are produced by the adrenal cortex: glucocorticoids (e.g., cortisol), mineralocorticoids (e.g., aldosterone), and sex steroids (e.g., testosterone, DHEA, and androstenedione). Conversion of cholesterol to pregnenolone is the rate-limiting step for steroidogenesis. Pregnenolone diffuses out of mitochondria and enters the endoplasmic reticulum. The subsequent reactions that occur are zone-dependent. In the *zona glomerulosa*,

pregnenolone is converted to progesterone. Progesterone is converted to 11-deoxycorticosterone by steroid 21-hydroxylase. In the mitochondria, deoxycorticosterone is then converted to aldosterone by aldosterone synthase. Aldosterone synthase also performs three successive oxidations: 11β-hydroxylation, 18-hydroxylation, and further oxidation of the 18-methyl carbon to an aldehyde. In the zona fasciculata, pregnenolone and progesterone are converted by 17α-hydroxylase to 17-hydroxy-pregnenolone and 17-hydroxyprogesterone, which is converted to 17-hydroxyprogesterone and 11-deoxycortisol by 3β-hydroxysteroid enzymes. 11-deoxycortisol is converted to cortisol by steroid 11β-hydroxylase. In the zona reticularis and, to some extent, in the zona fasciculata, 17-hydroxy-pregnenolone is converted by 3βHSD to androstene-dione.

The major regulator of glucocorticoid secretion is by ACTH that is produced in the anterior pituitary. The normal diurnal rhythm of cortisol secretion is established after infancy. In children and adults, the pulses of ACTH and cortisol are the highest in the early morning hours, become lower in late afternoon and evening, and reach their nadir 1 or 2 hrs after sleep begins. ACTH secretion from the anterior pituitary is stimulated mainly by CRH. The secretion of ACTH and CRH is predominantly regulated by cortisol through a negative-feedback effect.

Aldosterone secretion is regulated mainly by the renin-angiotensin system and by serum potassium levels. Predominantly in response to decreased intravascular volume, as in dehydration, renin is secreted by the juxtaglomerular apparatus of the kidney. Renin is a proteolytic enzyme that cleaves an *angiotensinogen*. This cleaving results in the formation of angiotensin I, which is cleaved further by angiotensin-converting enzyme in the lungs yielding the biologically active angiotensin II. Angiotensin II is cleaved further to produce the angiotensin III. Angiotensins II and III are potent stimulators of aldosterone secretion.

ADRENAL STEROID ACTION

Glucocorticoids have regulating effects on carbohydrate, lipid, and protein metabolism. They increase hepatic gluconeogenesis, glycolysis, proteolysis, and lipolysis. Glucocorticoids can result in increased insulin levels, which will inhibit peripheral tissue glucose uptake, leading to hyperglycemia. In addition, glucocorticoids may work in parallel with insulin by stimulating glycogen deposition and production in the liver, which provides protection against starvation. An increase in free fatty acid levels is associated with glucocorticoid administration and results from glucocorticoid enhancement of lipolysis, decrease in cellular glucose uptake, and decrease in glycerol production. Glucocorticoids also exert a direct inhibitory effect on the epiphyses which results in delayed skeletal maturation and decreased linear growth in children. Although excess glucocorticoids can impair growth, they are also essential for normal growth and development. In the fetus and neonate,

they accelerate the differentiation and development of various tissues (e.g., the hepatic and gastrointestinal systems) as well as the production of surfactant in the fetal lung.

Glucocorticoids suppress the inflammatory process by depletion of monocytes, eosinophils, and T lymphocytes. T lymphocytes are reduced more than B lymphocytes, leading to a predominantly humoral immune response. Glucocorticoids inhibit immunoglobulin synthesis and stimulation of lymphocyte apoptosis. Glucocorticoids have a positive inotropic effect on the heart that leads to an increase in left ventricular output. They also increase blood pressure by mechanisms that involve the vascular system and the kidneys. In the vascular smooth muscles and the heart, glucocorticoids have a permissive effect on the actions of epinephrine and norepinephrine. They also increase the sensitivity to pressor agents such as catecholamines and angiotensin II, while reducing nitric oxide–mediated endothelial dilatation. Hypertension is often observed in patients with glucocorticoid excess. Glucocorticoids increase excretion of renal calcium and inhibit calcium absorption by the intestine. Long-term use of glucocorticoids can lead to osteopenia and osteoporosis, as they also inhibit the osteoblastic activity. Glucocorticoids have been associated with appetite stimulation, insomnia, and mood changes. The major role of mineralocorticoids is to maintain intravascular volume, which is achieved by sodium retention coupled with the elimination of potassium and hydrogen ions. The main target tissues for the action of mineralocorticoids are the kidney, gut, and salivary and sweat glands.

Stress can lead to increased secretion of ACTH, which involves an immune-endocrine cascade that results in the activation of the hypothalamic-pituitary-adrenal (HPA) axis. The CRH-ACTH-cortisol axis is activated, leading to increased plasma cortisol concentration, which then results in a negative feedback on the macrophages. IL-6, tumor necrosis factor-α, and IL-1 are other cytokines that have been shown to stimulate CRH release and to be inhibited by cortisol. Aldosterone secretion is increased in the presence of the hyperkalemia that is associated with renal failure. In patients with heart failure, renin-angiotensin-aldosterone is secreted in response to inadequate systemic perfusion.

ADRENAL MEDULLA

The catecholamines dopamine, norepinephrine, and epinephrine are the main hormones produced by the adrenal medulla. The biosynthesis of catecholamines is illustrated in **Figure 70.1**. Catecholamine metabolites are excreted in the urine.

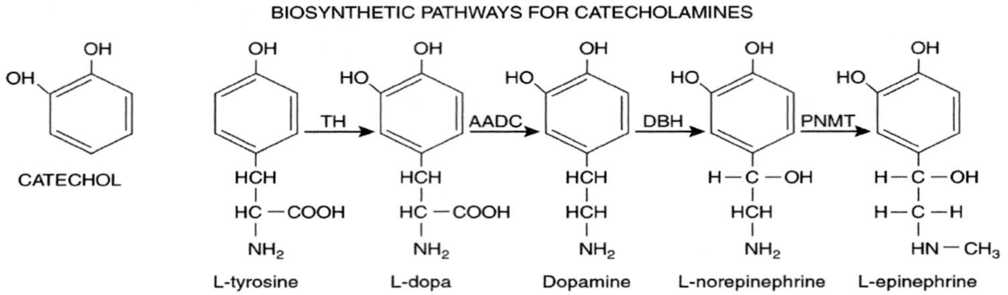

BIOSYNTHETIC PATHWAYS FOR CATECHOLAMINES

FIGURE 70.1. Biosynthetic pathway for catecholamines (*left to right*). All catecholamines contain the catechol nucleus. L-tyrosine is converted to L-3, 4-dihydroxyphenylalanine (L-dopa) in the rate-limiting step by tyrosine hydroxylase (TH). Aromatic L-amino acid decarboxylase converts L-dopa to dopamine. Dopamine is hydroxylated to L-norepinephrine by dopamine β-hydroxylase (DBH). L-Norepinephrine is converted to L-epinephrine by phenylethanolamine N-methyltransferase (PNMT).

They include 3-methoxy-4-hydroxymandelic acid, metanephrine, and normetanephrine. Loss of basal epinephrine secretion, as well as the response to upright posture, cold pressor, and exercise, has been reported in patients with glucocorticoid deficiency due to ACTH unresponsiveness.

CLINICAL PRESENTATION AND DIFFERENTIAL DIAGNOSIS OF ADRENAL INSUFFICIENCY

Primary adrenal insufficiency (AI) can result from the reduced production of cortisol and occasionally aldosterone that is caused by congenital or acquired lesions of the adrenal cortex. Lesions in the anterior pituitary gland or hypothalamus may cause a deficiency of ACTH (*secondary AI*) or CRH (*tertiary AI*) and lead to insufficient production of cortisol by the adrenal cortex (**Table 70.1** and **Table 70.2**).

In infancy, the salt-wasting forms of congenital adrenal hyperplasia are the most common causes. These patients usually have CYP21 deficiency; lipoid adrenal hyperplasia. The inability to synthesize cortisol and/or aldosterone is present in these patients and can lead to symptoms of salt-wasting (shock and vascular collapse) in the newborn period. Females with CYP21 deficiency or 3βHSD deficiency are easier to diagnose owing to virilization of the external genitalia. Adrenal hypoplasia congenita with AI occurs in conjunction with Duchenne muscular dystrophy, glycerol kinase deficiency, and mental retardation. The combination of these conditions has been termed a *contiguous gene defect*.

Familial glucocorticoid deficiency is another form of inherited AI, and patients present with hypoglycemia, seizures, and increased pigmentation. These symptoms commonly present in the first decade of life, and patients usually have an isolated

deficiency of glucocorticoid, elevated levels of ACTH, and normal aldosterone production. Triple A syndrome, an autosomal recessive disorder, is another syndrome of ACTH resistance that occurs in association with achalasia of the gastric cardia and alacrima. Patients with Smith-Lemli-Opitz syndrome have been reported to have AI.

The term *Addison disease* is used to describe primary AI that is mainly due to autoimmune adrenalitis, the most common cause of acquired AI. Addison disease has also been described in association with two syndromes: type I autoimmune polyendocrinopathy (APS-1), which is known as autoimmune polyendocrinopathy/candidiasis/ectodermal dystrophy syndrome, and type II autoimmune polyendocrinopathy (APS-2), which consists of Addison disease associated with autoimmune thyroid disease (Schmidt syndrome) or type 1 diabetes (Carpenter syndrome).

Adrenoleukodystrophy is a potential cause of AI. Patients have demyelination of the CNS due to the accumulation of high levels of very long-chain fatty acids in different tissues including the adrenal gland, as a result of impaired β-oxidation in the peroxisomes. The most common infection that causes AI is meningococcemia, which can present as adrenal crisis and is referred to as the *Waterhouse-Fredrickson syndrome*. Drugs such as rifampicin, phenytoin, and phenobarbital induce steroid-metabolizing enzymes in the liver and reduce the effectiveness and bioavailability of corticosteroid replacement therapy. Ketoconazole, by inhibiting adrenal enzymes, can cause AI. Mitotane is cytotoxic to the adrenal cortex. It is used in the treatment of refractory Cushing syndrome and adrenal carcinoma. In children, hypoadrenalism can occur after severe adrenal hemorrhage in the neonatal period, which can be observed after breech presentation and/or difficult labor. These patients may present with an abdominal mass, anemia, unexplained jaundice, or scrotal hematoma.

TABLE 70.1

ETIOLOGY OF ADRENAL INSUFFICIENCY

Primary adrenal insufficiency
  Adrenal hypoplasia or aplasia
    X-linked
      Duchenne muscular dystrophy and glycerol kinase deficiency (Xp21 deletion)
      Hypogonadotropic hypogonadism (*DAX1* mutation)
    Familial glucocorticoid deficiency
    Corticotrophin-receptor mutations/ACTH unresponsiveness
      Alacrima, achalasia, and neurologic disorders (triple A syndrome)
  Defects of steroid biosynthesis
    Lipoid adrenal hyperplasia (StAR mutation)
    3β-hydroxysteroid dehydrogenase deficiency
    21-hydroxylase (P450C21) deficiency
    Isolated aldosterone (P450C18) deficiency
  Pseudohypoaldosteronism (aldosterone unresponsiveness)
  Adrenoleukodystrophy (peroxisomal membrane protein defect)
  Acid lipase deficiency
    Wolman disease
  Destructive lesions of adrenal cortex
    Granulomatous lesions (e.g., tuberculosis)
  Autoimmune adrenalitis (idiopathic Addison disease)
    Isolated
    Associated with hypoparathyroidism or mucocutaneous candidiasis (type I autoimmune polyglandular
      syndrome/AIRE gene mutation), or both
    Associated with autoimmune thyroid disease and insulin-dependent diabetes (type II autoimmune polyglandular
      syndrome)
  Neonatal hemorrhage
  Acute infection (Waterhouse-Friderichsen syndrome)
  Mitochondrial disorders
  Acquired immunodeficiency syndrome

Secondary adrenal insufficiency (ACTH deficiency)
  Isolated
  Autosomal recessive
  Multiple deficiencies
    Pituitary hypoplasia or aplasia
    Destructive lesions (e.g., craniopharyngioma)
    Autoimmune hypophysitis

Tertiary adrenal insufficiency
  Isolated
  Multiple deficiencies
    Congenital defects (e.g., anencephaly, septo-optic dysplasia)
    Destructive lesions (e.g., tumor)
    Idiopathic (e.g., idiopathic hypopituitarism)

Secondary/tertiary/combined forms of adrenal insufficiency
  Iatrogenic
    Abrupt cessation of exogenous corticosteroids or corticotropin
    Removal of functioning adrenal tumor
    Adrenalectomy for Cushing disease
    Drug administration: Aminoglutethimide, mitotane (o, p′-DDD), metyrapone, ketoconazole
  Fetal adrenal suppression—maternal hypercortisolism

In early infancy, the most common causes include sepsis, inborn errors of steroid biosynthesis, adrenal hypoplasia congenita, and adrenal hemorrhage. In older children with Addison disease, the onset is usually more gradual and is characterized by muscle weakness, malaise, anorexia, vomiting, weight loss, and orthostatic hypotension. Hyperpigmentation is often but not always present. Hypoglycemia, hyponatremia, and ketosis are common. Hyperkalemia occurs later in the course of the disease, is more frequent

TABLE 70.2

SIGNS AND SYMPTOMS OF ADRENAL INSUFFICIENCY

Glucocorticoid deficiency	Mineralocorticoid deficiency	Adrenal androgen deficiency
Fasting hypoglycemia	Weight loss	Decreased pubic and axillary hair
Increased insulin sensitivity	Fatigue	Increased β-lipotropin levels
Nausea	Nausea	Hyperpigmentation
Vomiting	Vomiting	
Fatigue	Salt-craving	
Muscle weakness	Hypotension	
	Hyperkalemia, hyponatremia, metabolic acidosis (normal anion gap)	

Adapted from Donohue PA. The adrenal gland and its disorders. In: Kappy MS, Allen DB, Geffner ME (eds.). *Principles and Practice of Pediatric Endocrinology*. Springfield: Charles C. Thomas, 2005:395.

in younger than in older children, and may not manifest in patients who also have significant vomiting and diarrhea.

Electrocardiographic signs of hyperkalemia should be sought. The blood urea nitrogen level is elevated if the patient is dehydrated. Cortisol levels may sometimes be at the low end of normal range but are invariably low when the patient's degree of illness and stress are considered. In primary AI, ACTH levels are high. Aldosterone level may be within the normal range but inappropriately low in relation to the level of hyponatremia, hyperkalemia, and hypovolemia and is usually associated with markedly elevated levels of plasma renin activity. Hypercalcemia is associated with Addison disease. A blood sample should be obtained before therapy for determination of electrolytes, glucose, ACTH, cortisol, aldosterone, and plasma renin activity to establish the etiology of AI. If possible, specifically in infants, a 17α hydroxyprogesterone level should be obtained. An ACTH-stimulation test can be performed even while initial fluid resuscitation is underway. A bolus of 20 mL/kg of 5% dextrose with 0.9% sodium chloride should be given, and IV fluid can be continued to correct hypoglycemia, hypovolemia, and hyponatremia. Hyperkalemia can be very severe and may necessitate specific treatment with calcium, sodium bicarbonate, potassium-binding resin (sodium polystyrene sulfonate), or IV infusion of glucose and insulin. Stress doses of hydrocortisone, preferably a water-soluble form, such as hydrocortisone sodium succinate, should be given intravenously. An acute dose of 10 mg for infants, 25 mg for toddlers, 50 mg for older children, and 100 mg for adolescents should be administered immediately and then every 6 hrs for the first 24 hrs. These doses may be tapered during the next 24 hrs if the patient has satisfactory

progress. Fluid and electrolyte balance is typically achieved by continuous IV saline administration, aided by the mineralocorticoid effect of high doses of hydrocortisone. Most patients require chronic replacement therapy for their cortisol and aldosterone deficiencies. Hydrocortisone may be given orally in doses of 10 mg/m²/day in 3 divided doses. During stressful conditions, such as infection or minor operative procedures, the dose should be increased 2–3-fold. Major surgery under general anesthesia requires high IV doses of hydrocortisone similar to those used for acute AI. If aldosterone deficiency is present, fludrocortisone, a mineralocorticoid, is given orally in a doses of 0.05–0.30 mg daily and often is started empirically pending steroid results.

Secondary AI is due to ACTH due to pituitary or hypothalamic dysfunction, often associated with deficiencies of other pituitary hormones such as growth hormone and thyrotropin. Craniopharyngioma and germinoma are the most common causes of corticotrophin deficiency in childhood. Surgical removal or radiotherapy of tumors in the midbrain leads to damage of the pituitary and/or the hypothalamus, resulting in secondary AI. Congenital lesions of the pituitary alone or with additional midline structure defect may be involved, as in septo-optic dysplasia. More severe developmental anomalies of the brain such as anencephaly and holoprosencephaly can also affect the pituitary.

Tertiary AI implies a hypothalamic decrease in CRH secretion or production, most commonly due to prolonged administration of high doses of a potent glucocorticoid that is withdrawn suddenly or tapered too rapidly. Patients at risk for this problem are those undergoing treatment for leukemia, asthma, and collagen vascular disease or other autoimmune conditions that require massive doses of potent glucocorticoids and those who have undergone tissue transplants or neurosurgical procedures. The maximum duration and dose of glucocorticoid that can be administered before encountering this problem is not known, but it is assumed that high-dose glucocorticoids (e.g., prednisone 2 mg/kg/day to a maximum of 60 mg/day) can be administered for up to ~1 week without requiring a subsequent slow taper of dose. On the other hand, when high doses of dexamethasone are given to children with leukemia, return of the integrity of the HPA axis may take more than a month after therapy is stopped. These patients, when subsequently subjected to stress such as severe infections or additional surgical procedures, should be presumed adrenally incompetent for up to 1 year unless normal cortisol response to provocative stimulation is documented (e.g., ACTH stimulation test). However, even with a normal peak stimulated cortisol response to ACTH, any sign of vasomotor instability during a surgical procedure warrants immediate glucocorticoid coverage.

Because the adrenal gland is intact in secondary and tertiary AI and the renin angiotensin system is not involved, aldosterone secretion is unaffected. Therefore, the signs and symptoms of secondary and tertiary AI are hypoglycemia, orthostatic hypotension, or weakness. Electrolytes usually remain in the normal range. Hyponatremia may be observed due to the decreased glomerular filtration rate and decreased free water clearance associated with cortisol deficiency. When secondary AI is due to an inborn or acquired anatomic defect that involves the pituitary, signs of associated deficiencies of other pituitary hormones may be seen, including microphallus and jaundice in infancy or poor growth after the first year of life.

Deficiencies in CYP11B2 are associated with two related genetic disorders of aldosterone synthesis without compromising glucocorticoid production. In pseudohypoaldosteronism, the kidneys do not respond to aldosterone. Administration of heparin may exacerbate relative hypoaldosteronism by inhibiting its synthesis and thereby precipitating significant salt wasting and volume loss.

Critically ill patients may develop glucocorticoid insufficiency at some point in the course of their illness. Critical illness can result in an increase in serum cortisol, changes in the circadian rhythm of serum cortisol, decrease in corticosteroid binding proteins, and changes in the number and sensitivity of tissue glucocorticoid receptors. Changes in cortisol levels in significant systemic illness are described in **Table 70.3**, and the effects of drugs on total cortisol concentration are described in **Table 70.4**.

The initial response to stress causes an early increase in CRH and ACTH, and cortisol levels are usually proportional to the degree of illness. However, due to multiple mechanisms, prolonged illness can lead to impairment of the glucocorticoid rise, resulting in acute AI. This phenomenon has been called *functional AI* to denote that a "functional" and not a "structural" defect is responsible for the AI. Another term that describes perturbations of the HPA axis during severe illness is *relative* AI, which is used by some to describe situations when, although high absolute cortisol levels are present, they are "relatively" insufficient to overcome the degree of physiologic stress put upon the patient. Moreover, the patient often cannot mount an additional response to subsequent stress. Attempts to define relative AI may require assessing the response to exogenous administration of ACTH. Many factors and illnesses can contribute to relative AI, including trauma, hemorrhagic shock, and following traumatic brain injury.

Diagnosis of relative AI is suggested by hemodynamic instability in a critically ill patient despite adequate fluid resuscitation. An inadequate response to empirical treatment in cases of ongoing inflammation can provide clues to the diagnosis. Cortisol levels and cortisol response to corticotropin were studied in adult patients with septic shock (**Fig. 70.2**). A high baseline cortisol level was the most prognostic factor. It was reported that a <9-mcg/dL increase from the baseline 60 mins after ACTH administration is associated with an increased death risk. A high baseline cortisol with low incremental rise probably means that the patient is maximally stressed and not that the patient has AI, per se. Another group compared a low-dose (1 mcg) corticotropin stimulation test with the standard (250 mcg) test for the diagnosis of relative AI. The ACTH-stimulation tests were performed consecutively with a minimum of 4 hrs between the low- and the standard-dose tests. Serum cortisol was measured at baseline, 30, 60, and 90 mins after ACTH administration, and an adequate response was considered if the increment in cortisol response was >9 mcg/dL. Nonresponders to the low-dose test had a higher mortality rate than responders to both tests, which suggests that the low-dose test can identify patients in septic shock with inadequate adrenal function. These patients had poorer outcomes and would have been missed by the high-dose test. The authors suggested that this subgroup may benefit from steroid replacement.

ADRENAL HYPERFUNCTION

The principal causes of Cushing syndrome in childhood are listed in **Table 70.5**. In the PICU setting, Cushing syndrome is most often seen in children who have received exogenous glucocorticoids.

TABLE 70.3

ILLNESSES AFFECTING MEASURED SERUM TOTAL CORTISOL CONCENTRATIONS IN CRITICALLY ILL PATIENTS

Illness	Hepatitis/liver disease	Septic shock	Malnutrition	Nephrotic syndrome	Dilutional	Illness severity
Mechanism	Increased transcortin	Possible glucocorticoid resistance; significant inflammatory response	Lower transcortin and albumin	Lower transcortin and/or albumin	Lower transcortin and albumin	Increased production
Impact	Generally higher levels	Increased levels despite symptoms suggestive of adrenal insufficiency	Relatively lower total but appropriate free cortisol	Relatively lower total but normal free cortisol	Relatively lower total cortisol but normal free cortisol levels	Generally proportionate to stress
Clinical Examples	Patients with hepatitis	Patients with septic shock	Patients with malnutrition	Patients with nephrotic syndrome	Cardiopulmonary bypass, excess IV fluids	Patients with septic shock

Adapted from Arafah BM. Review: Hypothalamic pituitary adrenal function during critical illness limitations of current assessment methods. *J Clin Endor Metab* 2006;91:3725–45.

TABLE 70.4

DRUGS THAT EFFECT MEASURED SERUM TOTAL CORTISOL CONCENTRATIONS IN CRITICALLY ILL PATIENTS

Drug	Estrogens	Ketoconazole	Spironolactone	Aminoglutethimide	Etomidate
Mechanism	Increases transcortin	Decreases synthesis of cortisol	Interferes in the assay, depending on antibody specificity	Inhibits cortisol synthesis	Decreases synthesis due to 11β hydroxylase-inhibition
Impact	Higher total cortisol; low free cortisol	Lower serum cortisol levels; low free cortisol	Generally higher cortisol levels; variable influence, depending on assay specificity	Lower serum total and free cortisol	Lower serum cortisol levels; decreased responsiveness to cosyntropin
Clinical examples	Estrogen, oral contraceptives, pregnancy, hepatitis	Patients receiving the drug	Patients receiving the drug	Patients receiving the drug, e.g., medical adrenalectomy for metastatic breast cancer	Use of the drug

Adapted from Arafah BM. Review: Hypothalamic pituitary adrenal function during critical illness limitations of current assessment methods. *J Clin Endocr Metab* 2006;91:3725–45.

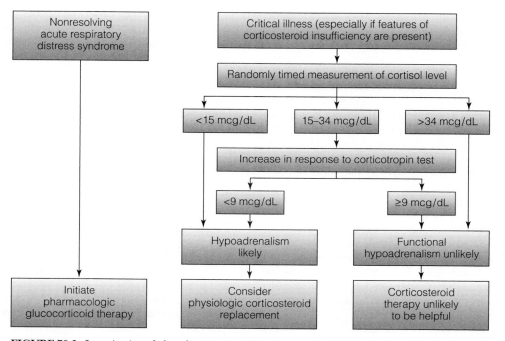

FIGURE 70.2. Investigation of adrenal corticosteroid function in critically ill patients on the basis of cortisol levels and response to the corticotropin stimulation test. The scheme has been evaluated for patients with septic shock. However, it must be remembered that no cut-off value will be entirely reliable. Adapted from Cooper M, Stewart P. Corticosteroid insufficiency in acutely ill patients. *N Engl J Med* 2003;348:727–34.

TABLE 70.5

ETIOLOGIES OF DIFFERENT TYPES OF ADRENAL HYPERFUNCTION

Disorder	Etiology
Cushing disease	Pituitary adenoma
Cushing syndrome	Adrenal adenoma
	Bilateral micronodular adrenal hyperplasia (e.g., McCune-Albright syndrome)
	Primary pigmented adrenal hyperplasia (e.g., Carney complex)
	Bilateral macronodular adrenal hyperplasia
	Adrenal carcinoma
	Ectopic ACTH (CRH): non-pituitary ACTH (CRH)-producing tumor
Pseudo-Cushing syndrome	Depression, alcoholism (increased CRH secretion)
Iatrogenic Cushing syndrome	Pharmacologic glucocorticoid therapy

ACTH, adrenocorticotropic hormone; CRH, corticotrophin-releasing hormone

Glucocorticoids can be administered for chronic steroid replacement in states of AI or as a part of high-dose or bolus steroid therapy for renal or rheumatologic disorders. In these instances, the patient may present with physical and biochemical signs of glucocorticoid excess, including cushingoid appearance, with moon-like facies, centripetal obesity, short stature, thin extremities with fragile capillaries, hirsutism, and acne. They may also present with delayed puberty and amenorrhea. Hypertension, hyperglycemia or glucose intolerance, and osteopenia are also observed. Patients who receive chronic treatment with glucocorticoid should not have abrupt cessation of their glucocorticoid therapy and should receive stress doses of glucocorticoid during the peri-, intra- and postoperative periods.

The diagnosis of Cushing syndrome in the ICU can be made on clinical grounds using the history and the physical examination. The most common cause of Cushing syndrome in children is of adrenal origin. In adolescents who have Cushing disease, a CNS lesion such as an ACTH-secreting pituitary adenoma is most likely the cause of Cushing syndrome. The treatment of choice for pituitary-related Cushing disease in children is transsphenoidal pituitary microsurgery. Patients with benign cortical adenoma can benefit from adrenalectomy. Such adenomas are occasionally bilateral and may require subtotal adrenalectomy.

Virilizing tumors of the adrenal gland are the most common adrenal tumors in children. Virilization is the most common presenting symptom and includes accelerated growth velocity, acne, muscular development, precocious development of axillary and pubic hair, and penile enlargement without testicular enlargement in males. In females, signs include hirsutism, musculinization with clitoral enlargement and the precocious development of axillary and pubic hair, with rapid growth. Ultrasonography, CT, and MRI can be used to diagnose the tumor and the presence of any metastases.

The hypertension associated with increased aldosterone is due to the increase in sodium, chloride, and water reabsorption. In familial hyperaldosteronism type-1, secretion of aldosterone and the 18OH corticosteroid metabolites is under ACTH regulation. In this condition, elevated levels of aldosterone suppress renin. Diagnosis can be made with a dexamethasone suppression test, which will cause virtual suppression of urinary aldosterone within 48 hrs. In familial hyperaldosteronism type-II, a trial of dexamethasone does not cause aldosterone suppression. Treatment of involves use of potassium-sparing diuretics such as spironolactone.

MANAGEMENT ISSUES DURING ANESTHESIA, INTUBATION, AND THE PERIOPERATIVE PERIOD

In patients with acute glucocorticoid or complete AI, treatment consists of supportive care, treatment of the underlying disease, and hydrocortisone replacement. Supportive care includes administration of fluids, appropriate electrolyte supplementation (to treat hyponatremia, hyperkalemia, hypercalcemia, and acidosis), nutritional supplements, medications,

TABLE 70.6

PHARMACOLOGIC CHARACTERISTICS OF VARIOUS STEROIDS RELATIVE TO CORTISOL

Steroid	Anti-inflammatory glucocorticoid effect	Salt-retaining mineralocorticoid effect	Growth-retarding glucocorticoid effect	Plasma half-life (mins)	Biologic half-life (hrs)
Cortisone (hydrocortisone, cortef)	1.0	1.0	1.0	80–120	8
Cortisone acetate (oral)	0.8	0.8	0.8	80–120	8
Cortisone acetate (intramuscular)	0.8	0.8	1.3		18
Prednisone	3.5–4	0.8	5	200	16–36
Prednisolone	4	0.8		120–300	16–36
Methylprednisolone	5	0.5	7.5		
Dexamethasone	30		80	150–300	36–54
9α-Fluorocortisone		200			
Aldosterone	0.3	200–1000			

Adapted from Miller WL. The adrenal cortex. In: Sperling MA (ed.). *Pediatric Endocrinology Textbook*, 2nd ed. Philadelphia: Saunders, 2002:413.

antibiotics, and organ support. It is important to maintain body temperature and glucose levels. Hyperkalemia is a contraindication to the use of succinylcholine. Etomidate has an inhibitory effect on adrenal function. Etomidate use in these patients results in depression of the adrenal cortical stress response, with reduction of cortisol and aldosterone production. Thiopental, propofol, and midazolam do not depress the adrenocortical response to stress. In Cushing syndrome, after surgical resection of the pituitary or adrenal tumor, most patients have transient suppression of the normal CRH/ACTH/adrenal axis, necessitating corticosteroid replacement therapy for several months.

Children who have been exposed to high doses of endogenous (Cushing syndrome or disease) or exogenous steroids are susceptible to osteoporosis and may be at risk for pathologic fractures. Therefore, care should be taken during positioning for procedures in the operating room or the PICU. As patients may have muscle weakness, neuromuscular-blocking drugs should be used with caution and at lower doses.

Patients who receive long-term steroid therapy need appropriate supplemental glucocorticoid therapy in the perioperative period. Although protocols vary, the following protocol has been useful: a dose of 25 mg/m^2 of hydrocortisone sodium succinate given IV immediately prior to anesthesia, followed by a dose of ~50 mg/m^2 as a constant infusion for the period of the surgical procedure; finally, a third dose of ~25–50 mg/m^2 hydrocortisone sodium succinate given as a constant IV infusion for the remainder of the first 24 hrs of the surgical day. These doses total 100–125 mg/m^2 over a 24-hr period, or ~10 times replacement therapy, and should be followed on the first postoperative day by 3–4 times replacement therapy (50 mg/m^2/day) of constant IV infusion.

Various derivatives of steroids are available and can be given via multiple routes (**Table 70.6**). In the ICU setting, the most commonly used corticosteroids are those that are administered intravenously and include dexamethasone, methylprednisolone, prednisolone, and hydrocortisone. Hydrocortisone has the highest mineralocorticoid activity, whereas dexamethasone has none. Thus, in patients with adrenal crisis and hypovolemia, hydrocortisone is the favored steroid, whereas in patients with intracranial tumors or increased intracranial pressure, dexamethasone is the most appropriate steroid to be used.

CHAPTER 71 ◼ DISORDERS OF GLUCOSE HOMEOSTASIS

STUART A. WEINZIMER • MICHAEL F. CANARIE • EDWARD VINCENT S. FAUSTINO • WILLIAM V. TAMBORLANE • CLIFFORD W. BOGUE

DIABETIC KETOACIDOSIS IN CHILDREN

Diabetic ketoacidosis (DKA) is defined as a blood glucose concentration >200 mg/dL, with ketonemia/ketonuria, and a pH of <7.3. The primary abnormality is insulin deficiency, which results in hyperglycemia by three mechanisms: increased gluconeogenesis, accelerated glycogenolysis, and impaired peripheral glucose utilization. Progressive dehydration and acidosis further stimulate the release of counter-regulatory hormones, which accelerates the production of glucose and ketoacids (**Fig. 71.1** and **Table 71.1**).

DKA is not difficult to recognize in a child with known diabetes who is dehydrated, hyperventilating, and obtunded. In the child whose diabetes has not yet been diagnosed, however, it may be confused with gastroenteritis, pneumonia, sepsis, toxic ingestion, or a CNS lesion. The diagnosis of diabetes is suggested by a history of polyuria, polydipsia, polyphagia, nocturia, weakness, unexplained weight loss, or enuresis in a previously toilet-trained child. Abdominal

pain, tenderness, and guarding is frequently present in DKA and may be of sufficient intensity to mimic an acute surgical abdomen. Other nonspecific symptoms of DKA, such as mental obtundation, vomiting, and abnormal breathing, are related to the dehydration and acidosis. DKA in children must be differentiated from such commonly occurring childhood illnesses as urinary tract infection, gastroenteritis, more severe conditions that result in a "surgical abdomen," asthma, and pneumonia. Extreme hyperglycemia, due to stress hormone excess, and acidosis, due to dehydration and/or fasting, may closely mimic DKA in infants and toddlers with a febrile illness associated with poor oral intake. However, in these children, (a) the absence of history of polyuria, (b) polydipsia, and (c) rapid clinical improvement with rehydration alone and without insulin easily differentiate these episodes of stress hyperglycemia from true DKA.

The physical examination findings in DKA are predominantly those of dehydration: tachycardia, delayed capillary refill, dry mucous membranes, and poor skin turgor. Severe acidosis and dehydration may impair cardiac contractility, resulting

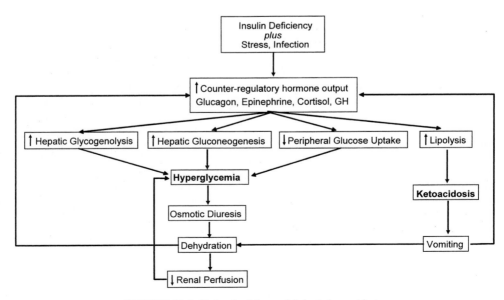

FIGURE 71.1. Pathophysiology of diabetic ketoacidosis.

TABLE 71.1

MAJOR ACTIONS OF COUNTER-REGULATORY HORMONES AND CYTOKINES
IN MEDIATING STRESS HYPERGLYCEMIA

Hormone	Mechanism
Glucagon	Increased gluconeogenesis Increased hepatic glycogenolysis
Epinephrine	Skeletal muscle insulin resistance by altering postreceptor signaling Increased gluconeogenesis Increased skeletal muscle and hepatic glycogenolysis Increased lipolysis, increased free fatty acids Direct suppression of insulin secretion
Norepinephrine	Increased lipolysis Increased gluconeogenesis, but hyperglycemia not marked except at high concentrations
Glucocorticoids	Skeletal muscle insulin resistance Increased lipolysis Gluconeogenesis increased through provision of substrate
Growth hormone	Skeletal muscle insulin resistance Increased lipolysis Increased gluconeogenesis
Tumor necrosis factor	Skeletal muscle insulin resistance, altered post-receptor signaling Hepatic insulin resistance

in hypotension. Respiratory compensation for the metabolic acidosis induces hyperventilation, which may appear as deep sighing respirations (Kussmaul breathing) and may initially suggest a primary respiratory illness. Acetone on the breath yielding a fruity odor may be present but is not always reliably detected. Mental status may vary from full alertness to frank coma; most patients with severe metabolic derangements are lethargic but do not have severe CNS depression and are able to protect their own airway. The primary survey should focus initially on the adequacy of the airway, breathing, a thorough assessment of the circulatory status (heart rate, blood pressure, description of mucous membranes, capillary refill, distal pulses, and warmth of extremities), degree of dehydration (including weight if possible), and mental status.

The laboratory evaluation of patients suspected to have DKA includes determination of the blood glucose, plasma or urinary ketones, serum electrolyte concentration, blood urea nitrogen, creatinine, osmolarity, baseline calcium and phosphorus, and if infection is suspected, complete blood count and blood culture. Bedside determination of the blood glucose with a glucose monitoring device and evaluation of the urine for glucose and ketones should be performed as quickly as possible, and treatment should be initiated without waiting for the results of the laboratory assessment to become available. A

baseline blood gas measurement should also be made to determine the pH and pCO_2. Venous blood gas measurements may suffice in most episodes of DKA. The initial blood glucose level is characteristically but not invariably elevated. Hyperglycemia beyond the renal threshold for glucose filtration indicates reduced glomerular filtration. Although the definition of DKA presupposes hyperglycemia, ketoacidosis with normal or even low glucose levels may occur in patients with known diabetes who have taken insulin recently. Poor oral intake and/or vomiting may also present with near-normal glucose concentrations.

Measurement of serum electrolytes in DKA reveals a low bicarbonate level and increased anion-gap metabolic acidosis, primarily due to the unmeasured ketoacids, including β-hydroxybutyrate and acetoacetate, as well as lactate in situations of severe tissue hypoxia. Most urine dipsticks detect only acetoacetate. In DKA, the ratio of β-hydroxybutyrate to acetoacetate may increase to 10:1 or more. Therefore, while useful to diagnose ketosis, these strips are not helpful in gauging the severity of DKA or response to treatment. The serum sodium will be reduced with the actual sodium determined by adding 1.6 mEq/L for each 100 mg/dL rise in glucose concentration >100 mg/dL. Furthermore, extreme hypertriglyceridemia may cause the serum sodium concentration to be spuriously lowered (pseudohyponatremia). A normal or elevated sodium level in the setting of severe DKA suggests extreme free water losses. The degree of elevation of the blood urea nitrogen and creatinine, as well as the hematocrit, may also indicate the extent of dehydration (and the possibility of renal damage).

The initial serum potassium may be low, normal, or high, depending on the degree of acidosis and the quantitative urinary losses. Potassium moves from the intracellular to extracellular and intravascular compartments in exchange for hydrogen ion in the setting of metabolic acidosis, typically leading to elevated serum potassium levels. However, total-body potassium stores are almost always depleted from excessive urinary losses, and normal or low potassium levels at presentation may be associated with severe hypokalemia once treatment for DKA is initiated. Phosphate, like potassium, is depleted in the setting of DKA, and serum phosphate levels may not accurately reflect total body stores. Serum phosphate level may also decrease during therapy.

As in other forms of hypertonic dehydration, too rapid fluid administration should be avoided. Fluid replacement in excess of 4 L/m^2/24 hrs has been associated with the development of potentially fatal cerebral edema in DKA. For this reason, an initial fluid bolus is usually advised to expand the vascular compartment and improve peripheral circulation, but once the patient has been stabilized, subsequent rehydration is accomplished with caution. Typically, the fluid defect should be corrected gradually, over 36–48 hrs. Serial calculations of actual (as opposed to measured) serum sodium concentrations are recommended, as sodium levels that fail to rise with treatment may signify excessive free water accumulation and an increased risk of cerebral edema. Generally, fluid replacement with 0.9% normal saline is provided for at least the first 6 hrs. Early potassium replacement is also important to correct the potassium depletion; with the initiation of insulin therapy and correction of acidosis, serum potassium levels may drop precipitously as potassium shifts back from the extracellular to the intracellular compartment. Potassium should be administered only after adequate renal function is determined. Electrocardiographic monitoring facilitates early recognition of either hyperkalemia (peaked T waves) or hypokalemia (flat or inverted T waves) and the development of potentially dangerous cardiac dysrhythmias. Potassium is usually given at a dose of 30–40 mEq/L of fluid, either as potassium chloride or in combination with potassium phosphate, which has the additional advantage of replacing the phosphate deficit.

Insulin therapy should be initiated immediately after the patient has been stabilized with an initial fluid bolus, at a dose of 0.1 unit/kg/hr. As with fluid replacement, the aim of therapy is gradual correction: reduction of the blood glucose by 50–100 mg/dL/hr.

However, the serum glucose concentration often falls significantly with initial rehydration alone due to increased glomerular filtration from improved renal perfusion. Because continuous insulin infusion often results in lowering of the blood glucose concentration before the decrease in ketoacidosis, it is important to add dextrose to the rehydration fluids, not to decrease the rate of insulin infusion, but to prevent hypoglycemia. Dextrose should be added to the IV solution when the serum glucose level falls below 300 mg/dL and should then be titrated to provide a continued gradual decline in blood glucose to target levels; this may be easily accomplished with the simultaneous use of two IV solutions that differ only in the dextrose concentration (10% and 0%); independent manipulation of each infusion allows the dextrose infusion to be varied quickly and efficiently (the so-called "two-bag" system).

Bicarbonate, once considered routine therapy in severe DKA, is no longer thought to be beneficial and is no longer recommended in the treatment of uncomplicated DKA. Bicarbonate administration may lead to a paradoxical worsening of CNS acidosis because carbon dioxide (but not bicarbonate) diffuses across the blood-brain barrier. During the hyperosmolar state of DKA, the brain produces "idiogenic osmoles" as a compensatory measure to increase intracellular osmotic pressure and prevent cerebral dehydration. If these idiogenic osmoles dissipate from the brain parenchyma at a slower rate than the plasma osmolality is being reduced by the treatment for DKA, the osmotic pressure gradient will favor fluid reaccumulation in the brain, leading to cellular swelling and increased intracranial pressure. Factors associated with greater risk of cerebral edema included younger age, new onset, longer duration of symptoms, lower pCO$_2$, more severe acidosis, increased blood urea nitrogen, use of bicarbonate, greater volumes of rehydration fluids, and failure of serum sodium to rise with treatment. However, a subsequent population-based, case-controlled study of cerebral edema complicating DKA found that early administration of insulin and high volumes of fluid, not bicarbonate therapy, were important predictors of cerebral edema. Therefore, until the precise mechanisms that underlie the development and progression of cerebral edema are elucidated, it appears prudent to avoid hypotonic fluids, correct dehydration evenly over 48 hrs, and monitor laboratory parameters including venous blood sugar concentrations hourly and electrolytes and venous pH every 2–4 hrs until normal. Blood urea nitrogen and creatinine levels should be followed until they are normal, and calcium should be monitored, particularly if potassium is given with phosphate.

Treatment of cerebral edema is aimed at lowering intracranial pressure: prompt administration of IV mannitol (0.25–1 g/kg), an osmotic diuretic, may be beneficial if given early in the course of cerebral edema. Tracheal intubation to mechanically hyperventilate and surgical decompression with ventriculostomy are less successful at preventing mortality or severe disability. Intracranial imaging to exclude other pathologies such as cerebral infarction or thrombosis should be obtained but not at the expense of timely therapeutic interventions.

Other less common complications of DKA include thrombosis, a particular concern in children who require a central venous catheter for access; cardiac arrhythmias, usually related to electrolyte disturbances; pulmonary edema; renal failure; pancreatitis; rhabdomyolysis; and infection, such as aspiration pneumonia, sepsis, and mucormycosis. Frequent iatrogenic complications include hypoglycemia and hypokalemia, which are rarely problematic if detected and treated promptly.

HYPERGLYCEMIC HYPEROSMOLAR SYNDROME

Hyperglycemic hyperosmolar syndrome (HHS) is a potentially lethal disorder of decompensated glucose homeostasis. Patients with this syndrome, known formerly as HONK (hyperosmolar, nonketotic crisis) or HHNS (hyperglycemic, hyperosmolar nonketotic syndrome), suffer from the dangerous consequences of marked hyperglycemia and hyperosmolarity. In HHS, insulin levels may be sufficient to suppress the full-blown lipolysis and ketogenesis seen in DKA, but they are inadequate to promote normal anabolic function and inhibit the creation of glucose through gluconeogenesis and glycogenolysis. In HHS, ketoacidemia is generally neither the underlying nor most extreme pathophysiologic disturbance. Due to the duration of symptoms and the extreme hyperosmolarity of patients with HHS, a much greater degree of volume depletion may be present. Thus, it is estimated that DKA patients are 10% dehydrated, whereas patients with HHS are felt to be 15–20% volume-depleted.

Patients with HHS commonly present with a history of weight loss, complaints of polydipsia/polyuria of variable duration, and gastrointestinal distress. On exam, patients are lethargic and often present with neurologic impairments that range from slightly altered sensoria, to focal neurologic deficits, to frank coma. These patients are dehydrated and in varying—and often tenuous—states of cardiovascular compensation. The duration of these symptoms and the ability of the patient to compensate for the prodigious osmotic diuresis dictate how they ultimately present. However, the diagnosis and treatment of HHS can be clouded by a number of factors. First, the onset of symptoms is likely insidious, with an indolent prelude to decompensation and a correspondingly vague history. An altered sensorium may further shroud the history (and a workup for mental status changes may not include HHS). Second, the frequent absence of the symptomologic and objective hallmarks of ketoacidemia may obscure the diagnosis; the abdominal discomfort and nausea and vomiting have been reported to be less severe, and acetone breath and Kussmaul breathing pattern are not present. Lastly, assessing the volume status of an obese patient can be considerably difficult, which may obscure both the gravity of illness and the correct diagnosis. The diagnostic criteria for HHS complement those for DKA, namely, a glucose of >600 mg/dL, $HCO_3 \geq 15$ mEq/L, serum osmolarity of >320 mOsm/L, and a pH ≥ 7.3 without evidence of significant ketosis.

The early goals of treatment should target airway protection and mechanical ventilation based on the Glasgow Coma Scale and compensatory response and the restoration of hemodynamic stability and tissue perfusion. The placement of appropriate cardiovascular monitoring (including arterial and central venous pressure monitoring as indicated) may be required. Electrolytes should be rigorously repleted based on frequent sampling and conservative correction of hyperglycemia. Finally, vigilant monitoring for neurologic or other complications, detection and treatment of precipitating causes, and appropriate prophylactic measures should be undertaken. Volume resuscitation is the mainstay of therapy for HHS. The American Diabetes Association guidelines for the management of DKA and HHS in patients younger than 20 years old suggest boluses of normal saline at 10–20 mL/kg (repeating as necessary to reverse shock), with replacement of the remaining volume deficit over 48 hrs. The adult critical care literature advocates a more aggressive degree of volume resuscitation (2–3 liters of normal saline over the first 2 hrs) with replacement of 50% of the deficits in the first 12 hrs. Although insulin may have salutary, antiinflammatory benefits, in the absence of significant ketoacidemia, it is felt by many to play a secondary role in the initial management of HHS. In fact, hyperglycemia can often be corrected by reestablishing renal perfusion and glomerular filtration rate and thereby ensuring a more gradual correction of hyperosmolarity without rapid fluid and electrolyte shifts. The American Diabetes Association currently recommends an insulin infusion at 0.1 U/kg/hr without bolus titrating and transitioning, as clinically indicated.

Theoretically, the absence of a large ketotic diuresis should lessen the cationic urinary loss. Estimated electrolyte deficit ranges in adults with HHS are

3–7 mmol/kg for phosphate, 4–6 mEq/kg for potassium, and 5–13 mEq/kg for sodium. Hyperglycemia predisposes to thrombogenesis, and HHS predisposes to deep-vein thromboses in patients with central venous catheters. Appropriate prophylaxis for deep vein thromboses should be employed.

HYPERGLYCEMIA IN CRITICALLY ILL CHILDREN

Threshold glucose values used for the initiation of insulin therapy in children range from 110 mg/dL to >200 mg/dL. Despite the lack of uniformity in defining hyperglycemia, elevated glucose levels have consistently been associated with increased morbidity and mortality in children. The intensity, timing, and duration of hyperglycemia substantially affects outcome. Tight control of glucose between 80 and 110 mg/dL resulted in a reduced risk of mortality by as much as 34% in mechanically ventilated adults admitted to a surgical ICU. In an adult medical ICU, tight glycemic control prevented the development of kidney injury, accelerated weaning from mechanical ventilation, and accelerated discharge from the ICU and the hospital.

Cellular glucose transport is facilitated by the glut proteins: glut1, glut2, and glut4 are thought to play major roles in glucose metabolism. While nearly all cells are involved in glucose uptake, glucose production occurs only in the liver and the kidneys. Two processes contribute to glucose formation: breakdown of glycogen in the liver and production of new glucose molecules from both liver and kidneys. Glycogenolysis provides most of the glucose after an overnight fast. However, with prolonged starvation, glycogen stores become depleted and other sources of energy are utilized. Insulin, glucagon, catecholamines, cortisol, and growth hormone are the major hormones involved in glucose metabolism. Insulin decreases blood glucose levels by enhancing glucose uptake and glycogenesis and conversely inhibiting gluconeogenesis. In contrast, the other hormones, which are also known as *counter-regulatory hormones*, have the opposite effect of elevating blood glucose by inhibiting glucose uptake and enhancing glycogenolysis and gluconeogenesis.

During stress, the hypothalamic-pituitary-adrenal axis and sympathetic system are activated, leading to increased cortisol and catecholamine secretion. Other counter-regulatory hormones and cytokines are secreted as well. The combination of these factors leads to insulin resistance and elevated blood glucose. Other gluconeogenic precursors, including lactate, alanine, glycerol, and glutamine, are produced during stress. Major sources of lactate are the lungs (in acute lung injury), intestines, and wounds—a reflection of increased rates of glycolysis and possible downregulation of pyruvate dehydrogenase. The liver avidly extracts lactate from the circulation and converts it to glucose via the Cori cycle.

HYPOGLYCEMIA IN CHILDREN

The brain in particular utilizes glucose at a rate, per gram, that is 20 times that of the rest of the body, primarily because it cannot use free fatty acids as a fuel source. The brain, therefore, derives >99% of its energy from glucose metabolism, and in neonates, whose brain constitutes a relatively greater proportion of body weight, glucose requirements are 5–10-fold greater than in older children and adults (8–10 mg/kg/min vs. 1–2 mg/kg/min). Recommendations consider any blood glucose <55–60 mg/dL as abnormal. The elements of fasting include the four alternative fuel pathways: (a) hepatic glycogenolysis, (b) hepatic gluconeogenesis, (c) adipose tissue lipolysis, and (d) hepatic fatty acid oxidation and ketogenesis. These systems are under hormonal control, primarily by insulin, which suppresses the fasting systems and the "counter-regulatory" hormones glucagon, cortisol, epinephrine, and growth hormone, which act to stimulate them.

Symptoms and signs of hypoglycemia can be divided into those that arise from autonomic responses to hypoglycemia (adrenergic) and those that arise from neurologic dysfunction (neuroglycopenic). Adrenergic symptoms/signs include tremors, diaphoresis, tachycardia, hunger, weakness, and nervousness. Neuroglycopenic symptoms/signs include lethargy, confusion, unusual behavior, and with more severe decrements in blood glucose, seizures and coma. Autonomic activation usually occurs earlier and at a glucose threshold higher than would cause neuroglycopenia, although with repeated episodes of hypoglycemia, the threshold for adrenergic responses decreases, leading eventually to the development of serious neurologic symptoms with little or no warning. This "hypoglycemia unawareness" or "hypoglycemia-associated autonomic failure" is more frequently encountered in patients with insulin-treated diabetes.

A normal child should not become hypoglycemic until all available fuel sources are depleted and counter-regulatory hormone stimulation is maximized, at which time (a) glycogen stores will be depleted and no glycemic response to glucagon will occur; (b) lactate will be low, reflecting exhaustion of gluconeogenic stores; (c) free fatty acids and ketones will be elevated; and (d) insulin will be undetectable in the serum. Studies to be obtained are summarized in

TABLE 71.2

CRITICAL SAMPLE FOR EVALUATION OF HYPOGLYCEMIA IN CHILDREN

Test	Sample requirements	Normal values @ hypoglycemia (Glu <55)
Glucose	1 mL serum or plasma	
Electrolytes	1 mL serum	Bicarbonate >18 mEq/L
Lactate	1 mL plasma	<2.5 mmol
Insulin	1 mL serum	<2 mcU/mL
Cortisol	1 mL serum	>20 mcg/dL
Growth hormone	1 mL serum	>7–10 ng/mL
Free fatty acids	1 mL plasma	>1.5 mmol/L
β-hydroxybutyrate	1 mL plasma	>2 mmol/L
Acetoacetate	1 mL plasma	>2 mmol/L
Ammonia	1 mL plasma	<35 mcmol/L
C-peptide	1 mL EDTA plasma	<0.5 ng/mL
Acylcarnitine profile	1 mL EDTA plasma	*
Urine organic acids	5–10 mL urine, frozen stat	*
Urine ketones	1–2 mL	Positive

*Requires specialist interpretation.

Table 71.2. The duration of fasting tolerance (i.e., time to hypoglycemia from last carbohydrate consumed), amount of glucose required to restore and maintain euglycemia, serum bicarbonate, urinary ketones, and response to glucagon suggest the etiology of the hypoglycemia until the confirmatory critical sample results are known. The presence of acidosis with hypoglycemia indicates an accumulation of either ketones or lactate. Ketoacidosis is a normal response to prolonged fasting, while lactic acidosis generally indicates a block in the gluconeogenic pathway (failure to convert lactate to glucose).

Fasting tolerance of <4–6 hrs, significant ketosis, and fatty acid breakdown in a child with hepatomegaly suggest one of the glycogen-storage diseases (GSDs), which are all characterized by the absence of glycemic response to glucagon (<30 mg/dL rise in blood glucose) and normal parenteral glucose requirements to restore and maintain euglycemia. Supraphysiologic glucose replacement, low or absent ketones, and glycemic response to glucagon (>30 mg/dL) are the hallmarks of hyperinsulinism (HI), in which excessive insulin action inhibits glycogenolysis and promotes excessive peripheral glucose uptake. Disorders of fatty acid oxidation are also associated with low or absent ketones, but glucose requirements are normal, and glycemic response to glucagon is absent. Hypopituitarism, either simple growth hormone deficiency or multiple pituitary hormone deficiency, is difficult to classify in this framework, as glucose requirements may be supraphysiologic and glycemic response to glucagon inconclusive. The GSDs are a family of autosomal recessively inherited disorders characterized by defects in the formation and/or degradation of glycogen. Certain subtypes of GSD are associated with hypoglycemia: debranching enzyme deficiency (type III GSD), liver phosphorylase deficiency (type VI), and phosphorylase kinase deficiency (type IX). Other associated features include hepatomegaly and failure to thrive. As hepatic gluconeogenesis is intact and some functional glycogenolysis occurs, these forms of GSD are typically associated with only mild defects in fasting tolerance. Muscle-specific forms of GSD, while associated with myopathy, do not cause hypoglycemia.

Defects in gluconeogenesis are characterized by hypoglycemia, hepatomegaly, lactic acidosis, and hyperlipidemia. The most severe disorder of gluconeogenesis is glucose-6-phosphatase deficiency (GSD type I). Other disorders of gluconeogenesis, such as fructose-1,6-diphosphatase deficiency, hereditary fructose intolerance, and galactosemia, are distinguished from GSD type I by a longer fasting tolerance, as glycogenolysis is intact.

Defects in fatty acid oxidation manifest when the fasting tolerance of ~12 hrs is exceeded or when a significant stress calls upon adipose tissue stores. Under normal fasting conditions, free fatty acids are mobilized by the hormone-sensitive adipose tissue lipase and utilized as alternative fuel, as a substrate for the production of ketone bodies, and as an energy source for gluconeogenesis. Children with a disorder of fatty acid oxidation have impairments either in transport of fatty acids across the mitochondrial membrane or metabolism within the mitochondrial β-oxidation cycle. The most common fatty acid oxidation disorder, medium-chain acyl-coenzyme A deficiency, presenting with hypoglycemia, hyperammonemia, liver dysfunction, myopathy, coma, and sudden death. Definitive diagnosis may be made by the demonstration of an abnormal acylcarnitine profile by mass spectrometry.

Hypoglycemia may occur in children with hypopituitarism, as both growth hormone and cortisol are required for optimal counter-regulation and fasting adaptation. Most commonly, hypoglycemia in adrenal insufficiency occurs during periods of intercurrent illness with vomiting or poor oral intake and inadequate replacement of cortisol. Hypoglycemia with isolated growth hormone deficiency is limited primarily to newborns.

HI may be transient or permanent. Transient dysregulated insulin secretion occurs in the newborn period, typically in the setting of some physiologic perinatal stress such as asphyxia, maternal hypertension, or precipitous delivery. Such hypoglycemia occurs within the first few hours of life and can last weeks unless treated. More familiar is the infant of the diabetic mother, in which the fetus upregulates insulin secretion in response to maternal hyperglycemia. At birth, the infant is large for gestational age due to the growth factor effects of insulin and suffers from hypoglycemia when the excessive glucose supply is acutely withdrawn. The time course to normalization of blood glucose in an infant of a diabetic mother may be several days to several weeks.

One of the most common causes of hypoglycemia in hospitalized children is the acute interruption of high-concentration IV dextrose infusion, particularly seen in sick newborns who are treated with total parenteral nutrition. By far the most common cause of drug-induced hypoglycemia in children (aside from insulin in diabetics) is alcohol. Sources of alcohol include parents' supply, mouthwash, and transdermal exposure of rubbing alcohol. The amount of alcohol required to induce hypoglycemia is frequently less than that required to cause drunkenness. Other drugs/medications that may induce hypoglycemia include sulfonylureas and other antidiabetic drugs, quinine, pentamidine, disopyramide, β-blockers, and salicylates. Factitious hypoglycemia due to Munchausen syndrome, in which children or their caregivers surreptitiously administer insulin or an oral secretagogue, may mimic true HI. Ketotic hypoglycemia is a poorly understood condition of blunted fasting tolerance that generally occurs in underweight children who are 1–6 years of age. Symptoms occur after a prolonged overnight fast or during intercurrent illness with vomiting or poor feeding. Reactive (or postprandial) hypoglycemia, either alone or in conjunction with other symptoms of the dumping syndrome, may rarely be seen in children with dysregulated intestinal transit or after fundoplication. Lastly, neonatal disorders such as sepsis and hyperviscosity syndrome are noted to cause hypoglycemia in sick newborns.

In the acute setting, the immediate goal in the treatment of hypoglycemia is to increase the plasma glucose to at least 70 mg/dL. Rapid improvement in blood sugar is normally seen after administration of 10% dextrose, 2 mL/kg by IV push, followed by continuous IV dextrose at a rate of at least 8 mg/kg/min. Some infants with HI require 20 mg/kg/min dextrose to maintain euglycemia; in fact, the requirement of supraphysiologic amounts of glucose indicates elevated glucose utilization, a reliable sign for HI. Children with mutations in glucokinase or glutamate dehydrogenase may respond well to diazoxide, given at a dose of 5–15 mg/kg/day. Octreotide, a long-acting somatostatin analog, may be administered subcutaneously every 6–8 hrs at a dose of 5–20 mcg/kg/day. However, tachyphylaxis frequently develops to octreotide, so that most children with potassium channel-sulfonylurea receptor complex mutations require subtotal or complete pancreatectomy for long-term control of hypoglycemia. Continuous IV infusion of glucagon, 1 mg/day, may be used to stabilize the glucose levels prior to surgery.

CHAPTER 72 ■ DISORDERS OF WATER, SODIUM, AND POTASSIUM HOMEOSTASIS

ANDREA KELLY • THOMAS MOSHANG, JR.

The kidney is the primary site for disposal of sodium, potassium, and water (**Fig. 72.1**). The glomerular filtration rate, the amount of renal blood flow that enters the nephron, dictates the maximum amount of fluid that can be delivered to the tubules. The glomerular filtration rate is heavily influenced by renal blood flow through the afferent and efferent arterioles. Vasoconstriction of afferent arterioles decreases glomerular blood flow, thereby decreasing glomerular pressure and filtration, while

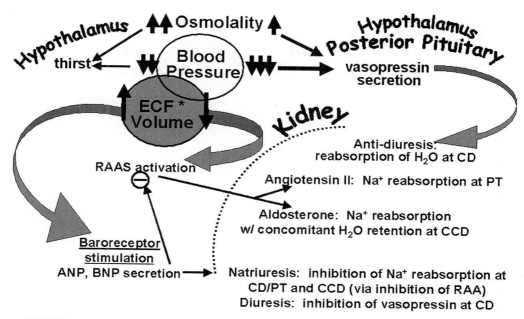

FIGURE 72.1. Regulation of extracellular fluid osmolality and volume. Vasopressin secretion is primarily responsible for preserving plasma osmolality. Secretion of vasopressin by the hypothalamus occurs with as little as a 1% increase in plasma osmolality. Much larger increases in plasma osmolality are required to trigger thirst, the center for which is also located in the hypothalamus. This offsetting likely occurs to avoid simultaneously activating thirst and vasopressin secretion at the lower end of normal plasma osmolality, which would result in overcorrection. Significant decreases in blood pressure/effective extracellular fluid (ECF) volume, communicated to the hypothalamus via cardiovascular baroreceptors, are required to trigger vasopressin secretion. Vasopressin recruits aquoporin-2 water channels in the renal collecting ducts (CD) to promote reabsorption of water and concentration of urine. ECF volume is primarily maintained through sodium homeostasis. Decreases in blood pressure/effective ECF volume also activate the renin angiotensin aldosterone system (RAAS). Aldosterone promotes reabsorption of sodium and water at the renal cortical collecting duct (CCD), and angiotensin II stimulates sodium reabsorption at the proximal tubules (PT). Hypertension/fluid overload activate cardiovascular baroreceptors, leading to atrial natriuretic peptide (ANP) and brain natriuretic peptide (BNP) release. These peptides promote sodium and water excretion at the level of the kidney.

vasoconstriction of efferent arterioles, to an extent, increases glomerular pressure and filtration. When the macula densa "senses" a low glomerular filtration rate, vasodilatation of afferent arterioles (and vasoconstriction of efferent arterioles mediated by angiotensin II) increases glomerular perfusion, thereby increasing the glomerular filtration rate to effect urine output. Conversely, with increased glomerular filtration, the macula densa again provides negative feedback to the afferent and efferent arterioles: vasoconstriction of afferent arterioles (and vasodilatation of efferent arterioles) occurs, decreasing glomerular filtration, slowing fluid transport through the nephron, and allowing increased filtrate reabsorption and, ultimately, decreased urine output.

Following filtration at the level of the glomerulus, the fluid is delivered to the tubules, where solute absorption varies depending upon the segment. The proximal tubule accounts for 65% of filtrate

reabsorption, including that of sodium, potassium, and water. The descending thin limb of the loop of Henle is permeable to water, urea, and other solutes, while the ascending thin limb is relatively impermeable to water. The thick ascending limb and the initial segment of the distal tubule avidly absorb sodium and other solutes but are impermeable to water regardless of the status of vasopressin and, hence, are referred to as the *diluting segment of the kidney.* The late distal tubule and cortical collecting duct mediate the sodium-retaining and potassium-wasting effects of aldosterone. In addition, like the collecting duct, they are permeable to water only in the presence of vasopressin. Sodium absorption occurs through an active process and facilitates absorption of many other solutes. Na^+, K^+-ATPase, expressed on the basolateral membrane of tubular epithelium, pumps sodium into the renal interstitium and ultimately to the peritubular capillaries.

WATER HOMEOSTASIS

The human body is composed of 42%–75% water, with the exact content dependent upon age, gender, and amount of body fat. Two-thirds of the water is located intracellularly. The remaining estimated one-third is located extracellularly and is divided between the interstitium (three-fourths) and plasma (one-fourth). Potassium is the primary constituent of intracellular fluid (ICF) and sodium being the major electrolyte in ECF. The normal range for blood osmolality is 280–290 mOsm/kg H_2O. ECF osmolality can be estimated based upon the equation:

$$2 \times Na^+ + [\text{urea nitrogen (mg/dL)}]/2.8 + [\text{glucose (mg/dL)}]/18$$

Water output is primarily regulated by vasopressin at the level of the kidney. In fact, >99% of water in the glomerular filtrate is reabsorbed by the renal tubules. However, unregulated (and potentially substantial) water loss can occur through the skin, gastrointestinal tract, and lungs.

Vasopressin

Vasopressin production and secretion are regulated by serum osmolality, ECF volume, and blood pressure Plasma osmotic pressure is the major determinant of vasopressin release Activation of neural stretch-sensitive sensors in the cardiac atria, aorta, and carotid arteries leads to tonic inhibition of vasopressin secretion. Pathways for baroreceptor-mediated vasopressin secretion are distinct from those of osmoreceptors; these pathways converge at the level of the vasopressin-secreting cells. The primary antidiuretic activity of vasopressin occurs through recruitment of renal water channels (aquaporin-2) in the collecting duct. In the absence of vasopressin/aquaporin channels, urine is dilute—$\sim$50 mOsm/kg H_2O—reflecting the obligate solute losses by the kidney. With the provision of aquaporin along the tubular side of the collecting ducts, water is absorbed along the concentration gradient.

Thirst

As with vasopressin, thirst is regulated by plasma osmolality and blood pressure/volume status. Cardiovascular baroreceptors transmit their signals to the thirst center through the vagal and glossopharyngeal nerves via the medulla, while angiotensin II directly stimulates thirst. Hypoosmolality, increased arterial blood pressure, and increased gastric water all inhibit thirst. The threshold for activating thirst

may be higher than that for vasopressin secretion, $\sim$295 mOsm/kg H_2O.

Renin-angiotensin System

Two distinct renin-angiotensin systems (RAS) exist: one in the brain and the other in the periphery, the latter of which only has access to the central nervous system (CNS) at sites where the blood-brain barrier is absent, such as the posterior pituitary and the circumventricular structures (Fig. 72.2). Decreases in circulating blood volume/blood pressure detected by baroreceptors in the renal arterioles, extrarenal baroreceptors, and the renal macula densa stimulate renin release from the renal juxtaglomerular cells. Renin release is inhibited by angiotensin II, vasopressin, and atrial natriuretic factor. A proteolytic enzyme, renin converts hepatically derived angiotensinogen to angiotensin I. Angiotensin-converting enzyme, located throughout the vasculature endothelium (particularly the lung), then converts angiotensin I to the active hormone angiotensin II, a potent vasoconstrictor (Fig. 72.2).

Aldosterone

Angiotensin II stimulates aldosterone secretion by the adrenal zona glomerulosa, the outermost zone of the adrenal cortex. In addition to angiotensin II, the major regulator for aldosterone secretion, increased plasma potassium, and decreased plasma sodium also stimulates aldosterone release. Coupled with vasopressin, aldosterone increases ECF: aldosterone-mediated sodium reabsorption increases plasma osmolality, triggering vasopressin secretion, and, hence, water reabsorption.

Natriuretic Peptides

A number of natriuretic peptides have been identified, the prototype of which is A-type natriuretic peptide (ANP), and include B-type natriuretic peptide (BNP), C-type natriuretic peptide (CNP), and urodilatin (**Fig. 72.3**). ANP, previously referred to as atrial natriuretic peptide, is produced both by the hypothalamus and the cardiac atrial myocytes. Atrial myocytes release ANP in response to distention of the cardiac atria, as occurs in the setting of fluid overload. β-adrenergic stimulation also promotes ANP release. ANP lowers circulating volume and, hence, blood pressure through a variety of mechanisms. Through its effects on the renal vasculature, ANP increases the glomerular filtration rate, thereby promoting fluid

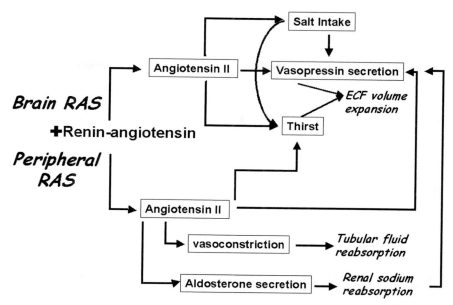

FIGURE 72.2. Effect of the renin-angiotensin system. Both brain and peripheral renin angiotensin systems exist, and both act to preserve ECF volume. Stimulation of both of the systems generates angiotensin II. In the brain, angiotensin II stimulates thirst, salt appetite, and vasopressin secretion. An increase in salt further stimulates thirst and vasopressin secretion. Angiotensin II, generated in the periphery, stimulates thirst, vasopressin secretion, vasoconstriction, which stimulates fluid absorption from the renal tubules, and aldosterone secretion, which promotes renal salt retention. The ultimate result of these intertwined and redundant pathways is an expansion of ECF volume. RAS, rennin-angiotensin system; ECF, extracellular fluid.

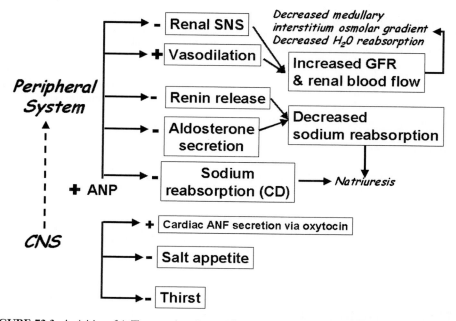

FIGURE 72.3. Activities of A-Type natriuretic peptide (ANP). ANP acts both centrally and peripherally to mediate its effects. Centrally, ANP suppresses thirst and salt appetite while promoting additional ANP release by the heart. Peripherally, ANP promotes vasodilation and inhibits the renal sympathetic nervous system (SNS) to increase glomerular filtration (GFR) and, ultimately, urine output. In addition, it directly inhibits renin and aldosterone secretion and sodium reabsorption at the collecting duct (CD), to promote natriuresis.

excretion. It decreases renal sodium reabsorption by the distal convoluted tubules and collecting ducts, thereby promoting natriuresis. In addition, it inhibits renin secretion. Given that angiotensin II stimulates ANP secretion, ANP provides negative feedback for the renin-angiotensin system. ANP also directly inhibits aldosterone secretion by the adrenal glomerulosa and relaxes vascular smooth muscle. ANP participates in water metabolism by inhibiting thirst. BNP, formerly referred to as brain natriuretic peptide, is secreted by the ventricular myocardium in response to excessive stretching (i.e., fluid overload). Its mode of action is similar to that of ANP, though it binds to the natriuretic peptide receptor with much lower affinity. Its half-life is only 22 mins, allowing it to reflect dynamically the state of the heart. Consequently, plasma BNP concentrations are used in the diagnosis and management of heart failure. CNP is produced by vascular endothelial cells and does not directly induce natriuresis and is thought to have an autocrine/paracrine effect at the level of the endothelium.

CELLULAR RESPONSES TO DISTURBANCES IN PLASMA OSMOLALITY

In response to an increase in plasma osmolality, water is shifted from the ICF to ECF in an attempt to maintain a balance in osmolality. Significant hyperosmolality occurring abruptly can be accompanied by cellular shrinkage and likely accounts for the abrupt clinical symptomatology that accompanies such perturbations. Conversely, for many cell types, additional mechanisms are operative to respond to chronic hyperosmolar states. For instance, in the brain, idiogenic osmoles are generated to offset increased plasma osmolality and reestablish normal intracellular volume without further increasing intracellular sodium and chloride that can interrupt normal metabolism. These "compatible" (idiogenic) osmoles include inositol, glycine, and taurine and do not interfere with cellular metabolism. However, the generation of these osmoles presents a therapeutic dilemma for clinicians, as rapid correction of the hyperosmolar state in their presence can lead to cellular swelling (i.e., cerebral edema).

POTASSIUM HOMEOSTASIS

Increases in ECF potassium stimulate aldosterone secretion, thereby indirectly stimulating potassium excretion in urine. Aldosterone interacts with the mineralocorticoid receptor in renal principal cells, which comprise the majority of the tubular epithelium in the late distal tubules and cortical collecting ducts. Stimulation of the mineralocorticoid receptor upregulates Na^+,K^+-ATPase activity at the basolateral membrane, thereby effecting an increase in intracellular potassium. Because the luminal border of the principal cells is highly permeable to potassium (unlike other renal tubular cells), potassium can flow down its concentration gradient into the tubular lumen for excretion. Aldosterone also acts upon the colon to stimulate sodium reabsorption and potassium secretion. Other nonrenal regulators of potassium include insulin, catecholamines, and acid-base balance. Stimulation of β_2-adrenergic receptors activates Na^+, K^+-ATPase, thereby lowering plasma potassium concentrations. This activity may prevent excessive ECF potassium concentrations due to exercise-induced potassium release by muscles. Stimulation of α-adrenergic receptors triggers movement of potassium to the ECF. Acidosis causes a shift in potassium to the extracellular space in exchange for hydrogen ions.

CLINICAL PRESENTATION AND DIFFERENTIAL DIAGNOSIS

Differential Diagnosis of Hypernatremic Conditions

The disorders that can result in hypernatremic states are noted in **Table 72.1**. Primary hyperaldosteronism is unlikely to occur in children, whereas Cushing syndrome may occur (often due to primary adrenal tumors and less commonly due to pituitary adenoma). The more common cause of Cushing syndrome in PICU patients is iatrogenic (i.e., due to prolonged use of high-dose glucocorticoids in patients admitted because of worsening of the primary

---

TABLE 72.1

HYPERNATREMIC CONDITIONS

Clinically normal hydration (or mild hypervolemia)
  Hypothalamic hypodipsia
  Iatrogenic
  Hyperaldosteronism
  Cushing syndrome

Clinically dehydrated (or mild dehydration to normal hydration)
  Diabetes insipidus (central or nephrogenic)
  Hypertonic dehydration—gastrointestinal losses (infection, fistulas)
  Skin loss—burns, fever, excessive sweating (over heating)
  Drugs—alcohol ingestion, diuretics

TABLE 72.2

CAUSES OF CENTRAL DIABETES INSIPIDUS

Genetic
 Autosomal dominant inheritance
 Autosomal recessive inheritance
 Wolfram syndrome (DIDMOAD syndrome)
  autosomal recessive
 X-linked recessive inherited (associated with Xq2B)

Anatomic congenital malformation
 Septo-optic dysplasia
 Holoprosencephaly
 Pituitary agenesis

Acquired
 CNS tumors that involve hypothalamus or pituitary
  stalk (germinoma, craniopharyngioma)
 Trauma—severing pituitary stalk
 Surgery involving pituitary stalk (removal of
  craniopharyngioma or optic glioma)
 Hypophysitis
 Granulomatous disease—histiocytosis, sarcoid
 Infection—meningitis, encephalitis
 Vascular injury

DIDMOAD—DI, diabetes insipidus; DM, diabetes mellitus;
OA, optic atrophy; D, deafness; CNS, central nervous system

TABLE 72.3

HYPONATREMIC CONDITIONS

**Associated with clinically normal hydration (or mild
 hypervolemia)**
 SIADH
 Iatrogenic—water overload
 Protein loss
 Renal disease
 Skin loss
 Central adrenal insufficiency
 Hypothyroidism

Associated with clinical dehydration
 Salt-wasting (cerebral, renal tubular)
 Primary adrenal insufficiency
 Non-ketotic hyperosmolar coma
 Drugs—diuretics

morbidity for which they are receiving glucocorticoid treatment). Diabetes insipidus (DI) can arise from vasopressin deficiency (central DI) or vasopressin insensitivity (nephrogenic DI). The causes of central DI are listed in **Table 72.2**. Vasopressin deficiency follows severing of the pituitary stalk/injury. In some children, a phase of excessive, although temporary, vasopressin release can follow this initial deficient state. This second phase reflects release of stored vasopressin from necrotic vasopressin-secreting neurons. Varying degrees of vasopressin deficiency then ensue. Alcohol will inhibit vasopressin release and cause excessive loss of free water.

Differential Diagnosis of Hyponatremic Conditions

Disorders associated with hyponatremia can be separated into those with clinically normal hydration (or mild overhydration) and those with clinical dehydration as outlined in **Table 72.3**. As a result of plasma expansion during syndrome of inappropriate antidiuretic hormone (SIADH), ANP may be elevated and exacerbate the hyponatremic condition by causing renal salt wasting. This compensatory response has led to the misdiagnosis of SIADH as cerebral salt wasting, a hyponatremic condition associated with polyuria and natriuresis from inappropriate secretion of BNP. Renal disease, both acute and chronic

renal failure, with reduced glomerular filtration and loss of tubular function, is a known cause of hyponatremia. Hyponatremia is also associated with postrenal transplant. Loss of sodium through skin occurs in patients with cystic fibrosis, adrenal insufficiency, and significant burns. Salt loss is concerning in patients with cystic fibrosis, salt-wasting congenital adrenal hyperplasia, and other forms of adrenal insufficiency. Hyponatremia can develop if thirst is treated by ingestion of nonelectrolyte fluids during periods of excessive heat and excessive perspiration.

Central adrenal insufficiency (i.e., secondary or tertiary corticotrophin-releasing hormone or ACTH deficiency) results in insufficient glucocorticoid production, especially during stress. Because glucocorticoids (a) have an adjunctive role in aldosterone production, (b) suppress production of nitric oxide, and (c) suppress vasopressin production, mild hyponatremia without hyperkalemia can occur with central adrenal insufficiency; this is true, as well, in the syndromes of ACTH insensitivity. Affected patients do not have the marked water and electrolyte problems of primary adrenal insufficiency because the adrenal zona glomerulosa is regulated by the renin-angiotensin system and not affected by ACTH deficiency.

Severe hyponatremia in the setting of persistent urine output raises questions as to whether the patient has (a) SIADH and compensatory ANP production from fluid overload, (b) cerebral salt wasting (CSW), or (c) vasopressin insufficiency in the setting of a salt-losing process. The child with CSW will be dehydrated; the child with SIADH has normal-to-expanded blood volume. The clinical picture becomes more complicated in the child with DI who also develops CSW as a result of underlying CNS pathology or radiation therapy. The clinical and biochemical differences between these often coexisting

TABLE 72.4

TABLE 72.4

CLINICAL AND BIOCHEMICAL FINDINGS IN PATIENTS WITH DI AND INADEQUATELY TREATED DIABETES INSIPIDUS, IATROGENIC FLUID OVERLOAD OR VASOPRESSIN EXCESS, SIADH, AND SALT WASTING

Disorder	Clinical and biochemical findings			
	Serum sodium	Urine sodium	Urine output	Hydration
DI—inadequate treatment	High	Low	High	Dehydrated
Excess DDAVP or water excess	Low	Low	Normal or Low	Normal or mild edema
SIADH	Low	High	Low	Normal or mild edema
Salt wasting	Low	High	High	Dehydrated

DI, diabetes insipidus; DDAVP, 1-deamino(8-D-arginine) vasopressin; SIADH, syndrome of inappropriate antidiuretic hormone

conditions are listed in **Table 72.4**. Prolonged use of diuretics, especially in the presence of concomitant salt restriction, can cause volume-contracted hyponatremia. The "loop" diuretics, such as furosemide, inhibit salt absorption in the medullary ascending limb of the loop of Henle, causing sodium loss but rarely causing hyponatremia. The thiazide diuretics inhibit the sodium chloride cotransporter reabsorption at the cortical diluting segments (the early distal convoluted tubule).

Differential Diagnosis of Hyperkalemic Disorders

Though the disorders of hyperkalemia are separated into mild, moderate, and severe hyperkalemia in **Table 72.5**, the clinical disturbances might not be reflected by serum concentrations of potassium. Mild hyperkalemia refers to plasma K^+ in the 5–6 mE/L range without ECG changes or with only tall T waves, moderate hyperkalemia refers to plasma K^+ in

TABLE 72.5

HYPERKALEMIC CONDITIONS

Mild increase
  Spurious hyperkalemia
  Dietary intake of potassium
  Fasting

Moderate (to severe) increase
  Drugs
  Cell death—tumor lysis
  Hyperkalemic periodic paralysis

Severe hyperkalemia
  Chronic and acute renal failure
  Adrenal insufficiency
  Low renin hyperkalemia

the 6–7 mE/L with ECG changes that reveal absent P waves and wide QRS complexes, and severe hyperkalemia refers to plasma $K^+ > 7$–8 and ventricular arrhythmias. It is the intracellular content of potassium that is of major concern. The acid-base status, serum calcium, and sodium concentrations, and rate of change in potassium concentrations all influence the clinical threat of hyperkalemia. The complaints vary from fatigue to muscle weakness, disorientation, paresthesias, and palpitations. The major concern is cardiac dysfunction due to the hyperkalemia, with asystole being the most serious outcome. Initially, hyperkalemia is demonstrated by tall-peaked T waves, then by a prolonged P-R interval, and then flattened or absent P waves. Concern for major cardiac disturbances and asystole is heightened by ECG findings that demonstrate widening QRS intervals, merging ST waves, and then bradycardia, all of which precede ventricular tachycardia.

Routine serum electrolyte determinations often find mild elevations of potassium secondary to hemolysis of RBCs during the blood sampling. A form of spurious hyperkalemia (also referred to as pseudohyperkalemia) is found, especially in hyperviscosity syndromes. The list of drugs that have resulted in mild hyperkalemia include β blockers, angiotensin-converting enzyme inhibitors, nonsteroidal anti-inflammatory drugs, potassium-sparing diuretics, such as spironolactone, and drugs that interfere with the renin-angiotensin system (including losartan). Massive cell death, such as occurs with tumor lysis or rhabdomyolysis, can cause hyperkalemia. Massive blood transfusion and red-cell lysis during mechanical dialysis can similarly cause red-cell breakdown and increase serum potassium levels. Hyperkalemic periodic paralysis includes a group of genetic disorders with mutations in sodium, calcium, and potassium channels. Hyperkalemic periodic paralysis presents with attacks of disabling weakness and elevated serum potassium levels. Precipitants for these attacks include cold, exercise, and hunger.

Renal disease, including chronic renal insufficiency, acute renal failure, and end-stage renal failure can be associated with significant hyperkalemia. In acute renal failure, the increase in potassium levels may be rapid and tolerated poorly. In more chronic situations, despite potassium levels of 7–8 mEq/L, cardiac function and ECG findings remain normal. Patients with primary adrenal crisis present in shock, dehydration, cardiac arrhythmias, hyponatremia, severe hyperkalemia, and a nonanion gap metabolic acidosis. Type IV renal tubular acidosis occurs in states of aldosterone deficiency or insensitivity and manifests as persistent hyperkalemia, reduced bicarbonate reabsorption, and potentially mild-to-moderate glomerular insufficiency.

Differential Diagnosis of Hypokalemic Disorders

Hypokalemia is generally less threatening than hyperkalemia. Nevertheless, low potassium levels can be associated with cardiac arrhythmias, particularly in the setting of preexisting cardiac problems. In general, no symptoms or only mild weakness are present. Certainly, muscular weakness can be associated with ileus or respiratory difficulties. The disorders of hypokalemia are listed in **Table 72.6**. Hypokalemic periodic paralysis are characterized by intermittent muscular weakness (particularly of the shoulders and hips) or generalized paralysis that lasts <24 hrs; weakness that compromises breathing and swallowing has also been described. Bartter syndrome is clinically recognized by failure to thrive, developmental delay, increased renin, hypokalemia, and alkalosis. Muscle weakness, muscle cramps, and salt craving may also be present. Hypertension and edema are absent. Hyperplasia of the juxtaglomerular cells, with elevated urinary excretion of prostaglandin E_2 is present. All 4 subtypes of Bartter syndrome are autosomal recessive in inheritance and are characterized by abnormal sodium chloride reabsorption in the ascending limb of the loop of Henle. Pseudo–Bartter syndrome describes those children with hypokalemic alkalosis, normotensive hyperreninism, and hyperaldosteronism, in whom these abnormalities arise as a result of chronic loop diuretic use or sodium chloride loss by other means, such as vomiting. Gitelman syndrome arises from mutations in the thiazide-sensitive sodium chloride cotransporter. Affected children do not have growth failure or developmental delay. This condition often presents later in childhood with hypokalemia, hypocalciuria, and, frequently hypomagnesemia. Prostaglandin E_2 excretion is normal. These children characteristically have carpopedal spasm.

TABLE 72.6

HYPOKALEMIC CONDITIONS

Drugs—diuretics, chemotherapeutic agents (cis-platinum), amphotericin B, penicillin derivatives and licorice
Gastrointestinal disease—severe diarrhea
Adrenal cortical excess, primary Aldosteronism and other hyporeninemic syndromes
Hypokalemic periodic paralysis
Bartter syndrome
Pseudo-Bartter syndrome
Gitelman syndrome

ASSESSMENT AND MANAGEMENT OF SODIUM AND POTASSIUM DISORDERS

In addition to a through history and physical examination, basic metabolic panel, ionized calcium, serum magnesium, blood urea nitrogen, and creatinine help to evaluate both the potential degree of dehydration and renal function. A spot urinary sodium is extremely useful, with urinary sodium >30 mmol/L, indicative of high urinary sodium excretion. Direct measurements of plasma and urine osmolalities can be extremely useful in DI and helpful in documenting salt-wasting polyuria. Urine output must be measured and recorded. Dependent upon a number of variables, including age, urine output >2–3 mL/kg/hr in children (outside of infancy) is excessive. CT scan of the brain in those patients with potential cerebral edema or brain injury may be indicated. ECG, especially in those patients with disorders of potassium, is necessary for evaluation and for monitoring progress of all patients with water and electrolyte disturbances. Central venous pressure determination might be indicated in assessing the degree of dehydration in certain patients.

Regardless of the underlying electrolyte abnormality (hypo- or hypernatremia, hypo- or hyperkalemia), the dehydrated child requires fluid resuscitation. The initial volume to be administered will depend upon the extent of cardiovascular compromise and generally consists of 0.9% NaCl solution. While a mildly dehydrated child may require only a 20 mL/kg bolus of normal saline solution, repeated boluses may be required for the severely dehydrated child. Isotonic saline is continued until the cardiovascular status is stabilized. Continued fluid therapy will then depend upon the child's cardiovascular status, remaining fluid deficit, and nature of the electrolyte abnormality.

Hypernatremia

Hypernatremic dehydration arises from excessive free water loss, as occurs with DI, or water loss that is disproportionate to electrolyte loss. Following initial resuscitation with boluses and continuous infusions administered to restore perfusion and correct volume depletion, replacement therapy is required and must address the free-water deficit in the child with persistent hypernatremia due to pure water loss or the sodium and water deficit, as occurs with hypotonic sodium loss. With the use of typical resuscitation fluids (0.9% NaCl), the plasma sodium is likely only to decrease slightly [for instance, 1 L of 0.9% NaCL in a 30-kg child with total body water of 18 L (30 × 0.6) and plasma sodium of 165 will decrease the plasma sodium by $(165 - 154)/(18 + 1) = 0.6$ mEq/L]. Continued use of isotonic saline will not correct the hypernatremia, and a hypotonic solution must be introduced. In the child with known or presumed chronic hypernatremia, the subsequent goal of therapy is to decrease plasma sodium by ~0.5 mEq/L every hour (12 mEq/L/24 hrs) to reduce the risk of cerebral edema.

$$\text{Free water deficit} = \text{Total body water} - \text{Total body water at time of hypernatremia} =$$
$$(\text{TBWD}) \times (\text{weight kg}) -$$
$$\frac{[(\text{normal } P_{Na} = 140 \text{ mEq/L}) \times (\text{TBWD}) \times (\text{weight kg})]}{(\text{current } P_{Na} \text{ mEq/L})}$$

where TBWD = total body water distribution and

$$P_{Na} = \text{plasma sodium.}$$

The TBWD depends upon the age, gender, and weight of the child. An extremely obese adolescent may have a water distribution of 0.5; 0.6 is frequently used for the adult male, 0.5 for the adult female, 0.7 for infants. If possible, this free water should be delivered via the gastrointestinal tract. Continued losses must also be addressed. For the child with central DI, institution of vasopressin by continuous infusion (starting dose 0.5 mU/kg/hr) will curb excessive losses. The continuous vasopressin infusion allows quick titration and avoids excessive urine output associated with "breakthroughs." DDAVP is avoided in the initial management because of its long half-life, preventing fine-tuning of fluid therapy. The use of vasopressin may dictate a recalculation of maintenance fluids (normally 1500 mL/m^2).

For children with hypotonic sodium loss, the above free water deficit formula may underestimate their losses. The Androgue-Madias formula calculates the amount that plasma Na will drop following infusion of 1 liter of fluid of varying components:

$$\frac{(\text{NaCl of infusate}) - (\text{current } P_{Na} \text{ mEq/L})}{\text{TBWD} \times \text{WT(kg)} + \text{infusate volume}}$$

For a 30-kg child with a total body water distribution of 0.6 and plasma sodium of 170 receiving 600 mL (0.6 L) of normal saline solution: $(154-170)/[(0.6 \times 30) + 0.6] = -0.86$; the plasma sodium will decrease by 0.86 mEq/L, whereas use of 600 nL of 1/2 normal saline solution (77 mEq/L) will decrease plasma sodium by 5 mEq/L. Additional loss must be addressed. For the child with severe diarrhea, vomitus, or nasogastric output, these losses will include water and other electrolytes, and additional fluid supplementation should reflect this fluid composition.

Hyponatremia

With hyponatremic dehydration, the sodium deficit exceeds the free water deficit. Treatment considerations should include administration of 3% NaCl to raise plasma sodium by ~3–5 mEq/L over several hours. If symptoms primarily reflect dehydration, normal saline solution should be administered; the plasma sodium will also increase with this step but to a much lesser extent. Again, following initial resuscitation, further correction of the fluid and sodium deficits must be addressed. Additionally, sources of free water should be discontinued. In general, a conservative approach is to assume that the development of hyponatremia has occurred over an extended period of time and, thus, should be corrected slowly (0.5 mEq/L/hr). Maintenance sodium and water requirements should be calculated; sodium and water deficits should be estimated. The total sodium deficit can be calculated as:

$$(140 \text{ mEq/L} - P_{Na} \text{ mEq/L}) \times (\text{TBWD} \times \text{WT in kg})$$

Generally, half of the deficit is replaced at a rate of 0.5 mEq/hr. Thus, the 30-kg child with a P_{Na} of 120 and a distribution of water of 0.6 will have a sodium deficit of $(140 - 120) \times (0.6 \times 30) = 360$ mEq. The initial correction of 10 mEq/L will be replaced at a rate of 0.5 mEq/hr (i.e., over 20 hrs). If 0.9% NaCl solution is used (154 mEq/L = 0.154 mEq/mL), the infusion rate necessary to correct half of the deficit is (360 mEq/0.154 mEq/mL)/20 hr = 117 mL/hr. Following institution of specific fluid rates and types, the effect of these therapies upon hydration and biochemical parameters must be reviewed.

For the child with DI who has been overtreated with vasopressin and water, the salt wasting reflects a normal response to fluid overload, and withholding of fluids and additional vasopressin will permit diuresis and correction of the hyponatremic state. For the child with DI and either concomitant cerebral salt wasting or natriuresis due to drug toxicity, the approach to hyponatremia can be more problematic. After initial resuscitation, the sodium deficit should be determined and ongoing urinary sodium losses should be calculated by measuring urine sodium and volume. Vasopressin is withheld because it can potentiate hyponatremia. However, a vasopressin drip should be readily available at the bedside, as the waning effect of previously administered vasopressin/DDAVP and resolution of the salt-wasting state may be accompanied by excessive free water losses and rapid increases in plasma sodium.

As with hyponatremic dehydration, initial management depends upon clinical symptoms. The child with symptomatic hyponatremia, such as significant lethargy, seizures, or coma, will require infusion of hypertonic saline. Following initial resuscitation in the symptomatic child, water restriction alone or in combination with hypertonic sodium chloride and furosemide will increase sodium without exacerbating the fluid overloaded state. In addition, the underlying cause of the hyponatremia must be addressed. Excessive free water intake due to primary polydipsia or to overdiluted infant formula may respond to fluid restriction. However, caution must be taken so that withdrawal of the free water source does not cause over-rapid correction of the plasma sodium.

Hyperkalemia

Hyperkalemia is treated with 10% calcium gluconate, 1 mg/kg IV over 2–3 mins as well as rapid IV infusion of glucose (0.25–0.5 g/kg, 2–5 mL/kg of 10% dextrose solution) and regular insulin (0.3 units/g glucose). Treatment with inhaled β-adrenergic agonists is recommended in adults. Kayexalate, 1 g/kg orally or by rectum in sorbitol solution is indicated if not contraindicated by bowel pathology. In the setting of renal failure, dialysis may be required. Treatment of hyperkalemia with sodium bicarbonate has recently been revisited, and the adult literature recommends that it not be used as initial or monotherapy, although it may have a role in the setting of severe metabolic acidosis.

Hypokalemia

The child with hypokalemia-induced paralysis or with hypokalemia-induced ECG changes requires urgent IV treatment (0.5 mEq/kg over 30–60 mins), continuous IV infusion. The child who is on digoxin or has an underlying cardiac defect is at increased risk of arrythmias and may require IV treatment at higher doses (1 mEq/kg) and at higher plasma potassium concentrations. Magnesium replacement may also be necessary to treat hypokalemia.

The child with hypokalemia in the setting of DKA also requires aggressive attention, as glucose and insulin administration will drive potassium intracellularly and aggravate hypokalemia. Potassium is delivered at higher-than-usual rates (provided that the child is urinating) in the setting of normal plasma potassium concentrations because, despite significant total body potassium deficits, the plasma potassium is normal or elevated as a result of insulin deficiency. The potassium can be administered as a combination of potassium chloride and potassium phosphate, as the child with DKA also has a phosphorus deficit. If hypokalemia develops during the course of DKA treatment and hyperglycemia and acidosis have nearly resolved, lowering the insulin infusion rate will help to address the hypokalemia.

CHAPTER 73 ■ DISORDERS OF CALCIUM, MAGNESIUM, AND PHOSPHATE

KENNETH J. BANASIAK • THOMAS O. CARPENTER

REGULATION OF CALCIUM, MAGNESIUM, AND PHOSPHATE HOMEOSTASIS

Unbound calcium and magnesium are the physiologically important forms. Plasma phosphorous exists in the ionized forms of phosphate, HPO_4^{2-} and $H_2PO_4^-$. The remaining plasma phosphate is complexed to cations, primarily Ca^{2+}, Mg^{2+}, and Na^+, or is bound to plasma proteins. The extracellular concentrations of calcium, magnesium, and phosphate are maintained within a normal range through (a) absorption of ingested calcium, magnesium, and phosphate through the intestinal tract, (b) absorption and excretion via the kidney, and (c) mobilization from the bone.

Dietary calcium is passively absorbed in a concentration-dependent fashion by mechanisms regulated by 1, 25-dihydroxyvitamin D. Dietary magnesium is absorbed by both active and passive mechanisms. Phosphate is absorbed by passive processes and active mechanisms regulated by 1, 25-dihydroxyvitamin D. Absorption of phosphate is impeded by the presence of polyvalent cations (e.g., Ca^{2+}, Mg^{2+}, and Al^{3+}) in the intestinal lumen or by deficiency of vitamin D.

Approximately 60%–70% of total plasma calcium, chiefly in its ionized and complexed forms, is filtered by the kidneys. Most (~70%) of filtered calcium is reabsorbed along with sodium and water in the proximal convoluted tubule by a concentration-dependent mechanism. Approximately 70%–80% of plasma magnesium, is filtered in the glomerulus, the bulk of which (60%–70%) is reabsorbed. Phosphate is filtered in the glomerulus, 80% of which is reabsorbed and is attenuated by PTH. Multiple factors can alter renal reabsorption or excretion of calcium, magnesium, and phosphate (**Table 73.1**). Administration of a saline infusion for volume expansion leads to increased calcium, magnesium, and phosphate excretion. During acute hypercalcemia, reduction in glomerular filtration rate, formation of calcium-phosphate-protein complexes (which prevents ultrafiltration of phosphate), and suppression of PTH release contribute to decreased phosphate excretion. During chronic hypercalcemia, phosphate excretion increases. Hypocalcemia and hyperphosphatemia each induce PTH secretion, which in turn, reduces renal excretion of calcium.

Both acute and chronic metabolic acidosis induce calciuria. Metabolic alkalosis reduces calcium excretion. Metabolic alkalosis reduces renal losses of magnesium. Acute metabolic acidosis does not seem to have any significant effect on phosphate excretion, while chronic metabolic acidosis causes phosphaturia. Respiratory acidosis enhances both calcium and phosphate excretion. Respiratory alkalosis decreases renal phosphate excretion but has no effect on calcium excretion. Thiazide diuretics enhance calcium reabsorption and induce phosphaturia. Loop diuretics augment calcium and magnesium excretion. Other medications such as aminoglycosides, cisplatin, and cyclosporine have been shown to increase magnesium excretion.

The plasma concentrations of calcium, phosphate and, to a lesser degree, magnesium are regulated by parathyroid hormone, 1,25-dihydroxyvitamin D, and calcitonin (**Table 73.2**). PTH stimulates the conversion of 25-hydroxyvitamin D to $1,25(OH)_2D_3$ in the proximal tubule. PTH secretion is decreased in response to high blood concentrations of ionized calcium and increased in response to low concentrations. Vitamin D is obtained from two primary sources: the skin and dietary supplementation. In the skin, the precursor of vitamin D undergoes photochemical cleavage to form previtamin D. Previtamin D then undergoes a temperature-dependent molecular rearrangement to form vitamin D. In the liver, vitamin D undergoes 25-hydroxylation. Subsequently, the 25-hydroxyvitamin D undergoes 1-hydroxylation in the kidney to form the biologically active 1,25-dihydroxyvitamin D. 1,25-dihydroxyvitamin D enhances calcium and phosphate absorption primarily in the intestine and, to some extent, in distal renal tubules. Calcitonin inhibits renal tubular reabsorption of calcium and osteoclast-mediated bone resorption. The secretion of calcitonin is stimulated by increased blood calcium levels and by glucocorticoids, calcitonin gene-related peptide, glucagon, enteroglucagon, gastrin, pentagastrin, pancreozymin, and β-adrenergic agents.

DISORDERS OF CALCIUM, MAGNESIUM, AND PHOSPHATE HOMEOSTASIS

Published normal values for total serum calcium range from 8.8–10.8 mg/dL. Normal values for ionized calcium range between 4.2 and 5.5 mg/dL (1.0–1.4 mmol/dL). Reported normal values of magnesium are 1.5–2.3 mg/dL. Normal phosphate levels vary with age, with values ranging from 4.8–8.2 mg/dL in newborns to 2.7–4.7 mg/dL in older adolescents.

Hypocalcemia

Hypocalcemia can occur as the consequence of inadequate calcium intake or malabsorption, hormonal imbalance or dysfunction, chelation by anions, or other causes (**Table 73.3**). Physiologic deficiency of PTH secretion occurs in neonates ("early neonatal hypocalcemia") during the first 4 days of life. This disorder most commonly occurs in premature infants, low-birth-weight infants, infants of diabetic mothers, and infants born after prolonged difficult deliveries. Congenital agenesis or dysgenesis of the parathyroid glands occurs in the family of disorders that are associated with deletions in the chromosome 22q11 region, the locus for DiGeorge syndrome, velocardiofacial syndrome, and conotruncal face syndromes. Antibody-mediated destruction of

TABLE 73.1

FACTORS AFFECTING RENAL EXCRETION OF CALCIUM, MAGNESIUM AND PHOSPHATE

Factor affecting excretion	Calcium		Magnesium		Phosphate	
	Effect on renal excretion	Mechanism(s)	Effect on renal excretion	Mechanism(s)	Effect on renal excretion	Mechanism(s)
Volume expansion	↑	↓ reabsorption in PCT	↑	↓ reabsorption in PCT	↑	↓ reabsorption in PCT
ELECTROLYTE DISTURBANCES						
Hypercalcemia	↑	↓ reabsorption in PCT, TALH, DCT (↓ PTH)	↑	↓ tubular reabsorption	↓ (acute) ↑ (chronic)	↓ ultrafiltration, ↓ GFR and ↓ PTH (acute); ↓ tubular reabsorption via unknown mechanism (chronic)
Hypocalcemia	↓	↑ reabsorption in DCT due to ↑ PTH	↓	↑ reabsorption TALH	↑ or ↓ (chronic hypocalcemia)	↓ tubular reabsorption secondary to ↑ PTH
Hypermagnesemia	↑		↑	↓ reabsorption in TALH		
Hypomagnesemia	↑		↓	↑ reabsorption in TALH		
Hyperphosphatemia	↓	↓ reabsorption in DCT due to ↑ PTH	↓		↓	↑ tubular reabsorption due to ↓ Na-P activity
Hypophosphatemia	↑	↓ reabsorption in DCT	↑	↓ reabsorption in TALH	↓	↑ tubular reabsorption due to ↑ Na-P activity
ACID-BASE DISTURBANCES						
Metabolic acidosis	↑	↓ reabsorption in DCT due to ↓ ECaC1 conductance	↑		↑ (chronic metabolic acidosis)	↓ tubular reabsorption due to ↓ gate of Na-P activity
Metabolic alkalosis	↓	↑ reabsorption in DCT due to ↑ ECaC1 conductance	↓	↑ reabsorption in TALH	↓	↑ tubular reabsorption due to ↑ gate of Na-P activity
Respiratory acidosis	↑		↑			
Respiratory alkalosis			↑			
MEDICATIONS						
Thiazide diuretics	↓		minimal ↑	↓ reabsorption in DCT due to inhibition of Na-Cl cotransporter		
Loop diuretics	↑	↓ reabsorption in DCT due to altered inhibition of Na-K-2Cl cotransporter	↑	↓ reabsorption in DCT due to altered inhibition of Na-K-2Cl cotransporter		
Aminoglycosides	↑		↑	↓ reabsorption in TALH		
Cisplatin	↑		↑	↓ reabsorption in TALH		
Cyclosporine	↑		↑	↓ reabsorption in TALH		

PCT, proximal convoluted tubule; TALH, thick ascending limb of the loop of Henle; DCT, distal convoluted tubule; PTH, parathyroid hormone; GFR, glomerular filtration rate
Modified from Suki WN, Lederer ED, Rouse D. Renal transport of calcium, magnesium, and phosphate. In: Brenner BM (ed). *Bremner and Rector's The Kidney*, 6th ed. Philadelphia: WB Saunders, 2000:520–74.

TABLE 73.2

HORMONAL REGULATION OF CALCIUM AND PHOSPHATE

Hormone	Effect on serum level			
	Calcium	Mechanism of action	Phosphate	Mechanism of action
PTH	↑	↑ reabsorption in DCT and TALH	↓	↓ reabsorption in PCT and DCT
Vitamin D	↑	↑ absorption in intestine and reabsorption in DCT	↑	↑ absorption in intestine and reabsorption in DCT
Calcitonin	↓	↓ bone reabsorption ↓reabsorption in renal tubules		

PTH, parathyroid hormone; DCT, distal convoluted tubule; TALH, thick ascending limb of the loop of Henle; PCT, proximal convoluted tubule

the parathyroid glands has been detected in autoimmune polyglandular syndrome type 1, also known as the autoimmune polyendocrinopathy-candidiasis-ectodermal dystrophy syndrome. End-organ resistance to the action of PTH, or pseudohypoparathyroidism, is associated with high PTH levels in the face of hypocalcemia.

Hypocalcemia as the result of low 1,25-dihydroxyviatmin D can occur due to inadequate vitamin D intake or production, increased vitamin D catabolism, decreased 25-hydroxylation in the liver, decreased 1-hydroxylation in the kidney, and vitamin D resistance. Inadequate intake of fatty fishes, mild or other vitamin D–containing foods, exclusive breast feeding (without vitamin D supplementation), and inadequate sun exposure can lead to vitamin D deficiency and rickets. Inadequate intestinal absorption of vitamin D has been observed in patients with gastrectomy, celiac disease, extensive bowel surgery, inflammatory bowel disease, hepatic, or pancreatic insufficiency due to cystic fibrosis. Hepatic 25-hydroxylation of vitamin D is mildly impaired in severe liver disease or dysfunction. Decreased 1-hydroxylation of 25-hydroxyvitamin D occurs in patients with renal disease.

Hyperphosphatemia as a consequence of massive tissue lysis (e.g., tumor lysis syndrome and rhabdomyolysis) or phosphate administration can induce hypocalcemia due to formation of calcium phosphate precipitates in soft tissues. Administration of lipids or excess release of free fatty acids, as seen in pancreatitis, may also cause hypocalcemia.

The signs and symptoms of hypocalcemia are summarized in **Table 73.4**. Patients may report myoclonic jerks and paresthesias of the perioral region, fingers, and toes. In more severe cases, patients may present with seizures, apnea, cyanosis, laryngospasm, tachypnea, tachycardia, and vomiting. On physical examination, percussion of the facial nerve below the zygomatic arch may result in facial muscle contrac-

tion (Chvostek sign). Compression of the arm or leg with a blood pressure cuff may result in carpopedal spasm (Trousseau sign).

Total serum calcium and, often, ionized calcium and albumin are useful, as are phosphorus, magnesium, blood urea nitrogen, creatinine, alkaline phosphatase activity, PTH, 1,25-dihydroxyvitamin D, and 25-hydroxyvitamin D. On a random "spot" urine collection, urinary calcium excretion is best interpreted as a calcium/creatinine (mg/mg) ratio.

Urinary phosphorous excretion is very dependent upon diet and body phosphorous status. The ideal assessment is obtained with a fasting 2-hr urine collection, with a concomitant serum sample obtained midway through the urine collection. The tubular reabsorption of phosphate (TRP) is expressed as a percentage of the filtered phosphate load and is calculated by the formula:

$$\text{TRP} = 1 - \left[\frac{[P]u \times [Cr]s}{[P]s \times [Cr]u} \right] \times 100\%$$

where [P]u is the concentration of phosphate in urine, [P]s is the concentration of phosphate in serum, [Cr]u is the concentration of creatinine in urine, and [Cr]s is the concentration of creatinine in serum. All units should be identical (e.g., mg/dL).

Serum phosphorus is usually low in patients with vitamin D deficiency and is elevated in renal failure, hypoparathyroidism, and pseudohypoparathyroidism. In vitamin D-dependent rickets type I, the serum 25-hydroxyvitamin D level is normal, and the 1,25-dihydroxyvitamin D is low. Serum alkaline phosphatase activity may be elevated in patients with long-standing vitamin D deficiency but usually not in early disease. A low or normal circulating PTH in the presence of hypocalcemia indicates an inappropriate parathyroid response to hypocalcemia or, therefore, functional hypoparathyroidism. Increased PTH secretion is a normal physiologic response to hypocalcemia, so that elevated serum PTH would

TABLE 73.3

CAUSES OF HYPOCALCEMIA

Inadequate intake or malabsorption
PTH-related
    Impaired parathyroid gland formation
        Congenital agenesis or dysgenesis of the
            parathyroid glands
        DiGeorge syndrome
        X-linked hypoparathyroidism
    PTH gene mutations
    Parathyroid gland destruction
        Autoimmune polyglandular syndrome type 1
        Inadvertent surgical destruction
        Hemochromatosis
        Thalassemia major
        Wilson disease
    Impaired secretion of PTH
        Hypomagnesemia
        Maternal hypercalcemia
        Calcium-sensing receptor mutations
        Cytokine release
        Respiratory alkalosis
    End-organ resistance to PTH
        (pseudohypoparathyroidism)

Vitamin D related
    Inadequate intake or absorption
        Breast-feeding (without vitamin D
            supplementation)
        Gastrectomy
        Small-bowel surgery
        Celiac disease
        Inflammatory bowel disease
        Cystic fibrosis
    Increased catabolism
        Phenobarbital
        Phenytoin
        Carbamazepine
        Isoniazid
        Rifampin
        Theophylline
    Decreased 25-hydroxylation (hepatic disease)
    Decreased 1-hydroxylation (renal disease)
    Vitamin D resistance

Chelation by anions
    Hyperphosphatemia
    Red blood cell transfusions (citrate)
    Lipid administration
    Pancreatitis (fatty acids)

Other
    Fluoride intoxication
    "Hungry-bone" syndrome
    Critical illness

TABLE 73.4

SIGNS AND SYMPTOMS OF HYPOCALCEMIA

Neuromuscular
    Paresthesias
    Chvostek sign (facial muscle spasm)
    Trousseau sign (carpopedal spasm)
    Bronchospasm
    Laryngospasm
    Apnea
    Seizures

Cardiac
    Prolonged QT interval
    Nonspecific ST-T wave changes

Rickets (radiographic findings)
    Epiphyseal widening
    Costochondral widening ("rachitic rosary")
    Widening of the wrists
    Genu varum or valgum
    Osteopenia

occur in nonparathyroid-related hypocalcemia such as in vitamin D deficiency or impaired vitamin D action. Increased PTH levels are usually seen in pseudohypoparathyroidism.

Calcium may be given intravenously or orally. For patients who present with acute symptomatic hypocalcemia, (i.e., tetany, muscle twitching, carpopedal spasm, laryngospasm, or seizures), a bolus dose of calcium gluconate (100–200 mg/kg or 9–18 mg/kg elemental calcium to a maximum of 1–3 g in adults) should be administered over 10–20 mins. Repeat bolus doses of 100–200 mg/kg/dose of calcium gluconate can be given every 6–8 hrs until the ionized calcium level stabilizes. Alternatively, a continuous infusion of calcium gluconate infusion may be administered at a starting dose of 10–30 mg/kg/hr. The rate of the infusion can then be titrated based on serial calcium measurements (or ionized calcium if necessary). Calcium chloride and calcium gluconate have similar bioavailability and are equally effective in correcting ionized hypocalcemia. We recommend administering IV calcium through a central venous catheter because of a significant risk of tissue necrosis with peripheral administration. Cardiac telemetry or electrocardiograms should be used during IV calcium administration to detect cardiac rhythm disturbances. In hypocalcemic patients with hypomagnesemia, magnesium should be replenished with IV magnesium sulfate or oral magnesium oxide. In patients with concurrent hyperphosphatemia, the elevated phosphate should be corrected with phosphate binders, due to the risk of tissue deposition of calcium phosphate if the calcium-phosphate product [(Ca)s × (PO$_4$)s] exceeds 80. This figure is the product of total serum calcium (mg/dL) and the serum phosphorous levels (mg/dL). In patients with hypocalcemia secondary to vitamin D deficiency or resistance, vitamin D replacement and adequate dietary calcium intake are the mainstays of therapy. The formulation and dosage of vitamin D required are dependent on the cause of the disorder.

Hypercalcemia

Hypercalcemia generally occurs as the consequence of excessive dietary calcium intake or increased intestinal absorption. These alterations may be related to hormonal imbalance or dysfunction, increased renal reabsorption, or increased bone resorption (**Table 73.5**). In addition to primary and secondary, "tertiary" hyperparathyroidism is seen in children with chronic renal failure. This entity refers to the development of autonomous PTH secretion

TABLE 73.5

CAUSES OF HYPERCALCEMIA

Excessive intake
  "Milk-alkali syndrome"
  Oral calcium supplements
  Parenteral nutrition

PTH-related
  Hyperparathyroidism (primary and secondary)
  Calcium-sensing receptor mutations
  Multiple endocrine neoplasia type 1
  Multiple endocrine neoplasia type 2a
  Parathyroid adenoma
  Transient neonatal hyperparathyroidism (parathyroid gland hyperplasia)
  Chronic lithium toxicity
  Chronic renal failure
  Hyperparathyroid-jaw tumor syndrome

Humoral hypercalcemia of malignancy (PTHrP-, TNF-, cytokine-mediated)

Vitamin D intoxication

Increased renal reabsorption
  Thiazide diuretics
  Calcium-sensing receptor mutations

Increased bone resorption
  Thyrotoxicosis
  Vitamin A intoxication
  Primary and metastatic tumors
  Cytokine release
  Immobilization

Other
  William syndrome
  Subcutaneous fat necrosis

TABLE 73.6

SIGNS AND SYMPTOMS OF HYPERCALCEMIA

Neuromuscular
  Fatigue
  Weakness
  Lethargy
  Confusion
  Coma
  Hallucinations
  Psychosis

Gastrointestinal
  Poor feeding
  Failure to thrive
  Nausea
  Vomiting
  Constipation
  Pancreatitis (rare)

Cardiac
  Shortened QT interval
  Ventricular dysrhythmias

Renal
  Polyuria
  Hyposthenuria
  Dehydration
  Hypernatremia
  Renal stone formation
  Nephrogenic diabetes insipidus
  Renal failure

after chronic "secondary" or physiologic parathyroid gland hyperfunction, for example, due to prolonged hypocalcaemia. A number of childhood malignancies, including rhabdoid tumors of the kidney, congenital mesoblastic nephroma, neuroblastoma, medulloblastoma, leukemia, Burkitt lymphoma, dysgerminoma, and rhabdomyosarcoma, are associated with hypercalcemia of malignancy.

Signs and symptoms of hypercalcemia are varied, and the severity of the symptoms is correlated with the degree of hypercalcemia (**Table 73.6**). Severe symptoms are observed in patients with serum calcium levels >15 mg/dL. Patients with serum levels of <15 mg/dL may be asymptomatic. Infants tend to present with gastrointestinal symptoms such as poor feeding, emesis, and failure to thrive. Laboratory investigation should include total serum calcium, serum phosphorus, blood urea nitrogen, creatinine, alkaline phosphatase, urinary calcium, urinary phosphorus, urinary creatinine (for calculation of the calcium/creatinine ratio and the tubular reabsorption of phosphorus), PTH, 1,25-dihydroxyvitamin D, and 25-hydroxyvitamin D. If malignancy is suspected as a cause, a PTHrP level may be useful. An elevated PTH in the presence of hypercalcemia is diagnostic for primary hyperparathyroidism, unless the history and physical examination suggest familial hypocalciuric hypercalcemia, malignancy, or lithium therapy. When distinguishing between primary hyperparathyroidism and familial hypocalciuric hypercalcemia, a urinary calcium:creatinine ratio of <0.01 (mg/mg) raises suspicion for the familial disorder, although the distinction may be difficult to make on clinical grounds. A low or normal PTH level should prompt investigation of malignancy-related or other non–PTH-dependent causes of hypercalcemia.

The treatment of hypercalcemia is dependent on its severity. The initial basic tenets of therapy are to restore intravascular volume (as hypercalcemic patients are typically dehydrated) and to enhance renal excretion, which can be accomplished by administration of normal saline at 2–3 times maintenance fluid rate. If the patient is adequately rehydrated and calcium levels do not decrease, loop diuretics may be administered to enhance renal excretion of calcium but should be done judiciously to avoid intravascular volume depletion. Calcitonin and bisphosphonates, which inhibit bone resorption, are useful adjuncts in severe hypercalcemia. Reasonable success has been achieved with IV pamidronate in treating selected cases of childhood hypercalcemia. In severe cases in which hydration and medications fail to reduce serum calcium levels, hemodialysis using a low-calcium dialysate can be performed. Glucocorticoids have been useful in treating hypercalcemia secondary to sarcoidosis and vitamin D deficiency (through inhibition of intestinal actions of vitamin D). Indications for surgery for primary hyperparathyroidism include total calcium level >12 mg/dL, hyperparathyroid crisis (discrete episode of life-threatening hypercalcemia), marked hypercalciuria, nephrolithiasis, impaired renal function, osteitis fibrosa cystica, reduced cortical bone density (measured with dual x-ray absorptiometry or similar technique), bone mass >2 standard deviations below age-matched controls, classic neuromuscular symptoms, proximal muscle weakness and atrophy, hyperreflexia, gait disturbance, and age younger than 50.

Hypomagnesemia

Hypomagnesemia generally occurs as the consequence of decreased dietary magnesium intake or malabsorption, its decreased renal reabsorption, or its redistribution from the extracellular to the intracellular space (**Table 73.7**). The movement of magnesium from the extracellular to the intracellular compartment occurs in a variety of disorders, including insulin therapy for diabetic ketoacidosis and hyper-

TABLE 73.7

CAUSES OF HYPOMAGNESEMIA

Decreased dietary intake or malabsorption
    Protein-calorie malnutrition
    Parenteral nutrition
    Alcoholism
    Diarrhea
    Celiac disease
    Inflammatory bowel disease

Decreased renal reabsorption
    Inherited disorders
        Isolated familial hypomagnesemia
        Primary hypomagnesemia with hypercalciuria
        Primary hypomagnesemia with hypocalcemia
        Bartter syndrome
        Gitelman syndrome
    Medications
        Loop diuretics
        Cisplatin
        Pentamidine
        Cyclosporine
        Aminoglycosides
        Foscarnet
        Amphotericin

Redistribution from the extracellular to the intracellular space
    Insulin therapy
    Hyperinsulinism
    Pancreatitis
    Hyperaldosteronism
    Respiratory alkalosis
    Catecholamines

insulinism associated with the "refeeding syndrome" in chronically malnourished children. Hypomagnesemia has been observed in patients who undergo cardiopulmonary bypass or require massive transfusion and in those with extensive burn injury or excessive sweating.

The signs and symptoms of hypomagnesemia are often due to the hypocalcemia from impaired PTH release and hypokalemia, which are also associated with hypomagnesemia. Presenting neurologic signs include muscle weakness and tremors, tetany, Chvostek sign, Trousseau sign, and seizures. Hypokalemia consequent to hypomagnesemia manifests in nonspecific T-wave changes, U waves, a prolonged QT interval, and ventricular arrhythmias. Hypomagnesemia per se can predispose to cardiac dysrhythmias, particularly those of ventricular origin. However, the degree of risk for dysrhythmias in patients with hypomagnesemia in general and the relative importance of Mg^{2+} deficiency alone versus hypomagnesemia with coexisting hypokalemia or intrinsic cardiac disease in the pathogenesis of the dysrhythmia remain controversial.

Serum magnesium, serum calcium and potassium levels should be measured. If the cause of hypomagnesemia is unknown, measurement of plasma and urinary magnesium and creatinine concentrations and calculation of the fractional excretion of magnesium (FE_{Mg}) using the following equation can assist in the differentiation between renal and nonrenal causes of hypomagnesemia.

$$FE_{Mg} = [(U_{Mg} \times P_{creatinine})/(0.7 \times P_{Mg} \times U_{creatinine})] \times 100$$

Normal values for the fractional excretion of magnesium range from 1% to 8%. In patients with hypomagnesemia due to nonrenal causes, the FE_{Mg} is <2%. In patients with renal magnesium wasting, the FE_{Mg} is >4%. If a renal cause of hypomagnesemia is suspected, an arterial blood gas should be obtained to assess for metabolic alkalosis.

Symptomatic patients or asymptomatic patients with magnesium levels <1 mg/dL require IV replacement with a magnesium salt. Magnesium sulfate at a dose of 25–50 mg/kg (2.5–5.0 mg/kg of elemental magnesium) given as a slow IV infusion is recommended. Serum magnesium levels should be closely monitored, and the dose should be repeated every 6 hrs until levels stabilize.

Hypermagnesemia

Hypermagnesemia can be the consequence of increased intake or administration of magnesium, decreased renal excretion, massive cellular release, or other causes (**Table 73.8**). The signs and symptoms

TABLE 73.8

CAUSES OF HYPERMAGNESEMIA

Increased intake
Laxatives
Enemas
Parenteral administration
Magnesium supplementation
Decreased renal excretion (renal failure)
Cellular release
Shock
Trauma
Burns
Other
Hypothyroidism
Hypoaldosteronism

Modified from Hastbacka J, Petilla V. Prevalence and predictive value of ionized hypocalemia among critically ill patients. *Acta Anesthesiol Scand* 2003;47:1264–9.

TABLE 73.9

SIGNS AND SYMPTOMS OF HYPERMAGNESEMIA

Neuromuscular
Muscle weakness
Muscle paralysis
Respiratory depression
Lethargy
Coma
Cardiac
Prolonged PR interval
Prolonged QT interval

of hypermagnesemia usually do not manifest until the serum level is >4.0 mg/dL (**Table 73.9**).

The basic tenets of therapy for hypermagnesemia are to interrupt magnesium intake and promote magnesium excretion. Hypermagnesemia may affect calcium levels. Patients with significant neuromuscular or cardiac toxicity require measures to enhance magnesium excretion, which can be achieved by hydration with normal saline and administration of a loop diuretic. Alternatively, non–magnesium-containing enemas or a cathartic may be administered. Patients with refractory hypermagnesemia or with renal failure and severe hypermagnesemia may require hemodialysis or peritoneal dialysis to effectively reduce serum magnesium levels. Hypocalcemia should be corrected by calcium replacement.

Hypophosphatemia

Hypophosphatemia occurs as the consequence of (a) decreased dietary phosphate intake or malabsorption, (b) decreased renal reabsorption, (c) increased bone formation, or (d) redistribution of phosphate from the extracellular to the intracellular space (**Table 73.10**). Critically ill, malnourished patients, in particular those who require mechanical ventilation, may develop hypophosphatemia during refeeding. Increased renal excretion of phosphate may occur by PTH-dependent and PTH-independent mechanisms. Signs and symptoms of severe hypophosphatemia occur when serum phosphate levels are <1–1.5 mg/dL. The signs and symptoms are believed to be the consequence of intracellular ATP and resultant cellular energy depletion (**Table 73.11**). The signs and symptoms are variable. Patients may present with hemolysis, leukocyte dysfunction, platelet dysfunction, muscle weakness and paralysis, muscle atrophy, respiratory failure, rhabdomyolysis, and lethargy.

CAUSES OF HYPOPHOSPHATEMIA

Decreased dietary intake or malabsorption
    Protein calorie malnutrition
    Disorders of the duodenum and jejunum
    Chronic diarrhea

Decreased renal reabsorption
    PTH-dependent mechanisms
      Hyperparathyroidism
      Tumor release of PTH-related peptide
    PTH/PTH-related peptide-independent
    mechanisms
      X-linked hyperphosphatemic rickets and other
        FGF23-related disorders
      Intravascular volume expansion
      Fanconi syndrome
      Vitamin D deficiency
      Medications/ toxins
        Acetazolamide
        Glucocorticoids
        Ifosfamide
        Cisplatin
        Pamidronate
        Heavy metal ingestion

Increased bone formation ("hungry-bone" syndrome)

Redistribution from the extracellular to the
    intracellular space
    Insulin therapy
    Catecholamine administration
    Theophylline
    Respiratory alkalosis

PTH, parathyroid hormone; FGF, fibroblast growth factor
Modified from Hastbacka J, Petilla V. Prevalence and
predictive value of ionized hypocalcemia among critically ill
patients. *Acta Anesthesiol Scand* 2003;47:1264–9.

**SIGNS AND SYMPTOMS OF
HYPOPHOSPHATEMIA**

Muscle weakness

Paralysis

Coma

Seizures

Respiratory depression

Hemolysis

Leukocyte dysfunction

Platelet dysfunction

Rhabdomyolysis

CAUSES OF HYPERPHOSPHATEMIA

Increased intake
    Phosphate supplements
    Phosphate-containing enemas

Decreased renal excretion
    Acute and chronic renal failure
    Hypoparathyroidism
    Acromegaly
    Heparin
    Tumoral calcinosis
    Vitamin D intoxication

Redistribution from the extracellular to the intracellular
    space
    Tumor lysis syndrome
    Rhabdomyolysis
    Hemolysis
    Crush injuries
    Hyperthermia
    Respiratory acidosis
    Metabolic acidosis

Modified from Hastbacka J, Petilla V. Prevalence and
predictive value of ionized hypocalcemia among critically ill
patients. *Acta Anesthesiol Scand* 2003;47:1264–9.

Patients with serum phosphate levels <1.5 mg/dL and/or symptomatic hypophosphatemia should be treated with IV phosphate. It has been recommended that patients with severe asymptomatic hypophosphatemia should receive 2.5 mg/kg body mass of elemental phosphorus over a 6-hr period, while symptomatic patients should receive 5 mg/kg body mass of elemental phosphorus over a 6-hr period.

Hyperphosphatemia

Hyperphosphatemia is the result of increased intake of phosphate, or its decreased renal excretion or redistribution from the extracellular to the intracellular space. Increased intake is an uncommon cause of hyperphosphatemia (**Table 73.12**). Hyperphosphatemia, in and of itself, generally does not result in acute physiologic manifestations. Hyperphosphatemia, however, may serve to increase the Ca × P product, which when >80, promotes soft-tissue calcification. Acute increases in serum phosphate levels will also result in a hypocalcemic response. The basic tenets of treatment are to improve renal filtration and excretion of phosphate through intravascular volume expansion with normal saline and to stop intake of excess phosphate. Dialysis is effective in decreasing phosphate in renal failure patients with severe hyperphosphatemia.

CHAPTER 74 ■ THYROID DISEASE

ORI EYAL • SUSAN R. ROSE

INTRODUCTION

Thyroid hormones play a key role in the regulation of energy expenditure and substrate metabolism and are essential for normal growth and development. A classic feedback control loop exists between the thyroid gland and the hypothalamus and pituitary (**Fig. 74.1**). In the blood, thyroid hormones are mainly associated with carrier proteins: thyroxine-binding globulin (TBG), prealbumin or transthyretin, and albumin.

CRITICAL NONTHYROIDAL ILLNESS

A decrease in serum T3 and an increase in rT3 levels are characteristic of the fasting state. These are also the most common changes in nonthyroidal illness (NTI) in response to a variety of acute and chronic illnesses, a condition that is referred to as the euthyroid sick syndrome, NTI, or the low-T3 syndrome. The most rapid and consistent findings in NTI are decline in circulating total T3 and free T3 and an increase in the inactivated rT3 concentrations. The concentrations of TSH typically remain within the low-to-normal range, but the circadian variation of TSH may be lost, and response of TSH to TRH is blunted. Various agents, such as dopamine and steroids, may further decrease TSH levels (**Table 74.1**). Patients with prolonged critical illness show diminished TSH pulsatility, characterized by an absent nocturnal TSH surge and decreased TSH pulse amplitude. In severe prolonged illness, the changes in thyroid function may be accompanied by decline in secretion of growth hormone, gonadotropins, and adrenocorticotropic hormone. During the recovery phase, the TSH levels may rise slightly above the normal range. The treatment of NTI is controversial. An argument may be made for using T3 therapy rather than T4 because of the decreased conversion of T4 into T3 that occurs in NTI. However, administration of T3 alone will not have an effect on the brain, as the cells in the

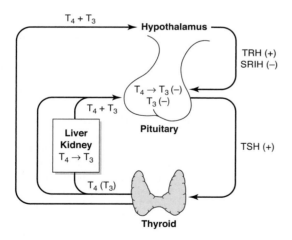

FIGURE 74.1. Basic elements in the regulation of thyroid function. Thyrotropin-releasing hormone (TRH) stimulates thyroid-stimulating hormone (TSH) synthesis and release. TRH synthesis is regulated directly by thyroid hormones. TSH stimulates the thyroid gland to synthesize and secret thyroid hormones. T4 is the predominant secretory product of the thyroid gland, with peripheral deiodination of tetraiodothyronine (T4) to triiodothyronine (T3) in the liver and kidney, supplying ~80% of the circulating T3. Both circulating T3 and T4 inhibit TSH synthesis and release independently; T4 via its rapid conversion to T3. SRIH, somatostatin.

TABLE 74.1
MEDICATIONS ASSOCIATED WITH HYPOTHYROIDISM

Decreased TSH secretion
    Dopamine
    Glucocorticoids
    Octreotide

Decreased thyroid hormone secretion
    Lithium
    Iodide
    Amiodarone

Decreased T4 absorption
    Colestipol
    Cholestyramine
    Aluminum hydroxide
    Ferrous sulfate
    Sucralfate

Increased thyroid hormone metabolism
    Phenobarbital
    Rifampin
    Phenytoin
    Carbamazepine

From Sugino K, Ito K, Mimura T, et al. Surgical treatment of Graves' disease in children. *Thyroid* 2004;14:447–52.

TABLE 74.2

CHANGES IN THYROID FUNCTION TESTS IN HYPOTHYROIDISM AND DURING CRITICAL ILLNESS

	TSH	T4	FT4	T3	rT3
Primary hypothyroidism	↑↑	↓	↓	↓ or =	↓
Central hypothyroidism	= or ↓	↓ or =	↓ or =	=	↓
NTI, acute phase	=	= or ↑	= or ↑	↓	↑
NTI, prolonged phase	↓	↓	↓	↓↓	↑ or =
Recovery phase	= or ↑	↓ or =	↓ or =	↓ or =	V

NTI, nonthyroidal illness; V, variable; ↑, increased; ↓, decreased; =, normal range

brain depend on T4 uptake and intracellular conversion of T4 to T3. In addition, treatment of critically ill patients with T3 has the potential hazardous effect of increasing metabolic rate and energy expenditure. Thyroid hormone therapy should not be initiated in the critical care setting in the absence of clear clinical and laboratory evidence for hypothyroidism. However, it is important to distinguish between patients with primary hypothyroidism and patients with NTI (**Table 74.2**). The former will benefit from therapy, and the latter will not.

Hypothyroidism

Congenital hypothyroidism might be due to thyroid dysgenesis, thyroid dyshormonogenesis, and hypothalamic-pituitary hypothyroidism. In parts of the world where salt is not iodized, iodine deficiency may be the most common cause. Hashimoto's (autoimmune) thyroiditis is the most common cause of acquired hypothyroidism in children older than 6 years of age in North America. The onset of the disease is insidious, with the thyroid gland enlarged and firm (goiter). Occasionally, the goiter causes local pressure and difficulty in swallowing. Most patients have detectable circulating autoantibodies against the thyroid. Hypothalamic or pituitary disorders are frequently associated with TSH deficiency, producing central hypothyroidism. All patients with hypothalamic or pituitary disease should have thyroid function tests performed. Isolated central hypothyroidism is uncommon and associated with subclinical hypothyroidism and short stature. In central hypothyroidism, the TSH is inappropriately low (below normal range, within normal range, or only slightly above normal) in relationship to low thyroid hormone concentrations. In children with central hypothyroidism, the FT4 concentrations are below the normal range or

in the lowest third of the normal range. These children manifest an abnormal circadian pattern of TSH concentrations, with absence or blunting of the normal nocturnal TSH surge. An increased frequency of primary hypothyroidism is associated with several chromosomal disorders, including Turner syndrome, Down syndrome, Klinefelter syndrome, and 18p or 18q deletions. The most common cause of hypothyroidism in these disorders is autoimmune thyroiditis.

Clinical Manifestations

Hypothyroidism should be considered in any child with subnormal growth and delayed bone age. In most children with hypothyroidism, pubertal development is delayed. Affected girls may present with primary or secondary amenorrhea. The onset of hypothyroidism is usually insidious. Signs and symptoms include lethargy, cold intolerance, bradycardia, weight gain, slow and husky speech, dry coarse skin, spare dry and coarse hair, constipation, muscle pain, anorexia, and delayed deep tendon reflexes (**Table 74.3**). In severe cases, the patient may exhibit myxedematous features that consist of edema of periorbital tissues and hands and feet, macroglossia, and cool and dry skin. In addition, pleural effusion, pericardial effusion, or bowel obstruction may be the first presenting symptom in previously unrecognized long-standing severe hypothyroidism. In primary hypothyroidism, serum TSH is usually elevated (>3 mU/mL), and is often the earliest laboratory finding. In secondary or tertiary (central) hypothyroidism, the TSH levels are low, normal, or slightly elevated (<10 mU/L). T4 and FT4 concentrations are low or low-normal (it is not useful to measure T3, as levels are preserved). When the FT4 is in the lowest third of the normal range and the TSH is low or normal, a TSH surge test is needed to confirm the

TABLE 74.3

MANIFESTATIONS OF HYPOTHYROIDISM

Symptoms	Signs
Fatigue	Thyroid enlargement
Lethargy	Cool, pale skin
Headache	Brittle nails
Weight gain	Bleeding tendencies
Cold intolerance	Alopecia; coarse, spare hair
Somnolence	Macroglossia
Decreased appetite	Bradycardia
Dry skin	Constipation
Hoarseness of voice	Muscle hypertrophy
Constipation	Slowed speech
Menstrual irregularities	Dementia
Myalgias	Slowed reflexes (with
Paresthesias	delayed relaxation phase)
Depression	Psychosis
	Diminished libido
	Memory defects

From Sugino K, Ito K, Mimura T, et al. Surgical treatment of Graves' disease in children. *Thyroid* 2004;14:447–52.

diagnosis of central hypothyroidism. In central hypothyroidism, the TSH surge test shows blunting of the normal nocturnal surge. Most children require therapy with ~100 mcg/m² body surface levothyroxine. A child with hypothyroidism who is admitted to the ICU should continue thyroid hormone therapy. If the patient cannot take oral medication, T4 should be given intravenously in a dose that is approximately two-thirds of the oral dose (if the patient is unable to take oral intake for only a day or two, thyroid the treatment can be omitted for this short period).

Hyperthyroidism (Thyrotoxicosis)

The term *thyrotoxicosis* is often used to describe the hypermetabolic state that results from elevated circulating levels of thyroid hormones. Hyperthyroidism in childhood and adolescence is most commonly the result of Graves disease. Graves disease is an autoimmune disease. Autoantibodies against the thyroid gland can be found in the majority of the patients, of which the autoantibodies against the TSH receptor play a key role. Graves disease involves hyperthyroidism, elevated metabolic rate, eye manifestations, and dermopathy. Other causes of hyperthyroidism include toxic multinodular goiter, toxic nodular goiter, exogenous thyroid hormone, iodine-induced thyrotoxicosis, excess release of thyroid hormone, struma ovarii, molar pregnancy, thyroid adenoma, destruction of thyroid tissue with

excess hormone release as a result of trauma, subacute thyroiditis, chronic thyroiditis, or postradiation thyroiditis. In rare cases, hyperthyroidism can be caused by increased TSH secretion as a result of pituitary adenoma. Generalized resistance to thyroid hormone involves tissues throughout the body being resistant to the effects of thyroid hormone. In resistance to thyroid hormone, T4 is high. The onset of thyrotoxicosis is usually insidious, with a period of increasing nervousness, palpitations, increased appetite, and muscle weakness. A cardinal sign is loss of weight in the face of increased appetite. Other symptoms include fatigue with sleep disturbance, emotional instability, heat intolerance, excessive sweating, tremor, diarrhea, dyspnea, tachycardia, atrial arrhythmia (**Table 74.4**). On physical examination, findings may include thyroid enlargement; thyroid bruit; ophthalmopathy; retraction of the eyelids and lid lag, tremor; hyperactive reflexes; increased precordial activity; tachycardia; atrial fibrillation; warm, smooth, and moist skin; and

TABLE 74.4

MANIFESTATIONS OF HYPERTHYROIDISM

Symptoms	Signs
Nervousness	
Anxiety	
Heat intolerance	Tachycardia
Palpitations	Thyroid enlargement[b]
Fatigue	Tremor
Weight loss	Thyroid bruit
Tachycardia	Eye signs[a]
Dyspnea	Hyperactive reflexes
Weakness	Atrial fibrillation
Increased appetite	Hot and moist skin
Eye complaints[a]	Thin and fine hair
Swelling legs	Onycholysis
Hyperdefecation	Muscle weakness
(without diarrhea)	Hyperactive precordial pulse
Diarrhea	Splenomegaly[c]
Anorexia	Gynecomastia
Personality change	Liver palms
Emotional lability	
Impaired concentration	
Insomnia	
Difficulty swallowing	
Menstrual irregularities	

[a] These manifestations are much more common in patients with Graves disease.
[b] Enlargement of the thyroid may be lacking in <5% of patients with thyrotoxicosis.
[c] Exclusively present in patients with Graves disease.
Adapted from Davies TF, Larsen PR. Thyrotoxicosis. In: Larsen PR, Kronenberg HM, Melmed SM, Polonsky KS (eds.). *Williams textbook of endocrinology*, 10th ed. Philadelphia: Saunders, 2003:374–421.

separation of the end of the fingernail from the nail bed (onycholysis). Proximal muscle weakness is common and may be the dominant manifestation in some individuals. Cardiovascular manifestations of thyrotoxicosis are common. The hemodynamic changes of thyrotoxicosis mimic a hyperadrenergic state. Supraventricular tachyarrhythmias are common. Severe hyperthyroidism may lead to cardiac failure. Uncontrolled hyperthyroidism with large goiter secondary to Graves disease may cause edema of the upper airway, a potentially life-threatening situation that requires a high degree of vigilance. Laboratory findings in patients with hyperthyroidism include increased serum concentrations of T3 and/or T4. Measuring the active thyroid hormone concentrations, free T3 (FT3) and FT4, and verifying that either or both are elevated are of more value. The TSH is low and usually undetectable (except in the extremely rare cases of TSH-secreting tumors, TRH-secreting tumors, and selective pituitary resistance to thyroid hormone). Quantitative human chorionic gonadotropin, which can cross-react at the TSH receptor level, is elevated in molar pregnancy. Management of hyperthyroidism includes medical treatment, radioactive iodine, or surgery. Most children with hyperthyroidism would initially be treated with antithyroid agent. The initial dose of propylthiouracil (PTU) varies from 300–600 mg (4–6 mg/kg) daily, divided to 3–4 doses. An initial dose of methimazole or carbimazole varies from 30–60 mg (0.4–0.6 mg/kg) daily, divided into 2–3 doses. In the initial state (before a euthyroid state is achieved), a β-adrenergic blocking agent, such as propranolol, may be added. Patients with hyperthyroidism admitted to the ICU should be monitored carefully for possible development of thyroid storm (see below). Medical treatment should be continued and adjusted according to the thyroid function tests. As no parenteral preparations of these drugs are available, they must be administered orally or via a nasogastric tube. Rectal administration has also been used. Radioactive iodine has been used relatively infrequently in childhood due to the potential risks of leukemia, thyroid cancer in the patient, and genetic mutations in the offspring of the patient. The main complication is primary hypothyroidism and thyroid storm. Surgical treatment is an effective treatment option for hyperthyroidism. With proper preparation and if performed by an experienced surgeon, the complication rate is relatively low (see Thyroidectomy). Surgery should be considered in patients with a large thyroid gland, severe ophthalmopathy, and a lack of remission with medical treatment. With proper surgical management most patients achieve a rapid remission; some may have recurrence of thyrotoxicosis or may develop hypothyroidism.

CRITICAL HYPOTHYROIDISM: "MYXEDEMA COMA"

The term *myxedema coma* is often used to describe clinically severe hypothyroidism. However, this term is a misnomer, because most patients who have severe hypothyroidism do not present with myxedema or in a comatose state. Critical hypothyroidism is characterized by progressive dysfunction of the cardiovascular, respiratory, and CNS. Myxedema is related to organ hypofunction (e.g., cardiac, gastrointestinal, skin, renal) and occurs with prolonged or severe hypothyroidism. If not recognized and treated, the mortality rate is exceedingly high. Myxedema coma is rare in the pediatric population. Typically, patients are older and have known hypothyroidism; however, it can be the initial presentation of hypothyroidism. Myxedema coma occurs most commonly in winter. Common precipitants include infection, trauma, hypothermia, and medications (**Table 74.5**). Cardinal findings include hypothermia and altered mental status. Additional features include bradycardia, hypotension, and hypoventilation. A reduction in hypoxic ventilatory drive causes a reduction in respiratory rate, leading to carbon dioxide narcosis and progressive somnolence, which compound the slow mental status of the patient. Respiratory muscle weakness may also occur, further compromising the ability to ventilate. Presence of ascites, pleural effusion, or pericardial effusion may further impede

TABLE 74.5

PRECIPITATING FACTORS FOR MYXEDEMA COMA

Infections
Pneumonia
Sepsis
Urinary infections
Influenza
Surgery
Burns
Trauma
Hypothermia
Drugs
Sedatives (narcotics, tranquilizers, barbiturates)
Cardiac medications (amiodarone, β blockers)
Lithium
Phenytoin
Rifampin
Stroke
Gastrointestinal bleeding
Congestive heart failure

From Sugino K, Ito K, Mimura T, et al. Surgical treatment of Graves' disease in children. *Thyroid* 2004;14:447–52.

TABLE 74.6

CLINICAL MANIFESTATIONS OF MYXEDEMA COMA

Organ system	Clinical features
Skin and soft tissues	Generalized swelling
	Edema
	Periorbital edema
	Ptosis
	Cool, dry skin
	Coarse, sparse hair
	Macroglossia; hoarseness
Neurologic	Hypothermia
	Lethargy
	Altered mental status
	Psychosis
	Seizures
	Delayed reflex relaxation
Cardiovascular	Bradycardia
	Hypotension
Respiratory	Depressed ventilatory drive
	Hypoventilation
	Hypoxia
	Hypercapnia
Gastrointestinal	Constipation
	Abdominal distention
	Paralytic ileus
	Megacolon
Hematologic	Anemia
	Leukopenia
Renal	Decreased glomerular filtration rate

From Fraser T, Green D. Weathering the storm: Beta-blockade and potential for disaster in severe hypothyroidism. *Emerg Med* 2001;13:376–80.

effective ventilation. Cardiac contractility is reduced, resulting in a reduction of stroke volume and cardiac output. Cardiac output can be further limited by significant pericardial effusion. If present, myxedema is characterized by decreased metabolic clearance of all substances, reduced intravascular volume with fluid retention in tissues, generalized skin and soft-tissue swelling, often with associated periorbital edema, ptosis, macroglossia, and cool, dry skin (**Table 74.6**). The diagnosis of myxedema coma requires low levels of T3 and of T4 (total and free). TSH levels are usually elevated but may be normal or low in the setting of hypothalamic-pituitary disease or critical illness. Additional laboratory findings include anemia, hyponatremia, hypoglycemia, azotemia, elevated liver enzymes, hypercholesterolemia, and elevated creatinine phosphokinase levels. Hypoxia, hypercapnia,

and respiratory acidosis are common. Pericardial effusion may be a frequent manifestation in myxedema at an advanced severe stage, but it is rare in hypothyroidism at an early mild stage. A chest radiograph may reveal cardiomegaly and pleural effusions. Echocardiography (ECG) can reveal septal hypertrophy and hypertrophic subaortic stenosis in addition to the pericardial effusion. ECG findings include sinus bradycardia, decreased voltage with electrical alternans if a pericardial effusion is present, and nonspecific ST and T wave abnormalities. Other ECG abnormalities include prolongation of the QT interval and conduction abnormalities of varying degrees. A lumbar puncture may be indicated to exclude meningitis. An increased opening pressure and elevated protein levels in the cerebral spinal fluid are nonspecific findings associated with myxedema coma. The treatment of myxedema coma involves general supportive measures, correction of physiologic derangements, and immediate intravenous replacement of thyroid hormone. Patients should be treated in the ICU setting with careful monitoring. In patients who have severe hypotension, vasopressor therapy should be considered. Warm room temperature and blankets and/or heating pad should be used to correct hypothermia. Rapid correction of hypothermia may cause hypotension and cardiovascular collapse due to peripheral dilation. Severe hyponatremia may be treated with hypertonic saline. Hypoglycemia should be treated with continuous dextrose infusion. Precipitating factors should be pursued and treated. Broad-spectrum antibiotics should be considered until infection has been excluded. Treatment is with intravenous T4 alone, with a loading dose of 200–500 mcg (4 mcg/kg), followed by 50–100 mcg/day (1–2 mcg/kg). We recommend using doses in parentheses for children who weigh <50 kg. Using T4 alone allows a slow conversion of T4 to T3 in the periphery, thereby reducing the possible adverse cardiac effects that may occur with a large dose of T3, especially in those with preexisting heart disease. If the combination of T3/T4 is used, a loading dose of 4 mcg/kg of T4 and 10 mcg of T3 (0.2 mcg/kg) may be used, followed by maintenance doses of T4 (50–100 mcg daily; 1–2 μg/kg) and T3 (10 mcg; 0.2 mcg/kg) every 8 hrs until oral therapy is initiated. If intravenous T3 alone is used, initial dose should be 10–20 mcg (0.2–0.4 mcg/kg), followed by 10 mcg (0.2 mcg/kg) every 4 hrs for the first 24 hrs, then 10 mcg (0.2 mcg/kg) every 6 hrs for another day or two. Rapid onset of action of T3 can lead to adverse cardiovascular effects. The intravenous route involved high peaks of plasma T3 and T4 within 3 hrs. IV administration of T4 at the proposed doses causes an abrupt rise in serum T4 to a supraphysiologic level and then a fall to the normal range in 24 hrs. Serum T3 levels rise slightly, and serum TSH levels fall sharply and substantially. With the IV route, the peak level is reached within 3 hrs, with subsequent gradual decline over a few days. Cortisol response to stress is blunted during severe hypothyroidism. Most investigators recommend the concurrent administration of "stress dose" corticosteroid therapy, in case of concurrent adrenal insufficiency. Hydrocortisone, 100 mg/m^2 IV, should be administered initially, followed by 25 mg/m^2 IV every 6 hrs. Cortisol levels should be drawn before initiation of corticosteroid therapy. If the levels are appropriately elevated, the steroid therapy may be safely discontinued. If the cortisol levels are low (<25 mcg/dL), steroid therapy should be continued until the critical illness phase is resolved.

CRITICAL HYPERTHYROIDISM: "THYROID STORM"

Thyroid storm (or thyrotoxic crisis) is a life-threatening condition caused by the exaggeration of clinical manifestations of thyrotoxicosis. Thyroid storm most commonly occurs in Graves disease. The progression from thyrotoxicosis to life-threatening thyroid storm involves high fever, mental status changes, and evidence of multiorgan dysfunction, including adrenergic crisis (tachycardia, hypertension) and gastrointestinal hypermotility. Early diagnosis and intervention are crucial to prevent morbidity and mortality. Precipitating factors include thyroid surgery, withdrawal of antithyroid drugs, radioiodine therapy, or the administration of iodinated radiocontrast dyes (**Table 74.7**). In patients who have preexisting thyrotoxicosis, thyroid storm can also be precipitated by systemic insults, including surgery, trauma, severe infection, and diabetic ketoacidosis. The sympathetic nervous system has been implicated in the pathogenesis of thyroid storm, as many of the manifestations are similar to those seen in conditions of catecholamine excess; administration of β-blockers causes a marked relief of these signs and symptoms. Thyroid storm is characterized by four major features: fever, tachycardia, CNS dysfunction, and gastrointestinal symptoms. The fever can progress to frank hyperpyrexia. Sinus tachycardia is usually seen, though a variety of supraventricular arrhythmias may also be present, such as atrial fibrillation. CNS manifestations can range from agitation, restlessness, and emotional lability, to confusion, frank psychosis, and coma. GI symptoms include nausea, vomiting, and diarrhea. A useful scoring system for recognition of thyroid storm is presented in **Table 74.8**. Laboratory findings include elevated serum total and free thyroid

TABLE 74.7

PRECIPITATING FACTORS FOR THYROID STORM

Infection
Surgery (thyroidal and non-thyroidal)
Therapy with radioactive iodine
Administration of iodinated contrast dyes or ingestion of large stable iodine loads
Withdrawal of antithyroid medication
Amiodarone therapy
Ingestion of excessive amounts of exogenous thyroid hormone
Diabetic ketoacidosis
Congestive cardiac failure
Hypoglycemia
Toxemia of pregnancy
Parturition and the immediate postpartum state
Severe emotional stress
Acute manic crisis
Pulmonary embolism
Cerebral vascular accident
Bowel infarction
Acute trauma
Tooth extraction
Vigorous palpation of thyroid gland

From Rose SR. Thyrotropin above 3 is not usually normal. *Endocrinologist* 2006;16:189–90.

hormonal levels (free T3 and/or free T4), with undetectable TSH. The aims of the treatment are to reduce the production and secretion of thyroid hormones, to antagonize the peripheral action of the thyroid hormones, to alleviate signs and symptoms, and to treat the precipitating factor. Supportive therapy includes respiratory support and management of hyperthermia. Phenobarbital may be used for sedation because it stimulates metabolic clearance of thyroid hormone by the liver. Hyperthermia may be treated with cool IV fluids, antipyretics, or cooling blankets. An early step in the treatment must include complete blockade of new thyroid hormone synthesis. PTU is the drug of choice because of its inhibition of peripheral conversion of T4 to T3 in addition to its inhibition of synthesis of thyroid hormone. PTU is administered as a 600–1000-mg (12–20 mg/kg) loading dose, followed by 200–300 mg (4–6 mg/kg) every 4–6 hrs orally. Methimazole is an acceptable alternative and is given as a loading dose of 60–100 mg (1.2–2 mg/kg), followed by 20–30 mg (0.4–0.7 mg/kg) every 6–8 hrs orally, but it does not provide inhibition of conversion of T4 to T3. Both PTU and methimazole can be administered rectally. As thyrotoxicosis improves, the doses should be gradually lowered to the standard dose ranges. In order to block the release of preformed thyroid hormone from the

TABLE 74.8

THE PREDICTIVE CLINICAL SCALE FOR THYROID STORM (BURCH AND WARTOFSKY)

Parameter taken into consideration	Scoring points
Thermoregulatory dysfunction, Temperature (oral; in °F)	
99–99.9	5
100–100.9	10
101–101.9	15
102–102.9	20
103–103.9	25
104	30
CNS effects	
Absent	0
Mild (agitation)	10
Moderate (delirium, psychosis, extreme lethargy)	20
Severe (seizures, coma)	30
GI-hepatic dysfunction	
Absent	0
Moderate (diarrhea, nausea/vomiting, abdominal pain)	10
Severe (unexplained jaundice)	20
Tachycardia (beats/min)	
99–109	5
110–119	10
120–129	15
130–139	20
140	25
Congestive cardiac failure	
Absent	0
Mild (pedal edema)	5
Moderate (binasal rales)	10
Severe (pulmonary edema)	15
Atrial fibrillation	
Absent	0
Present	10
Precipitating event	
Absent	0
Present	10

A cumulative score of ≥45 is highly suggestive of thyroid storm, 25–44 is suggestive of "impeding" storm, and <25 is unlikely to represent thyroid storm.
From Rose SR. Thyrotropin above 3 is not usually normal. *Endocrinologist* 2006;16:189–90.

thyroid gland, inorganic iodine should be used. Ideally, iodine therapy should be administered 2 hrs after initial thiourea dosing, to allow for initial blockade of iodine organification. Formulations for oral inorganic iodine that can be used include saturated solution of potassium iodide (children, 5 drops, 250 mg,

TABLE 74.9

INDICATIONS FOR THYROIDECTOMY

Thyroid cancer

Prophylactic thyroidectomy in children with MEN-2

A large multinodular goiter

Graves disease (including young children, not responding to antithyroid drugs, in whom radioactive iodine is contraindicated)

2–4 times a day; infants, 2 drops 4 times a day) and Lugol's solution (4–8 drops 3 times a day). Iodinated contrast dyes given intravenously, including ipodate and iohexol, are also effective. In addition to blocking thyroid hormone release, these radiocontrast agents interfere with peripheral conversion of T4 to T3 and may antagonize the binding of thyroid hormone to its receptors. Lithium therapy (300 mg or 6 mg/kg every 6 hrs) may be used in addition to iodine to block thyroid hormone release. High-dose corticosteroids (hydrocortisone 50–100 mg, IV, every 6–8 hrs or 25–50 mg/m^2 body surface) are also effective in blocking peripheral conversion of T4 to T3. Blocking the action of thyroid hormone is another mainstay of the treatment. Beta blockers (e.g., propranolol, 40–80 mg, 0.5 mg/kg, orally, every 4–8 hrs) are effective in reducing tachycardia, hypertension, and adrenergic symptoms associated with thyrotoxicosis. In life-threatening cases in which medical therapy has been proven ineffective, plasmapheresis, plasma exchange, charcoal plasma perfusion, and peritoneal dialysis have all been used successfully to remove circulating thyroid hormone. After initiation of therapy for thyroid storm, clinical and biochemical improvement should occur within 24 hrs, although full recovery may take several days to weeks. In rare cases, definitive therapy with thyroidectomy may be considered during the acute phase of thyroid storm. Radioactive iodine has no role in the acute management due to therapeutic administration of inorganic iodine, antithyroid drugs, and concerns over excess thyroid hormone release.

TABLE 74.10

COMPLICATIONS OF THYROIDECTOMY

Transient hypocalcemia

Permanent hypocalcemia

Transient recurrent laryngeal nerve palsy

Permanent recurrent laryngeal nerve palsy

Thyroid storm

Hemorrhage

THYROIDECTOMY

Thyroidectomy may be indicated in children and adolescents with Graves disease who have had adverse reaction to antithyroid drugs or who relapse after antithyroid drug therapy (**Table 74.9**). Surgical complications were more frequently observed in children than in adolescents (**Table 74.10**). After thyroid surgery, it is crucial to monitor serum calcium by frequent measurements of ionized calcium (every few hours), to monitor for signs and symptoms of hypocalcemia and to begin IV administration of calcium gluconate as soon as indicated. After the acute phase, calcitriol (20–60 ng/kg/day) and supplemental calcium may be needed. In addition, it is crucial to watch for upper-airway obstruction that may occur secondary to edema, hemorrhage, or vocal cord paralysis.

CHAPTER 75 ▪ ACUTE RENAL FAILURE AND END-STAGE RENAL DISEASE

RICHARD M. HACKBARTH • NORMA J. MAXVOLD • TIMOTHY E. BUNCHMAN

ACUTE RENAL FAILURE

Acute renal failure (ARF) is defined as an abrupt reduction in glomerular filtration rate (GFR) of at least 50% from baseline that is characterized by $\geq 50\%$ increase in serum creatinine, rising levels of nitrogenous wastes, and disturbances in the regulation of fluid, electrolyte, and acid-base homeostasis by the kidney. A useful classification is to divide causality into prerenal, renal, and postrenal categories (**Table 75.1**). Processes that decrease extracellular fluid volume or cause extravascular redistribution of that fluid (dehydration, burns, nephrotic syndrome), processes associated with decreased cardiac output (cardiogenic shock, myocarditis, tamponade), or those associated with vasodilatation or renal vasoconstriction (sepsis, drugs, anaphylaxis) are all causes of prerenal ARF. Renal blood flow is ~25% of total cardiac output. Approximately 90% of renal blood flow is to the renal cortex and, hence, the glomeruli. Renal blood flow is autoregulated between mean arterial blood pressures of 80 mm Hg and 180 mm Hg in adults (**Fig. 75.1**).

Acute tubular necrosis (ATN) can be divided into 3 phases: initiation, maintenance, and recovery. The initiation phase entails the time period in which the ischemic or toxic insult occurs, as well as the postischemic-reperfusion period. The next phase is a protracted period of maintenance in which ongoing inflammation causes further injury, cell necrosis, and apoptosis. Finally, the third phase is a recovery period in which tubular cell regeneration and clearance of tubular debris take place.

Evaluation and Treatment of ARF

The definitive laboratory diagnosis of prerenal azotemia is based on the fractional excretion of sodium (FE_{Na}):

$$FE_{Na} = (U_{Na}/P_{Na})/(U_{Cr}/P_{Cr}) \times 100$$

where $\quad U_{Na}$ = urine sodium concentration
$\qquad P_{Cr}$ = plasma creatinine concentration
$\qquad P_{Na}$ = plasma sodium concentration
$\qquad U_{Cr}$ = urine creatinine concentration

The calculation requires simultaneous urine and plasma values to be meaningful. As a rule, an FE_{Na} of <1% is compatible with prerenal azotemia. However, the accuracy of this assay can be influenced by confounding therapies, the most common being diuretic use. Fractional excretion of urea [FE_{UN}] which is calculated in the same manner as FE_{Na}:

$$FE_{UN} = [(\text{urine urea nitrogen/blood urea nitrogen})/ \\ (\text{urine creatinine/blood creatinine})] \times 100\%$$

Prerenal oliguria and azotemia are associated with an FE_{UN} of <35%; intrarenal disease, including ATN, produces an FE_{UN} of >50%. This effect may be influenced by the use of diuretics but should be considered, even if diuretics are being used. An alternative method by which to differentiate between prerenal and intrarenal processes is Doppler ultrasound, which in addition to being noninvasive, is unaffected by changes in sodium or creatinine after diuretics or hemodialysis and can be formed in complete anuria.

TABLE 75.1

CATEGORIES OF ACUTE RENAL FAILURE IN CHILDREN

Prerenal causes	Intrinsic renal causes	Postrenal (obstructive) causes
Intravascular volume depletion	**Acute tubular necrosis (ATN)**	Posterior urethral valves
Dehydration	**Ischemic Injury**	Obstruction of a solitary kidney
Gastroenteritis	Prerenal causes	Bilateral ureteral obstruction
Hemorrhage	**Exogenous toxins**	Neurogenic bladder
Diabetes Insipidus	Nephrotoxic antibiotics	Trauma
Burns	Chemotherapeutic agents	
Diuretics	NSAIDs	
Redistribution of fluid/vasodilation	ACE inhibitors and ARBs	
Sepsis	Radiographic contrast	
Pancreatitis	Venoms	
Intestinal obstruction	Heavy metals	
Peritonitis	Ethylene glycol	
Nephrotic syndrome	**Endogenous toxins**	
Hepatic failure	Myoglobinuria/hemoglobinuria	
Decreased cardiac output	Tumor lysis syndrome	
Congenital heart failure	**Acute interstitial nephritis**	
Cardiogenic shock	Drug-induced or idiopathic	
Myocarditis	**Acute glomerulonephritis**	
Cardiac tamponade	Postinfectious (Streptococcal)	
	HSP, SLE, Goodpasture syndrome	
	Vascular Pathology	
	Renal artery/vein thrombosis	
	HUS/TTP	
	Cortical necrosis	
	Congenital	
	Renal dysplasia/hypoplasia	
	Polycystic kidney disease	

NSAIDs, nonsteroidal anti-inflammatories; ACE, angiotensin-converting enzyme; ARBs, adrenergic receptor binders; HSP, Henoch-Schönlein purpura; SLE, systemic lupus erythematosus; HUS, hemolytic-uremic syndrome; TTP, thrombotic thrombocytopenic purpura

The evaluation of intrarenal disease in general, and ARF in particular, should start with the urinalysis. If the urine is bland without any evidence of protein, hemoglobin, concentrating defect, or white cells, acute interstitial nephritis should be considered. If the urine contains eosinophils, the cause may be drug-related. If the urine contains protein, the protein should be quantified using either a spot urinary protein/creatinine ratio, or a 24-hr urine collection. A protein/creatinine ratio of 2 is equivalent to a 2-gram collection in 24 hrs. If the urinary sediment contains blood and protein and hypertension is present, glomerulonephritis (GN) should be suspected. Blood work should include electrolytes, blood urea nitrogen (BUN), creatinine, calcium, phosphorus, albumin and complement C3 and C4 levels (**Table 75.2**). Obtaining other serology, including antinuclear antibody, anti-DNA (more specific), and antineutrophil cytoplasmic antibody may be helpful. In the event of a concomitant finding of pulmonary involvement, especially pulmonary hemorrhage, Wegener granulomatosis, systemic lupus erythematosus

(SLE), Churg-Strauss syndrome, and Goodpasture syndrome should be considered. In the case of a normal complementemic GN or an unknown etiology of ARF, a renal biopsy is in order.

Pos-renal disease is evaluated with ultrasound, IV pyelogram, CT imaging, or radioisotope studies. The problem with IV pyelogram and CT scan is the potential for contrast nephropathy. Nuclear medicine studies do not show anatomic detail well. Therefore, the standard diagnostic imaging modality is bedside ultrasound. Ultrasound evaluates kidney size and assesses for hydronephrosis, ureteral or bladder dilatation, and the presence of debris or echogenicity in the kidneys or bladder.

Treatment of Acute Renal Failure

Prevention of Acute Renal Failure and Renal Protection Strategies

Prerenal causes of renal insufficiency should be aggressively treated by optimizing intravascular volume

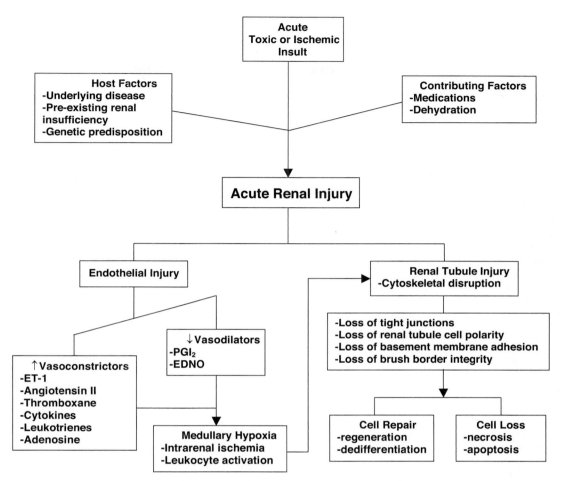

FIGURE 75.1. Changes in renal vascular pressure will trigger compensatory mechanisms to maintain a constant glomerular filtration rate by modifying afferent and efferent arteriolar tone. Decreased renal perfusion pressure leads to afferent arteriole dilation via prostacyclin or endothelium-derived nitric oxide (EDNO). Efferent arteriole tone is increased by angiotensin II. The combined effect is to maintain the transcapillary hydrostatic pressure and, therefore, glomerular filtration rate. ET-1, endothelin-1; EDNO, endothelium-derived nitric oxide.

TABLE 75.2

COMPLEMENT PATTERNS IN GLOMERULAR NEPHRITIS

Diagnosis	C3	C4
Postinfectious glomerular nephritis	Decreased	Normal Limits
Systemic lupus erythematous	Decreased	Decreased
Membranoproliferative glomerular nephritis	Decreased	Decreased or normal limits
IgA nephropathy	Normal limits	Normal limits
Henoch Schönlein purpura	Normal limits	Normal limits
Anti-GBM disease	Normal limits	Normal limits
Insulin-dependent diabetes mellitus	Normal limits	Normal limits
Membranous nephropathy	Normal limits	Normal limits
Focal segmental glomerulosclerosis	Normal limits	Normal limits
Wegener granulomatosis	Normal limits	Normal limits
Churg-Strauss syndrome	Normal limits	Normal limits

and cardiac output. Regardless of the cause of renal insufficiency, ensuring adequate perfusion pressure to the kidney is key to supporting the renal function. Vasopressin improves systemic perfusion, though it has not been shown to improve the renal-perfusion gradient. The use of "renal dose" dopamine (0.5–3 mcg/kg/min) has found wide acceptance for decades despite poor evidence of any real advantage in patients with ARF. Early implementation of low-dose dopamine prior to the development of renal insufficiency may ease management of fluid balance in patients. Fenoldopam, a DA-1 receptor agonist, causes a rise in GFR and renal plasma flow, though it's utility is unclear. Atrial natriuretic peptide (ANP) and its synthetic analogs cause vasodilatation of the afferent glomerular arteriole and constriction of the efferent arteriole, thereby increasing GFR independent of the renal blood flow. ANP also increases tubular flow rate and natriuresis. However, protection of renal function has not been demonstrated. Of all of the agents that affect vascular tone, only norepinephrine has been shown to improve GFR under the circumstances of experimentally compromised renal perfusion.

Mannitol and furosemide theoretically exert beneficial effects by inducing an osmotic diuresis, which clears tubular debris and prevents compensatory preglomerular vasoconstriction. As an inhibitor of active transport in the ascending thick limb, furosemide lessens the energy expenditure of injured cells, thus reducing substrate depletion and tubular damage in the ischemic kidney. Loop diuretics carry the risks of ototoxicity and nephrotoxicity, which can be potentiated by other agents (e.g., aminoglycosides). Continuous (versus intermittent) dosing of loop diuretics demonstrates greater effectiveness and less toxicity. Improved response to diuretics can be seen when hypoalbuminemia is corrected. Calcium-channel blockers added to the infusate of the donor kidney prior to transplant and given to the recipient as well, result in a significant drop in posttransplant ATN.

Estimation of Glomerular Filtration Rate by Creatinine Clearance and the Impact of Acute Renal Failure on Drug Dosing

The most utilized and accurate measurement of renal dysfunction is the GFR. The preterm infant at 30-week gestation has a GFR of <10 mL/min/1.73 m^2; at term, the GFR is $\sim$10–40 mL/min/1.73 m^2, and by 2 yrs of age, the GFR reaches adult levels of 110–120 mL/min/1.73 m^2.

Although multiple methods for calculating GFR are available, the most commonly used is creatinine clearance (CrCl). Creatinine is water-soluble and distributed throughout total body water compartments.

In addition to being filtrated at the glomerulus, it is secreted by the tubules. Therefore, CrCl gives somewhat of an overestimation of the GFR. For this reason, some centers prefer to use a filtered substance (e.g., inulin) that is neither secreted nor absorbed. For children 1–18 years of age:

$$CrCl \ (mL/min/1.73 m^2 BSA) = (0.48)(H) \ / \ S_{Cr}$$

where

$$BSA = \text{body surface area}$$
$$H = \text{height (cm)}$$
$$S_{Cr} = \text{measured serum creatinine}$$

To attempt a more accurate assessment of GFR, a timed CrCl can be measured, the standard interval being a 24-hr collection.

$$CrCl = U_{Cr} \times V_U/S_{Cr} \times t$$

where
$$U_{Cr} = \text{urine creatinine concentration}$$
$$\text{(mg/dL)}$$
$$V_U = \text{urine volume (mL)}$$
$$S_{Cr} = \text{serum creatinine concentration}$$
$$\text{(mg/dL) at the midpoint of the}$$
$$\text{collection}$$
$$t = \text{time interval of the collection}$$

Measuring levels of aminoglycosides provides help in pharmacokinetic dosing based on the elimination half-life of the drug in patients with renal dysfunction as well as a greater appreciation of the true degree of GFR impairment.

Nutrition and Energy Requirements in Acute Renal Failure

In addition to an impaired renal clearance of nitrogen, the rate of protein catabolism is exceptionally high in children with ARF, on the order of 180–250 mg/kg/day, which further exacerbates uremia. In ARF, there are alterations in the clearance of specific amino acids as well as impairment of the normal interconversion of amino acids by the kidneys. Glutamine balance in ARF is critical in that this amino acid is the primary metabolite for ammonia genesis by the kidney and accounts for $>50\%$ of total renal amino acid metabolism. In all critical illness, a great efflux of glutamine from muscle occurs, which provides the amino acid substrate for gluconeogenesis in the liver due to altered substrate utilization. Glutamine becomes a conditionally essential amino acid during critical illness or catabolic stress and that glutamine supplementation limits nitrogen loss. During acute renal dysfunction, an attempt must be made to adequately support the protein requirements, which are often >2 g/kg/day, in an effort to limit the large nitrogen losses, even if a net positive nitrogen balance cannot be achieved. Overfeeding is detrimental during acute illness; patient energy requirements are 0.20–0.26 mJ/kg/day, or 50–60 kcal/kg/day.

Lipid metabolism is likewise altered in ARF, with total cholesterol and high-density lipoprotein cholesterol being decreased and low-density lipoprotein being increased. These abnormalities are a result of impaired lipolysis. Electrolyte disorders due to impaired renal clearance include those of potassium, magnesium, calcium, and phosphorus.

Dietary vitamins and trace elements are also altered by renal dysfunction. In ARF, plasma levels of water-soluble vitamins are often low. Additional supplementation of these vitamins is often necessary if the ARF becomes extended. Ascorbic acid is an exception; the intake recommended for vitamin C is to be no >200 mg/day due to the risk of causing oxalosis. Vitamin A and vitamin E are often low during ARF. As renal failure extends beyond the acute phase (>4 weeks), adjustment of vitamin A to prevent accumulation may be necessary. Vitamin K seems to be stable during ARF. Vitamin D activation in the kidney is severely depressed in ARF; therefore, supplementation is required as the active form—calcitriol. Selenium concentrations are often low in critically ill patients, and this is also seen in ARF. Chromium, is elevated in uremia. As trace elements tend to be highly protein bound, supplementation with them will not be eliminated by dialytic therapies; therefore, supplementation with trace elements should be accompanied by caution for potential accumulation.

Specific Diseases that Lead to or Present with Acute Renal Failure

Glomerulonephritis

The glomerulonephritides are a group of diseases characterized by an immune-mediated injury to the glomerulus. Poststreptococcal GN, Henoch-Schönlein purpura nephritis, and lupus nephritis are examples. Alternatively, antibody production may be directed against the glomerular basement membrane (as in Goodpasture syndrome), or immune complexes may not be discernable (Wegener granulomatosis). GN can lead to ARF, or it can follow a more indolent course and lead to chronic renal insufficiency and end-stage renal disease (ESRD). Any GN, regardless of cause, is characterized by hematuria and proteinuria, which is often accompanied by oliguria, hypertension, and fluid overload.

Postinfectious GN presents with symptoms of GN ~7–21 days following the initial insult. The most common cause of postinfectious GN is due to group A β-hemolytic streptococci. Less common causes include atypical mycobacteria, mycoplasma, staphylo-

cocci, and viruses. The diagnosis is usually made clinically without need for biopsy. Treatment is primarily supportive, with fluid and salt restriction and diuresis as needed. Antihypertensive medications are frequently required to control blood pressure.

Henoch-Schönlein Nephritis

Henoch-Schönlein nephritis is a vasculitic process characterized by a purpuric rash mostly on the lower extremities and buttock, abdominal pain, and arthritis. Peak age of onset is 4–6 yrs, and the renal pathology manifests within a month of diagnosis. Renal biopsy shows crescent formation with mesangial IgA deposition. The pathology is very similar in appearance to IgA nephropathy. Treatment includes corticosteroids and other immunosuppressive agents. Angiotensin-converting enzyme inhibitors and angiotensin receptor blockers may also be useful.

Systemic Lupus Erythematosus

SLE is seen in teenagers. Renal disease occurs in as many as 82% of affected individuals, and can progress to ESRD. Serology showing markedly decreased C3 and C4 in a patient with GN is highly suggestive of lupus nephritis. Treatment includes corticosteroids and other immunosuppressive agents, such as cyclophosphamide, azathioprine, or mycophenolate mofetil, as well as control of hypertension and management of fluid overload.

Hemolytic Uremic Syndrome

Hemolytic uremic syndrome (HUS) is the most common cause of intrinsic ARF in children worldwide. The syndrome is manifest by microangiopathic hemolytic anemia, thrombocytopenia, and acute, usually oliguric, renal failure. HUS in children most commonly follows a diarrheal prodrome often due to toxin-producing *E. coli*, but it can be associated with other bacterial pathogens, bone marrow transplant, SLE, hereditary factor H deficiency, or certain drugs. An atypical form also exists. In North America, the most common cause of the diarrheal form is the verotoxin-producing strain of *E. coli* 0157:H7. Other pathogenic strains are more common in other areas of the world. The illness typically starts as hemorrhagic colitis that precedes HUS by several days. The toxin is essentially the same as Shiga toxin (*Shigella dysenteriae* serotype 1). Neurologic involvement occurs in 20%–30% of patients and manifests as seizures, altered mental status, or cerebral infarction.

The management of HUS consists of control of fluid overload and hypertension, nutritional support and dialysis if uremia or fluid and electrolyte abnormalities cannot be controlled with more conservative measures. Red cell transfusions may be necessary for symptomatic anemia. Platelet transfusion may promote the pathologic process and should be reserved for procedures associated with significant bleeding risk or for profound thrombocytopenia. Corticosteroids, prostacyclin, anticoagulants, and thrombolytics have not been shown to be helpful. Plasmapheresis is usually unnecessary in the diarrheal form of HUS but may be helpful in the nondiarrheal (atypical) form of HUS. Plasmapheresis is warranted for HUS following bone marrow transplant, or the adult counterpart of HUS, namely, thrombotic thrombocytopenic purpura.

Contrast Medium-induced Nephropathy

Contrast medium-induced nephropathy (CIN) is defined as a 25% rise in creatinine 48–72 hrs following contrast that has no alternative explanation. Renal function usually returns to baseline within 2 wks of the insult. The incidence is higher in patients with preexisting renal insufficiency, dehydration, or diabetes mellitus. The treatment of CIN should focus on prevention. Non-ionic iso-osmolar contrast should be used in the minimum volume necessary to achieve a quality study. Hydration is the only therapeutic intervention proven to minimize the risk of developing CIN. As a general guideline, hydration with IV isotonic saline should begin 6–12 hrs prior to contrast injection. Sodium bicarbonate-containing fluids may be superior to saline. N-acetylcysteine has been promoted as a preventative agent for its antioxidant properties. Mannitol, fenoldopam, furosemide, and dopamine have not been shown to reduce the risk of CIN. Prophylactic hemofiltration has been used and may be effective, but it is invasive, and for most patients, the risk outweighs the benefits.

ARF Secondary to Rhabdomyolysis

Rhabdomyolysis is caused by trauma, hyperosmolar diabetic coma, drugs, malignant hyperthermia, infection, certain inherited metabolic disorders, and autoimmune diseases such as polymyositis. Rhabdomyolysis results from myocyte injury that causes a rapid influx of calcium, sodium, and fluid into the cytoplasm. Myoglobin, potassium, phosphate, and lactate are released to the extracellular fluid space, resulting in hypocalcemia, hyperkalemia, and acidosis. The diagnosis of rhabdomyolysis is supported by high serum creatine kinase levels and dark, tea-colored urine that tests heme-positive without evidence of red blood cells. Although a urine myoglobin level may be helpful, it is often not readily available, and the diagnosis and treatment should not be delayed while awaiting the result. Patients with creatine kinase levels of >20,000 ng/mL are likely to be at greatest risk of developing ARF. Vigorous hydration with IV fluids

to maintain intravascular volume and urine output is the mainstay of therapy. Bicarbonate-containing fluids, although not shown to be superior to saline alone, theoretically offer the advantage of decreasing systemic acidosis and facilitating urine alkalinization. Using these fluids will help to treat hyperkalemia that may be present, discourage myoglobin cast formation, and inhibit free radical formation and lipid peroxidation. Using mannitol as an osmotic diuretic with IV hydration may be helpful. Compartment syndrome may develop from muscle injury and additional tissue swelling due to hydration. Intractable hyperkalemia and acidosis unresponsive to hydration and alkalinization requires renal replacement therapy.

END-STAGE RENAL DISEASE IN THE PICU

Glomerular-based renal disease is associated with fluid retention, hypertension, and blood and protein in the urine. Tubular interstitial renal disease is often associated with polyuria and polydipsia. Classically, these children have a history of recurrent dehydration, for they have no ability to concentrate their urine. Therefore, at the time of progressive loss of kidney function or at the time of inter-current illness (i.e., vomiting, diarrhea), new-onset ESRD may be discovered. Patients with uremia and hypernatremia present a very unique problem in terms of hyperosmolality. Osmolality can be calculated as

$$\text{Osms} = 2 \times \text{Na} + (\text{BUN}/2.8) + (\text{glucose}/18)$$

In a dialysis setting, the osmolality of a dialysate bath is roughly 280 mOsm. Therefore, in patients with osmolality ≥350 mOsm, if aggressive dialysis (such as with hemodialysis) is begun, a rapid osmolar shift could occur, which may result in seizures, referred to as *dialysis disequilibrium*. Therefore, improving hydration status and electrolyte imbalance prior to dialysis will lower BUN, and sodium, and, consequently, osmolality, which will often make the first dialysis less problematic.

As with other forms of ESRD, patients often will have a combination of hypocalcemia and hyperphosphatemia. They also present with anemia secondary to loss of their natural erythropoiesis compounded by iron deficiency. Low calcium is often seen in the absence of hypomagnesemia or hypoalbuminemia. If hyperphosphatemia coexists, reduction of phosphate by use of phosphate binders, phosphorous restriction, or dialysis is indicated. Aluminum-based phosphate binders and calcium carbonate are no longer recommended. Newer phosphate binders, including sevelamer (rINN), are the current therapeutic choice.

Phosphate binders are used at the end of meals to bind the phosphate load during the time of dietary intake. Calcium stores are improved with calcium supplementation and vitamin D. Vitamin D can be given orally as 25-hydroxy D3 or 1,25-dihydroxy D3, or it can be given IV as 1,25-dihyroxy D3. The regulation of calcium and phosphorous is done slowly over time to minimize the risk of seizures and to prevent ongoing metabolic bone disease.

The anemia of ESRD is due to iron deficiency and lack of natural erythropoiesis. Iron can be supplemented either orally or intravenously. The newer forms of IV iron are safe. In combination with short-acting erythropoietics (erythropoietin) or long-acting erythropoietics (darbepoetin alfa [(rINN)], IV iron can improve the hemoglobin levels in these patients. Erythropoietin products will not work effectively in the face of inflammation, such as infection or severe secondary hyperparathyroidism.

In patients with ESRD, the primary cause of hypertension is fluid retention, and one of the causes of fluid retention in ESRD is overestimation of dry weight in malnourished patients. In this case, very aggressive dialysis to achieve the true dry weight and eliminate volume overload will result in improved blood pressure control. Certain antihypertensives may cause hyperkalemia (angiotensin-converting enzymes, adrenergic receptor binders, β blockers); therefore, in situations that are risky for hyperkalemia, these should be avoided. Further, certain medications such as sodium nitroprusside are contraindicated in ESRD due to poor renal clearance and the potential for thiocyanate toxicity. Calcium-channel blockers, either orally or intravenously, offer a safe method of blood pressure control with minimal side effects.

In hemodialysis patients, infectious complications are usually related to vascular access. Access in the majority of children is an external double-lumen venous access. Broad-spectrum antibiotics such as vancomycin and aminoglycosides should be used in ESRD patients. The advantage of using these medications is that a single dose can be given initially, with subsequent doses based on dialysis clearance. In patients on peritoneal dialysis, peritonitis can be treated with intraperitoneal instillment of antibiotics. Occasionally, patients with many exposures to antibiotics may develop fungal peritonitis. The risk of fungal peritonitis is particularly high in patients who are malnourished. The therapy of choice for fungal peritonitis is removal of the peritoneal dialysis catheter, treatment with antifungal medications, and converting the patient to hemodialysis.

Morbidity and mortality in patients with ESRD are often related to the patient's nutritional state. An adult with an albumin of <2.5 has a 100% mortality rate within 5 years. Malnutrition is often related to the anorexia of chronic illness, certain food restrictions by the medical service, and lack of taste sensation by the patient. The malnutrition may be exacerbated in patients on peritoneal dialysis who are typically in negative nitrogen balance because of protein losses across the peritoneal membrane. The typical patient on peritoneal dialysis may lose 0.5–1 g/kg/day of protein. It is not unusual for these patients to have albumin levels of <3 g/dL secondary to negative nitrogen balance, resulting in severe protein malnutrition, which constitutes a medical emergency and requires either transpyloric feedings or, less preferably, total parenteral nutrition. There are a number of enteral formulas (Similac PM 60/40, Suplena, Renalcal, Nepro, and Nutren Renal) which can be used. In patients with severe electrolyte disturbances who cannot be dialyzed but require ongoing nutritional support, formulas such as Renalcal can be used. In the setting of the malnourished ESRD patient on phosphate binders, the clinician should very wary of the potential for refeeding syndrome with low phosphate formulas. It is not unusual that these patients will present with normal-to-high phosphorus levels, and once adequate nutrition is established, the phosphorous will plummet. Monitoring the phosphorous level routinely in this patient population is an essential component of management.

Preoperative Care of End-stage Renal Disease

It is important to optimize the volume status of all patients so that they are euvolemic or hypervolemic at the time of surgery. If these patients are on dialysis, they are dialyzed preprocedure for solute clearance, avoiding hypovolemia from excessive fluid removal. Optimum hemodynamic status at the time of anastomosis of the transplanted kidney is essential to good graft perfusion. The typical blood volume of a transplanted kidney is ~250 mL. In a child who weighs ≥40 kg, this volume is insignificant. In a 10-kg child, it could account for 30% of their blood volume being perfused the transplanted that kidney at the time of immediate perfusion.

Intraoperative Care of End-stage Renal Disease

A patient who is hypovolemic at the time of transplantation will experience hypotension and have suboptimal allograft perfusion. Many programs would prefer a postoperative patient to be intubated and hypervolemic after transplantation, as opposed to extubated and dehydrated. Whereas the latter approach may appear to facilitate postoperative pulmonary management, it may also result in poor allograft perfusion and potentially adversely affect graft survival. Urine output in the first 1–2 hrs after the transplant can be reflective of allograft function but can be reflective of native urine output. Therefore, a patient who produces a liter of urine per day from the native kidney (40 mL/hr) pretransplant and 200–300 mL/hr posttransplant shows evidence of immediate allograft function.

In the face of no urine output or low urine output, urgent assessment of the cause is essential. The most important determination to be made is whether blood flow is reaching the kidney, which can be evaluated either by Doppler flow ultrasound or a nuclear medicine renal blood flow study. Ultrasonography can assess for both vascular flow to the kidney and the presence of fluid around the kidney. Furthermore, an ultrasound allows for bladder evaluation. If the bladder is full, the Foley catheter is blocked. Foley patency is often an issue after kidney transplantation because the urine is usually bloody. Gently flushing the Foley with 20–30 mL of either sterile saline or sterile water will maintain patency and may be necessary every 1–2 hrs until consistent urine flow is achieved. If the catheter cannot be cleared, it must be replaced. If the bladder is empty, it must be determined whether blood flow to the kidney is compromised or if urine is leaking outside the bladder or the kidney. Urine leak may be associated with abdominal pain, fevers or decreased urine output, and increasing ascites. A simultaneous analysis of urinary creatinine, plasma creatinine, and the perinephric fluid for creatinine will help to discriminate the source of the fluid. Urinary leaks must be immediately fixed surgically, and prolonged Foley drainage maintained.

Fluid Management

Fluid management in the immediate postoperative period is crucial and has 3 components. The first is maintenance IV fluids, typically D5/0.45% normal saline with or without sodium bicarbonate and with or without potassium, based on the patient's needs. The second is urine replacement with 0.45% normal saline without dextrose. Many programs would use 1-to-1 urine output replacement for the first 6 hrs to maintain euvolemia. The final component would be any sort of bolus fluid, whether normal saline, lactated ringer solution, or 5% albumin used to optimize preload. In the face of a low central venous pressure (CVP) and low urine output, it is imperative to improve the CVP and establish adequate urine output.

Conversely, a low CVP and good urine output are reassuring that the transplanted kidney is doing well. High CVP with poor urine output warrants diuretic therapy. Finally, if CVP is high and urine output is good, reducing the replacement fluid is in order. Typically 36 hrs after surgery, extravascular volume will recirculate into the intravascular space. If the patient is making good urine, spontaneous diuresis will occur. If, however, the patient is oliguric or anuric, development of pulmonary edema and hypertension should be considered. Hypertension in this setting can best be treated with antihypertensives and either (a) with diuretics if the patient is making urine or (b) dialysis if the patient is anuric. Calcium-channel blockers are the preferred drugs of choice in transplant patients because of the renal protective mechanisms they offer in the face of the patient being on calcineurin inhibitors (tacrolimus, cyclosporin, sirolimus).

Immunosuppressive Agents

T-cell induction is used at many programs immediately after transplantation. T-cell induction agents, such as antithymocyte globulin, lymphocyte immune globulin, basiliximab, and daclizumab, as well as other agents can be used at the time of induction. These drugs have a very low risk of causing anaphylaxis. The polyclonal agents (e.g., antithymocyte globulin, lymphocyte immune globulin) should be infused through a central venous catheter in order to avoid peripheral vessel irritation. Other immunosuppressive regimens often employ a combination of steroids (prednisone or methylprednisolone), calcineurin inhibitors (tacrolimus or cyclosporin), an antiproliferative agent (mycophenolate or azathioprine), and, in some cases, sirolimus as an alternative to either the calcineurin inhibitors or to the antiproliferative agent. The side effects of these drugs are primarily related to fluid retention and hypertension (steroids and calcineurin agents) and hyperkalemia (calcineurin inhibitor agents). Other preventative therapies are often used in the posttransplantation period. These include the use of trimethoprim sulfa for both *Pneumocystis carinii* pneumonia and urinary tract prophylaxis, antifungal agents, and antiviral agents, depending on the patient's cytomegalovirus or Epstein-Barr virus.

Patients who are cytomegalovirus or Epstein-Barr virus–naïve and receive a cytomegalovirus or Epstein-Barr virus–positive kidney may be at risk for infection from these viruses. The peak time of onset of cytomegalovirus or Epstein-Barr disease is roughly 8–12 weeks after transplantation. Therefore, prophylactic antivirals are used for the first 3 months posttransplant. Some programs will also use immunoglobulin products such as cytomegalovirus immune globulin IV for additional antiviral protection. Antifungal prophylaxis is often used, which would typically include nystatin swish and swallow. Many of the newer-generation antifungals interfere with calcineurin-inhibitor kinetics and may cause calcineurin-inhibitor toxicity.

Fever in the Immediate Posttransplant Period

Evaluation of fever in the patient who is 0–7 days posttransplant includes assessment in 3 areas: exclusion of atelectasis or other pulmonary pathology (necessary but may not be the only cause), evaluation for urinary tract infection, and assessment of the wound. In the first week after transplant, fever is often related to bacterial infection. Fungal and viral infections typically occur later (6 and 12 weeks posttransplant, respectively).

Rejection

Rejection is a very rare event in the immediate posttransplant period. Acute rejection caused by humoral or T-cell rejection can be treated with the use of polyclonal agents, plasmapheresis, or an increase in the total amount of immunosuppression. The use of noninvasive therapies such as ultrasound or scan is not diagnostic and may lead to either over- or undertreatment with immunosuppression. Biopsy of the kidney in the first weeks posttransplant has a high yield for identifying the cause of allograft dysfunction.

CHAPTER 76 ◼ HYPERTENSIVE CRISES

GEORGE OFORI-AMANFO • ARTHUR SMERLING

Blood pressure (BP) homeostasis is achieved by a fine relationship between blood flow and resistance across the vascular bed. This relationship is defined as:

$$Pressure = Flow \times Resistance$$

Hypertensive emergency is defined as sudden, severe hypertension complicated by acute end-organ damage; *hypertensive urgency* is characterized by severely elevated BP without end-organ damage (**Table 76.1**).

TABLE 76.1

MANIFESTATIONS OF HYPERTENSIVE CRISES

Hypertensive crises
Hypertensive encephalopathy
Acute stroke
Retinopathy
Acute myocardial ischemia
Acute left ventricular failure with pulmonary edema
Dissecting aortic aneurysm
Acute renal failure
Microangiopathic hemolytic anemia

Malignant hypertension describes a syndrome of severe hypertension associated with encephalopathy or acute nephropathy, but this condition is best referred to and treated as a hypertensive crisis. The diagnosis of this entity requires the presence of papilledema on funduscopy. Hypertensive crisis can develop either de novo or as a complication of preexisting essential or secondary hypertension (**Table 76.2**). Activation of the rennin-angiotensin system, nitric oxide, endothelin, vasopressin, and catecholamines all have been postulated to play important roles in the pathophysiology of hypertensive crises.

CEREBRAL AUTOREGULATION

Autoregulation of cerebral blood flow (CBF) is governed by the relationship between cerebral perfusion pressure (CPP) and cerebrovascular resistance (CVR).

$$CBF = CPP/CVR$$

CPP is defined as mean arterial pressure (MAP)—intracranial pressure (ICP) (or central venous pressure [CVP]).

In normotensive adults, CBF is maintained over a wide BP range (MAP between 60 and 150 mm Hg).

TABLE 76.2

CAUSES OF HYPERTENSIVE CRISIS

Disorder	Associated clinical conditions and drugs
Essential hypertension	
Renal parenchymal disorders	Glomerulonephritis Interstitial nephritis Hemolytic uremic syndrome Systemic lupus erythematosus Vasculitides
Renovascular disorders	Fibromuscular dysplasia Acute renal artery occlusion Polyarteritis nodosa
Endocrine disorders	Renin secreting tumors Pheochromocytoma Thyroid crisis Cushing syndrome Conn disease
Ingestions/Drugs	Cocaine Amphetamines Phencyclidine Cyclosporine Tacrolimus
Cardiovascular disorder	Coarctation of the aorta Midaortic syndrome
Pre-eclampsia/ eclampsia	Pregnancy

The range of autoregulation shifts to the right in chronically hypertensive patients (**Fig. 76.1**), a phenomenon that is reversible with long-term BP control. This autoregulation is maintained by the appropriate adjustments in CVR. Hypertensive en-

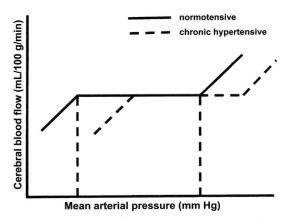

FIGURE 76.1. Chronic hypertension is associated with a rightward displacement of the cerebral autoregulation curve.

cephalopathy occurs when MAP exceeds the upper limit autoregulation. The absolute BP is often not as important as the rate of elevation. Acute elevations in BP are less well tolerated and more likely to produce symptoms than are chronic elevations. In the neonate, symptoms and signs related to hypertension are lethargy and irritability, whereas in the older child, they include severe headache, dizziness, blurred vision, and epistaxis. Typically, the headache is occipital and more prominent in patients with hypertensive encephalopathy.

BLOOD PRESSURE

It is difficult to apply an absolute BP level to define hypertensive emergencies and urgencies. Normal and abnormal BPs vary widely with age and body size. The Fourth Task Force has defined stage II hypertension as systolic or diastolic BP that is >5 mm Hg >99th percentile for age and height, and this condition requires prompt evaluation and pharmacologic therapy. Systolic and diastolic BP levels for children and adolescents by age and height percentiles are defined in the Fourth Report on the Diagnosis, Evaluation, and Treatment of High Blood Pressure in Children and Adolescents, published in *Pediatrics*.

Neurologic Manifestations

Hypertensive encephalopathy is defined as an acute, organic brain syndrome characterized by profound headache, severe nausea and vomiting, blurred vision, and altered mental status. These symptoms may progress to focal or generalized seizures, focal neurologic deficits, and cortical blindness. If not appropriately treated, hypertensive encephalopathy may progress rapidly to cerebral hemorrhage, coma, and death. It occurs as a result of failure of the upper limit of cerebral vascular autoregulation (autoregulation breakthrough), cerebrovascular endothelial dysfunction, microhemorrhage, or blood–brain barrier disruption, with cerebral edema and intracranial hypertension. It is associated with untreated or inadequately treated hypertension and other known causes and associations of severe hypertension, such as renal disease, immunosuppressive therapy (e.g., tacrolimus, cyclosporine), erythropoietin administration, and thrombotic thrombocytopenic purpura. In the pregnant adolescent, hypertensive encephalopathy may occur in the setting of preeclampsia and eclampsia. In some cases, funduscopy may reveal evidence of malignant hypertension: papilledema, retinal hemorrhages, and exudates. These manifestations occur as a result of failure of cerebral autoregulation and are completely reversible with appropriate BP management. In chronic hypertensive patients, adaptive mechanisms allow cerebral autoregulation to occur at relatively higher MAPs and thereby provide some protection against the development of hypertensive encephalopathy during sudden increases in BP (**Fig. 76.1**).

In acute stroke with concomitant severe hypertension, the hypertension may be a reflex response to maintain cerebral perfusion, or it may be the cause of the stroke. In many patients in whom hypertension is secondary to stroke, the BP tends to resolve spontaneously within 48 hrs. The clinical presentation includes acute onset of severe headache, altered mental status, or loss of consciousness associated with focal neurologic findings (e.g., hemiparesis, hemiplegia).

Cardiovascular Manifestations

Acute hypertensive crisis subjects the left ventricle to a sudden increase in afterload, intraventricular pressure, and myocardial oxygen demand. Ischemia results if an increase in myocardial blood flow does not occur in parallel. Sustained increase in myocardial work load leads to failure of the left ventricle, elevated left ventricle end-diastolic pressure, and pulmonary edema. These pathophysiologic events manifest as acute chest pain, tachypnea, dyspnea, orthopnea, cough, and hemoptysis and potential for myocardial infarction. Physical examination reveals diffuse, fine crackles at the lung bases, and possibly an S_3 gallop on cardiac auscultation.

Severe acute hypertension can cause aortic dissection, especially in patients with predisposing syndromes such as Marfan syndrome. Severe chest or abdominal pain is the most common symptom of acute aortic dissection. Syncope, paralysis, and blindness may result from carotid or innominate artery involvement. Dissection of the thoracic aorta may be associated with hemoptysis, orthopnea, and dyspnea, while involvement of the abdominal aorta may cause a variety of gastrointestinal and genitourinary disturbances. The diagnosis of acute aortic dissection should be suspected in a hypertensive patient with abrupt onset of pain, pulse deficits, and signs of end-organ circulatory compromise.

Renal Manifestations

The most common etiology of severe hypertension in pediatric patients is renal or renovascular disorders. Renal diseases, such as poststreptococcal glomerulonephritis and hemolytic uremic syndrome, are common causes of de novo acute hy-

pertension. Mild proteinuria and elevated serum creatinine can be the result of a primary renal disease or may be secondary manifestations of severe hypertension, and such cases may be difficult to differentiate.

Clinical Evaluation

BP should be obtained in all 4 extremities to exclude coarctation of the aorta. Funduscopic examination is particularly useful because it can distinguish a true hypertensive emergency from hypertensive urgency (the presence of new hemorrhages, exudates, or papilledema, indicating hypertensive emergency). The cardiovascular assessment should focus on the presence of heart failure, and neurologic examination should evaluate level of consciousness, signs of meningeal irritation, visual fields, and focal neurologic deficits.

Initial laboratory investigations include serum electrolytes, urea, and creatinine, full blood count with peripheral smear (for evidence of hemolysis), urinalysis, electrocardiogram, and chest x-ray. Measurement of plasma renin and aldosterone activity may be helpful in making a retrospective diagnosis of hypertension. Once the patient is stabilized, investigations for secondary causes of severe hypertension should be performed, as guided by clinical presentation and laboratory findings (**Table 76.2**). Brain MRI, though not part of the initial workup, may reveal the characteristic posterior leukoencephalopathy that predominantly (but not exclusively) affects the white matter of the parieto-occipital regions, which are best appreciated on T_2-weighted images. Pregnancy must be ruled out in female adolescents who present with hypertensive crisis, as this may impact on the approach to treatment and the choice of antihypertensive agents.

Differential Diagnoses

Hypertensive encephalopathy must be differentiated from other acute neurologic events that may be associated with hypertension, such as cerebral infarct or hemorrhage. Reflex elevation of systemic BP in response to cerebral ischemia (e.g., brainstem ischemia can induce hypertension) or hypertension as a component of the Cushing triad must be recognized. Pseudotumor cerebri, when associated with severe hypertension, may mimic hypertensive encephalopathy. Other diagnoses to be considered include primary renal disease with severe hypertension and uremic encephalopathy, as well as hepatic encephalopathy with hepatorenal syndrome and hypertension.

Postcoarctectomy Hypertension

Severe paradoxic hypertension commonly occurs in the first week after relief of coarctation of the aorta. Provided the repair is satisfactory, the hypertension usually resolves after several days, though intensive antihypertensive therapy during the early postoperative period is frequently required. Both the sympathetic and renin-angiotensin systems have been implicated in the pathogenesis of paradoxic hypertension. Aggressive treatment of the hypertension is crucial if end-organ damage and risk of rupture of surgical suture lines are to be avoided. Treatment with esmolol infusion or sodium nitroprusside has been successful.

Treatment

The recommended aim is to reduce MAP by 20%–25% within a period of 15 mins to 2 hrs. Subsequent rate of reduction of the BP is dictated by clinical status and the rapidity with which the hypertension may have evolved. Too rapid a reduction in BP is to be avoided, as that can worsen end-organ dysfunction. An exception to this guideline is the treatment of hypertensive crisis associated with aortic dissection. Aortic dissection is the most dramatic and most rapidly fatal complication of severe hypertension. Appropriate treatment requires rapid reduction of systolic BP. Rapid minimization of aortic wall stress is imperative and can be accomplished by lowering both BP and heart rate. Volume depletion is common in patients with hypertensive crises and may lead to excessive fall in BP during treatment. Volume repletion with IV crystalloid often restores organ perfusion.

Pharmacologic Therapy

Drugs such as clonidine and methyldopa that significantly affect the central nervous system should be avoided in patients with hypertensive encephalopathy. Drugs that act by predominant β-receptor blockade must be avoided in pheochromocytoma crisis, as unopposed α-receptor stimulation may cause a paradoxic worsening of the hypertension. From the wide array of IV antihypertensive drugs available, the most commonly used in the pediatric population are sodium nitroprusside (SNP), fenoldopam, labetalol, and nicardipine, although esmolol has been favored in postcoarctectomy hypertension. The most commonly used oral agents are the calcium-channel blockers (e.g., nifedipine), ACE inhibitors (enalapril, captopril), and ganglion blockers (clonidine).

Sodium Nitroprusside

SNP has been used as first-line medication in most cases of hypertensive crisis. A nonselective vasodilator that affects both arterioles and venules, it decreases both systemic and pulmonary vascular resistance. Once infused, SNP interacts with oxyhemoglobin, dissociating immediately to form methemoglobin, while releasing free cyanide and nitric oxide. Nitric oxide activates guanylate cyclase in the vascular smooth muscle, triggering an increase in intracellular cGMP, followed by relaxation of vascular smooth muscle and vasodilation. The free cyanide radicals (CN^-) bind to methemoglobin to form cyanomethemoglobin. Each molecule of SNP metabolized results in the release of 5 cyanide radicals, some of which bind to methemoglobin, with the remainder available to be converted to thiocyanate by rhodanese enzyme in the liver and kidneys. Any free cyanide that is not rapidly converted to thiocyanate can bind to and inactivate tissue cytochrome oxidase and manifest as tissue hypoxia. Because the conversion of SNP to cyanide is a nonenzymatic process, the amount of CN^- released from SNP depends entirely on the total dose of the drug administered. The subsequent rate at which CN^- is converted to the less toxic thiocyanate by rhodanese enzyme is dependent on the availability of a sulfur donor for the enzyme, usually endogenous thiosulfate derived from the amino acid cysteine. Thiocyanate is cleared by the kidneys with an elimination half-life of 4–7 days. The presence of renal failure or prolonged SNP therapy can cause accumulation of thiocyanate.

SNP acts within 30 secs, peak antihypertensive effect occurs within 2 mins, and its effects persist for 2–4 mins after cessation of infusion. Most patients respond to a starting dose of 0.3–0.5 mcg/kg/min, and the dose may be escalated as needed to rates not exceeding 5 mcg/kg/min. Occasionally, doses as high as 10 mcg/kg/min may be necessary for adequate BP response, but they must be administered for no longer than 10 mins to minimize toxicity. Reflex tachycardia can occur with SNP therapy, which may be accompanied by inadequate BP response. In such situations, the addition of a small dose of β-blocker will result in significant improvement in BP control. When used in the treatment of aortic dissection, prior institution of β-blocking agent is imperative, as the reflex tachycardia could be extremely deleterious in such patients.

The most common adverse effect of SNP is precipitous hypotension, with or without reflex tachycardia, due to its potent vasodilator effect on both the venous and arterial beds. This reaction is accentuated in the hypovolemic patient. SNP has been shown to cause increased intracranial pressure. Cyanide accumulation (i.e., cyanide poisoning) accounts for the rare but fatal toxic effects of SNP. Toxic accumulation of cyanide that leads to severe lactic acidosis can occur if SNP is infused at a rate >5 mcg/kg/min over a period of hours to days, assuming normal rhodanese activity. Patients receiving SNP who demonstrate any evidence of tissue hypoxia must be investigated for methemoglobinemia and cyanide poisoning. Antidotes for cyanide poisoning include sodium thiosulfate and hydroxocobalamin (vitamin B_{12}). Methemoglobinemia is another important toxic effect of SNP. Severe methemoglobinemia causes tissue hypoxia and subsequent acidosis. The total SNP required to generate 10% methemoglobinemia exceeds 10 mg/kg ($\sim$10 mcg/kg/min for >16 hrs). The most common clinically observed toxicity of SNP is thiocyanate accumulation, which results in nausea, confusion, and muscle weakness. This toxicity occurs predominantly in patients with concomitant renal dysfunction.

Fenoldopam

Fenoldopam is a selective DA_1 receptor agonist causing vasodilation, diuresis, and natriuresis. During reduction of severely elevated BP, fenoldopam significantly increases creatinine clearance, urinary flow, and sodium and potassium excretion. These unique effects on the kidneys make fenoldopam a particularly attractive drug in the treatment of hypertensive emergencies with renal impairment. It is not metabolized by the cytochrome P450 pathway and, therefore, has no significant drug interactions; furthermore, its pharmacokinetics is not altered by hepatic or renal insufficiency. Fenoldopam has a short half-life (5 mins) and predictable dose response, is easily titrated, and is not associated with precipitous decline in BP. The onset of BP response occurs within 15 mins of initiation (3 half-lives); therefore, it is recommended that the drug be titrated no more frequently than every 15 mins. Steady state is reached within 30 mins, and elimination half-life is $\sim$10 mins. The recommended starting dose is 0.1 mcg/kg/min, titrated to effect to a maximum of 1.6 mcg/kg/min. Most adverse effects associated with fenoldopam are attributable to the vasodilator action of the drug. These include headache, flushing, dizziness, and reflex tachycardia. Most of the adverse effects occur in the first 24 hrs of treatment. Electrocardiographic changes (flattening T waves in anterior and lateral leads) have been reported with fenoldopam, but these have not been shown to have any clinical significance. Elevation of intraocular pressure has also been reported. Fenoldopam must be used with caution in patients with increased intracranial pressure because of the risk of worsening intracranial hypertension.

Nicardipine

Nicardipine is a calcium-channel blocker that is 100 times more water-soluble than nifedipine. Nicardipine acts by blocking calcium influx through voltage-sensitive channels in vascular smooth-muscle cells, resulting in smooth-muscle relaxation and vasodilation. It can be given as a continuous IV infusion and is easily titratable. The pharmacokinetic characteristics of nicardipine include onset of action of 5–15 mins, peak hypotensive effect at 30 mins to 2 hrs, half-life of 2–4 hrs, and duration of action of 4–6 hrs. It is administered as a loading dose of 5–10 mcg/kg, given over 1 minute, followed by a continuous infusion of 1–3 mcg/kg/min. Adverse effects include orthostatic hypotension, tachycardia (reflex), and peripheral edema. It can be used alone or in conjunction with other antihypertensive agents.

Labetalol

Labetalol is a competitive α_1-adrenergic and β-adrenergic receptor antagonist. When given intravenously, the β-blocker effect is 7 times greater than the α-blocker effect. The hypotensive effect of labetalol begins 2–5 mins after an IV dose, peaks at 5–15 mins, and persists for $\sim$2–4 hrs. The recommended dose in children is an initial dose of 0.25 mg/kg bolus, followed by continuous infusion of 0.25 mg/kg/hr, titrated up to 3 mg/kg/hr. The most common adverse effects associated with labetalol are precipitous hypotension and orthostatic hypotension. Bradycardia, heart block, and bronchospasm may also complicate its use.

Esmolol

Esmolol is an IV, ultra-short-acting, selective, β_1-adrenergic antagonist. It has virtually no intrinsic sympathomimetic activity; therefore, significant bradycardia can be associated with its administration. Peak hemodynamic effect occurs in 6–10 mins following an appropriate loading dose; it has a half-life of 8 mins, and a rapid offset of effect occurs within 15–30 mins following discontinuation. Esmolol is administered as a bolus of 300–500 mcg/kg IV over 1–3 mins, then 25–200 mcg/kg/min. An infusion dose may be titrated by 25–50 mcg/kg/min every 5–10 min for optimal antihypertensive effect to a maximum infusion dose of 1000 mcg/kg/min. Adverse effects include bradycardia, hypotension, congestive heart failure, and bronchoconstriction. Esmolol is contraindicated in second- or third-degree heart block and in cardiogenic shock.

Nifedipine

Nifedipine is administered either orally or sublingually. Following its administration, nifedipine reduces BP abruptly and therefore has an important role in the management of hypertensive urgencies. The usual dose is 0.25–0.5 mg/kg/dose; however, the lower end of this range is the preferred starting dose due to the risk of precipitous hypotension. The dose may be repeated as needed to a daily maximum of 3 mg/kg. Onset of action is observed within 15–30 mins, and the elimination half-life may be as short as 1.5 hrs. Even though its rapid onset of action is viewed as a major advantage, nifedipine must be used with caution, as the peripheral vasodilation that follows its administration can trigger an intense reflex adrenergic stimulation with tachycardia, as well as activation of the renin-angiotensin system.

Captopril

Captopril, an ACE inhibitor, which works by reducing the levels of circulating angiotensin II, represents an important component of the treatment of hypertensive crises. Captopril lowers BP promptly without causing tachycardia and, therefore, offers distinct hemodynamic advantage over other vasodilator drugs. Captopril has an antihypertensive effect within 15 min of administration and can last for up to 2 hrs with an elimination half-life of 4–6 hrs. The initial dose of 0.3–0.5 mg/kg may be repeated to a maximum daily dose of 6 mg/kg. Patients must be closely monitored after the first dose, as an exaggerated hypotensive effect may be observed in patients who present with acute severe hypertension associated with a high renin state. Adverse effects include cough, hyperkalemia, neutropenia, and rarely, angioedema. In patients with renovascular hypertension, the glomerular filtration rate is maintained by an increased postglomerular arteriolar resistance caused by angiotensin II. Therefore, in patients with bilateral renal artery stenosis or stenosis in a solitary kidney, captopril and other ACE inhibitors are contraindicated. Autoimmune renal disease with hypertension (e.g., scleroderma) is often associated with high renin states, and ACE inhibitors are to be used with utmost caution. Captopril is also contraindicated in severe renal failure.

CHAPTER 77 ■ INBORN ERRORS OF METABOLISM

MICHAEL WILHELM • WENDY CHUNG

INTRODUCTION

Inborn errors of metabolism (IEMs) are inherited predominantly in an autosomal recessive fashion. The mitochondrial genome is maternally inherited, and thus some mitochondrial disorders are maternally transmitted. Features of the family history may suggest a metabolic disease, including parental consanguinity, ethnicity of the patient (hepatorenal tyrosinemia in French Canadians and maple-syrup urine disease in Pennsylvania Amish, Old Order Amish and Mennonites, and Ashkenazi Jewish populations). Also implicated are a history of sudden, unexplained death such as SIDS, developmental delay, seizures, failure to thrive, or other unexplained chronic illness in a sibling or other family member.

These diseases manifest either as a result of the lack of products of the deficient enzyme, accumulation of upstream metabolites, shunting of accumulated metabolites into other pathways, or some combination of the above. Pathophysiologically, IEMs presenting in the PICU can be categorized into one of the following processes: (a) intoxication from a metabolite such as ammonia, amino acid derivatives, or ketoacids, (b) reduced fasting tolerance, (c) derangements of energy metabolism, (d) derangement of neurotransmission, or (e) storage of nonmetabolizable substrates in vital organs or tissues. **Table 77.1** lists disorders associated with each of these categories.

CLINICAL PRESENTATION

Commonly, IEMs present with changes in mental status (lethargy, irritability, seizures, and coma) with or without overt cardiorespiratory compromise and can be easily confused with sepsis. Furthermore, infection often exacerbates metabolic derangements and precipitates metabolic decompensation due to increased energy requirements and the frequent association with decreased food intake. Certain IEMs

TABLE 77.1

CATEGORIES OF INBORN ERRORS OF METABOLISM WITH ACUTE PRESENTATIONS

Pathophysiology	Likely disorders
Intoxication (encephalopathy)	Urea cycle,* organic acidemias,* aminoacidopathies*
Reduced fasting tolerance	Glycogen storage disease type 1, disorders of gluconeogenesis, fatty acid oxidation defects
Impaired energy production	Mitochondrial disorders, fatty acid oxidation disorders, and disorders of the pyruvate dehydrogenase complex
Altered neurotransmission	Pyridoxine- or folinic acid-dependent epilepsy, nonketotic hyperglycinemia, sulfite oxidase deficiency
Storage disorders/complex macromolecules	Mucopolysaccharidoses, sphingolipidoses, glycogen storage diseases, peroxisomal biogenesis disorders, congenital disorders of glycosylation

*Denotes diseases that may require emergent dialysis.

make patients more susceptible to infection such as *Escherichia coli* sepsis in galactosemia and due to neutropenia associated with many organic acidurias. Therefore, empiric treatment for suspected sepsis should be initiated after obtaining appropriate cultures. Neonates may present with failure to regain birth weight by the second week of life. The older child may present with recurrent episodes of lethargy and difficulty recovering from minor illnesses. Children of all ages often demonstrate failure to thrive.

In rare cases, the specific dietary intake may suggest the diagnosis. Particular foods such as a high protein meal may induce symptoms, including nausea in urea cycle defects. Children with partial enzymatic deficiencies and milder disorders may even unknowingly alter their diet to avoid foods that make them feel lethargic or ill.

A history of developmental delay, hypotonia, and/or seizures is associated with many of the IEMs. A history of developmental regression is particularly concerning and should prompt a careful search for an IEM, particularly the lysosomal storage disorders and mitochondrial disorders.

Though the prenatal history is often unremarkable, a history of maternal liver disease or hemolysis, elevated liver enzymes, and low platelets (HELLP) syndrome may suggest a long-chain fatty acid oxidation disorder. The gender of the patient is relevant in a small number of IEMs that are X-linked such as the urea cycle defect ornithine transcarbamylase deficiency, the carbohydrate defect pyruvate dehydrogenase deficiency E1α, and the defect of the nucleotide salvage pathway Lesch-Nyhan disease.

On physical examination, the presence of an unusual body or urine odor might suggest a specific organic acidemia (**Table 77.2**), but these odors can be subtle, and their absence should not dissuade pursuit of an IEM. Careful attention should be paid to the respiratory pattern; although tachypnea may

herald sepsis with ARDS, Kussmaul respirations occur with metabolic acidosis. Hypothermia may be associated with metabolic decompensation, especially in the urea cycle defects.

The baby who is large for gestational age and hypoglycemic suggests an infant of a diabetic mother. Macrosomia, hemihypertrophy, macroglossia, umbilical hernia, and ear pits or creases in a neonate suggest *Beckwith-Wiedemann syndrome*. Midline defects with a cleft lip and/or palate or a small penis may suggest panhypopituitarism. Hepatomegaly suggests a glycogen storage disorder or nonspecific liver disease. Inverted nipples and decreased gluteal fat suggest a *congenital disorder of glycosylation* that may be associated with hyperinsulinemia.

Progressive hepatosplenomegaly occurs in a number of IEMs as nonmetabolizable substrate accumulates in glycogen storage disorders and lysosomal storage disorders. Dysmorphic features are present at birth in a number of peroxisomal biogenesis disorders, fatty acid oxidation disorders, congenital disorders of glycosylation, and pyruvate dehydrogenase

TABLE 77.2

ODORS ASSOCIATED WITH METABOLIC DISEASES

Odor	Associated inborn error(s)
Sweaty feet	Glutaric acidemia (type II), isovaleric academia
Maple syrup	Maple-syrup urine disease
Mousy	Phenylketonuria
Boiled cabbage	Hypermethioninemia, tyrosinemia type I
Swimming pool	Hawkinsinuria
Rotten fish	Trimethylaminuria, dimethylglycinuria

TABLE 77.3

LABORATORY EVALUATION OF A SUSPECTED IEM

	Blood tests	Urine tests	CSF tests
Intial studies	Blood gas, dextrose stick, electrolytes, basic metabolic panel, ammonia, lactate, pyruvate, β-hydroxybutyrate, transaminases, blood count, coagulation profile, creatinine kinase	Ketones, pH, reducing substances	As indicated
Further workup	Plasma amino acids, plasma acylcarnitine profile, carnitine	Organic acids, amino acids	

deficiency while they develop progressively over time in the mucopolysaccharidoses as storage material accumulates. Smith-Lemli-Opitz syndrome, a defect in sterol biosynthesis, may present with ambiguous genitalia. Ophthalmologic examination may also provide clues to an IEM, with cataracts observed in disorders such as galactosemia and retinal pigmentary changes in Tay Sachs disease and some mitochondrial disorders.

Myopathy demonstrated by hypotonia or cardiomyopathy (hypertrophic or dilated) possibly detected by heart murmur or signs of heart failure may herald a disorder of fatty-acid oxidation, mitochondrial derangement, glycogen storage disorder, or rarely a congenital disorder of glycosylation. IEMs are important causes of cardiomyopathy to exclude in children since these can be treated and in some cases cured.

Routine laboratory test results may suggest an IEM as well (**Table 77.3** and **Table 77.4**). A primary respiratory alkalosis may be found with hyperammonemia caused by a urea cycle defect. A metabolic acidosis, particularly with an elevated anion gap (AG) or elevated lactate also occurs in certain IEMs, though this may also occur in other diseases such as sepsis or hypoperfusion. However, while patients with elevated lactate due to hypoperfusion appear quite ill, patients with an IEM may have lactate elevations out of proportion to their degree of illness. Subtracting the lactate level (in mMol/L) from the anion gap yields the lactate-adjusted AG. In diseases of energy metabolism or hypoperfusion, the lactate-adjusted AG is normal while it is elevated in the organic acidemias owing to the presence of other anions besides lactate. The lactate-to-pyruvate ratio is also helpful, with normal levels being ~20 when both concentrations are expressed in mMol/L. A consistent ratio of <10 suggests a pyruvate dehydrogenase deficiency, which has important therapeutic implications, while a consistent ratio of >25 occurs in tissue hypoxia, pyruvate carboxylase deficiency and mitochondrial disorders.

Hypoglycemia may also occur in sepsis, liver disease, or any other severe illness, particularly in the

TABLE 77.4

RESULTS OF INITIAL LABORATORY TESTS IN IEMS

	Urea cycle defect	Amino acidopathy	Organic aciduria	Fatty acid oxidation disorder	Carbohydrate metabolism	Electron transport chain
Blood pH	↑	↓/−	↓	↓/−	↓	↓
Anion gap	WNL	↑/−	↑	↑/−	↑	↑
Glucose	WNL	+/−	WNL	↓↓	↓↓	+/−
Ammonia	↑↑	WNL	↑	↑	WNL	WNL
Lactate	WNL	WNL	↑/−	WNL	↑	↑↑
Ketones	Neg	↑	↑	↓↓	↑	Neg
LFT's	WNL	WNL	WNL	↑	↑	WNL
Serum amino acids	Abnormal	Abnormal	Abnormal	WNL	WNL	Alanine high
Urine organic acids	Some abnormal	Abnormal	Abnormal	Abnormal	WNL	Lactate in urine
Urine reducing substances				+/−		

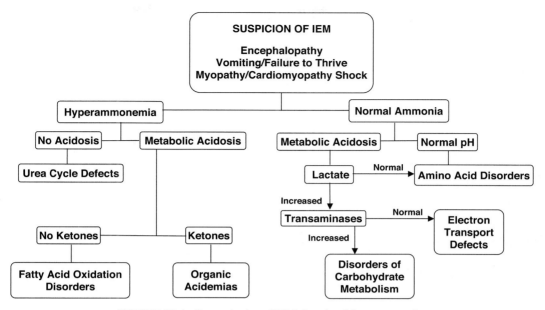

FIGURE 77.1. Categorization of IEMs based on laboratory results.

neonate when the ability to mobilize glycogen stores is limited. However, in the setting of other clinical and laboratory findings listed here, hypoglycemia is much more likely to indicate an IEM. The relationship of hypoglycemia to feeding can be helpful in identifying a specific disease. Hypoglycemia occurring immediately after ingestion of fructose (fruits or sweet foods containing sucrose), usually when an infant begins eating solid foods, suggests hereditary fructose intolerance. Hereditary fructose intolerance can be further suggested by the presence of reducing substance in the urine. In most other IEMs, including the glycogen storage diseases, fatty acid oxidation defects, disorders of gluconeogenesis, and some organic acidemias, hypoglycemia occurs with fasting. In the setting of hypoglycemia, the liver mobilizes ketone bodies as an alternative energy substrate. Therefore, nonketotic hypoglycemia suggests a defect in fatty acid oxidation or ketogenesis. Although normal neonates effectively generate 3-hydroxybutyrate, they have a limited capacity to generate acetoacetate. Because urine dipsticks detect only acetoacetate, *serum 3-hydroxybutyrate* levels must be evaluated in the hypoglycemic infant. Conversely, a positive urine dip for ketones in the first month is always abnormal and suggests an organic acidemia or inability to utilize ketone bodies. Elevated ketone levels in the nonfasting/nonhypoglycemic patient suggest an organic acidemia or maple syrup urine disease (MSUD).

Although individually each of the above historical, physical, or laboratory findings may occur in a number of disease states, the combination of several of these features increases the likelihood that a given patient has an IEM. In addition to supporting the diagnosis of an IEM, these initial labs help point to specific etiologies (**Figure 77.1**). Once an IEM is suspected, specific metabolic tests should be performed, including urine organic acids, plasma amino acids, the plasma carnitine levels and acylcarnitine profile, and other specific tests depending on the suggested diagnoses. These samples should preferably be obtained before therapy because pathognomonic metabolites may clear rapidly with resuscitative therapy. Definitive diagnosis beginning with the biochemical signature of the above tests often requires tissue for enzymatic assays and/or molecular genetic testing and may require several weeks to months for complete evaluation.

CLINICAL MANAGEMENT PRINCIPLES

As in all cases, initial management begins with provision of adequate respiratory and circulatory support. A number of complications of IEMs may require respiratory support. Encephalopathy may render a patient unable to protect the airway. With profound metabolic acidosis, even with adequate energy production, patients may not maintain an adequate minute ventilation, particularly during infancy. In older children capable of generating large tidal volumes, it may be difficult to maintain an equivalent minute ventilation after administering neuromuscular blockade. Acute worsening of acidosis may necessitate treatment of its complications (i.e., hyperkalemia, worsened cardiovascular function).

Because many of these diseases are associated with emesis and anorexia, patients often present with dehydration. Care must be exerted, however, in volume resuscitation of patients who may have a complicating cardiomyopathy or cerebral edema. Rapid correction of hypoglycemia requires a bolus of dextrose (2–4 cc/kg of 25% dextrose solution). Furthermore, if an IEM is strongly suspected, all patients should be made NPO and given sufficient intravenous glucose (~10 mg/kg/min) to prevent catabolism of amino acids and fatty acids that may increase the production of abnormal metabolic products. Rarely, glucose will exacerbate a lactic acidosis, suggesting an error in the pyruvate dehydrogenase complex, in which case changing to a ketogenic diet will improve the metabolic acidosis. Older patients with intoxication syndromes may present with cerebral edema and are at greater risk for intracranial hypertension during therapy than neonates since their sutures are closed. (Management of the cerebral edema is discussed more extensively in Chapter 35.) Intravenous fluids must provide adequate sodium to prevent hyponatremia, which could exacerbate this situation.

Disease-specific therapies must also sometimes be initiated empirically prior to obtaining a specific metabolic diagnosis. In diseases where symptoms result from toxic metabolic intermediates (see **Table 77.1**), direct elimination of these toxins must be done quickly to prevent irreversible brain damage. Initial approaches included exchange transfusion with or without peritoneal dialysis. Continuous venovenous hemofiltration and dialysis in children has become the method of choice when available. Rapid elimination of ammonia or leucine correlates with improved neurodevelopmental outcome.

Neonatal epileptic encephalopathy warrants a trial of intravenous pyridoxine and folinic acid. Given the low toxicity of these agents, they should be initiated before confirmation of a definitive diagnosis if the specific disease is within the differential diagnosis. General recommendations for empiric therapy based on suspected disease category are given in **Table 77.5**.

Unfortunately, some patients with a suspected IEM will die despite aggressive therapy prior to establishing a specific diagnosis. In this setting, making a postmortem diagnosis can have significant implications for the patient's siblings and for genetic counseling of the parents

Neonatal Screening

Many disorders are screened in the newborn period. Information can be obtained from http://www.mchb. hrsa.gov/screening and http://genes-r-us.uthscsa. edu/.

Specific Metabolic Disturbances

Lactic Acidosis

Symptoms of lactic acidosis include poor feeding, failure to thrive, lethargy, change in mental status, seizures, hypotonia, ataxia, developmental delay, optic nerve atrophy, deafness, and dysfunction of the most energy dependent organs, including the brain, heart, muscle, kidney, and liver. As a general rule, the greater the number of systems involved, the greater the likelihood of a mitochondrial disorder of oxidative phosphorylation. The family history may suggest an IEM when there have been previously affected children within the nuclear family, or similarly but more or less severely affected individuals on the maternal side of the family due to mutations in the maternally transmitted, mitochondrial encoded genes.

Lactic acidosis results from accumulation of pyruvate, which is converted into lactic acid and alanine. *Primary* lactic acidemia results from either defects in gluconeogenesis or defects in oxidative phosphorylation. *Secondary* lactic acidemia results from either anaerobic metabolism or other IEMs that produce less significant degrees of lactic acidosis. Many conditions in the PICU promote tissue hypoxia or hypoperfusion sufficient to cause lactic acidosis. In addition, liver injury or malperfusion prevents the normal conversion of lactate into pyruvate. One must, however, be cautious because severe metabolic decompensation due to an IEM can also be associated with cardiopulmonary failure. Therefore, IEMs should always be considered when the underlying cause of tissue hypoxia is unknown. The differential diagnosis of IEMs causing secondary lactic acidosis includes many of the organic acidemias (propionic and methylmalonic acidemia), which can be readily identified by analyzing urine for organic acids.

The levels of lactic acid can be artifactually elevated by use of a tourniquet, difficulty obtaining the blood sample, or prolonged time between sample collection and analysis. A primary lactic acidemia occurs when serum lactate is twice the normal level (3 mM/L). Consideration should be given to measuring lactic acid from the cerebrospinal fluid if any neurologic symptoms are present even without elevated plasma lactate. Fluctuations in levels of lactate with feeding may suggest the underlying etiology. Lactate

TABLE 77.5

SUPPLEMENTAL THERAPY FOR METABOLIC EMERGENCIES

Suspected category of IEM	Empiric Therapy	Rationale
Urea cycle	L-Arginine 600 mg/kg over 90 mins and 200–600 mg/kg/24 hrs	Essential amino acid in all but arginase deficiency
	Sodium benzoate 250 mg/kg over 90 mins and 250 mg/kg/day	Condenses with glycine to enhance nitrogen excretion
	Sodium phenylacetate 250 mg/kg over 90 mins and 250 mg/kg/day	Condenses with glutamine to enhance nitrogen excretion
	Sodium phenylbutyrate 100–200 mg/kg PO TID	Source of phenylacetate to enhance nitrogen excretion once patient is stabilized
Biotinidase deficiency and Multiple carboxylase deficiency	Biotin 10–15 mg/kg/d PO	Replace biotin that is not adequately recycled
Methylmalonic academia and methionine synthase deficiency	Hydroxycobalamin 1–5 mg/d IM/IV	Enzymatic cofactor
Organic acidurias, carnitine transport defects, and fatty acid oxidation disorders	L-Carnitine 50–100 mg/d divided b.i.d. IV/PO	Replace carnitine losses
Propionic acidemia	Metronidazole 15 mg/kg q 8–12 hrs PO/IV	Inhibit production of propionate by intestinal bacteria
MSUD	Thiamine 150 mg/d IV/PO; >3 yrs, 300 mg/day	Enzymatic cofactor
Mitochondrial disorders	Coenzyme Q10 25 mg t.i.d.	Cofactors and antioxidants
	Carnitine 50 mg/kg b.i.d.	
	αlipoic acid 100 mg q.d.	
	B complex vitamins (100 mg each q.d.)	
	Vitamin E 50 units q.d.	
Ketotic hyperglycinemia	Sodium benzoate 250 mg/kg over 90 mins and 250 mg/kg/day	Condenses with glycine to enhance nitrogen excretion

is most elevated after a prolonged fast in disorders of gluconeogenesis (*fructose bisphosphatase deficiency*), and provocative, carefully monitored fasting studies may be necessary to evaluate these diagnoses. In the setting of fasting lactic acidosis, measurement of biotinidase can identify readily treatable cases of *biotinidase deficiency*. In other cases of gluconeogenic defects, the patient should be treated by avoiding fasting.

In defects of oxidative phosphorylation, lactate levels may fluctuate significantly in the blood or may only be elevated in the cerebrospinal fluid. The ratio of lactate to pyruvate reflects the redox potential of the cell, and ratios >25 suggest a defect in mitochondrial oxidative phosphorylation. Repeated simultaneous measurements of lactate and pyruvate and their

relative ratios are often helpful to establish a consistent ratio. Measuring alanine in the blood and cerebrospinal fluid also allows for an independent, indirect measurement of defective pyruvate metabolism and is not subject to the same difficulties in measurement as lactate. If a defect in mitochondrial oxidative phosphorylation is suspected, a muscle biopsy should be performed to look for ragged red fibers as well as biochemically assess the respiratory chain complexes. In addition, specific genetic tests for conditions such as *MELAS* (*Mitochondrial Encephalopathy, Lactic Acidosis and Stroke*) and *MERRF* (*Mitochondrial Encephalopathy with Ragged Red Fibers*) are available. Defects of the *pyruvate dehydrogenase complex* should be treated with a high-fat, low-carbohydrate diet and supplementation with thiamine and lipoic acid. Most of the other mitochondrial defects of oxidative phosphorylation are difficult to treat but can be empirically treated with thiamine, riboflavin, nicotinamide, vitamin K, and coenzyme Q10 while a definitive diagnosis is being established (see **Table 77.5**). Sodium bicarbonate can be used to correct the metabolic acidosis, but will not decrease lactic acid production.

Metabolic Acidosis without increased Lactate

Although any metabolic disease may present with lactic acidosis during an acute decompensation because of the associated dehydration or hypoperfusion, the organic acidemias and aminoacidopathies typically present with an anion gap acidosis due to accumulation of the abnormal organic acids or ketoacids but *not* predominantly due to elevated lactate. The lactate-adjusted AG is abnormal in these conditions. Many of these disorders present with significant ketoacidosis, Classically, the organic acidurias present as massive ketosis and metabolic acidosis in a vomiting or lethargic neonate. The most common disorders within this category are MSUD, methylmalonic acidemia, and propionic acidemia. Most of these disorders present as intoxication syndromes with episodes of encephalopathy and vomiting, particularly during periods of catabolic stress. Thus, they tend to present during the early neonatal period in an infant that initially appears well or during an intercurrent illness. The age-specific differential diagnosis for metabolic acidosis without elevated plasma lactate is given in **Table 77.6**. Because intoxication plays a central role, extracorporeal toxin removal with hemodialysis or hemofiltration may be useful in the

TABLE 77.6

AGE-SPECIFIC DIFFERENTIAL DIAGNOSIS OF METABOLIC ACIDOSIS WITHOUT INCREASED LACTATE

Age at presentation	Metabolic derangement
Neonate	MSUD, isovaleric acidemia, glutaric acidemia type II, multiple carboxylase deficiency
Infant	MSUD, methylmalonic acidemia, propionic acidemia, ketotic hyperglycinemia, biotinidase deficiency
Older children	Biotinidase deficiency, dietary biotin deficiency

MSUD, maple syrup urine disease

acute management of some of these conditions including maple syrup urine disease.

MSUD is a disorder of metabolism of the essential, branched-chain amino acids, valine, leucine, and isoleucine. Infants with the *classic* form present in the first few days of life with vomiting, encephalopathy, and severe metabolic acidosis. The characteristic odor of urine, sweat, and cerumen can provide an important clue to the diagnosis. Milder forms, with greater residual enzyme activity may present later in life during stress (infection, surgery) in a child with mild developmental delay or failure to thrive. Some patients respond dramatically to thiamine supplementation, which should be started empirically in all patients upon presentation.

Isovaleric acidemia results from a deficiency of *isovaleryl CoA dehydrogenase*, which is further down the leucine degradative pathway. The acute form presents much like MSUD, though these patients have a characteristic odor of sweaty socks and may have associated neutropenia.

Propionic acid and *methylmalonic acid* are sequential catabolic products of isoleucine and valine as well as threonine, methionine, cholesterol, and odd-chain fatty acids. Deficiency of the enzymes responsible for their catabolism (*propionyl CoA carboxylase* and *methylmalonyl CoA mutase*, respectively) result in *ketotic hyperglycinemia*. These conditions all present with vomiting, severe ketoacidosis, encephalopathy progressing to coma, and neutropenia. Due to secondary inhibition of the urea cycle, moderate to severe hyperammonemia may also occur. In addition to supportive care, constipation should be prevented or treated, and sterilization of the intestinal tract with metronidazole should be initiated to minimize production of propionic acid by intestinal bacteria. Carnitine supplementation (50–100 mg/kg/24 hr IV or orally) replaces losses due to propionyl-carnitine formation and hastens resolution of metabolic acidosis. Because propionic acidemia may occur as part of *multiple carboxylase deficiency*, biotin (10 mg/24 hr) should be provided until a definitive diagnosis is established. Similarly, large doses of cobalamin (1–2 mg IV /24 hr) should be provided to patients with suspected methylmalonic acidemia.

Disorders affecting the four *biotin-dependent carboxylases* present with metabolic acidosis, ketosis, and an intoxication syndrome. Deficiency of *holocarboxylase synthetase* results in the most severe disorder and presents in the first few weeks of life. These patients have rashes that mimic eczema and a tomcat-urine odor in addition to the above metabolic derangements. *Biotinidase deficiency* presents with an eczematoid rash. Dietary biotin deficiency may occur in short-gut syndrome, inadequate supplementation in parenteral nutrition, prolonged anticonvulsant

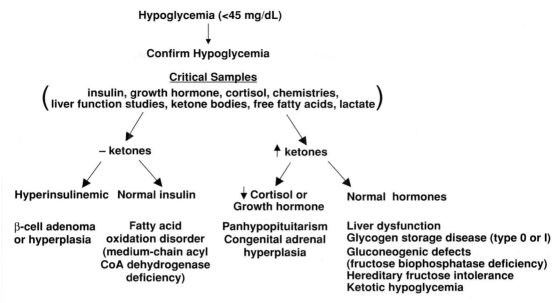

FIGURE 77.2. Evaluation of hypoglycemia and examples of disorders within each diagnostic category.

therapy, and significant raw egg consumption. Biotinidase deficiency and acquired biotin deficiency both respond well to biotin supplementation (10 mg/24hr) and can be cured with this simple therapy.

Hypoglycemia

Children with hypoglycemia present with diaphoresis, pallor, irritability, decreased feeding, jitteriness, temperature instability, lethargy, coma, or seizure. Hypoglycemia must be promptly recognized and treated to prevent damage to the brain. Severe and/or recurrent hypoglycemia can result in permanent brain damage, producing a range of injuries including global mental retardation, behavioral problems and attention deficit disorder, and occipital blindness.

Hypoglycemia is defined as a serum concentration of <50 mg/dL or a whole-blood concentration of <45 mg/dl. A patient can appear artifactually hypoglycemic if the blood has been sitting for several hours. Therefore, hypoglycemia should be confirmed with the bedside glucometer reading and a stat measurement.

Hypoglycemia must be treated promptly and continuously reassessed. Acute treatment in the intensive care setting consists of a bolus of intravenous dextrose, 0.5–1 g/kg given as a 10%–25% solution followed by continuous dextrose infusion to maintain a glucose concentration >70 mg/dl (usually 3–5 mg/kg/min in older children and 5–10 mg/kg/min in neonates). An intravenous line should be in place at all times, and glucose should be monitored at least every 4 hrs to ensure normoglycemia.

Though sometimes difficult, it is diagnostically ideal to evaluate the etiology at the time of hypoglycemia (**Fig. 77.2**). **Table 77.7** lists common etiologies of hypoglycemia. It is essential to evaluate the metabolic status during the time of derangement to produce the maximal diagnostic yield. The timing of the hypoglycemia in relationship to meals may offer clues to the etiology. Hypoglycemia immediately after a meal suggests provocation by some component of the ingested substance. Infants with *hereditary fructose intolerance* typically present at ~6 mos of age when transitioning from breast milk or formula to solid foods, including introduction of fruits and vegetables. Within ~30 mins of ingesting foods containing fructose or sucrose, they will become acutely hypoglycemic and have transient elevations of transaminases and lactic acid. Treatment for hereditary fructose intolerance consists solely of eliminating fructose and sucrose from the diet and is compatible with normal health, growth, and development. Hypoglycemia associated with a high-protein diet can be provoked by high levels of leucine in disorders such as a deficiency of *glutamate dehydrogenase*, resulting in *hyperinsulinemic hyperammonemia*. Hypoglycemia and liver dysfunction in infancy can also be caused by ingestion of breast milk– or cow's milk–based formulas in *galactosemia*, but most cases are now diagnosed by newborn screening and readily treated with a soy-based formula.

TABLE 77.7

COMMON CATEGORIES AND CAUSES OF HYPOGLYCEMIA

Endocrinopathies
  Growth hormone deficiency
  Cortisol deficiency
  Hyperinsulinism
  ▪ Infants of diabetic mothers
  ▪ Beckwith-Wiedemann syndrome
  ▪ Surreptitious insulin

Defective hepatic glucose release and/or utilization of available gluconeogenic substrate
  Ketotic hypoglycemia
  Enzymatic defects
  ▪ Glycogen storage diseases (Glycogen synthetase deficiency, glucose-6-phosphatase deficiency)
  ▪ Galactosemia (galactose-1-phosphate uridyltransferase deficiency)
  ▪ Hereditary fructose intolerance (fructose-1-phosphate aldolase)

Fatty acid oxidation or ketogenesis disorders
  Carnitine acyl transferase deficiency
  Long-chain fatty acid acyl-CoA dehydrogenase deficiency
  Medium-chain fatty acid acyl-CoA dehydrogenase deficiency
  Short-chain fatty acid acyl-CoA dehydrogenase deficiency
  Hydroxymethylglutaryl CoA lyase deficiency

Toxic
  Salicylate
  Acetaminophen
  Alcohol
  Oral hypoglycemic agents (biguanides, sulfonylureas)

Hypoglycemia can also be associated with ingestion of toxins or medications. Oral hypoglycemic agents such as the sulfonylureas can produce acute, rapid hypoglycemia. Other agents such as aspirin, acetaminophen, ethanol, and any hepatotoxic agent can cause hypoglycemia.

Hypoglycemia associated with fasting for ~8 hrs is most characteristic of *glycogen storage disorders* such as *glycogen storage disorder type I* (*glucose 6 phosphatase deficiency*) or *glycogen storage disorder type 0* (*glycogen synthase deficiency*). These disorders frequently present as infants begin to sleep through the night with increased fasting intervals and/or during periods of intercurrent illness associated with anorexia or vomiting. Children with *type I glycogen storage disease* have a biochemical profile of lactic acidosis, hyperalaninemia, hyperuricemia, and hyperlipidemia associated with their hypoglycemia. Hypoglycemia associated with fasting for ~16 hrs is more characteristic of defects in gluconeogenesis (*fructose 1,6 bisphosphatase deficiency, glycerol kinase deficiency, pyruvate carboxylase deficiency,* or *pyruvate kinase deficiency*) or *fatty acid oxidation disorders*. After ~16–24 hrs, all the glycogen reserves have been utilized and the body begins to rely on gluconeogenesis and fatty acid oxidation.

Hyperinsulinemia causing hypoglycemia can be due to exogenous or endogenous insulin. An insulin value of >10 U/mL simultaneous with hypoglycemia is always abnormal. Levels of C-peptide can differentiate the source of insulin because C-peptide is produced only with *endogenous* insulin. Endogenous hyperinsulinemia typically presents within the neonatal period and can produce the most severe, persistent, and difficult hypoglycemia to manage. Persistent dextrose requirements of 10 mg/kg/min suggest underlying hyperinsulinemia. Hyperinsulinemia may ultimately require treatment with diazoxide to inhibit insulin secretion, partial pancreatectomy if there is evidence of an islet-cell adenoma or near-complete pancreatectomy for diffuse islet-cell hyperplasia.

Hypoglycemia is more common in neonates who are small for gestational age or the preterm infant in the first few days of life. Additionally, maternal diabetes may lead to perinatal hyperinsulinemia and hypoglycemia in the neonate. Hypoglycemia in these situations is always associated with ketosis and usually resolves within the first few days to weeks of life.

Patients with liver disease are also more susceptible to hypoglycemia due to the decreased capacity of the liver to supply glucose through glycogenolysis and gluconeogenesis. This may be a nonspecific manifestation of liver dysfunction and is best treated symptomatically by supplying glucose intravenously.

A common and relatively benign cause of hypoglycemia is *ketotic hypoglycemia* often seen in toddlers and young children. These children appropriately mobilize fats and have massive ketosis during periods of hypoglycemia. Children are most often symptomatic during an intercurrent illness associated with anorexia or a vomiting. This condition can be treated simply by avoiding fasting for >12 hrs and is usually outgrown by the age of 5–10 yrs.

Hyperammonemia

Newborns often present with rapidly progressive decreased feeding, hypothermia, lethargy, apnea, coma, and death within a period of hours in the most severe cases. Severe hyperammonemia can be rapidly progressive and associated with respiratory depression. Therefore, prophylactic intubation is indicated with ammonia levels >500 μM/L.

Hyperammonemia is defined as ammonia >150 μM/L in the neonate or >100 μM/L in the older child. Blood samples should be placed on ice and analyzed immediately to avoid artifactual elevations. Mild hyperammonemia (<~300 μM/L) can be associated with *transient hyperammonemia of the newborn* as well as with several inborn errors of metabolism, including the *organic acidurias, fatty acid oxidation defects, lysinuric protein intolerance*, and *hyperammonemia, hyperornithinemia, and homocitrullinuria syndrome*. More severe degrees of hyperammonemia are typically observed with *urea cycle defects* with depression of the blood urea nitrogen due to the inability to produce urea. These patients often initially demonstrate a respiratory alkalosis on their arterial blood gas. Secondary hyperammonemia can also be associated with liver failure and/or overwhelming viral hepatitis.

Initial treatment should consist of making the child NPO and keeping the child anabolic with infusion of only dextrose and electrolytes to meet the age dependent metabolic demands. Diagnostic laboratory tests should include arterial blood gas, serum chemistries, liver function studies, urine organic acids (specifically tested for orotic acid), urinalysis, serum amino acids, acylcarnitine profile and repeated and frequent measures of ammonia until the rate of rise can be determined. Metabolic acidosis or an increased anion gap suggests that the diagnosis is not a urea cycle defect. Urinary ketosis with mild hyperammonemia suggests an organic aciduria. *Fatty acid oxidation disorders* should not be associated with urinary ketones but are often associated with hypoglycemia and elevated CPK with *mild* hyperammonemia.

Urea cycle defects are associated with the greatest and most rapid rise in ammonia. Elevations of ammonia rapidly rising beyond 500 μM/L should be treated with hemodialysis if available. Peritoneal dialysis and exchange transfusion with such severe hyperammonemia are much less efficacious. While awaiting the results of diagnostic studies, in addition to initiation of hemodialysis, patients with suspected urea cycle disorders should be started on intravenous L-arginine to maintain the urea cycle and given loading doses and continuous infusions of sodium benzoate and phenylacetate that can be used to remove ammonia via alternative metabolic pathways utilizing glycine and glutamine to eliminate nitrogen (see **Table 77.5**). Mannitol should be utilized to decrease cerebral edema if present.

Females heterozygous for the X-linked *ornithine transcarbamylase deficiency* or patients with partial urea cycle defects may demonstrate only periodic metabolic crises with normal intervening metabolic evaluations. In these cases, metabolic crises are associated with ingestion of large amounts of protein and/or a catabolic state induced by an intercurrent illness.

Liver Failure

Liver failure associated with elevated transaminases, jaundice, bleeding, and edema and/or hepatomegaly is a common presentation for inborn errors of metabolism. Because the liver is the metabolic center of the body, most processes causing severe hepatic impairment can also cause alterations in metabolic pathways and produce mild hyperammonemia or hypoglycemia. Some inherited disorders cause direct hepatocyte damage, including *hepatorenal tyrosinemia, galactosemia, Wilson disease,* α1-antitrypsin deficiency, peroxisomal disorders (*Zellweger syndrome* and *Refsum disease*), and defects in cholesterol and bile acid synthesis. Initially, it may be difficult to distinguish these inborn errors of metabolism from infectious causes such as sepsis, hepatitis A, B, or C, cytomegalovirus, Epstein-Barr virus, herpes simplex, toxoplasmosis, or HIV. The size of the liver may aid in differentiation between IEMs and infectious etiologies; hepatomegaly occurs more commonly with inborn errors of metabolism.

Liver function should be assessed with a liver function panel including albumin, transaminases, direct and indirect bilirubin, alkaline phosphatase, γ glutamyltranspeptidase, α-tfetoprotein, glucose, ammonia, blood urea nitrogen, prothrombin time, and partial thromboplastin time. If liver disease is suspected, titers and viral cultures of stool and urine should be performed to rule out viral etiologies of hepatitis A liver biopsy may be necessary to identify storage material within the liver followed by specific enzymatic testing using fibroblasts or liver tissue for definitive diagnosis.

Many children with liver disease present initially with jaundice. As neonates, most babies with inborn errors of hepatic metabolism present with conjugated hyperbilirubinemia. Unconjugated hyperbilirubinemia, in contrast, suggests the diagnosis of *Crigler-Najjar* or a hemolytic anemia. Crigler-Najjar is treated with phototherapy and plasmapheresis acutely and ultimately by liver transplantation. *α1-antitrypsin deficiency* presents as cholestasis in a minority of infants. *Progressive familial intrahepatic cholestasis, Dubin-Johnson,* and *Rotor syndromes* usually present as conjugated hyperbilirubinemia after 3 mos of age. *Hepatorenal tyrosinemia, Niemann Pick type C,* and *peroxisomal disorders* can also initially present as conjugated hyperbilirubinemia, but all usually progress rapidly to severe liver failure.

In the older child, hepatocellular necrosis and encephalopathy suggest a Reye-like syndrome that may be due to an underlying inborn error of metabolism, chronic viral hepatitis, autoimmune disease, or acute intoxication. The differential diagnosis of inborn errors of metabolism presenting with Reye-like syndrome includes *fatty acid oxidation disorders, urea cycle disorders, hepatorenal tyrosinemia, hereditary fructose intolerance, Wilson disease,* and *α1-antitrypsin deficiency. Wilson disease* is characterized by choreoathetoid movements and dystonia, Kayser-Fleischer rings around the cornea, reduced levels of serum ceruloplasmin, and increased urinary copper. The age of presentation for some of these disorders depends on the degree of the enzymatic deficiency, with less severe deficiencies presenting at older ages.

In many of the *lysosomal storage disorders,* liver function is intact, although the liver can become extremely enlarged. Lysosomal storage disorders are further suggested by short stature, failure to thrive, or coarse facial features, and developmental delay, hypotonia, or seizures. Many of the *glycogen storage diseases* can also produce hepatomegaly with or without associated hypoglycemia and are often diagnosed by findings of abnormal quantity and/or quality of glycogen on a liver biopsy. *Hemochromatosis* is a rare cause of hepatomegaly resulting from excess storage of iron.

Treatment for many liver disease caused by inborn errors of metabolism is supportive therapy to treat associated coagulopathies with vitamin K and fresh-frozen plasma, edema due to hypoalbuminemia with diuretics and albumin infusion, unconjugated hyperbilirubinemia with phototherapy, and deranged

metabolism producing hypoglycemia and hyperammonemia. A lactose-free, soy-based diet is a simple cure in *galactosemia.*

Nonmetabolic Critical Illness in IEMs

Many IEMs present in the PICU not in metabolic crisis but due to the effects on specific vital organ systems. Effects on the hepatic, renal, pulmonary, cardiovascular, and hematologic systems may all have significant implications for the pediatric intensivist. Lactate-containing fluids should not be administered to patients who may not metabolize exogenous lactate (mitochondrial disorders and pyruvate dehydrogenase complex deficiency). Although propofol has been used successfully in mitochondrial disorders, it should probably be avoided in fatty acid oxidation defects because of possible predisposition to propofol infusion syndrome. Several IEMs place patients at significant risk of *hyperkalemia* and *rhabdomyolysis* leading to myoglobinuria after depolarizing neuromuscular blockers, including glycogen storage diseases V (*McArdle disease*), and VII (*Tauri disease*). The absence of acidosis distinguishes this phenomenon from malignant hyperthermia (MH). The mitochondrial disorders, however, may predispose to true MH after use of depolarizing agents and volatile anesthetics.

The mucopolysaccharidoses (MPS) can affect both the myocardium and the endocardium (valvular disease). Type I (*Hunter/Scheie*) and Type II (*Hurler*) MPS result in varying degrees of myocardial and valvular disease. Although the mucolipidoses (MLS), *I-cell disease,* and *pseudo-Hurler polydystrophy* share many features with the MPSs such as valvular disease, reports of cardiomyopathy are rare. Together with Pompe disease, these lysosomal storage disorders also affect a variety of systems involved in respiratory management in the PICU. The associated dysmorphisms and tracheal narrowing can make endotracheal intubation extremely challenging. Atlanto-axial instability, particularly in MPS IV (*Morquio syndrome*), must be considered during laryngoscopy as well. These patients are also at high risk of airway obstruction during induction. Therefore, these patients may require fiberoptic intubation or even tracheotomy and should be intubated awake whenever possible. Muscle relaxants are contraindicated before successful intubation unless an easy mask airway can be established.

CHAPTER 78 ■ CANCER THERAPY: MECHANISMS, TOXICITY, AND ETHICS IN THE PICU

DAVID M. LOEB • DAVID G. NICHOLS

MECHANISMS

Most pediatric malignancies are treated with multimodal therapy, traditionally consisting of chemotherapy, radiotherapy, and surgery. More recently, biologically based therapies have been developed, including small-molecule kinase inhibitors, cytokine therapies, differentiation therapies, and antiangiogenic therapies. Chemotherapy drugs are classified by their mechanism of action. **Table 78.1** lists the commonly used constituents of each major drug class. **Table 78.2** lists some commonly used regimens to treat certain pediatric malignancies.

Alkylating Agents

Most alkylating agents commonly used in pediatric oncology are derivatives of nitrogen mustard, including cyclophosphamide and ifosfamide, or derivatives of methylnitrosourea, such as lomustine and carmustine (BCNU). These drugs contain highly reactive alkyl groups that form covalent bonds with DNA and other intracellular macromolecules. In addition to the nitrogen mustard and nitrosourea derivatives, platinum-based antitumor compounds also create DNA cross-links. While not true alkylating agents, these compounds have a similar mechanism of action and are, therefore, sometimes referred to as "non-classical alkylating agents." The two commonly used platinum-based compounds are cisplatin and carboplatin.

Antimetabolites

Methotrexate was developed as a clinically useful chemotherapeutic agent that acts by competitively inhibiting the enzyme dihydrofolate reductase. Inhibition of this key enzyme for synthesis of thymidine leads to depletion of intracellular thymidine triphosphate and eventually to arrest of DNA synthesis. There are also reports that high doses of methotrexate lead to decreased purine synthesis and ultimately to cell death. Another potential mechanism of action of methotrexate is its toxicity to endothelial cells. There is mounting evidence that methotrexate is effective therapy for autoimmune diseases in part

---

TABLE 78.1

CHEMOTHERAPEUTICS ORGANIZED BY CLASS

Class	Drugs
Alkylating agents	Cyclophosphamide, ifosfamide, BCMU, CCNU, cisplatin, carboplatin
Antimetabolites	Methotrexate, 6-mercaptopurine, 6-thioguanine
Topoisomerase inhibitors	Etoposide (VP16) and teniposide (VM26) inhibit Topo II
	Irinotecan and topotecan inhibit Topo I
Anthracyclines	Doxorubicin, daunorubicin, idarubicin
Antimicrotubule agents	Vincristine, vinblastine, vinorelbine, paclitaxel, docetaxel

BCMU, carmustine; CCNU, lomustine

TABLE 78.2

COMMONLY USED CHEMOTHERAPY REGIMENS IN PEDIATRIC ONCOLOGY

Diagnosis	Chemotherapy
Acute lymphoblastic leukemia: induction	Prednisone or dexamethasone, vincristine, L-asparaginase (and daunorubicin for high risk patients)
Acute myelogenous leukemia: induction	Daunorubicin, cytarabine, etoposide
Osteosarcoma	Methotrexate, cisplatin, doxorubicin (ifosfamide and etoposide added for some patients with poor response to neoadjuvant therapy)
Ewing's sarcoma	Vincristine, doxorubicin, cyclophosphamide alternating with ifosfamide and etoposide
Rhabdomyosarcoma	Vincristine, dactinomycin, cyclophosphamide
Hodgkin's disease	**Low risk:** doxorubicin, prednisone, vincristine, cyclophosphamide **Intermediate and high risk:** doxorubicin, bleomycin, vincristine, etoposide, prednisone, cyclophosphamide
Neuroblastoma	**Intermediate risk:** carboplatin, etoposide, cyclophosphamide, doxorubicin **High risk:** cyclophosphamide, topotecan, cisplatin, etoposide, doxorubicin, vincristine
Wilms tumor	**Low risk:** vincristine, dactinomycin **Intermediate risk:** vincristine, dactinomycin, doxorubicin **High risk:** vincristine, doxorubicin, cyclophosphamide, etoposide

through inhibition of angiogenesis, and this mechanism may also play a role in the antineoplastic effects of methotrexate as well. 6-mercaptopurine and 6-thioguanine are thought to act primarily by being incorporated into growing DNA strands and thus inhibiting DNA synthesis. Other mechanisms by which these drugs exert their cytotoxicity include inhibition of the activity of enzymes necessary for the synthesis of natural purines (adenine and guanine).

Topoisomerase Inhibitors

Topoisomerases are enzymes involved in the maintenance of supercoiling of the DNA double helix. These enzymes are essential for DNA replication, transcription, and chromosomal segregation—critical processes for cell division and therefore for tumor growth. There are two classes of topoisomerase inhibitors: type I enzymes, which make single-strand cuts in DNA, and type II enzymes, which make double-strand cuts. There are two types of topoisomerase II inhibitors: podophyllotoxins and anthracyclines. Etoposide (VP16) is the more commonly used podophyllotoxin. Etoposide poisons topoisomerase II by increasing the steady-state concentration of their covalent DNA cleavage complexes. Antibiotics such as doxorubicin, daunorubicin, and idarubicin also inhibit topoisomerase II. Other activities of anthracycline antibiotics include effects on nuclear helicases and the generation of iron free radicals. Inhibitors of topoisomerase I represent a newer class of chemotherapeutic agents. The agents in

common use, irinotecan and topotecan, are derivatives of camptothecin, a plant alkaloid obtained from the *Camptotheca acuminata* tree. These drugs target the DNA-topoisomerase I complex, preventing the reannealing of the nicked DNA strand. This leads to the accumulation of drug stabilized nicked DNA strands, causing an arrest of DNA replication and subsequent cell death.

Antimicrotubule Agents

Vincristine, vinblastine, and vinorelbine are vinca alkaloids that produce cytotoxicity through interaction with tubulin, the major protein component of microtubules. This interaction disrupts the structure of the microtubules, leading to dissolution of the mitotic spindle and metaphase arrest of dividing cells. The importance of microtubules in other cellular functions explains the noncytotoxic effects of these compounds. In particular, neurons require intact microtubules for axonal transport, and disruption of this function causes the well-known peripheral neuropathy associated with vincristine treatment. Docetaxel and paclitaxel are the two most commonly used taxanes, and they act by binding to tubulin at sites distinct from those bound by the vinca alkaloids. Taxanes function by stabilizing microtubules against depolymerization, primarily through an effect on tubulin dissociation rates at both ends of the microtubule. This affects dynamic instability of the microtubules, which is critical for normal microtubule dynamics during both mitotic and nonmitotic phases of the cell cycle. Ultimately, this disruption of microtubule dynamics leads to induction of apoptosis. Interestingly, taxanes also inhibit angiogenesis at concentrations below those which are cytotoxic.

Other Cytotoxic Drugs

L-asparaginase hydrolyzes asparagines to aspartic acid and ammonia. In sensitive tumor cells that lack adequate levels of asparagine synthetase, this enzyme depletes the cells of a critical amino acid, thus rapidly inhibiting protein synthesis. DNA and RNA synthesis are eventually also inhibited, and cell death ensues. Asparaginase is particularly used to treat pediatric acute lymphocytic leukemia (ALL). Cytarabine, or Ara-C, is serially phosphorylated to generate ara-CTP by deoxycytidine kinase. Cytarabine decreases intracellular concentrations of deoxycytidine by competition for enzymes responsible for the activation of cytidine and thereby inhibits DNA synthesis. DNA polymerase is also inhibited by incorporation of ara-CTP into nascent DNA strands, and incorporation of ara-CTP into DNA correlates with cytotoxicity. In addition to these effects, ara-C also causes cells to synthesize small reduplicated segments of DNA, increasing the possibility of crossovers and recombination. Gemcitabine is another cytidine analog that has recently been introduced into pediatric oncology practice. Like ara-C, gemcitabine is phosphorylated by nucleoside kinases. Gemcitabine triphosphate competes with dCTP for incorporation into DNA and inhibits DNA polymerase and thus inhibiting DNA synthesis.

Radiotherapy

General Principles of Radiotherapy

Radiotherapy is the delivery of packets of energy to a target tissue with the intention of causing lethal damage to malignant cells while minimizing damage to normal cells. Radiation energy comes in different packets, the most commonly used being photons (for example, from x-rays), as well as protons or electrons. Different packets of energy have different properties, including the amount of energy per packet and penetration through tissue, and these properties determine the mode of treatment. As the packets deposit their energy, ionization events occur in biologically important molecules, and it is these events that lead to tissue damage and death. These events can occur directly (as when a photon causes the release of electrons from a target biological molecule, and this electron directly damages the molecule) or indirectly (as when a released electron interacts with a neighboring water molecule to generate free radicals which then damage macromolecules). The dose of energy delivered is measured in Gray (Gy), and 1 Gy = 1 J/kg. An older dose term, rad, is still sometimes used, and 1 rad = 1 cGy = 0.01 Gy. While multiple biologic macromolecules can be affected by ionizing radiation, it is thought that induction of double-strand DNA breaks is the proximate cause of cell death. Ionizing radiation initiates a complex cascade of cellular responses that can result in cell cycle arrest, induction of stress response genes, induction of apoptosis, or repair of DNA damage. Hypoxic tumors are more resistant to ionizing radiation than are normally oxygenated tumors. As cancer cells die within the tumor mass, anoxic regions can "reoxygenate," and cells that had been relatively protected can become more sensitive. Cells in the G2 and M phases of the cell cycle are most sensitive to radiation, while cells in late S phase are relatively resistant. This differential sensitivity can lead to a relative synchronization of tumor cells.

Types of External Beam Radiation

Typical external beam radiotherapy is delivered from a ^{60}Co source and is composed of photons. In order to minimize dose delivery to normal tissue, perpendicular beams are used to deliver the radiation, with the area of overlap corresponding to the target. Because the beams are rectangular, but most tumors are irregularly shaped, devices known as collimators in the head of the radiation source shape the beam to more closely conform to the shape of the tumor. The beam can be further shaped with the use of individually constructed blocks that shield body regions that are not in the target area. Modern multileaf collimators provide additional precision to the shape of the beam. Photons typically deposit energy relatively deep in tissue, with higher energy photons penetrating more deeply than lower energy photons. Electrons, in contrast, deposit their energy in a relatively shallow range, with a rapid drop-off of energy with increasing depth. Thus, a superficial tumor (such as leukemia cutis) will be more appropriately treated with electron beam therapy, rather than standard photons. Like electrons, protons have a very rapid drop-off of energy in the last few millimeters of penetration. Unlike electrons, protons penetrate relatively deeply into tissue. Thus, a proton beam can treat a target deeper than an electron beam but with similar precision in the deposition of energy. Thus, proton beam radiation is valuable when the target is located deep but adjacent to particularly sensitive normal tissue. Whereas photons and electrons are commonly available, there are a limited number of centers capable of delivering proton beam radiotherapy.

Targeted Radiotherapy

Physiologic targeting includes the use of ^{131}I-MIBG to treat neuroblastoma and ^{153}Sm-EDTMP to treat osteosarcoma. Metaiodobenzylguanidine is a catecholamine precursor that, when labeled with ^{123}I, has been used as a diagnostic imaging tool for neural crest tumors like neuroblastoma. Samarium-153 ethylene diamine tetramethylene phosphonate (EDTMP) is a bone-seeking radiopharmaceutical that has been used to treat high-risk osteosarcoma. Just as the MIBG targets ^{131}I to neuroblastoma cells, EDTMP targets ^{153}Sm to osteosarcoma cells, essentially sparing surrounding normal tissue. Like ^{131}I-MIBG, ^{153}Sm-EDTMP is being delivered in the context of autologous peripheral blood stem cell support.

Biological Therapy

Differentiation Therapy

The best-known example of differentiation therapy is the use of all-trans retinoic acid (ATRA) in the treatment of acute promyelocytic leukemia (APML). APML is well known to the intensivist because of the characteristic profound bleeding diathesis seen at presentation. Pharmacologic doses of ATRA overcome the block to differentiation caused by PML-RARα, and the malignant promyelocytes differentiate into granulocytes. A second common example of differentiation therapy in pediatric oncology is the use of 13-cis-retinoic acid to treat neuroblastoma.

Immunotherapy

Immunotherapy includes allogeneic hematopoietic stem cell transplantation with or without infusion of donor lymphocytes and treatment with various recombinant cytokines. Cytokine administration remains a rare event in pediatric oncology, but this approach was pioneered by the National Cancer Institute's efforts at inducing an immune response to metastatic melanoma and to renal cell carcinoma by infusions of interleukin-2.

Small-Molecule Kinase Inhibitors

The advent of Gleevec for the treatment of chronic myelogenous leukemia (CML) heralded the era of targeted therapy based on a molecular understanding of tumorigenesis. CML is defined by the presence of a distinctive chromosomal translocation, t(9;22) or the Philadelphia chromosome. This translocation leads to the production of a fusion protein tyrosine kinase called BCR-ABL, and this kinase drives the neoplastic process. Gleevec is a competitive inhibitor of the BCR-ABL tyrosine kinase and causes complete hematologic response

Monoclonal Antibodies

Rituximab is an antibody against CD20, a marker of B lymphocytes, and is used to treat non-Hodgkin's lymphoma and autoimmune disorders such as ITP and hemolytic anemia. Response to Rituximab can be monitored indirectly by measuring CD20-positive cells in the circulation, and these often become undetectable within a day of just a single dose of the antibody. Another commonly used monoclonal antibody is alemtuzumab, which is anti-CD52. CD52 is a panlymphocyte marker, and treatment with alemtuzumab results in a rapid, profound, and longlasting depletion of circulating T cells, B cells, NK cells, and monocytes. Patients become lymphopenic within 2 weeks and remain lymphopenic for as long as a year after treatment. In adult oncology, alemtuzumab is primarily used as therapy for lymphomas, but in pediatric oncology its primary use is in the context of bone marrow transplantation—either as part of an immunoablative preparative regimen or in the prevention or treatment of graft-versus-host disease.

TOXICITIES

Table 78.3 lists common toxicities caused by the commonly used chemotherapy drugs.

Fever in the Neutropenic Patient

The most common side effect of cytotoxic chemotherapy is myelosuppression, leading to periods of absolute neutropenia. A fever in a neutropenic cancer patient represents a true emergency, as there is a significant rate of bacteremia that can rapidly lead to septic shock.

Toxicities Related to Bone Marrow Transplantation

Children who have undergone bone marrow transplantation (BMT) are subject to a number of unique toxicities, including veno-occlusive disease, cytokine storm/engraftment syndrome, and graft-versus-host disease (GVHD). BMT patients may also develop fever while they are neutropenic, and many of the immunosuppressive drugs used as prophylaxis or treatment of GVHD can cause significant, difficult-to-control hypertension. Finally, pneumonitis is a common problem encountered in the post-BMT setting.

TABLE 78.3

COMMON TOXICITIES OF COMMONLY USED CHEMOTHERAPY DRUGS

Drug	Toxicities
Ifosfamide	Renal tubular dysfunction, encephalopathy, hemorrhagic cystitis
Cyclophosphamide	Renal tubular dysfunction, hemorrhagic cystitis, myocardial necrosis
Cytarabine	Cerebellar syndrome, myelopathy, leukoencephalopathy, pulmonary edema, pneumonitis
Methotrexate	Skin sloughing, nephrotoxicity, seizures, hepatic dysfunction
Anthracyclines	Severe mucositis, congestive heart failure
Bleomycin	Pneumonitis
ATRA	Capillary leak syndrome
L-asparaginase	Pancreatitis
Cisplatin	Renal tubular dysfunction, cardiotoxicity
Vincristine	Peripheral neuropathy, ileus, neuropathic pain

ATRA, all-trans retinoic acid.
Note: Most chemotherapeutic agents cause nausea, vomiting, mucositis, and pancytopenia, so these are not included in the table above. This table is *not* intended to be a comprehensive listing of chemotherapy side effects but rather to highlight the most common toxicities that may be encountered by the pediatric intensivist.

Toxicities of the Central Nervous System

A number of commonly used chemotherapeutic drugs cause distinct CNS toxicities. The greatest culprit in the pediatric population is ifosfamide. Ifosfamide causes encephalopathy, which can range from mild (somnolence) to severe (coma or seizure), occurring between 2 and 48 hrs after drug administration. The management of ifosfamide-induced encephalopathy includes discontinuation of the drug and standard supportive measures. There have been several reports of the use of methylene blue for the treatment of ifosfamide-induced encephalopathy. The other chemotherapy drug that commonly causes acute CNS toxicity is cytarabine (Ara-C). The neurologic toxicities depend on dose and route of administration. Intrathecal Ara-C has been associated with a rapid-onset myelopathy (though this might be related to the use of benzyl alcohol as a diluent) or a slower-onset myelopathy, with symptoms beginning 2 days to 6 months after treatment. Other CNS toxicities have also been reported more rarely after intrathecal Ara-C, including seizures and leukoencephalopathy. Seizures have also been described in patients being treated with intravenous high-dose Ara-C. In general, these have been self-limited and do not recur once therapy is stopped. Cerebral dysfunction, usually accompanying cerebellar syndrome, has also been described and usually takes the form of generalized encephalopathy. Cerebral dysfunction usually resolves spontaneously as well. The acute cerebellar syndrome is the most prominent and common neurologic toxicity associated with cytarabine. The

syndrome is seen only after treatment with high-dose systemic cytarabine and occurs 3–8 days after treatment; manifestations include dysarthria, dysdiadochokinesia, dysmetria, and ataxia. Possible risk factors include age, renal dysfunction, and cumulative exposure to drug. There is no effective therapy for this disorder other than discontinuation of the drug and institution of supportive care as indicated.

Cardiac Toxicities

The best-known cardiotoxic chemotherapy drugs are the anthracyclines: doxorubicin, daunorubicin, and idarubicin. The mechanism of cardiotoxicity involves the generation of oxygen-free radicals that ultimately lead to irreversible loss of myocardiocytes and the development of cardiomyopathy. Anthracycline cardiotoxicity can be acute or delayed. Acute effects include transient arrhythmias and acute left ventricular failure. The acute effects are usually transient and will attenuate after discontinuation of therapy. Cardiac injury can also present in a delayed fashion, years or decades after treatment, as new-onset congestive heart failure. The most significant risk factor for serious cardiotoxicity is cumulative dose. Limiting total exposure, administration of liposome-encapsulated anthracyclines, and the use of cardioprotectants such as dexrazoxane (Zinecard) are strategies to limit toxicity. Dexrazoxane acts as an iron chelator, prevents the formation of an anthracycline-iron complex that is thought to be a critical mediator of myocardiocyte injury, and thus prevents cardiac damage. Once patients exhibit symptoms of cardiotoxicity, standard treatments should be administered, aimed at decreasing afterload and increasing contractility. Anticoagulation is useful in the setting of severe left ventricular dysfunction and persistent dysrhythmia. Cyclophosphamide has also been associated with severe cardiotoxicity at high doses such as are employed in BMT. Risk factors include prior anthracycline chemotherapy and chest irradiation. Clinically, cardiotoxicity presents as congestive heart failure or myocarditis. Symptoms may be delayed by up to 2 weeks after administration. There is no specific treatment for cyclophosphamide-induced cardiotoxicity, so standard supportive measures are indicated. Paclitaxel has been associated with asymptomatic bradycardia, as well as second- and third-degree heart block. These bradyarrhythmias are reversible. Several cases of acute myocardial infarction after cisplatin therapy have also been reported. Amsacrine, an acridine derivative with activity against hematologic malignancies, can affect cardiac electrophysiology and cause a wide range of EKG changes, including ventricular tachycardia. The arrhythmias can occur within minutes or days of treatment. 5-fluorouracil has also been reported to induce cardiotoxicity (including arrhythmias, silent ischemia, and even sudden death). This occurs mostly in the setting of continuous infusion, rather than bolus dosing, and risk factors include preexisting coronary artery disease and concurrent radiotherapy.

Pulmonary Toxicities

Bleomycin is the chemotherapeutic most frequently thought of in the context of pulmonary toxicity, but other cytotoxic treatments can cause pulmonary fibrosis or edema, including gemcitabine, cytarabine, and radiotherapy. Additionally, a number of drugs have been linked with a hypersensitivity pneumonitis syndrome, including BCNU, methotrexate, procarbazine, and bleomycin. Also referred to as inflammatory interstitial pneumonitis, this syndrome is characterized by an insidious progression of nonproductive cough, dyspnea, and low-grade fevers. Eosinophilia is noted in the peripheral blood and on lung biopsy, which often also reveals bronchiolitis obliterans with organizing pneumonia. This syndrome resolves with removal of the offending agent, although sometimes oral corticosteroids speed recovery. Bleomycin toxicity is primarily limited to lungs and skin because these organs lack bleomycin hydrolase. Most commonly, bleomycin causes an interstitial pneumonitis (BIP). BIP usually begins during therapy and is initially indolent, with a cough and dyspnea on exertion being the primary symptoms. The disorder can progress to dyspnea at rest, tachypnea, and cyanosis. Radiographic findings are nonspecific and may be

unilateral, may be focal, but may also be bilateral and diffuse. Interstitial or alveolar infiltrates can be seen on plain film, and CT scan often shows small linear and subpleural nodular lesions in the lung bases. Lung biopsy may show characteristic lesions such as squamous metaplasia of bronchiolar epithelium, inflammatory cells infiltrating into alveoli and alveolar septa, edema plus focal collagen depositions in these septa, and fibrotic areas. Decrease in diffusion capacity and vital capacity (with concomitant administration of other agents) is seen in patients with bleomycin pneumonitis. High-dose corticosteroids are frequently used to treat clinically significant BIP. A vascular leak syndrome, leading to significant, sometimes life-threatening, pulmonary edema has been described with infusions of Ara-C or interleukin-2. The vascular leak is usually reversible with discontinuation of therapy and is treated with diuresis and oxygen. Acute onset of pulmonary edema, often mimicking ARDS, can occur in patients previously treated with bleomycin and exposed to high concentrations of inspired oxygen, as may occur in conjunction with a surgical procedure, even years after chemotherapy is completed. This complication can be minimized by administering the lowest possible concentration of oxygen to patients with a history of treatment with bleomycin. Other chemotherapeutic agents associated with pulmonary toxicity include mitomycin-C, which causes a delayed-onset interstitial pneumonitis; actinomycin D, which acts as a radiation sensitizer; and rarely cyclophosphamide or ifosfamide. Radiotherapy can damage capillary endothelial cells and type I pneumocytes, which eventually leads to a pneumonitis syndrome. Radiation pneumonitis is rare in patients treated with <20 Gy but is highly likely in patients who receive >60 Gy. Symptoms become evident 2–3 mos after completion of therapy and include primarily complaints of dyspnea and a nonproductive cough. Physical findings are usually minimal. Permanent changes of fibrosis evolve over 6–24 mos but usually stabilize after this time period. Clinical symptomatic relief has been reported in patients with pulmonary fibrosis who were treated with pentoxifylline and vitamin E.

Retinoic Acid Syndrome

The major complication of ATRA treatment is the retinoic acid syndrome. The diagnosis is established by the presence of at least three of the following signs and/or symptoms in the absence of alternative explanations: fever, weight gain, respiratory distress, pulmonary infiltrates, pleural or pericardial effusions, hypotension, and renal failure. The syndrome most commonly manifests ~10 days after the start of chemotherapy but has been reported as rapidly as 2 days into treatment. The pathogenesis is related to tissue infiltration with newly differentiated granulocytes and cytokine production by these cells. The final pathway is endothelial damage leading to edema, hemorrhage, fibrinous exudates, and respiratory failure. The only specific therapy available for retinoic acid syndrome is dexamethasone.

Pancreatitis

It has long been recognized that treatment with L-asparaginase may cause acute pancreatitis. Management of asparaginase-induced pancreatitis is identical to the management of idiopathic pancreatitis, including gut rest. Asparaginase-induced acute pancreatitis can progress to hemorrhagic pancreatitis, and chronic pancreatitis is also seen in some patients.

Urinary Tract Toxicities

Both ifosfamide and cyclophosphamide can cause hemorrhagic cystitis. Both drugs are broken down to produce, among other degradation products, acrolein. Ifosfamide is a more potent urotoxin than cyclophosphamide. Acrolein has been incriminated as the major cause of hemorrhagic cystitis after treatment with these drugs. Prophylaxis against hemorrhagic cystitis includes aggressive hydration (alkaline intravenous fluids at twice maintenance) and the use of mesna (sodium-2-mercaptoethanesulfonate). Mesna is orally bioavailable (as well as being administered intravenously) and is rapidly oxidized to dimesna, which is taken up by the kidneys. Between 30% and 50% of glomerularly filtered dimesna is reduced back to mesna in the renal tubular epithelium by glutathione reductase. Mesna collects in the bladder where it detoxifies acrolein and other oxazaphosphorine metabolites. Uncontrolled hemorrhagic cystitis can be life-threatening, and exsanguination can occur. If prophylaxis fails, management includes cystoscopy and clot evacuation, aggressive bladder irrigation, and intravesicle instillation of formalin. In addition to cystitis, cyclophosphamide and ifosfamide can also cause renal dysfunction, both tubular and glomerular. Ifosfamide is a far more potent nephrotoxin, although nephrotoxicity is seen after very high doses of cyclophosphamide. Proximal tubular dysfunction is the most common form of nephrotoxicity observed and frequently manifests as Fanconi's syndrome, with hypophosphatemia, renal tubular acidosis, hypokalemia, hypocalcemia, or hypomagnesemia. Distal tubular dysfunction is less common, but nephrogenic diabetes insipidus has been reported.

Glomerular toxicity, though more rare, can be severe enough to require dialysis and may become chronic. Hypertension is also seen. Risk factors for ifosfamide nephrotoxicity include age (increased risk in children <5 years old), total dose of ifosfamide (increased risk with total dose >60 g/m^2), prior or concurrent treatment with cisplatin (which increases the risk), and preexisting renal impairment. Cisplatin is also nephrotoxic and accumulates in the proximal tubules, with intracellular concentrations fivefold higher than plasma concentrations. Cisplatin administration results in a dose-dependent reduction of glomerular filtration rate, hypomagnesemia, hypokalemia, and polyuria. There is evidence that aggressive hydration, including the use of mannitol, can attenuate the toxicity of cisplatin. The renal toxicity of cisplatin is usually reversible but can become chronic and progressive.

Radiation Recall

Radiation recall is an inflammatory reaction in a previously irradiated body area. Most commonly, radiation recall manifests as an acute dermatitis. Reactions can range from a mild maculopapular erythematous skin rash to severe necrosis. Reactions occur in a sharply demarcated area corresponding to the prior irradiation field. The reaction can occur weeks to years after radiation exposure. Although skin is the most common organ involved, radiation recall has been reported in lung, esophagus, gut, and the CNS. In visceral organs, this manifests as inflammation of the target organ within a previous radiation field. Treatment is straightforward, with the mainstays of therapy being corticosteroids and withdrawal of the offending agent. Topical steroids are appropriate for skin reactions, and systemic steroids are necessary for visceral involvement.

Management of Chemotherapy Overdose

There are few reports in the literature of the effects of accidental chemotherapy overdose and even fewer reports of successful, specific treatments. Most reports document the efficacy of aggressive supportive care allowing the patient to recover. There are reports of specific therapies administered to patients who received an overdose of cisplatin, including plasmapheresis, and the administration of sodium thiosulfate. Hemodialysis has not been found to be effective, probably because cisplatin is extensively protein-bound and deposits in tissues where it is unable to be cleared by hemodialysis. Plasma-pheresis is expected to be more effective by virtue of removing circulating plasma proteins to which cis-platin is bound. The other reported specific treatment for cisplatin overdose is the administration of N-acetylcysteine to replete glutathione and allow the usual detoxification reactions to function. Ifosfamide overdose has been treated with the use of methylene blue. Another recently developed "antidote" to chemotherapy overdose is carboxypeptidase G2. Carboxypeptidase G2 is a bacterial enzyme that hydrolyzes methotrexate to its inactive metabolites, 4-deoxy-4-amino-N10-methylpteroic acid and glutamate. Carboxypeptidase G2 has been administered intravenously to patients with delayed methotrexate clearance after being given appropriate high-dose methotrexate therapy. Hemodialysis is a nonspecific intervention often employed in the treatment of drug overdose. The effects of hemodialysis on the pharmacokinetics of antineoplastic drugs are summarized in **Table 78.4**.

Paclitaxel pharmacokinetics are unaltered in anephric patients undergoing hemodialysis. Dialysis is effective in clearing cisplatin and carboplatin only within a relatively short time after drug administration due to rapid and stable binding to proteins in

TABLE 78.4

USE OF HEMODIALYSIS FOR OVERDOSE OF CHEMOTHERAPY

Readily cleared by hemodialysis	Not cleared by hemodialysis
Ifosfamide Methotrexate Cyclophosphamide	Etoposide Dactinomycin Vinca alkaloids Anthracyclines

Platinum agents are cleared only if dialysis is initiated rapidly after drug administration. These drugs become protein-bound (carboplatin) or distribute into tissue (cisplatin) quickly and are no longer dialyzable. Paclitaxel pharmacokinetics are unaltered in anephric patients undergoing hemodialysis.

serum (carboplatin) or peripheral tissues (cisplatin). Methotrexate and cyclophosphamide are readily dialyzable, with an increased rate of elimination compared to renal clearance. Ifosfamide is also readily removed by hemodialysis, whereas etoposide, dactinomycin, vinca alkaloids, and anthracyclines are rapidly and extensively protein-bound and not cleared effectively by hemodialysis.

CHAPTER 79 ■ ONCOLOGIC EMERGENCIES AND COMPLICATIONS

RODRIGO MEJIA • JOSE A. CORTES • DEBORAH L. BROWN • GERARDO QUEZADA • MICHAEL E. RYTTING • CARROLL J. KING • ALAN I. FIELDS

Earlier published reports indicated poor outcomes for oncology patients admitted to the PICU. As a result, pediatric oncology units, especially those that offered stem cell transplants, developed a very broad therapeutic repertoire. These units started to treat patients with a severity-of-illness, which would have ordinarily dictated a PICU admission. In some, this included attempts at hemodynamic support for early septic and/or hypovolemic shock and renal replacement therapies, reserving admission to the PICU for those children requiring mechanical ventilation, usually for acute respiratory failure. More recent studies noting improved outcomes for pediatric cancer patients admitted to the PICU suggest that a more aggressive therapeutic approach with earlier applica-

tion of invasive therapies may be responsible. Early intervention for patients with a lower Pediatric Risk of Mortality Score upon PICU admission are associated with better outcomes, and mortality increases as more organ systems fail. It seems reasonable that intervention before end-organ failure has occurred is a prudent therapeutic goal, as once three or more organ systems fail, survival markedly decreases.

SHOCK IN THE CHILD WITH CANCER

Septic shock or sepsis in the pediatric cancer patient presents special challenges because these patients are usually immunocompromised and frequently profoundly neutropenic with impaired mucosal barriers, and they may have preexisting end-organ dysfunction and are more vulnerable to multiple organ system failure (MOSF). Aggressive fluid resuscitation, prompt administration of appropriate antibiotics and antifungals, use of inotropic support, and ventilator strategy designed to minimize lung injury and optimize oxygenation are critical. Renal replacement therapies should be applied early to maintain fluid balance, avoiding the lung injury and breakdown of integument associated with fluid overload and diminished renal function. In addition to the aggressive fluid resuscitation (60 mL/Kg in the first hr) and the goal-directed therapy commonly employed in critically ill patients with sepsis syndrome, physicians caring for cancer patients with sepsis should be mindful that preexisting complications of chemotherapy present special risks and also opportunities for intervention (**Table 79.1**). The practitioner caring for a critically ill pediatric cancer patient should be aware that steroids are used frequently in these patients as part of their chemotherapy as well as for control of complications such as vomiting and graft-versus-host disease. The ACCM's Practice Parameters for Pediatric Shock suggest that the use of steroids be limited to patients with catecholamine-resistant shock and proven or suspected adrenal insufficiency. The neutropenia common in PICU patients with cancer predisposes them to acquire sepsis or septic shock as well as to have a longer and potentially more complicated course than other children. Cultures should be frequently reviewed and antibiotics tailored appropriately. The *transfusion of granulocytes* has been used in the treatment of disseminated infection in neutropenic patients with unclear benefit. *Colony-stimulating factors* are being utilized to shorten the duration of neutropenia and for patients who have neutropenia and MOSF, sepsis or septic shock, or invasive fungal disease that shows promise.

TABLE 79.1

EVALUATING A CHILD WITH CANCER AND SEPTIC SHOCK

1. Consider *early admission* to the PICU.
2. Consider *preexisting organ dysfunction* from chemotherapy or its complications.
3. Consider *resistant bacterial or fungal infections* in these patients who have frequently had multiple courses of broad-spectrum antibiotics.
4. Consider that prior use of steroids places these patients at increased *risk of adrenal insufficiency.*
5. Consider aggressive search for *infectious source.*
6. Consider early evaluation for *cardiac dysfunction.*

CARDIOGENIC SHOCK

Cardiac tamponade is defined as the significant compression of the heart by accumulating pericardial contents, including effusion fluid, blood clot, pus, or air. In cancer patients, such effusions are most frequently either malignant or hemorrhagic (as the result of erosion of pericardial vessels by tumor or secondary to thrombocytopenia). If the reserve pericardial volume is exceeded, cardiac tamponade is life-threatening. Classic signs of cardiac tamponade include tachycardia, jugular venous distension, pulsus paradoxus, Kussmaul's sign (respiratory variation of JVD), muffled heart sounds on auscultation, electrical alternans on ECG, and chest radiograph findings of cardiomegaly, water-bottle heart, and no venous congestion. The evaluation of any patient in whom a pericardial effusion is suspected should include an echocardiograph (ECHO). The diagnosis cannot be excluded on the basis of a normal chest radiograph, and ECG changes may be nonspecific. A cardiac ECHO is helpful in assessing both the extent of hemodynamic compromise by evaluating diastolic collapse of the atria and the effectiveness of interventions. The management of cardiac tamponade may include the use of inotropes to support cardiac output, but careful attention should be given to fluid status, as hypovolemia will exacerbate the pathophysiology of this condition and lead to a relatively greater reduction in cardiac output. Definitive treatment for tamponade requires drainage accomplished by surgical pericardiotomy, pericardiocentesis, or the placement of a percutaneous pericardial catheter.

RESPIRATORY EMERGENCIES

Respiratory emergencies are frequent in the pediatric cancer patient and may have a dramatic presentation in patients after bone marrow transplantation. The immune deficiency that results from the primary disease, the toxicity of the therapy or both, makes these patients susceptible to a wide range of infectious and noninfectious problems that may progress rapidly to respiratory failure (**Table 79.2**). Initiation of broad-spectrum antimicrobial therapy (to address *Pseudomonas, Cytomegalovirus, Pneumocystis, and Aspergillus*) is often indicated in patients with rapid clinical or radiologic deterioration. Bronchoscopy with bronchoalveolar lavage or open-lung biopsy should be carried out early in the course of the illness. The former may help differentiate infection from diffuse alveolar hemorrhage (DAH), a common complication after stem cell transplantation. High-resolution CT should be considered in patients with respiratory symptomatology and normal plain radiographs.

PULMONARY COMPLICATIONS AFTER BMT

Phase	Infectious	Noninfectious
Neutropenic phase (0–30 days)	Bacteria (20%–50%) Fungal (12%–45%)	Pulmonary edema Drug toxicity Diffuse alveolar hemorrhage
Early phase (30–100 days)	CMV pneumonitis (40%) PCP	Idiopathic pneumonia syndrome
Late phase (>100 days)	Uncommon except in GVHD	Bronchiolitis obliterans Cryptogenic organizing pneumonia Chronic GVH

CMV, cytomegalovirus; GVHD, graft-versus-host disease; PCP, pneumocystic pneumonia

Stem cell transplant recipients with respiratory failure require endotracheal intubation, especially in the presence of pneumonia or DAH. Lung-protective strategies with low tidal volumes or high-frequency oscillatory ventilation have improved the outcome.

Massive hemoptysis is defined as a volume of blood >240 ml (in adults) and can lead to rapid asphyxiation and death. The most common cause of massive hemoptysis is invasive pulmonary aspergillosis (IPA). IPA usually presents after myeloablative chemotherapy for bone marrow transplantation or during the recovery phase of prolonged neutropenia after chemotherapy. Other etiologies include mucormycosis, tuberculosis bacterial necrotizing pneumonia, primary endobronchial tumors, bronchiectasis, and foreign bodies. Neutropenic patients with fever >96 hrs despite adequate antibiotic therapy should be evaluated for IPA. Chest pain and cough are common symptoms. The highest risk for hemoptysis occurs during recovery from prolonged neutropenia. The inflammatory process includes a focal cavitary lesion surrounded by collateral vessels. The presence of increasing neutrophils leads to focal necrosis and enhanced risk for vessel perforation and bleeding. CT scan is the most sensitive radiologic test available for the early diagnosis of IPA. The halo sign, a dense nodular lesion surrounded by ground-glass attenuation (>180°) is consistent with IPA. The air crescent sign indicates necrosis and cavitation. Tissue diagnosis is required to conclusively exclude or confirm IPA. Tissue may be obtained by CT-guided percutaneous lung biopsy, trans-bronchial biopsy, or open-lung biopsy. The treatment of massive hemoptysis should be directed at the prevention of asphyxia. Early intubation and mechanical ventilation should be considered. Aggressive treatment of any associated coagulopathy, thrombocytopenia, and anemia is warranted. Combination antifungal therapy with Caspofungin and liposomal amphotericin B with voriconazole should be initiated for patients with invasive mycosis. Bronchoscopy should be considered in patients in whom endoluminal therapy for control of the bleeding is feasible. Fiberoptic bronchoscopy is helpful as a diagnostic tool for confirmation of the bleeding site only when radiologic confirmation cannot be obtained. Bronchial arteriography with transcatheter embolization may be effective in nonsurgical candidates. Wedge resection of the affected lung segment or lobectomy carries a low mortality risk and offers a lower recurrence rate when compared with nonsurgical options.

Superior Mediastinal Syndrome

Superior mediastinal syndrome (SMS) results from the compression of the superior mediastinum structures. SMS is almost synonymous with superior vena cava syndrome (SVCS), which refers to the symptoms resulting from compression or obstruction from invasion or thrombus of the superior vena cava's normal venous flow. SVCS is most often associated with congenital heart lesions or lymphomas. Dyspnea, orthopnea, and wheezing are common symptoms. Progressive venous congestion and airway compression will lead to the usual symptoms found in SVCS and SMS: facial engorgement, headache, plethora, cyanotic facies, cough, dyspnea, orthopnea, hoarseness, and dysphagia. Less common symptoms include pleural and/or pericardial effusions. Most patients at this stage may not tolerate the supine position. Chest radiograph and CT scan may confirm shape distortion of the superior mediastinal structures. Echocardiography is indicated in patients with suspected thrombus or pericardial effusion. Pulmonary function tests may also be obtained to evaluate pulmonary reserve. Elevation of lactate dehydrogenase may be present with non-Hodgkin's lymphoma and leukemia. Alpha-fetoprotein may be elevated in yolk sac tumors.

Patients with anterior mediastinal masses are at particular risk of rapid cardiopulmonary collapse when sedated or placed under general anesthesia. Bone marrow biopsy, lymph node biopsy, or CT-guided percutaneous mediastinal biopsies may be safely performed with local anesthesia if tolerated. Pericardial and or pleural collections should be drained under ultrasound or CT guidance for therapeutic and diagnostic purposes. General anesthesia should not be administered if the tracheal cross-section area and the peak expiratory flow rate are <50% of predicted values. In some situations, it is impossible to obtain a tissue sample before beginning treatment. Most of these tumors, particularly lymphomas, may prove to be very sensitive to irradiation or chemotherapy and will dissolve rather quickly, making a tissue diagnosis later in the course impossible. Surgical resection may be unavoidable in patients with tumors not sensitive to cytoreductive therapy (e.g., large-cell lymphomas, teratomas, germ cell tumors).

NEUROLOGIC EMERGENCIES

Increased Intracranial Pressure

Increased intracranial pressure (ICP) may occur in pediatric cancer patients as a result of a mass effect exerted by a primary or a metastatic brain neoplasm on normal brain structures, spontaneous bleeding of a tumor mass, or obstruction of normal cerebrospinal fluid (CSF) flow causing hydrocephalus frequently requiring early ventricular drainage. Early management includes conventional ICP measures and dexamethasone 2 mg/kg followed by 0.5 mg/kg q6h is helpful in reducing the edema surrounding the tumor.

Spinal Cord Compression

Spinal cord compression most frequently results from metastatic spread of sarcomas, neuroblastoma, germ cell tumor, lymphoma/leukemia, or metastatic CNS tumors. Back pain is a red flag. The pain can start weeks to months before the diagnosis is made, but once neurologic signs appear, the progression is rapid and may be irreversible. Other common symptoms include lower extremity weakness, sphincter dysfunction, and sensory abnormality. All patients with progressive neurologic signs or symptoms should be treated with high-dose steroids (dexamethasone 1–2 mg/kg). Craniospinal T_1- and T_2-weighted MRI allows demonstration of epidural involvement, in-

traparenchymal spread, and compression of nerve roots. CSF studies are necessary to evaluate for subarachnoid disease, CNS leukemia, or carcinomatosis. Further treatment addresses three different scenarios: (a) radiotherapy, if the diagnosis is known and the tumor is radiosensitive; (b) chemotherapy, if the diagnosis is leukemia/lymphoma or neuroblastoma; or (c) surgery, if the diagnosis of the tumor is unknown or if symptoms progresses despite radiation therapy.

Convulsions can occur with primary CNS tumors, metastatic CNS lesions, CNS leukemia, antineoplastic therapy, metabolic abnormalities, hemorrhage, or infection. Treatment of the seizure is to provide supportive care, conduct appropriate studies including blood tests, EEG and/or CT, and treat any known or discovered abnormalities. It may be wise to avoid starting valproic acid or carbamazepine, as these agents are known to cause marrow suppression.

Stroke can occur with leukemia and hyperleukocytosis. The majority of strokes in children are due to arterial or venous thrombosis, intraparenchymal hemorrhage, local or metastatic tumor spread, or hematologic abnormalities. Embolic events are uncommon.

Table 79.3 lists the etiology of the stroke in relation to the stage of the oncologic process. Patients with any form of leukemia and hyperleukocytosis are at high risk for stroke at diagnosis and early in the treatment phase. In acute promyelocytic leukemia, stroke may result from enhanced thrombin activation and increased production of plasmin secondary to annexin II expression. L-asparaginase, alone or in combination with vincristine and prednisone, is associated with an increased risk of venous thrombosis (acquired antithrombin III, protein S and protein C deficiency). Radiotherapy may cause stroke even

TABLE 79.3

ETIOLOGY OF STROKE

Time of presentation	Likely diagnosis
At presentation of malignancy	Malignancy Coagulopathy Intratumoral hemorrhage
During treatment of malignancy	Drug toxicity Malignancy
At the end stage of the malignancy	Infection Disseminated intravascular coagulation Progressive malignancy
Months to years after therapy	Radiation-induced vascular damage

years after treatment, and the risk is related to the total dose of radiation. Large-vessel occlusions are associated with doses in excess of 50 Gy. The adjuvant use of intrathecal or parenteral MTX and cytosine arabinoside potentiates this risk. CT or MRI with and without contrast is useful in evaluating the nature and extent of a stroke. The management of stroke is supportive. The use of isotonic fluids and correction of any coagulopathy or electrolyte abnormality is recommended. If stroke is the presenting symptom, treating the underlying malignancy with cytotoxic therapy may prevent additional strokes. In hemorrhagic stroke, platelet levels should be maintained >75 thousand/mL.

Coma

Occasionally, a pediatric cancer patient may present with significant obtundation or in coma. Infratentorial tumors can produce obstructive hydrocephaly, elevated intracranial pressure, and herniation. The intensivist should focus on the stabilization of the patient's airway, breathing, and circulation and on the management of impending herniation. A contrast/noncontrast CT or MRI is often helpful in determining the etiology. Common causes of coma in pediatric oncology include tumor, bleeding, infection, or therapeutic agents.

METABOLIC EMERGENCIES

Syndrome of Inappropriate Antidiuretic Hormone Secretion

The syndrome of inappropriate antidiuretic hormone secretion (SIADH) evinces an excessive secretion of antidiuretic hormone in the presence of low sodium levels and normal or low plasma osmolal-

ity. SIADH may occur in the pediatric cancer patient (medulloblastoma, lymphoma, ovarian teratoma) and in the setting of cerebral insults (intracranial surgery, trauma), neck surgery, mechanical ventilation, infections and lung disease. SIADH has been recognized to occur with several medications, including anticonvulsants (carbamazepine) and chemotherapeutic agents (vincristine, iphosphamide and cyclophosphamide). SIADH-related hyponatremia may be aggravated by the aggressive fluid hydration strategy used in patients receiving chemotherapy. The late manifestations of SIADH (confusion, seizures, and coma) are usually the reason for admission to the PICU. Confirmation of the diagnosis is based on the presence of increased total body water and hyponatremia in the setting of low serum osmolality <280 mOsm/L with an elevated urine osmolality, usually >500 mOsm/L (urine to serum osmolality ratio >1), elevated urinary sodium concentration, and decreased urine output (<1 mL/kg/hr). The treatment of SIADH should include fluid restriction to 30%–50% maintenance until the serum sodium levels normalize. Hypertonic saline (3% saline solution) infusion 3–5 mL/kg or normal saline infusion 20 mL/kg is indicated in severe symptomatic patients with coma and/or seizures until symptoms resolve. Once symptoms have subsided, the rate of correction of hyponatremia should be limited to 12 mmol/L/day. Rapid correction of hyponatremia may lead to central pontine myelinolysis.

Cerebral Salt-Wasting Syndrome

Patients with cerebral salt-wasting (CSW) syndrome may share similar intracerebral diseases and laboratory criteria with those patients with SIADH (**Table 79.4**). CSW in children typically occurs 2–7 days after CNS injury and is probably the result of abnormal secretion of natriuretic peptides. Patients with

TABLE 79.4

DIAGNOSIS OF SIADH, CSW, AND DI

	SIADH	CSW	DI (central)
Body water	Increased	Decreased	Decreased
Sodium	Low	Low	High
Serum osmolality	<280 mOsm/L	Decreased	>300 mOsm/L
Urine osmolality	>500 mOsm/L	Increased	Low
Urine-to-serum osmolality ratio	>1	>1	<1.5
Urine output	Low	High	High
Urine sodium concentration	Increased	Increased	Decreased

SIADH, syndrome of inappropriate antidiuretic hormone secretion; CSW, cerebral salt wasting; DI, diabetes insipidus

CSW syndrome have volume contraction and hyponatremia in the setting of polyuria and increased urine sodium losses. The differentiation between SIADH and CSW is made by observing urine volume patterns during the development of hyponatremia and natriuresis. The treatment of CSW should be directed to vigorous extracellular fluid and sodium replacement. Treatment with high-dose fludrocortisone (0.2–0.4 mg/day) has proven to be beneficial in some patients.

Diabetes Insipidus

Diabetes insipidus (DI) typically presents in the pediatric cancer patient as a result of a direct injury, compression or infiltration of the hypothalamic supraoptic or paraventricular nuclei, or the supraoptic-hypophyseal tract. DI is most often caused by surgical resection of a hypothalamic-pituitary tumor (craniopharyngioma, germinoma) or by local tumor infiltration or destruction (histiocytosis, leukemia, lymphoma). The diagnostic confirmation is based on the presence of elevated serum osmolality >300 mOsm/L, low urine osmolality (urine-to-serum osmolality ratio <1.5), and increased urine output. DI most often presents in a triphasic pattern after surgical resection of a suprasellar mass: During the initial phase typically lasting 2–5 days, the patient may develop DI as a consequence of a deficient secretion of arginine vasopressin or secretion of a biologically inactive form. The second phase is characterized by an inappropriate arginine vasopressin (AVP) release lasting 1–14 days, during which time the signs and symptoms of DI may disappear. A recurrent and very often permanent form of DI characterizes the third phase. The treatment of DI should be directed to fluid and AVP replacement. Patients in shock should receive fluid replacement with large volumes of isotonic solutions in order reverse the shock state. Subsequent matching of the urine output up to a maximum of 4 L/m^2/24 hr with hypotonic solutions (0.25%–0.45% normal saline in 5% dextrose) requires close monitoring (every 2–4 hrs) of the serum sodium, serum osmolality and urine osmolality. Hypernatremia should be corrected over 48–72 hrs. Desmopressin acetate (DDAVP) or arginine vasopressin (AVP) should be used cautiously, bearing in mind the risk of developing hyponatremia. The recommended dose for DDAVP is 2–4 mcg/day IV or SC in two divided doses. Recommended doses for AVP start at 0.5 mU/kg/hr with a 30-minute titration interval to a maximum of 10 mU/kg/hr.

Hypercalcemia associated with malignancy can be found in patients with leukemia, lymphoma, hepatoblastoma, rhabdomyosarcoma, Ewing's sarcoma, or brain tumors. The most common cause of malignancy-associated hypercalcemia is a humoral hypercalcemia, caused by solid-tumor production of a parathyroid hormone-related peptide, resulting in a systemic osteoclast-mediated bone resorption, increased renal calcium resorption, and increased renal phosphorus excretion. The second most common cause of hypercalcemia is osteolysis secondary to cytokine-mediated osteoclast activation at the site of bone metastasis. The third category is calcitriol-mediated hypercalcemia, the most frequent form of hypercalcemia in Hodgkin's and non-Hodgkin's disease. Patients with malignant hypercalcemia will usually present with bradyarrhythmias, coma, muscle weakness, and renal insufficiency. The basic principles for the management of severe hypercalcemia (>14 mg/dL) are monitoring electrocardiographic changes (prolonged PR, broad T waves), vigorous hydration with saline solution (saline 10–20 mL/kg/bolus), forced diuresis with furosemide (1–2 mg/kg/dose) to induced calciuresis, decreased calcium mobilization with calcitonin 4 IU/kg IM or SC every 24 hrs in combination with prednisone 1 mg/kg/day IV, treatment of the underlying malignancy.

Pamidronate, a bisphosphonate, binds hydroxyapatite crystals and blocks osteoclast-mediated resorption. The recommended dose is 1 mg/kg/dose IV. The side effects include hypocalcemia, hypophosphatemia, and hypomagnesemia. Combined treatment with calcitonin and pamidronate may be used in refractory cases not responding to conventional treatment with hydration and forced diuresis with loop diuretics.

Tumor Lysis Syndrome

Tumor lysis syndrome (TLS) is a constellation of metabolic abnormalities resulting from the rapid destruction of tumor cells overwhelming usual metabolic pathways. TLS usually occurs after chemotherapy, steroids, hormones, or radiotherapy. It is typically characterized by hyperuricemia, hyperkalemia, and hyperphosphatemia. Precipitation of calcium phosphate in the microvasculature results in symptomatic hypocalcemia. If left untreated, the precipitation of the urate cry‍‍‍‍ phosphate crystals in the renal t‍ lead to acute renal failure. Lab‍ TLS includes a dramatic rise ‍ uric acid, urea nitrogen, phosph‍ overwhelming the normal hom‍ A rapid rise in serum potassi‍ in severe arrhythmias and de‍

TABLE 79.5

TREATMENT OF TLS

5% dextrose in 0.25% normal saline + 60–100 mEq sodium bicarbonate/L at 2–4 × maintenance
Keep urinary pH 7–7.5, SG 1.010.
Restrict potassium and phosphorus. Replace calcium in symptomatic patients only.
Urate oxidase (Rasburicase): 0.15 or 0.2 mg/kg once daily in a 30-min intravenous infusion for 5 days
Allopurinol: 10 mg/kg/day or 200 mg/m^2/day starting 24–48 hrs prior to initiation of chemotherapy

ionized form at normal serum concentrations and normal pH. The presence of metabolic acidosis and high uric acid plasma concentrations increases the risk of uric acid crystal formation and precipitation in the renal collecting ducts and tubules (sites of urinary acidification). Metabolic acidosis exacerbates the already elevated serum phosphate concentration by shifting intracellular phosphate to the extracellular space. Secondary hypocalcemia results from calcium phosphate precipitation when the solubility product factor is reached (Ca × P = 60). Risk factors for acute renal failure include primary tumor infiltrates, obstruction of urine flow, preexisting renal pathology, and dehydration. Risk factors for TLS are Burkitt's lymphoma/leukemia (B-ALL), acute leukemias (ALL, AML), non-Hodgkin's lymphoma, tumors with rapid growth rate, large tumor burden, elevated serum lactate dehydrogenase (LDH) >500 U/L, dehydration, and elevated uric acid. Symptoms in TLS include anorexia, malaise, weakness, vomiting, hiccups, paresthesia, tetany, carpopedal spasm, and seizures. ECG changes associated with hyperkalemia include prolonged PR, flattened P, widened QRS, peaked T wave, and/or hypocalcemia (prolonged QT interval). A summary of TLS treatment is presented in **Table 79.5.** Early and aggressive hydration is crucial in the management of TLS. Rapid and aggressive alkalinization should be discouraged since it may worsen the hypocalcemia by shifting the calcium to a nonionized from its ionized form.

Management of Severe Electrolyte Disturbances

Patients with hyperkalemia should have dietary as well as supplemental potassium restricted. Patients with potassium levels >6.5 mEq/L or with ECG alterations should receive insulin, glucose, bicarbonate, and calcium. Diuretics (potassium wasting) should be used with caution in volume-depleted patients. Kayexalate (sodium polystyrene sulfonate), a potassium exchange resin, should be given early to help the potassium rebound after the transient acute hyperkalemia treatment. The usual

dose is 1 g/kg orally, mixed in water or sorbitol. Renal replacement therapy should be considered early in patients with rapid renal deterioration or in those with refractory hyperkalemia. Calcium replacement is indicated only in patients with neuromuscular irritability secondary to hypocalcemia: seizures, arrhythmias, or positive Chvostek or Trousseau signs. Calcium replacement in hyperphosphatemic non-symptomatic hypocalcemic patients may aggravate calcium phosphate precipitation in the renal tubules. Hyperphosphatemia is managed with oral phosphate binders such as sevelamer hydrochloride, calcium carbonate, calcium acetate, or aluminum hydroxide.

Renal Replacement Therapy

The goals of dialysis are treatment of obstructive nephropathy by rapid removal of uric acid and phosphorus and treatment of acute renal failure and the associated metabolic abnormalities or early initiation of chemotherapy in the oliguric patient. Continuous venovenous hemofiltration has a potential role if used prospectively in addition to conventional preventive measures before chemotherapy initiation. Cytoreductive chemotherapy should be delayed if indicated in patients with high risk of TLS until the preventive treatment measures are initiated.

HEMATOLOGIC EMERGENCIES

Febrile Neutropenia

Febrile neutropenia requires hospitalization with empiric antimicrobial therapy. Fever is defined as a single oral temperature ≥38.3°C or a temperature of ≥38°C that persists for >1 hr. A rectal temperature should never be taken in a neutropenic pediatric patient. Neutropenia is defined as an absolute neutrophil count <500 cells/mm^3 or <1000 cells/mm^3 with a downward trend. The risk of sepsis or invasive bacterial infections increases with the degree and duration of neutropenia. The risk for bacteremia and septicemia increases with an absolute

TABLE 79.6

CLINICAL AND LABORATORY HIGH-RISK FACTORS IN FEBRILE NEUTROPENIA

Clinical risk factors	Laboratory-based risk factors
Evidence of shock (hypotension, delayed capillary refill >3 sec) Near-myeloablative chemotherapy (leukemia induction or delayed intensification) Allogeneic hematopoietic stem cell transplant recipient Relapsed leukemia Pneumonia Neutropenic enterocolitis Invasive fungal infection Oropharyngeal mucositis Prolonged neutropenia (>7 days) High presenting temperature (>39°C)	Elevated C-reactive protein >90 mg/dL Absolute neutrophil count <200 cells/mm3 Absolute monocyte count <100 cells/mm3 Gram-negative bacteremia

neutrophil count of <200 cells/mm^3. Neutropenia that lasts longer than 7 days results in a worse outcome. Hematologic malignancies (including relapsed leukemia) as well as those who have undergone an allogeneic hematopoietic stem cell transplant (HSCT) are at increased risk of prolonged periods of neutropenia. **Table 79.6** lists the clinical as well as laboratory risk factors that may place a pediatric cancer patient at a higher risk for a serious infection. Furthermore, a presenting temperature of >39.5°C, capillary refill time >3 seconds, a low diastolic blood pressure (defined as DBP <2 standard deviations below the mean), and the presence of oral mucositis were identified as significantly associated with implementation of critical care therapies in febrile neutropenic children with cancer.

Specific Complications

Bacteremia

Catheter-related infections are the most common cause of bacteremia. While the rate of gram-positive infections has increased, the rate of infections caused by gram-negative organisms has remained unchanged. While most gram-positive infections are less virulent than gram-negative ones, an exception is α-hemolytic streptococcal infections. Certain groups, such as AML patients, are at a higher risk. Mucositis also places these patients at risk for streptococcal viridans infections. For this reason, adequate antimicrobial coverage for Streptococcus viridans should be instituted for any AML patient admitted with fever and neutropenia. **Table 79.7** lists commonly used antimicrobials for the management of febrile neutropenia. Strong evidence exists that monotherapy with a broad spectrum antimicrobial with antipseudomonal coverage is appropriate for neutropenic patient presenting with a fever without infectious focus.

Neutropenic Enterocolitis

Neutropenic enterocolitis is a complication seen in patients with prolonged neutropenia. It is referred to as *typhlitis* when it involves the cecum. The classic triad of fever, abdominal pain, and diarrhea may not always be present and is not highly specific, making the clinical diagnosis difficult. Imaging with either ultrasonography or an abdominal CT scan is essential. CT allows for differentiation of other diagnosis and is usually the modality of choice.

TABLE 79.7

SELECT ANTIMICROBIALS FOR MANAGEMENT OF FEBRILE NEUTROPENIA

Broad-spectrum antibiotics	Gram-positive coverage	Gram-negative coverage	Anaerobic coverage

Cefepime
Ceftazidime
Carbapenems (meropenem,
  imipenem)
	Vancomycin
	Ampicillin/sulbactam
	Linezolid
		Aminoglycoside
		  (gentamicin, tobramycin)
		Aztreonam
			Metronidazole
			Clindamycin

Ultrasonography may also prove useful as a prognostic tool based on the degree of bowel thickness. Sepsis and perforation are the most common complications. A conservative approach that includes bowel rest, nasogastric suction, total parenteral nutrition, and broad antimicrobial coverage is appropriate. Surgical intervention may be needed in some cases but is not universally recommended and may be unnecessary even in high-risk pediatric patients.

Invasive Fungal Infections

Periods of prolonged neutropenia as well as steroid use are two well-known risk factors for the development of invasive fungal infections. Populations at risk include patients with an acute leukemia and those patients who have undergone an allogeneic hematopoietic stem cell transplantation. The immunosuppression involved in treating graft-versus-host disease also places the transplant population at high risk for invasive fungal infections. Mortality from disseminated fungal infections is high. *Candida* and *Aspergillus* are the two most frequently isolated organisms, but the advent of fluconazole prophylaxis has resulted in a shift toward non-albicans species as well as invasive aspergillosis. The neutropenic patient with persistent fever for >3–5 days should have empiric coverage expanded to include fungal organisms. Amphotericin, caspofungin, and voriconazole are used in the empiric management of fungal infections.

Lower Respiratory Tract Infections

Pneumonia is an uncommon complication of febrile neutropenia. Although routine chest radiography is not warranted, febrile neutropenic patients presenting with cough or respiratory distress require immediate imaging due to the potential for rapid progression in these patients. *Pneumocystis carinii* pneumonia (PCP) is now rare thanks to widespread use of trimethoprim-sulfamethoxazole prophylaxis in our patients. PCP should be in the differential of any immunocompromised patient presenting with respiratory symptoms and diffuse patchy infiltrates on chest radiography. First-line treatment is with intravenous trimethoprim-sulfamethoxazole (pentamidine is an alternative). Corticosteroids should be initiated within 72 hrs of initiating therapy for any patient with moderate or severe PCP (PaO$_2$ <70 mm Hg on room air).

Community acquired infections well known to the general pediatric population (influenza, respiratory syncytial virus (RSV), and parainfluenza) can have devastating effects in immunocompromised hosts, especially in transplant patients. While therapy is available for influenza (neuraminidase and M2 inhibitors), there is no effective therapy for parainfluenza pneumonia. Ribavirin, palivizumab, and RSV–immunoglobulin may benefit HSCT patients with RSV pneumonia. Preemptive therapy is indicated when a patient has an active CMV antigenemia. Either intravenous ganciclovir or foscarnet are adequate for preemptive therapy depending on what prophylactic agent was used prior to detection of CMV antigenemia.

Hyperleukocytosis

Hyperleukocytosis is defined as a white blood cell (WBC) count of ≥100,000/mL in the peripheral blood. It is seen mainly in patients with acute leukemia or occasionally chronic myelogenous leukemia. Children with hyperleukocytosis often develop a consumptive coagulopathy. The platelet count, protime, partial thromboplastin time, fibrinogen, and d-dimers should be evaluated at diagnosis and followed for abnormalities. To avoid bleeding problems, the fibrinogen should be maintained over 100 g/dL, if possible, and the platelet count should be maintained over 50,000/mL until the patient is stable. Finally, hyperleukocytosis can lead to hyperviscosity and microvascular complications. Leukapheresis or exchange transfusion should be considered in patients with symptoms of leukostasis or with very high WBCs. However, more invasive interventions may not be superior to hydration, alkalinization, and allopurinol. Equally important to any of the above therapies is the prompt start of cytotoxic therapy. In patients with AML, the occurrence of microvascular complications is more frequent and occurs at lower WBC counts. If apheresis is not available, exchange transfusion may be attempted. Since patients with hyperleukocytosis may have problems with blood viscosity, infusions of packed red blood cells (PRBC) should be avoided.

Hemorrhage and thrombosis in childhood malignancy are potentially life-threatening complications of cancer treatment for patients who may otherwise be cured of their disease. The approach is summarized in (**Table 79.8**). Localization of bleeding vessels or mucosal injury is important to identify potential surgical or mechanical remedies. Topical treatment of bleeding is an important first line approach to mucosal or cutaneous bleeding sites. Topical thrombin or tissue sealants applied with pressure dressings to bleeding sites in the oral cavity or nasopharynx may lessen the requirement for transfusions. A 1-hr and 6-hr posttransfusion platelet count can differentiate between immune and nonimmune

TABLE 79.8

CAUSES OF BLEEDING IN PEDIATRIC CANCER PATIENTS

Cause	Diagnostic test	Treatment	Monitoring
Local anatomic causes	Visual inspection Unexplained drop in hemoglobin	Surgical control and pressure dressings	Hemoglobin, dressing inspection
Thrombocytopenia: Chemotherapy-induced	Post-transfusion platelet increase	1 random donor platelet (RDP) unit/10 kg of body weight or 1 single donor platelet unit/50 kg will increase platelets by 40K	Platelet count daily
Thrombocytopenia with alloimmunization	No increase with 1-hr posttransfusion platelet count	ABO-type specific or HLA-matched platelets	1-hr posttransfusion platelet count
Thrombocytopenia with sepsis	Drop in platelet count between 1 and 6 hrs after transfusion	1 RDP unit/10 kg of body weight as often as needed to maintain platelets >20K	Platelet count 6 hrs after transfusion
Coagulopathy: DIC	Prolonged PT/INR Elevated d-dimer or FDPs Low fibrinogen	FFP to control bleeding Cryoprecipitate for fibrinogen <100 ng/mL	PT/INR, fibrinogen, d-dimer every 6 hrs
Coagulopathy: Hepatic dysfunction	Prolonged PT/INR Factors II, V, VII, IX, X are low. Factor VIII and fibrinogen are normal.	FFP to maintain INR <1.5	PT/INR 6 hrs after FFP and daily
Coagulopathy: Vitamin K deficiency	Prolonged PT/INR Factors II, VII, IX, X are low. Factors V and VIII are normal.	FFP if bleeding Vitamin K PO/SQ	PT/INR 6 hrs after vitamin K and daily
Fibrinolytic disorder	Consider if bleeding out of proportion to coagulopathy in appropriate clinical setting (APL, ALL). Diagnostic laboratory tests of limited utility: Euglobulin lysis test TAT/roTEG (research).	Consider antifibrinolytic therapy for life-threatening bleeding.	None

RDP, random donor platelet; SDP, single donor platelet; HLA, human leukocyte antigen; DIC, disseminated intravascular coagulopathy; PT/INR, prothrombin/International Normalized Ratio; FDP, fibrin degradation products; FFP, fresh frozen plasma; SC, subcutaneously; APL, acute promyelocytic leukemia; ALL, acute lymphoblastic leukemia; TAT, thrombin-antithrombin complex; roTEG, rotational thromboelastography causes of a poor response to platelet transfusion. If random donor platelet transfusions are no longer achieving a therapeutic goal, ABO-type specific or HLA-matched single donor units may be requested from the blood bank. Acute promyelocytic leukemia is associated with DIC in >50% patients at diagnosis and up to 40% of patients with DIC develop CNS or pulmonary hemorrhage in the first few weeks of treatment. A prolonged prothrombin time with elevated d-dimer or FDPs and low fibrinogen is suggestive of DIC and should be treated with replacement therapy of fresh-frozen plasma, cryoprecipitate, and platelet transfusions prior to onset of major bleeding symptoms is indicated. Antineoplastic agents may also induce coagulopathies. L-asparaginase significantly decreases plasma concentrations of coagulation proteins although it does not appear to impair thrombin generation. Methotrexate-associated hepatotoxicity may reduce synthesis of factors II, V, VII, IX, and X, while factor VIII and fibrinogen are usually spared. Prednisone use has been associated with hypofibrinogenemia. Vitamin K deficiency as a result of inadequate dietary intake, malabsorption, or prolonged antibiotic use will cause decrements in factors II, VII, IX, and X, sparing factor V. Replacement therapy with fresh-frozen plasma and/or cryoprecipitate is needed to treat bleeding symptoms associated with hepatic dysfunction and vitamin K deficiency, as specific factor concentrates are not available for most coagulation factors. Use of recombinant factor VIIa has been used for patients with liver failure when volume restrictions impose limitations on FVII replacement through plasma, but rFVIIa should be used guardedly in patients with DIC and malignancy, as thrombotic complications have been described. Central venous catheters are a common factor for thrombosis during treatment for cancer. The chemotherapeutic agent L-asparaginase, which is used during induction therapy for ALL, causes reduction of the endogenous anticoagulants antithrombin, protein C, and protein S, leading to thromboembolic events during the first 30 days of ALL induction. Symptomatic thrombosis most often occurs in the CNS or upper central venous system. Headaches, seizures, decreased level of consciousness, with papilledema or cranial nerve palsies, are presenting signs and symptoms of cerebral venous thrombosis in children. Asymptomatic thrombosis occurs predominantly in the upper central venous system and may result in extensive collateralization or symptoms of the postphlebitic syndrome as well as limit future sites for venous access. Thromboprophylaxis for adult cancer patients with indwelling catheters has been shown to reduce the incidence of thrombosis, but these studies have not been replicated in children.

ABDOMINAL EMERGENCIES

Acute Abdomen

Acute appendicitis is one of the most common abdominal surgical conditions in childhood with a peak incidence at age 12. The use of steroids may mask the symptoms of appendicitis in some patients making the diagnosis more difficult. The differential diagnosis of appendicitis includes typhlitis, abdominal obstruction, intussusception, gastroenteritis/constipation, urinary tract infection/renal colic, pelvic inflammatory disease, and lower lobe pneumonia. CT or ultrasound should be performed in all patients suspected of typhlitis.

Bowel obstruction may be the presenting symptom of certain diseases such as non-Hodgkin's lymphoma, rhabdomyosarcoma, metastatic disease, carcinomatosis, and colonic neoplasias. It is most commonly seen in children who have received adjuvant therapy for their primary malignancy and/or have had abdominal surgery. Increased risk of bowel obstruction is encountered in children who have had surgery, radiotherapy, narcotic use, prolonged bed rest, malnutrition, and electrolyte abnormalities. CT is superior to plain radiographs in identifying the level and sometimes the cause of the obstruction.

Patients with partial obstruction (i.e., those with plain radiographs showing the presence of intraluminal air in the small and large bowel) and those without mechanical obstruction may be managed medically. Surgery is indicated for patients with complete mechanical obstruction, partial mechanical obstruction not responding to medical treatment, or developing signs of peritonitis and frank perforation. Palliative measures such as the use of a venting gastrostomy or jejunostomy are appropriate in patients with end-stage disease presenting with inoperable bowel obstruction.

Intussusception may be caused by primary intestinal neoplasms or intestinal metastatic lesions occurring in the jejunum and the ileum. Nausea, vomiting, abdominal distension, and lethargy are the most consistent presenting symptoms. Ultrasonography is more accurate than abdominal radiographs and can also detect the lead point and other intra-abdominal pathology. The treatment of choice in the cancer patient is surgical reduction of the intussusception and resection of the inciting pathology rather than radiologic reduction using contrast enema.

Abdominal compartment syndrome is a life-threatening condition characterized by elevation of intra-abdominal pressure affecting the viability and function of the tissues within. Organ dysfunction may occur if the abdominal pressure is >10 mm Hg. Higher pressures, between 15 and 25 mm Hg, may also cause an increase in intrathoracic pressure and intracranial pressure. Reduced cardiac output and diminished flow to the celiac, superior mesenteric, and renal arteries predispose these patients to bacterial translocation and sepsis. Possible precipitating factors include septic shock requiring large-volume resuscitation, ascites (veno-occlusive disease), bowel distension from ileus or mechanical obstruction, peritonitis or peritoneal bleeding, tumor load, and complication of surgery.

The diagnosis can be confirmed by measuring bladder pressure. Timely surgical decompression of abdominal compartment syndrome using a prosthetic silo, mesh, or plastic bag will produce an immediate improvement of cardiopulmonary and renal function. A prophylactic prosthetic mesh may be indicated in high-risk surgical patients to prevent abdominal compartment syndrome.

CHAPTER 80 ■ HEMATOLOGIC EMERGENCIES

R. BLAINE EASLEY • KENNETH M. BRADY • JOSEPH D. TOBIAS

The normal pediatric ranges for red cell, white cell, platelet, and coagulation values in children are detailed, respectively, in **Table 80.1**, **Table 80.2**, and **Table 80.3**.

RED BLOOD CELL ABNORMALITIES IN INFANTS AND CHILDREN

The most common anemia etiologies that require emergent evaluation and care are acute blood loss, acute hemolysis, and acute splenic sequestration. Common symptoms of anemia are pallor, nausea, vomiting, weakness, fatigue, irritability, tachycardia, tachypnea, and edema. The differential diagnoses of anemia based on mean corpuscular volume (MCV) are summarized in **Figure 80.1**.

Iron-deficiency anemia is the most common nutritional abnormality worldwide and is the leading cause of anemia in early childhood. Additional iron studies (serum iron, ferritin, total iron-binding capacity, and transferrin) are rarely necessary in young children with a typical history and characteristic CBC findings. Recommendations to prevent iron-deficiency anemia include iron supplementation (1–2 mg/kg/day) for all breast-fed infants after 3 mos of age, use of iron-fortified formulas (containing 12 mg iron as ferrous sulfate per liter) and cereals, iron supplement (2–3 mg/kg/day) to preterm infants after the first month of life, and delaying the introduction of cow's milk until after 1 yr of age. In differentiating between iron deficiency and Thalassemia, the Mentzer index (MCV/RBC count) can be a useful bedside tool. Mentzer index values of >13.5 suggest iron deficiency, while a value of <11.5 suggests thalassemia minor.

Children with multifactorial anemia (nutritional, malaria, hemoglobinopathy, etc.) have improvements in mortality with blood transfusion therapy, regardless of age. Children with or without cardiorespiratory symptoms when Hb is ≤4 g/dL should be transfused. In infants and children who have Hb values >4 and ≤6 g/dL, the decision to transfuse is largely based on symptoms, available resources, and comorbid conditions (malaria, fever, hypotension). If transfusion therapy is undertaken in either severe or moderate anemia, slow, monitored transfusion of packed RBCs should be performed, with continuous cardiorespiratory monitoring to avoid congestive heart failure. Typically, 5 mL/kg over 4 hrs, followed by another 5 mL/kg transfusion over 4 hrs is adequate. Diuretics may also be required.

Hemolytic anemia can be caused by either intracellular or extracellular disorders. Tests that are useful in the diagnosis of a hemolytic process include evaluation of peripheral blood smear for Heinz bodies (denatured Hb) or irregular RBCs (spherocytes), elevated reticulocyte count, positive Coombs test (direct and indirect), elevated serum aspartate aminotransferase, lactate dehydrogenase, and serum bilirubin, with lowered serum haptoglobin.

G6PD catalyzes the reduction of nicotinamide adenine dinucleotide phosphate (NADP) to NADPH in the hexose-monophosphate shunt. NADPH

TABLE 80.1

NORMAL VALUES AND RANGES FOR RED BLOOD CELL INDICES

Age	Hemoglobin (g/dL) Mean	Hemoglobin (g/dL) ± 2SD	Hematocrit (%) Mean	Hematocrit (%) ± 2SD	Reticulocytes (%) range	MCV (fL)
Cord	16.8	13.7–20.1	55	45–65	3.0–7.0	110
2 wk	16.5	13.0–20.0	50	42–66	0.1–1.7	98–116
3 mos	12.0	9.5–14.5	36	31–41	0.7–2.3	a
6 mos–6 yrs	12.0	10.5–14.0	37	33–42	0.5–1.0	70–74
7–12 yrs	13.0	11.0–16.0	38	34–40	0.5–1.0	76–80
12–18 yrs					1.6	
Female	14.0	12.0–16.0	42	37–47		80–96
Male	14.5	14.0–18.0	43	36–50		80–96
Adult					1.6	
Female	14.0	12.0–16.0	42	36–47		80–96
Male	16.0	14.0–18.0	47	42–52		80–96

MCV, mean corpuscular volume; fL, femtoliters
[a] Approximate MCV ranges in ages >1 month to ≤9 years: low MCV = 70 + (age in years), high MCV = 90 − (age in years).
Adapted from Dallman PR, Siimes MA. Percentile curves for hemoglobin and red cell volume in infancy and childhood. *J Pediatr* 1979;94(1):26–31.

TABLE 80.2

NORMAL VALUES AND RANGES FOR WHITE BLOOD CELL COUNT AND DIFFERENTIAL

Age	Leukocytes (WBC/mm³) Mean	Leukocytes (WBC/mm³) Range	Neutrophils (%) Mean	Neutrophils (%) Range	Lymphocytes (%) Mean	Eosinophils (%) Mean	Monocytes (%) Mean
Cord	18,000	9000–30,000	61	40–80	31	2	6
2 wks	12,000	5000–21,000	40		63	3	9
3 mos	12,000	6000–18,000	30		48	2	5
6 mos–6 yrs	10,000	6000–15,000	45		48	2	5
7–12 yrs	8,00	4500–13,500	55		38	2	5
Adult	7500	5000–10,000	55	35–70	35	3	7

WBC, white blood cell
*Relatively wide range.
Adapted from Cranendonk E, van Gennip AH, Abeling NG, et al. Reference values for automated cytochemical differential count of leukocytes in children 0–16 years old: Comparison with manually obtained counts from Wright-stained smears. *J Clin Chem Clin Biochem* 1985;23(10):663–7.

TABLE 80.3

NORMAL VALUE AND RANGE FOR PLATELET COUNT AND COAGULATION PARAMETERS

Age	Platelets (10³/mm³)	PT (sec)	aPTT (sec)	Fibrinogen (g/dL)	BT (min)
Preterm	180–327	15.4 (14.6–16.9)	108 (80–168)	243 (150–373)	
Birth	290	13.0 (10.1–15.9)	42.9 (31.3–54.3)	283 (167–309)	
1 mo	252				
1 yr–7 yrs	150–350	11 (10.6–11.4)	30 (24–36)	276 (170–405)	6 (2.5–10)
7 yrs–18yrs	150–350	11.2 (10.2–12.0)	32 (26–37)	300 (154–448)	5 (3–8)

PT, prothrombin time (extrinsic pathway); aPTT, activated partial thromboplastin time (intrinsic pathway); BT, bleeding time (clot formation)
Adapted from Andrew M, Paes B, Milner R, et al. Development of the human coagulation system in the full-term infant. *Blood* 1987;70(1):165–172; Andrew M, Paes B, Milner R, et al. Development of the human coagulation system in the healthy premature infant. *Blood* 1988;72(5):1651–7; and Andrew M, Vegh P, Johnston M, Bowker J, et al. Maturation of the hemostatic system during childhood. *Blood* 1992;80(8):1998–2005.

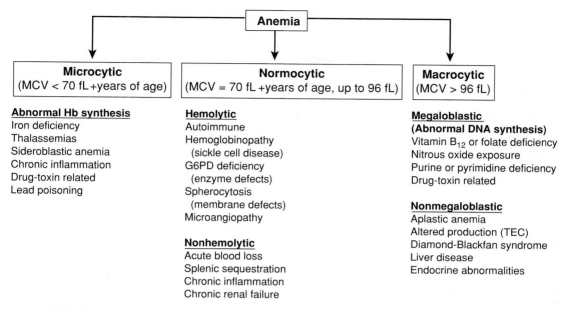

FIGURE 80.1. The differential diagnosis of anemia. MCV, mean corpuscular volume; fL, femtoliter; TEC, transient erythropenia of childhood. Adapted from Sadowitz PD, Amanullah S, Souid AK. Hematologic emergencies in the pediatric emergency room. *Emerg Med Clin North Am.* 2002;20(1):177–98, vii.

converts glutathione disulfide to reduced glutathione. Glutathione, in turn, inactivates hydrogen peroxide (H_2O_2) and protects protein sulfhydryl groups from oxidation. Lack of this enzyme allows for the rapid depletion of protective antioxidants and subsequent denaturation of the Hb unit. Oxidative stressors attack Hb sulfhydryl groups, releasing heme, the protein chain of which then unfolds and precipitates as insoluble aggregates (Heinz bodies). Unripened peaches, fava beans, methylene blue, naphthalene, phenazopyridine, sulfamethoxazole and stress (e.g., infection and surgery) can cause hemolysis in G6PD-deficient patients. Salicylates do not pose a risk for hemolysis, except in high doses.

Antibody-mediated (autoimmune) hemolytic anemia is an extracellular process of RBC destruction. The laboratory findings reveal a rapidly falling Hb, low haptoglobin, increased bilirubin metabolites in the urine, positive Coombs tests, and spherocytes on the smear. The direct Coombs test confirms the diagnosis of antibody bound to the patient's RBCs. The indirect Coombs test detects free antibody in the patient's serum. Typically, IgG antibodies do not agglutinate RBC in vitro and react at 37°C; therefore, they are termed *warm (incomplete) antibodies*. IgM antibodies cause in vitro agglutination at ≤20°C and are termed *cold (complete) antibodies*. The antibody-coated RBCs are destroyed in the reticuloendothelial system of the spleen making intravascular hemolysis

rare. The treatment involves high-dose steroids, and if necessary, RBC transfusion using the most compatible blood.

Transient erythrocytopenia of childhood is characterized by gradual onset of a normocytic anemia and reticulocytopenia. It usually occurs in children between 1 month and 6 yrs of age and is commonly preceded by a viral illness. Blood transfusions are necessary if Hb concentration is <5 g/dL. Transient erythrocytopenia of childhood must be distinguished from *pure red cell aplasia* or *Diamond-Blackfan syndrome*. Patients with Diamond-Blackfan syndrome typically have macrocytic erythrocytes (elevated MCV), dysmorphic features, and persistent anemia. Bone marrow recovery is the hallmark of transient erythrocytopenia of childhood and rules out Diamond-Blackfan syndrome.

Bone marrow infiltration can result from malignant cells or be the result of other processes such as inherited metabolic disorders or infections (fungus, tuberculosis). Regardless of the primary process, the result is a normocytic anemia (normal MCV) with a low reticulocyte count. These patients can have lymphadenopathy, hepatomegaly, and splenomegaly on physical examination, although laboratory abnormalities can include reticulocytopenia, neutropenia, thrombocytopenia, and circulating immature cells (e.g., nucleated RBCs, promyelocytes, metamyelocytes, and myelocytes). Bone marrow examination is essential in this setting to establish the

TABLE 80.4

COMMON AGENTS THAT CAUSE APLASTIC ANEMIA

Acetazolamide	Ibuprofen
Antineoplastic[a]	Mephenytoin
Alkylating	Oxyphenbutazone[a]
Antimetabolite	Paramethadione
Antibiotics	Phenothiazines
Benzene[a]	Phenylbutazone[a]
Captopril	Phenytoin
Carbamazepine	Propylthiouracil
Chloramphenicol[a]	Quinacrine
Chlorpheniramine	Radiation (ionizing)[a]
Colchicine[a]	Sulfonamides[a]
Gold salts[a]	

[a] Toxic mechanism.

correct diagnosis. *Acquired aplastic anemia* is defined as peripheral blood pancytopenia with variable bone marrow hypocellularity in the absence of underlying malignant or myeloproliferative disease. Causes of drug-induced aplastic anemia are summarized in **Table 80.4**.

Megaloblastic anemias result from decreased vitamin B_{12} and folate. Agents that impair vitamin B_{12} gut absorption include metformin, colchicine, neomycin, para-aminosalicylic acid, and slow-release potassium chloride. Causes of these anemias (especially folate deficiency) include: sepsis, pregnancy, malignancy, chronic hemodialysis, and drugs including chronic ethanol ingestion, nitrous oxide anesthesia (5-hr exposure to $\geq 50\%$) and some anticonvulsant drugs. Approximately 50% of patients on long-term phenytoin therapy have low serum folate concentrations, and ~30% have red cell macrocytosis and early megaloblastic changes in the bone marrow. Folate replacement therapy improves the anemia.

Hemoglobinopathies

In normal human maturation, HbA ($\alpha 2\beta 2$) becomes the dominant form, taking over from the HbF ($\alpha 2\gamma 2$) during the first year of life. Presence of abnormal Hb species, as in SCD (HbS) and its variants (HbSC, HbAS, etc.), can result in persistence of HbF. The thalassemias are the most common worldwide genetic disorder. Unstable Hb forms result in denaturation and formation of Heinz bodies on peripheral smear in the RBC.

Secondary hemoglobinopathies include methemoglobinemia, carboxyhemoglobinemia, cyanohemoglobinemia, and sulfhemoglobinemia. All dyshemoglobinemias result in shifting of the oxygen disassociation curve, impairment of binding of O_2 by Hb, and impairment of O_2 delivery to the tissues. Diagnosis is often made with routine co-oximetry, which measures the elevated fraction of the abnormal Hb. Iatrogenic causes include inhaled nitric oxide therapy (methemoglobinemia) and nitroprusside infusions (cyanohemoglobinemia). Exchange transfusion and hyperbaric oxygen therapy are considerations for acute and life-threatening causes of dyshemoglobinemia with clinically impaired O_2 delivery. MetHb will cause chocolate-brown discoloration of blood, cyanosis, and functional "anemia" if present in high enough concentrations. Cyanosis becomes obvious at a concentration of MetHb of 1.5 g/dL (~10% of total Hb). Levels of 35%–50% result in mild symptoms, such as exertional dyspnea and headaches, and levels exceeding 70% are probably lethal. Therapy with ascorbic acid or methylthioninium chloride (methylene blue) will reduce the level of oxidized Hb. CyanoHb forms when Hb combines with cyanide. Cyanide is present in many forms and can be inhaled, absorbed transcutaneously, or ingested. Toxic effects of cyanide arise because of the greater affinity of Hb for cyanide than for O_2, which leads to decreased O_2 delivery, and because of the inhibition of mitochondrial cytochrome oxidase, which leads to decreased cellular oxidative metabolism. Sodium nitroprusside contains an iron molecule bound to 5 cyanide molecules and 1 molecule of nitric oxide. The nitric oxide molecule is rapidly released during infusion from the iron moiety, creating significant arteriolar dilatation, whereas the cyanide molecules are liberated gradually. In most patients, cyanide release from sodium nitroprusside is slow enough that the body's innate detoxification mechanisms (thiosulfate to thiocyanate formation via the rhodanese enzyme) can eliminate the poison before it interferes with cellular respiration. Treatment for cyanide toxicity has classically involved inducing MetHb (with nitrites) to attract the cyanide ion from cytochrome oxidase, as MetHb has a high affinity for cyanide and readily combines to form CyanoMetHb, a safe but non–oxygen-carrying form of Hb.

Hb has the capacity to combine with CO with an affinity 210 times greater than for O_2, which means that CO will bind with Hb. COHb will build up until typical symptoms of CO poisoning appear (headache, dizziness, muscular weakness, and nausea). COHb shifts the Hb-oxygen dissociation curve increasingly to the left, thus adding to the anoxia. If a patient poisoned with CO receives pure O_2, the conversion of COHb to O_2Hb is greatly enhanced. COHb is light-sensitive and has a typical "cherry red" color, and patients demonstrate high values on pulse oximetry.

TABLE 80.5

DIFFERENTIAL DIAGNOSIS OF ERYTHROCYTOSIS IN CHILDREN

Primary erythrocytosis (Epo level normal or low)

Congenital	Epo receptor mutations (primary familial congenital erythrocytosis)
Acquired	Polycythemia vera

Secondary erythrocytosis (Epo level elevated)

Congenital	Hemoglobinopathy with increased O_2 affinity 2,3-DPG deficiency
	Chuvash polycythemia (rare VHL mutation)
	Sporadic or familial erythrocytosis secondary to VHL mutation
Acquired	Physiologic elevation of Epo secondary to:
	Right-to-left shunting cardiac lesion
	Pulmonary disease
	Renal disease
	Hepatic disease
	Abnormal elevation in Epo synthesis:
	Renal: malignancy
	Liver: malignancy
	CNS: hemangioblastoma
	Endocrine tumor: pheochromocytoma
	Uterine tumor

Epo, erythropoietin; VHL, von Hippel-Lindau disease; CNS, central nervous system

TABLE 80.6

SEQUENTIAL EVALUATION OF ERYTHROCYTOSIS

1. CBC, including differential WBC count
2. Rule out plasma volume decrease
3. Diagnose *secondary erythrocytosis*:
   Arterial oxygen saturation (rule out hypoxia)
   Co-oximetry (rule out dyshemoglobinemias)
   Renal ultrasonography
   Abdominal/cranial CT
   Erythropoietin level (if elevated suggests secondary etiology)
4. Special studies for *primary erythrocytosis*:
   (See **Table 80.5** for diagnostic evaluation for *polycythemia vera*)
   Leukocyte alkaline phosphatase
   Serum vitamin B_{12} level and binding capacity
   Red blood cell colony formation

CBC, complete blood count; WBC, white blood cell

Erythrocytosis

Apparent increases in red cell mass and Hb content (>2 SD of appropriate normal) can occur from a variety of causes, such as dehydration, chronic hypoxia, and overtransfusion. Relative or "spurious" causes of erythrocytosis are the result of serum volume loss, such as in dehydration from diarrhea or aggressive diuretic therapy. Direct and indirect complications of elevated RBC mass include hyperviscosity, hypercoagulability, and thrombosis. The approach to polycythemia is summarized in **Table 80.5** and **Table 80.6**.

Neonatal Polycythemia and Hyperviscosity

Clinical symptoms may include lethargy, cyanosis, respiratory distress, jitteriness, hypotonia, feeding intolerance, hypoglycemia, and hyperbilirubinemia. Treatment of neonatal polycythemia (Hct rises above 65%), and hyperviscosity is either symptomatic therapy or partial exchange transfusion (PET). In the polycythemic newborn, the total exchange volume for PET is generally calculated using the following formula:

$$\text{PET volume} = \text{Circulating blood volume} \times [(\text{Hct current} - \text{Hct desired})/\text{Hct current}]$$

In term infants, the circulating blood volume is estimated at 80–90 mL/kg; and in preterm infants, intravascular volume is usually estimated at 100 mL/kg. In clinical practice, the exchange procedure is performed through removal and administration of 5–10 mL aliquots. Typically, arterial and venous line access is required. Attention to thermoregulation, glucose homeostasis, and vital signs is imperative. Both during and up to 4 hrs following PET, feedings should be withheld. In addition, monitoring should be continued until the infant is asymptomatic. Typical Hct goals from PET are <55%.

WHITE BLOOD CELL ABNORMALITIES (NONMALIGNANT) IN INFANTS AND CHILDREN

Leukopenia is defined as a total white blood cell (WBC) count <4000/mm^3. Lymphopenia (<1000/mm^3 in adults and 4500/ mm^3 in infants) results transiently from viral, fungal, or parasitic infections. However, it can result from chronic illness or reflect more serious inherited or acquired disease. Human immunodeficiency virus, with or without AIDS, is the most common globally relevant

TABLE 80.7

DIFFERENTIAL DIAGNOSIS OF LYMPHOPENIA IN CHILDREN

Infection	Mycobacteria	*Mycobacterium tuberculosis*
		Atypical mycobacteria
	Viral	Cytomegalovirus
		Epstein-Barr virus
		Hepatitis B virus
		Human immunodeficiency virus
		Human T-cell lymphotropic virus 1 and 2
		Influenza
		Respiratory syncytial virus
Malignancy		Non-Hodgkin lymphoma
		Mycosis fungoides
		Aplastic anemia
		Myelodysplastic syndrome
Autoimmune diseases		Sjögren's syndrome
		Systemic lupus erythematosus
		Rheumatoid arthritis
Drugs		Corticosteroids
		Chemotherapy and cytotoxic immunosuppressants (cyclophosphamide, azathioprine, methotrexate)
		Others (cephalosporin, IFN-α)
Primary immunodeficiency		Common variable immunodeficiency
		Severe combined immunodeficiency
		Bare lymphocyte syndrome, type I
Miscellaneous conditions		Severe burns
		Radiotherapy
		Malnutrition

infectious disease associated with lymphopenia (**Table 80.7**).

An absolute neutrophil count <1500/mm^3 is defined as neutropenia. Increased risk for a life-threatening infection occurs when the absolute neutrophil count is <500/mm^3 (**Table 80.8**). The standard approach for managing a neutropenic patient who develops fever with no discernable focus of infection has been combination therapy to cover Gram-positive and Gram-negative bacteria. Ceftazidime and vancomycin are often used as initial therapy. Other centers choose to use an aminoglycoside in combination with a β-lactam antibiotic. Children with pneumonia or perirectal infections require antibiotics to cover pathogens such as *Pneumocystis* and *Clostridium*. Most simple catheter infections can be cleared with antibiotics without catheter removal. Despite appropriate antibiotics, many catheters must be removed to clear the infection. Recombinant human granulocyte colony-stimulating factor (rhGCSF or GCSF) stimulates the production of neutrophils from committed progenitor cells in the marrow. The dose is 5–10 mcg/kg (maximum dose = 480 mcg) administered subcutaneously.

Autoimmune neutropenia is usually self-limited, with return of a normal neutrophil count over a 5- to 7-week period. Appropriate antibiotics and rhGCSF should be given to febrile, neutropenic patients. Alternative treatments are corticosteroids (prednisone, 1–2 mg/kg/day for 1 week) and IV immunoglobulin (IVIG) (a single dose of 1 g/kg over 3 hrs). Congenital cyclical neutropenia is characterized by chronic periodic oscillations in the neutrophil count from normal to profound neutropenia and is associated with oral ulcers, stomatitis, pharyngitis, tonsillitis, lymphadenitis, cellulitis, otitis media, and sinusitis. All infectious episodes should be treated with appropriate antibiotics and rhGCSF (5 mcg/kg daily subcutaneous injections until WBC count is ≥10,000/mm^3).

Hemophagocytic lymphohistiocytosis (HLH) is a multisystem disease process that results from hyperinflammation from the phagocytosis of blood cells and their precursors (**Table 80.9**). Bone marrow aspiration and lumbar puncture are recommended early in the evaluation. The Histiocyte Society (www.histio.org) helped to establish the current diagnostic guidelines and treatment protocol for HLH (HLH-2004), which includes dexamethasone,

<table>
<tr><td>

TABLE 80.8

DIFFERENTIAL DIAGNOSIS OF NEUTROPENIA

Congenital Neutropenic Disorders
  Kostmann's agranulocytosis-severe congenital
    neutropenia
  Reticular dysgenesis (absence of thymus,
    lymphocytes, and neutrophils)
  Cyclic neutropenia (autosomal dominant)
  Shwachman syndrome (neutropenia, pancreatic
    insufficiency, growth failure, and skeletal
    anomalies)
  Neutropenia with abnormal B or T lymphocytes
    (e.g., X-linked agammaglobulinemia)

Transient Neonatal Neutropenia
  Prematurity/sepsis/asphyxia
  Pregnancy-induced maternal hypertension
  Periventricular hemorrhage
  Congenital cytomegalovirus infection
  Maternal antineutrophil antibodies
    (alloimmune-isoimmune neutropenia)

Immune-mediated Destruction
  Autoimmune neutropenia

Postinfectious
  Influenza A, Hepatitis A and B, varicella, respiratory
    syncytial virus, Epstein-Barr Virus,
    cytomegalovirus (counts recover spontaneously
    over several days)

Drug-induced
  Chemotherapy, anticonvulsants, cimetidine,
    ranitidine, phenothiazines, semisynthetic
    penicillins, cephalosporins, NSAID

Acquired/Decreased Production
  Aplastic anemia
  Marrow infiltration (malignant cells, inborn
    metabolic errors)

Sequestration
  Splenomegaly

</td><td>

TABLE 80.9

DIAGNOSTIC GUIDELINES FOR HEMOPHAGOCYTIC LYMPHOHISTIOCYTOSIS

The diagnosis of HLH requires either criteria 1 or 2 to
  be present:
1. A molecular diagnosis consistent with HLH (e.g.,
   PRF gene mutations, SAP gene mutations, etc.)
   OR
2. Having 5 of 8 of the following findings:
   a. Fever
   b. Splenomegaly
   c. Cytopenia ($\geq$2 cell lines)
   d. Hypertriglyceridemia ($\geq$265 mg/dL) and/or
      Hypofibrinogenemia ($\leq$150 mg/dL)
   e. Hyperferritinemia ($\geq$500 ng/mL)
   f. Hemophagocytosis in the bone marrow, lymph
      node, spleen, or CSF
   g. Low or absent NK cell cytotoxicity
   h. Elevated soluble CD25 ($\geq$2400 U/mL)

HLH, hemophagocytic lymphohistiocytosis; CSF,
cerebrospinal fluid; NK, natural killer
Adapted from Treatment Protocol of the 2nd International
HLH Study, 2004.

</td></tr>
</table>

etoposide, cyclosporine A, and intrathecal methotrexate (in select cases). Hyperinflammation is treated with immunosuppression. Etoposide may have significant benefit in Epstein-Barr virus–associated HLH.

Abnormally high (>2 SDs) circulating levels of age-appropriate WBCs counts are regarded as "leukocytosis." WBC counts >50,000/mm^3 are classified as *leukemoid reactions* because of the similarity of features to leukemia. Stress-induced demargination in the setting of trauma, burns, surgery, hemolysis, and hemorrhage will typically result in an elevation of multiple WBC subtypes (neutrophils, monocytes, lymphocytes). However, acute leukocytosis with a

neutrophil predominance is highly suggestive of a serious bacterial infection, while elevation in WBC with a majority of eosinophils is suggestive of an allergic reaction or parasitic infection.

Neutrophilia is an elevation in the age-appropriate amount of neutrophils in the serum. In adults and older children, neutrophil counts >8000/mm^3 are usually significant for neutrophilia. Common medications that induce neutrophilia are epinephrine, corticosteroids, and rhGCSF. Chronic inflammatory diseases (autoimmune, tuberculosis, sarcoidosis, etc.), and chronic drug exposure (corticosteroids) can result in a more chronic neutrophilia.

Eosinophilia has been related to a number of acute and chronic disease processes in adults and children and is arbitrarily classified as mild (351–1500/mm^3), moderate (>1,500–5000/ mm^3), or severe (>5000/mm^3). The most common cause of eosinophilia worldwide is helminthic infections, and the most common cause in industrialized nations is atopic disease (**Table 80.10**).

Leukemia and lymphoma are the most common cause of lymphocytosis in children. However, the most common, isolated, nonmalignant elevation is related to an acute transient increase of circulating T cells (lymphocytes) brought on by infection. Pertussis infections result in lymphocytosis in up to 25% of infants <6 months of age.

TABLE 80.10

CAUSES OF EOSINOPHILIA

Differential diagnosis	Examples
Reactive Eosinophilia	
Allergic	Rhinoconjunctivitis, asthma, eczema
Infection	Bacterial and fungal
Parasitic infection	Helminth
Drug reaction (iatrogenic)	Granulocyte colony-stimulating factor
Secondary (Disease-associated) Eosinophilia	
Autoimmune disorders	Rheumatoid arthritis, eosinophilic fasciitis
Vasculitis	Polyarteritis nodosa, Wegner granulomatosis
Gastrointestinal disorders	Inflammatory bowel disease, eosinophilic gastroenteritis, eosinophilic esophagitis, allergic colitis
Pulmonary disorders	Churg-Strauss syndrome, Loeffler syndrome
Endocrine disorders	Adrenal insufficiency (Addison disease)
Clonal Eosinophilia	
Cytogenetic	FIP1L1-PDGFRA fusion gene positive
Leukemia	Acute and chronic eosinophilic leukemia
Mastocytosis	Systemic mastocytosis with eosinophilia, myeloproliferative disorder
Idiopathic Persistent Eosinophilia (Diagnosis of Exclusion)	
Idiopathic	Idiopathic hypereosinophilia syndrome

PLATELET ABNORMALITIES IN INFANTS AND CHILDREN

The definition of thrombocytosis varies between platelet counts of 400,000 and 1,000,000/mm^3.

Children with reactive thrombocytosis (RT) have viral or bacterial respiratory illness. Pharmacotherapy that creates or contributes to RT in children includes epinephrine, corticosteroids, vinca-alkaloids, penicillamine, imipenem, and meropenem. Risk factors for thromboembolic disease in children are young age (neonate/infant), central venous catheter, cardiac malformations, and septicemia. Prophylactic treatment with antiplatelet drugs (e.g., aspirin) has not proven beneficial in preventing thromboembolic complications in asymptomatic children.

The approach to thrombocytopenia is summarized in **Table 80.11** and **Table 80.12**. Spontaneous bleeding rarely occurs until the platelet count is <10,000/mm^3. In comorbid medical illness, such as trauma or surgery, maintaining higher platelet counts is often clinically indicated to reduce bleeding risk. In surgical patients, especially with postbypass bleeding,

TABLE 80.11

PREVALENT INHERITED THROMBOCYTOPENIAS: DIFFERENTIATION BASED ON PLATELET FEATURES

Small platelets (MPV <7 fL)	Normal platelets (MPV 7–11 fL)	Large/giant platelets (MPV >11 fL)
Wiskott-Aldrich syndrome	Familial platelet disorder	Bernard-Soulier syndrome
X-linked thrombocytopenia	Congenital amegakaryocytic thrombocytopenia	DiGeorge syndrome
	TAR syndrome	Grey platelet syndrome
		GATA 1 mutation
		Paris-Trousseau thrombocytopenia

AR, autosomal recessive; AD, autosomal dominant; TAR, thrombocytopenia and absent radii; AML, acute myeloid leukemia; MPV, mean platelet volume
Adapted from Drachman JG. Inherited thrombocytopenia: When a low platelet count does not mean ITP. *Blood* 2004;103(2):390–8.

TABLE 80.12

COMMON AGENTS THAT CAUSE THROMBOCYTOPENIA

Increased destruction or usage	Decreased production
Amitriptyline	Alkylating agents
Amphotericin B	Anthracyclines
Amrinone	Antimetabolite agents
Asparaginase	Cytarabine
Benzene	Epipodophyllotoxins
Bleomycin	Ethanol
Carbamazepine	Procarbazine
Chloroquine	Radiation, ionizing
Chlorpheniramine	Thiazides
Cimetidine	Vinblastine
Cocaine (i.e., DIC)	
Colchicine	
Crotalidae envenomation (i.e., DIC)	
Cyclosporine	
Furosemide	
Ganciclovir	
Glyburide	
Gold salts	
Heparin	
Indomethacin	
Meprobamate	
Mesoridazine	
Methyldopa	
Penicillin	
Pentamidine	
Quinidine	
Quinine	
Rifampin	
Sulfonamides	

DIC, disseminated intravascular coagulation
Adapted from Drachman JG. Inherited thrombocytopenia: When a low platelet count does not mean ITP. *Blood* 2004;103(2):390–8.

we will attempt to keep the count >100,000/mm^3. The differential diagnosis of acquired thrombocytopenia is summarized in **Figure 80.2.**

Idiopathic thrombocytopenic purpura (ITP) is caused by the production of antibodies against platelet antigens. The typical history is sudden onset of petechiae and bruising in a previously healthy child; often, the child has a history of a preceding viral illness. Physical findings of lymphadenopathy and/or hepatosplenomegaly are atypical of ITP. In the diagnostic evaluation of ITP, the CBC and blood smear are normal except for isolated thrombocytopenia. Additional laboratory tests include antinuclear antibody, anti-DNA antibody, and human immunodeficiency virus tests. The need for bone marrow examination to confirm the diagnosis is controversial; many specialists perform this test before initiating prednisone therapy. Typically, the bone marrow shows a normal hematopoietic system with increased number of megakaryocytes. In many children with ITP, the thrombocytopenia resolves within 6 weeks. Therapies are summarized in **Table 80.13**.

Almost all conditions that lead to portal hypertension and enlargement of the spleen have been associated with reduction of circulating platelet counts. The spleen can empty its reservoir to create a transient thrombocytosis. Hypersplenism is associated with thrombocytopenia. Peripheral smears may demonstrate burr cells but are typically normal except for thrombocytopenia. Patients with low starting platelet (~100,000/mm^3) counts developed dilutional thrombocytopenia and bleeding after blood loss of only 1–2 blood volumes. In this scenario, patients often require platelet treatment at ≤50,000/mm^3. In addition, certain surgeries associated with higher bleeding complications (e.g., neurosurgery, cardiac surgery, or organ transplantation), may require a higher threshold for treatment.

Neonatal thrombocytopenia that occurs in a sick infant from birth to 2 months of age is likely related to the primary disease process and will resolve as the primary process improves. Most of these infants develop platelet counts of <50,000 at >48 hrs of age. Causes include abnormalities of decreased production, increased consumption, and immune-mediated destruction. When platelet counts are <30,000/mm^3, head ultrasounds to evaluate and monitor for intraventricular hemorrhage are common practice. Of these various neonatal causes, alloimmune thrombocytopenia represents a unique and potentially treatable newborn cause of low platelets. In this disease, maternal antibodies are attacking and destroying the neonatal platelets. This process often begins in utero and may necessitate fetal therapy in future pregnancies. If platelets cannot be maintained at >20,000/mm^3 with platelet transfusion, consideration should be given to IVIG (1 g/kg/day) and/or methylprednisone (1 mg/kg IV q8h) therapy until the platelet counts improve (>30–50,000/mm^3). If an intracranial bleed is detected, random platelet transfusions should be performed emergently until antigen-negative platelets are available.

Described functional abnormalities of platelets are both inherited and acquired (**Table 80.11** and **Table 80.14**). Aspirin permanently inhibits cyclooxygenase and causes decreased platelet aggregation causing a prolonged bleeding time. The drug effects are worsened in the face of an underlying platelet dysfunction (von Willebrands and vitamin K deficiency). Treatment with desmopressin in some cases, may be beneficial, as desmopressin increases

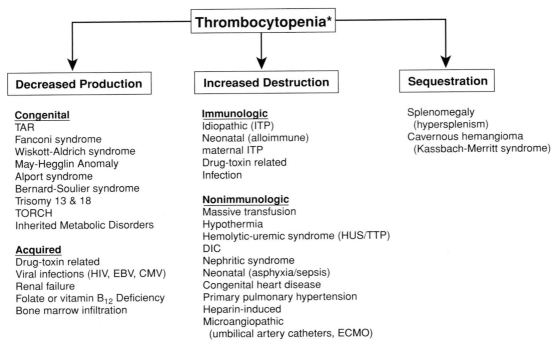

FIGURE 80.2. Differential diagnosis of thrombocytopenia. Note: "Pseudo-thrombocytopenia" occurs with platelet clumping, either spontaneously or from collection-tube preservatives (EDTA or citrate). TAR, thrombocytopenia with absent radius; TORCH, toxoplasmosis, other infections, rubella, cytomegalovirus infection, and herpes simplex; HIV, human immunodeficiency virus; EBV, Epstein-Barr virus; CMV, cytomegalovirus; ITP, idiopathic thrombocytopenic purpura; DIC, disseminated intravascular coagulopathy; ECMO, extracorporeal membrane oxygenation. Adapted from Sadowitz PD, Amanullah S, Souid AK. Hematologic emergencies in the pediatric emergency room. *Emerg Med Clin North Am.* 2002;20(1):177–98, vii.

von Willebrand factor levels and promotes platelet aggregation.

THROMBOTIC DISEASES IN INFANTS AND CHILDREN

Normal coagulation function involves not only the production of adequate amounts of thrombin and fibrin to stop bleeding but also mechanisms to prevent pathologic clot formation. Through these processes, the coagulation process attempts to confine thrombin generation to the site of the injury and avoid thrombotic events. Endothelial-dependent inhibition of coagulation includes protein C (and its co-factor, protein S) and tissue factor pathway inhibitor (TFPI). Thrombin formed either on the surface of platelets or at the site of tissue injury binds to the endothelium via thrombomodulin. TFPI is produced and released from the vascular endothelium. It is the major inhibitor of the tissue factor pathway that regulates the conversion of factor VII to VIIa after tissue factor has been exposed at the site of tissue injury.

Hepatic-dependent aspects of the antithrombotic cascade include antithrombin III (AT-III), heparin cofactor (HC) II, and plasminogen. The two physiologic activators of plasminogen are tissue plasminogen activator (TPA) and urinary-type plasminogen activator, as known as *urokinase*. Thrombin generated from the coagulation cascade stimulates the release of TPA from endothelial cells. Exogenously produced forms of TPA, urokinase, and streptokinase, have been used as therapeutic agents in the treatment of thrombotic disease.

The two principal inhibitors of fibrinolysis in the circulation are plasminogen activator inhibitor (PAI-1), which inhibits both urinary-type plasminogen activator (urokinase) TPA and α_2-antiplasmin, a specific plasmin inhibitor. A summary of some of the commonly encountered risk factors for thrombosis in children is presented in **Table 80.15**. CVCs represent the single most commonly identified acquired risk factor for thrombotic events in infants and children. Antiphospholipid antibody syndrome (APAS) is characterized by the formation of autoantibodies to phospholipids. Anticardiolipin antibodies may

TABLE 80.13

TREATMENT OF ACUTE CHILDHOOD IDIOPATHIC THROMBOCYTOPENIA PURPURA

Corticosteroids – one of the following:
Prednisone, 1–5 mg/kg/day in 3 divided doses for 1–2 weeks, followed by tapering and discontinuation by day 21
OR
Methylprednisolone, 30 mg/kg (maximum, 1 g/dose) IV over 30 mins every 24 hrs for 3 doses. Then return to maintenance steroid therapy. This option is reserved for hospitalized patients with severe bleeding.

IgG Concentrates
IVIG 1 g/kg/day for 2 consecutive days
Anti-D (for Rh-positive patients)
IV anti-D, single dose of 40–80 mcg/kg IV over 5 mins

Combination Therapy
Corticosteroids in combination with either IgG or anti-D (using the previously cited dosages). This option is used for patients with significant mucocutaneous bleeding in a hospital setting in consultation with a pediatric hematologist.

Platelet Transfusion
Not routinely needed. Indicated for life-threatening hemorrhage and in conjunction with above medical management.

TABLE 80.14

DRUGS THAT INHIBIT PLATELET FUNCTION (THROMBOCYTOPATHY)

Nonsteroidal anti-inflammatory drugs
Aspirin, ibuprofen, indomethacin, naproxen, and others
Antibiotics
Penicillins, cephalosporins, nitrofurantoin
Cardiovascular drugs
Amrinone/milrinone, dipyridamole, diltiazem, propranolol, nitroprusside, nifedipine, nitroglycerin, procainamide, verapamil
Anticoagulants, fibrinolytics, and antifibrinolytics
Aprotinin, ε-aminocaproic acid, heparin, protamine, alteplase
Anesthetics
Propofol, ketamine, benzocaine, cocaine, lidocaine, procaine, tetracaine, halothane, heroin
Anticonvulsants/psychotropic drugs
Valproate, amitriptyline, haloperidol, imipramine, nortriptyline, chlorpromazine
Chemotherapy
Carmustine, daunorubicin, vincristine, L-asparaginase
Antihistamines
Chlorpheniramine, diphenhydramine, ranitidine, cimetidine
Herbal/alternative medicines
Garlic, ginseng, gingko biloba
Other drugs/toxins
Guaifenesin, dextran, pseudoephedrine, hetastarch, mustard gas

predispose patients in renal failure to thrombotic complications, including fistula thrombosis. The co-existence of SLE and APAS remains a significant risk factor for thrombotic complications. Treatment strategies aimed at reducing the antiphospholipid antibody levels include the administration of corticosteroids, immunosuppressive agents, IVIG, and plasmapheresis. Perioperative measures may include the use of low-dose heparin protocols, maintenance of adequate hydration, early ambulation, and antiembolic intermittent compression devices for the lower extremities.

HIT can develop after exposure to unfractionated heparin or low-molecular-weight heparin (LMWH). Exposure to heparin can occur from a bolus or an infusion, through the intravenous or subcutaneous route, as a flush solution for invasive monitors, or on heparin-impregnated catheters. HIT type 1 is a less severe form of the disease in which patients experience a mild, early decrease in platelet count that improves even with the ongoing administration of heparin. Thrombotic complications generally do not occur. HIT type 2 results in a more severe degree of thrombocytopenia, which does not resolve without cessation of heparin therapy and includes

the potential for thrombotic complications that involve both the arterial and venous vasculature. The diagnosis of HIT is based on the identification of heparin antibodies. Common treatment of HIT includes the immediate cessation of heparin administration of any type or route, including LMWH, heparin-coated catheters, and heparin flushes of invasive catheters. Several alternative anticoagulants are available for patients with HIT who require ongoing anticoagulation (danaparoid sodium, warfarin, LMWH hirudin, recombinant hirudin-lepirudin, bivalirudin, argatroban, and ancrod).

Homozygous states of S and C deficiency result in severe disease, including purpura fulminans, during infancy, while the heterozygous state increases the risk of spontaneous thrombotic events.

A prothrombotic state may be the result of alterations in factor-V molecule. Factor V Leiden confers a relative risk of thrombotic complications. Antithrombin concentrates are available, and their use is considered when oral anticoagulants are not feasible (prior to a major surgery and during pregnancy). AT-III concentrates may also be used in AT-III

TABLE 80.15

RISK FACTORS FOR HYPERCOAGULABILITY IN CHILDREN

Physiologic alterations	Clinical conditions
Blood Flow	
Hypovolemia	Shock, dehydration
Hyperviscosity	Erythrocytosis, leukocytosis, thrombocytosis, sickle cell disease
Mechanical stasis	Immobilization after surgery
Foreign body	CVC, cardiac prosthesis
Vasculature	
Anatomic defects	Congenital heart disease, arteriovenous malformation
Endothelial disorders	Vasculitis, inflammation (meningitis, mastoiditis, or otitis media), trauma, SLE, Takayasu arteritis, Kawasaki disease
Blood coagulation	
Increased and/or abnormal	Malignancy, dysfibrinogenemias, procoagulants, inflammatory bowel disease
Decreased anticoagulants	AT-III deficiency, protein S or C deficiency, APC resistance (factor V Leiden) Plasminogen deficiency
Decreased fibrinolysis	Hereditary defects
Increased platelet-vessel reactivity	Atherosclerotic disease, inherited dyslipidemia, diabetes mellitus
Mixed or idiopathic	HIT, HUS, TTP, oral contraceptives, nephrotic syndrome, recurrent idiopathic DVT
Metabolic diseases	Diabetes mellitus, homocystinuria, increased lipoprotein A, and galactosemia

CVC, central venous catheter; APC, activated protein C; HIT, heparin-induced thrombocytopenia; HUS, hemolytic uremic syndrome; TTP, thrombotic thrombocytopenic purpura; DVT, deep vein thrombosis
Adapted from Hathaway WE. Congenital and acquired defects in coagulation: Diagnosis and treatment. *Mead Johnson Symp Perinat Dev Med* 1986;(28):45–54.

deficient states to allow for therapeutic heparinization during cardiopulmonary bypass. Homocystinuria is an inherited defect of amino acid metabolism that results in a syndrome of mental retardation, skeletal involvement, and visual problems related to lens dislocation and arterial/venous thrombosis. Administration of pharmacologic doses of vitamin B_{12} or B_6 may provide effective therapy and control plasma levels. Prothrombin gene mutation results in the increased production of prothrombin. Unlike factor V Leiden and deficiencies of proteins C and S, which tend to lead to venous thrombotic disease, the prothrombin mutation in children is often associated with arterial thrombosis and CNS events.

CLINICAL SIGNS, RADIOLOGIC IMAGING, LABORATORY STUDIES, AND TREATMENT

On the arterial side, the clinical signs and symptoms are relatively straightforward when total occlusion is present and include a painful, cold, pulseless extremity. Loss of patency of a CVC may be the first

indication of thrombotic disease. The development of collateral circulation may be the primary manifestation of the disease process when bleeding occurs from esophageal varices with splenic, portal, or hepatic vein thrombosis.

On the venous side, the manifestations are frequently more subtle and may remain asymptomatic, with the diagnosis made only by radiologic imaging. Although the venogram remains the gold standard for the diagnosis of thrombotic disease, ultrasound or echocardiography remain the primary techniques used to identify thrombotic disease. A diagnosis of thrombus is made by Doppler ultrasonography by identification of the following features: an echogenic filling defect, noncompressibility of the vein, loss of respiratory variability and vessel pulsation, and lack of flow or abnormal Doppler waveforms distal to the occluded segment. MR venography has become the most sensitive and specific test, especially for venous disease of the lower extremities and pelvis. The diagnostic approach to thrombosis in children is summarized in **Table 80.16** and www.med.unc.edu/isth/.

Therapy includes the elimination of comorbid diseases or associated conditions that exacerbate the prothrombotic state. These may include early

TABLE 80.16

DIAGNOSTIC EVALUATION OF HYPERCOAGULABILITY IN CHILDREN

LEVEL I—Basic Evaluation
Basic hematologic test
   CBC with differential
      PT, PTT, fibrinogen
      Antithrombin III activity[a]
      Protein C activity[a]
      Protein S – free and total antigen[a]
      Anticardiolipin (antiphospholipid) antibodies[a]
      APC resistance (factor V Leiden)[b]
      Homocysteine level[a]
      Lupus anticoagulant[a]
      Lipoprotein (a)[b]
      [HIT type 2][a]

LEVEL II—Extended Evaluation
   Dysfibrinogenemia Evaluation[b]
   (FDP, fibrinogen activity, thrombin and reptilase time, consider immunoelectrophoresis)
   Heparin cofactor II[c]
   Plasminogen activity[c]
   PAI: plasminogen activator inhibitor[c]
   If not previously performed:
      ESR, CRP
      Hemoglobin electrophoresis
      Fasting homocysteine level
      Functional APC resistance (modified assay for factor V Leiden)

LEVEL III—Under Investigation
   Factor VIII[b]
   Factor XII[c]
   Factor XI[c]
   Von Willebrand factor level[c] and multimers [ADAMTS13[a]]
   Spontaneous platelet aggregation
   Tissue plasminogen activity
   Tissue factor pathway inhibitor

CBC, complete blood count; PT, prothrombin time; PTT, partial thromboplastin time; APC, activated protein C; HIT, heparin-induced thrombocytopenia; FDP, fibrin degradation products; ESR, erythrocyte sedimentation rate; CRP, C reactive protein; [ ], studies to be done when clinical scenarios implicate their involvement
Level I tests are recommended in all children with thrombosis. Level II tests are recommended in those children with normal Level I values and/or in the settings of recurrent thrombosis or strong family history of thrombotic disease. Level III tests are recommended in those patients with normal Level I and Level II tests with a history of recurrent thrombosis.
[a] Indicates high risk factors with therapeutic and/or prognostic relevance.
[b] Indicates lower risk factors.
[c] Potential thrombotic risk factors.
Adapted from Manco-Johnson MJ, Grabowski EF, Hellgreen M, et al. Laboratory testing for thrombophilia in pediatric patients. On behalf of the Subcommittee for Perinatal and Pediatric Thrombosis of the Scientific and Standardization Committee of the International Society of Thrombosis and Haemostasis (ISTH). *Thromb Haemost* 2002;88(1):155–6; and Schneppenheim R, Greiner J. Thrombosis in infants and children. *Hematology Am Soc Hematol Educ Program* 2006:86–96.

ambulation, maintenance of adequate hydration, or the use of physical maneuvers such as sequential lower extremity compression devices. Additionally, elimination of medications such as oral contraceptive pills, avoidance of provocative factors (e.g., heparin in patients with HIT), avoidance of hyperlipidemia, and weight reduction may be beneficial. In the perioperative period, the use of adjunctive regional anes-

thetic techniques may be considered. No guidelines exist for the use of intravascular coagulation filters in pediatric patients with risk factors that preclude anticoagulation. In the adult population, therapeutic anticoagulation with Coumadin carries the risk of hemorrhage of ~3% per year, with one-fifth of the hemorrhages being fatal. Recommendations from the International Society on Thrombosis and

TABLE 80.17

TREATMENT OF CENTRAL CATHETER OCCLUSION

Age/Weight	Type of catheter and no. of lumens	Urokinase dose and volume	Alteplase (TPA) dose and volume
Newborn (birth-4 wks)	Single-lumen Hickman	0.5 mL/2500 U	0.5 mg/0.5 mL
10 kg	Single-lumen Hickman	1 mL/5000 U	1 mg/L mL
10 kg	Double-lumen Hickman	1 mL/5000 U each lumen	1 mg/1 mL each lumen
10 kg	Single-lumen Hickman	1.5 mL/7500 U	1.5 mg/1.5 mL
10 kg	Double-lumen Hickman	1 ml/5000 U each lumen 1.5 mL/7500 U in large lumen	1 mg/1 mL small lumen 1.5 mg/1.5 mL large lumen
Any weight	Small/low-volume Infusaport	1.5 mL/7500 U	1.5 mg/1.5 mL
Any weight	Large/high-volume Infusaport	3 mL/15,000 U	3 mg/3 mL
Any weight	3.0 & 4.0 Fr. PICC	1 mL/5000 U	1 mg/1 mL
Any weight	2.0 Fr. PICC	Manufacturer does not recommend declotting	

PICC, peripherally inserted central catheter
General recommendations: Urokinase or Alteplase (TPA) are the drugs of choice for bolus administration to indwell in the catheter. Length of time urokinase or TPA should indwell in catheter: First dose of urokinase or TPA should indwell for at least 2 hrs before blood withdrawal is attempted. After 2 hrs, attempts to withdraw blood may be made every 2 hrs for 3 attempts. The second dose of urokinase or TPA should indwell in the catheter for 3–4 hrs before blood withdrawal is attempted. After 3–4 hrs, blood withdrawal should be attempted every 2 hrs for 3 attempts. If the catheter remains difficult to flush after 2 bolus urokinase doses or 2 bolus TPA doses, a 24-hr continuous urokinase infusion can be considered.
Urokinase and streptokinase continuous infusion doses: (a) The dose of streptokinase for a continuous infusion is 80 U/kg/hr (per lumen) and (b) the dose of urokinase for a continuous infusion is 200 U/kg/hr (per lumen).
Note: TPA is not routinely utilized as a continuous infusion for catheter clearance due to limited data in pediatrics. The urokinase and streptokinase should be mixed in solutions of normal saline or dextrose and water for IV infusion. In patients with a recent *Streptococcal* infection or signs and symptoms of an allergic response to streptokinase, an alternative agent is selected. Unsuccessfully declotted catheters should be considered for removal.
Adapted from Children's Center Care Protocol, Johns Hopkins Hospital.

Haemostasis for the treatment of venous thromboembolic disease in infants and children is similar to that recommended for adults and includes unfractionated heparin (bolus dose of 75 units/kg, followed by a continuous infusion of 20 units/kg/hr for children and 28 units/kg/hr for infants). The PTT is measured 4–6 hrs following the initiation of therapy and maintained at 1.5–2.5 times the normal range. When long-term anticoagulation therapy is planned, oral coumadin is started at 0.2 mg/kg (maximum dose of 10 mg) and adjusted according to the International Normalized Ratio (INR) of the PT. Once a therapeutic level is achieved with warfarin (INR = 2–3), heparin is discontinued. Problems with unfractionated heparin include variability in bioavailability and age-related pharmacokinetics, requirements for ongoing IV access for administration, delays in achieving the desired level of anticoagulation, repeated blood draws to monitor the PTT, and adverse effects, including hemorrhage. Unlike unfractionated heparin, the benefits of LMWH include: the option of subcutaneous administration, predictable pharmacokinet-ics, a decreased incidence of HIT, minimal monitoring, and a decreased risk of bleeding. Argatroban hirudin lepirudin, and bivalirudin are alternatives to heparin.

The currently available thrombolytic agents include tissue plasminogen activator TPA, streptokinase, and urokinase. Given the high probability of recent streptococcal infections in pediatric patients and the risk of allergic phenomena, streptokinase is rarely used in infants and children. Urokinase and TPA, are used for clearing of central-line occlusions (**Table 80.17**). Dosing of TPA has been suggested as 0.5 mg/kg/hr and limited to 6 hrs for most patients. The most important complications of antifibrinolytic therapy is bleeding. In general, thrombolytic therapy may be indicated when the risks of morbidity and morality from the thrombotic process outweigh the risks of thrombolytic therapy. Such instances may include arterial occlusions, especially in the CNS or where loss of limb is imminent, and thrombi within the cardiac chambers, which may necessitate a major surgical intervention with CPB for removal.

CHAPTER 81 ■ BONE MARROW AND STEM CELL TRANSPLANTATION

KATHERINE BIAGAS • M. BRIGID BRADLEY • MITCHELL S. CAIRO

Blood and marrow transplantation have been successfully utilized in a variety of childhood and adolescent diseases, including malignant conditions, immune deficiencies, inborn errors of metabolism, genetic disorders, hematopoietic disorders, and autoimmune conditions including: acute lymphoblastic leukemia, acute non-lymphoblastic leukemia, chronic myelogenous leukemia, non-Hodgkin lymphoma, Hodgkin disease, severe aplastic anemia, Fanconi anemia, SCID, severe combined immunodeficiency disorder, Wiskott-Aldrich syndrome, sickle cell disease, β thalassemia and adrenoleukodystrophy. Autologous hematopoietic committed progenitor cells (HPCs) have been successfully utilized to (a) rescue patients from prolonged bone marrow (BM) pancytopenia, (b) correct BM aplasia, (c) induce a graft-versus-tumor effect, (d) induce a graft-versus-autoimmune effect, (d) serve as gene replacement therapy for genetic disorders, and (f) serve as a vehicle for gene transfection and gene therapy. HPCs may be collected and obtained from BM, peripheral blood, or cord blood (CB). Autologous HPCs are progenitor cells obtained from the recipient (self). Syngeneic HPCs are obtained from an identical twin. Allogeneic HPCs are cells obtained from a human being other than a genetically identical twin.

Histocompatibility leukocyte antigens (HLAs) are critical to both immunocompetence and self-tolerance. The two major classes of HLA antigens include HLA class I antigens (A, B, C) and class II antigens (DR, DQ, DP). The preferred allogeneic donor source is a genotypic-matched sibling donor who usually matches at HLA A, B, and DR (6 of 6 match). Additional good allogeneic donor sources include related mismatched family members, including parents and other siblings who match at 6 of 6 or 5 of 6 antigens at HLA A, B, and DRB1. If a closely matched family donor is not available, 2 large sources of unrelated donors exist—unrelated adult donors and unrelated CB donors. The National Marrow Donor Program has a computerized registry of potential adult donors. Additionally, a number of umbilical CB banks have been established.

Prior to infusion of HPCs, most patients receive some form of conditioning or preparative therapy, usually consisting of myeloablative therapy, which commonly includes total-body irradiation with additional high-dose chemotherapy (chemoradiotherapy) or in some settings of AlloSCT, a nonmyeloablative conditioning regimen is used. The HPC infusion is usually used to rescue the patient from hematopoietic toxicity and to reduce the time to hematopoietic reconstitution. Common acute complications following myeloablative conditioning include mucositis, infection, bleeding, pain, nausea and vomiting, and aggravation of graft-versus-host disease (GVHD). However, some centers have initiated the use of nonmyeloablative conditioning to reduce the acute and long-term effects that usually follow the myeloablative approach.

HPCs sometimes require processing before infusion into the recipient. All autologous stem cell transplantation (AutoSCT) requires previous collection of HPCs from the recipient before myeloablation. HPCs derived from CB almost always require prior cell processing and cryopreservation, as they are most commonly collected from unrelated maternal donors who are located at distant sites. Traditionally, CB HPCs are depleted of red blood cells and then incubated with DMSO for long-term cryopreservation.

Most recipients are premedicated with diphenhydramine and acetaminophen prior to HPC infusion. Usually, HPCs are infused through a central venous catheter. Infusion of HPCs may result in acute reactions, including fever, chills, tachycardia, bradycardia, hypotension, respiratory distress, allergic reactions, and on rare occasions, anaphylaxis. Furthermore, if the HPCs are contaminated with microbial organisms, HPC infusion may result in overwhelming infection. In the setting of ABO incompatibility, hemolytic reactions may occur.

GRAFT-VERSUS-HOST DISEASE PROPHYLAXIS

The setting of AlloSCT is associated with a measurable risk of the patient developing acute and/or chronic GVHD. GVHD most commonly occurs after AlloSCT; however, it can develop following AutoSCT, although the incidence is well under 10%. In the case of an AlloSCT, the development of GVHD requires the following 3 underlying risk factors: the recipient must have a depressed or abnormal immune system, the donor cells must be immunocompetent, and an HLA disparity must exist between the donor and the recipient. Previous GVHD prophylaxis regimens have utilized tacrolimus, mycophenolate mofetil, and sirolimus. The delicate balance between the prevention of GVHD and an increased risk of developing serious opportunistic infections presents a serious challenge. Another GVHD prophylaxis approach is T-cell depletion of allogeneic HPC donor sources, which results in extremely low incidence of GVHD after significant T-cell depletion.

Hematopoietic reconstitution is accelerated using hematopoietic growth factors, either granulocyte colony-stimulating factor or granulocyte macrophage colony-stimulating factor, and is performed after AutoSCT and AlloSCT.

RESPIRATORY FAILURE ASSOCIATED WITH TRANSPLANTATION

Dyspnea, impaired gas exchange, and respiratory system dysfunction are common presenting signs in an HPC recipient who is admitted to the PICU. The many possible causes are generally classified as infectious and noninfectious etiologies. Pulmonary function testing usually reveals that the dysfunction is restrictive in nature, often with a reduction in diffusion capacity and sometimes obstruction to ventilation (**Table 81.1**).

In the early posttransplant period, usually up to 3 weeks, patients are neutropenic and susceptible to

TABLE 81.1

CAUSES OF PULMONARY DISEASE

Early recovery period
  Bacterial and fungal infections
  Sepsis
  Mucositis and upper airway obstruction
  Acute pulmonary edema
  Pulmonary vascular disease
    Diffuse alveolar hemorrhage

Mid-recovery period
  Cytomegalovirus pneumonitis
    Primary or reactivation
  Opportunistic infections
  Interstitial pneumonitis

Late recovery period
  Common childhood infections
  Cytomegalovirus reactivation
  Adenovirus infection
  Chronic graft-versus-host disease
  Bronchiolitis obliterans

bacterial and fungal infections, especially *Aspergillus* and *Candida* species. *Aspergillus* infections in this early phase may be particularly severe, with angioinvasive disease. Isolation from respiratory specimens, including bronchoalveolar lavage (BAL) is specific but not sensitive. High-resolution CT is usually the study of choice. If CT lesions are peripheral, a lung biopsy may be considered. Noninfectious complications of this early posttransplant period, such as pulmonary edema and fluid overload, drug reactions, and diffuse alveolar hemorrhage, may be superimposed on infection and worsen pulmonary function. Clinical presentations of transplant-associated pulmonary infections include: fever, increased work of breathing, progressive respiratory insufficiency, and progressive hypoxemia with eventual respiratory acidosis.

From 3 weeks to 3 months after HPC transplantation, viral infections predominate, particularly CMV infection. CMV pneumonitis has a very high fatality rate that is higher in recipients of HPC than in those with solid-organ transplants. Increased incidence of the disease is seen in certain subpopulations, namely, patients who are seropositive, are older, have received total-body irradiation, or suffer from more severe GVHD. Patients are also at risk for *Pneumocystis carinii* in the first few posttransplantation months. The use of low-dose TMP-SMX (5 mg TMP/kg/day in divided doses every 12 hrs, 3 days/week on consecutive days) or pentamidine (4 mg/kg given IV every 14 days) provides effective prophylaxis and greatly reduces the incidence of PCP in this patient population. For true infection, TMP-SMX is the treatment of choice (15–20 mg TMP/kg/day in divided doses every 6–8 hrs). Pentamidine can be used in patients unable to tolerate TMP-SMX.

In the late posttransplant phase, >100 days after HPC infusion, noninfectious pulmonary complications predominate, such as bronchiolitis obliterans (BO) and chronic GVHD (cGVHD). The hallmarks of noninfectious pulmonary diseases are interstitial disease, restrictive changes of respiratory system components, and chronic airflow obstruction consistent with BO. These result from host responses to irradiation and previous cytotoxic therapy, especially as a consequence of the same techniques used at the time of transplantation. Noninfectious respiratory diseases include mucositis with upper-airway inflammation and obstruction, pulmonary edema, pulmonary vascular disease, interstitial pneumonitis and BO.

Pulmonary edema is associated with large volumes of fluids needed to administer medications, minimize their toxicity, and provide parenteral nutrition. Cardiac dysfunction may be present, including congestive cardiomyopathy associated with the use of anthracyclines and mediastinal irradiation.

The necessary use of large fluid volumes in patients with such dysfunctions is often poorly tolerated, and pulmonary edema results. Patients may have concurrent processes that promote systemic inflammatory response syndrome, such as systemic infection, pneumonia, or recent irradiation, exacerbating pulmonary edema. The clinical manifestations are impaired gas exchange, especially hypoxemia, and increased work of breathing. Pulmonary vascular involvement includes thromboembolism, thrombus in situ, pulmonary VOD, and diffuse alveolar hemorrhage. Clinical signs are those of acute, congestive right-heart failure with hepatic engorgement, jugular venous distention, tachycardia, and right ventricular heave. High doses of corticosteroids (>100 mg/day of methylprednisolone or equivalent) may be effective in reducing mortality from diffuse alveolar hemorrhage. Interstitial pneumonitis occurs predominately in patients who undergo total-body irradiation, although it may occur with conditioning regimens that do not contain total-body irradiation at all. The clinical hallmarks are fever, restrictive lung disease (tachypnea, dyspnea, retractions and grunting, and gas exchange abnormalities), and diffuse interstitial infiltrates on chest x-ray.

Chronic GVHD plays an important role in the development of BO. Patients present with progressive dyspnea on exertion, nonproductive cough, and breathing patterns of obstructive disease, so-called *braking respirations* or *pursed-lipped breathing*. Pulmonary function tests reveal nonreversible obstructive airflow. Chest x-ray shows hyperinflation with or without infiltrates. Biopsy material shows occlusion of the lumens of respiratory and terminal bronchioles with inflammatory and fibrous material. In extreme cases, termed *constrictive obliterative bronchiolitis*, cicatricial scarring is present, with obliteration of distal airways. Reversal of airway obstruction is usually only partial, and associated lung infection may worsen with the increase in immunosuppressive therapy. BAL is necessary to target antimicrobial therapy appropriately. Repeated studies may be required to follow the course of disease in severe cases.

MANAGEMENT OF RESPIRATORY FAILURE

Volutrauma, barotrauma, oxygen toxicity, atelectotrauma and ventilator-associated pneumonia contribute to morbidity and mortality. Noninvasive ventilatory support with either continuous positive-airway pressure or bilevel positive-airway pressure may avoid some of these complications. Normalization of gas exchange is not necessary; respiratory acidosis (generally pH $\geq$7.15) and moderate hypoxemia (SaO$_2$ $\geq$90) are usually tolerated. Intubation is reserved for patients with severe or progressive respiratory failure. Intubation may also be required to safely perform diagnostic studies such as BAL.

Treatment of cardiac failure, supportive care for renal and liver failure, and management of fluid overload are important adjunctive therapies. Fluid management should be targeted to render the patient 10% dehydrated as long as cardiac output is maintained. An "open-lung" strategy that limits ventilator peak pressures to 25 torr and tidal volumes to 6–8 mL/kg should be employed to minimize ventilator-induced injury. Positive end-expiratory pressure should be used liberally, and the fraction of inspired oxygen should be limited. Permissive hypercapnia with respiratory acidosis and moderate hypoxemia (SaO$_2$ $\geq$80%) are tolerated. If adequate oxygenation cannot be achieved with such measures, consideration should be given to the use of high-frequency oscillatory ventilation. Alternative modes of pulmonary support include surfactant, nitric oxide, and extracorporeal membrane oxygenation.

RENAL FAILURE ASSOCIATED WITH TRANSPLANTATION

Renal dysfunction and acute renal failure (ARF) are common sequelae after HPC transplantation. Some children will require renal replacement therapy, usually to control fluid imbalance. An increase of serum creatinine by twofold or greater is associated with doubling of mortality for all types of HPC transplantation. Mortality is $\geq$80% in patients who require dialysis for correction of severe acidosis or electrolyte disturbances.

The causes of ARF in the early period (first 3 months) include preexisting renal dysfunction due to cytotoxic therapy for their primary disease as well as sepsis. While infection of the kidney is rare, renal abscesses, with fungal or Gram-negative bacterial species, occur. Infection with adenoviruses, especially BK virus, can cause primary nephritis. Hepatitis B or C infection may cause membranous glomerulonephropathy. Additional deleterious effects on the kidney are seen with nephrotoxic side effects of antimicrobial therapies. Although often required, antimicrobials such as vancomycin, aminoglycosides, amphotericin B, and β-lactam antibiotics require careful consideration when used in patients with already reduced renal function.

The most severe form of renal disease in the early phase of transplantation is hepatorenal syndrome, characterized by hepatic dysfunction with poor GFR and sodium retention with peripheral edema, weight gain, and ascites. Hepatic failure usually accompanies sepsis, GVHD, or veno-occlusive disease (VOD) and is heralded by hyperbilirubinemia with mild elevations in serum transaminase levels. Patients also demonstrate a high urea/creatinine ratio. Patients have pulmonary edema, hypotension, and preserved urine output, especially in the early phase of the condition. Urine output falls later, and hypotension worsens. Hemorrhagic cystitis, though not generally nephrotoxic, may cause bladder obstruction and postrenal failure. Maintenance of brisk urine output is essential in such cases, and aGVHD, while not involving the kidney primarily, may require treatment, which may be nephrotoxic.

Late renal dysfunction, termed *BMT nephropathy*, is similar to hemolytic uremic syndrome or thrombotic thrombocytopenic purpura syndrome, with hypertension, peripheral edema, and microangiopathic hemolytic anemia. Renal dysfunction may be rapidly progressive with accompanying proteinuria and, sometimes, hematuria. Plasma exchange and immunoadsorption have been attempted for fulminant cases of BMT nephropathy, although efficacy of such therapies has not been proved. Efforts should be made to identify underlying treatable conditions, such as sepsis, GVHD, or VOD.

In patients with normal urine output, especially those with requirements for large volumes of IV fluids, frequent doses of diuretics may diminish fluid overload while maintaining normal intravascular volume (**Table 81.2**). Continuous infusion is better tolerated in patients with hemodynamic compromise. In the oliguric patient, a trial of larger-than-standard-dose furosemide (2–4 mg/kg to a maximum dose of 200 mg) may be made; however, the potential for toxicity is greater. Loop diuretics may improve renal

blood flow and may reestablish adequate urine flow. Peritoneal dialysis and intermittent hemodialysis are possible but not popular. Extracorporeal continuous venovenous hemofiltration (CVVH) can be tailored to achieve primarily fluid removal, hemofiltration, dialysis, some degree of solute removal, or any combination of these goals. Indications for CVVH in this population are anuria or severe oliguria, severe metabolic acidemia (pH <7.1), hyperkalemia (serum K >6.5 mmol/dL or rapidly rising), progressive dysnatremia, or coagulopathy that requires administration of large volumes of blood products. Early initiation of CVVH should be considered for patients with underlying electrolyte disorders, anuric ARF, Fanconi syndrome, or renal tubular acidosis.

FLUID AND ELECTROLYTE PROBLEMS

Indications for parenteral nutrition include anorexia, mucositis, and enteritis, and aGVHD. Total parenteral nutrition is associated with high cost, need for ongoing central venous access, fluid overload, hyperglycemia, biliary stasis, hepatic dysfunction, and enterocyte atrophy with loss of gut mucosal barrier. Even small-volume, non-nutritive feedings may ameliorate barrier dysfunction.

GRAFT-VERSUS-HOST DISEASE

The incidence and severity of GVHD following AlloSCT depends on donor source, HLA disparity between donor and recipient, type of graft-versus-host prophylaxis, CMV status of donor and recipient, and age of donor, among others. The pathophysiology of

---

TABLE 81.2

INTRAVENOUS DIURETIC THERAPY IN FLUID OVERLOAD STATES

Medication	Dose	Comment
Furosemide	Intermittent dosing: 0.5–1.0 mg/kg/dose every 6–12 hrs	May be ototoxic, especially at extremely large doses noted here.
	Trial of extremely large dose: 50–200 mg/dose Infusion: 0.3–1.0 mg/kg/hrs	May increase RBF.
Bumetanide	Intermittent dosing: 0.5–2.0 mg/dose every 6–12 hrs	Similar to furosemide.
Ethacrynic Acid	Intermittent dosing: 0.5–1.0 mg/kg/dose every 8–12 hrs	Increases RBF and venous capacitance. Potentially ototoxic.
Chlorothiazide	Intermittent dosing: 1.0–2.0 mg/kg/dose every 12 hrs	Usually not useful when GFR <30 mL/min.

RBF, renal blood flow; GFR, glomerular filtration rate

TABLE 81.3

CONSENSUS GRADING OF ACUTE GRAFT VERSUS HOST DISEASE

	Organ/extent of involvement		
	Skin	**Liver**	**Intestinal tract**
Stage			
1	Rash on <25% of skin[a]	Bilirubin 2–3 mg/dL[b]	Diarrhea >500 mL/day[c] or persistent nausea[d]
2	Rash on 25%–50% of skin	Bilirubin 3–6 mg/dL	Diarrhea >1000 mL/day
3	Rash on >50% of skin	Bilirubin 6–15 mg/dL	Diarrhea >1500 mL/day
4	Generalized erythroderma with bulla formation	Bilirubin >15 mg/dL	Severe abdominal pain with or without ileus
Grade			
0	None	None	None
I	Stage 1–2	None	None
II	Stage 3	or Stage 1	or Stage 1
III	—	Stage 2–3	or Stage 2–4
IV[e]	Stage 4	or Stage 4	—

[a] Use the "rule of nines" to determine body surface area involvement.
[b] Range given as total bilirubin. Downgrade one stage if an additional cause of elevated bilirubin has been documented.
[c] Volume of diarrhea applies to adults. For pediatric patients, the volume of diarrhea should be based on body surface area.
[d] Persistent nausea with histologic evidence of GVHD in the stomach or duodenum.
[e] Grade IV may also include lesser organ involvement but with extreme decrease in performance status.
From Przepiorka D, Weisdorf D, Martin P, et al. 1994 Consensus Conference on Acute GVHD Grading. *Bone Marrow Transplant* 1995;15(6):825–8, with permission.

aGVHD following AlloSCT is a 3-step process in which interaction between innate and adaptive immunity occurs. Acute GVHD involves 3 target organs: skin, liver, and GI tract (**Table 81.3**). Rarely is skin aGVHD, by itself, sufficient to require admission to the PICU; however, stage 4 disease requires management using burn protocols with support of fluids, electrolytes, and cardiovascular function. The differential diagnosis of skin GVHD includes skin reactions secondary to (a) conditioning regimens or antibiotics or (b) histopathologic skin manifestations of disseminated infections. In fact, severe skin aGVHD may be difficult to distinguish from Stevens-Johnson syndrome and/or toxic epidermal necrolysis. A major difference is the lack of involvement of the conjunctiva in skin aGVHD. A skin biopsy is required to document dermal-epidermal junction damage with evidence of epidermal and basal cell vascular degeneration, disorganization of epidermal cell maturation, or evidence of apoptosis.

The biomarker of acute hepatic GVHD is an increase in the serum bilirubin level, with staging based entirely on this level. The differential diagnosis of acute hepatic GVHD includes hepatic VOD secondary to intensive conditioning, drug toxicity, infection, cholelithiasis, and other sinusoidal obstructive syndromes. On occasion, a liver biopsy is required.

Gastrointestinal GVHD presents as secretory or watery diarrhea, abdominal pain, nausea, vomiting,

and anorexia. Severe intestinal GVHD may lead to significant mucosal damage with electrolyte abnormalities, protein-losing enteropathy, bloody diarrhea, and massive losses of fluid to the extravascular space. In stages 1–3, staging of GI GVHD is based on the amount of diarrhea per day. Stage 4 GI GVHD is defined as severe abdominal pain with or without ileus and large amounts of secretory diarrhea.

In addition to supportive care, specific treatment usually requires systemic immunosuppression, most commonly with systemic corticosteroids.

VENO-OCCLUSIVE DISEASE

VOD usually presents with the triad of hepatomegaly, weight gain, and jaundice. It is heralded with the appearance of right upper-quadrant tenderness and hepatomegaly within 7–20 days after myeloablative HPC transplantation. Fluid retention usually manifests as peripheral edema, ascites, pleural or pericardial effusions, and measurable weight gain. Additional signs of liver dysfunction include hyperbilirubinemia, portal hypertension, and clotting abnormalities. Ultrasound and CT of the liver demonstrate hepatomegaly, ascites, and, most important, attenuated hepatic venous flow. VOD should be differentiated from direct drug toxicity, liver failure from parenteral nutrition or infection, cholelithiasis, and systemic conditions such as sepsis. If symptoms are severe or when the diagnosis is uncertain, liver biopsy may be helpful in differentiating the etiology. However, percutaneous liver biopsy is associated with a high risk of bleeding due to the usual coagulopathy. Transjugular biopsy has a lower morbidity and is the procedure of choice, especially in the early posttransplant period.

Identification of high-risk patients and the initiation of prophylactic measures are important in the prevention and amelioration of hepatic VOD. Prophylactic therapies include the use of ursodeoxycholic acid, a hydrophilic water soluble bile acid to prevent bilirubin and stone formation, and low-dose, low-molecular-weight heparin to treat microthrombosis. Mild VOD does not require medical intervention. Moderate VOD requires medical intervention but is reversible with little serious systemic toxicity. Severe VOD is associated with important systemic complications and a high mortality rate. The risk of developing severe VOD is based on the percent of weight gain, total serum bilirubin, and days posttransplant. The treatment for moderate and severe VOD includes close fluid and electrolyte monitoring, aggressive use of diuretics, reduction of weight gain, and nutritional support. Thrombolytic therapies with recombinant human tissue plasminogen activator and heparin have shown some efficacy in treating patients with moderate-to-severe VOD. These therapies are frequently limited by the risk of severe or fatal bleeding, especially in patients with disordered coagulation. Other anticoagulant therapies have included human antithrombin III concentrate or activated protein C. Defibrotide has been used with moderate success in patients with moderate-to-severe VOD. Surgically or radiologically placed peritoneal venous shunts or transhepatic and intrahepatic portal systemic shunting have had some success. The shunting procedure, which creates a channel between the hepatic vein and the portal vein by percutaneous catheter insertion, has resulted in significant improvement in patients with severe ascites and coagulopathy.

INFECTIONS

The risk of developing infection is influenced by the type of transplantation, conditioning regimen, donor source, underlying disease, intensity of previous therapy, and other complications. Fever, usually the main indicator of infection, may be blunted by immunomodulatory treatment. Other signs, such as tachycardia, tachypnea, and organ dysfunction, should be considered as signs of possible infection. Sites with known risk, such as the peri-anal area, lungs, skin, central venous catheter exit sites, and oropharynx, should be assessed for any sign of infection. Workup should include blood cultures and cultures from any suspected site of infection.

Bacteria account for >90% of infections during the neutropenic phase. Infections with Gram-positive organisms are mainly associated with central venous catheters and severe mucositis; infections with Gram-negative organisms occur with severe GI mucosal damage. In the neutropenic patient, infections with *Staphylococcus epidermidis*, *Staphylococcus aureus*, streptococcus species, *Pseudomonas aeruginosa*, *Escherichia coli*, *Klebsiella spp.*, *Corynebacterium jeikeium*, and *Bacillus spp.* often lead to serious sepsis. Alpha-haemolytic streptococci are increasingly recognized as a cause of sepsis in the neutropenic patient. *Streptococcus mitis* is associated with acute respiratory distress syndrome and septic shock. Infection caused by aerobic Gram-negative bacilli, such as *Enterobacteriaceae* and *P. aeruginosa*, can cause overwhelming sepsis and toxemia in the neutropenic patient. The most serious localized infection in the HPC recipient is ecthyma gangrenosum, often caused by *P. aeruginosa*.

Viral infection is the leading cause of morbidity and mortality following HPC transplantation. The herpes viruses, including HSV, CMV, varicella-zoster virus, Epstein Barr virus, and human herpes virus 6, account for the majority of posttransplant viral infection. Esophagitis is common, and pneumonia can develop. Isolation of the virus or positive direct immunofluorescence using monoclonal antibodies leads to diagnosis and aids in management. CMV commonly occurs 4–10 weeks after transplantation and can be life-threatening. With preemptive therapy, the disease is also seen after day +100. Pretransplant serology helps to identify patients at risk for CMV reactivation, but diagnosis is made by isolation of the virus or by detection of viral DNA by PCR. Active CMV infection manifests as fever, fatigue, leukopenia, hepatitis, colitis, myelitis, chorioretinitis, or pneumonia. Varicella-zoster virus infection, develops as a primary infection or as reactivation of latent virus and is potentially lethal. Reactivation of latent virus can present as shingles or as disseminated disease. Herpes virus 6 infection manifests as encephalitis, pneumonitis, or graft suppression. Infection with Epstein Barr virus, typically in the first 6 months, also develops as either primary disease or reactivation and can cause B-cell posttransplant lymphoproliferative disorder (PTLD). Patients present with high fever, lymphadenopathy, and sometimes diarrhea or elevated liver enzymes, depending on organ involvement. Adenovirus infection presents with diarrhea, hemorrhagic cystitis, and pneumonia. Diagnosis is made by viral culture from infected body fluids or tissue (excluding the GI tract) by direct antigen detection or by molecular methods. Adenovirus infection develops from reactivation of latent virus or, commonly, in young children with primary infection contracted by contact. Infections with respiratory syncytial virus, influenza A and B, or parainfluenza infection occur seasonally and coincide with community outbreaks.

Risk factors for invasive fungal disease include neutropenia, HLA-mismatched transplant, GVHD or its treatment, steroid therapy, and graft failure. Signs and symptoms of fungal infection are often absent or nonspecific and include fever unresponsive to antibiotics. Diagnosis relies on culture of the organism from a sterile site or identification by histologic methods. Serum antigens can be detected in select situations, such as detection of cryptococcal antigen. Galactomannan antigen can be detected in *Aspergillus* infection. A shift has occurred in the incidence of *Candida* infections, with a decrease in *Candida albicans* and an emergence of non-albicans species, such as *C. tropicalis*, *C. parapsilosis*, *C. glabrata*, and *C. krusei*. *C. albicans* and *C. tropicalis* are known causes of disseminated candidiasis. *C. parapsilosis*, a catheter-associated yeast, rarely disseminates systemically. Hepatosplenic candidosis commonly presents during neutrophil regeneration. *Aspergillus* is the leading cause of death from infection after AlloSCT. *Aspergillus* species such as *A. fumigatus*, *A. flavus*, and *A. niger*, cause invasive disease, predominately during the neutropenic period. The primary site for *Aspergillus* infection is the lung. Such infection often presents as invasive, pulmonary aspergillosis with thrombotic and hemorrhagic lung disease. Dissemination to the brain, liver, and skin is common. Cutaneous lesions, also known as ecthyma gangrenosum, are a common manifestation of disseminated disease. Cryptococcosis is rare and most often results in meningitis or pulmonary infection. Zygomycosis or mucormycosis often present as sinusoidal disease, but pulmonary and disseminated disease may occur.

Pneumocystis carinii pneumonia, a protozoan infection, occurs postengraftment. Patients present with progressive dyspnea with a dry cough but can also present with a fulminant course. Hypoxia is present and chest x-ray often shows interstitial acinar infiltrates. BAL is the preferred diagnostic test. Molecular diagnosis by PCR is highly sensitive and specific.

Tuberculous and non-tuberculous Mycobacterium infections are infrequent in HPC transplant recipients.

Prophylactic or preemptive therapies have reduced the incidence and the morbidity and mortality associated with most infections. Empiric therapy started at the onset of fever and new antimicrobial agents improve outcome. Acyclovir is the drug of choice in the treatment of HSV and varicella-zoster

virus infections. Immunocompromised patients exposed to varicella-zoster virus should receive zoster immunoglobulin to confer passive immunity. Ganciclovir, foscarnet, and cidofovir are effective therapies against infection with herpes virus 6. Treatment of Epstein Barr virus PTLD involves antibody therapy with rituximab and donor-derived cytotoxic T cells. No specific therapy has been identified for adenovirus infection; however, some have reported that cidofovir is successful. Prophylactic or preemptive approaches to those patients at risk for CMV reactivation has reduced the incidence of infection and disease and resulted in a significant reduction in mortality. For seronegative patients who receive transplants from seronegative donors, the use of CMV-negative blood products will suffice. For seropositive patients or seronegative patients who receive a transplant from a seropositive donor, intervention is required. CMV disease can be prevented by prophylactic administration of antiviral medication or preemptive early intervention in which treatment is started when antigenemia or evidence of viral replication is observed. Ganciclovir and foscarnet are effective in preventing and treating CMV. The use of ganciclovir in combination with foscarnet and high-dose IV immune globulin was associated with a 50% survival rate in patients with acute CMV infection. Prophylaxis with either ganciclovir or foscarnet has reduced the incidence and severity of CMV infection in CMV-seropositive patients. Lastly, it is the lack of CMV-specific T-cell responses that places the patient at risk for recurrence of CMV disease or persistent disease. Some centers have shown that the adoptive transfer of CMV-specific T cells restores immunity and is effective treatment. Adenovirus infection is associated with almost uniformly fatal disease.

With fungal infection, prevention is the goal. Amphotericin B has broad antifungal activity; liposomal amphotericin shows equal efficacy and reduced toxicity. The azoles have broad antimycotic activity. Fluconazole, used prophylactically, protects against candidiasis. It has no activity against some of the non-albicans species. Voriconazole has activity against *Aspergillus* species and is considered the treatment of choice in patients with proven *Aspergillus*, although it lacks activity against newer, emerging molds. The echinocandins, caspofungin and micofungin, are as effective as amphotericin B for the treatment of invasive candidiasis and have shown efficacy as salvage therapy in patients with invasive aspergillosis. The combination of caspofungin with a broad-spectrum azole or amphotericin B is effective.

Treatment of mycobacterium infection requires multidrug therapy. Testing for organism sensitivity is recommended to better tailor therapy, as resistant strains are seen. The usual course of recommended treatment is 3–6 months and should continue until evidence of immune reconstitution is observed.

MUCOSITIS

Oral and GI mucositis contribute significantly to morbidity and mortality and are severe complications of treatment. Approximately 75%–90% of HPC-transplantation recipients experience mucositis, with 50% developing grade III–IV mucositis (**Fig. 81.1**). For some, oral mucositis is the most common and most debilitating side effect reported. Severe mucositis causes pain and bleeding. Patients experience prolonged hospitalization, increased need for analgesics, increased need for total parenteral nutrition, reduced quality of life, and episodes of infection, especially bacteremia, invasive fungal disease, and typhlitis associated with mucosal-barrier breakdown. Bloodstream infections with *S. aureus*, *P. aeruginosa*, *Clostridium* species, and *Candida* occur and are associated with typhlitis. Mucositis involves the entire GI tract. Mucosal barrier injury is now viewed as a complex biologic process that consists of 5 phases (**Fig. 81.1**). Clinical assessment scales have been developed to classify the severity of mucosal damage. No single mucositis assessment scale is universally accepted. Most combine both subjective and objective measures of appearance, patient pain, and functional capabilities. One of these is depicted in **Table 81.4**. Differential diagnosis of mucositis includes oral hemorrhage, infection, GVHD, and local viral infections. Infection with HSV is often accompanied by extensive and deep ulcerations. Although uncom-

TABLE 81.4

WORLD HEALTH ORGANIZATION MUCOSITIS SCALE

Grade 0	No mucositis.
Grade 1	Irritation of the oral mucosa with pain; no overt ulceration; patient is able to eat a normal diet.
Grade 2	Sores are evident in the oral mucosa, but patient is still able to swallow solid food.
Grade 3	Patients need to be on a liquid diet, as they experience extreme sensitivity on swallowing solid food.
Grade 4	Patients are not able to swallow. Total parenteral nutrition or tube feeding is necessary.

mon, CMV infection can lead to mucosal tissue injury. It is important to distinguish mucosal tissue injury that results from infection so that appropriate antiviral therapy will be used. Biopsy may be required to make this determination.

Management is focused on supportive care to control symptoms. Basic oral care is important to reduce oral microbial flora, reduce symptoms of pain and bleeding, and prevent soft-tissue infections. Most oral regimens incorporate a combination of agents that collectively serve to coat and anesthetize the mucosa and to reduce the risk for mucosal infection. Saline and sodium bicarbonate rinses or mucosal coating agents can provide symptomatic relief for mild mucositis. As mucosal breakdown and pain increase, topical anesthetics, such as viscous lidocaine and benzocaine, and analgesics are added.

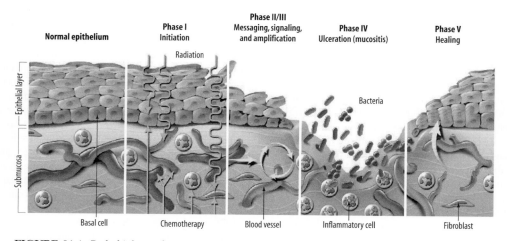

FIGURE 81.1. Pathobiology of mucositis: a 5-stage process. The biologic sequence of mucositis can be arbitrarily divided into 5 stages or phases: initiation, upregulation and message generation, amplification and signaling, ulceration, and healing. From Sonis ST. A biological approach to mucositis. *J Support Oncol* 2004; 2:21–32, with permission.

Additional ingredients in topical oral solutions include diphenhydramine, magnesium hydroxide/ aluminum hydroxide, pectin, sucralfate, nystatin, chlorhexidine, and corticosteroids. IV pain medication, especially with patient-controlled analgesia, may be required. For patients with severe-grade III/IV mucositis who are also often neutropenic and thrombocytopenic, treatment focuses on control of severe bleeding, tissue desquamation, and infection. Protection of the airway with either an oral airway or intubation may be required until the patient reaches the healing phase.

CHAPTER 82 ■ COAGULATION ISSUES IN THE PICU

ROBERT I. PARKER • JAN A. HAZELZET

While it was previously thought that the intrinsic pathway, beginning with the activation of factor XII in contact with some surface was physiologically the most important in the initiation of clot formation, it is now known that the activation of factor X to factor Xa through the action of the factor VIIa/tissue factor (TF) complex is paramount. *Tenase* refers to the action of F.VIIa /TF complex, along with the F.IXa/F.VIIIa complex on the activation of F.X to F.Xa, and *prothrombinase* describes the F.Xa/F.Va complex, which cleaves prothrombin (F.II) to form thrombin (F.IIa). "Crosstalk" occurs between the two arms of the clotting cascade, with F.VIIa being able to enhance the activation of F.IX (to F.IXa) and F.XI (to F.XIa), further highlighting the central role of F.VIIa and TF in vivo (**Fig. 82.1**). The activation of coagulation is initiated from TF. Clotting does not occur in free-flowing blood but rather on surfaces. Platelets, endothelial cells, the subendothelial matrix, and biologic polymers (e.g., catheters, grafts, stents, etc.) provide these surfaces for clot formation.

Platelets not only initiate the clot formation through the formation of a platelet plug but, more important, they bring specialized proteins that regulate the clotting response (e.g., F.VIII, inhbitors of fibrinolysis, etc.) to the area of bleeding and provide a surface for the co-localization of clotting factors for efficient clot formation. Platelets do not ordinarily adhere to the vascular endothelium, but when the endothelium is mechanically disrupted (e.g., cut) or activated by inflammation, platelets will bind to the endothelial cell or subendothelial matrix via a von Willebrand factor–dependent mechanism. Once adherent, the platelets become activated and secrete various molecules that further enhance platelet adherence and aggregation, vascular contraction, clot formation, and wound healing.

The normal endothelium produces inhibitors of blood coagulation and platelet activation and modulates vascular tone and permeability. Endothelial cells also synthesize and secrete the components of the subendothelial extracellular matrix, including adhesive glycoproteins, collagen, fibronectin, and von Willebrand factor. When this system is disrupted, bleeding occurs. The endothelium often becomes a prothrombotic rather than an antithrombotic organ, and unwanted clot formation may occur.

INTERACTION OF COAGULATION AND INFLAMMATION

The response of the coagulation system during acute inflammation has received wider attention owing to the recognition that coagulation is an integral part of the host immune response. Disseminated intravascular coagulation (DIC), when accompanied by sepsis and a systemic inflammatory response, results in a more severe clinical picture, higher degree of organ dysfunction, and a higher mortality. In DIC, coagulation pathways are activated, natural inhibitory pathways are dysfunctional, and the fibrinolytic system is dysregulated. During sepsis, TF expression is upregulated in activated monocytes and endothelial cells as a response to endotoxin and other pathogen-associated molecular patterns, with the consequence being the secretion of proinflammatory cytokines and activation of coagulation. The presence of thrombin will result in the activation, aggregation, and lysis of leukocytes and platelets, in the activation of

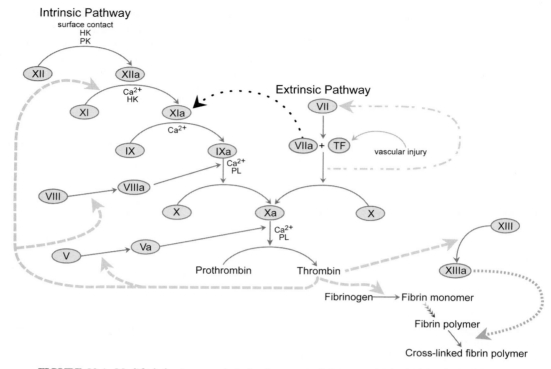

FIGURE 82.1. Modified clotting cascade indicating cross-talk between the intrinsic and extrinsic pathways by the action of factor VIIa/tissue factor (TF) enhancing the conversion of factor XI to activated factor XI (XIa)(dotted lines). HK, high-molecular-weight kininogen; PK, prekallikrein; PL, phospholipid. From Parker RI. Coagulation disorders. In: Civetta JM, Taylor RW, Kirby RR (Eds.), *Critical Care*, 4th ed. Philadelphia: Lippincott Williams & Wilkins, 2008, with permission.

endothelial adhesion molecules, and in the expression of a proinflammatory cytokine (IL-6). Thrombin increases endothelial permeability and also stimulates cellular proliferation. The net result of thrombin generation is production of a procoagulant state; it leads to the formation of fibrin, activates coagulation factors V, VIII, IX, XI, and leads to the expression of TF and von Willebrand factor and the aggregation of platelets. However, thrombin also has anti-inflammatory effects through the production of activated protein C (APC). Besides coagulation activation, two other crucial mechanisms occur during sepsis. One is the depression of natural anticoagulant systems, involving antithrombin and protein C (PC), and the second is the inhibition of fibrinolysis through the production of plasminogen activator inhibitor type-1 (PAI-1) and thrombin-activatable fibrinolysis inhibitor. The PC pathway is engaged when thrombin binds to thrombomodulin on the surface of the endothelium. Binding of PC to the endothelial cell PC receptor augments PC activation by the thrombin-thrombomodulin complex.

APPROACH TO THE PATIENT WITH AN ACTUAL OR SUSPECTED COAGULATION DISORDER

Specific questions regarding bleeding and thrombosis include spontaneous, easy, or disproportionately severe bruising; intramuscular hematoma formation (either spontaneous or related to trauma); spontaneous or trauma-induced hemarthrosis; spontaneous mucous membrane bleeding; prior problems with bleeding related to surgery (including dental extractions, tonsillectomy, and circumcision); the need for transfusions in the past; menstrual history; and, current medications. A prior history of significant thrombosis (e.g., deep venous thrombosis, pulmonary embolus, stroke) suggests the possibility of the presence of a hypercoagulable condition. Vasculitis associated with an autoimmune disorder such as systemic lupus erythematosus must be considered in the evaluation of a child with an unexplained pathologic clot. In all cases, the family history is important in attempting to separate congenital from acquired disorders.

Correction of the coagulopathy usually requires improvement in the patient's overall clinical status in critically ill children. The presence of an enlarged spleen coupled with thrombocytopenia suggests that splenic sequestration may be a contributor to the observed thrombocytopenia. Further, evidence of liver disease (e.g., portal hypertension, ascites), points to decreased factor synthesis as a possible etiology of a prolonged PT or aPTT. When lymphadenopathy, splenomegaly, or other findings suggestive of disseminated malignancy are detected, acute or chronic DIC should be suspected as the cause of prolonged coagulation times, hypofibrinogenemia, and/or thrombocytopenia. Purpura that are palpable suggest capillary leak from vasculitis, whereas purpura associated with thrombocytopenia or qualitative platelet defects are generally not elevated and cannot be distinguished by touch. Venous and arterial telangiectasia may be seen in von Willebrand disease and liver disease, respectively. When selective pressure is centrally applied to an arterial telangiectasia, the entire lesion fades, whereas a venous telangiectasia requires confluent pressure across the entire lesion (as with a glass slide) for blanching to occur.

Heparin is commonly present, either in solutions used to flush the cannula, to transduce a waveform, or as a component of the IV infusion. Depending on the concentration of heparin in the infusing fluid and the volume of blood withdrawn, several tests can be influenced. Several major categories of hemorrhagic disorders and the tests that are characteristically abnormal in each are summarized in **Table 82.1**. In most instances, measurement of the platelet count, fibrinogen level, PT, aPTT, and TT should provide sufficient information for determining the correct diagnosis. Patients who present with a thrombotic event will generally not display abnormalities of usual "clotting" studies; that is, their PT, aPTT,

TABLE 82.1

HEMORRHAGIC SYNDROMES AND ASSOCIATED LABORATORY FINDINGS

Clinical syndrome	Screening tests	Supportive tests
Disseminated intravascular coagulation	Prolonged PT, aPTT, TT; decreased fibrinogen, platelets; microangiopathy	(+) FDPs, D-dimer; decreased factors V, VIII, and II (late)
Massive transfusion	Prolonged PT, aPTT; decreased fibrinogen, platelets ± prolonged TT	All factors decreased; (–) FDPs, D-dimer (unless DIC develops); (+) transfusion history
Anticoagulant overdose Heparin	Prolonged aPTT, TT; ± prolonged PT	Toluidine blue/protamine corrects TT; reptilase time normal
Warfarin (same as vitamin K deficiency)	Prolonged PT; ± prolonged aPTT (severe); normal TT, fibrinogen, platelets	Vitamin K-dependent factors decreased; factors V, VIII normal
Liver disease Early	Prolonged PT	Decreased factor VII
Late	Prolonged PT, aPTT; decreased fibrinogen (terminal liver failure); normal platelet count (if splenomegaly absent)	Decreased factors II, V, VII, IX, and X; decreased plasminogen; ± FDPs unless DIC develops
Primary fibrinolysis	Prolonged PT, aPTT, TT; decreased fibrinogen ± platelets decreased	(+) FDPs, (–) D-dimer; short euglobulin clot lysis time
Thrombotic Thrombocytopenic purpura	Thrombocytopenia, microangiopathy with mild anemia; PT, aPTT , fibrinogen generally within normal limits/mildly abnormal	ADAMTS13 deficiency/inhibitor, unusually large von Willebrand factor multimers between episodes; mild increase in FDPs or D-dimer
Hemolytic uremic syndrome	Microangiopathic hemolytic anemia, ± thrombocytopenia; PT, aPTT generally within normal limits	Renal insufficiency; FDPs and D-dimer generally (–)

PT, prothrombin time; aPTT, activated partial thromboplastin time; TT, thrombin time; FDPs, fibrin degradation products

TT, and fibrinogen will usually be within normal ranges.

Several inherited or acquired abnormalities place an individual at increased risk for thrombosis. Prior to initiation of anticoagulation, plasma levels of PC (antigen and activity), protein S (antigen and activity; total and free), and antithrombin-III (antigen and activity) should be obtained. In addition, polymerase chain reaction analysis for mutations in the F.V [F.V Leiden; R(Arg)506Q(Gln)], prothrombin [G(Gly) 20210A (Ala)], and methylenetetrahydrofolate reductase (MTHFR); [C(Cys)677T(Thr)] genes should be performed. In addition, a baseline serum homocysteine may be obtained. Confounding clinical conditions, such as dehydration (in the case of central venous sinus thrombosis), indwelling catheters, vascular compression (e.g., cervical ribs), type-II heparin-induced thrombocytopenia, need to be evaluated in evaluating a patient with thrombosis.

CONDITIONS ASSOCIATED WITH SERIOUS BLEEDING OR A HIGH PROBABILITY OF BLEEDING

Disseminated Intravascular Coagulation

DIC results from the activation of blood coagulation, which then leads to excessive thrombin generation. The final result of this process is the widespread formation of fibrin thrombi in the microcirculation, with resultant consumption of certain clotting factors and platelets, which is responsible for the development of significant bleeding. Several specific conditions associated with the development of DIC are presented in **Table 82.2**. Fibrinolysis invariably accompanies thrombin formation in DIC, and thrombin generation or release of tissue plasminogen activator usually initiates this process. Plasmin is generated and then digests fibrinogen and fibrin clots as they form. In a given patient with DIC, either bleeding or thrombotic tendencies may predominate; in most patients, bleeding is usually the predominant problem (**Table 82.1** and **Table 82.2**). Infection, multiple trauma, hepatic insufficiency, and splenectomy are common conditions associated with the development of DIC. The tests most commonly employed in many of these scoring systems for the diagnosis of DIC are listed in **Table 82.3**. Differential diagnosis includes liver disease, massive transfusion, primary fibrinolysis, thrombotic thrombocytopenic purpura (TTP)/hemolytic uremic syndrome (HUS), heparin therapy, and dysfibrinogenemia. The D-dimer assay for the D-dimer fragment of polymerized fibrin has

TABLE 82.2
UNDERLYING DISEASES ASSOCIATED WITH DISSEMINATED INTRAVASCULAR COAGULATION
Sepsis Retained placenta Liver disease Hypertonic saline abortion Shock Amniotic fluid embolus Penetrating brain injury Retention of a dead fetus Necrotizing pneumonitis Eclampsia Tissue necrosis/crush injury Localized endothelial injury (aortic aneurysm, giant hemangiomata, angiography) Intravascular hemolysis Acute promyelocytic leukemia Thermal injury Freshwater drowning Disseminated malignancy (prostate, pancreatic) Fat embolism syndrome

been shown to be both highly sensitive and specific for patients with suspected DIC. Purpura fulminans is a systemic coagulopathy similar, if not identical, to DIC that classically accompanies meningococcal sepsis and is sporadically noted with other similarly severe infections.

While neither TTP nor HUS generally produces a coagulopathic state, both are characterized by marked microangiopathy and microvascular thrombosis. HUS is more commonly seen in children and is characterized by a prodrome of fever and diffuse diarrhea (often bloody). Endemic cases of HUS are generally caused by verotoxin expressing enteropathic strains of *Escherichia coli* (O157:H7) or Shigatoxin-expressing strains of *Shigella*. Sporadic cases are

TABLE 82.3
LABORATORY TESTS FOR THE DIAGNOSIS OF DISSEMINATED INTRAVASCULAR COAGULATION

Test	Discriminator value
Platelet count	<80–100,000 or a decrease of >50% from baseline
Fibrinogen	<100 mg/dL or a decrease of >50% from baseline
Prothrombin time	>3-sec prolongation above upper limit of normal
Fibrin degradation products	>80 mg/dL
D-dimer	"moderate" increase

generally not associated with diarrhea and may represent variant TTP or familial defects in complement factor H. Neither plasma infusion nor plasma exchange appears to be beneficial. TTP is characterized by the pentad of microangiopathic hemolytic anemia, thrombocytopenia, neurologic symptoms, fever, and renal dysfunction. This disorder is felt to be due to the absence of a von Willebrand factor–cleaving protease (ADAMTS13), resulting in the circulation of unusually large von Willebrand factor multimers that can induce or enhance the pathologic adhesion of platelets to the endothelium. The therapy of choice for TTP is plasma exchange by apheresis. Platelet transfusions are generally not recommended, except in the case of major bleeding.

The primary treatment for DIC is correction of the underlying problem that led to its development. Supportive therapy for DIC includes the use of several component blood products. Packed RBCs are given according to accepted guidelines in the face of active bleeding. Fresh whole blood (i.e., <24–48 hrs old) may be given to replete both volume and oxygen-carrying capacity, with the potential additional benefit of providing coagulation proteins, including fibrinogen and platelets. Cryoprecipitate contains a much higher concentration of fibrinogen than does whole blood or fresh-frozen plasma (FFP) and therefore is more likely to provide the quantity of fibrinogen necessary to replete fibrinogen that is consumed by DIC. FFP infusions may effectively replete other coagulation factors consumed with DIC. The goal of blood component therapy is not to produce normal "numbers" but rather to produce clinical stability. If the serum fibrinogen level is <75–50 mg/dL, repletion with cryoprecipitate to raise plasma levels to ≥100 mg/dL is the goal. A reasonable starting dose is 1 bag of cryoprecipitate for every 10 kg of body weight every 8–12 hrs. As cryoprecipitate is not a standardized component (i.e., its content varies from bag to bag), the fibrinogen level should be rechecked after an infusion to document the increase. The amount and timing of the next infusion is then adjusted according to the results. Platelet transfusions also may be used when thrombocytopenia is thought to contribute to ongoing bleeding. Platelet transfusions in patients with DIC should be considered to maintain platelet counts up to 40,000 to 80,000/mcL.

Recombinant APC, was shown to result in a 6% reduction in sepsis mortality in adults and possibly a reduction in the incidence of DIC. However, its use was associated with an increase in intracranial bleeding in older adults. A multi-institutional trial in pediatric sepsis failed to result in a recommendation for its use and was stopped because of a significant incidence of severe bleeding, particularly in infants and young children. Activated recombinant human F.VII (rhF.VIIa) may have a therapeutic role in bleeding disorders.

Liver Disease and Hepatic Insufficiency

In liver disease, synthesis of factors II, V, VII, IX, and X is impaired. Fibrinogen synthesis by the liver usually can be maintained at levels that prevent bleeding until terminal liver failure supervenes. Deficiencies in plasma coagulation protein synthesis in liver disease are associated with an increased fibrinolytic activity. Thrombocytopenia may be present to a variable degree in patients with hepatic dysfunction—usually ascribed to splenic sequestration. Patients with synthetic liver disease may also exhibit decreased synthesis of the vitamin K–dependent anticoagulant proteins PC and protein S, as well as antithrombin-III. Decreased levels of these natural anticoagulants may increase the risk of thrombosis. The PT, aPTT, and TT will not be affected by the levels of any of these naturally occurring anticoagulants.

In patients with liver disease and impaired synthetic capabilities, particularly those who are critically ill, F.VII activity levels are usually the first to decrease due to its short half-life. The D-dimer assay result should be negative in the patient who has liver disease. In patients with a prolonged PT who are in a postoperative state or are scheduled for an invasive procedure, correction of the PT should be attempted. FFP provides the most immediate source of specific coagulation factors (i.e., F.VII) and usually corrects an isolated mild PT prolongation. Cryoprecipitate is required only if fibrinogen levels are <50–100 mg/dL or if significant dysfibrinogenemia is documented. Vitamin K deficiency also is relatively common in this patient population, and replacement may be necessary. Patients with significant hepatic impairment may manifest a partial response or may not respond at all. The immediate use of FFP is therefore appropriate when rapid correction is necessary. rhF.VIIa infusions have been shown to control bleeding in severe liver disease. The use of F.IX concentrates (prothrombin complex concentrates) has been advocated for uncontrolled bleeding. The products produced from plasma pooled from multiple donors carry a significant risk of hepatitis (both types B and C). The use of prothrombin complex concentrates or rhF.VIIa should be reserved for patients with poorly controlled bleeding that is unresponsive to other, more established therapeutic modalities such as infusion of FFP. FFP, 10–15 mL/kg body weight every 6–8 hrs, or 2–4 mL/kg/hr may be given until bleeding slows significantly. rhF.VIIa or prothrombin complex concentrates may be used in those patients who are unresponsive to FFP infusions. Cryoprecipitate should be infused for fibrinogen levels <50–100 mg/dL. Platelet transfusions also may be required if the platelet count is <40–80,000/mcL, depending on the clinical situation. Vitamin K should be empirically administered. Many of the second- and third-generation cephalosporins directly interfere with vitamin K absorption from the gut lumen.

The differential diagnosis of an isolated prolongation of the PT, with or without bleeding, includes vitamin K deficiency, liver disease, vitamin K antagonist rodenticides (so-called "superwarfarin"), and warfarin administration. Infants who fail to receive vitamin K in the immediate postnatal period may develop a systemic coagulopathy manifested by bruising and gastrointestinal bleeding, generally occurring between 1 and 2 weeks of age. The first manifestation is often prolonged bleeding following circumcision. The laboratory findings of an isolated vitamin K deficiency, in addition to a prolonged PT, include a normal fibrinogen level, platelet count, and F.V level. F.V is not a vitamin K–dependent protein and should therefore be normal, except in cases of DIC (consumption) or severe liver disease (decreased production). Prolongation of the aPTT from vitamin K deficiency, warfarin therapy, or liver disease is a relatively late event and occurs initially as a result of F.IX depletion. This risk of anaphylactoid reactions is minimized when the drug is given as a piggyback infusion over 30–45 mins in a small volume of fluid rather than as a bolus or "slow-push" dose; the former is the preferred method of drug administration in hemodynamically unstable patients. The usual dose of vitamin K in children is 1–5 mg IV or subcutaneously (up to 10 mg in larger children). If the PT does not correct within 72 hrs after 3 daily doses of vitamin K, intrinsic liver disease should be suspected. Further administration of vitamin K is of no additional benefit in this setting. When the patient is actively bleeding, 10–15 mL/kg body weight of FFP is typically required. A similar approach is used in patients who were previously given warfarin. rhF.VIIa has been used with success to reverse the bleeding noted in vitamin K deficiency and in warfarin overdose.

As a general rule, residual plasma clotting activity after single-blood-volume exchange falls to 18%–37% of normal; after a double-blood-volume exchange, residual activity is only 3%–14% of normal; and after a triple-blood-volume exchange, <5% of normal clotting function remains. DIC may develop associated with major hemorrhage or massive transfusion. Exsanguinating hemorrhage sometimes requires blood replacement faster than a type and crossmatch of each unit can be performed, and unmatched

blood is given as a life-saving measure. Donor-recipient incompatibility—even when the mismatch is only of the minor blood group systems—can lead to DIC. The patient who is bleeding as a consequence of massive transfusion or washout presents with abnormalities, including prolonged PT, aPTT, and TT. Fibrinogen levels and platelet counts are typically decreased; FDPs are not usually increased unless concurrent DIC is present (**Table 82.1**). Platelets and FFP are given to replete the components of coagulation that are typically lacking. Severe bleeding associated with thrombocytopenia alone is uncommon, unless counts fall below 20,000–30,000/mcL of blood. Because of the complex nature of bleeding seen with massive transfusion, patients may benefit from platelet transfusion at counts even as high as 80,000–100,000/mcL. FFP is preferred over cryoprecipitate because it has a more complete coagulation protein composition. However, cryoprecipitate may be specifically given when fibrinogen depletion is thought to be a major contributor to the observed bleeding. In larger children (e.g., weight ≥30–40 kg or body surface area ≥1.0 m^2), 4 units of platelets (or half of a unit of apheresis-collected platelets) and 1 unit of FFP should be given for each 5 units of whole blood or packed cells transfused. In smaller children, 10 mL/kg of platelets and 10–15 mL/kg FFP should be given for each 40–50 mL/kg of blood transfused.

Anticoagulant Overdose

Anticoagulant therapy is not unusual in the PICU, and the possibility of errors in administration exists. Methods of prophylactic anticoagulant use, systemic anticoagulation, and thrombolytic therapy are sometimes poorly standardized and can lead to overdose.

Heparin

Heparin is currently found in two forms: unfractionated heparin (UH) and low-molecular-weight heparin (LMWH). Heparin is metabolized in the liver by the "heparinase" enzyme in a dose-dependent fashion, with excess heparin then being excreted through the kidneys. Serious bleeding associated with heparin overdose can be rapidly reversed by protamine sulfate. As a general rule, 1 mg of protamine neutralizes ~100 U of heparin. The dose of protamine required is calculated from the number of units of active heparin remaining in the patient's system. This, in turn, is estimated from the original heparin dose and the typical half-life for that infusion rate. The aPTT is used to gauge the residual effects of heparin. During and after cardiopulmonary bypass surgery, the activated clotting time is frequently used to measure heparin effect and to judge the effectiveness of and need for protamine neutralization. This methodology is sometimes employed in the ICU. However, the equipment used for this measurement is poorly standardized, with different systems giving different results. Protamine should be given by slow IV push over 8–10 mins. A single dose should not exceed 1 mg/kg (50 mg maximum dose). This dose may be repeated, but no >2 mg/kg (100 mg maximum dose) should be given as a cumulative dose without rechecking coagulation parameters. The dose of protamine should always be monitored by coagulation studies. The allergic reactions to protamine represent type I anaphylactic reactions between an antigen (protamine) and antibody (IgE or IgG) and result in histamine release. Consequently, H2 blockers have been shown to be effective in treating and minimizing these reactions. In that LMWH is not consistently neutralized by protamine, invasive procedures should not be performed within 24 hrs of administration. Bleeding following LMWH therapy has been treated effectively with rhF.VIIa.

Warfarin

When warfarin is present in sufficient plasma concentrations, the active forms of vitamin K–dependent factors are depleted. The PT is an accurate indicator of the effects of warfarin when its use has continued beyond 2 or 3 days. The PT becomes prolonged with F.VII depletion alone but does not reflect an overall state of anticoagulation until an equilibrium period of several days has passed. Over this time, the other vitamin K–dependent factors are depleted, and PT prolongation can then be used to assess the anticoagulant effects of warfarin. In severe cases of warfarin overdose, the aPTT also becomes prolonged as a result of depletion of the active forms of factors II, IX, and X. Many of the drugs known to prolong the effects of warfarin are listed in **Table 82.4**. A clinical syndrome referred to as "warfarin (Coumadin) necrosis" has been noted during the initial stages of anticoagulation with a vitamin-K antagonist. It is characterized clinically by the development of skin and subcutaneous necrosis, particularly in areas of subcutaneous fat, and pathologically by the thrombosis of small blood vessels in the fat and subcutaneous tissues. Individuals who are heterozygous for PC deficiency and have baseline PC levels of 50%–60% may develop a prothrombotic environment during the first few days of warfarin therapy. The risk of developing warfarin necrosis appears to be greater when an initial dose of warfarin >10–15 mg is administered. The development of this syndrome generally can be avoided if heparin and warfarin therapy are overlapped until "coumadinization" is complete and if large loading doses of warfarin are avoided.

TABLE 82.4

DRUGS THAT POTENTIATE THE ANTICOAGULANT EFFECTS OF WARFARIN

Antibiotics
  Broad-spectrum antibiotics (especially cephalosporins)
  Griseofulvin (oral)
  Metronidazole
  Sulfonamides
  Trimethoprim-sulfamethoxazole

Anti-inflammatory Drugs
  Steroids (anabolic, in particular)
  Acetylated salicylates
  Phenylbutazone (oxyphenbutazone)
  Sulfinpyrazone

Other Drugs
  Clofibrate
  Disulfiram
  Phenytoin
  Thyroxine (both D- and L-isomers)
  Tolbutamide

When over-anticoagulation with warfarin presents with bleeding, immediate reversal is usually mandated. The treatment of choice is FFP, which provides prompt restoration of the deficient vitamin K–dependent coagulation proteins, along with restoration of hemostatic function. Ten to 15 mL/kg of FFP is usually sufficient to produce significant correction of the PT, although repeat infusions of FFP may be necessary to effect continued correction of the PT owing to the short half-life of F.VII. Vitamin K also may be administered, particularly in situations that are less acute. For severe bleeding or bleeding not controlled by FFP infusions, rhF.VIIa has been used successfully.

Platelet Disorders

An overview of platelet disorders based on this classification scheme is presented in **Table 82.5**. The prototypic example of immune thrombocytopenia is ITP. Acute ITP is usually self-limited, with life-threatening bleeding occurring only rarely. In contrast, chronic ITP generally requires immunosuppressive therapy. Steroids may be given (2–4 mg/kg day of prednisone or its equivalent). High doses of IV γ-globulin (1–2 g/kg given over 2–5 days) and infusions of anti-RhD antigen antibody (WinRho; 25–60 mcg/kg) are equally efficacious in producing at least transient elevations in platelet counts. Splenectomy may be required to avert serious bleeding complications in patients who do not respond to medical management, though this approach is chosen much less often in children than in adults. In

TABLE 82.5

PLATELET DISORDERS SEEN IN THE ICU

Quantitative	Qualitative
Increased destruction	**Drugs**
Immune	Anti-inflammatory agents
Idiopathic thrombocytopenic purpura	Aspirin (irreversible)
Systemic lupus erythematosus	Nonsteroidal anti-inflammatory agents
Acquired immunodeficiency syndrome	Corticosteroids
Drugs (gold salts, heparin, sulfonamides,	Antibiotics
quinidine, quinine)	Penicillins (e.g., ampicillin, carbenicillin, ticarcillin,
Sepsis	penicillin-G)
Nonimmune	Cephalosporins (e.g., cephalothin)
Thrombotic thrombocytopenic purpura/	Nitrofurantoin
hemolytic uremic syndrome	Chloroquine, hydroxychloroquine
Mechanical destruction (e.g., cardiopulmonary	Phosphodiesterase inhibitors
bypass, hyperthermia)	Dipyridamole
Consumption (i.e., disseminated intravascular	Methylxanthines (e.g., theophylline)
coagulation)	
	Other drugs
Decreased Production	Antihistamines
Marrow suppression	α-blockers (e.g., phentolamine)
Chemotherapy	β-blockers (e.g., propranolol)
Viral illness (e.g., cytomegalovirus,	Dextran
Epstein-Barr virus, herpes simplex, parvovirus)	Ethanol
Drugs (thiazides, ethanol, cimetidine)	Furosemide
Marrow replacement	Heparin
Tumor	Local anesthetics (e.g., lidocaine)
Myelofibrosis	Phenothiazines
Other conditions	Tricyclic antidepressants
Splenic sequestration	Nitrates (e.g., sodium nitroprusside, nitroglycerin)
Dilution (see massive transfusion syndrome)	
	Metabolic causes
	Uremia
	Stored whole blood
	Disseminated intravascular coagulation
	(i.e., fibrin degradation product-mediated inhibition)
	Hypothyroidism

ITP, the degree of bleeding attributed to thrombocytopenia is generally less than that noted when thrombocytopenia results from decreased production. In general, severe bleeding is not noted until the platelet count is <10,000/mcL, although levels below 40,000–50,000/mcL may increase the risk of bleeding associated with invasive procedures.

Heparin-induced Thrombocytopenia

Acute non-idiosyncratic, heparin-induced thrombocytopenia (HIT)-1 causes a mild thrombocytopenia and usually remits despite continued use of the drug. Heparin need not be stopped in these patients. Idiosyncratic HIT is of much greater clinical consequence. Arterial thrombosis is the most significant risk of this form of HIT (type II HIT) and may be life-threatening, causing myocardial infarction, cerebrovascular accident, pulmonary embolism, or renal

infarction. Clinical bleeding is an infrequent problem in these patients. The diagnosis of HIT is one of exclusion. When type II HIT is suspected or confirmed, all exposure to heparin, including heparin flushes, heparin in total parenteral nutrition, and heparin-coated catheters, must be removed, and anticoagulation with an alternate agent must be initiated because of the risk of delayed thrombosis, which can occur up to 30 days after removal of heparin exposure. Patients with type II HIT should receive continued anticoagulation with direct thrombin inhibitors (argatroban, lepirudin) or with the heparinoid danaparoid. The direct thrombin inhibitors are preferred, as they carry no risk of cross-reacting with the heparin-dependent antibodies already present. Argatroban is cleared by the liver and lepirudin by the kidney. Warfarin alone is not adequate therapy for suspected type II HIT because of the risk of thrombosis from depression of PC levels. However, warfarins can be utilized in conjunction with a direct thrombin inhibitor and subsequently continued as a single agent once therapeutic suppression of vitamin K–dependent clotting factors has been achieved.

An abbreviated list of the drugs that can affect at least in vitro platelet function is presented in **Table 82.5**. Aspirin irreversibly inhibits platelet cyclooxygenase, resulting in a defect that lasts for the duration of the platelet life span (8–9 days). Ideally, all aspirin ingestion should be avoided for at least 7 days prior to an elective invasive procedure. The effect of nonsteroidal anti-inflammatory agents is reversible, and normal platelet function is usually restored within 24 hrs of the last dose. Under most circumstances, the degree of platelet inhibition produced by these agents is not clinically significant, and patients can receive these drugs for analgesia and fever control. Several conditions, such as massive transfusion syndrome and DIC, may respond to empirical platelet transfusion at counts as high as 80,000 or even 100,000 platelets/mcL, although bleeding in the presence of a platelet count of 80,000/mcL (or greater) is unlikely to be a result of the thrombocytopenia. With other causes, such as thrombocytopenia seen with cancer chemotherapy and bone marrow aplasia, therapy may not be required until counts fall below 10,000–20,000/mcL. rhF.VIIa has been used to reverse the hemostatic defect caused by aspirin or clopidogrel.

Uremia

Uremia causes a reversible impairment of platelet function. The primary therapy in this setting is dialysis. Cryoprecipitate, 1-deamino-8-D-arginine vasopressin (DDAVP; 0.3 mcg/kg, maximum dose 21 mcg), and conjugated estrogens (10 mg/day in adult patients) have been given with good results to patients with severe uremia and an acquired defect in primary hemostasis. The benefit derived by treatment with cryoprecipitate or DDAVP appears to be related to the consequent increase in the plasma concentration of the large multimeric forms of von Willebrand factor, thus greatly improving platelet adhesion. However, the durations of action of these agents are limited, with them reaching their zenith at between 2 and 6 hrs. Additional doses of DDAVP during the same 24-hr period may result in a diminished response to the drug (tachyphylaxis) with little or no further benefit. Patients who exhibit tachyphylaxis to DDAVP may require 48–72 hrs before again responding to this agent.

THROMBOTIC SYNDROMES

Thrombosis is associated with deep venous thrombosis (specifically in association with a central venous catheter), HIT, pulmonary embolism syndrome, TTP/HUS, thrombotic DIC, stroke, and CNS venous sinus thrombosis (most commonly seen in infants in association with marked dehydration). Thromboprophylaxis measures should be considered for postpubertal pediatric patients, as their risk of thrombosis may more closely conform to that of the adult population. The initial management approach for a child with a documented (or highly suspected) thrombotic event is generally anticoagulation with either UH or LMWH. An adult or older child might be started on UH with a bolus dose of 50 U/kg followed by a continuous infusion of 10 U/kg/hr, the dose for a young child is a bolus of 75 U/kg followed by 15–20 U/kg/hr, and the dose for an infant is 100 U/kg bolus followed by a continuous infusion of 25 U/kg/hr. Irrespective of the age of the patient, anticoagulation is adjusted to keep the aPTT roughly 1.5–2.5 times baseline values. Dosing of LMWH does not appear to be age related. Warfarin (Coumadin) therapy is weight related, with a loading dose of ~0.2 mg/kg/day for 2–3 days followed by a maintenance dose of ~0.1 mg/kg/day. The dose of warfarin is titrated to maintain an international normalized ratio of the PT between 1.5 and 4.0, depending on the intensity of anticoagulation desired. Thrombolytic therapy is generally not recommended as first-line therapy for thrombosis in newborn infants because of the high risk of hemorrhage; however, thrombolytic therapy may be appropriate in older infants and children, depending on the clinical presentation.

SELECTED DISORDERS

Amyloidosis, Gaucher disease, and the nephrotic syndrome may have one or more associated factor deficiencies that may complicate patient management and result in bleeding. Patients with either amyloidosis or Gaucher disease may develop F.IX deficiency. F.X deficiency has also been associated with amyloidosis. In the nephrotic syndrome, F.IX deficiency may develop. The deficiency typically remits with corticosteroid therapy. Finally, antithrombin III deficiency can be seen along with the nephrotic syndrome and may lead to thrombosis.

CHAPTER 83 ◼ SICKLE CELL DISEASE

KEVIN J. SULLIVAN • NIRANJAN "TEX" KISSOON • SALVATORE R. GOODWIN

NORMAL HEMOGLOBIN

Normal hemoglobin (Hb) quantity, structure, and function are essential for adequate oxygen delivery to tissues. Normal human Hb is a tetrameric protein composed of two alpha (α) chains and two beta (β) chains. Hemoglobin A$_2$ is a component of normal adult hemoglobin and is composed of two α and two delta (δ) chains (HbA2, $\alpha_2\delta_2$). Fetal hemoglobin, which is the predominant hemoglobin in fetal development and gradually declines during the first half of the first year of life, is composed of two α and two gamma (γ) chains (HbF, α_2, γ_2). At birth, our erythrocytes contain 70%–90% HbF, which predominates until 2–4 months of age in normal patients. The persistence of HbF production exists in many conditions and offers a protective effect when present in patients with certain hemoglobinopathies.

ABNORMAL HEMOGLOBIN

Sickle cell disease (SCD) refers not to a specific disease but to a variety of genotypes that share a common phenotype characterized by the production of sickled erythrocytes on Hb deoxygenation, chronic hemolysis, recurrent vaso-occlusion, and ischemic end-organ injury to virtually every organ system. All patients with a SCD phenotype share in common the inheritance of a mutant β-globin allele in which the sixth codon is altered, resulting in the substitution of valine for glutamine at the sixth amino acid position of the β-globin chain. The various diseases are summarized in **Table 83.1**. SCD is inherited in an autosomal recessive fashion with standard mendelian inheritance so that two heterozygote (HbAS) parents will have a 25% chance of producing either a normal (HbAA) or abnormal [sickle cell anemia (SCA), HbSS] homozygote offspring and a 50% chance of producing a heterozygote (SCT, HbAS).

PRINCIPLES OF CLINICAL MANAGEMENT

The fundamental defect in SCD is an abnormality of the β globin gene that results in a tendency for hemoglobin to irreversibly polymerize and form a gel that decreases the flexibility of the erythrocyte, resulting in microvascular occlusion, hemolysis, and chronic anemia. Factors that contribute to the pathogenesis of SCD-related complications include (1) hemoglobin and erythrocyte, (2) platelets, (3) coagulation cascade, (4) endothelium, (5) nitric

TABLE 83.1

SEVERITY AND DIAGNOSTIC TESTING FOR RELEVANT SICKLE CELL SYNDROMES

Syndrome	Genotype	Severity	Neonatal[a] screening[a]	Hemoglobin electrophoresis in older children (%)				
				HbA	HbS	Hb F	HbA$_2$	HbC
Sickle cell anemia (HbSS)	S-S	$++++$	FS	0	80–95	2–20	<3.5	0
Sickle β^0-thalassemia[d]	S-β^0	$+++$	FS	0	80–92	2–15	3.5–7	0
Hemoglobin SC disease (HbSC)	S-C	$++$	FSC	0	45–50	1–5	NA[c]	45–50
Sickle β^+-thalassemia[d]	S-β^+	$+$	FSA or FS[b]	5–30	65–90	2–10	3.5–6	0
Sickle cell trait (HbAS)	A-S	0	FAS	50–60	35–45	<2	<3.5	0

F, fetal hemoglobin; S, sickle hemoglobin; C, hemoglobin C; A, hemoglobin A.
[a] Hemoglobins reported in order of decreasing quantity (e.g., FS = F>S).
[b] Quantity of HbA at birth sometimes insufficient for detection.
[c] Quantity of HbA2 cannot be measured in the presence of HbC.
[d] β^0 indicates thalassemia mutation with absent production of β-globin; β^+ indicates thalassemia mutation with reduced production of β-globin.
Adapted from Lane PA.: Sickle cell disease. *Pediatr Clin N Am* 1996; 43:639–64, with permission.

TABLE 83.2

PRECIPITANTS OF COMPLICATIONS OF SICKLE CELL ANEMIA

Intrinsic patient factors
Erythrocytes
Endothelial cells
Platelets
Leukocytes
  Lymphocytes
  Neutrophils
Coagulation cascade
Aberrations in nitric oxide metabolism
Oxidant mediated injury
Systemic inflammation

TABLE 83.3

FACTORS THAT MAY PROMOTE SICKLING

1. Hemoglobin desaturation
   a. Failure to oxygenate in the lungs
      i. Atelectasis
      ii. Infection
         1. Bacterial
         2. Viral
      iii. Chronic lung disease
      iv. Pulmonary vascular disease
      v. High altitude
   b. Diminished tissue oxygen delivery
      i. Diminished cardiac output
         1. Hypovolemia (dehydration, sequestration, sepsis)
         2. Septic Shock
         3. Diminished cardiac contractility
         4. Pericardial disease
         5. Increased systemic vascular resistance
         6. Anesthetics/drugs
      ii. Severe anemia
      iii. Hypoxemic cardiac output (see 1.a.)
   c. Increased tissue extraction of oxygen
      i. Increased tissue demands
         1. Vigorous exercise
         2. Thyrotoxicosis
         3. Malignant hyperthermia
         4. Seizures
         5. Sepsis
         6. Shivering
      ii. Factors accelerating tissue oxygen extraction
         1. Acidosis
         2. Hyperthermia
2. Increased microvascular transit time
   a. Increased viscosity
      i. Excessive transfusion
      ii. Dehydration
   b. Vasoconstriction
      i. Hypothermia
      ii. Vasoconstrictor drugs
      iii. Tourniquet use (orthopedic surgery)

oxide, (6) systemic oxidant-mediated injury, (7) environmental factors, and (8) hypoxemia (**Table 83.2** and **Table 83.3**).

Close monitoring of arterial oxygenation and administration of supplemental oxygen to keep arterial oxygen saturation in the normal range is recommended. The consequences of hemoglobin deoxygenation may be mitigated if the transit time of the erythrocyte through the microcirculation to the pulmonary circulation is rapid. As such, avoidance of clinical circumstances in which both significant desaturation and slow transit time to the lungs are present is critical. Significant hemoglobin desaturation occurs when oxygen delivery to the tissues is impaired by diminished cardiac output, severe anemia, or arterial hypoxemia. Patients with SCD are accustomed to moderately severe anemia and preserve oxygen delivery with increased cardiac output, altered erythrocytic 2, 3-diphosphoglycerate concentrations, and preserved arterial oxygenation. Transit time through the circulation is adversely affected by dehydration, systemic hypotension, occlusive tourniquet use, and physiologic or pharmacologically induced vasoconstriction. Preservation of arterial oxygenation, oxygen-carrying capacity, and cardiac output are essential to minimize excessive and prolonged hemoglobin deoxygenation. Dehydration may be a precipitant of SCD-related complications, though this is not a consistent finding. Nevertheless, it seems prudent to tailor perioperative fluid management to provide generous intravascular hydration that at least preserves euvolemia. Hypothermia restricts oxygen unloading, promotes cutaneous vasoconstriction, increases red cell tissue-lung transit time, and may promote erythrocyte sickling. Although controversial, the basic tenet of anesthetic and critical care management is to try to preserve normothermia in SCD patients in the perioperative period. The benefits of mild therapeutically induced hypothermia used in the critical care setting for neu-

rologic protection would have to be weighed against the potential for hypothermia to work synergistically with other physiologic and environmental perturbations to promote SCD-related complications. Hyperthermia also occurs in the perioperative period and may be due to many causes, including atelectasis, infection, and systemic inflammation. Hyperthermia shifts the hemoglobin-oxygen dissociation curve to the right, favoring release of oxygen to the tissues and hemoglobin desaturation and may be associated with vasoconstriction or vasodilation in core and peripheral compartments. As such, it could theoretically promote vaso-occlusive phenomena.

Systemic acidosis shifts the hemoglobin-oxygen dissociation curve to the right, facilitating oxygen delivery and hemoglobin desaturation and may theoretically potentiate erythrocyte deformation in the microvasculature.

Methods of identifying a patient with sickle hemoglobinopathy include neonatal screening, solubility tests, and Hb electrophoresis In the presence of high concentrations of HbF, solubility testing lacks the sensitivity required to detect HbS, and cannot be relied upon for testing in children younger than 6 months. Hb electrophoresis is required in this age group to exclude the presence of a sickle hemoglobinopathy.

Vaso-occlusive crisis (VOC) is a painful condition that usually does not require ICU admission but may precede the development of more serious complications. The most common type of VOC is bony crisis affecting the long bones, ribs, and vertebrae. Patients with bony VOC will present with symptoms of ischemic pain from the bony cortex or marrow compartment of the extremities, chest, and back and is often associated with fever, leukocytosis, and malaise. In children younger than 3 years old, the distribution of VOC may be confined to the small bones of the hands and feet and is referred to as *hand-foot syndrome*, or dactylitis. The clinical presentation of bony VOC is fairly characteristic and usually very familiar to the patient and physician. The differential diagnosis of bony VOC when accompanied by fever, focal bone tenderness, or overlying erythema and tenderness includes local trauma, and osteomyelitis, a condition common in SCD patients owing to their susceptibility to bacteremia. Differentiation of the two conditions can be difficult but can be aided by cultures of the blood and involved bone and a combination of plain radiographs, MRI, and bone scan. The white blood cell count and differential are not helpful in making the distinction between infection and infarction. If osteomyelitis is suspected on clinical grounds, therapy should be initiated with antimicrobials effective against *Staphylococcus aureus* and *Salmonella* spp. while arrangements are made for bone biopsy, if necessary. VOC involving the abdominal vasculature (mesenteric vessels and blood vessels supplying the solid abdominal organs) produces abdominal pain, fever, malaise, anorexia, and nausea. Patients will demonstrate diminished bowel sounds and nonspecific abdominal tenderness, making differentiation of VOC from a surgical cause of abdominal symptoms difficult. As noted for bone VOC, the nature and distribution of the abdominal crisis pain may be typical of previous crises, but other causes for abdominal pain should always be considered. Children with SCD have an increased frequency of cholelithiasis and cholecystitis due to chronic hemolysis. On the basis of history and physical examination, the clinician may elect to exclude non-SCD abdominal

pathology through plain radiographs, CT of the abdomen, and liver function tests including total and fractionated bilirubin, amylase, lipase, and urinalysis. Serial examinations of the abdomen and surgical consultation are recommended if the diagnosis remains in question after initial evaluation.

Treatment

Treatment is largely supportive, with emphasis placed on the provision of adequate analgesia, supplemental oxygen, antibiotics to treat any precipitating infections, and hydration provided liberally (at 1.5 × maintenance fluid requirements). For VOC that is refractory, many pediatric hematologists will provide simple transfusion to break the VOC cycle.

The acute chest syndrome (ACS) is a clinical syndrome characterized by fever, cough, pleuritic chest pain, tachypnea, hypoxemia, and a new or rapidly progressive pulmonary infiltrate on chest radiograph. It is not uncommon for a patient with ACS to also demonstrate an abrupt decrease in platelet count and hematocrit. ACS may develop de novo, in the perioperative period, or in the setting of VOC or an otherwise innocuous pulmonary infection. Risk factors for the development of ACS include younger age, higher steady-state Hb level, lower fetal Hb percentage, and increased neutrophil count. ACS is of clinical significance to hematologists and intensivists because the mortality associated with an episode of ACS has been reported to be as high as 25%. Treatment is focused on both acute pulmonary infection and pulmonary vaso-occlusion. Hydration is instituted liberally and modified as clinically indicated on the basis of cardiovascular status, renal function, and measured atrial filling pressures. Supplemental oxygen is administered with a goal of keeping arterial partial pressure of oxygen (PaO_2) >80–100 mm Hg and hemoglobin saturation (SaO_2) >95%. For milder disease, incentive spirometry and ambulation can be encouraged to improve ventilation/perfusion matching, preventing atelectasis, and slow the progression of pulmonary injury. Analgesia should also be provided to minimize pleuritic chest pain, and exercises promoting pulmonary toilet are encouraged. Analgesia can be delivered by administration of narcotics and scheduled acetaminophen doses during the acute illness. In the absence of significant renal disease or gastrointestinal bleeding, nonsteroidal anti-inflammatory medications such as ibuprofen or ketorolac may be offered as well. Finally, dexamethasone (0.3 mg/kg/dose every 12 hours for 4 doses) may be administered in mild and moderate ACS. ACS can progress in severity to severe acute lung injury or acute respiratory distress syndrome, requiring positive-pressure airway support in the form of non-invasive continuous positive airway pressure, bi-level positive airway pressure, or more commonly with standard endotracheal intubation. In keeping with minimizing pulmonary injury secondary to mechanical ventilation, efforts should be made to minimize plateau pressure and tidal volume while positive end-expiratory pressure is adjusted to provide optimal lung compliance and inflation. In order to minimize iatrogenic lung injury while optimizing ventilation-perfusion matching, pressure-limited or airway pressure release or high-frequency oscillatory ventilation can be used. Inhaled nitric oxide given to patients with severe ACS may inhibit pulmonary artery hypertension, right ventricular function, severe V/Q mismatch, and systemic oxygenation. Children with SCD are very susceptible to infection due to deficiencies in splenic function and opsonization of bacterial pathogens. Broad-spectrum antibiotic therapy with third-generation cephalosporin and a macrolide antibiotic is instituted while appropriate diagnostic interventions are implemented. Blood is sent for bacterial culture, and Mycoplasma serologies, sputum for bacterial and viral culture, and nasopharyngeal aspirates are sent for detection of viral antigens of common respiratory pathogens (respiratory syncitial virus, adenovirus, parainfluenza virus, and influenza viruses). In critically ill patients with extensive lung disease, bronchoalveolar lavage is performed, and specimens are sent for opportunistic pathogens (fungi, protozoa) in addition to the more commonly encountered pathogens. Aggressive empiric antibiotic therapy is instituted with consideration given to local antibiotic resistance patterns of commonly encountered pathogens. In those patients considered to be at risk for infection with nosocomial or resistant pathogens, antistaphylococcal and antipseudomonal antibiotics (nafcillin or vancomycin, ceftazidime, and an aminoglycoside) are added. When culture results are known, the spectrum of antibiotic coverage can be appropriately narrowed. The most effective therapeutic modality available to the intensivist in the treatment of ACS is transfusion therapy. Blood transfusion is not offered to correct anemia but is offered in the setting of ACS to dilute the HbS-containing erythrocytes with HbA-containing erythrocytes in the hope that microvascular occlusion of the pulmonary circulation will be attenuated. During critical illness, systemic oxygen delivery may be compromised by impaired cardiac output or decreased arterial oxygen saturation, so simple transfusions are initiated with a goal hemoglobin concentration of 10 g/dL. For more severe disease, or disease that is rapidly progressive, exchange transfusion is provided to rapidly decrease the percentage of HbS to <30%, with a total hemoglobin and hematocrit of 10 g/dL and 30%,

respectively. Extracorporeal membrane oxygenation has been used in the most severe disease.

Stroke or cerebrovascular accident (CVA) patients have angiographic abnormalities specifically proximal intracranial arterial stenosis, particularly of the internal carotid artery. Occlusion of the vessel may, therefore, result from intimal hyperplasia, secondary thrombosis, distal thromboembolization, or any combination of these factors. Most cerebrovascular accidents in children are due to ischemic infarcts. SCD patients with CVA may present to the ICU with sudden onset of neurologic symptoms, Flow velocity in the middle cerebral artery (MCA) and terminal internal carotid artery (ICA) utilizing transcranial Doppler ultrasonography can detect elevated flow velocity in the MCA or ICA resulting from local stenosis in the blood vessels. The diagnosis of CVA is made on the basis of the usual clinical signs and symptoms of CVA. In the presence of acute contralateral hemiplegia and aphasia (left-sided CVA), there should be little diagnostic dilemma. However, in many cases the presentation may not be straightforward, and stroke may present simply as altered or depressed mental status. In these cases, in addition to stroke other causes for acute alteration in mental status will need to be considered. Focal seizures may be the presenting symptom of focal cerebral ischemia and may progress to a generalized tonic-clonic convulsion. In patients with SCD, the new onset of seizure activity should be considered to be indicative of cerebral ischemic injury until proven otherwise. Seizure control should be implemented as described for status epilepticus, with particular care taken to ensure arterial oxygenation. In the appropriate age groups, acute alteration in mental status may be secondary to toxic ingestion and should be pursued and treated accordingly. In the presence of fever, acute alteration in mental status may also be indicative of meningitis due to bacterial or viral pathogens. Lumbar puncture should be performed, and antibiotics implemented, if the clinical picture suggests meningitis and physical examination and imaging studies have excluded intracranial hypertension or neurosurgical catastrophes. SCD patients presenting with signs or symptoms of CVA or other intracranial pathology should undergo emergent CT scan or MRI of the brain to define any CNS abnormalities and to exclude the presence of lesions amenable to neurosurgical intervention (parenchymal, epidural or subdural hematoma). Advantages of MRI over CT scan in acute CVA include the ability to clearly define the CNS vasculature using magnetic resonance angiography and increased sensitivity of MRI for early detection of ischemic parenchymal changes. When selecting the most appropriate neuroimaging procedure for a given patient, the clinician must weigh the benefits of increased diagnostic potential of MRI against the need for sedation to facilitate longer MRI studies in uncooperative or physiologically unstable pediatric patients. The most urgent therapeutic intervention for the SCD patient presenting with CVA is an immediate exchange transfusion to reverse, or prevent progression of ischemic CNS injury. Exchange transfusion is provided to decrease the HbS percentage to below 30% while keeping the hemoglobin concentration at or about 10 g/dL. Therapy for children with SCD and CVA is otherwise supportive, with careful attention to protection of the airway, suppression of seizure activity, and preservation of respiratory and hemodynamic function. In the setting of a large cerebral infarction, the patient is monitored for the development of intracranial hypertension, and neurosurgical consultation is obtained when clinically indicated. The goal is to maintain normothermia and to institute a normoglycemic protocol to minimize secondary neuronal ischemic injury. At this time, no role for thrombolytic therapy has been defined by a large clinical study in the management of CVA in the setting of SCD.

Splenic sequestration and aplastic crisis occasionally cause life-threatening decreases in hemoglobin concentration. Viral suppression of bone marrow function from parvovirus B19, for instance, may result in severe anemia. Acute sequestration crisis (ASC) refers to a sudden drop in hemoglobin concentration associated with development of splenomegaly, reticulocytosis, intravascular volume depletion, and shock. Platelet and leukocyte counts may decrease as well. ASC is a disease of toddlers and infants and is not seen in older children, presumably owing to auto-splenectomy. Treatment of aplastic crisis is supportive with erythrocyte transfusion to restore hemoglobin concentration to levels sufficient to support systemic oxygen delivery until marrow function recovers and reticulocytosis resumes. Therapy of ASC involves restoration of circulating blood volume with crystalloid solutions and sickle-free packed red blood cells. With resolution of ASC, spleen size decreases and sequestered blood elements may return to the circulation.

Sepsis

Children with SCD are at increased risk for serious bacterial infections due to impaired splenic function and decreased opsonic activity. This results in susceptibility to infection with a variety of bacterial pathogens, especially encapsulated organisms such as *Streptococcus pneumoniae* and *Neisseria meningitidis*. Early identification of patients at risk through newborn screening sickle cell screening programs, use

of penicillin prophylaxis, availability of vaccinations against *S. pneumoniae, N. meningitidis,* and *Hemophilus influenzae,* and aggressive antibiotic therapy in febrile SCD patients have had a beneficial effect on sepsis related mortality in such patients. Therapy for patients with sepsis includes early, aggressive administration of broad-spectrum antibiotics in all febrile SCD patients and in afebrile SCD patients who demonstrate other clinical signs of systemic bacterial infection. In patients with infection, hypotension, and organ dysfunction, supportive therapies include early goal directed therapy, mechanical ventilation, vasopressor support, steroid therapy (when appropriate), and other sepsis therapies.

Chronic Lung Disease

Sickle cell chronic lung disease has been well documented in SCA, and its etiology is not completely understood. It is marked by progressive episodes of chest pain, progressive dyspnea, and progressive pulmonary fibrosis on chest radiograph. The mechanism that underlies the development of disabling lung disease in SCA is not clear but is thought to involve repetitive episodes of pulmonary injury that result in pulmonary parenchymal fibrosis, and/or an ongoing obliterative pulmonary vasculitis. SCD patients may present to the PICU with preexisting pulmonary abnormalities that include restrictive lung disease, obstructive lung disease, airway smooth-muscle hyperreactivity, and significant ventilation-perfusion mismatch. Preexisting respiratory system injury may compromise the physiologic reserve of the SCD patient.

Cardiovascular System

Cardiac dysfunction is understood in the context of high-output left ventricular failure. Due to severe anemia, cardiac output must necessarily increase to provide adequate systemic tissue oxygen delivery in the setting of SCD. This results in left ventricular dilation to augment stroke volume and cardiac output. More ominous, however, is the presence of pulmonary artery hypertension and right ventricular dysfunction.

Renal

While children rarely experience such disorders, older patients may suffer anatomic and functional impairment of renal function requiring dialysis or renal transplantation. SCD patients demonstrate isosthenuria, a progressive impairment to concentrate the urine and preserve free water, making the SCD patient more susceptible to dehydration. The potential for presence of renal dysfunction in SCD patients must be considered for fluid management, acid-base, electrolyte, and pharmacologic considerations.

Principles of Transfusion Therapy

Transfusion therapy is employed to decrease the percentage of erythrocytes in the circulation containing HbS so that vaso-occlusion can be minimized and to increase systemic oxygen delivery (DO_2). Transfusion therapy can be administered in the form of simple transfusion or exchange transfusion. Simple transfusion refers to the intravenous administration of sickle-free, packed red blood cells, whereas exchange transfusion involves the intravenous administration of sickle-free packed red blood cells with simultaneous removal of the patient's whole blood. Great care must be taken when providing transfusion support to SCD patients to carefully monitor the hemoglobin concentration and hematocrit, as abrupt elevations in hematocrit >33% are associated with increase in blood viscosity and potential for CNS ischemic injury. Exchange transfusion therapy can be accomplished in infants after placement of an arterial catheter for blood withdrawal and suitable venous access for infusion of blood. Alternatively, a large-bore central venous catheter can be used for both withdrawal and infusion of blood during exchange transfusion. Exchange transfusion can be carried out manually by clinicians at the bedside or, in larger children, can be accomplished through automated erythrocytapheresis. In order to quickly reduce HbS percentage to <30% in smaller infants and children, roughly twice the circulating blood volume is replaced with a solution of reconstituted sickle free erythrocytes and fresh frozen plasma over 4–6 hours while closely monitoring the hematocrit. If the hematocrit increases to >30%–33% at any time during the transfusion, a non-erythrocyte volume expander (i.e., fresh-frozen plasma) is substituted for the packed red blood cells until the hematocrit falls to an acceptable level. With rapid transfusions and in the setting of hepatic dysfunction, ionized hypocalcemia may result from citrate toxicity and must be closely monitored and treated when necessary. In erythrocytapheresis, sickle erythrocytes are separated from the patient's circulating blood volume and replaced with sickle-free erythrocytes.

Perioperative Management of the SCD Patient

In most states in the United States, newborns are screened for hemoglobinopathy along with other inborn errors and endocrine disorders before leaving the nursery. In many instances, these results can be retrieved with a phone call to the state laboratory during regular business hours, which offers a definitive diagnosis of the hemoglobin or hemoglobinopathy present in a given patient. This screening test, however, can be erroneous in infants and children who are transfused in the NICU prior to the performance of neonatal screening.

For children presenting for surgery in which neonatal screening has not been done or the results cannot be found, a suitable screening algorithm is needed, such as Hb electrophoresis. Sickling complications do not occur in children younger than 4 months of age due to the protective effects of HbF. For children 4–6 months of age, hemoglobin electrophoresis is sent, and the surgery is delayed pending the results. For children older than 6 months of age, sickle prep solubility testing is sent, and, if positive, Hb electrophoresis is performed to define the type of sickle hemoglobinopathy present.

Preoperative Preparation

Once the diagnosis of a SCD phenotype is made, a pediatric hematologist may help in the preoperative preparation of the SCD patient. Preoperative preparation includes careful attention to preoperative hydration, optimization of vital organ function, and consideration to the administration of prophylactic preoperative packed red blood cell transfusion. Patients with SCD should be well hydrated. The patient should be screened and treated for infection, a potent stimulus for many systemic inflammatory complications. Major organ systems should be evaluated for dysfunction that may adversely impact the intraoperative and postoperative course. Finally, a thorough preoperative evaluation and discussion with the parents is required to delineate risk, explain the anesthetic plan, and provide for postoperative analgesia and prevention of postoperative SCD complications. Perioperative transfusion therapy is a common, sometimes controversial topic of discussion among surgeons, anesthesiologists, hematologists, and intensivists. The reasons for provision of perioperative transfusion therapy would be to correct anemia and improve oxygen-carrying capacity. This is an uncommon indication, however, as the anemia associated with SCD is a chronic, compensated anemia. The other reason for the provision of preoperative transfusion therapy would be to dilute the erythrocytes containing HbS with erythrocytes containing HbA to minimize the extent of hemoglobin gel formation and erythrocyte sludging in the microvasculature. Prophylactic therapy of this nature should be effective in decreasing postoperative SCD complications. Conservative transfusion strategy using simple transfusion to a target Hgb of 10 gm/dl is effective in the prevention of SCD complications. The benefit from such a strategy must be weighed against the potential for transfusion related complications which include hemolytic reactions, transfusion-associated acute lung injury, alloimmunization, iron overload, allergic reaction to leukocyte antigens, and transmission of viral pathogens.

Operative Management

There is wide variation in the reported incidence of SCD-related complications in the perioperative period, and an individual patient's risk of developing SCD complications is probably determined by many factors. The type of operation performed has been described to impact the probability of development of SCD complications in the perioperative period with high-risk procedures variously described as obstetrical procedures, thoracotomy/laparotomy, intracranial procedures, and operations related to the airway. Other considerations in operative management of SCD patients include the presence or absence of significant major organ system dysfunction, recent patterns of SCD-related activity, and precipitants of SCD complications, particularly infection. Anesthetic technique has not been shown to be related to the development of perioperative SCD complica-

tions, with successful application of general anesthesia, regional anesthesia, or combined techniques to the care of these patients. Additionally, regional anesthetic techniques have been safely employed, with variable efficacy to assist in the management of SCD crises, including refractory vaso-occlusive crisis and priapism.

Postoperative Management

Patients are admitted to the ward for perioperative management wherein aggressive analgesia is provided in the form of peripheral nerve blocks, neuraxial blockade, patient-controlled opioid analgesia, and nonsteroidal anti-inflammatory drugs (when not contraindicated). Analgesia is optimized to facilitate respiratory function without excessively depressing respiratory drive. Pulmonary toilet is optimized with incentive spirometry for older children, bubble-blowing games for younger children, supplemental oxygen administration where it is required, and getting out of bed to chair and early ambulation wherever possible. Intravenous hydration is continued postoperatively, with careful attention to fluid intake and output, including insensible losses, urine output, and all losses from drains and catheters.

■ INDEX

Page numbers followed by f indicate figures; page numbers followed by t indicate tabular material.

Herpes virus type 6, 551–552
Heulitt, Mark J., 108–116
High-frequency flow interrupters, 115
High-frequency jet ventilation, 115
High frequency oscillatory ventilation (HFOV), 62, 115
High-frequency ventilation, 115
Highly active antiretroviral therapy (HAART), 487–488, 496, 555
Hippocampus, 250
Hirschsprung disease, 573
Histoplasma spp., 514t, 515t
Histoplasmosis, 554–555
HIV (human immunodeficiency virus), 487, 493–498, 494t, 495t, 496t, 497t
Hodgkin disease, 661t, 662t
Hoffman, Julien I., 344–350
Homocystinuria, 690
Hormonal control of circulation, 346–347
Horner syndrome, 257
Howell, Joy D., 59–66
HSP70, 253
Human African trypanosomiasis (HAT), 535
Human DNAse, 197
Human immunodeficiency virus. *See* HIV
Human metapneumovirus (hMPV), 194
Human tetanus immunoglobulin (HTIG), 540
Hurler syndrome, 660
Husain, S. Adil, 424–426
Hydration, bronchiolitis and, 196
Hydrocortisone, 455, 456t, 600, 636
Hydroxy butyrate, 88
Hydroxychloroquine, toxicity levels of, 74t
Hydroxycobalamin, 655t
Hyoscyamine, 82t
Hyperaldosteronism, 604
Hyperammonemia, 323, 659
Hyperbaric oxygen, 487
Hypercalcemia, 567, 626–627, 626t
  cancer patients and, 673
Hypercapnic respiratory failure, 128–129
Hyperglycemia, 567, 607t, 610
  brain injury and, 256
  sepsis and, 486
Hyperglycemia hyperosmolar syndrome (HHS), 609–610
Hyperglycolysis, 254
Hyperhomocysteinemia, stroke and, 306
Hyper IgE syndrome (Job syndrome), 464t–465t, 466
Hyper IgM syndrome, 462, 464t–465t
Hyperinsulinism, 611
Hyperkalemia, 91
Hyperkalemic disorders, 618–619, 618t
Hyperlactatemia, 328t, 331t
Hyperleukocytosis, 148, 676–678
Hyperlipemia, 567
Hypermagnesemia, 628, 628t
Hypernatremia, 325, 567
Hypernatremic conditions, 616–617, 616t, 617t
Hypernatremic dehydration, 592
Hyperparathyroidism, 627
Hyperphosphatemia, 629, 629t
Hypersensitivity pneumonitis syndrome, 666
Hypertension, stroke and, 306
Hypertensive crises, 645, 645t, 646t
  blood pressure, 646
  cardiovascular manifestations, 647
  cerebral autoregulation, 645–646, 646f
  diagnosis of, 647
  evaluation of, 647
  manifestations of, 645t, 646t
  neurologic manifestations, 646–647
  renal manifestations, 647
  treatment for, 648–650
Hypertensive emergency, defined, 645
Hypertensive encephalopathy, 646

Hypertensive urgency, defined, 645
Hyperthermia, 89–90
  brain injury and, 255
  defined, 89
  syndromes, 89–90, 93–94
Hyperthyroidism (thyrotoxicosis), 326, 632–633, 632t
Hypertrophic cardiomyopathy (HCM), 373, 373f, 383
Hyperuricemia, 91
Hyperventilation, 160, 683
Hyperviscosity syndromes, 148
Hypoalbuminemia, 62, 590
Hypocalcemia, 91, 567, 622–627, 625t
Hypoglycemia, 91, 324, 486, 567, 610–612, 611t
  brain injury and, 256
  etiology, 657–659, 657f, 658t
Hypokalemia, 91, 567
Hypokalemic disorders, 619, 619t
Hypomagnesemia, 91, 567, 627–628, 627t
Hypomotility, 589
Hyponatremia, 91, 325, 567
Hyponatremic conditions, 617–618, 617t, 618t
Hyponatremic dehydration, 591
Hypophosphatemia, 91, 567, 628–629, 629t
Hypoplastic left-heart syndrome, 344
Hypotension, brain injury and, 255–256
Hypothalamic hypodipsia, 616t
Hypothalamic-pituitary-adrenal axis, 427, 428
Hypothalamic-pituitary injury, 285, 294–295
Hypothermia
  cardiac arrest and, 320t
  cardiopulmonary bypass and, 425
  clinical features, 96, 97t
  defined, 94–96
  etiology of, 96, 96t
  neutrophil function and, 448
  pathophysiology of, 94–96
  response of organs to, 96, 95t
  rewarming methods, 96–97, 98f
  submersion injuries and, 55, 56
  treatment for, 96–98, 98f, 320t, 322
Hypothyroidism, 326, 630t, 631–632, 631t, 632t
Hypoventilation, 160, 161
Hypovolemic shock, 35
  management of, 45–47, 46t
Hypoxemia, 255–256, 406–407
Hypoxemic respiratory failure, 128–129, 128t
Hypoxia inducible factor (HIF), acute lung injury and, 153, 154t
Hypoxic gas mixtures, 120–121
Hypoxic-ischemic encephalopathy (HIE)
  biomarkers, 322, 322f
  defined, 317
  global and focal, 317–318, 318f
  neurologic imaging and monitoring and, 275–278, 276f, 277f, 320–322
  therapeutic hypothermia, 320t, 322
  treatment for, 319–322
  variables that affect cerebral blood flow after cardiac arrest, 318–319, 319t
Hypoxic pulmonary vasoconstriction, 168

Ibopamine, 380
Ibuprofen, 712
Idarubicin, 662
Idiopathic hypertrophic subaortic stenosis. *See* Hypertrophic cardiomyopathy (HCM)
Idiopathic thrombocytopenia purpura, 687, 687t
Ifosfamide, 661
  toxicities, 665, 665t, 666, 667, 668t
Ileus, 576
Imaging technology
  See also Neurologic imaging and monitoring
  heat stroke and, 91–92
Imidazolines, toxicity levels of, 74t